COOVADIA'S
PAEDIATRICS &
CHILD HEALTH

SIXTH EDITION

COOVADIA'S PAEDIATRICS & CHILD HEALTH

SIXTH EDITION

A manual for health professionals
in developing countries

DF Wittenberg

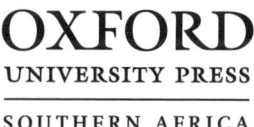

OXFORD

UNIVERSITY PRESS

SOUTHERN AFRICA

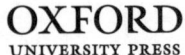

SOUTHERN AFRICA

Oxford University Press Southern Africa (Pty) Ltd

Vasco Boulevard, Goodwood, Cape Town, Republic of South Africa
P O Box 12119, N1 City, 7463, Cape Town, Republic of South Africa

Oxford University Press Southern Africa (Pty) Ltd is a subsidiary of
Oxford University Press, Great Clarendon Street, Oxford OX2 6DP.

The Press, a department of the University of Oxford, furthers the University's objective of
excellence in research, scholarship, and education by publishing worldwide in

Oxford New York

Auckland Cape Town Dar es Salaam Hong Kong Karachi
Kuala Lumpur Madrid Melbourne Mexico City Nairobi
New Delhi Shanghai Taipei Toronto

With offices in

Argentina Austria Brazil Chile Czech Republic France Greece
Guatemala Hungary Italy Japan Poland Portugal Singapore South Korea
Switzerland Turkey Ukraine Vietnam

Oxford is a registered trade mark of Oxford University Press
in the UK and in certain other countries

Published in South Africa
by Oxford University Press Southern Africa (Pty) Ltd, Cape Town

Coovadia's Paediatrics and Child Health
Sixth edition
ISBN 978 0 19 598843 7
© Oxford University Press Southern Africa (Pty) Ltd 2009

The moral rights of the author have been asserted
Database right Oxford University Press Southern Africa (Pty) Ltd (maker)

Sixth edition published 2009

Publishing Manager: Alida Terblanche
Assistant Commissioning Editor: Marisa Montemarano
Managing Editor: Lisa Andrews
Editor: Dr Bridget Farham
Designer: Judith Cross
Illustrator: Bronwen Lusted
Indexer: Ethné Clarke

Set in Utopia Std 9 pt on 11 pt by RO Theiner, Box 116, Aurora 7325
Printed and bound by ABC Press, Cape Town
111991

Acknowledgements
The authors and publisher gratefully acknowledge permission to reproduce copyright material
in this book. Every effort has been made to trace copyright holders, but if any copyright
infringements have been made, the publisher would be grateful for information that would
enable any omissions or errors to be corrected in subsequent impressions.

Contents

Foreword

It is especially satisfying to read through this 2009 version of Paediatrics and Child Health and come across substantial improvements from previous editions and positive changes over the period since its first publication 25 years ago.

The modern environment is hugely complex; it brings together the biomedical, social, economic and political determinants of well-being, disability and death in an intricate and often poorly understood matrix. Furthermore, the truly remarkable digital revolution, rapid advances in scientific medicine, and the numerous transitions in health, epidemiology, and disease patterns in children over the past few decades have vastly increased the scope and depth of information that is required by students, health professionals and their mentors in order for them to function and discharge their responsibilities effectively.

It is always going to be an unending and imperfect task to decide on priorities for teaching and learning in child health; priorities that are the minimum necessary for practising professionals. However, there may be a wider focus for some who may wish to go beyond these boundaries. Medical books should also attract and introduce such individuals to the mysteries of science and the precision of the scientific method. This edition has within its covers material to address both these ends of the learning spectrum; its highest priority has been to find a balance between theory for the practice of day-to-day medicine and knowledge, which offers glimpses of more profound truths.

The format of the chapters is similar to previous editions, but some sections have been reorganized to highlight specific themes and to refine content. This has been undertaken with the express purpose of reducing repetition and overlap between the problem-based approach, which can be directly utilizable in the clinic or field, and the more formal descriptions of organ systems.

Numerous new contributors have been recruited in an attempt to obtain a comprehensive coverage of perspectives from different institutions. There has been large scale rewriting of many chapters, and all chapters have been thoroughly reworked to bring the content up to date.

This book, I am hopeful, will be regularly consulted, kept on bookshelves and treasured by students and their teachers in the health sciences in this part of the world. This edition can serve as a gateway to understanding the rudiments of the dilemma of this continent, which simultaneously bears the heaviest burden of disease in the world and has the weakest health systems and woefully inadequate infrastructure (facilities and personnel).

I am honoured and grateful for the generous recognition of my long and close association with this book through the eponymous title of the current edition.

Hoosen Coovadia
Director: HIV Management
Reproductive Health and HIV Research Unit
University of the Witwatersrand;
Victor Daitz Professor of HIV/AIDS Research
Nelson Mandela School of Medicine
University of Kwazulu-Natal.

List of contributors

ADHIKARI, PROFESSOR M. MB.ChB. (UCT), FCP(SA), MD (Natal) Head, Department of Paediatrics and Child Health, University of Kwazulu-Natal, Durban

ARCHARY, DR M., MB.ChB. (Natal), FCP(SA), Department of Paediatrics and Child Health, University of Kwazulu-Natal, Durban

BOBAT, PROFESSOR R., MB.ChB. (Natal), FCP(SA), MD (Natal), Department of Paediatrics and Child Health, University of Kwazulu-Natal, Durban

BOY, PROFESSOR SC., BChD (Pretoria), MChD (Oral Pathology) (Pretoria) Department of Oral Pathology and Oral Biology, University of Pretoria

CHRISTIANSON, PROFESSOR A., MB.ChB. FRCP(Edin), Head, Division of Human Genetics, School of Pathology, National Health Laboratory Services and University of Witwatersrand, Johannesburg

COOKE, DR L., MB.ChB.(UCT), FCPaed(SA), Department of Paediatrics and Child Health, Tygerberg Hospital and University of Stellenbosch, Bellville

COOPER, PROFESSOR PA., MB.ChB. (UCT), DCH, FCP(SA), PhD (Wits), Head, Department of Paediatrics and Child Health, Charlotte Maxeke Academic Hospital and University of Witwatersrand, Johannesburg

COTTON, PROFESSOR M., MB.ChB.(UCT), MMed(Paed), FCPaed(SA), DTMH(Wits), DCH(SA), PhD (Stell), Department of Paediatrics and Child Health, Tygerberg Hospital and University of Stellenbosch, Bellville

ELEY, PROFESSOR B., MB.ChB.(UCT), FCP(SA), Department of Paediatrics and Child Health, Red Cross War Memorial Children's Hospital and University of Cape Town

ESSER, DR M., MB.ChB., MMed(Paed), Department of Paediatrics and Child Health, Tygerberg Hospital and University of Stellenbosch, Bellville

GIE, PROFESSOR R., MB.ChB., MMed(Paed), FCPaed(SA), Department of Paediatrics and Child Health, Tygerberg Hospital and University of Stellenbosch, Bellville

GODDARD, DR E., MB.ChB.(UCT), FCPaed(SA), Department of Paediatrics and Child Health, Red Cross War Memorial Children's Hospital and University of Cape Town

GREEN, PROFESSOR RJ., MB.BCh.(Wits), DCH(SA), DTM&H(Wits), FCP(SA), Dip Allerg (SA), FACCP, PhD(Wits), Department of Paediatrics and Child Health, Steve Biko Academic Hospital and University of Pretoria

GREGERSON, DR N., MB.BCh.(Wits), MSc(Med), DCH(SA), FCPaed(SA), Cert Med Genetics(SA), Division of Human Genetics, School of Pathology, National Health Laboratory Services and University of Witwatersrand, Johannesburg

GROTTE, DR R., MB.ChB. (UCT), FCOphth (SA), Department of Paediatric Ophthalmology, Red Cross War Memorial Children's Hospital and University of Cape Town

HADLEY, PROFESSOR GP., MB.ChB. (St Andrews), FRCS (Edin), Head, Department of Paediatric Surgery, Nkosi Albert Luthuli Central Hospital and University of Kwazulu-Natal, Durban

HAJINICOLAOU, DR C., MB.BCh.(Wits), FCP(SA), Department of Paediatrics and Child Health, Chris Hani Baragwanath Hospital and University of Witwatersrand, Johannesburg

KHUMALO, DR N., MB.ChB.(Natal), FCDerm(SA), PhD (UCT), Department of Paediatric Dermatology, Red Cross War Memorial Children's Hospital and University of Cape Town

KRUGER, PROFESSOR M., MB.ChB.(Pret), MMed(Paed), MPhil, PhD (Leuven), Head, Department of Paediatrics and Child Health, Tygerberg Hospital and University of Stellenbosch, Bellville

MACKENJEE, DR H., MB.ChB.(Natal), FCP(SA), Department of Paediatrics, Nkosi Albert Luthuli Central Hospital and University of Kwazulu-Natal, Durban

MADHI, DR S., MB.BCh.(Wits), FCPaed(SA), Department of Paediatrics and Child Health, Chris Hani Baragwanath Hospital and University of Witwatersrand, Johannesburg

MARAIS, PROFESSOR BJ., MB.ChB.(Stell), MMed(Paed), PhD., Department of Paediatrics and Child Health, University of Stellenbosch, Bellville

MCKERROW, DR NH., MB.ChB.(UCT), DCH, FCP(SA),MMed(Paed), Department of Paediatrics and Child Health, Greys Hospital, Pietermaritzburg, and University of Kwazulu-Natal

MOLYNEUX, PROFESSOR E., MB.BS.(London), FRCP(UK), FRCPCH(UK), FFAEM(UK), Head, Department of Paediatrics and Child Health, College of Medicine, Blantyre, Malawi

MOODLEY, DR T., MB.ChB.(Pret), FCPaed(SA), Department of Paediatrics and Child Health, Steve Biko Academic Hospital and University of Pretoria

NEL, DR E., MB.ChB.(Stell), MMed(Paed), BScHons (Epidemiol), Department of Paediatrics and Child Health, Tygerberg Hospital and University of Stellenbosch, Bellville

PARBHOO, DR K., MB. BCh. (Wits), FCPaed(SA), Department of Paediatrics and Child Health, Chris Hani Baragwanath Hospital and University of Witwatersrand, Johannesburg

PETTIFOR, PROFESSOR JM., MB.BCh. (Wits), FCP(SA), PhD (Wits), Head, Department of Paediatrics and Child Health, Chris Hani Baragwanath Hospital and University of Witwatersrand, Johannesburg

RABIE, DR H., MB.ChB.(Stell), MMed(Paed), FCPaed(SA), Department of Paediatrics and Child Health, Tygerberg Hospital and University of Stellenbosch, Bellville

RICHARDS, DR M., MB ChB.(UCT) FCPaed(SA), Department of Paediatrics and Child Health, Red Cross War Memorial Children's Hospital and University of Cape Town

ROBERTSON, DR T., MB.BCh. (Wits), FCOrth(SA), Department of Orthopaedic Surgery, Charlotte Maxeke Academic Hospital and University of Witwatersrand, Johannesburg

RODDA, PROFESSOR J., MB. BCh (Wits), DCH(SA), FCP(SA), FCPaed(SA), Department of Paediatrics and Child Health, Chris Hani Baragwanath Hospital and University of Witwatersrand, Johannesburg

ROLLINS, PROFESSOR NC., MB.BCh. BAO, (Queen's University of Belfast), MRCP(UK), DCH, MD, (Queen's University of Belfast), FRCPCh., Scientist, Department of Child and Adolescent Health and Development, World Health Organization, Geneva; Honorary Professor of Maternal and Child Health, University of KwaZulu-Natal, Durban

SALOOJEE, PROFESSOR H., MB.BCh (Wits), FCPaed (SA), MSc (Wits) Department of Paediatrics and Child Health, University of the Witwatersrand, Johannesburg

SCHAAF, PROFESSOR HS., MB.ChB.(Stell), MMed(Paed), DCM, MD (Stell)., Department of Paediatrics and Child Health, Tygerberg Hospital and University of Stellenbosch, Bellville

SMUTS, PROFESSOR I., MB.ChB.(Pret), MMed(Paed)., Department of Paediatrics and Child Health, Steve Biko Academic Hospital and University of Pretoria

SWINGLER, PROFESSOR GW., MB.ChB.(UCT), FCP(SA), MD(UCT). Head, Department of Paediatrics and Child Health, Red Cross War Memorial Children's Hospital and University of Cape Town

TAKAWIRA, PROFESSOR F., MB.ChB., DTM&H(Wits), MMed(Paed), FCPaed(SA), Cert Cardiol(SA), Department of Paediatrics and Child Health, Steve Biko Academic Hospital and University of Pretoria

THANDRAYEN, DR K., MB. BCh.(Wits), FCPaed(SA), Department of Paediatrics and Child Health, Chris Hani Baragwanath Hospital and University of Witwatersrand, Johannesburg

THEJPAL, DR R., MB.ChB. (Natal), FCP(SA), Department of Paediatrics and Child Health, Nkosi Albert Luthuli Central Hospital and University of Kwazulu-Natal, Durban

THOMSON, PROFESSOR P., MB.BCh.(Wits), FCP(SA) Paed., Paediatric Nephrologist, Donald Gordon Centre and University of Witwatersrand, Johannesburg

TSHIFULARO, PROFESSOR M., MB.ChB. (Medunsa) MMed(Otol), FCORL(SA), Head, Department of Otolaryngology, Steve Biko Academic Hospital and University of Pretoria

VENTER, PROFESSOR A., MB.ChB. (Wits), FCP(SA), PhD (Wits), Head, Department of Paediatrics and Child Health, Universitas Hospital and University of the Free State, Bloemfontein

WESSELS, PROFESSOR G., MB.ChB.(Stell), MMed (Paed), MD (Stell), Department of Paediatrics and Child Health, Tygerberg Hospital and University of Stellenbosch, Bellville

WITTENBERG, PROFESSOR DF., MB.ChB. (UCT), FCP(SA), MD (Natal), Formerly Head, Department of Paediatrics and Child Health, University of Pretoria

PART 1

Evaluation, growth and development

1 History-taking, physical examination, and evaluation of the sick child

Paediatrics is the study of the growth and development of the child from the moment of conception through to adolescence. It embraces the science and art of the prevention, diagnosis, and treatment of the disorders of childhood, whether these disturbances are physical, mental, or emotional.

Good history-taking and clinical examination are the essential tools for:

- Assessing whether or not the child is physically, intellectually, and emotionally normal
- Identifying children who are especially at risk
- Making an early diagnosis of conditions that need treatment.
- Appropriate counselling and support of parents.

Differences between children and adults

There are major differences between children and adults that must be taken into account during history-taking and examination. These differences include the following:

- The history is generally obtained indirectly from an adult.
- Physical examination can often not be done in a fixed order, depending on the child's apprehension and mood. To avoid omissions it is important to record the findings systematically.
- The impact of genetic, environmental, and social factors is often more pronounced in children.

- The major impact of disease may be on growth and development.
- The growth and developmental status of children may influence the expression of disease.
- Clinical norms in children differ with age and from those of adults.

The importance of child health surveillance at every contact

Child health surveillance involves detecting deviations from normal using screening, case-finding, and vigilance. It also includes the preventative and promotive aspects of growth monitoring, promotion of breastfeeding and nutrition, and the provision of appropriate immunizations at each opportunity.

During surveillance, history-taking is the key to the early detection of:

- Familial diseases
- Contact with infectious diseases
- Visual and hearing defects
- Developmental, behavioural, and psychological problems.

Clinical examination is the key to surveillance and detection of:

- Congenital abnormalities (e.g. squint, undescended testes, congenital dislocation of the hip, and cardiac murmurs)
- Abnormal nutritional state
- Growth and developmental abnormalities.

Health surveillance in childhood can only be successfully accomplished with an understanding of what is normal and the variations of this, and of the impact that growth and development have on normality.

Common errors in history-taking and examination

Some of the most common errors made by health professionals when examining children include:
- Inadequate history-taking and failure to listen to the parent or caregiver
- Failure to observe the child and inadequate inspection of the various organ systems before starting palpation, percussion, or auscultation
- Failure to plot height and weight on growth charts, and to measure head circumference in infants and younger children
- Failure to determine the blood pressure
- Failure to observe the gait
- Failure to examine the genitalia because of modesty on the part of the patient or reluctance on the part of the health professional.

The paediatric history

The ability to listen is the most important of the skills and attitudes necessary in good data collection. There is a tendency to hurry through the history-taking, to get on with the physical examination, and to depend unduly on laboratory procedures and other special investigations, but a good history is the launching pad to the diagnosis.

The doctor should be friendly, courteous, and non-judgmental. Doctors' cultural, educational, and social backgrounds are often very different from those of their patients, and the doctor has a special responsibility to recognise this and to listen carefully. If at all possible try to understand children and their carers using the language in which they are most proficient. Understanding people and appreciating why they act as they do is central to providing care.

Elements of a complete history

As in adults, the following information should be obtained:

- Name, age, birth date, gender, and population group
- Present illness
- Main complaint
- Systematic review of other organ systems
- Details of any treatment and response to treatment
- Details of any change in condition
- Past medical history including previous diseases and their sequelae, hospitalisations and any operations.

Additional details of the paediatric history include the following:
- Pregnancy and the mother's health during pregnancy
- Events of labour and delivery
- Condition of the baby in the neonatal period
- Growth and development
- Immunizations
- Diet and feeding history
- The child's emotional development and adjustment
- Family history of disease
- Social make-up of the child's carers and financial status.

Technical information on perinatal health, growth, immunisation and past medical history should be on the Road-to-Health Card.

Perinatal health

Prenatal history
Enquire about the pregnancy, all previous pregnancies, and the health of the mother during these pregnancies. Maternal illnesses acquired before or after conception may affect the child and thus the history should include data on any infections, illnesses such as hypertension or diabetes, vaginal bleeds, or toxaemia that occurred during pregnancy. Results of serological tests, as well as the blood group of the mother, should be recorded. Sensitively request the mother's HIV status and, if positive during pregnancy, her CD4 status and whether she and her child were enrolled in a PMTCT programme.

Birth history
The duration of the pregnancy, and the ease and duration of labour should be recorded. It is also important to know whether the delivery was spontaneous, forceps-assisted, or by Caesarean

section, and why this was so. The place, date of birth, birth weight, difficulty in initiating breathing, as well as the Apgar scores, are also pertinent.

Neonatal history

Important information includes the presence of cyanosis, difficulty in establishing feeds, convulsions, blood transfusions, medications, nursing in an incubator, assisted ventilation, necrotising enterocolitis and the length of stay in the nursery. A history of treated jaundice, the age of onset, duration, and treatment given (e.g. exchange transfusion or phototherapy), must be specifically asked for.

Growth and development

Growth and development are distinguishing features of infancy and childhood. It is important to enquire about physical growth, in particular height, weight, and head circumference. The child's Road-to-Health Chart should provide serial information.

The sequential acquisition of each of several functional milestones is the essence of development, and age-appropriate developmental milestones should be enquired about and recorded (*see* Chapter 2, Growth and development). For a child of school-going age, note the grades and marks achieved in school.

Immunization history

Obtain a record of immunizations from the Road-to-Health Chart, and whether any adverse reactions occurred. List the dates and number of immunizations.

Diet and feeding history

This history is especially important in the small baby and infant, including whether the baby was breastfed or bottlefed. Details concerning the use of vitamins and iron, and the introduction of solid foods are also important.

In a child with feeding difficulties or a nutritional problem, obtain information on the date of onset, feeding methods, types of formula or feeds, interval between feedings, weight changes, and any other relevant data. Twenty-four-hour dietary recall by the carer is the best way of obtaining an accurate reflection of the child's food intake.

Previous diseases and hospitalization

The history of each past disease should include the date of onset, symptoms, diagnosis, treatment, course, complications, and sequelae. Note all accidents, injuries, and poisonings.

Family history

Many disorders run in families or are inherited, and the family history is especially important in paediatrics. Record all medical conditions in blood relatives that may affect the health of the child.

Social make-up and financial status

Children's health is especially sensitive to social factors. The occupation of the mother and father, housing, access to clean water, school and play facilities are all relevant. Determine who provides financial support for the family and who cares for the child during the day. Also note access to grants.

The paediatric physical examination

Approach to the patient

Whenever possible, perform the examination with the parent present. If the child is frightened, sending the parent out of the room will frighten the child even more. Newborns and infants up to six months of age are not often apprehensive while being examined, while those aged between one and four years are the group who show most anxiety and lack of cooperation. A pre-school child may be reassured and distracted by interesting objects such as toys. With an older child gain cooperation by making complimentary remarks, engaging in suitable conversation, or discussing mutual interests.

The examination is best performed in the position most comfortable and non-threatening for the child. Infants are often best examined sitting on the mother's lap with the clinician sitting facing the mother. Older children may stand in front of the mother. In these positions the level of eye contact is equal. Children feel vulnerable and threatened when a clinician towers above them. If a child has a deformity do not focus on it initially. Most of the examination can be conducted satisfactorily without lying the patient down. When it is necessary to place a small child on the examining couch, do this last and permit the mother to stand next to and reassure the child.

The value of observation

The physical examination begins as soon as the patient enters the room. Starting palpation, percussion, or auscultation before making thorough inspection may cause you to miss the obvious in searching for the obscure. The child's attitude towards the parent and the health professional, and the disposition of the parent and family towards the child and the clinician reveal much of the emotional balance of the child and the parent–child relationship. A tentative diagnosis can frequently be made simply by observing the child while in the mother's arms or as he walks or stands in the room. A glance will uncover much detail about the child: whether the child seems well, sick, malnourished, pale, cyanosed, or jaundiced, or shows any other visible abnormalities. Inspection also gives an excellent opportunity to assess the neuromuscular status and developmental level of the small child.

Begin physical contact peripherally with the child's hands or lower leg as he sits on the mother's lap. It may help to examine the mother's fingers first, compare them with your own, and then examine the child's fingers together with the mother. The purpose is not just to examine the fingers, but also to make the first physical contact at a relatively remote spot and as gently as possible. Avoid looking directly into the child's eyes. Rather allow the child to watch you and hopefully decide that you are harmless.

If the child is not upset when the examination begins it is usually sensible to examine the site of suspected pathology first. For example, if the history indicates the presence of a heart problem, a gentle approach and auscultation of the heart may permit evaluation of a murmur before the child begins to cry. The same is true for suspected abdominal pathology. However, if the presenting complaint suggests a painful region, such as an inflamed joint, examining it first would not be advisable. The same is true for examination of oral or pharyngeal lesions as this is often the most dreaded part of the examination for the child.

During the course of the examination the child should be undressed so that the entire body may be examined. Mothers do this best. If the room is cool or if the patient is modest or frightened, only part of the clothing is removed at any one time. Modesty should be respected in the child regardless of age.

When the child's cooperation is necessary for more difficult procedures (e.g. examination of the throat), the patient should be told firmly but kindly what she is to do and what you are going to do. (A request for cooperation that is refused is hard to reverse.) The sight of instruments (e.g. stethoscope, otoscope) often frightens children. When using instruments, it may help if the clinician first demonstrates their use on the mother, or allows the patient to play with or touch them before use. Before any frightening or painful procedure the patient should be told what is going to happen and what is expected of her.

Regardless of how patient you are, some children will reject all attempts at examination. Such children can be at least partially examined in their mother's arms. For instance, if the child clings to the mother, the back and extremities may be examined in this position. The remainder of the procedure may have to be done later.

Measurements

The usual measurements taken at the physical examination include height, weight, blood pressure, temperature, pulse and respiratory rate. For the child less than two years of age measure the head circumference routinely. Growth charts and their interpretation are covered in Chapter 2, and blood pressure recording in Chapter 27. Measurements are frequently made before the child is seen by the clinician. Abnormal findings should be checked.

Weight

Weight should be taken to the nearest 10 g in infants and to the nearest 100 g in older children. Weigh children in minimal clothing, preferably at the same time of the day using the same scale. Record this on the child's Road-to-Health Chart. A single measurement tells little compared with the information obtained from serial measurements, which indicate the rate of growth.

Height

Length is best recorded from birth to two years using a firm, horizontal board with a fixed, vertical headpiece and a sliding, vertical foot piece. A scale is fixed along the length of the board. Two observers are required. Measure the infant in the supine position with the ankles gently pulled to stretch the infant, the knees flat, the head against the headpiece, and the sliding foot piece in firm contact with the soles of the feet held vertically. The head must be held firmly in line with the body and with the lower orbital border in the same vertical plane as the external auditory canal. Record the distance between the headpiece and foot piece.

Height is measured with a rule fixed to the wall, with a smooth sliding headpiece. (Make sure that the rule is fixed to the wall at the correct height!) The position of the child is important: feet together without shoes, back straight with the occiput, buttocks and heels lightly touching the measuring rod, head aligned so that the lower rim of the orbit and the auditory canal are in a horizontal plane. The child is told to stand straight, is stretched gently upwards by pressure under the mastoid process and instructed to relax the shoulders so that they are not shrugged. Take care that the heels are not lifted from the floor. The sliding headpiece is lowered to rest firmly on the head. The distance from the floor to the lower border of the headpiece is measured to the nearest 0.1 cm.

Head circumference

The head circumference is measured with a non-stretchable tape measure at its greatest fronto-occipital circumference and plotted on a centile chart. For greater accuracy use the average of three measurements. A head circumference that crosses centile lines is almost always abnormal.

Assessment of the nutritional state

Clinical nutritional assessment

It is important to determine:
- Whether the child's nutritional state is normal
- What abnormality or pattern of nutritional disorder is present
- The severity or chronicity of an underlying disease process causing malnutrition

- The likelihood of secondary immune deficiency
- The chance of delayed recovery or complications from infection.

For the interpretation of anthropometric measurements (weight for age, length for age, and weight for height) *see* Chapter 2, Growth and development.

Temperature

Axillary and groin temperatures are about 1 °C lower, and oral temperatures 0.5 °C lower, than rectal (core) temperature. In older children it is more suitable to take the oral temperature. Rectal temperatures are best avoided due to the real danger of perforating the bowel.

A temperature above 38 °C is defined as fever, and under 35.5 °C as hypothermia.

Systematic examination

It is outside the scope of this text to describe fully the examination of children and their different organ systems. The description below is not comprehensive and selective attention is given to aspects where the examination of children differs from that of adults.

General appearance

Does she look acutely or chronically ill, comfortable or uncomfortable, is he breathing easily or with difficulty? Is she alert, comatose, delirious, lethargic, dull, bright, responsive, hostile, or cooperative? Watch the interaction between the child and his parents during the examination.

Skin

The skin may be examined as a whole, or as each underlying part is exposed. **Rashes** are difficult to see in pigmented skin. Note the distribution, colour, and character of any skin lesions. Petechiae or purpura are better seen if the skin is stretched and tested for blanching. Purpuric lesions that are palpable and do not blanch with pressure indicate the presence of **vasculitis**. A tangential light shone on the skin will highlight papular rashes.

Peripheral **cyanosis** is most easily detected in the nail beds, while in central cyanosis the mucous membranes of the mouth are also discoloured. Cyanosis is caused mainly by pulmonary disease or congenital cyanotic heart disease. **Jaundice** is best seen in natural light and may be entirely missed in artificial light. It is visible in the newborn when the total serum bilirubin exceeds 90 µmol/l and in the older child 40 µmol/l.

Pallor or paleness should be noted. It is best seen in the palms of the hands. 'Some' pallor suggests a haemoglobin concentration of 10 g/dl or less, while 'severe' pallor suggests a concentration of less than 6 g/dl. Pallor should never be considered an accurate estimate of haemoglobin concentration. Pallor of the nail beds may be due to hypoproteinaemia, a low haemoglobin concentration, or shock.

A child's state of **hydration** can be assessed using a number of indicators of interstitial fluid volume. Skin turgor is best determined by pinching the patient's abdominal wall skin and subcutaneous tissues between the thumb and index finger, squeezing, and then allowing the skin to fall back into place. Normally the skin appears smooth and firm and, when released, falls back into place immediately without residual marks. In children with poor tissue turgor, the skin loses its elasticity and falls back into place more slowly. In severe cases it remains suspended and creased for a few seconds. This may not occur in obese infants. The skin feels thin and loose in children with chronic diseases and malnutrition. Oedema is demonstrated by firm pressure over the dorsum of the foot, anterior tibia, or lower spine. The presence of a sunken fontanelle when a child is lying prone, the absence of tears and dry mucous membranes in the mouth are also indicators of dehydration. No single sign must be interpreted in isolation.

In malnutrition **the hair** may be pale, lustreless, red or grey, easily broken, thinner, and lacking curl.

Clubbing in small children is best shown by looking at the fingers in profile to see if they are clubbed. The finger nails may show **koilonychia** (spoon-shaped deformity) or be brittle or discoloured.

Inspect **the hands** for single palmar creases, missing digits, clinodactyly (incurving of little finger) or other abnormalities. Terminal thickening of the radius at the wrist joint is found in rickets.

Head

Note shape, bossing, and the fontanelles (whether open or closed, either prematurely or normally).

The anterior fontanelle remains open to 18 months, closing prematurely in microcephaly and craniostenosis, and remaining open for longer than normal in hydrocephalus, rickets, and cretinism. Bulging of the fontanelle occurs with crying or straining, but in a relaxed child it is an extremely important sign and suggests raised intracranial pressure, the causes of which include meningitis, encephalitis, brain tumour, and subdural haematoma. A tense, bulging fontanelle is best noted if the patient is sitting up. It is most easily shown by holding the curved palm of the hand over the top of the skull, and feeling the bulge of the fontanelle above the level of the surrounding bone. Running the hand from behind forwards also gives the feel of a full fontanelle above the level of the cranial bones. A depressed anterior fontanelle suggests dehydration.

Face

The appearance of the face may be typical in many disorders, e.g. cretinism, Down's syndrome, and fetal alcohol syndrome.

Eyes

Squint, inflammation, cataracts, and conjunctival haemorrhages may be seen, as well as hypertelorism, slanted or small palpebral fissures, epicanthic folds and so on.

Nose

Discharge can be either watery, mucoid, purulent, bloodstained, or a combination of these. Check the patency of the nasal passages as well.

Ears

The long axis of the pinna is normally in line with the long axis of the body, and the superior upper insertion of the pinna is at or above a straight line extended posteriorly from the palpebral fissure. Note any discharge from the ear. The examination technique for the external ear canal and tympanic membrane differs in children. The direction of the ear canal in newborns and infants is upward, and in older children downward and forward. To visualize the tympanic membrane with the otoscope, gently pull the pinna up and back in older children, and downwards in infants and newborns. This can be done with the child in the prone position or sitting upright on the mother's lap.

Mouth and throat

Check the lips, gums, teeth, tongue, and palate, paying special attention to the soft palate to exclude a localized cleft. Examination of the throat is often resented by smaller children. Proper and secure immobilization of the head is essential and a bright light should be used to visualize the oropharynx and tonsils. Tonsillar exudate occurs in infectious mononucleosis and moniliasis, and rarely in diphtheria. Retropharyngeal abscess forms a unilateral swelling of the posterior pharyngeal wall. A postnasal drip and pharyngeal hyperplasia are often seen in nasal allergy or infection.

Neck stiffness

Exclude neck stiffness in all acutely ill children, although its absence does not exclude meningitis under two years of age. First look for active resistance to flexion before passive resistance (i.e. ask the child to follow a light, ask him to kiss his knees, or to flex his chin onto his chest, or place a bright toy into his lap). Always look at facial expression when looking for meningism. Free movement of the neck may be limited by inflamed lymph glands, muscular spasm (trauma), joint disease (rheumatoid arthritis), bony disease, or apical lobar pneumonia.

Lymph nodes

Feel for lymph nodes in the submental, tonsillar, cervical (deep and superficial), and supraclavicular regions. Systematic examination of all lymph nodes in other regions is essential, including the epitrochlear area.

The respiratory system

Inspection

Count the respiratory rate before the child is undressed or otherwise disturbed. During inspiration both the chest and abdomen expand, and the reverse occurs in expiration. In small children abdominal movement is more prominent than thoracic movement. During obstructive sleep apnoea there is intercostal muscle inhibition and some paradoxical movement of chest and abdomen. Careful inspection may be rewarded by seeing that one side of the chest moves less than the other, indicating underlying pleural disease, lobar collapse, or lung destruction. Flaring of alae nasi reflects increased work of breathing and respiratory distress. Deformity such as a barrel shape suggests chronic conditions like obstructive lung disease. Compliance or chest wall elasticity is reduced in the presence of fibrosis and restrictive lung disease. Inspection of the spine is essential to exclude any kyphoscoliosis that could cause restrictive lung disease.

Palpation

A deviated trachea indicates that it is either being pulled across by collapse or shrinkage of a lung or lobe; or being pushed by an effusion or tension pneumothorax. Deviation of the trachea may be difficult to assess in children and this sign must be interpreted in conjunction with palpation for the apex beat of the heart and findings on percussion and auscultation. Expansion of the chest is often best palpated.

Percussion

Percussion of the chest may frighten the child and should be done later in the examination. The chest wall in children is thinner and the chest more resonant than in adults. In newborns and infants with small chests, percussion of the last digit of the finger is the most useful. Hyper-resonance (airway obstruction, pneumothorax), dullness (consolidation, atelectasis, pleural thickening), stony dullness (effusion or empyema) are useful clinical signs. Important aspects to note are the position of the upper border of the liver and the size of the cardiac dullness. Remember that in a child most of the lung lies posteriorly so do not forget to percuss the back.

During **auscultation** listen for breath sounds and adventitious sounds. Warm the stethoscope before use and press it firmly against the chest wall, or artifacts will be heard. The entire chest, including the maxillary areas, should be auscultated. It is useful to allow the child to handle the end of the stethoscope prior to examination so that he or she is re-assured that it is not an instrument that will cause pain. Breath sounds in children are normally louder and heard for longer in the expiratory phase than in adults, because of the thin chest wall. These bronchovesicular sounds may be difficult to distinguish from bronchial breathing. Breath sounds may be normal, decreased (less air entry), absent (no air entry because of collapse or obstruction of airway), louder and normal (as in hyperventilation of acidosis), louder and abnormal (with air space consolidation). Vocal resonance is best appreciated when the baby is crying (every dark cloud has a silver lining), but is otherwise difficult to do in a young child.

Crackles are interrupted sounds associated with the movement of air through inflammatory secretions within the airways or air spaces. They are usually associated with airway conditions such as bronchitis, bronchiolitis, or bronchopneumonia. Stridor is most easily heard during inspiration but as the obstruction becomes more severe it is audible in both inspiration and expiration. This high-pitched inspiratory sound is mainly the result of extrathoracic airway obstruction. It is generally heard better at the mouth than in the chest during auscultation, with the bell of the stethoscope over the mouth. Croup is the most common cause of stridor. Wheezes are softer and higher pitched sounds made by obstruction to either small or large intra-thoracic airways. Small airways obstruction is distinguished from large airway obstruction by the fact that the wheeze is not as prominent (best heard with a stethoscope), the presence of associated crepitations (crackles) and air trapping. The most common small airway disease is acute viral bronchiolitis. In large airway obstruction, the wheeze is often so loud that it can easily be heard without a stethoscope and is often audible in both inspiration and expiration.

The cardiovascular system

The quality of peripheral perfusion can be checked by noting the warmth of peripheral tissues and the capillary filling time. The brachial pulse is usually the easiest to feel in children. Note the rate, rhythm, and volume. Feel the pulses in both arms and also the femoral pulses, to exclude coarctation of the aorta. The pulse rate is usually increased by 10 to 12 beats/min for each 1 °C rise in fever

External jugular vein distension, with the body inclined to 45°, is usually difficult to see in young children because of their short necks.

The apex beat of the heart is the most lateral and the lowest position at which an impulse can be easily palpated. Up to the age of seven years this is normally in the 4th intercostal space just to the left of the mid-clavicular line, and thereafter in the 5th intercostal space. The apex impulse may be difficult to feel in children less than two years, or in children with pericardial effusion, heart failure, or air trapping.

Thrills and pericardial friction rubs may also be palpated. Thrills at the apex are more easily felt with the child lying on his left side, and basal thrills with the child sitting upright.

Percussion dullness to the right of the sternum in the 3rd or 4th intercostal space usually indicates right-sided heart enlargement or mediastinal deviation.

The nature of the **heart sounds** is important in children. Splitting of the second sound is more easily heard in children than adults, is best heard in the pulmonary area, and is common in normal children. The split widens on inspiration. Absent splitting (a single second sound) suggests a lesion involving the pulmonary valve. Splitting heard throughout the respiratory cycle suggests the wide fixed splitting of an atrial septal defect. A third heart sound is common in children and is best heard at the apex. It is softer and with a longer interval between the second and third sound than in a gallop rhythm.

Determining the significance of **murmurs** is often difficult. Many children have innocent physiological murmurs without heart disease. Murmurs heard in systole are: early systolic, late systolic, or throughout systole (pansystolic). Diastolic murmurs may be heard early (proto-diastolic), mid-diastolic, or late in diastole (presystolic).

Record the quality of the murmurs as soft, harsh, blowing, or whistling. The intensity of the murmur is graded as follows:

- Grade I murmur is the softest possible murmur, only heard in a quiet room. It is not heard in all positions.
- Grade II murmur is the weakest murmur heard in all positions in the normal paediatric out-patients or a ward.
- Grade III murmur is a loud murmur, not accompanied by a palpable thrill.

- Grade IV murmur is a loud murmur with a palpable thrill.
- Grade V murmur is heard with the stethoscope barely touching the chest.
- Grade VI murmur can be heard without the stethoscope touching the chest.

Blood pressure measurement in children is frequently overlooked. (*see* Chapter 27, Renal and urinary tract disorders).

The abdomen

It is impossible to do a thorough examination if the child is crying or if the abdominal wall is tense, so it is important to take advantage of the right opportunity as it arises.

The **abdominal muscles** are thinner than those in adults, and the child normally has a lordotic posture, giving the appearance of a prominent 'pot-belly'.

Veins are rarely visible in small infants with good subcutaneous tissue and in dark-skinned children. Although visible but not distended veins are usually seen in normal older children until puberty, these veins are especially noticeable in malnourished children. Distended superficial veins are seen with heart failure, peritonitis, or may be collaterals associated with portal hypertension or obstruction of the inferior vena cava. Direction of flow of blood in distended veins should be established.

Visible peristalsis can be normal and can be seen through a thin abdominal wall in marasmic or premature infants. If limited to a fixed area or associated with vomiting it suggests intestinal obstruction. In infants up to two months of age, a visible gastric wave or peristalsis which passes from under the left costal margin to the right may indicate pyloric stenosis. Abnormal peristalsis occurs in surgical obstruction, in tuberculous adhesions, and when there is a bolus of worms, for example.

During **palpation**, first palpate gently and superficially, observing for tenderness, beginning in the left lower quadrant, and then proceeding to the left upper, right upper, and right lower quadrants. If a localized site of pain or tenderness is found, this area should be palpated at the end of the examination, after the other parts of the abdomen have been palpated. Rigidity of abdominal muscles may be due to a neighbourhood cause, such as lower lobe lobar pneumonia, but peritonitis and surgical causes must be excluded. If tenderness in the right iliac fossa prevents deep palpation of the posterior abdominal wall, it may be due to appendicitis or iliac lymphadenitis.

The **normal liver** is generally palpable as a superficial mass with a clear border 1–2 cm below the right costal margin during the first five years. It should be palpated along its entire margin, as the lobes may be unequally enlarged. Record size, consistency, tenderness, and pulsation. The normal liver edge is sharp and flexible so it can be bent slightly. Fatty infiltration of the liver gives a firm edge while a hard rounded edge indicates cirrhosis or malignant disease. An irregular surface suggests cirrhosis. Pulsation of the liver occurs in tricuspid incompetence. The upper border must be determined by percussion and the span recorded, particularly when there is apparent hepatomegaly, as it may be due to downward displacement by over-distended lungs. The normal liver span is dependent on age and increases from 4.5–5 cm at one week of age to about 6–7 cm by mid-childhood.

An **enlarged spleen** is felt as a superficial mass in the left upper quadrant, often laterally in the child, enlarging in the direction of the iliac crest. Its size should be recorded and tenderness noted. Soft splenic enlargement is found in children with diseases such as septicaemia, many of the common viral infections (such as measles and infectious mononucleosis), tuberculosis, malaria, bilharziasis, and leukaemia. A very large spleen with little hepatomegaly is seen with portal vein obstruction.

Kidneys are normally palpable only in young infants. If palpable outside this period it suggests abnormal enlargement or a tumour. They are bimanually palpated in the lumbar regions and have a lobular shape. They have no medial notch. The left kidney can be distinguished from the spleen by the ability to define its upper pole and movement late in inspiration.

The **bladder** may be seen as well as palpated, lying above the pubis. If it cannot be emptied some obstruction must be present. The anus should be examined for a fissure. The testes, epididymis, and especially the hernial orifices, must be examined; strangulation of gut in a hernial orifice can occur within the first few days of life.

A distended abdomen with little tympany suggests fluid or solid masses. When fluid is suspected, test for a fluid thrill and shifting dullness.

The central nervous system

The nervous system is huge and its disease manifestations vast in array. With a good approach, however, very few significant conditions will be missed. Children are tricky candidates for a formal neurological examination and so one must often rely first on observation in their natural state, which is usually play! Hence the need to be a systematic opportunist.

One of the challenges of paediatric neurology is to appreciate the normal evolution and maturation of the child's nervous system. The natural state of the neonate is one of irregular, poorly regulated movements in a body that is predominantly flexed, through to the infant who is becoming more extended, has lost primitive reflexes and is aware of the outside world, to a toddler who has fine dexterity in the hands, takes a few steps and is able to call her mother for attention. Synapse proliferation, myelination and memory loops are central to these processes.

The functional side of a child's neurological system is reflected in its state of development. Where significant alteration of function exists this disability can significantly alter the quality of life of both the child and those caring for it. Thus, it is essential to understand a child's nervous system as more than just a compendium of pupil sizes, muscle tones and Babinski's reflex.

The aim of the neurological examination is two-fold:

1 What is the anatomical location and pathological nature of the lesion?
2 How is the child impaired by the condition?

Here are some broad groups of abnormality that one might encounter and which it is important to describe accurately.

Alterations of consciousness describe the state of a child who is not responding appropriately to her environment. This includes confusion and agitation, drowsiness and various degrees of rousability through to the deeply comatose child. A coma score is useful, but easier perhaps is the AVPU scoring system, which is applicable to all ages of children. (A = alert, V = responds to verbal stimuli, P = responds to painful stimuli, U = unresponsive.)

Conditions causing altered levels of consciousness tend to involve more diffuse areas of the brain, although the primary pathology might be of very localized nature (e.g. a chemical encephalopathy from a failing liver). It is helpful to determine whether these problems arise:

- Outside the brain and skull, e.g. hepatic encephalopathy
- Within the skull, e.g. encephalitis or raised intra-cranial pressure from a brain tumour.

There are a number of different characterisations of **abnormal tone**:

- **Spasticity**. On examination you find increased tone in peripheral striated muscle, which is present in sleep, increasing resistance to more rapid stretch of a muscle (e.g. moving a joint slowly versus quickly), clonus, Babinski sign in the older child and, if severe enough, the persistence of abnormal reflexes such as a Moro or crossed adductors. This is classically a feature of an upper motor neurone lesion, where the normal moderating effect of the cerebral cortex and corticospinal tracts on spinal reflex arcs is lost.
- **Dystonia**. A state of abnormal increase in tone with altered posture and positions of limbs as a result of loss of control of muscles in opposition to one another. The tone is rigid and joint movement characteristically 'lead pipe' in nature (initially stiff and then constant resistance throughout movement). Movements are repetitive and writhing. Reflexes are normal and movements cease when sleeping when tone is normal. Typically disorders are located within the basal ganglia.
- **Hypotonia**. This can be difficult to distinguish from weakness, but it typically describes a muscle at rest. In infants the hypotonic state may exist before the onset of hyertonicity following cortical brain injuries.

Floppiness describes an infant who shows little resistance to passive movement. The infant is often seen flexed in ventral suspension or lying in a frog leg position on a bed. The phenomenon is common to conditions that cause low tone or muscle weakness.

Weakness should be described by location, i.e. proximal versus distal (e.g. a myopathy versus a neuropathy), left versus right, or upper limbs versus lower limbs. To understand weakness it is important to understand the motor system from the cerebral cortex to the muscle body itself.

Each component of the nervous system has typical modes of neurological presentation:

 * *Cerebral cortex* – discrete localization possible with hallmark spasticity, weakness, reduced muscle bulk and brisk reflexes, e.g. a child with spastic cerebral palsy following hypoxic ischaemic encephalopathy.
 * *Spinal cord* – typically findings as for cerebral cortex, but with manifestations only below the neurological level of the lesion. If a complete cord abnormality exists (e.g. traumatic transection), there will be abnormalities in sensation and autonomic control as well. The hallmark of these lesions is the presence of a discrete level above which normal neurology exists.
 * *Motor horn cell* – located at the junction between the descending motor tracts and the peripheral nerve. There are varying degrees of weakness that notably spare the muscles of facial expression. Reflexes are usually absent and there is muscle fasciculation, classically in the tongue. Typical examples are the spinal muscular atrophies (SMA) and polio.
 * *Peripheral nerve* – varying degrees of weakness with atrophy of muscles and absent reflexes, as in Guillain-Barré syndrome.
 * *Neuromuscular junction* – abnormalities are rare, and present with weakness, particularly on repetition (fatiguability).
 * *Muscle* – a predominantly proximal weakness (shoulder and pelvic girdles), which can sometimes be elicited by asking a child to get up from a sitting position on the floor (Gower's sign). There may be markedly atrophic muscle, or the calf muscle pseudohypertrophy of the Duchenne's muscular dystrophy.

Abnormal movements include:

 * *Chorea* – a rapid, jerky, irregular movement that cannot be controlled or anticipated by the patient.
 * *Athetosis* – similar to dystonia but of a slower more writhing nature
 * *Ataxia* – inability to coordinate voluntary bodily movements
 * *Tremor* – involuntary movements with a fixed frequency
 * *Tics* – involuntary, regular movements while awake. The movements are subconscious but can be consciously suppressed. They may be motor (e.g. eye blinking) or vocal (e.g. repetitive throat clearing)
 * *Myoclonus* – rapid, short lived, jerky movements of muscle groups.

The coordination and control of movement requires an array of working components from consciousness to working muscles, the ability to fine tune movement and position in space using proprioception, the vestibular apparatus and visual cues.

Useful tests to establish the cause of ataxia include getting a child to walk, reach for objects at the end of his reach or asking a cooperative child to do finger-nose movements.

Assessment of **development** is an integral part of the neurological examination of a child, and is covered in Chapter 2.

An **abnormality of gait** is one of the most reliable tests of neurological function in children. If a child is too young or too disabled to walk it might help to assess posture and position control when sitting. Walking is a neurologically demanding movement that sensitively elicits signs of abnormal tone, power and coordination. Never forget to ask a child to walk for you. Look for coordination difficulty, abnormal posture, limp, abnormal swings of the legs and asymmetry of stepping. Even more demanding is to ask a child to walk on her heels, when an abnormally flexed arm can sometimes unmask a subtle hemiparesis on that side.

Neck stiffness. See 'Systematic examination' above.

Head circumference. See 'Measurements' above.

Examine the **cranial nerves** in the following way:

 * **First** cranial nerve. It is seldom possible to test this in children.
 * **Second** cranial nerve. Does the child fix and follow a light? If there are pupillary responses but no behavioural responses

there is a high likelihood of cortical visual impairment.

- **Third, fourth and sixth** cranial nerves. Get the child to follow a bright object or toy, watching for nystagmus or strabismus during this procedure. Unilateral ptosis (droopy eye lid) usually indicates a third nerve palsy.
- **Fifth** cranial nerve. This nerve is very difficult to test in young children. Eliciting the corneal reflex is the only accurate way of testing this cranial nerve (but very unpleasant for the child).
- **Seventh** cranial nerve. Watch facial movements while the child is laughing or crying. Differentiate between an upper and lower motor neuron seventh palsy.
- **Eighth** cranial nerve. Children cannot localise the direction of sound before the age of six months. From six months to three years of age hearing is tested by the distraction test and, when speech has been acquired, by a response to whispered speech (the response can be emotional, non-verbal or verbal). Remember that mothers are very good at discerning whether or not their children are hearing impaired.
- **Ninth to twelfth** cranial nerves. Watch the child drinking or chewing. Children with chewing and swallowing abnormalities will often cough when drinking liquids but manage more solid foods. In older children excessive drooling or dysarthria may indicate problems with the lower cranial nerves.

Start the **motor examination** by observing posture, movement and hand function. Power is the main denominator in the motor examination.

In a young child who is **not yet walking**:
- *Supine.* Assess symmetry of movement, posture and quality of movements. The hypotonic/floppy child will assume a frog-like posture and there will be paucity of spontaneous movements.
- *Pull to sit.* Assess head control (at three months there should be little to no head lag).
- *Sitting position.* Supported or unsupported sitting, propping reflexes, straightness of back.

- *Vertical suspension.* Assess support on standing. The hypotonic child will have little or no support on standing. The spastic (hypertonic) child may have advanced standing, but will tend to stand on his toes and show scissoring. Also look for placing and stepping reflexes.
- *Horizontal suspension.* Assess the position of the child's head and buttocks in relation to the horizon. A hypotonic child will have an inverted 'U' position, while the hypertonic child will have increased extensor tone.
- *In prone position.* Assess whether the infant is able to lift and turn head and support herself on her elbows.

Valuable clues may be the 'frog position' with low muscle tone in the supine position, and 'palmar thumbing' and 'scissoring' of the legs with increased tone.

NB: Do not use these test positions in children with a decreased level of consciousness. They can be dangerous in the absence of head control.

When examing a child who is **already walking** a very useful 'screening test' for the power and tone in the upper limbs is the arm extension test with the arms fully extended and the palms up and eyes closed. This tests for power, tone, contractures, cerebellar function, proprioception in upper limbs, tremor and abnormal movements. Also ask the child to touch the fingers of each hand with the thumb while the hand is in this position. Synkinesis (mirror movements of the opposite side) can be normal in preschool infants but not in school-going children. Ask the child to walk and run. Look for specific abnormalities of gait, e.g. broad based (ataxic/cerebellar), waddling (weakness of the hip girdle), slapping (peripheral neuropathy) and antalgic (arthritis).

Power in the lower limbs is tested by heel and toe walking (distal muscles) and getting up from the floor (hip girdle muscles). Ask the child to balance and hop on one leg and to walk along a line. This tests cerebellar function as well as power.

Tone in a young child is tested on the mother's lap. Assess tone at each joint by passive movement (not by shaking the limbs). The definition of tone is resistance against passive movement. Children with cerebral palsy often have low axial and proximal tone with increased distal tone. This will be missed if the tone is not assessed at all the joints.

It is often difficult to elicit upper limb **reflexes** in the young child. Clues to abnormal lower limb reflexes include the presence of a crossed-adductor reflex and the ability to elicit the patella reflex with very light touch or distal to the insertion of the patella tendon on the shin. A few diminishing beats of **clonus** are normal in an infant, but no more than two beats are acceptable. Persistent clonus is always abnormal.

The intensity of the stimulus for a plantar reflex should not result in withdrawal of the foot. Extensor plantar responses are normal in young infants who are not yet walking, provided that they are symmetrical.

The value of the **primitive reflexes** in the neurological examination of infants can be summarized as follows:

◆ Primitive reflexes are present at birth, except for the tonic neck reflex, which often appears a few weeks after birth.
◆ They should be symmetrical.
◆ These reflexes start disappearing from the age of three months. At nine months of age only the plantar grasp may still be present in normal infants. Persistence of the other primitive reflexes, (e.g. Moro, palmar grasp etc.) after the age of nine months indicates an upper motor neuron lesion – usually cerebral palsy.

By this stage of the examination **cerebellar function** should already have been assessed, i.e. by looking for nystagmus when eye movements were assessed, balance and coordination when the child was sitting, walking, balancing on one leg, and toe-to-heel walking. Intention tremor should have been assessed when the child reached out for an object.

In the very young infant the only components of **sensory function** that can be assessed are touch and pain.

If motor function is normal, test touch by a withdrawal response to touch. The most accurate means of assessing touch in an older child is to ask the child to point with his finger to the point of touch with his eyes closed. Before testing for proprioception with the eyes closed first demonstrate what is meant by 'up, middle, and down' with the child's eyes open.

Children who have not yet been 'potty trained' are naturally incontinent. In these children inspection of the anal sphincter tone and anal 'wink' reflex may be the only indication of a problem with **autonomic function** in this area. If indicated, a rectal examination may be necessary to determine anal tone. A distended bladder or dribbling of urine when pressure is applied to the bladder is abnormal in all age groups and usually indicates a measure of autonomic dysfunction.

Recording information obtained during history-taking and examination

Once all the information has been gathered it needs to be synthesized into a cogent whole. A child might walk into a consulting room and the diagnosis is rapidly established by recognising a pattern or a very particular feature of a condition. More often though, a healthcare worker has to be methodical and systematic in the process of synthesizing all the history and clinical information into a comprehensive report. For example it might include the pathological diagnosis of bronchiolitis, but will also take note of the child's experience of hypoxia, the thirst from inability to feed properly and the child's poor growth as a result of the poor financial state of the home. The management plan will involve both active relief of discomfort (oxygen and fluid in this case), directing definitive antibiotic therapy and considering social and nutritional support for the child on discharge.

Disease processes constantly evolve and require constant adjustments to treatment. It is important then to constantly evaluate the assessments made in the light of new information or a child's condition changes.

Much of the examination of a child is necessarily opportunistic and not always in the same order. To avoid omissions, it is especially important to record findings systematically. Two important recording systems are the Road-to-Health Chart and the problem-oriented medical record (POMR). Both have their uses and are complementary.

Good record-keeping clarifies thinking and improves communication. It is an essential part of good patient care. A management plan is formulated after the health worker has completed the initial data gathering–understanding all the components of a child's environment and the abnormal physiology that may be contributing to the pain, discomfort or general ill health. This is often a dynamic process whose final point might be some hours or months away from completion.

Road-to-Health Chart

This is a patient-retained dynamic record that includes perinatal information, growth, development, immunizations, and a summary of illness or disease events (*see* Chapter 4, Community paediatrics, child health and survival). It is an extremely important record in early childhood and the first step in history-taking should be to examine the information on the chart. The last act is to make a brief note documenting the current visit and to hand it back to the mother. Updating the growth record and seizing the opportunity to administer immunizations when needed are important responsibilities at every patient contact.

The problem-oriented medical record

The main advantages of the POMR are:
+ It identifies and ensures attention to each of the patient's problems on an ongoing basis and provides a record of this.
+ It improves communication and audit of patient care.
+ It ensures that problems that may not be in the forefront of each visit are not forgotten.

The POMR comprises four elements:
+ Database
+ Problem list
+ Initial plan
+ Progress notes.

Basic information. A lot of the basic information needs to be recorded only once, whereas some is dynamic and requires regular updating. This includes demographic details (name, age, address, family size, housing, and income), family history, including medical history of parents, siblings and relatives, psychosocial and socio-economic situation, environmental influences and home circumstances, past history comprising antenatal and post-natal events and problems, immunization record, growth and development record, school history (when applicable), and important medical information, e.g. allergies, medications, and infections.

Information from the Road-to-Health Chart should be transcribed to the database.

Current episode. This section records the present history and physical findings of the current consultation. This usually starts with the reason for the consultation and the concerns of the patient or parents, followed by the specific and systematic history relating to these.

The problem list

Active problems that require immediate action and management are defined, and also problems that may be inactive and not in need of immediate attention.

The problem list is the key and index of the POMR and it may require revision on each occasion, i.e. active problems may have resolved and become inactive problems and new problems may be added.

Initial management plan

At this point, important decisions have to be made regarding the following:
+ How sick is the patient?
+ Where should she be managed?
+ Which problems need management?

For each active problem, a plan is formulated to solve that particular problem. This includes setting hypotheses and testing them. The plan includes treatment, investigation, monitoring, counselling, and follow-up.

Progress notes
These are organized systematically to keep track of all relevant information, to monitor the resolution of problems, and to identify new problems as they develop.

Progress notes for each problem are recorded in the SOAP (subjective, objective, assessment, plan) structure:

S *Subjective information* — information offered by the child, nursing staff, parents, and medical personnel.

O *Objective information* including:
- changes in physical examination
- monitoring information (pulse, BP, etc.)
- changes in flow charts
- results of investigations.

A *Assessment* – updated assessment of the position in the light of information obtained in S and O.

P *Plan* — further or revised plan of action structured in the format Dx, Mx, Rx, Ex.

Evaluation of the sick child

A functional approach to organ evaluation is vital in assessing the ill child. At present two widely held approaches include the WHO Integrated Management of Childhood Illness (IMCI) and the Advanced Paediatric Life Support (APLS©) system. The IMCI system is designed for primary care health professionals with a strong emphasis on recognising illness, in particular disease states and how to initiate immediate management. It is of particular relevance in low and middle income countries. The APLS approach has a greater emphasis on the management of the seriously ill or injured child and is more useful in the hospital setting. Both approaches have, at their core, the stress on recognising the signs of organ dysfunction rather than the particular pathological diagnosis.

> It is more important to recognize the signs of organ dysfunction in an ill child than to make a particular pathological diagnosis

Children rarely have sudden loss of a vital function, such as cardiac output, which an adult might experience after a myocardial infarction, for example. When a vital function in a child becomes compromised it is usually the culmination of processes that have existed for a few hours or days. When children do experience cardio-respiratory arrest, resuscitation is very rarely successful outside a hospital. Even when this occurs inside the hospital the outlook for complete neurological recovery is grim. It is crucial to recognise the signs of significant organ impairment and appreciate the antecedent pathways that lead to life threatening events. Programmes such as the Advanced Paediatric Life Support (APLS©) and the Advanced Life Support (ALS©) are examples of courses where a stress is laid on being able quickly to recognise the seriously ill or injured child.

The fundamental approach to the seriously ill child is the ABC approach, which is common to all first aid and advanced care algorithms.

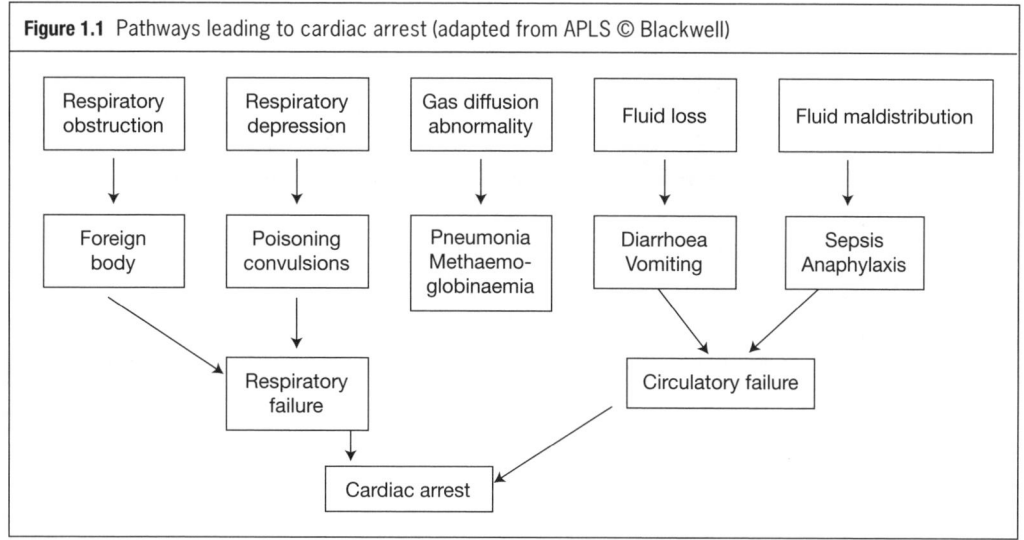

Figure 1.1 Pathways leading to cardiac arrest (adapted from APLS © Blackwell)

Table 1.1 The ABC approach

Airway and breathing compromise
Increased effort of breathing – this might be demonstrated by
    Tachypnoea
    Flaring of the alae nasi
    Inability to feed
    Recession
    Noisy breathing
    Grunting
    Gasping

Reduced efficacy of breathing
    Reduced chest or abdominal movement
    Quiet or silent breath sounds on auscultation
Effects of impaired respiratory function
    Tachycardia or bradycardia
    Mottling or cyanosis (beware the anaemic child who may never become cyanosed)
    An agitated, drowsy or unconscious child

    Note: these signs might be absent in the presence of severe respiratory failure, when a child is exhausted, neurologically depressed or where there are intrinsic neuromuscular disorders, e.g. Guillain-Barré syndrome.

Circulatory compromise
Compensatory mechanisms
    Age-adjusted tachycardia
    Reduced pulse volume or distal-central pulse volume discrepancies
    Delayed capillary filling of more than 3 seconds
    Hypotension (expected systolic BP = 80 + (age in years × 2). **This is a late and ominous sign.**

Organ effects of impaired circulation
    Tachypnoea
    Cold, mottled skin
    Abnormal consciousness – agitated, drowsy or unconscious
    Oliguria (<2 ml/kg/hr in infants and <1 ml/kg/hr in children)

Neurological impairment
Level of consciousness. A rapid assessment in all children can be made using the AVPU mnemonic:
    A Alert
    V Voice response
    P Pain response only
    U Unresponsive to all stimuli

Abnormal posture. Very unwell children are often hypotonic. Stiff posturing with either legs or arms in extension usually indicates serious brain abnormalities. A proviso is the child who may be convulsing. Note also signs of severe meningeal irritation such as opisthotonic posturing.
Pupillary signs. Widely dilated and unreactive, discrepant sizes and tightly constricted pupils.

Integrated management of childhood illness (IMCI)

The IMCI (integrated management of childhood illness) is a World Health Organization (WHO)-initiated process designed to improve the management of the most common causes of disease mortality in developing countries, namely acute respiratory illnesses, malaria, measles, malnutrition and diarrhoea. It is common for children in areas of high disease burdens to be suffering from more than one condition and so the thrust in diagnosis is directed at classification of the common manifestation of these diseases into mild, moderate, severe categories, with clear guidelines on their respective managements. It uses more global assessments of organ dysfunction or abnormality as classification tools to arrive at a management plan. Its purpose is to strike an appropriate balance between being both sensitive and specific in diagnosing disease, reliably recognising the ill child and using a rational and cost effective approach to care for the child in resource-limited settings.

In its comprehensive form it is also a method to improve health system function and to help manage children's health holistically. For example, aspects of a child's growth are also assessed and immunisation status is checked. A child's carers are counselled about nutrition and breastfeeding, and advice is given to the mother about basic illness management such as oral rehydration for diarrhoeal illness.

It has been widely adopted throughout the developing world, including South Africa.

Table 1.2 An example of an IMCI algorithm

Signs	Classify as	Immediate treatment
• Any general danger sign or • Chest indrawing or • Stridor in calm child	Severe pneumonia or very severe disease	• Give first dose of an appropriate antibiotic. • Refer URGENTLY to hospital.
• Fast breathing	Pneumonia	• Give an appropriate oral antibiotic for 5 days. • Soothe the throat and relieve the cough with a safe remedy. • Advise mother when to return immediately. • Follow-up in 2 days.
• No signs of pneumonia or very severe disease	No pneumonia: cough or cold	• If coughing more than 30 days, refer for assessment. • Soothe the throat and relieve the cough with a safe remedy. • Advise mother when to return immediately. • Follow-up in 5 days if not improving.

2

Growth and development

The normal processes of growth, development, and maturation of the healthy child from fetal life to adulthood are continuous and dynamically interrelated. They take place in tissues, organs, regions, and systems at different rates and velocities (*see* Figure 2.1).

Figure 2.1 Differences in growth curves of different parts and tissues of the body

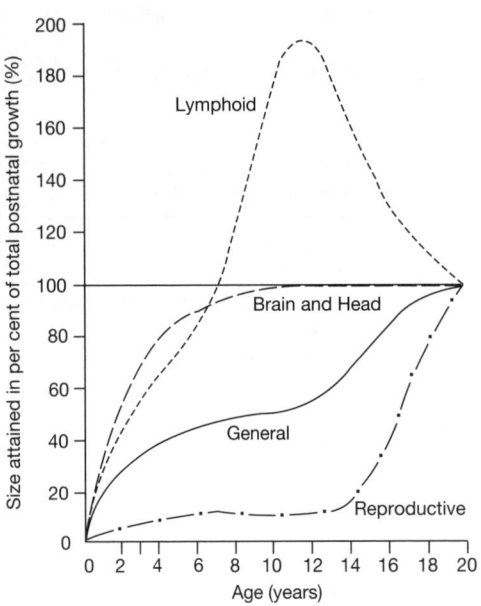

Source: Tanner, J. M. Growth at Adolescence, 2nd edn., Blackwell Scientific Publications, Oxford, 1962. Redrawn from Scammon, 1930.

The sequence in which these processes proceed is largely predictable and similar for all children as they progress from intra-uterine life through to infancy, the toddler period, pre-school childhood, pre-pubertal and pubertal childhood, adolescence, and adulthood (*see* Figure 2.2)

The health of adults is in part determined by their health and nutrition *in utero*, in infancy, and during childhood. This has been well illustrated by a number of studies where low-birth-weight infants were shown to be at increased risk for diseases such as type-2 diabetes and hypertension in later life. The well-being of the fetus, infant, and child is therefore central to optimal functioning in adult life.

♦ Growth is a function of several, often interrelated factors (genetic, nutritional, psychosocial, and medical).

♦ Standardized tables or charts are used to assess weight, length or height, skull circumference, and growth velocity.

♦ Normal development in early childhood is assessed according to achievement in the areas of locomotion, fine motor adaptation, language, and personal and social development.

♦ Preventive child health care consists of organized programmes for immunization, growth monitoring, and developmental screening.

♦ All those involved in child health care should ensure that growth and development are monitored by means of established tests that screen for deviations from the norm.

* Assessment of growth and development is an essential requirement at every contact with a health care provider, be it at primary care or at tertiary hospital level.

Normal progression from one stage to the next can take place only if specific biological, emotional, and social needs are met. Any interruption of growth or development may be completely or partially corrected by the process of adaptation termed 'catch-up'. This is a compensatory response. The potential to adapt during childhood diminishes with recurring insults and with age. It also varies according to the organ or system involved. For example, since brain growth is most rapid in the last trimester of pregnancy and the first year of life, inadequate brain growth during this period may have permanent consequences.

Definitions and terminology

Growth implies an increase in the size, composition, and distribution of tissues. It is associated with changes in their proportions, shape, and functions.

The **velocity** or speed at which the process takes place may be measured over a period of time and is expressed as the rate of change between measurements per unit of time. A **growth spurt** implies an increase in growth velocity. **Growth lag** refers to a decrease in the rate or velocity of normal expected growth. **Catch-up growth** is a return towards the size that would have been attained if the growth lag had not occurred.

Development is the increase in the complexity of structures and of their functions which takes place in the same time period and often in a parallel fashion. It is the product of the interaction between the processes of maturation and learning.

A **milestone** is designated as the usual age at which the ability to perform a specific activity is achieved. This varies considerably among children.

Chronological age is recorded as years, months, weeks, and/or days calculated from the birth date of the individual.

Corrected age is used to adjust for prematurity, particularly in very-low-birth-weight infants (<1 500 g) born two to three months prematurely. To correct age for prematurity, calculate the age from when the infant should have been born if the pregnancy had gone to term (40 weeks), e.g. an infant born after 28 weeks' gestation and assessed at 18 weeks' chronological age would be evaluated as a six-week-old infant rather than as an infant of 18 weeks. Correction is employed for at least the first year in very-low-birth-weight infants when assessing growth, and for at least two years when assessing development. Shorter periods are appropriate for larger premature infants.

Bone age is a measurement of the osseous maturation in long bones (usually the hand and wrist).

Mental age describes the functional age that has been reached, i.e. a child's performance on tests of cognitive function expressed in terms of the average age at which normal children would perform the same tasks.

Figure 2.2 Age periods of childhood

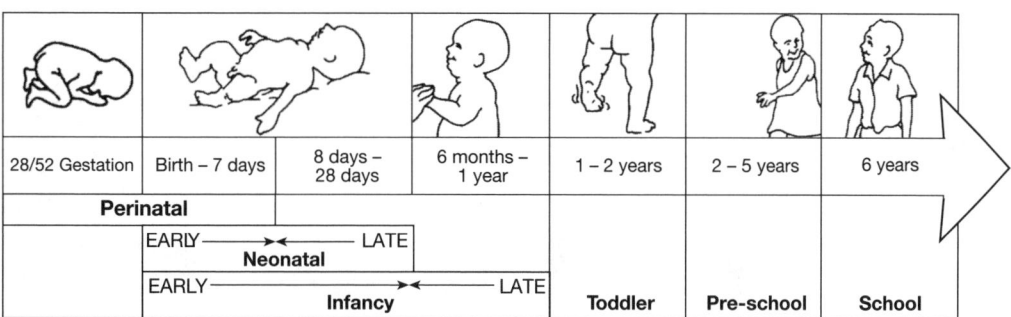

28/52 Gestation	Birth – 7 days	8 days – 28 days	6 months – 1 year	1 – 2 years	2 – 5 years	6 years
Perinatal						
	EARLY ——→◄—— LATE **Neonatal**					
	EARLY ——————————→◄—— LATE **Infancy**			**Toddler**	**Pre-school**	**School**

Puberty is the series of biological changes through which the individual is transformed into a young adult.

Adolescence is the period following puberty, during which all the dimensions of growth, development and maturity are completed.

Growth charts

These are constructed for boys and girls separately, using large populations of normal children living under near-optimal conditions and therefore representing the range of normal growth achieved by children at different ages. New growth standards have been developed by the World Health Organization (WHO) based on the growth of normal breastfed infants in various regions of the world.

The most important feature of growth charts is that they provide the health professional with a measure with which to compare and monitor the physical status of childhood populations or of an individual child on an ongoing basis. The Road-to-Health Chart (*see* Chapter 4, Community paediatrics, child health and survival)

has been introduced world-wide. One of its most significant features is that it enables the mother, as well as health workers to see at a glance whether the child is gaining weight appropriately.

Centiles

Normal children vary widely in length or height, weight, and head circumference at any age, and in the velocity of growth from one age to the next. This variation within the normal range at a given age is expressed conventionally by comparing the individual child's measurements to centiles or percentiles, i.e. 3rd, 15th, 50th, 85th, and 97th: WHO Growth Charts from birth to five years of age for boys and girls for weight-for-age, length/height-for-age, weight-for-length and head circumference are given in Figures 2.3–2.10. Since the WHO charts currently do not go beyond five years of age, adapted growth charts, produced for North American children from the National Center for Health Statistics and the Centers for Disease Control for boys and girls from two to 20 years of age are given in Figures 2.11 and 2.12.

Figure 2.3 Weight-for-age boys: Birth to 5 years (percentiles)

World Health Organization

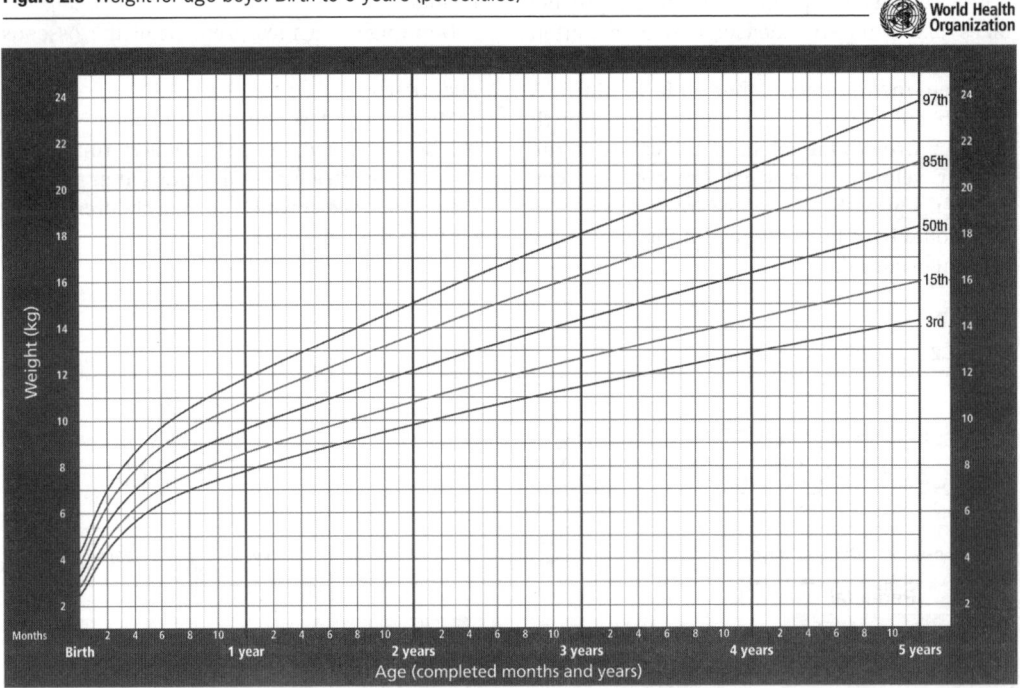

WHO Child Growth Standards

Figure 2.4 Weight-for-age girls: Birth to 5 years (percentiles)

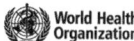

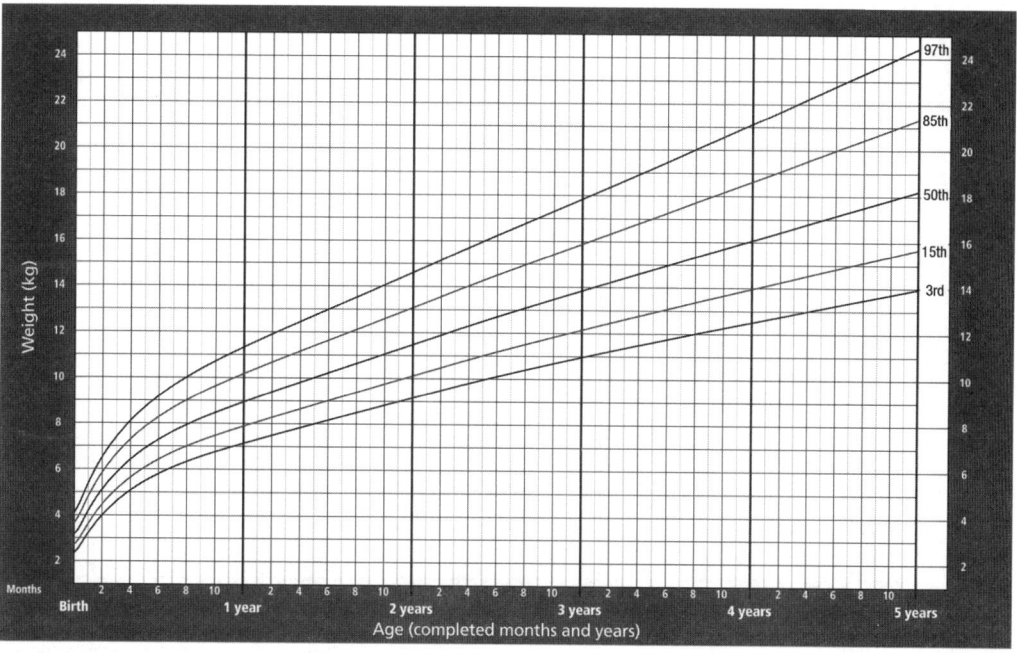

WHO Child Growth Standards

Figure 2.5 Length/height-for-age boys: Birth to 5 years (percentiles)

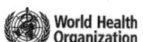

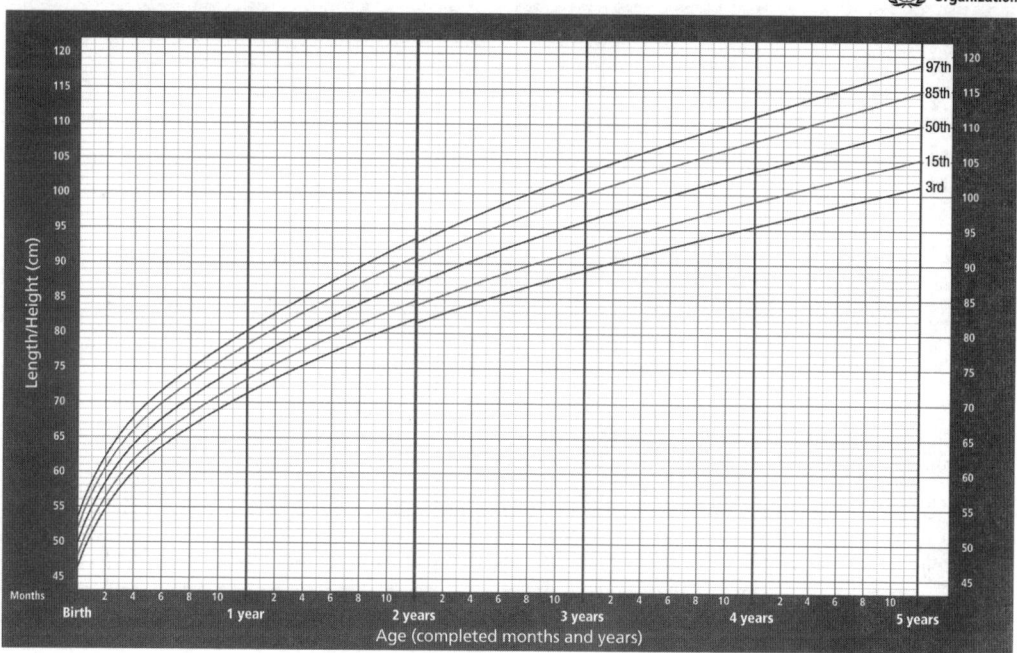

WHO Child Growth Standards

Figure 2.6 Length/height-for-age girls: Birth to 5 years (percentiles)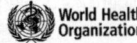

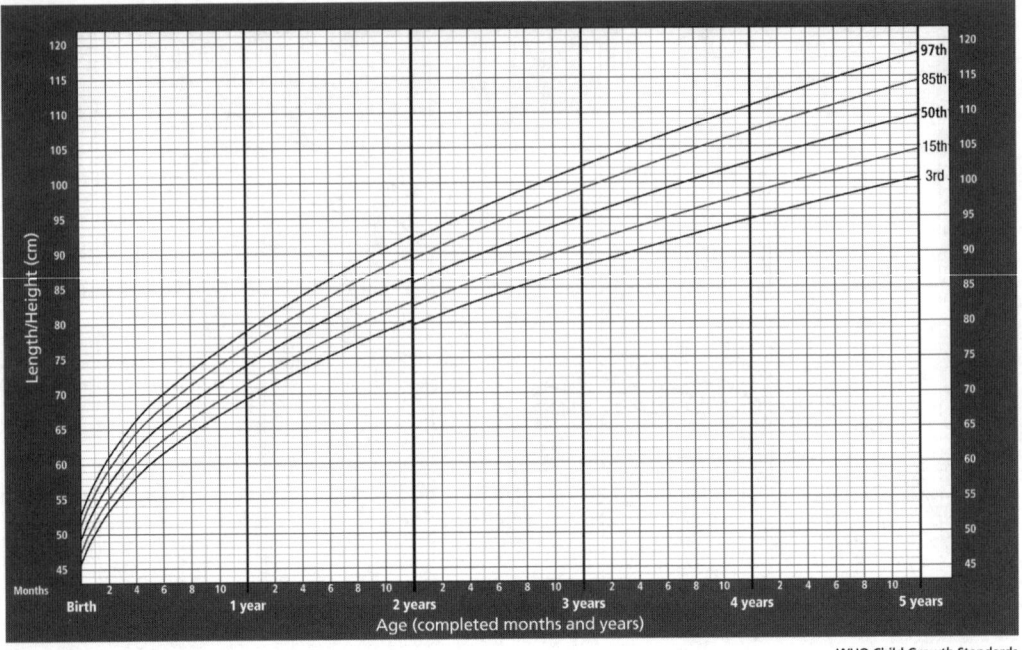

WHO Child Growth Standards

Figure 2.7 Head circumference-for-age boys: Birth to 5 years (percentiles)

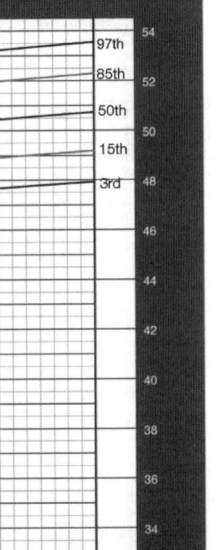

WHO Child Growth Standards

Figure 2.8 Head circumference-for-age girls: Birth to 5 years (percentiles)

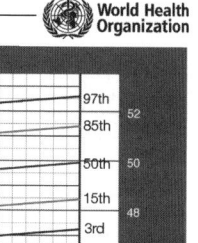

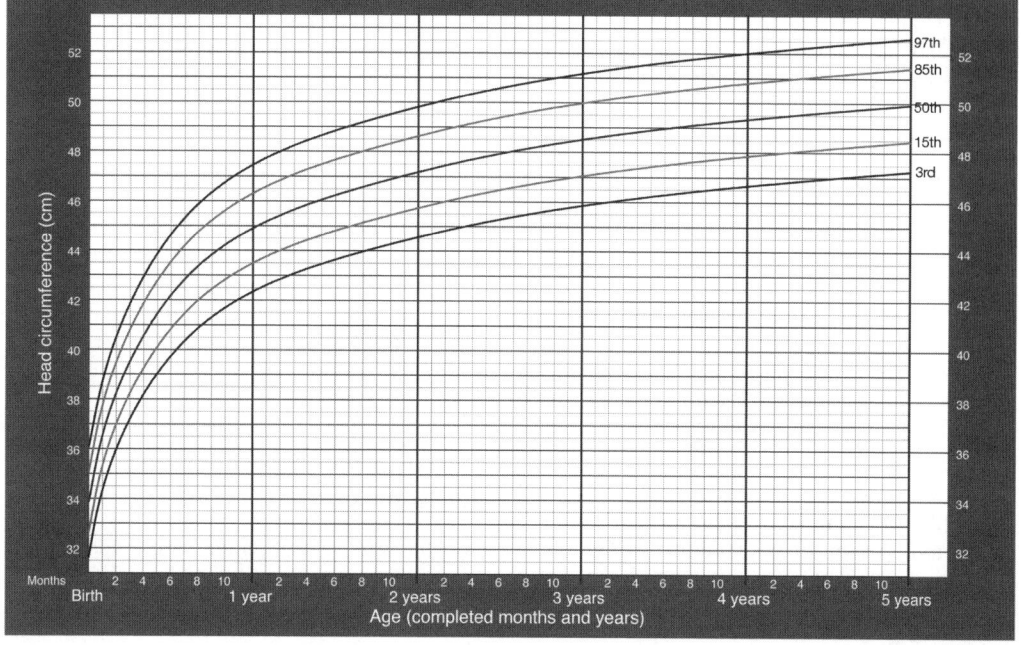

WHO Child Growth Standards

Figure 2.9 Weight-for-length boys: Birth to 2 years (percentiles)

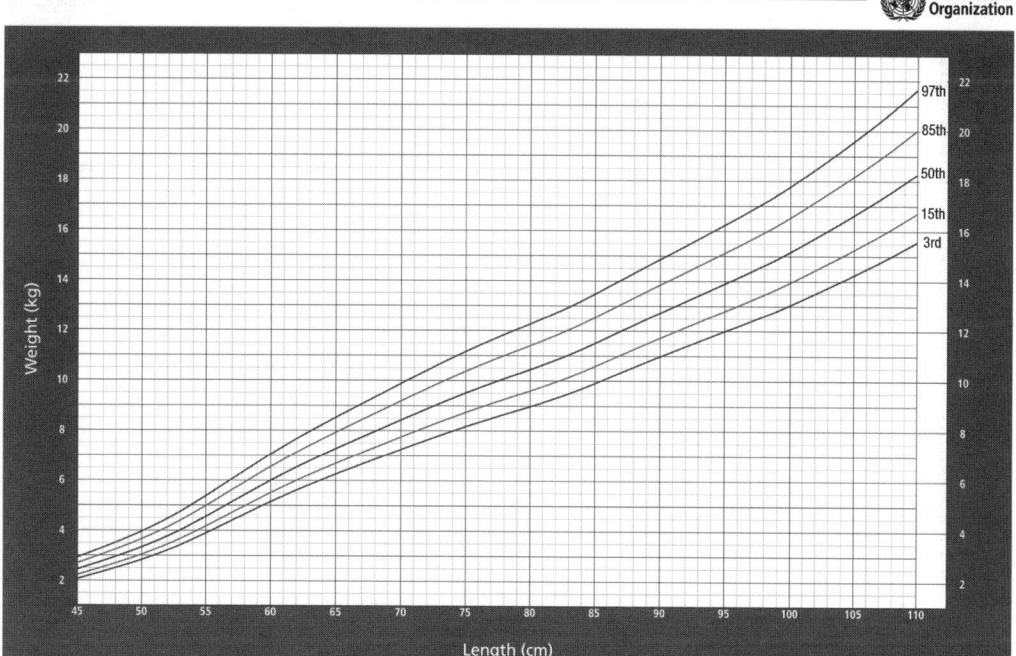

WHO Child Growth Standards

It is important to understand the meaning of a percentile. If the height or weight percentiles were constructed from a population of 100 healthy children at a given age, the smallest 3 per cent would have height or weight measurements less than the 3rd percentile, 15 per cent less than the 15th percentile, 50 per cent less than the 50th percentile, and so on. At the other end of the scale, 97 of 100 children would have measurements below the 97th percentile and only the three largest would have measurements above it. Height and weight have a normal (Gaussian) distribution and the 50th percentile measurement, therefore, corresponds to the mean and median height and weight of the population measured. Thus a weight or a length/height below the 3rd percentile is not necessarily abnormal as 3 per cent of the normal population will be below this centile.

Individuals tend to 'track' along the same percentile over time and repeat measurements are far more useful than single measurements. Visual inspection of a child's tracking will tell whether the child is progressing normally.

Progressive deviation from the centile line indicates a problem of growth and is a strong indication for early intervention. For example, a single measurement on the 3rd percentile may represent normal genetic potential on the one hand, or gross deviation on the other, if earlier measurements had been on the 50th or higher percentile.

Velocity charts provide standards with which to compare the rate of growth. Contrary to longitudinal or distance studies, where an individual child tends to follow the same centile from infancy to adulthood, even the healthy child will generally not stay on the same velocity centile throughout the growth period. An example of a velocity chart for boys is shown in Figure 2.13.

Factors affecting growth and development

Growth and development are products of constitutional and hereditary factors on the one hand, and the environment, experience, and

Figure 2.10 Weight-for-length girls: Birth to 2 years (percentiles)

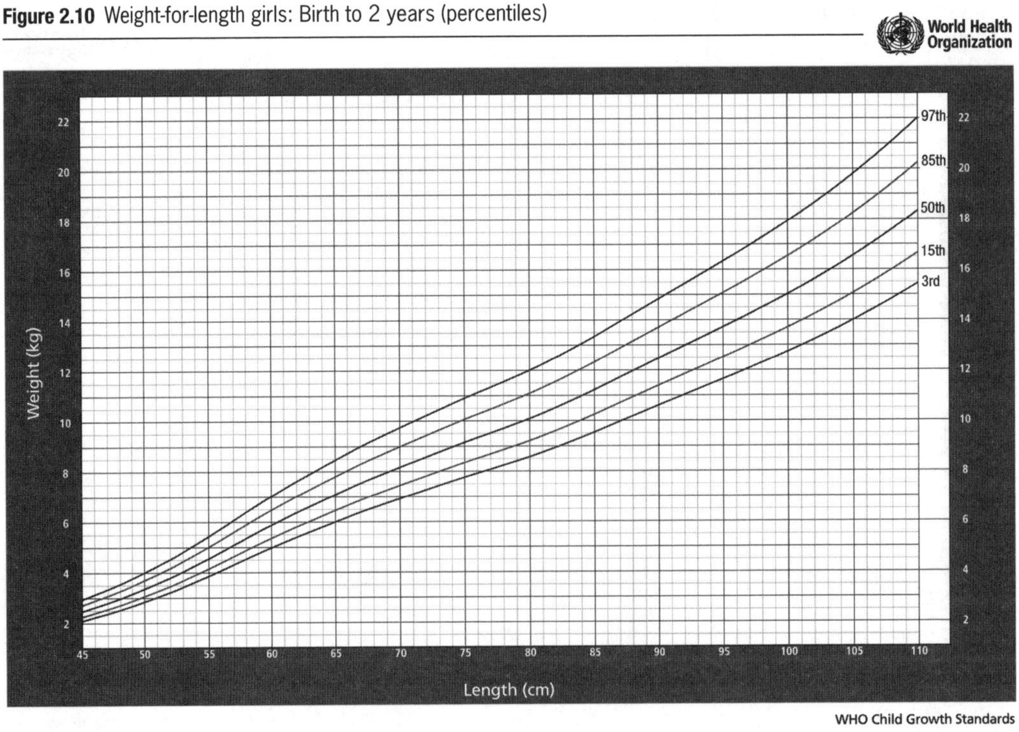

World Health Organization

WHO Child Growth Standards

Figure 2.11 Physical growth: NCHS percentiles
Boys: 2 to 20 years

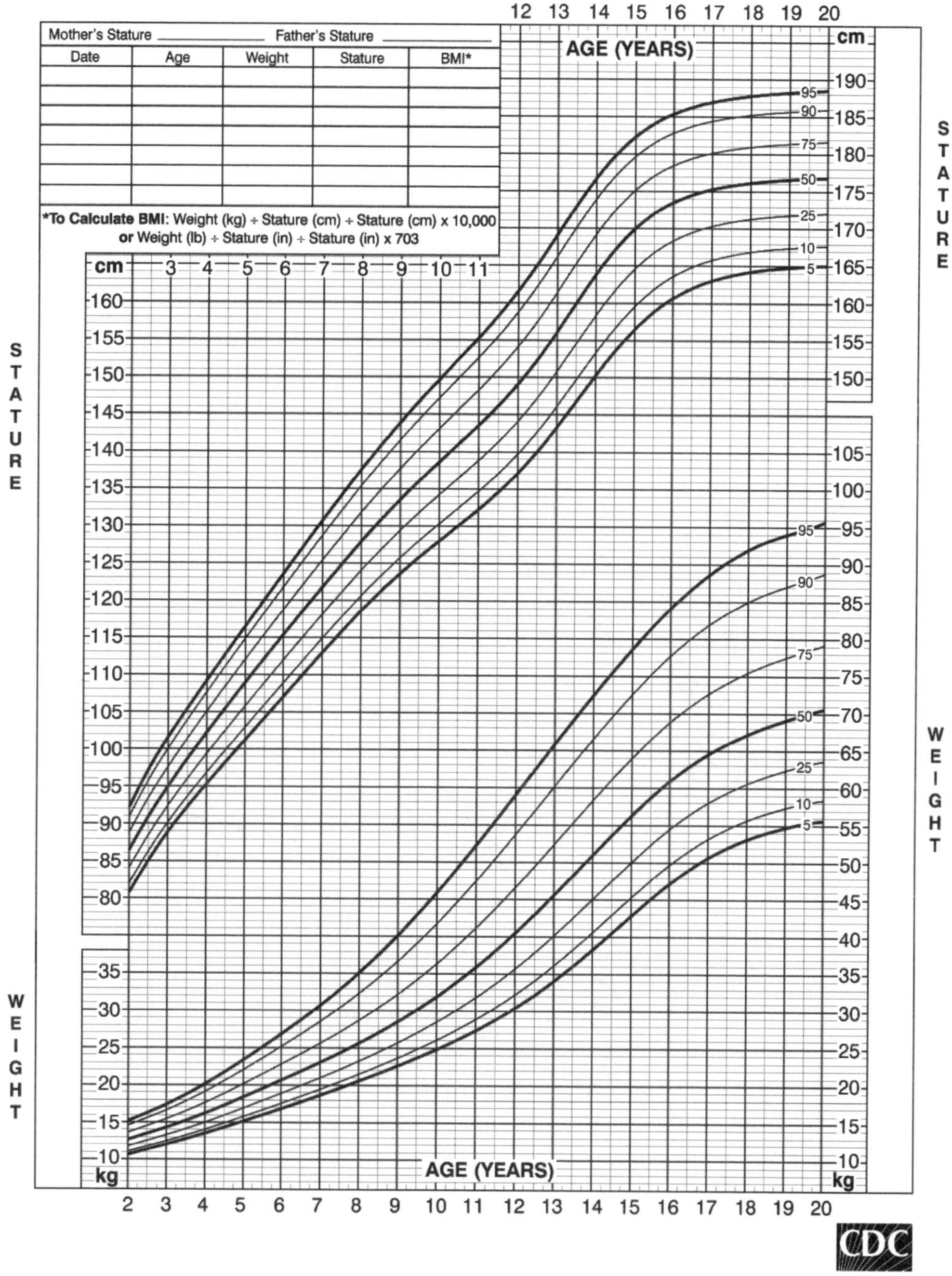
Mother's Stature
Father's Stature
Date
Age
Weight
Stature
BMI*
*To Calculate BMI: Weight (kg) ÷ Stature (cm) ÷ Stature (cm) x 10,000
or Weight (lb) ÷ Stature (in) ÷ Stature (in) x 703
AGE (YEARS)
STATURE
WEIGHT
cm
kg
2 3 4 5 6 7 8 9 10 11 12 13 14 15 16 17 18 19 20
95
90
75
50
25
10
5
CDC

Revised and corrected
November 28, 2000

Source: Developed by the National Center for Health Statistics in collaboration with the National Center for Chronic Disease Prevention and Health Promotion (2000). http://www.cdc.gov/growthcharts

Figure 2.12 Physical growth: NCHS percentiles
Girls: 2 to 20 years

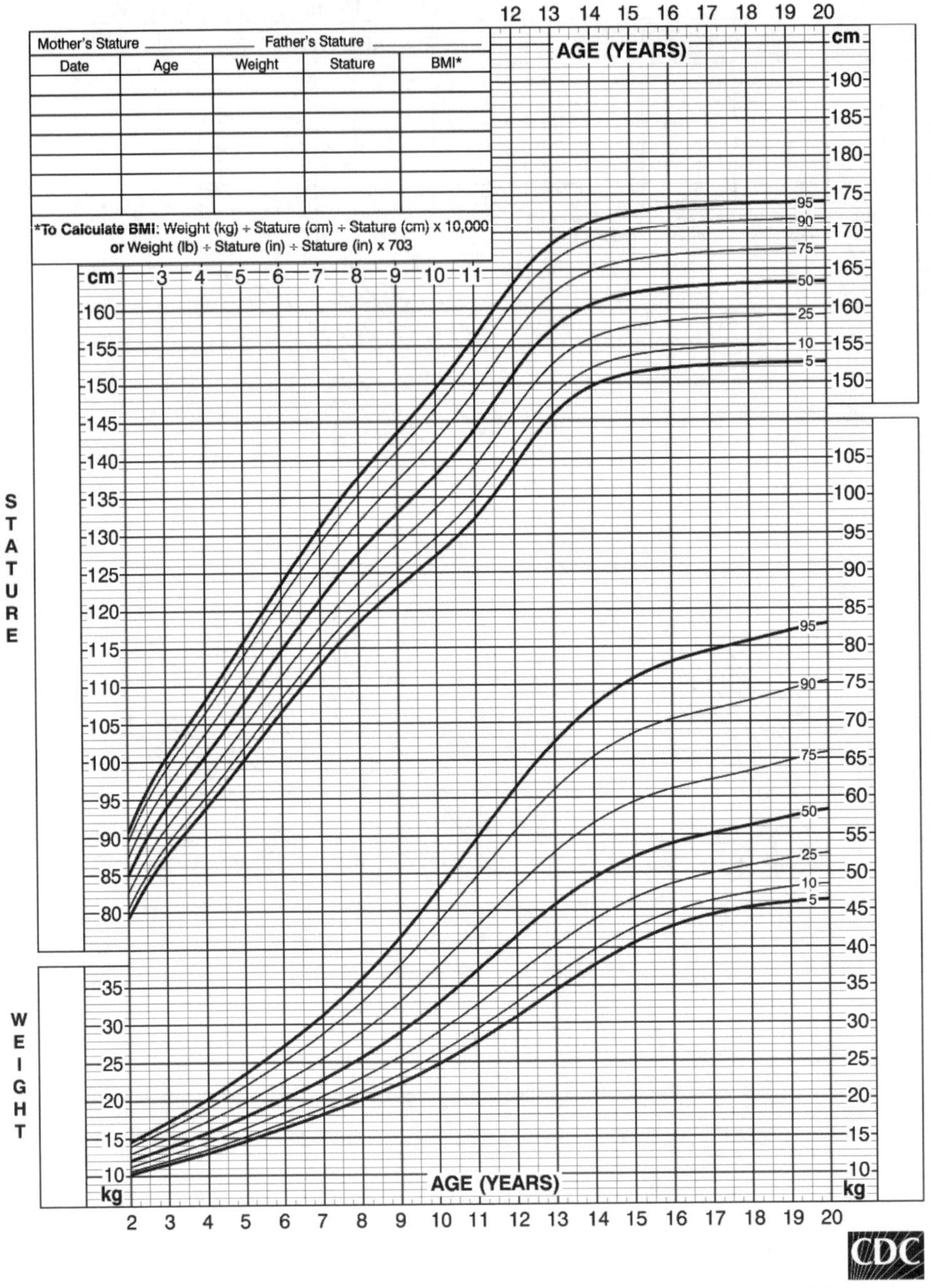

Revised and corrected
November 28, 2000

Source: Developed by the National Center for Health Statistics in collaboration with the National Center for Chronic Disease Prevention and Health Promotion (2000).
http://www.cdc.gov/growthcharts

Figure 2.13 Height velocity centile chart for boys

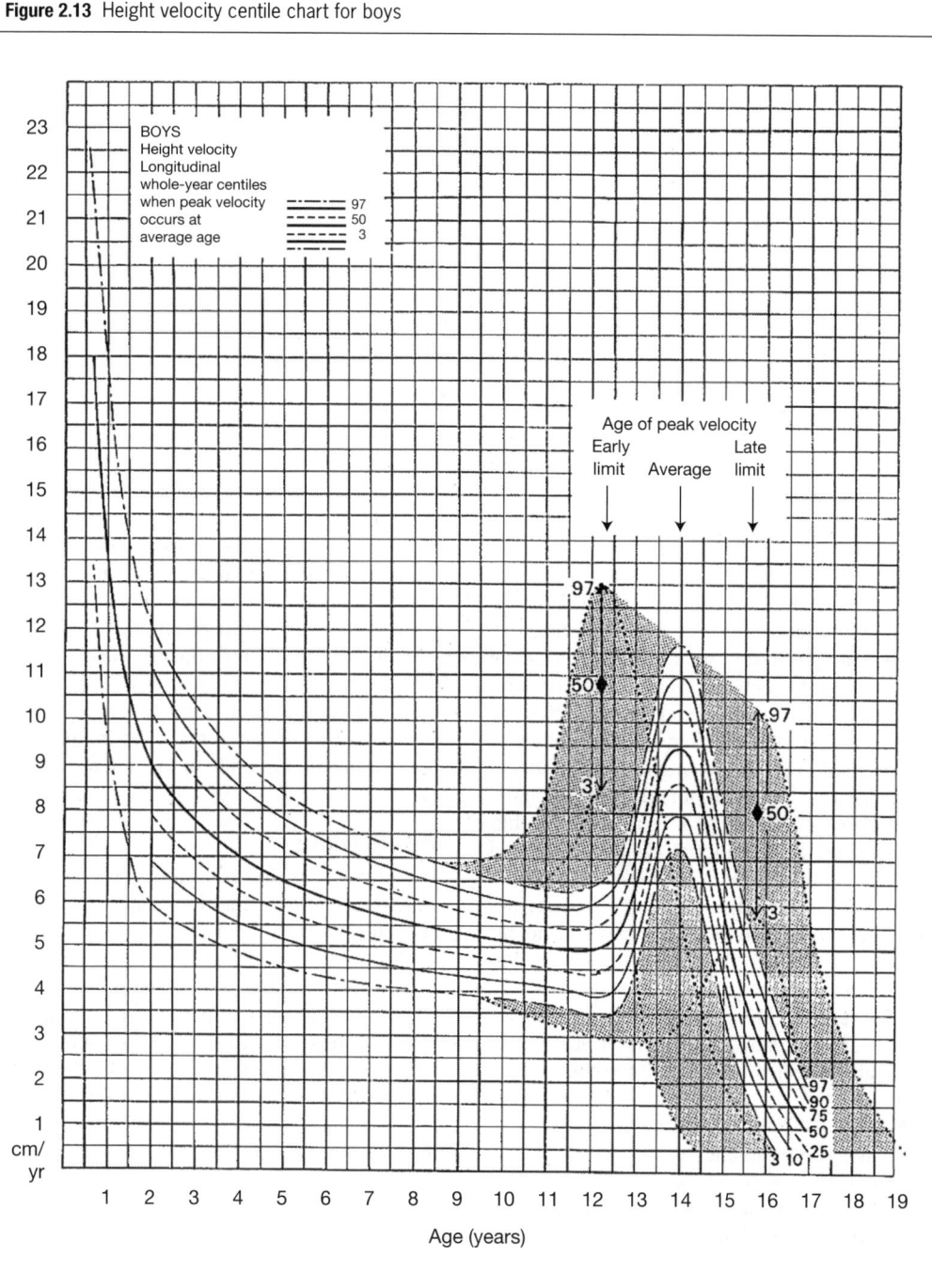

Source: Tanner, J. M. Growth at Adolescence, 2nd edn., Blackwell Scientific Publications, Oxford, 1962.

circumstances to which the individual is exposed on the other. The 'nature-nurture' controversy centres on the relative contributions of heredity and environment, but the complex interaction of the two makes it almost impossible to separate one clearly from the other.

Hereditary and constitutional factors

At conception every person is provided with a unique genetic and chromosomal composition, which is responsible for determining gender, ethnicity, and physical characteristics. Genetic inheritance also determines the individual's potential and limitations. Uni-ovular twin studies have indicated that heredity plays a major part in personality traits. However, temperament, manifested as the behavioural style of the child, is influenced by child-rearing practices, as well as by the continuous interaction between parents and children.

Intra-uterine period

During intra-uterine life, maternal influences play an important part in the growth of the fetus. The size of a full-term infant correlates to some extent with maternal size, weight, nutrition and socio-economic status. Fetal growth may be affected by maternal infections, smoking, alcohol use, or medical problems, such as hypertension or renal, cardiac, or respiratory disease. Placental insufficiency may occur as a result of many other causes. Small-for-gestational-age infants caused by placental insufficiency in the latter stages of pregnancy usually demonstrate a satisfactory catch-up growth period after birth, whereas this may not occur if placental insufficiency was present throughout pregnancy.

Babies of primiparous and grand multiparous women are generally smaller than normal, and male babies are heavier than female babies.

Postnatal period

The major part of infancy is characterized by a rapid growth rate, which becomes increasingly related to the genetic background. The infant at 12 months is more than 50 per cent longer and about three times heavier than at birth. This period of rapid growth is largely determined by nutritional rather than endocrine factors. It is then followed by a more consistent growth rate of 5–7.5 cm per year in the pre-school and pre-pubertal child, during which time endocrine factors become a major factor. The deposition of fat, which may be striking during infancy, becomes less marked, but increases two to three years before the onset of puberty. The latter is associated with an increased growth rate, which is then followed by deceleration, until cessation in linear growth occurs with the ossification of the epiphyses of the long bones.

Nutrition

Growth is profoundly affected by nutrition. Linear growth, expressed as length or height measurement, is a sensitive indicator of the physical health of an infant or child or, collectively, of the health of the children of a community or population. The adequacy of catch-up growth, which follows the correction of the cause of a growth deficiency, will depend on the age of the individual and on the aetiology, severity, and duration of such a deficiency prior to corrective therapy. When growth deficiency is of a postnatal onset, as occurs with malnutrition during infancy, there may be dramatic catch-up growth following the correction of the infant's nutritional status. Nutrition may also influence the pattern of growth. For example, exclusively breastfed infants commonly show a different pattern of growth than formula fed infants, tending to grow more rapidly in the first few months of life.

Health status

The physical health and emotional status of a child or of his family may have a direct or indirect effect on his growth and development.

Chronic illness often leads to disability and may result in handicap. In addition, chronic illness is usually accompanied by prolonged or repeated hospitalization. The problems faced by parents of such a chronically disabled child include uncertainty, chronic sorrow, stigma, and a 'burden of care', which may affect their attitude towards the child. Central nervous system dysfunction, as well as having effects similar to those of any chronic illness, is often associated with motor and intellectual retardation.

Socio-economic status

Poverty, poor education, and social adversity increase the possibility of having a complication of pregnancy and are associated with an increased risk of low-birth-weight infants.

Many long-term studies have shown that socio-economic status can have a major effect on various aspects of a child's growth, performance, and on the incidence of handicap. In a Johannesburg study, developmental scores of very-low-birth-weight infants at 18 months of age correlated with the birth-weight percentile which in turn reflects the interaction of maternal health, nutrition, and lifestyle — all markers of socio-economic status.

Cultural factors

Cross-cultural studies have shown variation in developmental patterns. For example, the motor precocity of African infants when compared with those in Europe or America is well documented. This raises the possibility of genetic differences in child development.

However, child-rearing beliefs and practices vary markedly from one culture to another. There is evidence to suggest that in the case of precocity among African infants, specific training in certain skills is responsible. In contrast, cultures in which swaddling is practised during the first year are associated with delay in gross motor development.

Physical growth

Normal growth patterns

In the normal child, values for height, weight, and skull circumference tend to conform and follow the same percentiles before puberty. Accurate longitudinal measurements plotted on a standard percentile chart are much more informative than single measurements. A gross difference between values, such as a head circumference below the 3rd percentile, with a height and weight in the region of the 75th percentile, may well be significant. Similarly, several measurements that deviate from a centile line require investigation to ascertain the cause.

In comparing the value of a measurement in a child with that of a standard, a measurement below the 3rd or above the 97th centile should alert one to the possibility of an abnormal state of health. However, before any deductions are made, certain sources of error should be checked:

- Incorrect method of measurement, e.g. in a six-month-old child, an error of 2.5 cm in length changes percentile ranking from 25th to 5th and vice versa
- Incorrect assessment of age, e.g. rounding off four and a half months to five months
- Failure to consider gestational age, i.e. to correct for prematurity.

In a child who is consistently below the 3rd percentile for weight and height, but who gains in these measurements at an acceptable rate, consider birth weight, parental size, and possible genetic factors.

Height and secular trend in growth

Height, or stature, is one of the most heritable traits recognized. Given an adequate environment, the height of an individual child bears a significant relationship to the genetic background of the individual, as exemplified by the height of the parents. Genetic background also influences the rate of maturation and therefore the length of time required to achieve adult size.

In developing countries, in contrast to developed countries, growth takes place over a longer period and final height attained may be reached at a later stage. This is an important factor when comparing the height or stature of childhood populations in developing countries with those in developed countries. The changing growth pattern over the past one to two hundred years is referred to as the secular trend. During this period there has been a profound change in the pace of maturation and, to a lesser extent, the ultimate size of individuals in developed countries. Faster maturation has resulted in greater increments of growth and a larger size-for-age during childhood, and an earlier advent of adolescence and final height attainment. A century ago the average male did not reach final height until the age of 23 years; he now reaches it by 17 to 19 years. These changes can probably be attributed to a decrease in growth-inhibiting factors, such as poor childhood nutrition, chronic childhood disease, and genetic outbreeding. In communities where socio-economic conditions are improving, a similar secular trend should be expected.

The child with abnormal growth

In a child in whom abnormal growth has been identified from the history and clinical examination, including measurements of body proportions, it is important to compare the child with immediate family members. Disturbed height and growth in the normal-looking child may be due to:

+ Extreme variations in normal growth
+ Genetic disorders
+ Environmental causes
+ Systemic or endocrine disorders.

Short stature

The child with short stature should be examined carefully for dysmorphic features, as many syndromes affect length/height. The upper to lower body segment ratio should also be measured since most skeletal dysplasias have predominantly long bone shortening and a consequent increase in this ratio (this is discussed in more detail in Chapter 18, Endocrine disorders).

Growth failure in poor communities

Children with weights below the 3rd percentile in a developing country should, for practical purposes, be regarded as being at risk both for morbidity and mortality. In this weight range, they are more likely to have a low serum albumin level, delayed bone age, and susceptibility to infection. In general, they come from homes with a poor social background. They have low body reserves to cope with the energy demands of stress and disease and they may progress to more severe forms of malnutrition, such as frank marasmus or kwashiorkor (*see also* Chapter 13, Nutritional disorders).

Growth in communities where obesity is common

In developed countries or in the wealthier socio-economic population groups of developing countries, nutrition may be excessive, resulting in obesity. In later life this is associated with hypertension, vascular disease, and premature mortality. There are no generally accepted definitions of obesity in children, but it is associated with excess fat. Methods used for attempting to classify obesity are all based on relationships between weight and height or on skinfold measurements, but none are satisfactory. It is difficult to detect those infants or children who will become obese adults. It should be noted, however, that there is only a weak correlation between obesity in infancy and adulthood, while the correlation becomes stronger as the child gets older. However, even obesity in the adolescent is still not a very strong predictor of adult obesity (*see also* Chapter 13, Nutritional disorders).

Development

Normal development in infancy and early childhood

Although normal development follows an orderly, coherent pattern, a problem-oriented approach to assessment is simplified if development is divided into:

+ Gross motor/locomotion
+ Fine motor/manipulation
+ Language/communication
+ Personal/social aspects.

Gross motor and locomotion

Definition. Gross motor development refers to the progression of abilities that ultimately enable the child to assume an upright posture and perform skilled activities while maintaining posture and equilibrium.

The newborn infant assumes a posture of general physiological *flexor hypertonus*, is relatively hypotonic, and has a number of primitive reflexes, e.g. the Moro-reflex, grasping, placing, stepping, rooting, and sucking. During the first few months of life, apart from a general increase in tone (which may be assessed by noting a decrease in head lag on 'pull to sit'), an *extensor facility* develops, which proceeds cephalocaudally or proximodistally. When lying prone at six weeks the infant can lift his chin off the bed; at three months can support himself on his elbows; and by six months can support himself on extended arms. The Landau response (ventral suspension) similarly demonstrates the extensor facility, so that by six months there is extension of all joints of the body. Thereafter, the infant has to develop the ability *to break up total patterns of extension or flexion*. For example, before he can sit, he needs to extend his back and at the same time flex his hips.

The primitive reflexes must be suppressed before voluntary movements can commence. For example, the palmar grasp must disappear before the baby can bear weight on his forearms in the prone position; the Moro reflex must go before the postural reactions, which are necessary for sitting, appear; the asymmetric tonic neck reflex must go before crawling can commence; and the placing and stepping reflexes must disappear to allow walking.

As the primitive reflexes fade there is a progressive development of *postural reactions.* The righting reactions enable the infant to maintain a normal position of the head in space, as well as to align the head, neck, trunk, and limbs. The *equilibrium reactions* are automatic responses to change in posture and act to restore balance. Once the child has righting reactions in sitting, kneeling, and standing, and equilibrium (parachute) responses sideways, forwards and backwards, he is equipped to walk and then run, jump, and climb.

Fine motor, manipulation, and adaptive behaviour

Definition. Fine motor development refers to a series of skills, which develop through a visually guided ability to grasp, thumb apposition, and the transition from unilateral to bimanual manipulation. Adaptive behaviour places these skills in the context of the environment and includes the ability to initiate new experience and profit from past experience.

In the newborn infant, the grasp reflex dominates and the hands are held in a fisted position. By two months this should be disappearing. The hands are open much of the time. Over the next three months, visually guided reaching matures, so that by five months, the infant can reach for and grasp an object and then bring it to her mouth. This mouthing is an automatic response. At six months she is able to transfer the object to the other hand. Reaching should be equally good with either hand. *Until seven months there is a midline barrier as far as hand use is concerned.* This means that the infant is unable to retain an object in each hand simultaneously. By about eight months this becomes possible. Mouthing continues, but is more exploratory in nature.

At six months there is a total (palmar) grasp. Over the next few months the grasp becomes more radial. The nine- to ten-month-old child will isolate and explore with her index finger. At the same time the pincer-grasp matures and by 12 months there is apposition of a thumb and terminal phalanx of the index finger. At this stage the infant can usually release an object on request and mouthing should be infrequent. Children of this age frequently enjoy throwing toys out of the cot. From 15 to 18 months, play becomes increasingly bimanual and manipulative skills develop. These can be tested by block construction, puzzles, and form boards. During the next three years *perceptual skills* and *sensory-motor integration* develop, laying the foundation for activities required for schooling. Handedness appears after the age of a year, but may change over the next few years.

Language and communication

Definition. Communication refers to the transmission of meaningful symbols. Language is the primary medium of communication and involves the formalization of thought.

The newborn infant cries and is able to produce only a few throaty sounds. By eight weeks she is capable of vowel sounds and vocalizes pleasure.

Thereafter, the infant initiates sounds to which her mother responds with sensitive timing. This is referred to as 'vocal contagion'. At 20 weeks guttural sounds are produced and by 32 weeks syllables are combined (babbling), e.g. 'baba, mama, dada'. Soon after this, early concept formation can be demonstrated by object permanence. The infant can retrieve hidden objects such as a block placed under a cup. Gradually the babbling sounds achieve meaning so that by a year the baby has two to three meaningful 'words'.

Language development slows down for the next few months, but between 15 and 18 months, the child shows the beginning of symbolization (inner language) by demonstrating definition by use, e.g. she will show by gesture that she understands the use of a brush, telephone, etc.

This heralds a new acceleration of language development and by 18 months, two-word utterances commence. At two years she is capable of short phrases and using pronouns. A three-year-old has an extensive vocabulary and chats incessantly. Immature articulation is common at this stage, but by five years articulation errors have disappeared and the child uses full sentences.

Personal and social

Definition. Personal development is assessed on culturally monitored skills of daily living, and social development is behaviour that is in accordance with social expectations. This is acquired through socialization.

The important bonding process between mother and child commences soon after birth. By six weeks the infant responds to his mother with a smile. He gradually becomes more sociable and a three- to four-month-old infant smiles and vocalizes freely with strangers. At six months he responds to his image in a mirror, usually by patting it. The age of eight to nine months, however, sees the onset of stranger anxiety.

Once on his feet, his world expands and he becomes increasingly explorative. Domestic mimicry commences between 15 and 18 months as he copies his mother's daily activities. A two-year-old plays alone or, if with other children, in parallel fashion. Group activities commence after three years and usually involve two to three children. By the age of five years, group play is frequent, although the size of the groups remains relatively small (three to five members). However, play is symbolic in that the child identifies himself as someone else, e.g. the postman or shopkeeper.

A newborn infant can drink from a cup if it is held, while a bottlefed three-month-old infant will attempt to hold the bottle. By six months old she can chew and by eight months can hold and eat a biscuit. At 15 months she will attempt to use a spoon, but will spill most of the food, whereas by 18 months very little is spilt. At 18 months a cup is handled well. Soon after she is one year old, the child will help in dressing by pushing her arm into a sleeve. At 18 months she can pull up her trousers.

An 18-month-old child indicates to his mother that his nappy is wet or soiled. By 24 months sphincter control enables him to be clean and dry during the day. Full toilet training is usually achieved by three years.

A three-year-old will dress alone but needs help with buttons. By four to five years she can dress without supervision.

Milestones of development

This term is used to refer to certain notable developmental achievements such as smiling, sitting, crawling, walking, talking and the typical age at which normal children demonstrate them. They are asked about in the history of a child's development. Any child who has not achieved the usual developmental milestones should be evaluated more closely. This could represent slow normal development or indicate significant delay.

The normal range of motor milestones can be seen in Figure 2.14. Of importance is that there is a wide age range or normality, e.g. it can be seen that walking alone may be achieved anywhere between 8 and 17 months of age.

Table 2.1 summarizes the ages at which milestones in the areas of gross motor, fine motor, hearing and speech and personal/social are typically achieved. Warning signs are also listed in this table and should be used as indications for referral.

Public health services attempt to promote and maintain normal health and development in childhood by organized programmes of well-baby care (*see* Chapter 4, Community paediatrics, child health and survival).

Different health services prescribe frequencies and ages of these visits that are appropriate for the particular country. At a minimum, the visits should coincide with the schedule of recommended immunizations.

Adolescent development

Early, middle, and late adolescence are characterized by different behavioural and developmental issues. The age at which each issue becomes manifest and the importance of the issue will vary widely among individuals, as will the rates of cognitive, psychosexual, psychosocial, or physical development.

Early adolescence (10–14 year olds)

This stage is characterized by maximal somatic growth and sexual growth. Thinking is focused on the present and on the peer group. Identity is focused primarily on the physical changes, and concern is about normality. Exploratory, undifferentiated sexual behaviour resulting in physical contact with peers of the same gender

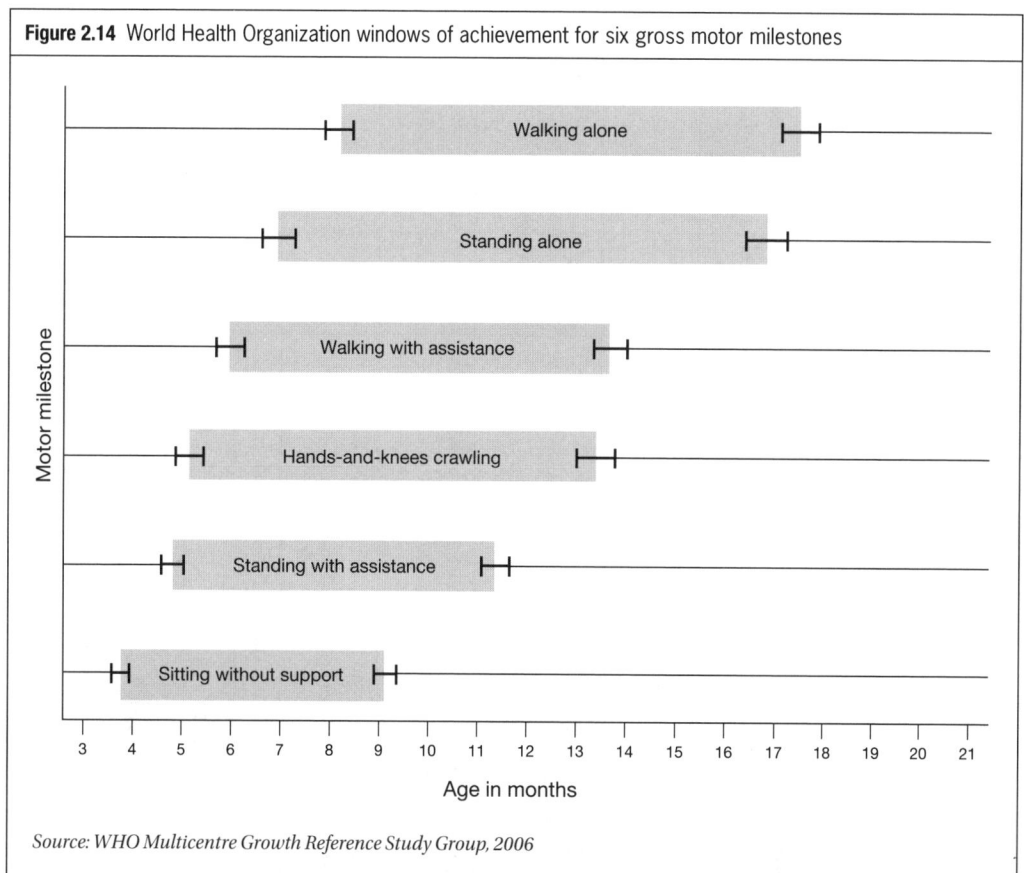

Figure 2.14 World Health Organization windows of achievement for six gross motor milestones

Source: WHO Multicentre Growth Reference Study Group, 2006

is normal during early adolescence, although heterosexual interests may also develop. Strivings for independence are ambivalent.

Middle adolescence (15–16 year olds)

This stage can be a most difficult time for both adolescents and the adults who have contact with them. Cognitive processes are more sophisticated. The stage is characterized by experimentation with ideas, consideration of alternative approaches to problems, development of insight, and reflection on personal feelings and those of others. As they mature cognitively and psychosocially, middle adolescents focus on issues of identity not limited solely to the physical aspects of the body. As middle adolescents socialize with peers, experiment sexually, engage in risk-taking behaviour, and develop employment and interests outside the home, they aug-

ment their unique, developing identities. As a result of experimental risk-taking behaviour, they may experience unwanted pregnancies, drug abuse, or motor-vehicle accidents. Middle adolescents' strivings for independence, testing of limits, and need for autonomy are maximal and often distressing to their families, teachers, or other figures in positions of authority.

Late adolescence (17–20 year olds)

This stage is usually characterized by full, formal operational thinking, including thoughts about the future (educationally, vocationally, and sexually). Late adolescents are usually more committed to their sexual partners than are middle adolescents. Unresolved separation anxiety from previous developmental stages may emerge at this time as the young person begins to move physically away from the family of origin.

Table 2.1 Developmental milestones in the first 10 years of life

Age	Gross motor	Fine motor/vision	Hearing and speech	Personal/social	Warning signs
Newborn	Ventral suspension: head droops, hips flexed, limbs hang downwards, Moro reflex; palmar/plantar grasp reflexes	Hands fisted; closes eyes to sudden bright light	Stills to sound, startles to sudden loud sounds	Alternates between drowsiness and alert wakefulness	Hyper-/hypotonia, asymmetrical reflexes; excessive head lag; poor sucking
6 weeks	Some head control; prone: head to side, buttocks moderately high; Moro reflex, ventral suspension	Stares; follows horizontally to 90°	Startle response	Smiles at mother	No visual fixation or following; asymmetry of tone or movement; floppy, excessive head lag; failure to smile; poor sucking
3 months	Pull-to-sit; little/no head lag; prone: support on forearms, lifts head, buttocks flat, rolls over	Follows through 180°; holds rattle when placed in hand	Coos, chuckles	Excited when sees mother; reacts to familiar situations	
6 months	Pull-to-sit; braces shoulders and pulls to sit, sits with support; prone: lifts head and chest well up, supports on extended arms	Reaches for and grasps toy; transfers toy from one hand to the other	Initiates conversation	Takes everything to mouth; response to mirror image	Floppiness; failure to use both hands; squint; failure to turn to sound; poor response to people
9 months	Sits without support, crawls on hands and knees, pulls to stand	Immediately reaches out, holds a cube in each hand	Vocalises deliberately, babbles	Stranger anxiety, holds bottle/cup	Unable to sit, hand preference; fisting, squint, persistence of primitive reflexes
10 months	Pulls to stand; walks with assistance	Picks up small object between thumb and index finger	Shakes head for no; waves bye-bye	Plays peek-a-boo with mother	
12 months	Bear walks; walks around furniture lifting one foot and stepping sideways, may walk alone	Pincer grasp, releases object on request	Knows own name; 2–3 words with meaning	Finger feeds, pushes arms into sleeves	Unable to sit or bear weight, abnormal grasp, failure to respond to sound
15 months	Walks alone – uneven steps, arms out for balance	2–cube tower	Jabbers with expression	Holds and drinks from cup; attempts feeding with spoon, spills most	

Age					
18 months	Walks well, arms down, pulls a toy, throws a ball; climbs onto chair	3–cube tower, scribbles	2-word utterances	Handles spoon and cup; indicates wet nappy	Failure to walk, no pincer grip, inability to understand simple commands, no spontaneous vocalisation, mouthing, drooling
24 months	Runs; up and down steps two feet per step	6–cube tower, train with cubes, imitates vertical line, hand preference usually obvious	Short phrases, uses pronouns	Spoon feeds without spilling, clean and dry by day	Unable to understand simple commands, tremor, in coordination
36 months	Rides a tricycle, up steps – one foot per step and down two feet per step	9–cube tower, bridge with cubes; copies circle	Knows name and sex, talks incessantly	Toilet trained; dresses without supervision	Ataxia; using single words only
48 months	Up and down stairs one foot per step, stands on one (preferred) foot for 3–5 seconds and hops on preferred foot	Copies cross, gate with cubes	Full name, home address and (usually) age; recognises colours	Eats with spoon and fork, washes and dries hands, dresses and undresses, make-believe play	Speech difficult to understand because of poor articulation or omission or substitution of consonants
60 months	Walks easily on narrow line, can hop on each foot separately	6–10 cube steps, copies square and triangle, draws a man with full features	Fluent speech; full name, age (usually)	Uses knife and fork competently, undresses and dresses alone, chooses own friends	Emotional immaturity
72 months	Sits up without help of hands; walks backwards along straight line (10 paces)	10 cubes steps, copies	and	Word definition (5),	compositions – door, shoes, spoon; knows birthday, address
7–8 years	Jumps 25cm feet together, throws ball up and catches	Writes name, draws a person, facial features, limbs correct, align to body, hands	Talks sentences of 10 syllables	One special friend, dresses, undresses completely without help	Poor pencil grip
9–10 years	Runs downstairs	Writes 3-word sentences	Produces all speech sounds including 's', 'z' and 'ng'	Takes full responsibility for personal care	Speech sound difficulty

Puberty

The age range for the onset of puberty has altered considerably over the past 150 years and secular trends indicate that the onset now occurs considerably earlier.

Local data is not available but American studies indicate that puberty normally commences at between 8.5 and 13 years in girls, and between 10 and 15 years in boys. Apart from a sexual variation, the time of onset of puberty may differ in race groups. In the United States puberty in blacks begins about six months later than in Latin Americans. Studies in South Africa indicate that rural black children have a somewhat later onset of puberty than their urban counterparts.

The physical changes of puberty are preceded by hormonal changes, leading to the appearance of secondary sex characteristics and an increase in growth velocity prior to the final cessation of growth.

Events at puberty can thus be divided into:
- Hormonal changes
- Appearance of secondary sex characteristics
- The change of growth velocity (secondary growth spurt).

Physical changes associated with puberty

Measurements of the changes taking place at puberty are based on the descriptions of Tanner, using standard ratings on a scale of one to five. Disorders of sexual development are discussed in Chapter 18, Endocrine disorders.

Boys

Genital development

Stage 1 Pre-pubertal: the testes, scrotum, and penis are of about the same size and proportions as in early childhood

Stage 2 Enlargement of the scrotum and testes. The skin of the scrotum reddens and changes in texture. Little or no enlargement of the penis

Stage 3 Lengthening of the penis. Further growth of the testes and scrotum

Stage 4 Increase in width of the penis and development of the glans. The testes and scrotum are larger; the scrotum darkens

Stage 5 Genitalia adult in size and shape.

Pubic hair

Stage 1 Pre-pubertal: no pubic hair

Stage 2 Sparse growth of slightly pigmented, downy hair, chiefly at the base of the penis

Stage 3 Hair darker, coarser and more curled, spreading sparsely over the junction of the pubes

Stage 4 Hair adult in type, but covering a considerably smaller area than in the adult. No spread to the medial surface of the thighs

Stage 5 Adult quantity and type, with spread to the medial surface of the thighs. Spread up the linea alba occurs later and is rated Stage 6.

Girls

Breast development

Stage 1 Pre-pubertal: elevation of the papilla only

Stage 2 Breast bud stage. Elevation of the breast and papilla as a small mound. Enlargement of the areola diameter

Stage 3 Further enlargement and elevation of the breast and areola, with no separation of their contours

Stage 4 Projection of the areola and papilla above the level of the breast

Stage 5 Mature stage: projection of the papilla alone due to recession of the areola.

Pubic hair

Stage 1 Pre-pubertal: no hair

Stage 2 Sparse growth of slightly pigmented, downy hair, chiefly along the labia

Stage 3 Hair darker, coarser and more curled, spreading sparsely over the junction of the pubes

Stage 4 Hair adult in type, but covering a considerably smaller area than in the adult. No spread to the medial surface of the thighs

Stage 5 Adult quantity and type, with distribution of a horizontal pattern and spread to the medial surface of the thighs.

3

Medical genetics and birth defects

Introduction

Biological variation refers to the differences in anatomy (body structure), morphology (body shape and form) and physiology (biochemical functioning) both between species and among individuals of a species. Genetics can be defined as the study of biological variation in plants and animals; medical genetics is the study of human biological variation as it relates to health and disease. Implicit is the study of underlying causes of biological variation.

Human biological variation embraces the whole range of physical, physiological and psychological characteristics that differentiate individuals. These are associated mainly with health and normality, but at the other end of the spectrum of biological variation are diseases or disorders, specifically birth defects and complex disorders.

Basic genetic concepts

The blueprint for life is carried as a triplet code within DNA. Human genetic material consists of nuclear and mitochondrial DNA. Unique

Clinical genetics is defined as the study, practice and art of the care and prevention of birth defects and complex disorders. In this context, care refers to diagnosis, treatment and genetic counselling with psychosocial support.

sequences of DNA are called genes, and these are separated by segments of repeated DNA. It is estimated that each person has about 25 000 genes. Long portions of the DNA helix are twisted and then looped around histones to form chromosomes. Each chromosome, and its genes, is unique. Chromosomes 1 to 22 are the autosomes, and the 23rd pair of chromosomes, X and Y, are the sex chromosomes. Each cell contains two copies of each autosome, but the sex chromosomes are represented differently in each person, depending on their sex. Females have two X chromosomes and no Y chromosome, while males have one X and one Y chromosome.

Each normal body (somatic) cell has a total of 46 chromosomes, the diploid number of chromosomes. Each gamete (ovum or sperm) formed by meiosis has 23 chromosomes, known as the haploid number of chromosomes. All somatic cells and ova contain mitochondria, and the mitochondria, in turn, contain mitochondrial DNA (mtDNA).

Each cell contains two copies of every gene, except the genes on the X chromosome (one copy in males and two copies in females) and genes on the Y chromosome (one copy in males and no copies in females). The gene locus refers to the site where a gene occurs on the chromosome. The different forms of the gene that occur at this locus are called the gene alleles. A person who has identical alleles at a locus is called a homozygote. A person with two different alleles at a locus is a heterozygote.

Natural variations between genes of individuals do not affect the function of the gene and are known as polymorphisms. Abnormalities in genes that result in abnormal function of the gene product are called mutations. The same condition can be caused by mutations in more than one gene, which is known as locus heterogeneity (e.g. tuberous sclerosis complex can be caused by mutations in either TSC1 on chromosome 9 or TSC2 on chromosome 16). Locus heterogeneity is more common in genetics than locus homogeneity, which makes genetic testing complex and costly.

Birth defects

Definition and epidemiology

Birth defects, also termed congenital disorders, are structural or functional abnormalities, including disorders of metabolism, which are present from birth. They may be clinically obvious at birth (e.g. cleft lip and palate) or manifest later in life (e.g. cystic fibrosis). Serious birth defects can cause death or disability.

Approximately 7 per cent of all births worldwide, an estimated minimum 9 million infants, are born annually with a birth defect that can kill them or result in disability. Of these, an estimated 7.9 million babies have a genetic birth defect and at least a million have teratogen-induced birth defects. A teratogen is an agent that causes birth defects in a developing fetus. The effect of the teratogen depends on the dose, duration and gestation of fetal exposure. Teratogens cause 5–10 per cent of birth defects in industrialized countries and 10–15 per cent in middle- and low-income countries.

In South Africa some 5.4 per cent of infants are born with a serious genetic birth defect, the common ones being congenital cardiac defects, neural tube defects (NTD), Down's syndrome and oculocutaneous albinism. More than 1 per cent of infants are born with a teratogen-induced birth defect, the vast majority with FASD.

Apart from a few specific disorders, the birth prevalence of individual serious genetic birth defects is considered to be similar worldwide. Birth defects with variable birth prevalence include sickle cell disorder, thalassaemia, glucose-6-phosphate dehydrogenase deficiency (G6PD deficiency), oculocutaneous albinism type 2 in sub-Saharan Africa, inborn errors of metabolism in countries where consanguinity is common, Down's syndrome and neural tube defects (NTD).

Congenital syphilis, congenital rubella syndrome, iodine deficiency disorder and fetal alcohol spectrum disorder (FASD) are the four commonest teratogenic birth defects.

Box 1. Factors influencing the birth prevalence of birth defects

- Malaria
  Heterozygote advantage of the haemoglobin disorders and G6PD deficiency against the lethal effects of malaria in endemic areas has, over the millennia, increased the carrier frequency of these disorders and therefore their birth prevalence.
- Parental consanguinity
  Parental consanguinity is prevalent in many parts of the world, in places occurring in over 50% of unions. It increases the birth prevalence of autosomal recessive disorders and thus spontaneous abortion, intrauterine death and postnatal mortality and morbidity.
- Advanced maternal age
  The risk of autosomal trisomies, particularly Down's syndrome, increases with advancing maternal age (AMA). Pregnant women 35 years or older are considered at significant risk. Populations with a high proportion of AMA women and no population screening and prenatal diagnostic services have a high birth prevalence of Down's syndrome. This is the case in most middle- and low-income nations.
- Level of health care service
  Poor maternal health care services increases the birth prevalence of birth defects like Down's syndrome, NTD, congenital syphilis and rubella. Good neonatal and child health services, particularly paediatric surgery, reduce mortality and morbidity from birth defects.
- Personal poverty
  This is associated with higher birth prevalence of certain birth defects like NTD and fetal alcohol syndrome (FAS).

These disorders contribute to the overall birth prevalence of birth defects being 20% higher in middle-and low-income nations than in industrialised nations. The factors underlying this difference are detailed in Box 1.

Globally, about 3.3 million children under five years of age with a birth defect will die each year. Additionally, an estimated 3.2 million of those who survive are disabled. The majority of affected individuals do not have access to appropriate care. More than 90 per cent of the births with a serious genetic birth defect and 95 per cent of the deaths of these children occur in middle-and low-income nations. Birth defects have a major influence on infant and childhood mortality and morbidity, the effects of which are consistently underestimated and neglected in efforts to improve child health and survival.

Causes of birth defects and complex disorders

An overview of the development of birth defects is presented in Figure 3.1.

- Pre-conception birth defects are genetic. They are caused by chromosome abnormalities, single gene defects or are multifactorial in origin.
- Post-conception birth defects are caused by teratogens or by fetal environmental abnormalities that deform or disrupt the developing embryo or fetus. The chromosomes and genes are therefore normal.

The mechanisms causing a structural birth defect include deformation, disruption, dysplasia and malformation.

Deformation

A deformation occurs when an external force changes the shape of the normal tissues of a developing fetus. The defect therefore occurs after the body has formed. Once the deforming force is removed, the deformation usually improves spontaneously as the tissues are allowed to grow

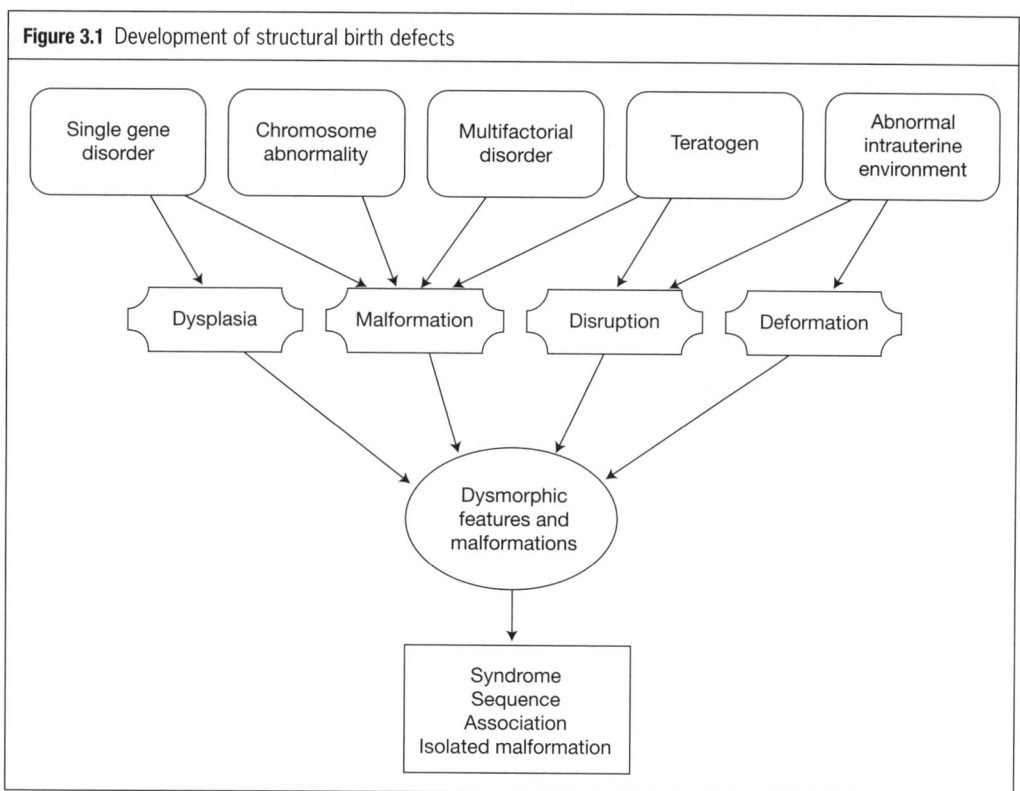

Figure 3.1 Development of structural birth defects

normally. The recurrence risks of deformations are low because there is no underlying genetic abnormality. An example is joint contracture secondary to fetal constraint in a twin pregnancy.

Disruption

A disruption occurs when an external agent destroys the normal tissues of a body part of a developing fetus. Since the tissues are destroyed, the defect is permanent. The recurrence risks of disruptions are low because there is no underlying genetic abnormality. An example is that of the amniotic band sequence, where multiple digit amputations and syndactyly result from the ischaemia caused by amniotic bands wrapped around the digits.

Dysplasia

A dysplasia refers to abnormal development of a single tissue type in the fetus. The abnormality is present for life because the tissue always grows abnormally. All dysplasias are caused by single gene mutations and the recurrence risks depend on the inheritance pattern of the particular condition. Examples include the skeletal and ectodermal dysplasias.

Malformation

A malformation is the result of abnormal embryonic development of an organ or body part. The defect is permanent because the underlying tissue is abnormal. Malformations can be caused by chromosome or single gene abnormalities, multifactorial conditions or teratogen exposure. The recurrence risk depends on the underlying cause.

Chromosome abnormalities

Chromosome abnormalities result in either an abnormal number of chromosomes or abnormalities in the structure of chromosomes. If genetic material is lost or gained by either of these mechanisms, physical and/or mental abnormalities result.

Numerical abnormalities

This is a loss or gain of a chromosome and is called aneuploidy. In general, the larger the chromosome that is lost or gained, the less likely the fetus is to survive. Results of aneuploidy include:

- Loss of a chromosome results in monosomy for that chromosome. Only monosomy X (Turner's syndrome) is compatible with life
- Gain of a chromosome results in trisomy for that chromosome. The commonest viable trisomies include trisomy 21 (Down's syndrome, see Box 2), trisomy 18, trisomy 13, and the sex chromosome trisomies (47,XXY or Klinefelter's syndrome, and 46,XXX)
- The presence of two different cell lines in one body, where the one cell line is derived from the other, is known as mosaicism (e.g. 46, XX/ 47, XX, +21).

Structural abnormalities

The commonest structural abnormalities are translocations, deletions, duplications, inversions, insertions, ring chromosomes, and isochromosomes. When part of a chromosome is lost or gained by one of these mechanisms, birth defects usually occur. Alternatively, the structural abnormality may disrupt a critical gene, which in turn results in birth defects. Some features of structural abnormalities are:

- Balanced translocations are common (an estimated 1 in 500 individuals), but the person carrying them is normal because the net genetic material remains normal. Carriers of balanced translocations are at risk of producing gametes with unbalanced amounts of genetic material. The resultant offspring may be incompatible with life or may be viable and have physical and/or mental defects.
- Some structural chromosome abnormalities can be diagnosed by standard testing techniques, but many require newer technology to be detected (e.g. microdeletions/duplications).

Single gene abnormalities

Gene mutations can be inherited in a variety of ways.

Box 2. Down's syndrome

Birth prevalence: 1 in 500 live births in South Africa

Cause: Trisomy 21. Non-disjunction (95%), translocation (4%), mosaicism (1%). Increased risk with increasing maternal age, especially in women >35 years (advanced maternal age (AMA))

Clinical features: hypotonia, mental retardation, brachycephaly, flat facial profile, up-slanting eyes, epicanthic folds, flat nasal bridge, small and low-set ears, protruding tongue, short stature, brachydactyly, 5th finger clinodactyly, single palmar crease, 'sandal-gap' between 1st and 2nd toes, congenital heart defect (40%), duodenal atresia

Complications: hypothyroidism (30%), acute leukaemia, Alzheimer's disease

Diagnosis: QF-PCR aneuploidy test, karyotyping

Treatment: Monitor growth and neurodevelopment, surgery as indicated, medical treatment of cardiac failure and hypothyroidism, neurodevelopmental interventions, genetic counselling

Prevention:
Primary: female education (AMA), family planning
Secondary: pregnancy screening for AMA, sonar and maternal serum screening
Tertiary: screening for hypothyroidism

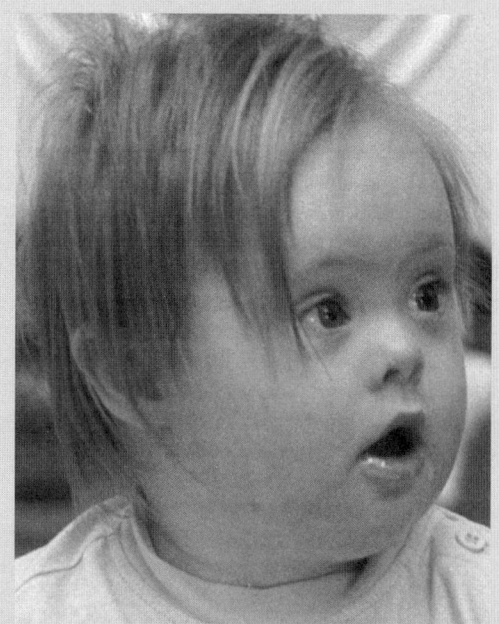

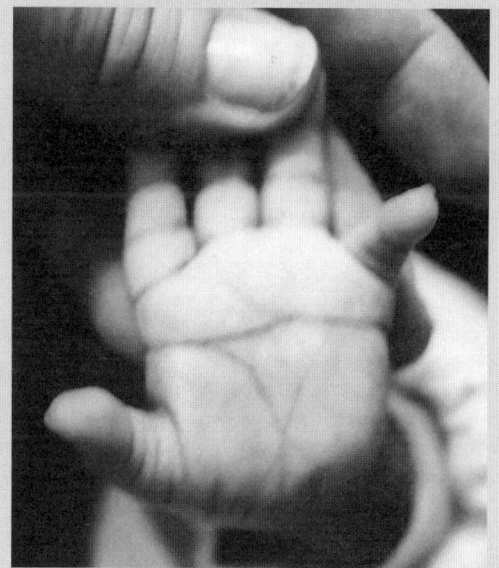

Box 3. Standard symbols used in pedigree drawing

Individuals

☐ Male	◯ Female
■ Affected male	◯ Affected female
4 (square) Four males	2 (circle) Two females
◇ Sex unknown	3 (diamond) Three persons, sex unknown
⬚ (slashed square) Deceased male	◯ (slashed) Deceased female
◼ (slashed filled square) Deceased affected male	● (slashed filled circle) Deceased affected female
■ (small) Prenatal death, male	● (small) Prenatal death, male
◇ (dashed diamond) Pregnancy	◆ Miscarriage
◧ Male carrier, autosomal recessive gene	◑ Female carrier, autosomal recessive gene
	◉ Female carrier, X linked recessive gene
☐ (arrow) Index (presenting) male	◯ (arrow) Index (presenting) female

Box 4. Relationships

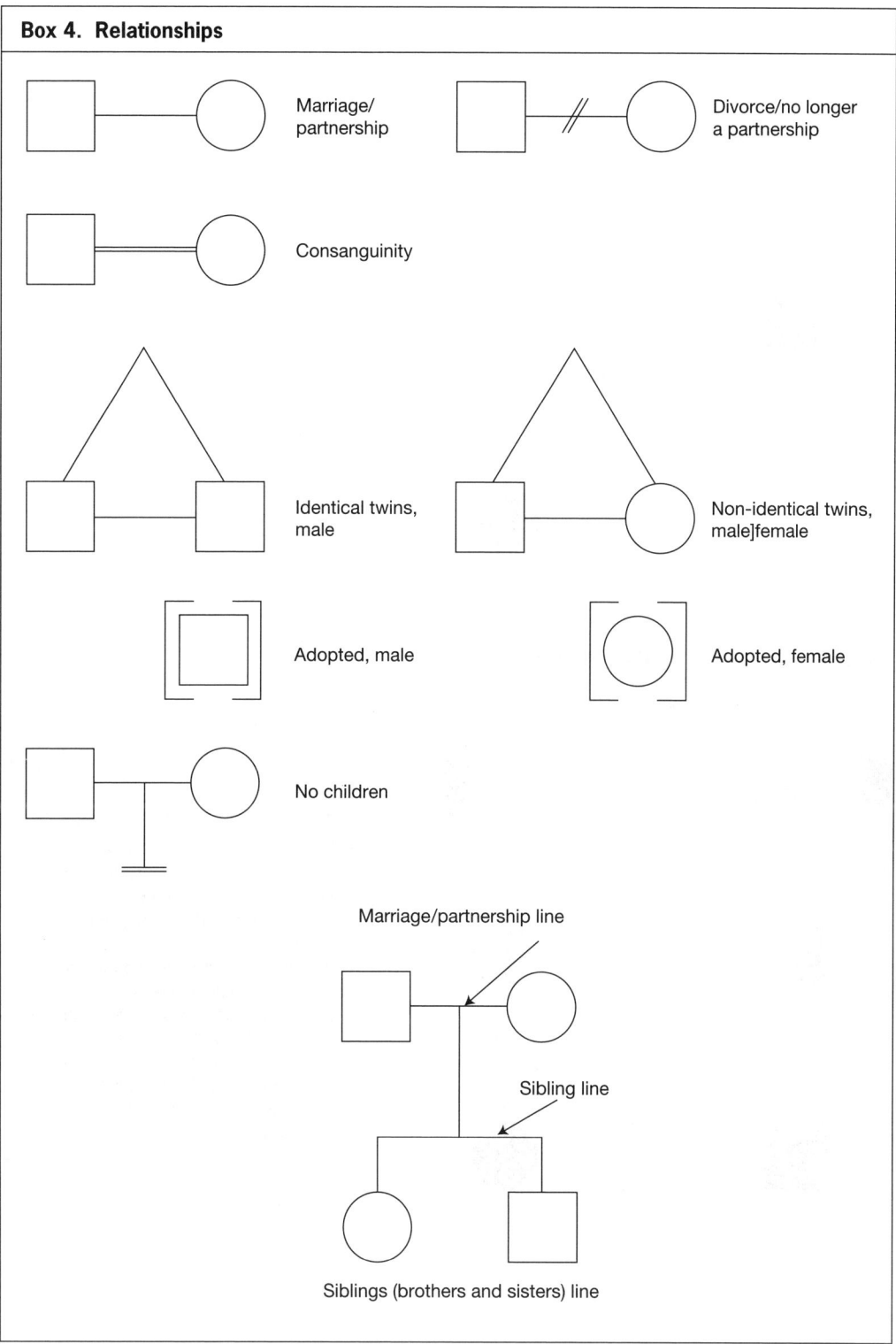

Marriage/partnership

Divorce/no longer a partnership

Consanguinity

Identical twins, male

Non-identical twins, male]female

Adopted, male

Adopted, female

No children

Marriage/partnership line

Sibling line

Siblings (brothers and sisters) line

Autosomal dominant (AD) inheritance

Figure 3.2 Autosomal dominant inheritance

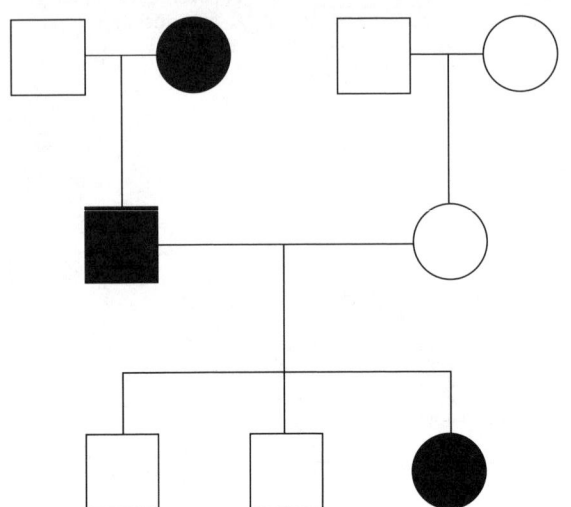

- Family history often positive
- Males and females equally affected
- Can be transmitted by males or females
- New mutations common
- Variable penetrance is usual
- Gonadal mosaicism occurs
- 50% recurrence risk to affected individuals
- Examples include achondroplasia, neurofibromatosis type 1, Marfan syndrome and Huntington disease.

Autosomal recessive (AR) inheritance

Figure 3.3 Autosomal recessive inheritance

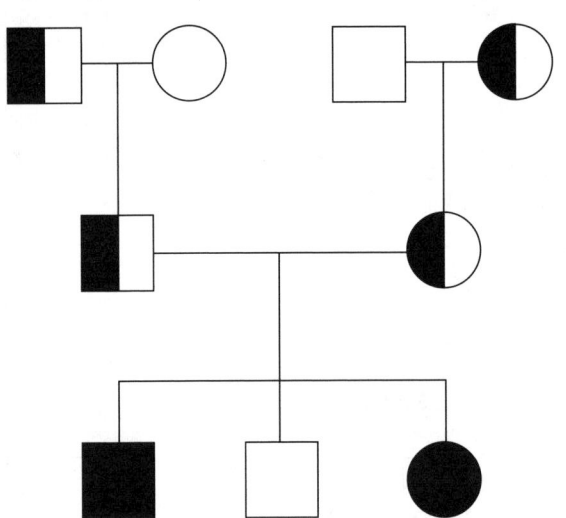

- Family history often negative
- More common with consanguinity
- Siblings may be affected
- Males and females equally affected
- Can be transmitted by males or females
- Parents of affected individuals are always (obligate) carriers
- 25% recurrence risk to carrier parents
- Examples include oculocutaneous albinism, spinal muscular atrophy, thalassaemia, sickle cell disease, cystic fibrosis and most inborn errors of metabolism.

Box 5. Oculocutaneous albinism type 2 (OCA2)

Birth prevalence: about 1 in 4 000–5 000 live births in sub-Saharan Africa

Cause: autosomal recessive single gene disorder. Mutations in P-gene, chromosome 15

Clinical features:
Depigmented hair (white to yellow), skin (milky white) and retina; reduced visual acuity and nystagmus

Complications: skin and eyes hypersensitive to sunlight; skin cancer

Diagnosis: clinical; DNA testing for common black South African gene mutations in P-gene

Treatment: sun protection (clothing, hats, sunscreen, sunglasses), genetic counselling

Prevention:
Primary: family planning; carrier testing after cascade screening by family history-taking
Secondary: prenatal DNA testing
Tertiary: screening for visual problems; screening for skin cancer

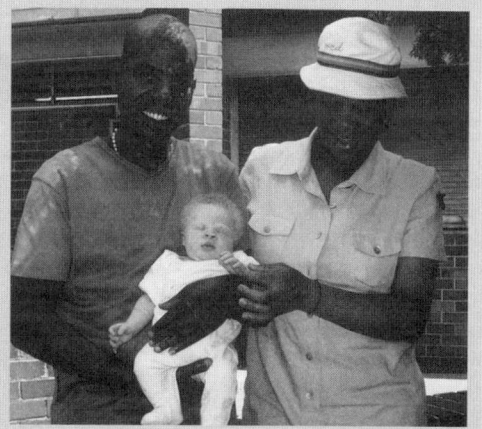

X-linked recessive (XLR) inheritance

Figure 3.4 X-linked recessive inheritance

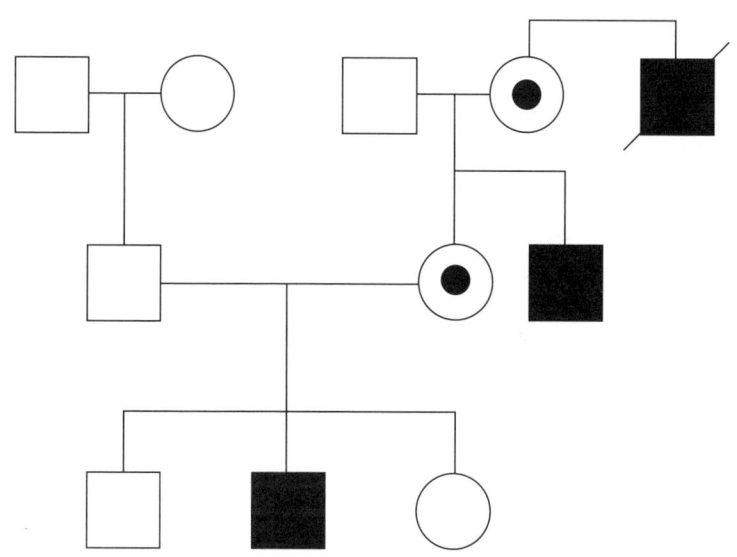

- Males are affected
- Females are usually normal or mildly affected
- Transmitted by females
- New mutations occur
- Gonadal mosaicism occurs
- Recurrence risk to carrier females: 50% of girls carriers; 50% of boys affected
- Recurrence risk to affected males: all daughters are carriers; sons normal
- Examples include Duchenne muscular dystrophy, haemophilia A and B, and fragile X syndrome.

X-linked dominant (XLD) inheritance

Figure 3.5 X-linked dominant inheritance

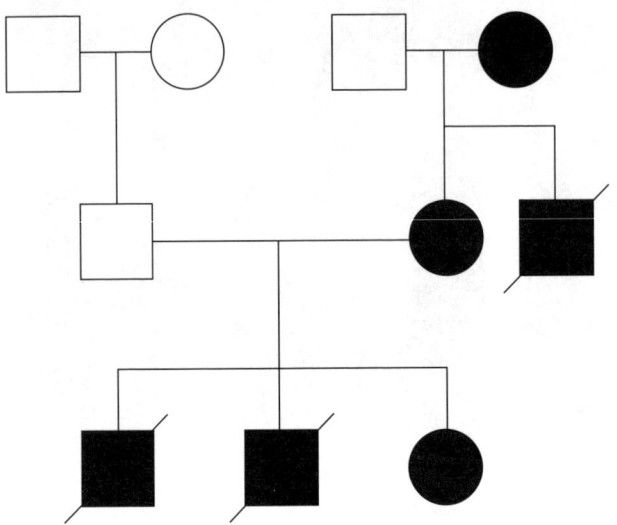

- Females are affected, ranging from mild to severe
- Males are usually severely affected or die
- Transmitted by females
- New mutations occur
- Gonadal mosaicism occurs
- Recurrence risk to carrier females: 50% of girls affected; 50% of boys severe or die
- Examples include Rett and Goltz syndromes

Triplet repeat disorders

This involves expansion of normally occurring nucleotide triplet repeats above a certain threshold. The triplet and thresholds are disease specific. Unaffected carriers have expanded triplet repeats in a pre-mutation range. The triplet can expand with each generation, depending on the parent carrying the triplet expansion. The disease occurs at a younger age and is more severe as the triplet expands, and this is called anticipation. Inheritance may be AD, AR or XLR, and examples are given in Table 3.1.

Imprinting disorders

Normally both genes of a pair are active (expressed), regardless of the parent of origin. However, certain regions on certain chromosomes (locus) are subjected to imprinting. This means that some genes at that locus are active while others are inactive, depending on the parent of origin of that chromosome region. If imprinted genes at a locus should normally be active, but are not present, or if two active copies of a normally inactive gene are present, abnormality results. Examples of imprinting

Table 3.1 Examples of triplet repeat disorders

Condition	Inheritance	Triplet repeat	Normal repeat size	Full mutation repeat size
Huntington's disease	AD	CAG	9–30	40–100
Friedreich's ataxia	AR	GAA	8–33	100–900
Fragile X mental retardation syndrome	XLR	CGG	10–50	>200

disorders include Prader-Willi and Angelman syndromes (chromosome region 15q11-13) and Beckwith-Wiedemann syndrome (chromosome region 11p15.5).

Mitochondrial inheritance

mtDNA is exclusively maternally inherited. However, conditions caused by mtDNA mutations can affect males and females, but mtDNA mutations can only be transmitted by a carrier or affected female. The offspring of males affected with a disorder caused by mtDNA mutations will be normal. It should be noted that mitochondrial conditions can be caused by both mtDNA and nuclear DNA mutations.

Box 6. Neural tube defects (NTD)

Birth prevalence: Overall 3 in 1 000 live births in South Africa. Higher in rural areas.

Cause: Most NTD can also occur with chromosome and single gene disorders and teratogen exposure. Multifactorial NTD has a higher occurrence if mother's diet is folate-deficient.

Clinical features:
Anencephaly: absent skull bones with brain destruction. Lethal.
Spina bifida:
Myelomeningocoele (95%). Involves meninges and spinal cord
Meningocoele (5%). Involves meninges only
Site: lumbar > lumbosacral > thoracolumbar
Encephalocoele (10%): localized skull defect with protrusion of brain

Complications: death, paralysis of legs, incontinence of bladder and/or bowel, hydrocephalus, developmental delay

Diagnosis:
Antenatal: sonar, raised maternal serum alphafetoprotein (AFP)
Postnatal: clinical features, CT or MRI scan (encephalocoele)

Treatment: surgical closure, ventriculoperitoneal shunt for hydrocephalus, management of urinary tract infections, monitor neurodevelopment, palliation, genetic counselling

Prevention:
Primary: food fortification with folate, periconception folate supplementation for women with previously affected child
Secondary: pregnancy screening with sonar, maternal serum AFP screen
Tertiary: screening for hydrocephalus, incontinence, urinary tract infection, developmental delay

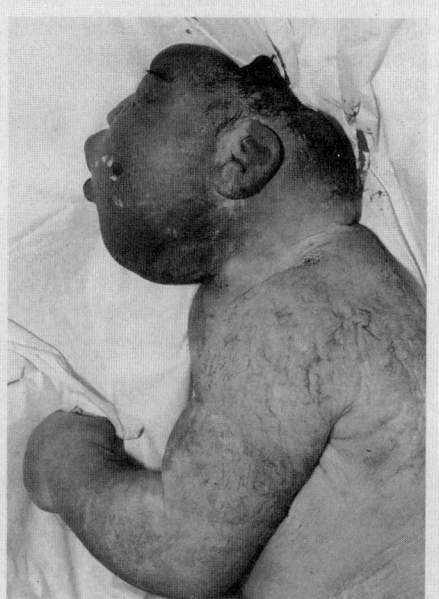
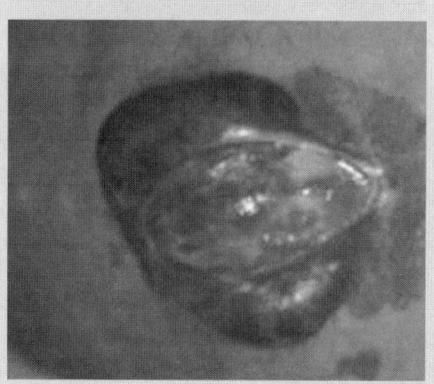

Multifactorial inheritance

Most physical traits such as height, intelligence, blood pressure and so on, are not determined by a single gene. Rather, they are the result of the interaction of many genes with each other and with the environment, and this is known as multifactorial inheritance. Certain birth defects and complex disorders follow multifactorial inheritance patterns. This means that a person's particular genetic make-up (genotype) interacts with specific environmental conditions to cause the condition.

Multifactorial malformations are present at birth and usually affect one organ, system or area of the body (e.g. neural tube defect, cleft lip and/or palate, clubfoot).

Teratogens

Teratogen exposure during the embryonic period (the first eight weeks of life) may result in fetal death or physical defects. Teratogen exposure after the embryonic period may affect fetal growth and brain development, which are ongoing throughout pregnancy. Teratogens include altered maternal metabolic states (diabetes mellitus, hypothyroidism, iodine deficiency), infectious agents, ingested substances (alcohol, illicit drugs and medications), hyperthermia, environmental pollutants and massive radiation exposure.

Fetal constraint

A fetus may be constrained due to oligo-

Box 7. Fetal alcohol syndrome (FAS)

Prevalence: 48–64 in 1 000 school-entry age children, Western Cape, South Africa

Cause: fetal exposure to teratogen (alcohol)

Clinical features:
Growth retardation: parameters less than 10th percentile for age
Typical facial features: short palpebral fissures, flat midface, underdeveloped philtrum, thin upper lip
Neurodevelopmental/cognitive effects: delayed milestones, poor concentration, hyperactivity
Associated birth defects: cardiac, skeletal, renal, ocular, deafness, neural tube defects

Complications: related to cognitive abnormality and structural defects

Diagnosis: clinical

Treatment: Monitor growth and neurodevelopment, surgery as indicated, neurodevelopmental interventions, assisted schooling, genetic counselling

Prevention:
Primary: eliminate alcohol from diet of women of reproductive age
Secondary: sonar screening in high-risk pregnancies
Tertiary: screening for cardiac and renal defects, neurodevelopmental and growth delay, hearing test

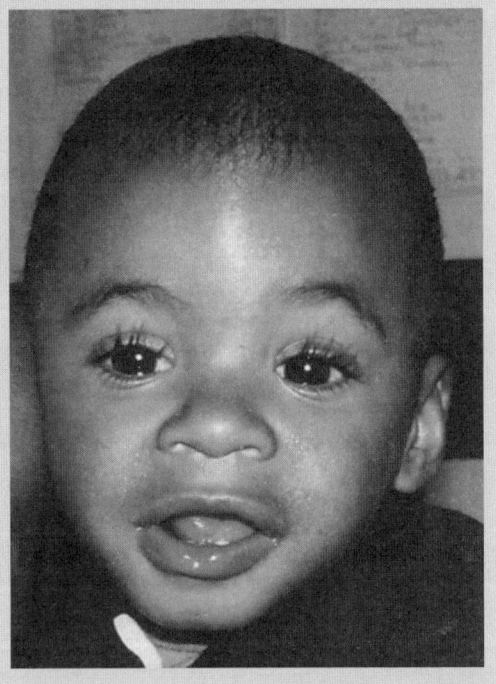

hydramnios, multiple pregnancy or a uterine abnormality (e.g. bicornuate uterus). Typically the features present at birth include joint contractures (including arthrogryposis), webbed fingers, micrognathia, cleft palate and other deformations. These features are the result of lack of fetal movement (fetal akinesia). Fetal akinesia sequence may be due to fetal constraint, but single gene disorders can also cause this sequence (e.g. congenital muscular dystrophy).

Complex disorders

These disorders develop after birth, some presenting in childhood, but most manifesting in mid or later life. Their aetiology requires an interaction between genes and, mostly postnatal, environmental factors. However, in some disorders it is postulated that prenatal environmental factors are also contributory. By comparison with multifactorial malformations, they are clinically complex, being systemic and involving different organs and systems. Common complex disorders include cancer, coronary artery disease, type-2 diabetes mellitus, hypertension, mental disorders and stroke.

In 2005 the WHO estimated that 35 million people (61 per cent of all deaths) died from cardiovascular disease, stroke, cancer and other complex disorders. Eighty per cent of these deaths occurred in middle- and low-income nations. If, between 2006 and 2015, just two per cent of complex disorder deaths are averted, 36 million deaths could be prevented and 500 million life years gained, most in middle- and low-income nations and almost half in people under 70 years old. This partly explains why resources are being allocated to determine the genetic components underlying these complex disorders. However, the known environmental factors contributing to these conditions should already be targeted as part of public health care strategies.

Clinical approach to medical genetics

The clinician faced with an individual with a birth defect or complex disorder, is asked to answer five questions:
- What is it?
- What caused it?

- What does it mean?
- Will it happen again?
- Can it be prevented?

A summary of the process of a medical genetic consultation, based on these questions, is presented in Figure 3.6.

What is it?

The aim of answering this question is to make a diagnosis. With a clear diagnosis, the other four questions can be answered accurately. To answer this first question, the process that is followed is that followed in all clinical medicine: history taking, physical examination and use of appropriate investigations. Each of these areas requires a specific emphasis.

History

- History of the main complaint and medical progress. Specifics to note include growth abnormalities (overgrowth or failure to thrive), seizures, cardiac or other organ dysfunction, recurrent infections and feeding difficulties.
- Family history. Note aspects such as similarly affected individuals, individuals with other birth defects or functional abnormalities (like mental retardation), possible patterns of inheritance, consanguinity, ethnicity, previous miscarriages and stillbirths. Construct a family pedigree. (Boxes 3, 4 and 8).
- Pregnancy history. Include information about maternal health (including diet and nutritional status), maternal illnesses (especially pre-existing diabetes mellitus and thyroid disease), maternal medication use, and pregnancy-related events that could result in birth defects such as maternal infections or other teratogen exposure (such as alcohol).
- Birth history must be detailed and complete. It should include birth parameters of weight, length and head circumference, details about presentation and resuscitation events.
- Developmental history is essential and should note specific age of achievement of motor and cognitive milestones (like speech), and specific or unusual behaviour

(including sleep, activity levels, unusual habits).

Examination

The aim of the examination is to detect all major and minor structural abnormalities. Where more than minor abnormalities are detected, a birth defect should be suspected. Where one major abnormality is found, a careful search should be made for other abnormalities. This may re-

quire special investigations to find less obvious abnormalities.

♦ Measurements. Growth parameters (weight, height, and head circumference) should be measured and plotted on appropriate growth charts at every examination. Other measurements like limb length or palpebral fissure length should be noted and plotted where considered helpful.

Figure 3.6 An approach to the medical genetic consultation

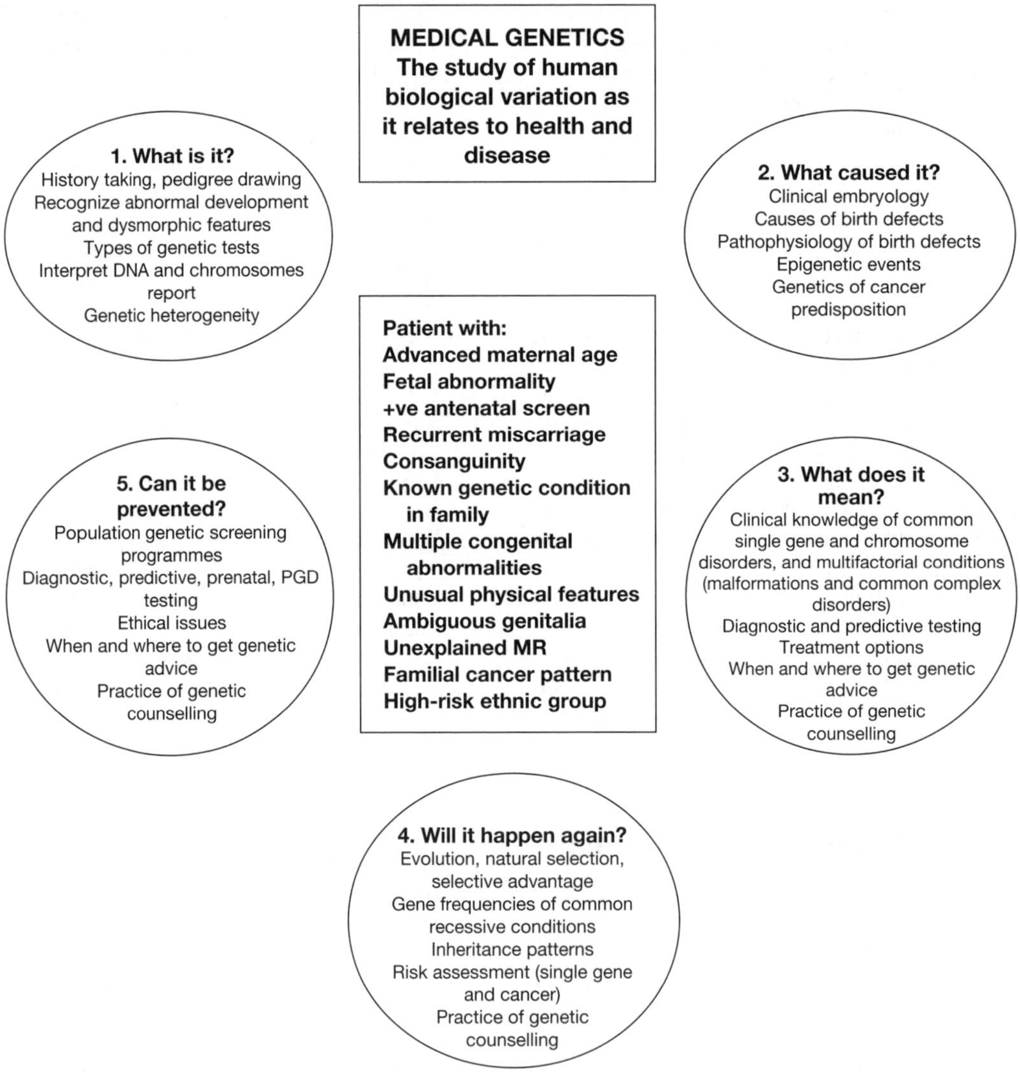

MEDICAL GENETICS
The study of human biological variation as it relates to health and disease

1. What is it?
History taking, pedigree drawing
Recognize abnormal development and dysmorphic features
Types of genetic tests
Interpret DNA and chromosomes report
Genetic heterogeneity

2. What caused it?
Clinical embryology
Causes of birth defects
Pathophysiology of birth defects
Epigenetic events
Genetics of cancer predisposition

Patient with:
Advanced maternal age
Fetal abnormality
+ve antenatal screen
Recurrent miscarriage
Consanguinity
Known genetic condition in family
Multiple congenital abnormalities
Unusual physical features
Ambiguous genitalia
Unexplained MR
Familial cancer pattern
High-risk ethnic group

5. Can it be prevented?
Population genetic screening programmes
Diagnostic, predictive, prenatal, PGD testing
Ethical issues
When and where to get genetic advice
Practice of genetic counselling

3. What does it mean?
Clinical knowledge of common single gene and chromosome disorders, and multifactorial conditions (malformations and common complex disorders)
Diagnostic and predictive testing
Treatment options
When and where to get genetic advice
Practice of genetic counselling

4. Will it happen again?
Evolution, natural selection, selective advantage
Gene frequencies of common recessive conditions
Inheritance patterns
Risk assessment (single gene and cancer)
Practice of genetic counselling

Box 8. Constructing a family pedigree

Aim: to create a clear, easy-to-read record of family relationships and relevant genetic information of individuals in the family

Important related information:
• First names and surnames
• Dates of birth (preferred to ages)
• Addresses: postal and physical
• Telephone numbers
• Occupations
• Ethnic group
• Religion, culture and language

Method:
Draw the presenting person first, males on left, females on right

Draw in the presenting person's partner next to him/her with a partnership line, noting consanguinity with a double line if needed

Draw in the descent line and record all pregnancies and their outcomes for the couple

Draw in siblings and parents for both partners. Be careful to note if brothers and sisters are full or half siblings

Draw in children of siblings. Shade affected individuals

- A detailed systematic examination is required so that abnormalities are not missed. Photographs provide accurate documentation of abnormalities and their evolution with time, and aid discussions with other clinicians. A minimum of a frontal and lateral face view, full body view, and views of the hands and feet should be taken. All other abnormal body parts should be photographed. Photographs should only be taken after obtaining written parental consent.

Investigations

Patients require investigations that are appropriate to their condition regardless of the genetic diagnosis.

Non-specific tests related to birth defects and complex disorders
- X-rays are essential when skeletal abnormalities are present (e.g. short limbs). The diagnosis of a skeletal dysplasia is impossible without X-rays. Skeletal abnormalities may occur as part of other genetic syndromes, and so any baby with abnormalities should have at least a chest X-ray. Where a skeletal dysplasia is suspected, appropriate films include AP and lateral skull views, AP and lateral views of the spine and pelvis, AP view of the chest, AP view of the arms, legs, hands and wrists. A whole body X-ray ('babygram') of the newborn, stillborn, or abortus can be very useful.
- Non-invasive imaging with ultrasound (cranial, abdominal, renal), echocardiography, and CT or MRI brain scanning may be required for a full evaluation of all abnormalities.

Specific genetic tests
These are tests that are aimed at making a genetic diagnosis, and will be discussed in the section on genetic testing.

What caused it?

The aim of answering this question is to decide whether or not the defect or condition has a genetic cause. Knowledge of a specific diagnosis allows for accurate recurrence risk counselling.

However, a diagnosis is not always made. It is then important to decide whether the abnormality is a deformation, disruption, dysplasia or malformation. Deformations and disruptions do not have a genetic cause; dysplasias always do; malformations have many causes, which are sometimes genetic. Based on this classification, genetic counselling can be refined.

What does it mean?

Answering this question requires discussion about prognosis, treatment, implications to relatives, reproductive choices and other psychosocial concerns. A firm diagnosis allows for these issues to be discussed accurately. Genetic counselling allows genetic information to be given in a way that is understandable and acceptable to patients and provides psychosocial support (*see* below). However, even without a diagnosis, appropriate care and discussions about the implications of the abnormality or condition can still be implemented.

Each person's unique situation will determine which medical, surgical, and neurodevelopmental treatments are needed. Some individuals may be cured with a single intervention while others will require multiple treatment methods. It is often the medical geneticist's role to act as coordinator for the multidisciplinary care of patients with birth defects.

The exact complications to be expected will depend on the diagnosis, what abnormalities are present, and which organ systems are involved. However, a few general comments can be made:
- Any baby with physical abnormalities should have regular neurodevelopmental follow-up because developmental delay may occur in individuals with physical abnormalities.
- Complications may result from the abnormalities themselves, or from treatments that are used.
- Certain conditions are known to be associated with specific complications, and these should be screened for (e.g. hypothyroidism in Down's syndrome).

Will it happen again?

The answer to this question relates to recurrence risks. If a definitive diagnosis is made, the underlying cause is usually known, and then accurate recurrence risks can be given according to the known inheritance pattern.

Sometimes it is clear that a condition has a genetic cause without making a specific diagnosis. In this case, only empiric recurrence risks can be given.

If a birth defect clearly does not have a genetic cause, the recurrence risks are usually low if the condition causing the birth defect is not present in future pregnancies. For instance, if a woman with a child with fetal alcohol syndrome does not drink in future pregnancies, she can have a normal baby. If the same conditions are present in a future pregnancy, the recurrence risks can also be determined (e.g. a woman on anti-epileptic medication can be given specific risks of birth defects depending on which drugs she takes).

Can it be prevented?

Peri-conception care seeks to enable the conception of a normal embryo and its wellbeing in the first eight weeks of pregnancy. This period, during most of which the mother is unaware of her pregnancy, includes the period of organogenesis when the embryo is most susceptible to damage from teratogens.

All couples who have had a child with a birth defect can minimise their risks in future pregnancies by following general advice with respect to folic acid supplementation, maternal serum screening and ultrasound scans. Women should take 0.4 mg folic acid every day from three months before they plan to fall pregnant, until three months into the pregnancy (periconceptional folate). In the case of a previous history of a NTD, higher doses are recommended. Detailed ultrasound scans should be done at 12 weeks of pregnancy and again at 18–20 weeks by an expert in fetal ultrasound.

In medical genetics there are three levels of prevention of birth defects:

♦ **Primary prevention**. This comprises basic reproductive health approaches that should be available through primary health care and should therefore be implemented in all countries (*see* Box 9). Once achieved, they result in a decrease in the birth prevalence of birth defects to a baseline level.

Box 9. Basic reproductive approaches for the prevention of birth defects

1. Family planning
This allows for:
- Reduction of the birth rate and thus the number of infants born with birth defects
- Decrease in the birth prevalence of Down's syndrome by reducing the number of mothers of advanced maternal age
- The introduction of the concept of reproductive choice, so that couples with affected children may chose not to have more children.

2. Optimising women's diet
Before and during a woman's reproductive years, ensuring a healthy, balanced diet that provides iodine through salt iodization and folic acid by food fortification and supplementation will:
- Prevent iodine deficiency in women during pregnancy and thereby prevent the cognitive impairment resulting from iodine deficiency disorder in their offspring
- Decrease neural tube defects and other malformations
- Also remove teratogens, notably alcohol and smoking.

3. Control infections in all women before and during pregnancy
- Test for and treat syphilis
- Prevent congenital rubella syndrome through immunization with rubella vaccine
- Test for and counsel HIV positive women*.

4. Optimize maternal health
Treat chronic illnesses associated with increased risk of birth defects including:
- Insulin-dependent diabetes mellitus
- Epilepsy and its control with anti-epileptic drugs
- Women with deep vein thrombosis and cardiac conditions on warfarin.

*By definition HIV can be considered a teratogen. The principles of MTCT of HIV are the same as for birth defects.

Table adapted from the report of a joint WHO-March of Dimes meeting on Management of Birth Defects & Haemoglobin Disorders. May 2006. Geneva, Switzerland.

- **Secondary prevention**. This seeks to reduce the birth prevalence of birth defects by reducing the number of infants born with a birth defect. It requires the implementation of medical genetic screening, prenatal diagnosis and the offer of therapeutic options, all with appropriate counselling.
- **Tertiary prevention**. Tertiary prevention aims to maximize the potential of children with birth defects. This requires early detection and treatment of clinical problems to minimize the development of complications or deterioration in health. The best possible care available in the circumstances must be offered. Interventions include newborn screening (if available), medical treatment of complications, surgical repair of congenital malformations and neurodevelopmental therapy for infants and children with disabilities. It also includes palliative care for children dying from the consequences of their birth defect. Ongoing screening for known complications in certain disorders is also required. In middle- and low-income countries as much as possible of the medical treatment, neurodevelopmental therapy and palliative care needs to take place in primary health care.

Medical genetic screening programmes apply to all levels of prevention. They can be expensive but can be introduced in a step-wise fashion according to a country's needs and circumstances, and are summarized in Box 10.

Genetic counselling

Genetic counselling is an education process that is used to fully inform individuals and families about the facts and implications of birth defects and complex disorders. The process is non-directive but also provides psychosocial support. It allows the individuals and families to come to terms with their condition and to make medical, reproductive and social choices. These principles are observed throughout the medical genetics consultation.

Box 10. Medical genetic screening that can be considered for implementation in middle-income countries

Preconception
- Use of family history as a screening tool for birth defects
- Carrier risk identification using family pedigrees and DNA analysis of identified individuals (cascade screening)
- Population carrier screening for common recessive disorders, the haemoglobin disorders (FBC and indices, electrophoresis, DNA) and cystic fibrosis (DNA).

Antenatal
- Rhesus negativity
- Down's syndrome (advanced maternal age, maternal serum, ultrasound)
- Neural tube defects (maternal serum screening, ultrasound)
- Major malformations (fetal anomaly scanning)
- Carrier screening for common recessive disorders, the haemoglobin disorders (FBC and indices, electrophoresis, DNA) and cystic fibrosis (DNA).

Postnatal
- Examination of all neonates by a trained healthcare practitioner before discharge from the hospital or clinic
- Neonatal screening (using Guthrie cards) Priority conditions to consider include:
  - Congenital hypothyroidism
  - Sickle cell disorders
  - G6PD deficiency
  - Common inborn errors of metabolism.

Additional conditions may be added when finances and priorities allow.

Table adapted from the report of a joint WHO-March of Dimes meeting on Management of Birth Defects & Haemoglobin Disorders. May 2006. Geneva, Switzerland.

Psychosocial support

Families and individuals with birth defects often have to deal with difficult issues such as accepting a birth defect, coping with the day-to-day burden of managing the condition, grieving for the loss of normality, and making complex decisions about future pregnancies. Some families and individuals require referral to psychological services for support. Many also appreciate the help they get from patient-parent support groups where they can discuss issues with families with similarly affected individuals. In addition, simple interventions like referral to the social welfare services to apply for a care-dependency or disability grant can lessen some of their problems.

Genetic testing

Broadly speaking, genetic tests are done to find either chromosome abnormalities or single gene mutations (DNA tests). Cytogenetics is the field of genetics that tests for chromosome abnormalities, and molecular genetics refers to DNA testing. Before genetic testing is offered, parents should have genetic counselling. Not only should they be clear about why they are having the test, but they need to consider the implications of both a positive or negative result, understand the limitations of DNA testing, and be aware of the cost of testing. Pre-test genetic counselling is particularly important for prenatal, presymptomatic and predictive testing.

Chromosome testing

Chromosome testing aims to identify numerical or structural chromosome abnormalities. In recent years, DNA technology has been used to test chromosomes in more detail, which has revolutionized the field of cytogenetics.

Chromosomes can be tested using the following methods:

- **Standard karyotyping**
  Live cells are required in samples like blood (lymphocytes), chorionic villus tissue, amniotic fluid (fibroblasts) or skin samples (fibroblasts) The cells are cultured in a special medium. Numerical abnormalities are easily identified, but structural abnormalities are only identified if they involve large pieces of chromosomes (3–5 megabases). Testing is labour-intensive and expensive, and results usually take 1–4 weeks. All chromosomes are screened in one test.

- **Fluorescent in situ hybridization (FISH)**
  FISH testing uses DNA probes to identify whether specific chromosome regions are present or absent. The condition to be tested for must be specified to the laboratory (e.g. velocardiofacial syndrome testing region 22q11). Testing is expensive and labour-intensive, but results are usually obtained sooner than they are in karyotyping.

- **Quantitative fluorescent polymerase chain reaction (QF-PCR)**
  This technique uses DNA testing to detect numerical abnormalities of chromosomes 13, 18, 21, X and Y. Because DNA is tested, live cells are not required and even post-mortem samples like skin snips can be used. The test is quick (72 hours) and can be semi-automated. It is particularly useful for prenatal testing. QF-PCR is not designed to detect mosaicism or structural chromosome abnormalities like translocation.

- **Multiplex ligation-dependent probe analysis (MLPA)**
  This technique uses DNA technology to detect very small deletions and duplications on chromosomes or even within genes. Various samples such as blood, skin, muscle and cancer tissue can be used.

- **Chromosome microarray analysis (CMA)**
  This test uses thousands of DNA probes scattered across all chromosomes, directed at chromosome regions of known and unknown pathological significance. Data from the probes is generated from controls and from the affected person. The data is statistically analyzed for ratio differences between the two samples. Simply stated, an over-representation of data suggests a duplicated region, and under-representation suggests a deletion.

Single gene testing

Various laboratory techniques can be used to detect mutations, including polymerase chain reaction (PCR), restriction fragment length polymorphism (RFLP) testing, Southern blotting,

DNA sequencing, and MLPA. The laboratory decides which test to use depending on the type of mutation to be looked for.

One advantage of DNA testing is that live cells are not required. DNA can be extracted from blood samples (lymphocytes), skin samples, biopsies of any description both ante- and post-mortem, and from prenatal samples (amniocytes in amniotic fluid, and chorionic villi). Non-blood samples requiring DNA extraction should always be submitted in saline and not formalin.

Before molecular testing can be done, the laboratory must know which genetic condition is suspected. If the gene to be tested is known, the laboratory tests for faults in that gene by direct mutation analysis. Linkage analysis is done when other DNA markers close to the gene are tested when direct mutation testing cannot be done. This gives information about the gene by association.

No gene test is 100 per cent accurate, and some of the reasons why gene faults may not be found include:

- Locus heterogeneity, where the wrong gene is being tested
- Technical limitations of the test
- Rare mutation present that is not routinely tested
- Incorrect diagnosis.

New genes are being found almost monthly and new laboratory techniques are always being developed. Doctors should therefore liaise with clinical geneticists and the molecular genetic laboratory on an ongoing basis about what tests can be offered.

Prenatal testing

Methods to detect birth defects before birth include:

- **Ultrasound scan**. This is a screening test, and further diagnostic tests are required to confirm a suspected diagnosis. Fetal anomaly scans should only be performed by persons trained in fetal medicine. In general, ultrasound scans only detect about 70 per cent of structural defects and will not detect functional abnormalities like mental retardation, deafness or metabolic abnormalities.

- **Chromosome testing**. This is indicated prenatally when:
  - Advanced maternal age (AMA) women choose the test after genetic counselling
  - Couples have had a child affected with a chromosome abnormality and are concerned about their recurrence risks
  - One partner in a couple is a known balanced-translocation carrier
  - Abnormalities are detected on ultrasound suggestive of a chromosome abnormality.

Chromosome testing can be done on samples of chorionic villi, amniotic fluid, or cord blood by standard karyotyping or by QF-PCR. Each technique has its advantages and disadvantages which should be discussed during pre-test genetic counselling.

- **Single gene testing**. This is indicated prenatally when:
  - A fetus is to be tested for a known genetic condition
  - Abnormalities are detected on ultrasound suggestive of a particular single gene condition
  - Fetal sexing is required.

Molecular testing can only be done for a single gene condition if the mutation causing that condition in the family is known, or if linkage analysis is informative. This usually means that DNA testing must have been completed in the family *before* the pregnancy. Prenatal DNA testing requires samples of chorionic villi, amniotic fluid, or cord blood. Maternal contamination testing must always be done on prenatal samples submitted for DNA testing.

Fetal samples required for chromosome or single gene tests are obtained by invasive procedures. Chorionic villus sampling (CVS) is usually done at 11–14 weeks of pregnancy and has a miscarriage rate of 1–2 per cent. Amniocentesis is performed from 15-20 weeks and has a miscarriage rate of less 1 one per cent. Cordocentesis is done from 18 weeks until term and has a miscarriage rate of 2–3 per cent.

- **Preimplantation genetic diagnosis (PGD)**. This involves testing one or two cells from an embryo at about the 8-10 cell stage for a *known* genetic condition, after *in vitro* fertilization. Chromosome and single gene disorders can be tested for. Unaffected embryos are then implanted into the uterus. Ideally the genetic test should be repeated later in the pregnancy by CVS or amniocentesis to confirm the initial result. This is recommended because of the chance that a genetic fault was missed after testing only a few embryonic cells. PGD requires considerable technical expertise and extensive pre-test work-up, and is very costly.

Predictive and presymptomatic testing

This type of testing is offered for late- or adult-onset disorders where genetic knowledge will alter the medical treatment of or decision-making by an individual. International guidelines should be followed before offering these tests, and a person may have to undergo a presymptomatic testing protocol of consultations before genetic testing is done. A predictive genetic test is done to refine a person's lifetime risk of developing a genetic condition (e.g. inherited breast cancer). A pre-symptomatic test is done on a healthy person to determine if they will develop symptoms of a genetic condition in the future (e.g. Huntington's disease, spinocerebellar ataxia).

Genetic testing of minors

Genetic testing of minors is a controversial topic requiring careful ethical debate. In general, a minor should only have genetic testing if the result has medical implications for that minor. For most genetic conditions, testing can be delayed until a person has attained majority or is ready to make reproductive choices. Although it is preferrable to test individuals 18 years or older, this guideline can not always be followed. For instance, a teenager who is at risk of passing on a genetic condition and who is at risk of a teenage pregnancy may have genetic testing after suitable genetic counselling. These guidelines are based on the principle of respect for individual autonomy. Testing of minors can be detrimental where the result has no medical implication for the minor. For example, parental knowledge of a child's carrier status can negatively influence how they treat that child. Further, it removes the child's right to choose to have knowledge about

his genetic make-up. Even in situations when it is thought best to do a genetic test in a child, that child's assent is usually required.

New genetics

The field of genetics moves rapidly, both at clinical and laboratory level. Only two recent developments in the field will be mentioned here.

Epigenetics

Epigenetics is the study of mechanisms that change DNA expression without causing changes in the DNA sequence. It is an area that will assume increasing importance over the next few years, particularly because of the interest in how epigenetics influences phenotypic traits and complex disorders, and how the environment influences epigenetics. Epigenetic mechanisms are important in certain well-recognized neuro-developmental and growth syndromes, and certain tumours and cancer. Further, epigenetic phenomena can vary with age, between populations and between individuals, and can be influenced by environmental factors like diet.

The best studied epigenetic mechanisms are DNA methylation and histone modification by methylation and acetylation. These mechanisms result in genes either being expressed or silenced.

Pharmacogenetics

Pharmacogenetics is the study of how drugs interact with specific genes, while pharmacogenomics is the study of how drugs interact with the entire genome. Individual variation in these genes may account for why individuals respond differently to drugs. Drug-gene interactions are usually multifactorial phenomena, but there are a few single genes that have been shown to interact with particular drugs.

If it is known which gene(s) variants alter a person's response to a drug, it may be possible to decide whether or not to use that drug, the dose to use, duration of use, and what side effects to expect. Most idiosyncratic drug reactions are the result of individual drug-gene interactions, so knowledge of a person's genotype may help to minimize such reactions in future.

PART 2

Psychosocial and community paediatrics

4 Community paediatrics, child health and survival

Why focus on children's health?

There is an increasing realization that it is in the national interest to have healthy children. Health must be viewed as a resource for everyday life, not the objective of living.

This definition elegantly captures the interaction of multiple influences such as genetics, behaviour and the environment in determining a child's health status. Basic pre-requisites for the health of children include food, shelter, education, household income, peace and a stable ecosystem. Children's body size and behaviours make them more susceptible than adults to environmental influences and they are also dependent on their families and communities to meet their needs.

Healthy children are more willing and able to learn, contribute to a society's sense of well-being, and may go on to become healthy adults who will raise healthy families, power the eco-nomy and contribute to the continued vitality of society. This creates an important ethical, economic and social imperative on society to ensure that all children are as healthy as they can be.

Figure 4.1 outlines the various determinants of children's health. Disadvantage in any of these areas, for example poverty, living in an under-resourced setting or unusual caregiver health-seeking behaviour could contribute to ill-health. A combination often has a compounding effect and may result in disability and death. Adequate health services for children and enabling child health policies can offset some of this disadvantage and contribute to the achievement of 'health' for all children.

Children's Health can be defined as 'the extent to which individual children or groups of children are able or enabled to:
- Develop and realize their potential
- Satisfy their needs, and
- Develop the capacities that allow them to interact successfully with their biological, physical, and social environments.'

(US National Academy of Sciences)

Figure 4.1 Determinants of child health

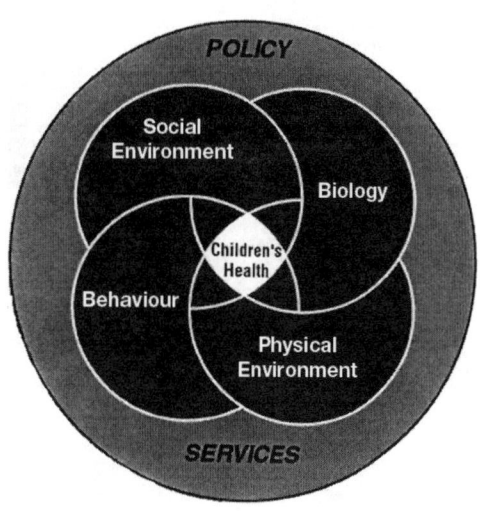

What is community paediatrics?

This term is usually used to encompass paediatrics practised in a community setting. In some resource-rich countries, paediatricians who provide mainly consultative services in a community setting and are skilled in the management of problems such as child abuse, learning or behavioural difficulties, or disability are known as community paediatricians.

In southern Africa, community paediatrics is much less about specialists managing individual children's health within a community, and

> Community paediatrics involves health professionals assisting and enabling the community to collectively fulfil its responsibility to children and their health

much more about child health practitioners (e.g. doctors, nurses, and allied health professionals) assisting with the delivery of preventive and promotive child health services (e.g. immunisation or developmental screening),

Table 4.1 Terms used in health care service delivery	
Levels of care	
Primary	Health services in a community that a patient makes contact with first. Provided by nurses, doctors at primary health care clinics, general practitioners, or hospital out-patient departments.
Secondary	Services provided by generalists or specialists to patients referred from a primary care level. Can be provided at a level one hospital, but more frequently available at level two and three hospitals.
Tertiary	Specialized services provided by specialists (e.g. paediatrician) or super-specialists (e.g. paediatric cardiologist). Provided at level two, or most often, at level three hospitals.
Quaternary	High specialized or expensive services such as organ transplantation offered at one or a few facilities in a country.
Hospital levels	
Level one (district)	District or non-specialist hospital to which patients from clinics or health centres may be referred. Staffed by medical generalists with access to basic diagnostic and therapeutic facilities. Offers 24-hour in-patient care.
Level two (regional)	Regional hospitals are the referral centres for patients from the district hospitals. Staffed by general specialists such as surgeons, paediatricians and anaesthetists. Also inevitably functions as a level one hospital for its own catchment area.
Level three (academic)	Super-specialist or academic hospitals staffed by general and super-specialists. Handle complex or uncommon conditions.
Level four (national)	Designated super-specialist (national) hospitals where particular procedures or kinds of interventions are offered, e.g. liver transplants.
Types of child care	
Primary health care (PHC) approach	The underlying philosophy for the provision of health care services that is based on the Alma Ata Declaration, i.e. comprehensive care that includes curative, preventive, promotive and rehabilitative care within the context of, among others, community participation and intersectoral collaboration.
Comprehensive care	The fullest possible range of, for example, primary health services; the provision of preventive, promotive, curative and rehabilitative care by a health care facility or authority.
Governance	
Health region	Geographic area into which a province is divided and within which secondary hospital services are available within the health districts that fall within its boundaries.
Health district	Geographic area that is small enough to allow maximal involvement of the community so that local health needs are met, but also large enough to effect economies of scale.

by their influence on child health policy development (e.g. health care provision in districts or regions), or through advocacy efforts for improving children's biological, physical, and social environments (e.g. food access, accident prevention, social grants).

Structure and organisation of child health services

South Africa has embraced the concept of district health services delivered within a three-tiered national health system framework. The three tiers are national, provincial and district. The National Health System refers to the organization of a country's health service, including services provided by government, non-governmental organizations (NGOs), community-based organizations (CBOs) and the private sector. Table 4.1 gives definitions of some of the terms used in describing health services.

The Constitution and the South African National Health Act (No. 61 of 2003) spells out the powers and functions of the three spheres of government and the division of functions within the national health system.

National health department responsibilities

The national health department has the power to make national legislation, set norms and standards, relate to international organisations and the Ministries of Health of other countries, monitor the delivery of services, and provide services that, because of economies of scale or financial constraints cannot be provided at provincial level. Its role includes developing national goals, objectives, indicators, and policies for monitoring programme implementation. They are, furthermore, responsible for providing support to provinces and districts in their implementation and monitoring of programmes. Several directorates in the South African Department of Health are responsible for programmes that affect the health of children, including maternal, child and women's health, nutrition, HIV/AIDS and other sexually transmitted infections, chronic diseases and disabilities; women's health and genetics, oral health, and mental health and substance abuse.

Provincial health department responsibilities

The provinces are charged with planning, regulating and providing effective support structures for health services with the exception of district/municipal health services. Responsibilities include the provision of level two and or three hospital services, coordination of emergency medical and forensic services, and facilitating research on health and health services. Strong provincial health structures are crucial for establishing districts and providing the support and oversight that are essential for their effective functioning.

District and metropolitan municipal health responsibilities

This level of the healthcare system is responsible for the provision and/or purchase of a full range of comprehensive primary health care services within its area of jurisdiction.

The district is responsible for the overall management and control of its health budget. Effective referral networks and systems are ensured through cooperation with other health districts. The district health system is responsible for all institutions and individuals, whether governmental, non-governmental, private or traditional, providing healthcare in the district, up to and including first-level hospitals. Most of the 52 districts in South Africa are divided into sub-districts to enable appropriate control and functioning.

Irrespective of the structure of decentralization and government adopted, there will always be an overlap of functions and responsibilities between different parts of the system. Setting a structure to the system is an attempt to help define some of the boundaries and rules by which the different actors and groups within the system are expected to work together to achieve the various health aims and objectives.

Many resource-poor countries experience a fragmented health system with ineffective links

> The responsibility for implementing all child health services and programmes lies with the district.

between levels, particularly between primary and secondary levels of care. Referral systems are also poor. Often the health system is centralised and lower-level managers, staff and the community have little say in how services are provided or run. This leads to inadequate resource allocation at the service point for clients (patients), demotivated health workers, no responsibility or accountability on the part of frontline health professionals and managers – and, inevitably, poor health services.

In low-income countries, particularly in sub-Saharan Africa, the decentralisation to, and strengthening of, district health systems has been the preferred strategy for structurally changing health services. Full decentralisation of responsibility for health services to local authorities has often been viewed as an ideal for district health systems – to establish strong local accountability and to bring health services closer to the people. However, experience across Africa has not been encouraging. Health services are technically complex and local authorities often find them very difficult to manage on their own.

Infrastructural and human resource norms

Developing and applying norms and standards can assist in highlighting deficiencies, and provide a basis for advocating for increasing resources together with more rational allocation.

Human resource norms developed by individual countries often are determined by the available human capital (i.e. doctors, nurses, etc) which in turn depends on factors such as the number of new graduates produced annu-

For maternal, child and women's health services, the following is a suggested minimum set of standards and norms for service delivery:
- 1 primary care clinic per 10 000 population
- 1 community health centre per 25 000 rural population and 50 000 urban population
- 1 first level (district) hospital per 250 000 rural population and 500 000 urban population
- 1 second level (regional) hospital per 1.2 million population
- 1 third level (tertiary) hospital per 3–3.5 million population.

ally, their location, brain drain (emigration) and retirement and death. The South African Health Department has elected not to develop human resource norms for fear of being held accountable if these are lacking in a particular setting.

Child health priorities

There are many approaches to establishing health priorities within a region, country, province or district. These are intimately linked to the country's economy, gross domestic product (GDP), disease profile (e.g. contribution of communicable and non-communicable diseases) and human resources, among others. In resource-poor countries, the major diseases contributing to under-five mortality are often targeted for priority intervention.

Millennium Development Goals

The global agenda for improving children's health has been dominated in recent years by the Millennium Development Goals (MDGs). In 2000, South Africa joined other nations in adopting the MDGs. These are:
- Goal 1: Eradicate extreme poverty and hunger
- Goal 2: Achieve universal primary education
- Goal 3: Promote gender equality and empower women
- Goal 4: Reduce child mortality
- Goal 5: Improve maternal health
- Goal 6: Combat HIV/AIDS, malaria and other diseases
- Goal 7: Ensure environmental sustainability
- Goal 8: Develop a global partnership for development.

The MDGs consist of eight goals, 18 targets and 48 indicators that all members of the United Nations agreed to attempt to achieve by 2015. At least four goals are directly relevant to child health, and have specific child health targets and indicators (e.g. a two-thirds reduction in the under-five mortality rate compared to that in 1990). Regrettably, based on progress made by 2009, it is predicted that more than half of the countries (including South Africa) will fail to meet most of the goals if they continue at their current rates of progress.

Child mortality

The mortality rate is a fundamental indicator of child health. Understanding the causes of child deaths provides insight into how these could be reduced. In general, infants are much more vulnerable than children, and causes of death patterns in the different age groups are very different. Monitoring child deaths in resource-poor settings is challenging owing to under-registration of births and deaths as well as misclassification of the causes of death. Table 4.2 presents definitions of some commonly used mortality indicators. In 2007, the countries with the lowest U5MR included Sweden and Singapore (3 per 1 000), while the highest was Sierra Leone (262 per 1 000).

Overall, the ten leading causes of death in low- and middle-income countries account for over 80 per cent of all child deaths in these

> HIV/AIDS is now responsible for 7 per cent of all child deaths in sub-Saharan Africa and more than a third of young child mortality in southern African countries.

countries. Infection remains the biggest killer, accounting for more than half of all deaths in children younger than five years of age globally (*see* Figure 4.2). The single greatest contributor is lower respiratory infections. The immense surge of HIV/AIDS in recent years in southern Africa means that HIV infection is now the commonest cause of death in young children in this region. The contribution of malnutrition to child mortality is well recognised – almost 60 per cent of young child deaths in poorer settings have under-nutrition as a contributing factor.

The contribution of perinatal conditions (such as perinatal asphyxia, preterm birth and sepsis) to child mortality has been under-appreciated

Table 4.2 Commonly described mortality rates and ratios, and statistics relating to a developing country, South Africa and Sweden (2007)

Rate	Definition	Developing countries average	South Africa	Sweden
Under-5 Mortality Rate	The number of children under 5 years who die in a year, per 1 000 live births during the year	74	72	3
Infant Mortality Rate (IMR)	The number of infants (children aged less than one year) who die in a year, per 1 000 live births during that year	51	49	2
Neonatal Mortality Rate (NMR)	Number of deaths within the first 28 completed days of life, in a year, per 1 000 live births during that year	31	17	2
Perinatal Mortality Rate (PMR)	The number of stillbirths and early neonatal deaths (≤7 days of age) per 1 000 total births (live and still births)	-	35	-
Maternal Mortality Ratio (MMR)	The number of women who die as a result of childbearing, during the pregnancy or within 42 days of delivery or termination of pregnancy in one year, per 100 000 live births during that year	450	170–400	3

Source: The State of the World's Children 2009

until recently. These are responsible for a quarter of under-five deaths worldwide, and account for almost half of all deaths in young children in high-income countries. In low-income settings most deaths from these causes occur in the first few days of life.

Over the past decade, progress has been made against respiratory, diarrhoeal, and measles mortality in most low- and middle-income countries. Although deaths from accidents and injuries have decreased worldwide, and while they occur more commonly in low- and middle income countries, their substantial contribution to child mortality is most noticeable in high-income countries.

Despite the inequities of the apartheid system, there was a significant reduction in infant and child mortality rates in South Africa between 1960 and 1994, mirroring gains achieved in other middle-income countries over the same period. This trend reversed around 1994; the infant mortality rate (IMR) and the under-five mortality rate (U5MR) increased similarly with both peaking around 2001 (IMR at 63 per 1 000, U5MR at 92 per 1 000). A single disease has been largely responsible for this reversal – HIV infection (Figure 4.3). Experts agree that child mortality rates are probably declining once again based mainly on the impact of the prevention of mother-to-child transmission (PMTCT) of HIV programme. Neonatal mortality rates have

remained relatively static in South Africa over the past 30 years, again mirroring trends in most other low- and middle-income countries.

Child morbidity

Recently, the focus of public health professionals has moved beyond a concentration on mortality to the effects of morbidity and resulting disability. The disability adjusted life year (DALY) is the internationally-accepted measure of death and disability, and is increasingly cited as a powerful tool for decision-makers in international health. In sub-Saharan Africa, HIV/AIDS is responsible for the highest burden of disease (responsible for 16.5 per cent of all DALYs), followed by malaria (10.3 per cent) and lower respiratory illnesses (8.8 per cent). Five other conditions that predominantly affect children (diarrhoeal disease, perinatal conditions, measles, pertussis, and protein-energy malnutrition) also feature in the top 10. Compared with the rest of Africa, South Africa has similar DALY rates for HIV/AIDS but lower rates for other communicable, maternal, perinatal, and nutritional conditions. The burden of non-communicable diseases is increasing worldwide, accounting for nearly half the global burden of disease for all ages.

Cost-effectiveness analyses are increasingly being used to establish if money spent on an intervention results in the expected health gain

Figure 4.2 Main causes of death among children under five years, worldwide, 2001

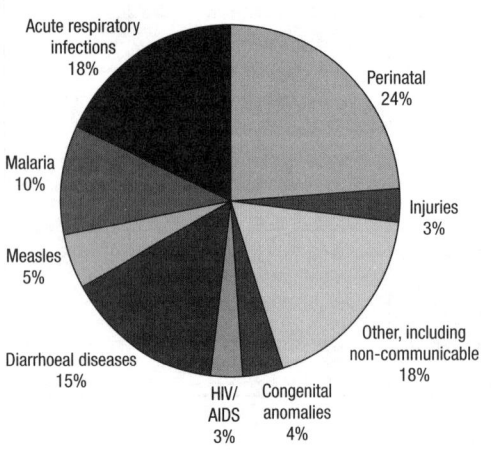

Figure 4.3 Main causes of death among children under five years, South Africa, 2000

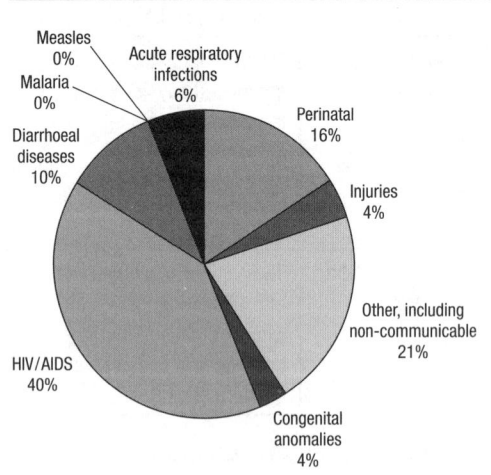

measured in natural units such as number of lives saved. One such WHO analysis of selected child health interventions found that food fortification with zinc or vitamin A was the most cost effective intervention, and that provision of supplementary food and counselling on nutrition were the least cost effective. Oral rehydration therapy, case management of pneumonia, vitamin A or zinc supplementation, and measles immunisation were ranked between these.

Priority child health interventions

In attempting to address the priority child health problems affecting its children, most countries select priority interventions to implement. The effectiveness of the intervention, feasibility, acceptability, cost effectiveness and intervention complexity (health system requirements for implementing the intervention) influences whether it is introduced or not. While some programmes or strategies are approved for national implementation, others may only be prioritised in a province, region, district or individual health centre. This is quite acceptable as the intention must be to target conditions that matter to that community. A few examples of interventions and strategies selected by the South African health system are discussed below.

Integrated Management of Childhood Illness (IMCI)

IMCI is the preferred strategy to deliver the primary level of health care to children younger than five years in developing countries. It is a WHO/UNICEF initiative that was launched globally in 1995 with the objective of reducing under-five mortality, morbidity and disability, and improving child growth and development. Its main challenge was to move from the vertical disease-specific approach of traditional programmes to a more integrated and horizontal approach, in line with the philosophy of primary health care. More than 100 countries worldwide, including South Africa, are implementing this approach on a large scale. It prioritises five conditions: pneumonia, diarrhoea, malnutrition, malaria and measles. In South Africa, the focus on the latter two conditions has been

downgraded while that on HIV and TB elevated. More than 10 000 health professionals (including medical and nursing students) have been trained to date, and all 52 districts in the country offer it (to a variable degree).

Prevention of Mother-to-Child Transmission (PMTCT) of HIV

Since HIV is the leading cause of under-five mortality in South Africa, it is not surprising that its prevention is a national priority. The key components of the PMTCT programme are voluntary counselling and testing for HIV; provision of advice on infant feeding choices; administration of combination therapy (including the use of nevirapine and zidovudine [AZT]) to pregnant women and their newborns soon after birth; provision of infant formula; and continuing counselling, education and support for mothers for 18 to 24 months.

Nutrition

An integrated nutrition programme was developed in 1994 to address children's nutritional needs at a health service, household, and community level. However, there has been limited implementation of the programme goals at a practical level. The **Baby Friendly Hospital Initiative** (BFHI) is UNICEF/WHO-led initiative to ensure that maternity hospitals and clinics provide mothers with the support necessary to encourage and establish breastfeeding. A maternity facility is designated 'baby-friendly' once it has implemented ten specific steps to support successful breastfeeding. More than 300 South African clinics and hospitals have acquired this status. **Kangaroo Mother Care** units in birthing centres ensure that preterm and low birth weight infants are offered appropriate warmth, feeding and earlier discharge. The **Primary School Nutrition Programme** provides one meal per day, comprising a snack and a drink, to over five million learners at 15 000 of the poorest schools in the country. There is evidence that this programme has promoted increased school enrolment and improved school performance by virtue of increasing alertness.

To satisfy the nutritional needs of undernourished children, three main public health strategies have been widely used. **Food diver-**

sification requires that children be exposed to a greater diversity in their diet. Diets of poor children can be both monotonous and nutritionally compromised. Food diversification programmes attempt to increase access to a variety of nutritious foods. The food vegetable garden project in Bangladesh, where over 70 per cent of households nationally now own a food garden, is the most remarkable success. **Food fortification** is highly cost-effective and requires that staple foods that are regularly consumed by children have essential or important nutrients artificially added to allow the recommended daily allowance of these nutrients to be met. In South Africa, all white and brown bread (wheat) flour and maize meal is fortified with vitamin A, thiamine, riboflavin, niacin, folic acid, vitamin B6, iron, and zinc. This allows for 10–40 per cent of the recommended dietary allowance of these nutrients to be met (for children between four and thirteen years of age consuming 100 g of flour or maize meal). All commercial salt is iodized. Finally, **food supplementation** is arguably the most effective, but difficult, alternative as it requires regular administration of micronutrients. The six-monthly vitamin A supplementation programme and daily or bi-weekly iron supplementation for preterm and low birth weight infants are the obvious examples.

Regular, **mass deworming** can be viewed as an extension of any nutritional strategy. Recognising the high worm burden present in pre- and school-aged children in poorer settings, and the negative consequences of this on growth and cognitive development in particular, regular (six monthly) administration of mebendazole or albendazole is offered to children to reduce the parasite burden.

Audit

An important component of any mortality reduction strategy is to continuously audit all deaths and identify preventable and modifiable contributors to a child's death. The **Child Health-care Problem Identification Programme** (Child PIP) is one such auditing programme, used at various hospitals in South Africa. Emerging evidence suggests that the programme has been successful in reducing the number of deaths as well as improving the quality of care delivered to children at hospitals.

Routine child health care (health promotion and prevention)

Ensuring that children develop into healthy adults requires more than access to health care services when the child falls ill. It demands that society take actions to promote healthy living and prevent disease. Much of this responsibility is trusted to the family, including what the child eats, where he/she plays, what environmental and other hazards are encountered, etc. Of pertinence to this chapter are the health service related health promotion and prevention activities.

Few health systems have successfully accomplished this, and in reality, while most of these services may be available they are provided in parallel rather than as an integrated package. Thus, the well-being of any single child depends more on the individual behaviour and idiosyncrasies of his or her caregiver and family rather than on a committed and easily accessible packaged schedule of health promoting activities.

Nevertheless, there are a number of child health promoting activities that are scheduled and universally provided and utilized. The best global example is **immunization** services. Worldwide, increased number of children are recipients of the WHO Expanded Programme on Immunization (EPI), which ensures that children are vaccinated against at least six major childhood infectious diseases. Many countries, including South Africa, have opted to expand the schedule to cover more microbes. Thus, the current South African public (EPI) immunization schedule includes ten vaccines and that in the USA, sixteen. Dramatic decreases in the incidence of vaccine-associated diseases have been achieved in the past decade – polio is close to eradication, as is neonatal tetanus elimination, with measles reduced by 75 per cent globally. However, there remains a need for

It is the intended goal of many health services to provide a comprehensive, integrated mother and child health (MCH) package in a continuum of care from pre-conception (e.g. genetic services), through antenatal care and birthing to the care of the well and the sick child.

more effective vaccines against diseases such as TB and malaria.

Growth monitoring and promotion is widely considered to be a core component of any child health promotion and prevention activity. Children are frequently weighed during routine and sick care visits to health services, and sometimes at crèches and schools as well. Despite this, the success of this strategy has been limited and frankly disappointing. The primary reason for this has been the limited capacity of health and other services to respond appropriately to growth retardation and failure by offering interventions such as nutrition counselling, community food support programmes (e.g. food gardens) and food supplementation. In practice, these are either too difficult or expensive for public services to promote and support. Consequently, growth monitoring has fallen somewhat into disrepute. Nevertheless, there are some excellent international examples of how properly implemented, community-based growth monitoring and promotion programmes can be extremely successful.

The **Road-to-Health Chart** is a very useful home-based personal child health record. Different versions are used in various countries. A new updated and improved chart is to be introduced in 2009 in South Africa. The new version is gender specific, and incorporates the new WHO growth standards and information related to the child's HIV status. Detail about the child's birth history, immunization, previous illnesses and their management, and development is also recorded.

Developmental screening of newborns, infants and young children for hearing, vision or critical developmental milestones offers an important opportunity for early intervention. Childhood disability receives low priority within resource-poor health care services despite its prevalence and significant impact on the lives of children, their caregivers and families. In well-resourced settings, such as the USA and the UK, children's development is monitored on a regular basis from birth. The preferred method for developmental monitoring in the resource-limited context is developmental screening, although this is not routinely carried out. Screening should coincide with health facility visits for immunization, caregivers should be fully involved, and screening should be linked to appropriate interventions. In South Africa, only the Western Cape has introduced this as a routine service with modest efficacy. It involves the use of standardized screening tools to screen children for moderate and severe disability when they visit the health facility for their immunizations at six weeks, nine months and eighteen months. The major obstacle has been the subsequent support services available for children identified via screening as requiring further investigation or care.

Health promoting activities for the individual child

In southern Africa it is recommended that, as a minimum, children are monitored at child health clinics during the first two years of life (*see* Table 4.3). Surveillance during this period should include a careful assessment at or soon after birth, monthly weighing in the first year of life (synchronized with the immunization schedule), two-monthly weighing in the second year of life, developmental screening at three to six months of age, six to nine months of age, and at 18 to 24 months of age. It is during these two years that child-rearing practices are established, most important preventive and promotive interventions take place, and most deviations in growth and development occur. Strategies for surveillance beyond two years will vary between different health care settings.

Community based child health care

There is increasing recognition that to achieve meaningful and sustainable improvements in child health, responsibility has to be devolved to the community and, ultimately, the household level. There are good reasons for this: ailing health systems are able to offer limited services and care and often ignore important aspects of care such as health promotion and prevention; much young child mortality is the result of inappropriate practices and delayed health seeking behaviour by caregivers; and community-based health care (CBHC) has the potential to offer an affordable, effective response to this situation.

Globally, the value of the community health promoter (worker) (CHW) is being re-

Table 4.3 Minimum child surveillance and health promotion activities during the first two years of life

Age	Growth Monitoring	Immunization	HIV	Developmental screening	Oral health	Vitamin A	Deworming	Health Promotion
Birth	Breast feeding support	BCG Oral polio						Use of Road to Health card
3–5 days	Breast feeding support							
6 weeks	Breast feeding support	OPV, DTaP-IPV/ HiB, hepatitis B, rotavirus, pneumo-coccus	PCR test Cotri-moxazole prophylaxis			50 000 IU (if not breast feeding)		
10 weeks	Breast feeding support	DTaP-IPV/HiB, Hepatitis B	PCR result and manage-ment					
14 weeks	Breast feeding support, 'weaning' and complemen-tary feeding advice	DTaP-IPV/HiB, hepatitis B, rotavirus, pneumo-coccus		Motor, Hearing, Vision				IMCI Danger Signs Oral rehydration solution preparation
6 months	'Weaning' and complemen-tary feeding advice			Yes	Yes	100 000 U		
9 months		measles pneumo-coccus		Yes		100 000 IU if not given in past 6 months		
12 months					Yes	200 000 IU	Yes	
18 months		DTaP-IPV/ HiB, measles	HIV Elisa			200 000 IU	Yes	
24 months (and 6-monthly thereafter till age 5 years)	Yes			Yes	Yes	200 000 IU	Yes	

appreciated and there is increasing evidence of the contribution they can make to improved child health. Usually, local women trained in basic health care serve this role. The best example is the role of the *arogyadut* (CHW) in managing neonatal sepsis in Maharashtra, India. Their ability to provide simple home-based newborn care reduced neonatal mortality by almost two-thirds and the incidence of neonatal illnesses by half. In Malawi CHWs assist in the earlier identification of malnourished children and supervise their rehabilitation at home when appropriate, while in Tanzania malaria eradication efforts such as home spraying and insecticide-impregnated net distribution is led by CHWs.

In South Africa, the role of the CHW has been poorly defined, with some being employed by the health service, others being paid by non-governmental organisations and many serving as unpaid volunteers. The majority of their effort has been directed at AIDS-related home-based care. A re-definition of their responsibility and training to address child health needs is needed. Likely areas of activity would include support for breastfeeding and good infant feeding practices at home, health promotion (e.g. use of oral rehydration therapy, immunization or injury prevention), counselling of caregivers on managing common child complaints, prescribing treatment for simple problems, and the identification of illnesses or conditions (such as a disability) warranting health centre intervention and facilitating the child's access to the service. They also offer the best possibility of a MCH package of services being implemented, i.e. care and support would be extended consistently to the pregnant mother and the new child subsequently.

CBHC is not the prerogative of community health workers only. Doctors and nurses need to regard the entire community they live and work in as their responsibility, not just those members (patients) who visit the health facilities. All health professionals need to be familiar with the principles and practice of CBHC while embracing a comprehensive approach to health care. CHBC cannot rely solely on staff with limited training and staff. Experienced and skilled managers, trainers and supervisors (often health professionals based at clinics and hospitals) are required to ensure that even basic community health programmes are effectively delivered.

Community participation is a vital component of CBHC. The needs and priorities of communities themselves need to be understood, and new interventions should obtain their support. Lack of consultation and consensus can result in wasted opportunities, frustration and ultimately failure. This does not imply that the community members are considered health experts, but their input can be critical for success.

Intersectoral collaboration

Intersectoral collaboration can be vital to achieving health goals. Intersectoral collaboration means that one sector, such as health, works with other sectors that influence child health, such as education, social development, justice and agriculture to achieve health outcomes in a way that is more effective, efficient or sustainable than could be achieved by the health sector acting alone. In its narrowest application the health sector will use other sectors to achieve health objectives, e.g. reducing the incidence or consequences of diarrhoea, malnutrition or child abuse. More appropriate would be for the different sectors to develop common objectives that mutually benefit all the sectors. Intersectoral action can occur at the global, sub-regional, national, sub-national and community levels. Political and civil society actors are often the key drivers of intersectoral action.

Intersectoral action has been used to address a wide range of health and socio-economic public policy challenges, including action on specific determinant(s) of health, populations, communities, diseases and health behaviours, health equity and risk factors. While a range of approaches have been used, at different levels of governance, there does not appear to be a 'one size fits all' model.

Two examples of the intersectoral approach are offered. At a global level, the Healthy Environments for Children Alliance facilitates intersectoral work on issues related to children's health and the environment. A few countries, such as New Zealand, have used the intersectoral approach to strengthen families, use collaborative case management, offer social workers in schools, provide family service centres, and to offer comprehensive services for children experiencing emotional, mental, and behavioural disturbances, and/or for children with multiple difficulties and needs. There are fewer good examplars of intersectoral collaboration in resource-poor settings. Nevertheless, Early Childhood Development (ECD) is an example of a programme being implemented in South Africa. Key government departments in the delivery of ECD services are Social Development, Education and Health. ECD sites or places of care include crèches, playgroups, after-school centres or a combination of the three.

Child health advocacy

An important, but underappreciated, role of any health professional dealing with children is to be a child health advocate. Advocacy is defined in the *South African Concise Oxford Dictionary* as 'the act of pleading for, defending, publicly supporting or recommending a cause.' Basically, advocacy is taking action to improve an existing situation.

The 1989 UN Convention on the Rights of the Child eloquently expresses many of the basic rights that every child is entitled to such as the right to a name, nationality, food, shelter or health. Many subsequent documents, such as the *Declaration on the Rights and Welfare of the African Child*, echo similar sentiments. The real challenge is to translate these 'pretty words' into action.

Opportunities for child health advocacy abound in every child health professional's daily life. Although the realisation of the right of access to antiretroviral prophylaxis for South African newborn infants required a Constitutional Court order (following an application by the Treatment Action Campaign and over 250 doctors and other health professionals), most advocacy efforts require action closer to home. Examples of such actions include a campaign to ensure that all sick newborns were adequately clothed while in incubators, improving pain management guidelines in children's wards, ensuring ongoing nutritional support for malnourished children on discharge, or simplifying the birth certificate acquisition process for children. All of these are real examples of activities recently undertaken by health and allied professionals in various settings. The message is clear; even minor advocacy efforts can result in substantial improvements.

5   Social paediatrics

The human infant is is, at birth, totally dependent on his mother and family for his immediate and long-term survival. Through a process of growth and development he attains varying degrees of independence until he is able to survive alone. The success of such growth and development is dependent not only on the inherent abilities of the individual but also on the nature of the physical and social environment in which he is nurtured. Social paediatrics is concerned with the social environment in which the infant or child is nurtured; with the consequences of both a normal and an abnormal social environment on the overall development and wellbeing of the child; and with strategies to maintain optimal family function and to protect children in abnormal or difficult social circumstances

The social environment

The social environment around any individual child is made up of four interacting systems:
- The most immediate environment of the mother's womb and subsequent care impinging directly on the senses of the fetus, neonate, and infant
- The family and home and the patterns of interaction between family members, parents and child
- Other settings in which the infant and child spends extended periods of time and which significantly influence development, e.g. day care, peer group, pre-schools and schools
- The environment provided by the local community and the wider world, including the political, social, and cultural influences that impinge directly or indirectly on children through their impact on the family and its members.

> The physical environment has its primary impact on physical health, while the social environment has the greatest impact on the child's psychological, emotional, and educational well-being.

The child's social environment is defined by the make-up of each of these components and the relationships between them.

The child. Every child has his own individual characteristics which reflect a sum of genetic, familial, and environmental factors. The overall growth, development, and wellbeing of each child is dependent on the balance between these positive and negative characteristics.

The family. The family is the single most important social environment capable of shaping and influencing the health and development of the child. Common genetic and familial factors and shared physical, social, and emotional environments often produce striking resemblances between children within a family unit. Physical wellbeing is determined by the physical environment of the home, and the health-risk behaviour and health-seeking practices of the parents. Emotional health is related to parental sensitivity to their children's needs, their expectations of their children, and the degree and

The classical, cultural definition of a family is based on kinship ties, but from a functional point of view, a family may be defined as any group of people living together, or in close proximity, who provide mutual care, support, and guidance.

quality of affective support children receive from their families. The ability to develop and maintain social relationships and to take on specific roles within a family or social unit are learnt by children from their experience of relationships within their own families or households.

This alternative definition is important, since the traditional extended family or the more isolated nuclear family are no longer the predominant family structures in South Africa or in many other developing countries. Single-parent families, multi-generation female-headed households, multiple family structures, and complex households are now more common than both nuclear and extended family households, and child-headed households are an increasing phenomenon throughout sub-Saharan Africa.

Whatever the composition of the household, the responsibilities of the family unit towards its children remains the same. These can be grouped into two broad categories:

- Material support and supervision — including the provision of food, clothing, shelter, safety, supervision, hygiene, health care, and education.
- Affective functions — including the provision of love, companionship, social support, socialization, and teaching coping and life skills.

The ability of parents to fulfil these roles is dependent on their standard of education, childhood and adult experiences, and innate and accessible resources, as well as on the level of support that they in turn receive from their immediate community.

The community. This macro-environment has an indirect impact on the child that is exerted through its influence on the family unit. Such influence, on both the child and the family unit, may be either negative or positive, depending on the nature of the community and its role as a source of stress or support.

The relationship between the family and the community is dependent on the tangible, such as child care, and recreational and healthcare facilities in the community, as well as the intangible, such as the attitudes, beliefs, and practices of the community. Those communities rich in resources are more likely to provide an adequate social network for families. Well-supported parents are, in turn, more able to fulfil their responsibilities towards their children.

Family functioning

A functioning or well-adapted family is one that has developed both the resources and coping mechanisms to deal effectively with the ordinary and extraordinary demands and stresses with which it is regularly faced (*see* Figure 5.1).

By achieving a balance between demands and capabilities, a family can minimize or eliminate the negative consequeces of stress and tension, and allow the children, other family members, and the family as a whole to thrive. Both the demands placed on a family and the capabilities available to the family to meet these demands can arise from the individual child, the family, or the community.

Demands. These demands may be acute, well-defined, single events over a discrete time period (stressors); chronic, vague, poorly defined circumstances which wax and wane in intensity (strains); or seemingly innocuous events of daily living (hassles). Table 5.1 provides a few examples of such stressors, strains, and hassles.

Capabilities. The capability of a family to meet these demands is dependent on the resources available to and the coping mechanisms of that family. Resources are the characteristics or competencies of an individual, the family, or the social system of a community, and may be tangible (e.g. money) or intangible (e.g. self-esteem) (*see* Table 5.2).

Coping mechanisms include the behavioural response of a family to stress. These activities may focus on reducing family demands, increasing family resources, maintaining or re-allocating resources, managing personal tension, or re-defining attitudes towards a problem.

The sequelae of an imbalance between the demands on family and its capabilities are stress, family malfunctioning, and, frequently, family breakdown. These in turn lead to increased levels

Table 5.1 Stressors, strains, and hassles

	Stressors	Strains	Hassles
Individual	Parent retrenched School closes Acute illness	Chronic illness Work deadlines Alcoholism	Loss of personal item Temper tantrum
Family	Divorce Family death	Poverty Large family size Marital conflict	Conflicting schedules Electricity cut off
Community	Natural disaster Poor services Lack of transport	Violence	

Table 5.2 Resources

Individual resources	Family resources	Community resources
Self-esteem Parent education Practical skills Sense of humour Empathy	Family income Parenting skills Adequate housing Communication skills Family size	Health services Friends Safe neighbourhood Recreational facilities Social services

Figure 5.1 Factors affecting family functioning

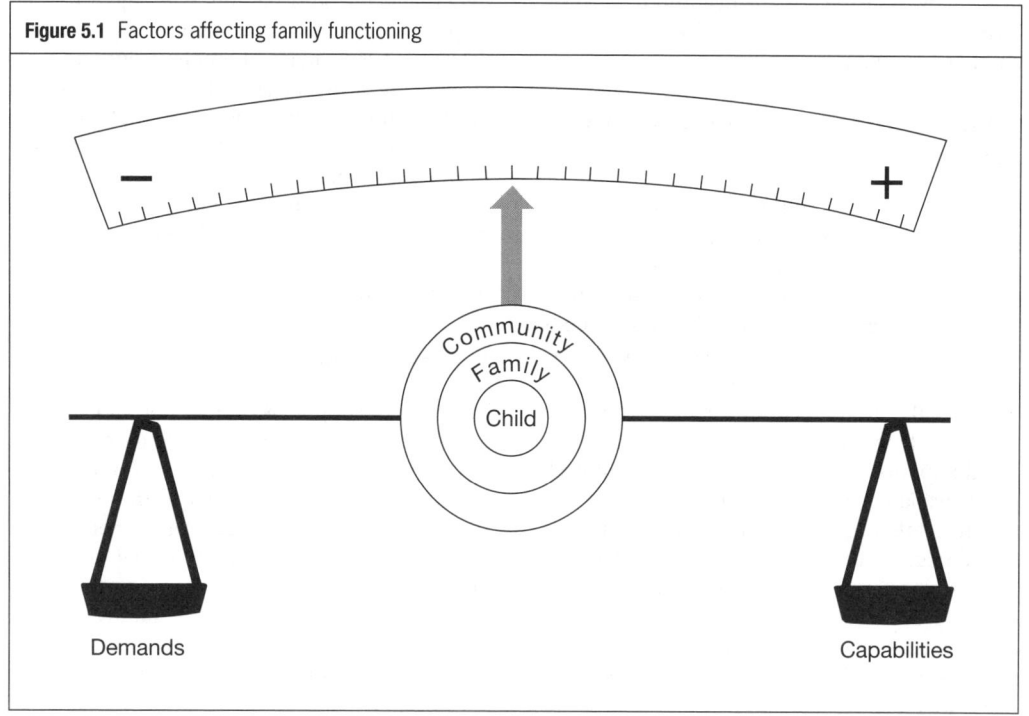

of physical illness, psychological symptoms, disruptive and destructive behaviour, depression, anxiety, and social and academic difficulties among individual members. The total breakdown of family function produces a category of children in especially difficult circumstances.

For the majority of South African families the greatest challenge is to survive the adversity arising from poverty. Close to 45 per cent of the population live below the minimum living level and just over 15 per cent live as informal settlers in impoverished, overcrowded, and dangerous settlements that lack basic services, such as electricity, water, and sanitation, and with inadequate health and education facilities and social support structures. Children living in such environments are at high risk for political, criminal, and family violence, as well as pervasive social and educational problems.

Families growing up under such circumstances not only experience a greater variety and intensity of demands, but simultaneously lack both the family and community capabilities of responding to them. The net result is increased perinatal morbidity, a higher prevalence of handicap, more childhood deaths, more child abuse, higher maternal mortality, and more children living in surrogate care. In addition, poverty is the single most powerful negative influence on child development.

Children's needs and social security networks

On a daily basis the ultimate responsibility for meeting a child's needs lies with the parents. This may be achieved alone or with the assistance of family members, friends, or various structures within the local community. The basic needs of all children can be categorized in the following way.

Physical. The physical needs of children are usually fully met by the parents. Apart from the Child Support Grant, a poverty alleviation cash grant available in South Africa to reduce the negative influence on children living in poor households, little alternative aid is available from state structures for those parents who cannot provide for their children's needs. Assistance is thus usually sought from the family network or local community. These physical needs include:

- Food
- Clothing
- Shelter
- Supervision
- Safety
- Health care.

Emotional. Emotional needs are best met by the parents and family, with limited input from additional caregivers. These emotional needs include:

- Security
- Love and affection
- Companionship.

Social and cognitive. Although social needs can only be fully met through interaction with peers and the broader community, many specific social skills and the basic patterns of socialization are learnt from within the household. These include:

- Socialization and peer interaction
- Coping skills
- Life skills.

The reality of family life in South Africa is that many households have a single parent and in those with two parents financial survival is often dependent on both parents working. The dual responsibilities of single parents and working mothers to their place of employment and their family may have a negative impact on their own physical, mental, and emotional wellbeing and, consequently, on the functioning of the family, in which they play a pivotal role. Under such circumstances the parent or parents are unable to meet all the needs of their children and various social networks need to be established or mobilized to assist.

Day care at home

This type of support is often found in extended families and in multiple-generation or multiple-family households. Pooling financial and human resources increases the capacity of the household to meet most of the children's basic needs.

In families with adequate financial resources, additional options include care of the child within the home by an employed nanny or babysitter. The advantages of such an arrangement are primarily the familiarity of the environment and the caregiver to the child. Disadvantages include difficulties in finding a suitable caregiver, the lack of back-up should the caregiver be absent, the lack of adequate supervision of the caregiver, and the lack of suitable peer group interaction for the child.

A particularly important problem experienced with household support networks, especially in rural and peri-urban communities, is the reliance placed on the elderly. They are often expected to contribute to the financial needs and daily running of the household and to fulfil a child-care role for numerous grandchildren. However willing they may be, their physical capabilities seldom allow them to act as effective caregivers for active toddlers and pre-school children.

Day care outside the home

In the absence of adequate support at home, assistance is required from the broader community. The commoner forms of community-based support include:

- Play groups
- Family day care
- Centre-based child care, consisting of a day-care centre, crèche, or pre-school.

These day-care options are found as formal and informal structures in most communities. Formal structures are those with more than six children, and that have registered with the Department of Welfare, the Department of Education, or with a local authority. In order to be registered these facilities need to conform to certain requirements with respect to their physical facilities, child-to-staff ratios, and staff training. Facilities catering for six or more children for a full day are registered with the Department of Welfare as crèches, and those caring for six or more children for a half day are registered with the Department of Education as pre-schools.

These formal facilities provide safe care and some degree of supervision for the child, and provide the opportunity for peer group interaction, socialization, stimulation, and skills training. The main drawbacks are their inability to address the individual needs of each child, the increased exposure to illnesses and, for working mothers, the lack of flexibility in the hours. Nevertheless, good-quality child care, characterized by small group size, low child-to-staff ratios, and training of the child caregivers,

is associated with improved social development by the child and so provides an acceptable alternative to home care.

The informal structures function outside the control or supervision of state structures and do not necessarily adhere to the various statutory requirements. They are being rapidly established in urban and peri-urban informal settlements, primarily as a response to the urgent need of working mothers for child care, but also as a channel for subsidized feeding in needy communities. They are also being seen by growing numbers of parents from disadvantaged communities as an opportunity for early education that will give their children access to good schools. They provide health authorities with a convenient way of reaching children between the ages of two and five years for health promotion activities.

Surrogate and alternative care

It is estimated that at least 20 per cent of children in this country do not live with their mothers. One-third of these children have been orphaned, one-tenth have been abandoned, and the rest have been placed in some form of alternative care because the mothers are unable, for some reason or another, to take care of the children themselves. These reasons include the mother's remarriage, her return to school, her need to live in at her place of employment, or her lack of resources. An additional unspecified number of children live with their mothers but under unsuitable and especially difficult circumstances. Surprisingly few of these children ever present to the formal health or welfare services for care or support. The vast majority are absorbed into the informal support networks in their communities. The mainstay of this support structure is the already overstretched extended family and, outside of the home, family friends, women's groups, and religious communities, which not only support but frequently replace the fragile extended family.

In the formal welfare sector the Children's Act makes statutory provision for children in need of care, who are defined as children without parents or guardians, or whose parents or guardians are considered unable or unfit to care for them adequately. The Act regulates the placement of such children into surrogate care. At present, four forms of surrogate or alternative care exist

– adoption, foster care, residential care, or a place of safety – and steps are in place for the development of places of secure care for children and youth in conflict with the law. Within each of these categories the Act caters for various models that recognize the need for surrogate care as well as the limited resources of both the state and most communities. These variations include leaving children in existing circumstance subject to suitable external supervision and support, shared care and cluster foster care.

Adoption

This is the legal procedure by which a child becomes the lawful child of a person or couple other than the biological parents. Such a step secures the permanent placement of the child in a family environment where it is hoped that the child will attain his or her full potential. Children suitable for adoption are those who have been orphaned or abandoned, those whose parents are unable to care for them effectively, or those whose parents wish, for various reasons, to give up all legal claim and responsibility for them.

Any adult is eligible to adopt a child as long as he or she has been screened by a social worker and found to be physically fit, reputable, and capable of maintaining and educating the child. In South Africa social workers are no longer bound by law to limit the placement of children to families of the same race or religious affiliation.

In all adoptions, consent has to be obtained from the natural parents of the child, from the child if he or she is over 10 years of age, and from the adopters. Exceptions to this requirement occur when the natural parents have died, have abandoned the child, are mentally incompetent to give consent, or have mistreated their child.

Adoptions may only be rescinded within two years of the placement and under the following circumstances: if the natural parent did not consent to the adoption; if the adopting parent was fraudulently induced to adopt the child; or if the child has a mental or physical problem, present at the time of adoption, which was not disclosed to the adopting parents.

Foster care and places of safety

Both foster care and places of safety are intended to act as temporary placements to protect children in need while steps are taken to improve their home circumstances.

Following investigation of such a child's circumstances by the police or a social worker, a Children's Court Inquiry is held to arrange for the appropriate care of the child. Pending completion of the investigation and the holding of a Children's Court Inquiry a child in need will be kept in a place of safety for a period of 14 days.

The outcome of such an inquiry might be to return the child to the care of his or her parent conditionally under the supervision of a social worker; to place the child into foster care under the supervision of a social worker; or to place the child into the care of a children's home. Parents whose children have been removed from their care lose custody of their children but retain their guardianship rights. From a medical perspective this means that their consent is still required for medical or surgical procedures.

Foster care entails the placement of a child in need into the care of a temporary parent or parents under the supervision of a social worker for up to two years at a time. This period may be extended by a commissioner of child welfare, following a Children's Court Inquiry, until such time as the child's home circumstances permit his or her return or the child turns 18.

Children in places of safety and foster care experience a number of problems. Since the majority of them come from homes where their parents were unable or unfit to adequately care for them, their physical, mental, and social well-being is poor and they demonstrate numerous physical, intellectual, and behavioural problems. Furthermore, they are frequently moved from one foster home or place of safety to another and during their period in care, despite the supervision of social workers, they are vulnerable to neglect, abuse, and exploitation.

Children's homes

Children's homes provide surrogate care in a residential facility. Although they provide a more permanent setting for the care of children than either foster care or a place of safety, they fulfil the same purpose and remain a temporary measure while a more permanent solution, such as improved home circumstances or adoption are explored.

In terms of the Children's Act all children's homes, both state and private, have to fulfil certain requirements with respect to their management, staff, and structure and must be registered with the Department of Welfare.

Legislative framework and social security provisions

A number of international conventions and charters have established the context within which individual nations can create a legal framework for the normal development, well-being and protection of their children. Two of these are of significance in South Africa:

- The United Nations Convention on the Rights of the Child, which was adopted in September 1990 and ratified by South Africa in June 1995. This convention includes a preamble and 54 articles. The preamble reaffirms the fact that children need special care, including legal and other protections before birth and throughout childhood. It places special emphasis on the role of the family in caring for children and the cultural values of a child's community. The convention defines a child as any person under 18 years of age and sets out a wide range of political, civil, cultural, economic and social rights. Provision is also made for the implementation of the convention.
- The Organization of African Unity (OAU) has developed an African Charter on the Rights and Welfare of the Child to better reflect African cultural concerns and to address other relevant issues not addressed in the UN Convention on the Rights of the Child. Although South Africa signed it in October 1997, this Charter is not yet in operation. It makes provision for protection against harmful social and cultural practices; children of imprisoned mothers; the responsibilties of the child to his or her family and the community at large; and education and armed conflict. It therefore addresses issues such as female circumcision, child soldiers, literacy, and the role of the family in adoption.

In line with these two international documents, the South African Constitution also recognizes that children require additional protection. Section 28 focuses on children and their various rights, specifically to a name and nationality from birth; to family or parental care or to appro-

priate alternative care when removed from the family environment; to basic nutrition, shelter, health care services and social services; to be protected from maltreatment, neglect, abuse or degradation; to be protected from exploitative labour practices; not to be detained except as a measure of last resort; and not to be used directly in armed conflict and to be protected in times of armed conflict. The most significant statute affecting children is the Children's Act, 2005 and the Children's Amendment Act, 2007. This new children's statute has broadened the scope of previous legislation to cover aspects such as parental roles and responsibilities, children in need of special protection, the age of majority, surrogacy, artificial insemination, prevention and early intervention, early childhood development, partial care, the health rights of children, and the rights of children as consumers.

The principles underpinning the new children's statute include the following objectives:

- To make provision for structures, services and means for promoting the sound physical, mental, emotional and social development of children.
- To utilize, strengthen and develop community structures that provide care and protection for children.
- To prevent, as far as possible, any ill-treatment, abuse, neglect, deprivation and exploitation of children.
- To provide care and protection for children who are suffering ill-treatment, abuse, neglect, deprivation or exploitation or who are otherwise in need of care and protection.
- Generally to promote the wellbeing of children.

Apart from the Children's Act, South Africa has a variety of statutes which, although not specifically focused on children, have an impact on their wellbeing. Some, like the Age of Majority Act, define the capacities of children at different ages. Others deal with particular services and rights that affect children (the National Health Act, 2007 and the Schools Act), or the family and care givers (the Marriage Act, the Mediation in Certain Divorce Matters Act,1987 and the Prevention of Domestic Violence Act, 1998).

In addition to the above legal framework, South Africa has a social security network to promote the family unit or to support children whose well-being is threatened. This network makes provision for support in two layers. The first layer is a general response focusing on poverty alleviation, while the second focuses more specifically on children with special needs. Apart from the development of communities, through establishing appropriate infrastructure and services, and job creation activities, poverty alleviation includes direct monetary transfers such as old age pensions, social relief and the Child Support Grant (CSG). The second layer of social security provision consists of two grants – the Foster Care Grant for children in surrogate care and the Care Dependency Grant for children with disabilities. Available security benefits for children include the following:

+ Social relief is a grant paid by the Department of Social Welfare and Development or the local Magistrates Court to persons who have absolutely no money and who would not survive without immediate help. It is issued for three months only in the form of either money or food.
+ The Child Support Grant is a poverty alleviation measure aimed at children. The primary caretaker of any child under the age of fourteen is eligible for the grant provided they live in a household with a total monthly income below the prevailing means test.
+ The Foster Care Grant is provided to the foster parent or parents of a child who has been placed in their custody in terms of a court order because their parents are unable to care for them or they have been abandoned or orphaned.
+ The Care Dependency Grant is paid to the parents of any severely handicapped child between the ages of one and eighteen years who pass a means test.

Affordable models of community care

The social conditions in many communities in southern Africa, which include rapid urbanization, high levels of unemployment, poverty and violence, and the escalating HIV/AIDS epidemic, have seriously undermined the social structure of all communities, the status of the family, and the wellbeing of children. Over the next decade these factors will produce an increasing population of children whose families will be unable to care adequately for them. There seems little prospect that state social security services will have the capacity to address the increasing needs of these children or their families. It is therefore essential that new models of social security are developed that spread the burden and responsibility of social security more widely between the public, private, and non-governmental sectors. Within the public sector greater collaboration is needed vertically, between the three levels of government and, at each level, between state departments, such as health, welfare, education, and public works (see Figure 5.2).

The state, through its Department of Social Development, has moved away from its traditional role of providing direct aid to a few fortunate individuals to a service model that focuses on facilitating the development of communities, thereby increasing their capacity to care for their own members. The state is to be responsible for developing the policy framework within which models of care can be developed and for the provision of financial or material aid to impoverished communities. Representatives of state welfare structures at district level need to work closely with and fund non-governmental service organizations and community-based organizations involved in training, social support, and delivery of care to needy communities, families, or individuals. They also need to enlist the support of private and international donors to finance these district-based activities. These resources must be used to identify and strengthen existing informal models of care and to develop new, innovative alternative models of care in consultation with the recipient communities.

At the district level specific emphasis must be placed on the development of community-based structures, such as child-care facilities and alternative residential care models. Central to such models is the concept of community child-care committees responsible for the monitoring and supervision of children in need or in especially difficult circumstances. The activities of these committees should include the creation of home-visiting networks for the early detection of high-risk families and children; the regular supervision of child-headed households by community volunteers; the running of community homes; the supervision of group rather than family foster care; and the implementation of various community rehabilitation services for the care and support of children with special needs.

Incentives need to be offered to families that care for children in need, such as eligibility for reduced municipal service charges, and provision of free education to both the children in need and the other children living in that household.

By shifting the responsibility for the care of children down to the community level while simultaneously supporting the community in the development of appropriate resources, there will be an increased likelihood of establishing sustainable, alternative models of care for this country's children which are both affordable and acceptable to communities.

Children with special needs

Children with mental or physical disabilities, learning disorders, or emotional and behavioural problems, invariably require greater physical care and supervision than average children.

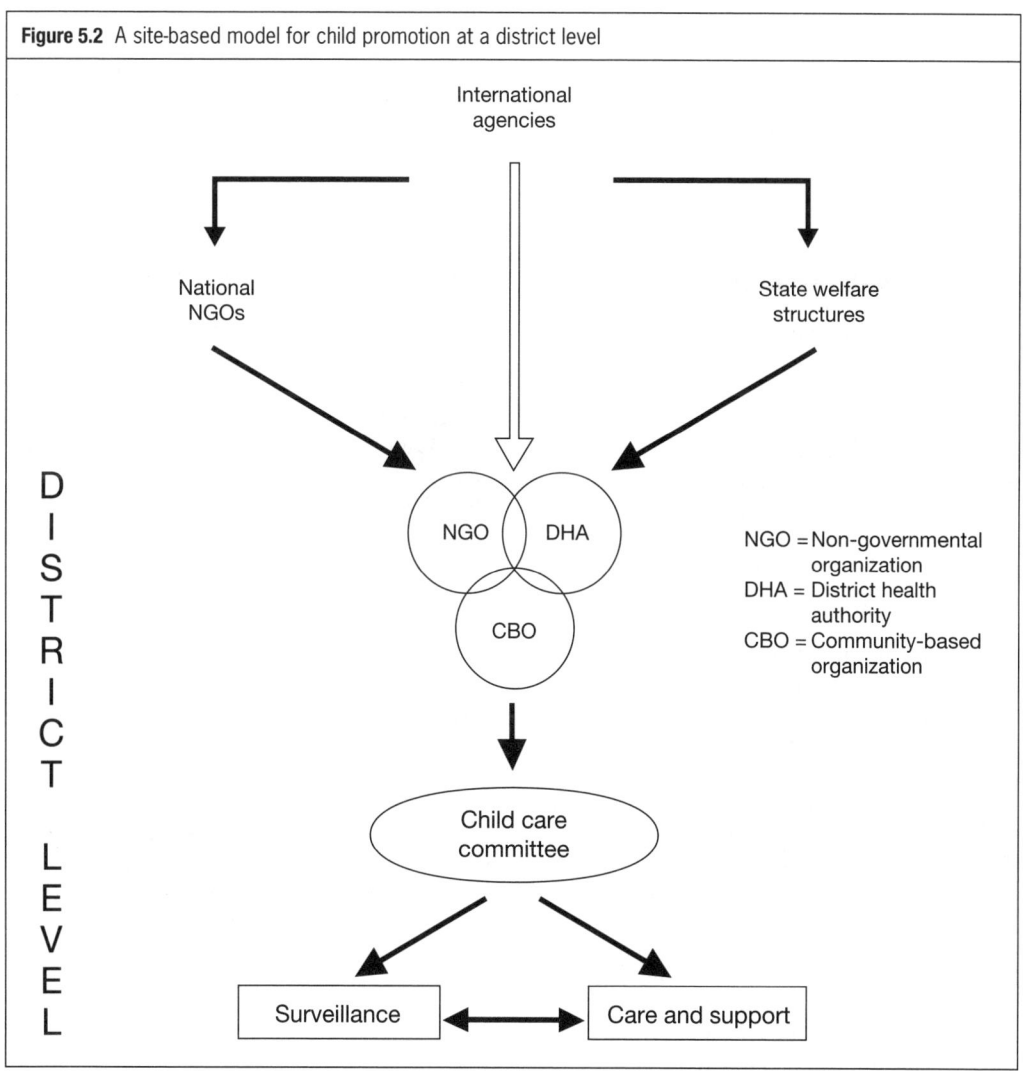

Figure 5.2 A site-based model for child promotion at a district level

Both they and their families need greater emotional and social support. These increased needs result in increased financial, physical, and social demands on the family.

To cope effectively with the increased demands associated with children with special needs, their families have to develop additional resources and coping skills. While many of these may be found within the immediate family or household, a supportive extended family and community network is usually required. Such networks include family friends, church groups, and support groups for specific problems, such as the Down's Syndrome Association, Cripple Care, and the Mental Health Society.

Limited state support is available for some children with special needs. This includes financial support in the form of a Care Dependency Grant for the needy families of mentally handicapped children, remedial classes in normal schools, special schools for various categories of handicapped children, training centres, and special residential care facilities.

The child with disabilities

The World Health Organization (WHO) makes a distinction between an *impairment*, which describes a pathological process such as spina bifida; a *disability*, which is the consequence of that impairment (e.g. someone who is unable to walk because of the paraplegia associated with spina bifida); and a *handicap*, which is the social consequence of impairment or disability (the way an individual responds to his or her impairment or disability). A person with an amputated arm who has adapted positively to a prosthesis may have a significant disability but be minimally handicapped. The WHO classification on which this categorization is based has recently been superceded by the International Classification of Functioning, Disability and Health, which places a much greater emphasis on the environment and its role in limiting the child's activities and restricting his or her full participation in society. This social model of disability argues against the previously dominant view that disability is a problem of the person, directly caused by a health condition, which requires medical care provided in the form of individual treatment by professionals. It rather views disability as a socially constructed problem requiring active

> Disability is the consequence of both a health condition that affects the individual, and of stigmatization and isolation of that individual by society as a result of their condition.

steps to combat stigma and to fully integrate children into society. What is ideally required is a systemic view that combines so-called medical and social models of childhood disability.

It has been estimated that 85 per cent of the world's disabled children under 15 years of age live in developing countries. However, services and programmes for these children are seldom a priority in these countries since services in general are undeveloped, health professionals are few in number, and more common conditions with high fatality rates are given greater prominence.

In an average community, approximately 8 per cent of children under the age of 10 years will suffer from some form of disability or another, but this figure may be higher in some disadvantaged communities. Among these children the largest group will be mentally handicapped as a result of both genetic and environmental factors (*see* Table 5.3).

The next largest group will be the physically handicapped, with conditions such as cerebral palsy, neural tube defects, and neuro-muscular disorders. The sensory handicaps – visual or hearing problems – are less common. Categories of handicap may overlap and a child may be mentally retarded, have cerebral palsy, a visual handicap, and also have behaviour problems.

Table 5.3 Estimated prevalence of common handicap

Number per 1 000	Handicap
70	Behavioural problems
20–30	Mental handicap (mild)
3–4	Mental handicap (severe)
2–2.5	Cerebral palsy
2	Deafness
1	Spina bifida
1	Speech problems
0.5	Blindness

In handicapped children an exact diagnosis with a clearly defined natural history and predictable outcome is the exception rather than the rule. The majority present with functional disturbances that vary widely in cause, severity, and clinical picture. Assessments therefore deal with two sets of questions – those that deal with diagnosis and establishment of a cause and those that are concerned with determining the child's functional disabilities. Both have an important bearing on the management plan. This distinction is important, especially for parents, who often have a great need to understand the reason for the handicap as they struggle to come to terms with their child's condition.

In providing care for handicapped children and their families the needs described below should ideally be addressed.

Early identification of the handicap. Early recognition of the handicap will increase the likelihood of effective treatment and amelioration of the handicap; will improve our understanding of causation; and will boost the confidence of the parents in the health professional and thereby improve the effectiveness of counselling.

Diagnosis. Although exact diagnoses are often elusive, an attempt should be made to use available diagnostic techniques to reach a diagnosis, since this may influence the risk of recurrence and the content of counselling.

Assessment. In planning a programme for a handicapped child, knowledge of his or her level of functioning is essential. Assessment is age-related and will need to be repeated periodically. This level of functioning should be reviewed in accepted categories, namely gross and fine motor functioning; vision; hearing; speech and language; perceptual and intellectual functioning; and emotional and social development. This assessment requires the skills of a number of health professionals, integrated to produce a global impression of the child.

Immediate advice and counselling. The parents' first need is for counselling as they cope with their stress and grief about the child's condition and, thereafter, for practical advice about how to deal with the child. They will need to understand that this child, like other children, has different needs at different ages but that these will often occur later than in a child who is not handicapped. In the early years, the child will need to attain daily living skills such as feeding and continence, to achieve mobility, and to acquire language. A programme must be followed to assist the child to achieve his or her maximum potential but the goals of this programme will need to be revised regularly.

Management programme. The aim of an ongoing management programme is to prevent or ameliorate secondary problems as far as possible. Certain problems, such as hip dislocation in cerebral palsy, may be anticipated and avoided by appropriate positioning and handling. Assistance with posture and mobility can be provided by occupational therapists and physiotherapists. Needs will change with age: the most important needs for the school-going child may be management of a learning disorder and for a child in high school, preparation for open employment.

Caregivers must specifically look for associated problems or disabilities that may be treatable, such as epilepsy, urinary tract infections, and visual acuity problems.

Advice about child-rearing. Parents of children with disabilities often find it hard to believe that there are difficulties in rearing normal children and attribute all their problems to the child's disability. They should be encouraged to see their children as going through developmental phases and encountering difficulties and frustrations in the same way as children without disabilities. The family should have access to the normal forms of support as well as the special support that may be needed because of the disability. Depending on the degree of disability, the child may be admitted to an ordinary school or to a special school for the physically handicapped.

Periodic reassessment. The clinical picture and the pattern of functional development are often unpredictable and therefore reassessment at periodic intervals is advisable. Timing may need to be adjusted to the emergent needs of the child but, at a minimum, assessments should occur at four to five years before entering school, at nine to ten years in anticipation of puberty, and at thirteen to fourteen years to assess post-school needs.

Reassessment may not only involve the needs of the child but of the whole family. Important events in the family, such as the birth of a child, a change in employment, marital problems, and the health problems of other family members may affect the status and care of the handicapped child and may require social interventions.

Community-based disability programmes

Many developed countries have multi-profes-sional teams at community level to provide support and care for disabled children and their families. This model links a team of disability professionals with child-care staff, teachers, and parents at medical and educational facilities. This arrangement coordinates a range of activities for children with handicaps that include assessment, training, surveillance, and research.

In developing countries simpler strategies, requiring fewer resources and involving com-munity members, have been promoted. This approach, referred to as community-based reha-bilitation (CBR), takes different forms in different locations, but generally requires the re-orienta-tion of services for the disabled away from insti-tutional care to a community-based approach. In this scheme professionals share their skills with disabled people, community workers, and parents. This attempts to address a number of difficulties that have arisen from the application of Western models based largely on institutional care. The most important of these difficulties are that these services reach only 5 per cent of dis-abled children and cause serious problems with the re-integration of disabled children into their communities.

Children and the HIV/AIDS epidemic

The socio-economic consequences of the HIV/AIDS epidemic have their greatest impact at the household level, leading to a marked increase in the vulnerability of children living in affected communities. Three categories can be defined within the relationship between children and the HIV/AIDS epidemic:

- HIV-infected children (discussed in greater detail in Chapter 18, HIV infection)
- Children living in an HIV-infected household – orphans and vulnerable children
- Children of uninfected households living in an affected society.

The true magnitude of orphaned and vulnerable children is hard to quantify. In the few sub-Saharan African studies that have been done some common observations have emerged:

- The peak national HIV seroprevalence among pregnant women should stabilize between 25 and 30 per cent five to ten years into the epidemic.
- The number of orphaned children will peak 10 to 15 years after the HIV seroprevalence peaks and then level out at a slightly lower plateau.
- The more rapid the progression from HIV to AIDS, the earlier the peak and the lower the plateau.
- Twenty years into the epidemic over 25 per cent of all children will have lost their mothers and will be maternal orphans.
- The mean age of children orphaned by AIDS is at least two years younger than children orphaned by other causes.

Effective antiretroviral programmes have the potential to reduce the number of orphaned children by up to a third of predicted figures.

During the early stages of HIV infection most adults are well and able to fulfil all their rou-tine family, social and economic obligations. As they become increasingly ill, their productiv-ity decreases at the same time as their personal need for physical and psychological support and health care increases. This frequently neces-sitates the restructuring of the household func-tioning and allocation of responsibilities with a significant impact on the children.

Prior to the death of their parents all children in the household begin to take on more and more of the adult household responsibilities. The older children frequently leave school to reduce household expenditure and work to supplement the household income or stay at home to care for their sick parent(s) or younger siblings. In order to generate income older, rural children may migrate to urban centres in search of work and frequently lose all contact with their homes as they merge with other children living on the city streets. The net effect on the children is a significant degree of physical and psychological trauma, which is often further aggravated by the social stigma so frequently attached to HIV-infected people and their households.

Unless suitable arrangements are made to cater to the needs of children before their parent's death, the trauma, grief and guilt so common among these children is compounded by the uncertainty of their future or their relocation within the extended family, often at the expense of breaking up the support offered by the sibling group.

In South Africa the formal welfare system battled to provide for the basic needs of children *prior* to the HIV/AIDS epidemic. Innovative shifts in welfare policy, an increase in social security grants, and greater recognition of the roles of non-governmental organizations and the extended family are all required to find alternative models of care to provide these additional vulnerable children with their basic needs, as well as love and nurturing.

It is important to note that all children and not only those in direct contact with an HIV-infected family member are affected by this epidemic. These children will be affected directly through day-to-day contact with peers experiencing personal tragedies, by sharing their homes with orphaned children or by participating in community programmes to address the needs of infected and affected community members. More pervasive is the indirect contact with the socio-economic sequelae of the epidemic. These include deteriorating levels of service provided within the education, health and welfare sectors secondary to reduced capacity resulting from staff losses and increased demands from orphaned and vulnerable children and their families.

It is crucial to recognize that all children will inevitably be affected by the HIV/AIDS epidemic and that the responsibility of minimizing the impact of the epidemic on children lies with each individual within our society.

Child abuse

With its initial recognition in the early 1960s, physical abuse emerged as a prominent medical, legal and social issue of childhood during the 1970s. It was subsequently displaced by the emerging awareness of childhood sexual abuse in the 1980s. There is no simple definition of child abuse, which is a broad term that embraces a variety of harmful interactions with children resulting in phsyical and emotional damage.

These activities include:
- Physical abuse or non-accidental injury (NAI)
- Emotional trauma
- Sexual abuse
- Neglect.

Prevalence

The deliberate physical abuse of children was first described as a medical entity by the radiologist Caffey over 50 years ago and characterized as the 'battered child syndrome' by Kempe in 1962. Since then, partly as a result of greater awareness on the part of medical practitioners but also because of an objective increase in its prevalence, increasingly large numbers of cases are being diagnosed and different manifestations of this problem are being described.

A problem reported in 447 children in the USA by 1960 has grown to the point that 2.3 million cases of suspected abuse and neglect are now reported each year – of these between 2 000 and 5 000 will die. Thus, a paediatric disorder unknown to most paediatricians who trained in the 1950s, thought to be rare by those who trained in the 1960s, and uncommon in the 1970s, has become an increasingly common problem in ambulatory settings today. Although figures are not generally available from developing countries, experience indicates that it is as common in these regions.

Risk factors

There are a number of recognized risk factors for child abuse, though each alone is of low predictive value. These include the following:

Families or parents 'at risk':
- Poor socio-economic circumstances
- Families under stress
- Young parents/teenage mothers
- Single self-supporting parent
- Psychiatric illness (chronic depression) in mother
- Parental drug dependence
- Parents who were abused or in institutional care as children
- Maternal illness
- Interference with mother-child bond at birth.

Children 'at risk':
+ Step or foster child
+ Premature baby
+ One of twins
+ Child with a mental or physical defect.

Physical abuse or non-accidental injury (NAI)

Non-accidental injury is any injury inflicted on a child by a responsible caregiver, irrespective of intent or justification, that produces anything more than erythema or redness and involves any area besides the buttock or hand. Included in this definition of NAI is any physical punishment administered to a child under the age of one year or to a child with a physical or mental disability. Clearly, any injury, within the context of the above definition, that results in bruising, breach of the skin, a burn, or disruption of a function is NAI.

This extreme definition deliberately sets out to state the acceptable limits of physical punishment at home and corporal punishment at school. It is essential to regard over-zealous punishment by parents and teachers as child abuse and to report these incidents to induce perpetrators to learn more acceptable, alternative modes of discipline.

Clinical picture

History. The history must include a complete and careful description of the injury including when, where, and how it occurred, who was present, and the time elapsed between injury and presentation. The child's age and development must be recorded, and current health status and past history of injuries documented. A social and family history describing the composition of the household, socio-economic conditions, and family support structures must be taken.

The following points on history should suggest the possibility of NAI:
- No or inadequate explanation of injuries
- Delay in seeking medical help
- Changing explanation for the injury
- Different explanations from different people
- Recurrent injuries in child or sibling.

Examination. In conducting the examination always try and answer the following two questions:
+ Is the injury compatible with the alleged cause or circumstances provided by the caregiver? For example, it is generally accepted that a child falling from a bed is highly unlikely to sustain a fracture or brain damage.
+ Is the injury compatible with the child's stage of development? For example, a child is unable to fall off a horizontal surface before being able to roll over; or unlikely to fall down stairs before being able to crawl.

Examination must include a precise description of all injuries: their length, shape, colour, position on the body, and degree of demarcation; and whether the injuries are bruises, scratches, abrasions, or burns. Comment on the child's general appearance, cleanliness, and state of the child's clothes. Note the child's mood and affect, e.g. apathy, frozen watchfulness, or irritability.

Also watch the interaction between the parent and child, and note whether there is apparent parental concern and whether there is a warm parent–child relationship. Note if there is a marked disparity between the state of hygiene, dress, or nutrition of the mother or caregiver and that of the child. Measure and plot the weight and length of the child against previous measurements if available. Examine the whole child and specifically look for hair loss, bruised or swollen ears and torn tympanic membranes, retinal haemorrhages, damage to the gums or torn frenulum, bruising of the neck, and evidence of injury to genitalia or anus.

The following points on examination should suggest the possibility of NAI:
+ Bruising or abrasions with any of the following characteristics:
  - Multiple bruises at different sites
  - Bruises of different ages
  - Well-demarcated linear bruises indicating imprint of well-known objects, such as a coathanger
  - Parallel 'tram-track' lesions from whipping with a stick or cord
  - Black eyes, especially when bilateral (blood from scalp injury may track down to soft tissues around the eyes)

- Teeth marks producing crescentic bruising
- Bruises on the legs of a child who is not yet walking
- Bruises to the face and neck
- Burns with any of the following characteristics:
  - Glove and stocking scalds to hands and feet (suggests forced immersion in hot water)
  - Well-demarcated, circular 'cigarette burns', usually on back of hands, wrists, and face
  - Any well-demarcated burn without an adequate explanation
- Multiple scars, abrasions, or scratches in different stages of development
- Circumferential injuries of ankles, wrists, and neck
- Sub-conjunctival, anterior chamber, and retinal haemorrhages
- Unexplained impaired level of consciousness
- Signs of a ruptured abdominal viscus
- Multiple or unusual fractures — children under one year of age cannot generate the momentum needed for a fracture.

All health professionals who deal with children should have a high index of suspicion when dealing with children who present with any of the above criteria. There are very few absolute diagnostic criteria for NAI and suspicion is a sufficient basis for reporting the case to the relevant authorities.

Investigation. Skeletal X-rays often provide supportive evidence for the diagnosis. Long bones are most commonly affected and diaphyseal fractures are four times more common than metaphyseal-epiphyseal fractures, although the latter are much more specific for NAI. Spiral fractures of long bones indicate torsional or rotational injuries, such as may occur when children are swung by their arms. Full skeletal surveys should be performed in children under the age of two suspected of NAI. In children with multiple bruises, bleeding disorders must be ruled out, but it must be noted that NAI can, of course, occur in children with bleeding disorders.

Management. The management of physical and sexual abuse will be discussed together as they share certain important principles.

Sexual abuse

Over the past three decades sexual abuse has emerged as the dominant form of child abuse throughout the world. Kempe has defined it on the basis of consent as the involvement of a child in sexual activity to which he/she does not consent; that he/she does not understand on the basis of his/her developmental age; and which violates the norms of society. Faller has produced an alternative definition, which considers the dynamic of the relationship and she describes sexual abuse as the involvment of a child in sexual activities in which there is a power imbalance. This imbalance, which may be on the basis of size, age, maturity, social position or financial status, facilitates the coercion or manipulation of the child.

Within these definitions there are four categories of sexual abuse:
- **Mild or non-contact abuse** – all activities that do not involve physical contact between a naked child and perpetrator such as sexual harassment, exhibitionism, exposure to pornography etc.
- **Moderate or contact abuse** – activities that involve physical contact of naked participants but without penetration of the body. This includes manipulation of the genitalia, anus or breasts of or by the child
- **Severe or penetrative abuse** – involving oral, anal or vaginal penetration of any body orifice, oral, anal or vaginal, by finger, penis, or any other object
- **Suspected abuse** – where behaviour, symptoms, signs or investigations suggest sexual activity but no corroborating history is available.

As only severe penetrative abuse is associated with the possibility of physical injuries, the diagnosis of sexual abuse is based on the story told by the child. This is unlike physical abuse where the diagnosis is based on clinical findings.

Disclosure of sexual abuse by children is a complex process rather than a simple event and invariably occurs days or weeks after the event. This is due the dynamics of the event and the role of coercion and manipulation, which frequently result in feelings of shame, guilt or fear. Partial disclosure is common, as children have poor memories and may not remember the details, may not appreciate the relevance of certain events or may be scared of a negative response to the disclosure.

It is estimated that one in three girls and one in six boys will be sexually abused before they reach 16 years of age.

Although girls form the bulk of sexually abused children, boys can account for up to 20 per cent of victims in some regions and have a different age incidence to girls. One-third of girls will be under six years of age and in the older ages there is a peak at 10 to 14 years, while boys have a single peak below 10 years of age. Boys are more commonly abused outside the home.

Most abuse results from the actions of a single perpetrator, usually a male. However, multiple perpetrators are occasionally involved and females may be involved directly as the perpetrator or facilitator of the abuse, or indirectly through failure to stop abusive activities of which they are aware. Perpetrators are found in all age groups and following the recent increase in juvenile offenders up to 40 per cent are under 18 years of age. When the identity of the perpetrator is known it is more often than not someone known to the child. The relationship between the perpetrator and the abused child falls into one of four categories:

  ◆ Unknown – where the child is too young or too frightened to disclose the identity of the perpetrator
  ◆ A family member – brother, father, grandfather, uncle or cousin
  ◆ A family acquaintance – a friend, lodger, neighbour, teacher, etc.
  ◆ A stranger.

Clinical picture

In view of absent, delayed or partial disclosure all healthcare workers need to have a high index of suspicion for sexual abuse. This should be precipitated by:

  ◆ What is heard – a story of abuse from the child, co-abuse, the perpetrator or a third party witness, or a variety of non-specific symptoms, including lower abdominal pain and genito-urinary complaints (dysuria, frequency, enuresis, discharge)
  ◆ what is seen – behavioural changes, developmental regression, deteriorating school performance, truancy, sexualized language and behaviour

  ◆ what is found on examination – anal or genital injuries, infections or structural changes.

History. Ideally the history should be obtained directly from the child. When speaking to the child it is essential to use the child's home language, to establish a common understanding of anatomy and to use terminology that the child is familiar with. For subsequent legal processes it is important to avoid unnecessary duplication and repeat interviews and to record the key point verbatim as described by the child.

The history is essential to guide the clinical assessment, the collection of forensic evidence and investigations and to assist in the interpretation of all findings.

Examination. The examination should only occur with the child's consent and in an appropriate child-friendly setting with both visual and auditory privacy. It should include a general examination to exclude non-genital injuries or provide an alternative diagnosis, a pubertal assessment to assist in the interpretation of the genital findings and to guide further management, as well as an ano-genital examaintion.

The examination should occur in two positions, supine and knee-chest, using two technigues, labial separation and labial traction. It is often easiest to examine infants and toddlers on their mother's lap. The examination needs to identify or exclude signs of acute genital or anal trauma (TEARS – tears or tenderness, ecchymoses, abrasions, redness and swelling or scars), structural changes to the hymen (enlarged hymenal orifice or acute/healed tears) or anus (distorted mucocutaneous appearance, venous engorgement or anal dilatation) and the sequelae of sexual intercourse (pregnancy or sexually transmitted infections).

An internal examination and the use of a speculum is totally unnecessary as is an examination under anaesthesia unless there are ano-genital injuries requiring surgical repair.

Investigation. Forensic specimens, to corroborate the story told by the child and to identify possible DNA of the perprtator, should be collected only when the child is assessed within 72 hours of the sexual assault, but medical specimens should be collected as indicated regardless of the interval between sexual assault and assessment.

Medical investigations include a pregnancy test for girls with Tanner stage 3 pubertal development, a swab of all discharges for microscopy and culture and blood to exclude syphilis, Hepatitis B and HIV infection. These infections can only be excluded if repeat specimens taken six and twelve weeks after the sexual assault are negative.

Management of child abuse

The management of all forms of child abuse should involve a wide range of professionals working together to address the needs of the abused child and his or her family. Traditionally, social workers have been responsible for coordinating the activities of these multidisciplinary teams. The management involves six basic steps with health practitioners having a role at each stage.

Detection of possible abuse

Since the diagnosis is often obscure, it is important to have a high level of suspicion (*see above*).

Investigation of possible abuse

Once child abuse has been suspected, this possibility must be investigated to ensure adequate management of the child, as well as protection from ongoing abuse. This entails the investigation of the physical or psychological state of the child and an investigation of the social circumstances of the child and family.

Physical abuse. The main goal is to document the nature and extent of the injuries and to exclude any possible organic cause for such injuries. These include nutritional disorders, blood disorders, and bone diseases such as osteogenesis imperfecta. Attention must be given to the emotional consequences of physical abuse, particularly post-traumatic stress disorder. The child's social circumstances should be assessed to ensure that precipitating factors and underlying family dynamics are addressed as part of the overall management of the child and family.

Sexual abuse. Since the minority of these children present to hospital within 48 hours of being abused, there is usually no urgency to examine them and examination can be deferred until someone who is competent to do so is available.

Validation

This process should take place as soon as possible after presentation and involves a team decision as to whether, based on all available information, the child has or has not been abused. At this stage the legal obligation of medical practitioners, in terms of section 42 of the Child Care Act, is to report all cases of suspected child abuse to a social worker and/or to the South African Police Services, usually through the Child Protection Unit, and to notify the regional director of the Department of Welfare.

Steps to protect the child

If child abuse is confirmed the continued safety of the child is the main priority. Ideally, the child is best left at home in the care of a responsible and caring parent. If this is not possible and places the child at risk of ongoing abuse, either the child or the abuser must be removed. As a temporary measure it may sometimes be necessary to admit the child to hospital while alternative solutions are pursued.

Treatment of the child

Treatment needs to focus on physical and emotional problems and must be both curative and preventive. Existing physical problems are easily identified and should be treated appropriately. Prophylactic treatment must be given for tetanus, secondary infections, sexually transmitted infections, and possible teenage pregnancy. All children presenting within 72 hours of the abuse should receive the following prophylaxis:

Physical abuse
- ATT 0.5 ml IMI stat (only if penetrating injuries are present).

Sexual abuse
- Metronidazole 15 mg/kg/day in divided doses for 7 days
- Ceftriaxone 125 mg IMI stat, erythromycin 50 mg/kg/day in four divided doses for 10 days
- If HIV negative on rapid testing, a 28-day course of antiretroviral therapy with AZT and 3TC should be prescribed
- Girls with Tanner stage 3 pubertal development, irrespective of whether or not they have started menstruating, are at risk of falling pregnant, which needs to

be excluded or prevented. They require a pregnancy test and if negative, must receive an abortifacient to prevent pregnancy: Ovral 28, 2 tablets stat and 2 after 12 hours.

Post-traumatic stress disorder is a common complication of all forms of child abuse and provision must be made for acute crisis intervention, follow-up, and long-term support should this be required. Such support should be left to professionals with the necessary skills.

Rehabilitation of the child and family

This is the final step in management. Family therapy and the re-integration of the child into the family is the responsibility of mental health professionals. The doctor is responsible for ensuring that these needs have been met before returning the child to his/her home.

Unusual manifestations of child abuse

Although these other manifestations are relatively rare they are worthy of mention since they illustrate the scope of the problem and highlight the need for vigilance among child health professionals. Examples include forced ingestion of drugs such as cocaine and alcohol; intentional microwave oven burns; forced ingestion of pepper, resulting in aspiration and fatality; and water deprivation, resulting in hypernatraemia.

Special passing mention must be given to a recently characterized condition that is being reported with increasing frequency in industrialized countries. In this condition, now known as *Munchausen syndrome by proxy*, a caregiver, usually the mother, induces factitious illness in her child, often with serious and even tragic consequences. In this perversion of mothering, mothers present repeatedly to hospitals and doctors with refractory complaints in their children that disappear when the child and mother are separated. The mothers who adopt this perverse pattern of behaviour derive gratification from the medical and nursing attention that results from placing their child under medical investigation. These women have a history of abusive experiences in their own childhood, have abnormal illness behaviour themselves, and possess a variety of unusual personality traits.

Child neglect and abandonment

This is the failure, on the part of parents or other caregivers, to meet the child's basic needs. It differs from abuse in that the harm to the child is a consequence of a parent's or caregiver's omission rather than commission.

In most situations where the child's needs are not met, this occurs as a result of the inability of the caregiver to provide the necessary conditions, through a lack of physical or personal resources, rather than from deliberate intent. Examples are parents who are extremely poor, who have low intelligence, or who have a particular cultural belief that has an adverse effect on the child's health. Seen in this way, neglect is an enormously pervasive problem, especially in developing countries. It is particularly difficult to manage, as large numbers of children may be affected, complex strategies are required, and substitute care is not a practicable solution except where malevolent neglect is demonstrated.

Neglect may take various forms, characterized by the failure of parents to meet the needs of their children for:

- Sufficient and nutritious food
- Warmth (clothes and housing)
- Cleanliness and personal hygiene
- Health care
- Protection from hazards in their environment
- Love and emotional support
- Stimulation and learning.

The impact of neglect in one or more of these areas on the growth, development, and well-being of the child may be profound. Recognized features of neglect include:

- Delayed development, especially of speech and language.
- Failure to thrive, characterized by objective evidence of growth failure in the absence of any organic cause.
- Characteristic physical features, such as:
  - dental caries
  - pallor
  - impetigo and contact dermatitis
  - chronic suppurative otitis media
  - hair loss over the occiput.
- Disorders of affect, such as:
  - avoidance of eye contact in infancy
  - lack of stranger anxiety as a toddler
  - poor interaction with peers at pre-school.

Situations that give rise to neglect may in their most extreme form result in abandonment of the child. There are clearly many additional reasons, besides those given earlier, for the decision to abandon the child, such as unwanted pregnancies and handicapped or chronically ill children. Given the poor outlook for these children, attempts must be made to prevent abandonment and neglect by:

- Promoting bonding and ensuring adequate support during the crucial postnatal period
- Identifying mother–child pairs who are at risk, as early as possible, for example a mother who displays little interest in her pregnancy or baby, is uncooperative during birth, or is loathe to breastfeed.

Special problems of the adolescent

Adolescence is a difficult and often confusing period of physical and emotional transition from childhood to adulthood, during which pre-existing problems may be exacerbated and many new problems may arise. These include impulsive and anti-social behaviour, depression and suicidal behaviour, eating disorders, drug dependency, sexual experimentation, and teenage pregnancies. Some of these will be dealt with in greater detail below.

Sexuality and adolescent pregnancy

To individual teenagers the most significant changes associated with adolescence are probably not the physical and psychological changes that take place but rather the increased awareness of their own sexuality.

Sexual activity among teenagers is becoming increasingly prevalent at younger ages in virtually all communities. In the USA, 70 per cent of 19-year-old girls are sexually active and the estimated teenage pregnancy rate is 95 per 1 000. The situation in South Africa is probably worse, with an estimated teenage pregnancy rate of 330 per 1 000 and up to 20 per cent of women giving birth in many state hospitals are below 19 years of age. The majority of such pregnancies occur within the first year of a teenager becoming sexually active.

Teenage pregnancies often occur in dysfunctional families in which there are low levels of education and inadequate supervision of the children. It is therefore closely related to a culture of poverty and deprivation and is closely associated with other high-risk behaviours, such as smoking and the use of alcohol. Additional factors include single-parent households; a family history of teenage pregnancy in the mother or an older sister; and an inadequate knowledge of sexuality, contraception, and pregnancy.

Problems

The sexual feelings that arrive with puberty are not in themselves harmful to health. However, the expression of these sexual urges is often greeted with anxiety or anger by adults, and frequently with fear, guilt, and shame by the young people themselves. These responses combine to drive sexual feelings and behaviour underground, making communication about the healthy development of sexuality within affectionate and responsible relationships more difficult. Sexual activity carries with it the inevitable risk of unwanted pregnancy and the possibility of contracting a sexually transmitted infection, including infection with HIV. Adolescents are understandably least prepared to prevent or deal with these consequences.

The consequences of early pregnancy for the teenage girl are multiple and serious. There is often late and erratic antenatal clinic attendance for a number of possible reasons — she may not recognize the signs of pregnancy, she may not know where to go for advice, and, if she is unmarried, may not want to believe she is pregnant or may be too ashamed to tell anyone. Young women who have not reached full physical and physiological maturity are almost three times as likely to die from complications in childbirth as older women. The risk for very young teenagers (10 to 14 years) is much greater than for older teenagers (15 to 19 years). Teenagers are known to be at a higher risk for infection, uncontrolled pregnancy-induced hypertension, and pre-term labour. Subsequent health problems include stunted growth following early epiphyseal closure and a 25 per cent likelihood of another pregnancy within a year.

Adolescent pregnancy also often causes serious psychosocial problems in the mother. It decreases the likelihood of finishing school, and causes an early entry into the workforce, at a lower level with fewer skills and poorer long-term prospects. There is also a higher rate of marital instability and the younger mother with less education, fewer financial resources, and less family support has an infant who is at greater risk for poor development and ill-health.

The adverse effects of early child-bearing on the mother are matched by disadvantages for her baby. Babies of adolescent mothers have a lower chance of survival. Low birth weight, which carries an increased susceptibility to illness and infection, is more common in babies of adolescent mothers. Perinatal and infant mortality rates, especially in developing countries, are consistently higher where mothers are under 20. There is also an increased rate of Sudden Infant Death Syndrome (SIDS), more hospitalizations, accidents, burns, poisonings, and superficial injuries. Most of these problems reflect inadequate supervision by an immature mother.

Not only are babies of very young mothers physically at risk during birth and throughout early life but their psychosocial and material wellbeing is compromised in a number of different ways. The child born outside marriage suffers, indirectly, from the social isolation and consequent stress suffered by the mother and, directly, from the material deprivation faced by mothers raising children by themselves with no support. The child born to a very young woman may be less well cared for because the woman still has some of the emotional needs of a child herself. These problems may be much less acute in an extended family, but where traditional family structures have been destroyed through migration and urbanization, the young woman often has to face these problems without any social support.

Interventions

Whereas health professionals may consider these issues outside their realm, the problem unquestionably impinges seriously on the life and health of the baby. It is imperative that the mother is armed with the basic knowledge of infant care; in cases where she is clearly unable to take on the demands of motherhood, the possibility of adoption must be offered to her (*see above*).

The role of the doctor in teenage pregnancy includes the need for an increased awareness of teenage sexuality and the need to enquire about sexual activity and contraceptive use. Health professsionals should promote early attendance at an antenatal clinic and provide increased support and nutritional supplements during the pregnancy. It is vital that the high risk of the babies, infants, and children of teenage parents is recognized and their wellbeing closely monitored.

Interventions must be considered at many levels, and provide ample opportunity for involvement by health professionals. Life and parenting skills should form an integral part of school curricula. In particular, sex education must be given high priority. Outside the school setting, religious institutions and other social structures can participate in educational camps, and by providing recreational activities. Contraceptive services must be geared to the needs of the adolescent. For the young mother, support groups and 'clubs' are a dire necessity.

Generally, health professionals should remain non-judgemental, while not condoning promiscuity. They should promote an understanding that the problem of adolescent pregnancy is a problem of the whole community, and that these large numbers of youngsters should not be allowed to enter premature parenthood by default.

Drug dependence

Drug dependence must be considered in a wide context, which includes the abuse of alcohol, solvent and glue-sniffing, and smoking marijuana (cannabis, dagga), and extending to the use of hard drugs such as heroin. There are very few children who are not exposed at some time or other to these risks. The child is particularly vulnerable, as traffickers tend to exploit the young and gullible.

Levels of drug abuse

The child may be involved in drug abuse at three levels:

- ◆ The infant born to a drug and/or alcohol-dependent mother enters the world with a profound handicap which, apart from physical and emotional neglect, may present as fetal alcohol syndrome or drug withdrawal symptoms (*see* Chapter 7, Care of the newborn).

- The families of those involved in illicit production or trafficking of drugs are frequently deprived of adequate education, nutrition, and domestic stability.
- The child or adolescent deprived of parental love and creative outlets is at risk of falling prey to this social disease.

Aetiological and epidemiological factors

Abusers can be grouped into:

- Those in search of an exciting experience because their life appears dull
- Those in search of oblivion because their life lacks any joy or lustre
- Those in search of a new personality because their life is filled with anxiety and indecision.

In communities in developing countries, urbanization and industrialization, together with migrant labour and high-pressure lifestyles, have disrupted families and eroded traditions and support structures. The younger generations are, therefore, deprived of stability and have scant resources to fall back on in the face of anxiety, conflicts, and temptations.

Generally, males are more frequently abusers, as are those who dwell in urban ghettos. The most important aetiological factors, however, are lack of parental love and understanding, as well as unrealistic expectations.

Clinical features

The drug scene is dynamic, varying with the socio-economic status of the family, the prevailing vogue, and the availability of different types of drug. The characteristics of the dependants are determined by the drug: thus alcohol produces a clinical picture very different from that of solvent-sniffing or smoking marijuana. Alcohol and marijuana are used by adolescents, while glue- and solvent-sniffing are widely practised among younger age groups.

Marijuana in moderate usage causes euphoria, inattentiveness, loss of memory for recent events, increased suggestibility, nausea, and vertigo. Examination shows tachycardia, conjunctivitis, dry mouth, and ataxia. In higher doses depersonalization, hallucinations, and anxiety states may be released. The most significant aspect is that habitual usage may replace social usage in an attempt to evade stress or confrontation. It interrupts the normal psychological growth process, thus preventing emotional maturation. While the abuser is using this escape mechanism, skills for coping with the stresses of everyday life are not developed.

Solvent- and glue-sniffing. The hydrocarbons in solvents and toluene in glue give rise to euphoria, hallucinations, and vertigo. These organic chemicals can cause appreciable liver, kidney, and nervous system damage. Permanent brain damage may occur, with ataxia and personality change, or there may be irreversible peripheral neuropathy.

The diagnosis should be considered when dealing with unexplained coma, seizures, ataxia, or behavioural disturbances. Sniffing is frequently the precursor to major drug dependence and is a sign of an emotionally distressed child.

Alcohol. The accessibility of alcohol is probably one of the main reasons why it is abused so frequently. Those who act as models for the child – parents and teachers – often contribute to the problem by drinking excessively themselves. Commercial promotion is a further powerful force urging the young to partake of a particular product, with the implied promise of a better life.

The dangers of dependence are no fewer with alcohol than with any of the other substances. As with solvent- or glue-sniffing, alcoholism in a child suggests emotional instability or distress.

The odour of the breath facilitates the diagnosis in the child, if seen within hours of imbibing. The clinical features may resemble those of the all-too-familiar presentation of alcohol intoxication. However, coma ensues earlier in the child and is a high risk in infants. Hypoglycaemia frequently results in coma because of the direct inhibition of gluconeogenesis by alcohol.

> Strategies to build self esteem, promote a healthy adolescence, minimize high risk behaviour and reduce adolescent suicide rates includes START:
> **S**ports promotion
> Addressing **T**eenage sexuality
> **A**lcohol avoidance
> **R**oad safety education
> **T**rauma avoidance.

Child rights and child advocacy

While the responsibility for ensuring the survival, development, and protection of a child resides primarily with the child's parents within the supportive structure of the family, civil society must ensure that this responsibility is adequately discharged. The first global attempt to entrench the rights of children in law was the Declaration of the Rights of the Child, adopted by the United Nations in 1959. This was given greater weight by the adoption of the Convention of the Rights of the Child by the same body in 1989 and all member countries were called on to ratify its terms, thus committing themselves morally and legally to its implementation.

The Convention establishes children as equal and vital members of families and communities with inalienable rights, rather than as passive and vulnerable beneficiaries of unpredictable and often patchy welfare services and institutional care. According to this view the needs of children should be met by addressing the underlying and often structural factors within society that result in the breakdown of care and nurture. This contrasts with the traditional approach of identifying the most vulnerable and providing them with social services such as shelter, food, and health care.

This approach requires child health professionals to take on the role of child health advocates, committed to the defence of children's rights and to social mobilization around the needs of children, particularly those in especially difficult circumstances, such as abused and neglected children, the disabled, children affected by HIV, and children in conflict with the law. These child advocates will need to support processes that contribute to changing people's attitudes concerning children and their rights and needs, both within the government and civil society. They will need to use the Convention as a tool to mobilize all levels of government, the media, communities, and families to influence changes in social policy which benefit children.

6

Developmental, psychological and behavioural disorders

Although child development includes social, emotional, behavioural, communication and physical progress with age, this chapter will deal only with some aspects of the first three.

All children, whether normal or abnormal, strive to develop. The tempo at which they develop may be delayed and the normal patterns of development may be disturbed. When children encounter developmental problems they may use differing strategies to overcome them. Not all these strategies are necessarily effective. Nevertheless, all children should be given opportunities, encouragement and assistance to develop.

Developmental problems are among the most common issues that general practitioners will come across. Statistically one out of every ten children will have a developmental problem, even if minor. For an optimal outcome, early identification and intervention is critical. Many children with developmental problems are referred too late.

General principles of development:
- Development takes place on a continuum. The concept of the 'developmental cascade' is applicable to all developmental modalities in children.
- The sequence of development is the same in almost all children, although the tempo may differ. The principle is that development is purposeful and that each milestone will follow a preceding milestone. Small deviations may occur, but the child who 'gets stuck' at a certain milestone, does not reach the next milestone,

or follows an aberrant developmental path should be examined thoroughly, preferably by a multidisciplinary team in order to make a diagnosis and develop a treatment plan.
- There is a wide normal variation for mastering specific milestones in children.
- Development is predetermined by hereditary (genetic) factors and environmental (stimulation) factors.
- Although we describe development as an age-dependent phenomenon, it is important to consider development as a continuous cascade of progressive learned skills.
- Quality of development is more important than quantity, in other words the 'how' is more important than the 'when'.

Remember:
- No child is so severely affected that nothing can be done.
- An attitude that children will 'outgrow' their problems is seldom beneficial.
- There are critical areas for development which, once lost, will lead to permanent deficits (e.g. language development).
- The parent's support, enthusiasm, commitment and perseverance are critical for the rehabilitation process to be successful.
- Ineffective or delayed intervention for one developmental difficulty may lead to secondary (e.g. social and emotional) disabilities.

The multidisciplinary professional team

Although the ideal would be for all developmental issues in children to be evaluated and managed by a multidisciplinary team, it is rarely possible in developing countries to assemble a team of experts, such as a paediatrician, developmental paediatrician, child psychiatrist, psychologist, remedial teacher, occupational therapist, physiotherapist, social worker and speech therapist. However, it is often possible and extremely useful to bring together a doctor, a nurse, and a teacher to form a basic team and to pool their information and expertise. Any member of the team may make the first contact and take a detailed history.

The **doctor**, paediatrician and developmental paediatrician contributes knowledge and expertise of physical illness or handicap and child development, and has knowledge of appropriate pharmacology.

The **nurse** is frequently the team coordinator and has a broad knowledge of physical problems and social factors.

The **teacher** is an expert in the cognitive and emotional aspects of education and is able to judge a child's performance in comparison to other local children.

The **child psychiatrist** is a medical doctor who has specialized in the psychological problems of children and thus combines knowledge of physical medicine with psychological and social aspects of mental distress.

The **psychologist** has an in-depth knowledge of psychology and is skilled in the administration of specific psychological tests and in various types of psychological treatment. The educational psychologist is trained in the psychological aspects of education and learning.

The **social worker** is trained to collect information from home visits and family interviews and may undertake a wide range of individual, group, and family therapy. The social worker also has wide knowledge of the law as it applies to children and families and is able to advise on grants, financial aid, or placement.

The **occupational therapist** (OT) has detailed knowledge of the physical development of children and is most useful in defining developmental problems of coordination or motor function.

The OT helps to clarify specific learning problems and performs individual and group therapy aimed at remediating deficiencies of function.

The **speech therapist** defines problems in the reception and expression of language (spoken and read). Since most education is language based, the speech therapist is a most important member of the team.

The **remedial teacher** has made a special study of learning disabilities and is able to recognize and treat specific problems.

All team members should have knowledge of the physical, emotional and social development of the children in the community they serve. Team members should be prepared to communicate with one another and learn from one another and from others.

The assessment procedure

Comprehensive assessment

In assessing a child with a possible developmental or behavioural problem, the following aspects require particular attention:

Child development

A comprehensive knowledge of the expected normal physical, social, and emotional development of the child is fundamental in the assessment of a patient.

The family environment

Children can be reared successfully within a nuclear or an extended family, provided primary caregivers are consistent. Permanent psychological and emotional scars are sustained by children who suffer disruption by frequent change of caregivers and by exposure to family violence.

However, children differ widely in temperament: some withstand great social and emotional deprivation successfully, while others are

> Apart from physical needs, the child has fundamental social and emotional needs that must be met in order that he or she develops into a balanced and mature person.

Table 6.1 The needs of the child

- Physical care
- Love, acceptance, and security
- Continuity and consistency of caregiving
- Behaviour controls
- Cultural identity
- Appropriate cognitive stimulation.

Table 6.2 Test kit for assessment of cognitive tasks

- Books
  - A simple picture book with good illustrations of familiar objects
  - Pages taken from three or four different graded reading books in English and local vernacular languages
  - Sets of maths calculations from three or four graded books
- Pencil, paper, and eraser for writing and drawing
- Tennis ball
- Toys: a few cars, doll, and animals
- Large beads and strings
- Set of basic blocks in various colours.

---

much more vulnerable to bad parenting and poor quality of family life.

Cultural environment

Many families are in a state of transition, moving away from the cultural and religious norms of their parents. High mobility between town and country, migration from country to informal peri-urban settlements, high social upward mobility, and the pressures of employment and unemployment are among factors that influence this transition. These in turn alter language, religion, family structure, and acceptable standards of behaviour. These external stresses have a marked bearing on child-rearing practices and family life. An analysis of the effect of these stresses on a specific family is recommended for every assessment but at the same time identifying the strengths and positive features, on which one will have to build.

Physical examination

A routine but thorough examination, with specific emphasis on the neurological system, hearing, and vision, is essential.

Testing basic cognitive tasks

This can be an extension of the physical examination. Reading, calculations, writing, and drawing are screened, and age-appropriate responses measured. More ingenuity is required to test children who have had little exposure to western culture. Bearing this in mind, an appropriate test kit could be put together (*see* Table 6.2)

The art of assessment is to use a few test items and gain experience by observing the responses of a number of children. Where available, the clinical or educational psychologist can verify test results if there is uncertainty. In most cases problems can be clearly identified and may be acted upon.

Tests for laterality and coordination

As a child matures, awareness of left- and right-sidedness and motor coordination develop. This is tested by observing which eye, hand, or foot the child prefers. Immaturity in these areas may indicate a specific learning disorder (*see below*) that can benefit from early remedial training. Exercises can be prescribed with the help of an occupational therapist, which can be supervised by a lay assistant or parent.

Drawing

Children usually love to draw. Both the way they draw and the content of the drawings can be most informative. The patient may be given drawing materials while the history is being taken. Subsequently the child is asked to draw a person. This should be done in pencil on plain paper for scoring by the occupational therapist or psychologist where appropriate. This draw-a-person (DAP) test gives a good indication of intelligence but culture and possible deprivation have to be considered. The example of a DAP shown in Figure 6.1 was done by a child who presented with disruptive behaviour at school and who was not coping. This was at the time of the 1986 school boycotts. The disturbance and distress are not difficult to diagnose; he is standing on an army personnel carrier. There is also evidence of a major learning problem in letter formation. This child was not mentally retarded.

Play

A play assessment is done by observing the child at play, which is especially useful in very young or grossly disturbed children. Even in the brief assessment that is being suggested, observations of the child's interaction with people, objects, and toys are very useful. Some children are anxious, afraid, and totally inhibited; some will not use equipment appropriately at all; others are disinhibited and explore everything in a very short time. The interaction between caregiver and child, the encouragement given, and the control exercised are all useful observations.

Problem analysis

The art and science of assessment lie in being able to collate a great deal of information and give priority to the main problem areas. The various aspects of the case should be discussed and correlated by the team before feedback is given. All findings are grouped under the following headings:

- **Problems in the child**
  - physical
  - psychological: intelligence, mental disorders
  - educational
- **Problems in the family**
- **Problems in the environment** (including school).

At the outset the healthcare worker must get a very clear idea of what the parents feel is the problem with the child. After assessment the parent's definition of the problem will be the starting point for discussing the child's problems.

Figure 6.1 Example of a person drawn by a disturbed schoolboy

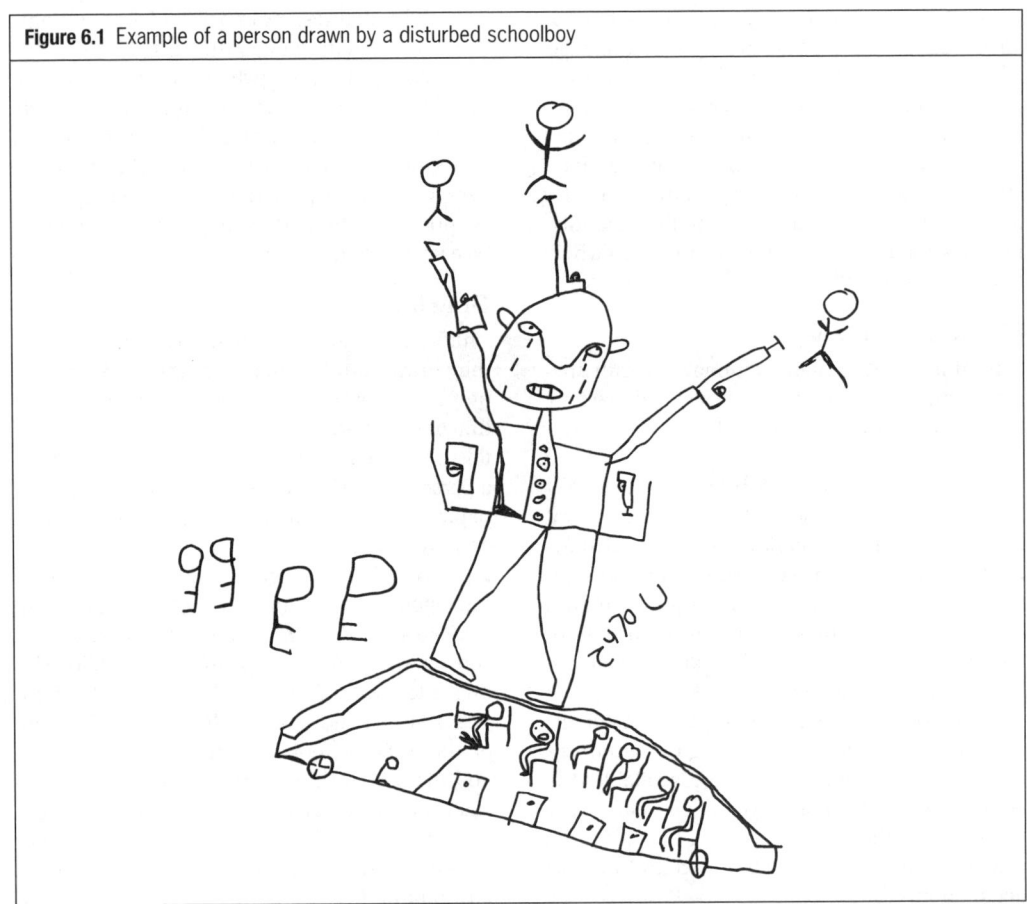

The issues to be highlighted include the strengths of the child, the family, and/or the school. The team should discuss the problems considered to be most important with the parents. Correctly labelling the child's problem often brings great relief to the family. The parents' expectations need to be analyzed and they need time to question and discuss the team's findings, especially if they differ from those of the parents. Authoritarian pronouncements should be avoided since these make the parents feel belittled or antagonized, which will not ultimately help the child.

> Assessment in itself should be recognized as a major intervention, which frequently leads to great improvement in the child's problem through insights gained by both the parents and the child.

A report to the school is usually necessary, especially if the child was referred by the school. Where the child is not being seen on a regular basis, organized follow-up is essential to monitor progress and to review the intervention.

Treatment

The team should decide whether treatment is really essential. Factors which determine the choice of treatment include accessibility and affordability in terms of time and cost, as well as the severity of the problem. A careful evaluation of the factors listed in Table 6.3 is recommended.

Possible treatment modalities may include medical treatment, occupational, speech and physiotherapy, psychotherapy, or special educational intervention (home programme), information or counselling for the parents, and family therapy.

Problems affecting children from the newborn to toddler age group

A few of the most common problems will be presented.

Colic

The clinical picture is that of recurrent bouts of uncontrollable crying in a baby who is healthy and feeding well. According to the Wessel criteria, a baby who cries more than three hours/day, for more than three days/week, for more than three

Table 6.3 Factors influencing the outcome of childhood psychosocial disorders	
Risk factors	**Ameliorating factors**
Family	*Parent and/or child*
Unstable	Stable temperament
Socio-economically deprived	Good coping skills
	Positive experience outside home
Parent	*Child*
Single	Good relationship with one parent
Immature	
Mildly retarded	
Displays conduct/behaviour disorder	
Rejects child	
In discord with other parent	
Other	*Other*
Unstable environment	Isolated nature of stress
Inadequate school and recreational activities	Improving socio-economic circumstances

weeks, suffers from colic. Colic occurs in 10–25 per cent of babies. Symptoms usually start at the age of two weeks and continue until three to four months. It typically starts in the late afternoon with a crying spell, fisting and flexion of the legs, as if in pain. The aetiology and pathophysiology is not known, but it probably represents an extreme variant of a normal neuro-developmental process. Both an immature central nervous system and gastrointestinal system may play a role. Although it is not caused by poor parenting, some parents have few resources and lack the resilience required to deal with the problem and become anxious or frustrated at the lack of response to medications.

Only 5 per cent of babies with excessive crying have an underlying organic cause. In these children the crying is not typically clustered at a particular time of day or in paroxysms.

After a full history and clinical examination, the parents should be reassured that the condition will improve. As the pathophysiology is not known there is no specific treatment.

The following may be of benefit:

- Breastfeeding mothers should avoid eggs, nuts, dairy products, caffeine and spicy food in their diet.
- Some bottle fed babies may benefit from lactose-free or hypoallergenic formulas.
- No medicine has been found to be beneficial, but simethicone may be tried.
- Non-harmful interventions such as massaging, a warm bath and white noise/ soft music can be tried.
- Over- and under-stimulation and feeding of the baby must be avoided

Thumb sucking

Thumb sucking starts usually in the newborn phase and is very common between 18–21 months. It may be related to hunger, teething, loneliness, boredom and sleep, and may indicate emotional neglect. It usually stops around five years of age. If thumb sucking persists after six years of age there is usually an emotional aetiology. It may be a sign of stress, anxiety or feelings of insecurity. These children may also suck their lips, teeth, blanket or nappy. Malocclusion may develop with prolonged thumb sucking. A pacifier (dummy) after feeding may prevent thumb sucking.

Temper tantrums

This is a common problem among toddlers in some communities. Tantrums occur mostly between age 15 months and three years – the so-called negative stage of child development, when parents do not allow the child to have his own way. During the attack the child usually lies on the ground kicking and screaming. Important factors are the child's and parent's temperament and inconsistency of the parent's behaviour towards the child.

Even though the physical examination is usually normal, it should be done if only to reassure the parents.

This usually is a passing phase with good response to counselling where parents are reassured and helped to cope with the tantrum. This becomes difficult where parental control is lacking and the lifestyle is chaotic. The child must never be allowed to have his/her way after such an attack.

The principles of managing tantrums are:

- Avoid frustrating situations by offering alternatives to the 'forbidden fruit'.
- Ignore the tantrum by walking away from the child.
- Avoid punishing the child for the tantrum. Parents should stay calm and not hit, scold or argue with the child.
- Give full attention and approval when behaviour is acceptable.
- Be consistent.

The parents need to be given constant reassurance and encouragement on subsequent visits.

Breath holding attacks

These attacks are closely related to temper tantrums. They start between 6–18 months and are rare after four years.

Two types are described:

Cyanotic type: The cyanotic type is more common than the pale type. A child who cannot have his/her way usually triggers the cyanotic type. He/she will cry lustily for whatever reason, hyperventilate and then develop apnoea and cyanosis. It lasts for 10-30 seconds and at the end the child may have increased tonus in the limbs, or clonic movement may occur. Once the child starts breathing normally the attack comes to an end. Afterwards the child is mostly apathetic but fully conscious.

Pale type: The pale type is usually associated with a minor injury or fear. The child becomes deathly pale and develops bradycardia, or may even become asystolic because of increased vagal tone.

Both attacks are precipitated by anoxia, the cyanotic type by apnoea and the pale type is caused by bradycardia and both types are associated with iron deficiency anaemia.

The treatment of the condition involves reassuring the parents that breath holding is a benign condition and has no relationship to epilepsy. A comprehensive medical history and full physical examination should be performed, and if iron deficiency anaemia is present it should be treated.

Sleep disorders

Most children develop sleeping problems at some time or another. Failure to sleep and excessive crying are common during the first years. The establishment of a good routine can be difficult with some children. Many of these develop because of parental ignorance and may lead to conflict between the child and the parents.

Aetiology

Organic causes are seldom the cause of sleeping disorders, except in infancy, when the following should be considered:

- Hunger
- Colic
- Urinary tract infections
- Teething
- Wet or dirty nappies
- Ear ache
- Nappy rash
- Too hot or too cold.

Important organic causes in older children include upper airway infections and allergies leading to obstruction and apnoea.

Duration of sleep. There may be large individual variations in the duration of sleep in childhood. After birth a baby sleeps almost continuously between feeds. A pattern of longer sleeping periods at night and two to three shorter periods during the day gradually develops. At two years the child sleeps approximately one to two hours in the afternoons and 12 hours at night. At three to four years of age most children are not interested in taking a nap in the afternoon. Parents often have a misconception of how long their children should sleep and may force the child to take a nap. A set bed-time is in order, but the system should be flexible.

Incorrect management of the child. This is a very common cause of 'sleeping problems'. Falling asleep on cue is a learned process, and does not happen instinctively. If a good routine is not set by six months the parents might experience problems with their child's sleep routine. Children develop set sleeping habits very rapidly. It is important to remember that the rituals and habits necessary for a child to fall asleep will be necessary every time he/she wakes up. For example, if a child is lulled in his mother's arms to go to sleep every night, he will not go to sleep if this action is not repeated every night. Rituals are not undesirable and indeed are helpful, but must be limited.

Test crying. Young babies usually cry for a few minutes after they have been put to bed. It is better not to respond to this. The baby will soon fall asleep.

Other causes for sleep disorders include

- Fear (e.g. darkness)
- Worries (e.g. weak school performance)
- Separation anxiety (18–30 months)
- Excitement (e.g. birthday)
- Negativism (18 months – three years)
- Social circumstances (crowded bed).

Management of sleep disorders should include the following steps:

- Take a detailed history, looking at feeding patterns, routine in the family, stresses on the child, and parents' attempts at coping with the problem.
- Exclude any physical abnormality (including epilepsy).
- Consider possible covert child abuse.
- Be supportive – reassurance is of paramount importance, particularly where the child is otherwise well and thriving.
- Find a way of getting the mother a few good nights' sleep to help her to cope.
- Involve the father or other members of the family.
- Assist in developing a bed-time routine.

- Develop a behavioural programme to teach the child to fall asleep.
- Arrange family therapy for chaotic and violent families.
- Hypnotics for the child are generally not useful.

Nightmares

These present with the child waking up scared at night, sometimes sobbing, because of a terrible dream. It occurs during REM sleep and usually after midnight and the incident (if not the dream) may be remembered the next morning.

It might follow after an upsetting incident or frightening story/film as well as separation anxiety, and occurs in most normal children.

Management. There is no specific treatment.

- Ensure that it is not an indication of an emotional disturbance.
- Let the child sleep with the light on.
- Use 'magic' to drive away 'monsters'.

Night terrors

The child does not wake up completely during a night terror and cannot remember the experience the next day. He/she is clearly very upset, with eyes wide open. He/she might be screaming, hitting in all directions, is disorientated and does not recognize anyone that comes to his/her aid. These children cannot be soothed and they fall asleep again later.

It starts during phase III non-REM (deep sleep) and usually occurs early in the night

There is no specific treatment. Do not try to wake the child up.

If the night terrors always take place at the same time every night (which is often the case) the child can be aroused (but not awoken) 15 minutes or so before that time to prevent the terror attack from occurring.

Pervasive developmental disorder (PDD)

This group of disorders includes children who have major impairment of social interaction and impairment of communication, and are markedly restricted in their activities and interests. The age of onset is during the first three years. Although some have normal intelligence, the majority are below average. These children

are particularly severely handicapped — more than can be attributed to the mental retardation alone. The prevalence rate is about two to four per 10 000 children.

Pervasive developmental disorder may be subdivided into infantile autism and non-specific PDD. The former is characterized by autistic aloneness (autism: lack of responsiveness to other people), delayed or abnormal speech, an obsessive desire for sameness, and unusually repetitive and sometimes inappropriate patterns of play.

Management. If the disorder is suspected, the child should be referred to a psychologist, psychiatrist, or paediatrician for diagnosis. These children can benefit from special intensive educational programmes, which should start early. The prognosis for independence in later life is not good.

Common developmental problems at age six to ten years

School failure

School failure is a very common presenting problem and the general practitioner is often the first professional that is consulted. There are many causes for a child failing or performing badly at school and they may co-exist in the same child. When a child's performance has suddenly deteriorated the cause is most likely to be physical or emotional. Consistently poor performance is more likely to indicate mental retardation or specific learning problems.

A detailed history is essential, and is probably the single most important factor in the initial management of these problems. A simple but effective approach to school failure is to consider the triad: school, child and parents (*see* Figure 6.2).

The school system

1 Poor attendance
   a Recurrent hospitalization
   b Truancy
   c Disrupted schooling – mobile parents, poor supervision etc.

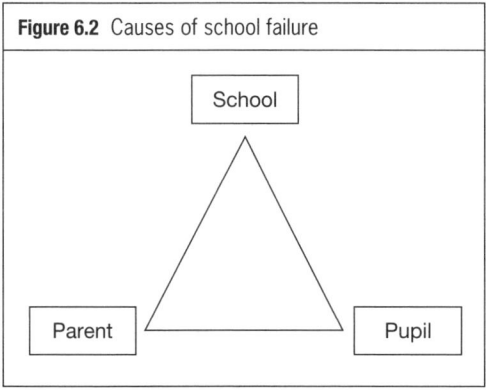

Figure 6.2 Causes of school failure

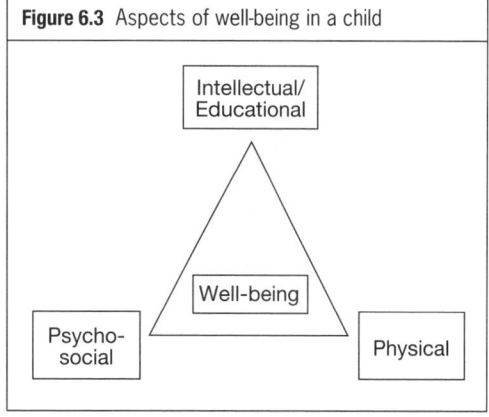

Figure 6.3 Aspects of well-being in a child

2 The school
   a Overcrowding
   b Poor learning ethos
   c Poor facilities.
3 The teacher
   a Absenteeism
   b Large learner allocations
   c Poor teaching methods
   d Poor learner/teacher relationships.

The parents

1 Inappropriate expectations
2 Poor home circumstances
   a Substance abuse
   b Family violence
   c Psychopathy
   d Disintegrating marriage etc.

The child

The approach to the child can also be considered as an interactive triad that includes physical well-being, psychosocial well-being and intellectual and educational development.

Physical well-being
1 The central nervous system
   a Sensory loss – hearing and vision
   b Epilepsy and associated complications
   c CNS diseases.
2 Systemic disease – this includes chronic conditions that may interfere with general well-being (e.g. asthma), pain (e.g. juvenile rheumatoid arthritis), poor oxygenation of the brain (cyanotic heart conditions) or poor sleep (chronic upper airway obstruction).

Psychosocial well-being
1 Affective (depression)/anxiety disorders
2 Personality/behavioural disorders
3 Substance abuse
4 School refusal/phobias
5 Deprived/unsupervised children
6 Hungry children
7 Children sent to school too young/not school ready.

School phobia

The main feature of school refusal is reluctance to attend school, associated with anxiety and often depressed mood. The child appears frightened to go to school (hence phobia). In a Western European setting it was found to occur in some 3 per cent of 10- to 11-year-olds. The anxious, school-refusing child must be distinguished from the delinquent child not attending school.

Management of school phobia requires an emphasis on the following:
   ♦ Full assessment of the child with parents and teacher cooperating.
   ♦ Establish areas of stress that may be remediated (at school, in the home, or within the child – physical, emotional, or educational factors).
   ♦ Get the child to go to school again with support and as soon as possible.
   ♦ Treat ongoing problems.
   ♦ Medication is rarely necessary.

The longer the child stays away from school the more difficult it may be to treat and the poorer the general prognosis. It may be necessary for someone to accompany the child to school each day in the early stages of treatment.

Intellectual development

Global mental handicap

This is a common disorder with a prevalence in the developing world of eight to twelve per 1 000 children aged between three and ten years.

Cognitive delay from an early age results in a deficient ability to learn and adapt socially and presents with a global delay in achieving milestones. Mild degrees of retardation are frequently not recognized. Causes include birth asphyxia, intra-uterine infections, intracranial infections, congenital abnormalities, and brain damage due to status epilepticus. Important causes of mental handicap with recognizable facial features include Down's syndrome, fragile X-syndrome, fetal alcohol syndrome and hypothyroidism. In 65–75 per cent of cases no organic cause may be found. Co-morbidity often includes sensory deficits, language delay, neuromuscular deficits, convulsions and emotional problems. Regression of development is an indication of a progressive disorder, such as lipid storage disease.

The subtypes are mild (IQ 50 to 70), moderate (IQ 35 to 49), severe (IQ 20 to 34), and profound (IQ below 20).

Examination. A thorough clinical examination is essential. Dysmorphic features might suggest a chromosomal abnormality or hypothyroidism. It is imperative that hearing and sight are assessed, as many impaired children have been erroneously labelled as being cognitively delayed. It may be difficult to be sure of the degree of mental retardation in a young child and a firm prognosis should be avoided.

Management of the mentally retarded child entails the following:

 • Treat the child for any physical problems (e.g. epilepsy, contractures).
 • Counsel parents about the condition and social benefits. The need for genetic counselling may be of particular relevance here.
 • Encourage appropriate stimulation of the child.

 • Discuss education, where appropriate.
 • Follow up.

Much emotional support for the parents is necessary, and the worker therefore needs to be able to walk the long road beside the parents of a retarded child. Each milestone can be a major obstacle, demanding support and counsel for the parents. Anticipating problems may be helpful. A handicapped child puts tremendous strain on the marriage relationship and many marriages fail as a result. Adequate professional support may help to prevent family disintegration.

In focusing on the child it is important to dispel unrealistic expectations, which many parents have, but at the same time to provide a step-wise programme that challenges the child to achieve. Toilet training, personal care, and basic social skills are among the most important achievements for which to aim. It involves reinforcement of the positive aspects of intellect and behaviour and hence guidance towards these modest yet rewarding achievements. The younger the child, the more effective the therapy will be. It must furthermore be emphasized that mentally retarded girls require protection against sexual exploitation. Behaviour problems may require special behaviour modification therapy or medication. Symptom-oriented medication used for short periods can be useful. Mentally retarded children can also suffer from anxiety, depression, psychosis, compulsions, and epilepsy. All of these may respond well to medication, but the tendency towards polypharmacy needs to be resisted.

Learning disabilities

'Pure' learning disorders (LD)

These disorders must be seen as maturational and developmental problems and may occur despite a good educational foundation in a child with normal intelligence. They may occur as discreet disorders limited to one or more learning modality: arithmetic, reading, expressive or receptive language coordination, and others. Reading disorder (so-called dyslexia) may occur in about 5 per cent of children. These disorders are missed unless a careful history is taken and assessment is performed. Teachers should suspect it when a child has very poor performance in certain areas but in general appears intelligent. The diagnosis should be considered in any pre-school child with a specific developmental delay. An unrecognized LD may cause profound emotional difficulties, which in turn aggravate the problem. Early intervention is essential.

Management. Always be on the alert for learning disorders, and manage them as follows:

- Preferably have the problem defined by a remedial teacher or psychologist.
- Explain it to the parents and class teacher.
- Introduce a remedial programme – preferably home-based.
- Support the child emotionally.
- Follow up and monitor.

Attention deficit/hyperactivity disorders (ADHD)

Prevalence figures vary between 2–8 per cent. The main problem is an inability to give sustained attention appropriate for the child's age. Although these children may be able to concentrate on activities they enjoy (such as watching television and playing computer games) they cannot concentrate on matters that they perceive as boring or repetitive or are able to attend on demand. The lack of attention (attention deficit) may occur with greatly increased activity (hyperactivity). The child presents with a short attention span and is distractible, disinhibited, and poorly organized with extreme overactivity.

Hyperactivity is not always present, particularly when the child is in a strange environment. The attention deficit disorder without hyperactivity can easily be missed, as the child is usually not troublesome in the class or at home. Children in these latter groups do badly at school, like their hyperactive counterparts, but they tend to be withdrawn, anxious, socially isolated, and poor at sport. The diagnosis of ADHD and its subgroups are made based on the criteria as set out in the DSM IV.

Management of attention deficit/hyperactivity disorders is based on the following:

- Early diagnosis, including identification of a possible learning disorder.
- Special education allowing for short attention and severe distractibility.
- Behaviour modification techniques.
- Medication with methylphenidate or atomoxitine

A distinction must be made between *enuresis*, defined as persistence of voluntary, normal voiding of urine during sleep beyond the age of five years, and *incontinence*, the involuntary loss of small amounts of urine during wakefulness or sleep.

Bedwetting (enuresis)

Most children achieve day and night control of the bladder by four years of age. Bedwetting at night (nocturnal enuresis) is considered a problem after the child has reached a mental age of four to five years. It may be an isolated developmental problem. It can also be a very disturbing symptom to the child and the family, often resulting in punishment. Primary enuresis implies that a child has never had total bladder control. Secondary enuresis occurs when a child starts bedwetting again after attaining bladder control for more than six months. Secondary enuresis is often the result of emotional stress or a physical problem, such as diabetes mellitus, urinary tract infection or renal disease causing polyuria. Enuresis tends to run in families. Roughly 10 per cent of five-year-olds wet their beds, 5 per cent of 10-year-olds and 1–2 per cent continue into their teens. The older the child, the more active the intervention has to be to attain bladder control.

Management. Enuresis can be assumed to be non-organic (benign) if it is exclusively nocturnal and there are no other urinary symptoms (frequency, urgency, dysuria) and the urine analysis is normal. There is a tendency to spontaneous cure. When enuresis is a symptom of a disturbed family setting or underlying psychopathology, symptomatic treatment is unlikely to be successful if the root cause does not receive attention.

Educating the parents on the nature of the problem often relieves the tension appreciably. Reaffirm that there is no disease present. Coercion and a punitive attitude must be replaced with an understanding and systematic approach. A simple home programme has been shown to have considerable success. The home programme is based on:

General measures:

+ Quiet bedtime routine
+ Restrict fluid 1–2 hours before bedtime
+ Avoid caffeinated beverages (causes polyuria)
+ Bladder voiding before retiring
+ Waking to urinate at regular intervals during the night
+ Protection of bedding
+ Night light (to facilitate arousal and voiding in the toilet)
+ Psychological evaluation if necessary.

Specific measures:

+ Motivation (reward dry nights and self arousal)
+ Record dry nights
+ Increasing bladder capacity: Bladder capacity can be readily increased by holding back the urine for as long as possible and then voiding into a container (30 ml per year of age is a good guide to a reasonable bladder capacity). The bladder capacity can be increased by drinking large quantities of fluids during the early part of the day and holding the urine in as long as possible. Other than an occasional word of encouragement, this is best left to the child
+ Dry bed training (waking children at longer intervals)
+ Self-training to wake up when there is an urge to urinate: A firm decision must be made by the child when he or she goes to bed to wake up should the bladder be full. Initially it may be of help if the parents wake the child, provided that he or she is fully conscious of what is happening and has recall of the event on the next day
+ Medication (not before six years of age)
  a Imipramine (Tofranil®): A dose of 25 mg on retiring usually suffices though this can be doubled in the older child.
  b DDAVP (desmopressin)
  c Oxybutinin (Ditropan®)

It must be stressed that drug therapy in isolation is unlikely to have a lasting cure. It may have to be continued for several months, then gradually tailed off and preferably replaced with a placebo before discontinuation.

+ Alarm therapy (reward cooperation) – bell and pad system.

Encopresis

Encopresis involves voluntary or involuntary passage of faeces in places that are inappropriate for the social and cultural background of the child. Although this is a distressing symptom it is very uncommon in the paediatric population.

According to the DSM IV the diagnostic criteria for encopresis are:

1   Repeated passage of faeces into inappropriate places (e.g. clothing or floor) whether involuntary or intentional.
2   At least one such event a month for at least three months.
3   Chronological age is at least four years (or equivalent developmental level).
4   The behaviour is not due exclusively to the direct physiological effects of a substance or a general medical condition, except through a mechanism involving constipation.

A detailed history is necessary to obtain a clear picture of exactly when and under what circumstances the encopresis occurs. In each instance a careful clinical examination must be undertaken to rule out organic causes such as megacolon, which causes chronic constipation with 'overflow' incontinence. A rectal examination is obviously essential in each case. Fecal overflow as a complication of constipation is much more common and will be dealt with in Chapter 24. Primary neurological deficits such as spina bifida or cord lesions must be excluded.

Tic disorders (stereotyped movement disorders)

These include transient tics, chronic motor tics, Tourette's disorder, and atypical tics and stereotyped movement disorder. The presenting features are rapid movements of a group of functionally related skeletal muscles or an involuntary production of noises or words. These characteristics distinguish them from other movement disturbances, such as choreiform movements. In some instances there may be an association with emotional disturbances.

Management. If the tic is of short duration, a trial with anxiolytics may be useful. Low doses of antipsychotics (haloperidol) are useful. Methylphenidate will frequently worsen tics. Focus on the tic should be minimized to prevent it from becoming worse. Parental counselling is important. The more severe form of this disorder requires specialist attention.

Atypical stereotyped movement disorders

These include conditions such as head banging, rocking, and repetitive hand movements. They are distinguished from tics in that they involve voluntary or non-spasmodic movement and the patient is not usually distressed by the symptoms. Incidence is high in children with mental retardation, pervasive developmental disorder, and markedly inadequate social stimulation. It may also occur in the absence of mental disorder.

Head rolling starts usually at 6–10 months, and seldom occurs in children older than two years. It is usually harmless, but may be a sign of emotional deprivation, or loss of special sensations (deaf or blind).

Head banging usually occurs in the second year and seldom continues after three years of age. It is found more often in children with developmental delay, pervasive developmental disorder and loss of special sensation. It is probably a form of auto-stimulation.

Management. This involves a detailed assessment of the interaction between parents and child. Increased contact between mother and child, and parent counselling are often indicated. Increased stimulation may help the child. Parents require reassurance about the favourable outcome of treatment. A useful technique for controlling rocking and hand movements is to try to make these rhythmic motor habits purposeful by using music, dancing, hobby-horses, see-saws, swings, and so on. Problems may arise if rocking occurs in a profoundly mentally retarded child, but even here increased stimulation and the introduction of some purpose into the movements may help.

Stuttering

Stuttering or stammering may be accompanied by jerks, blinks, or tremors. The onset is usually before the age of 12 years and there may be a family history. Over 50 per cent of milder cases make a spontaneous and complete recovery. The child is distressed because of teasing and social ostracism by peers, experiences academic difficulties, and displays a reluctance to speak in class.

Management. As there is no consensus on the long-term efficacy of the various treatment modalities, management remains controversial. Modern approaches are based on the concept that the disorder is a learned form of behaviour. Most patients can be helped significantly through use of techniques such as speech therapy, and behaviour and individual therapy directed at reducing fears, pressures, and feelings of inadequacy.

Childhood sexuality and masturbation

Sex roles in the young child are acquired with the understanding that males and females differ and are reinforced by differences between the sexes in appearance, dress, behaviour, attitudes, and by parental expectations. Parents are generally the main models of appropriate sexual roles. Although cultural influences play a major role in this process, most pre-school children experience a period of sexual curiosity when interest in the genitalia of siblings and friends is common. In some cultures children tend to be open and spontaneous in their sexual behaviour, whereas in others their sexual activity or curiosity is suppressed by parents.

Children quickly discover the gratification that results from stimulation of the well-innervated external genitalia. Touching the penis with consequent erection and rubbing the vulva against a firm object are common practices in young children. Masturbation should be viewed with concern only if it becomes a persistent habit. In most children it is a passing phase.

Masturbation may become a frequent preoccupation in the deprived or seriously retarded child, or when harsh punitive measures have overemphasized the undesirability of this practice.

Emotional deprivation occasionally leads to the child expressing an uninhibited and affectionate attitude to relative strangers which may be interpreted as sexual precocity and has resulted in sexual abuse.

Precocious and/or persistent aberrant sexual behaviour must raise the suspicion of sexual abuse (*see* Chapter 5, Social paediatrics).

Management. This must take into account the developmental level of the child. In the very young it tends to be effective because the habit is not well established. Spontaneous remissions are common in infants, most of whom grow up to be normal unless the situation is mismanaged. Parents' attitudes need to be assessed and they should be assured of the innocuousness of the habit. Boredom must be considered a contributory factor, as must be the possibility of irritations such as may be caused by tight clothing.

In young children, opportunities for masturbation should be reduced and the child's energy channelled into other physical activities. Sex education for the child may be necessary, during which it is useful to mention that masturbation is an infantile habit. Urethral irritation, urinary frequency, and pruritus may be present and require treatment. With correct management masturbation can be discouraged, particularly if a constructive pastime can be suggested. Whenever it is a presenting symptom, careful enquiry should be made into any contributory emotional factors. A simple explanation of the harmless nature of this habit with appropriate parental guidance is all that is required in the vast majority of cases.

The pre-school child often develops a natural interest in the genitalia of the opposite sex but parents are inclined to over-react and interpret this normal development as perversion or deviation. A matter-of-fact approach is sometimes all that is required.

During adolescence, sexual feelings constitute a period of renewed awareness and heterosexual interest. Many find it difficult to discuss these within the confines of the family, with the result that guidance and support are often not obtained. Lack of appropriate education in a community, particularly during cultural change, has resulted in a wave of adolescent pregnancies, giving rise to large numbers of unwanted infants.

Anxiety disorders (neurotic and emotional)

These are common disorders among children. Heightened anxiety varies according to the age of the child. Symptoms include fearfulness, misery, unhappiness, sensitivity, shyness, relationship problems, and separation anxiety. In adolescence, somatoform disorders with physi-cal symptoms are quite common. Anxiety may be severe and affect the child's performance socially and at school.

Management involves the following aspects:
- Detailed assessment is necessary, with careful exclusion of physical pathology.
- Therapy usually must involve both the parents and the child.
- Provide specific treatment of physical or educational problems.
- Medication – short term with anxiolytics or long term with antidepressants – may prove useful.
- Refer the child to a main centre for review if there is no improvement in a few months.

Depression

This is part of the group of mood disorders (affective disorders) not unlike those seen in adults. However, children may present with different symptoms and signs from adults. Mania is less common in young children than in adolescents.

Before puberty, the prevalence of depressive disorder ranges from about 2 to 4 per cent. After puberty it approaches the prevalence in adults. The cause may be hereditary with a biological vulnerability.

Depression may be precipitated by bereavement or environmental stress such as family break-up due to divorce. On the other hand, there may be underlying emotional problems such as anxiety.

The essential features are depressed mood, sadness, tearfulness, loss of energy, self-blame, and feelings of guilt. There are often changes in the sleep and appetite pattern, which may be increased or decreased. Misery may be expressed as physical symptoms. In adolescents, psychotic symptoms such as auditory hallucinations may occur.

Management must include the following:
- Make a detailed assessment with careful exclusion of physical pathology.
- Treat the child for specific areas of stress.
- Provide family counselling.
- Antidepressant medication may be useful and should be maintained for several months.

Caution – tricyclic antidepressants taken in overdose can be lethal.

◆ Where there is suicidal behaviour or if there is no significant response to treatment within five to six weeks, it is imperative to refer the child to an expert.

Child abuse and neglect

(*See* Chapter 5, Social paediatrics.)

Common psychological and behavioural problems at age eleven to fourteen years

Conduct disorders

Conduct disorders are characterized by anti-social behaviour. There is a persistent pattern of conduct in which the basic rights of others are violated or major age-appropriate societal norms or rules transgressed. The problems must have existed for six months or longer. Conduct disorders are the most common psychiatric disorders in older children. British statistics show the prevalence to be between 4 and 12 per cent of young adolescents with the condition being twice as common in boys.

Common features are aggressive behaviour, theft, vandalism, arson, truancy, drug abuse, and aberrant sexual behaviour.

Conduct problems may occur as a group activity or as solitary physical aggression.

Management. The only really useful forms of treatment are family and behaviour therapy, which call for expert guidance. The intervention will be long, trying, and arduous, but the prognosis is not hopeless. Conduct disorders frequently occur together with other problems, such as learning disorders or attention deficit disorders (*see above*), which must be treated at the same time. Medication has a small place, for instance in attention deficit disorder. Enforced institutionalization should only be a last resort.

Suicidal behaviour

Suicide threats or behaviour should never be taken lightly as just 'attention seeking' or 'a cry for help'. Depression and conduct disorders each account for approximately 50 per cent of these children and adolescents. Presentation ranges from a well-planned, potentially lethal, failed suicide attempt, through unplanned impulsive acts of low potential danger, to threats of suicide.

The assessment should always include an evaluation of the risk of a repeat, and possibly successful, attempt. Disorders such as depression, psychosis, and drug abuse should be identified and attended to. In the evaluation, predisposing, precipitating, perpetuating, and protective factors must be identified for which an interview with the parents is essential. A common scenario is a disagreement between the teenager and parent followed by the impulsive taking of tablets or a household cleaner. Simply facilitating communication may go a long way to restoring a positive relationship. Good supportive work can be done by lay people in this field and societal structures should be used.

Psychotic disorders

'Psychotic' means that a patient is out of touch with reality. The main features are disorientation, memory loss, and inability to do simple intellectual tasks. It is important to exclude organic causes, such as typhoid and other infections, brain tumours, substance abuse, and epilepsy. Apart from therapy for these specific causes, management of psychotic disorders is in the realm of specialists.

Substance abuse

(*See* Chapter 5, Social paediatrics.)

Teenage pregnancy and abortion

(*See* Chapter 5, Social paediatrics.)

Violence, children, and mental health

Children are unavoidably a part of this violent community. In no way can this be called a normal society. The evil effects of racism, educational deprivation, and more recently the 15 years of sporadic violence have taken a tragic toll on the mental health of a generation. These factors need to be considered for every disorder covered in this chapter, and for the treatment of many of them.

There is an urgent need to establish community-based, easily accessible, walk-in child and family help centres where preventive and rehabilitative mental health principles will be applied; where educational problems can be addressed; and where help can be given to people to restore stable family life and to maintain the integrity of the family. Present structures can be used for this purpose. Professionals can join with lay people and youth groups in mass action to provide dignity and hope.

PART 3

Neonatal paediatrics

7

Care of the newborn

The first 28 days of life constitute the newborn period. The baby is very vulnerable during this time when adaptations to extra-uterine life take place. This is seen in the respiratory and gastro-intestinal systems, in the haemodynamics of the cardiovascular system, and in the kidneys and the liver, which have to take on the full excretory and metabolic functions that were shared by the placenta during intra-uterine existence.

These illnesses are frequently associated with problems during the pregnancy, during delivery, or during neonatal care and can therefore be prevented. Furthermore, many neonatal illnesses present in a somewhat different way to those of older children. Early identification of possible illness, and appropriate and timely intervention decrease the risk of morbidity and mortality.

The high-risk pregnancy

There are a number of conditions during pregnancy, labour, and delivery in which serious neonatal problems must be anticipated. Early identification of these conditions is the first step in the prevention of neonatal illness, thus reducing morbidity and mortality. They include

Approximately 15 per cent of newborn babies require more than routine care as a result of illness after birth.

poor socio-economic conditions, an adolescent or single mother without a stable partner, and a history of abortions, stillbirths, low birth weight, complicated deliveries, neonatal deaths, and congenital abnormalities.

Evaluation of the current pregnancy includes: the duration of pregnancy; smoking and substance abuse during pregnancy; maternal blood group; counselling and testing for HIV with a plan of preventative management for the baby if necessary; syphilis serology; maternal diseases such as diabetes, cardiac, and renal; pregnancy-related illnesses such as hypertension, abruptio placentae, and placenta praevia; and abnormal maternal weight gain. Labour and birth details must include the duration of the stages of labour and of membrane rupture, the amount and character of liquor, drugs administered to the mother during labour and delivery, and the need for and extent of resuscitation of the baby.

Once a high-risk pregnancy and/or fetus are identified, the progress of labour and delivery must be carefully monitored, and appropriate action taken. Optimal management of these babies requires good communication between those caring principally for the mother and the delivery, and those responsible for the baby. Birth asphyxia is probably the most common neonatal condition associated with a high-risk pregnancy, and therefore skilled resuscitation and correct equipment and drugs are essential. Factors associated with, and which identify, the high-risk pregnancy are outlined in Table 7.1.

Delivery room management

Initial examination, resuscitation, and management in the delivery room

The temperature of the delivery room must be suitable for the baby, i.e. 23 to 28 °C, and must be free of draughts. If the liquor is meconium-stained on delivery of the head, the mouth is suctioned gently. Following a normal delivery, the cord is probably best clamped after the infant has uttered its first cry. On the other hand, early clamping facilitates rapid resuscitation of the asphyxiated newborn.

The aim of the immediate physical examination at this stage is to determine whether or not the baby needs to be resuscitated. This is assessed by using the Apgar score at one minute and at five minutes after birth (*see* Table 7.2).

The first score indicates the possible need for immediate intervention, and the second score, at five minutes, gives an indication of the response to resuscitation.

It must also be ascertained whether the baby is normal. The examination is restricted to gross physical abnormalities and is therefore rapid and simple.

If the baby is well at delivery, the cord is clamped and cut. The baby is then warmly wrapped and handed to the mother for the first feed. Vitamin K, 1 mg, is best given later together with the procedures of eye prophylaxis and identification of the baby.

Table 7.1 Factors identifying the high-risk pregnancy

Maternal	Labour and delivery	Fetal
Obstetric	Maternal hypertension	Oligohydramnios
Elderly primigravida	Maternal hypotension	Polyhydramnios
Anaemia	Maternal sedation	Multiple pregnancy
Poor weight gain, obesity	Prolonged rupture of membranes	Fetal distress (acidosis, meconium-
Previous abruption	Prolonged first or second stage	stained liquor, abnormal FHR)
Previous assisted delivery	Caesarean section	Growth retardation
Poor obstetric history (stillbirth,	Breech	Post-maturity
>2 abortions)	Cord compression	Malformations
Previous LBW	Precipitate delivery	
Neonatal birth	Preterm labour	
Illness: diabetes, cardiac, renal	Forceps or vacuum extraction	
Pregnancy-induced hypertension		
Social		
Age <16 >35 years		
Socio-economic deprivation		
Alcohol consumption		
Smoking		
Child with cerebral palsy		

Table 7.2 Apgar score

Sign/score	0	1	2
Heart rate	Absent	<100	>100
Respiratory effort	Absent	Slow, irregular	Good, crying
Muscle tone, movement	Limp	Some flexion	Active
Response to nasal catheter	Nil	Grimace or sneeze	Cry
Colour	Pale, central cyanosis	Body pink, extremities blue	All pink

Birth asphyxia and resuscitation

Failure to initiate spontaneous, sustained respiration after delivery is called birth asphyxia, and can result in severe hypoxia. Fetal hypoxia refers to inadequate oxygenation before delivery. This may predispose to birth asphyxia.

Hypoxia during labour in term babies is the most common cause of neonatal brain damage and is the leading cause of cerebral palsy in the developing world.

Consequences of severe hypoxia

Although the *clinical manifestations of perinatal hypoxia* are, in the first instance, neurological in nature, less obvious effects on other organs, such as the lungs and the kidneys, may manifest during the ensuing days. Hypoxia, hypercapnia, and acidaemia cause tissue injury. Clinical manifestations of the cerebral insult are those of hypoxic ischaemic encephalopathy (HIE). Acidaemia itself affects the myocardium, with a consequent drop in cardiac output. The combination of hypoxia, acidaemia, and hypotension can affect the lungs, kidneys, gut, and liver. Metabolic disturbances such as hypoglycaemia, hyperglycaemia, hypercalcaemia, and inappropriate antidiuretic hormone secretion may occur. There may also be clotting disturbances resulting in disseminated intravascular coagulation.

Neonates with severe asphyxia who have not established sustained respiration after 20 minutes almost always develop signs of severe HIE with a poor long-term outcome.

Less common causes include profound lung pathology as in hyaline membrane disease or meconium aspiration, severe anaemia, and some of the congenital malformations. Occasionally severe immaturity or primary muscle disease is responsible. Excessive suctioning may result in reflex apnoea.

Factors causing delay in the onset of respiration at birth are intra-uterine hypoxia, trauma to the brain, and drugs depressing the respiratory centre.

Labour ward management of resuscitation

Ideally, every birth should be attended by a health professional skilled in neonatal resuscitation. In order to effect rapid and efficient resuscitation, all the necessary equipment must be available and in working order at all times (*see* Table 7.3).

Furthermore, adequate facilities for keeping the neonate warm must be at hand. The resuscitation procedure is outlined in Figure 7.1.

Every attendant should be able to administer basic resuscitation by:
- Ensuring warmth and NOT allowing hyperthermia to occur
- Administering oxygen – 100% oxygen is given and as soon as colour improves the oxygen should be reduced to room air
- Applying gentle nasopharyngeal suction, if indicated
- Administering mask ventilation
- Administering naloxone, when indicated
- Commencing intravenous therapy for shock
- Undertaking external cardiac massage for bradycardia.

Table 7.3 Equipment required on resuscitation trolley

Laryngoscope – straight blade, plastic (e.g. Penlon®), infant size, spare batteries and bulbs

Magill's forceps – paediatric size

Endotracheal tubes sizes 2.5; 3.0; and 3.5 mm

Neonatal Ambu-bag® and mask

Suction catheters sizes 8 FG and 6 FG

Umbilical catheters sizes 8 FG and 6 FG – to be used only if peripheral intravenous line is not possible

Feeding tubes sizes 8 FG and 6 FG

Adhesive tape

Dextrostix®

Intravenous fluids 5% dextrose, 5% dextrose in 0.2% saline, 4% albumen

Syringes and needles of different sizes

Blood culture bottles, specimen containers and tubes

Ampoules of 50% dextrose

Ampoules of 4% sodium bicarbonate

Naloxone

Figure 7.1 Flow diagram of the resuscitation procedure

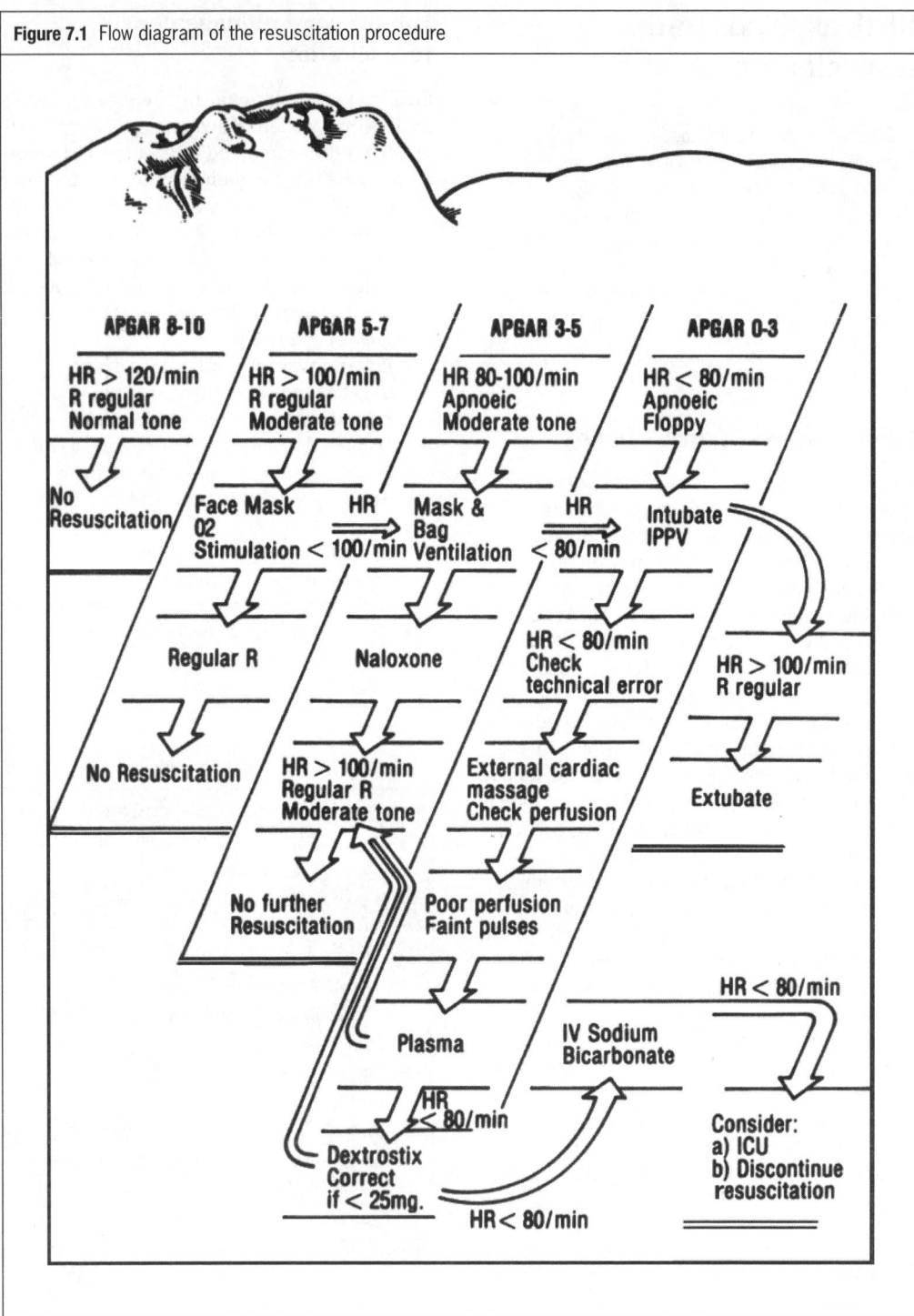

Advanced resuscitation skills require that staff are trained in intubating the newborn baby.

Immediate intermittent positive pressure ventilation (IPPV) by mask or via endotracheal tube is essential for the neonate who is floppy, pale, breathes poorly and has a heart rate of less than 80 beats per minute. Intubation must be preceded by clearing the airway of mucus, blood, or meconium, under direct laryngoscopy. The baby must be kept dry and warm during this procedure.

Routine suctioning of the pharynx is not indicated if there are clear secretions, as irritation by blind, vigorous suction may precipitate laryngospasm, apnoea, and bradycardia.

The infant who does not respond to resuscitation

If the response to resuscitation is poor but the baby is otherwise normal in appearance, technical or mechanical problems must first be excluded (*see* Table 7.4).

Whenever possible, a chest radiograph must exclude severe underlying lung disease. Only after all the above conditions have been excluded, and drug depression is not a possible contributing factor, is it appropriate to discontinue life-support.

Care following resuscitation

Ongoing care of the infant who required resuscitation is very important.
* Monitor the temperature (avoid hyperthermia).
* Monitor the blood sugar level.
* Maintain a clear airway by oropharyngeal suction.

> The infant who becomes pink and has a good cardiac output with IPPV, but is unable to maintain respiration after 20 minutes is suffering from severe hypoxic damage, drug depression, metabolic acidosis, and/or shock.

* Give oxygen when necessary.
* Tube feeding is advisable until the baby is stable.
* Observe for developing complications.

Persistent cyanosis in the presence of a metabolic acidosis suggests the development of persistent pulmonary hypertension.

Enlarging kidneys, decrease in urine output, and the presence of blood or protein in the urine suggest renal damage.

Disturbances of tone or subtle convulsions herald the onset of hypoxic ischaemic encephalopathy (HIE)

The normal newborn

Examination of the newborn

> The aims of the first routine physical examination of the baby are to:
> - Assess the baby's gestational age.
> - Ensure that the baby is not acutely ill.
> - Establish a baseline of normality and identify any abnormality of development.

Table 7.4 The infant who does not respond to resuscitation	
Technical problem	**Possible solution**
No air entry	Oxygen tube is disconnected, the endotracheal tube is kinked or blocked with secretions: must replace tube
Breath sounds are unequal in the lungs	Endotracheal tube is probably placed in the right main bronchus: withdraw tube till breath sounds symmetrical
Unequal breath sounds with a displaced apex beat	Pneumothorax: confirmed by an urgent chest X-ray or transillumination An intercostal drain must be inserted if the diagnosis is confirmed
Diminished breath sounds and chest movements	Misplaced endotracheal tube in the oesophagus: replace

A thorough physical examination is carried out at a convenient moment soon after birth, preferably in the presence of the mother. The examiner's hands should be warm and disinfected, and care must be taken to avoid hypothermia during the examination. After this examination, the normal baby need not be re-examined until just before discharge, when the weight and any unusual findings are noted.

Birth weight and gestational age

The routine physical examination of the various systems is best performed after the baby has been fed, and each system should be observed and examined. The examination can proceed systematically from the head downwards.

It is essential that all findings should be evaluated in terms of normal and abnormal, and it is also important to know and recognize the normal appearances and values for the newborn, which are as follows:

- *Low birth weight* is a birth weight of less than 2 500 g.
- *A preterm infant* is one born prior to 37 weeks' gestation (259 days).
- *Underweight for gestational age* (UGA) or *light for dates* (LFD) is a birth weight below the 10th centile for that period of gestation.
- *Overweight for gestational age* (OGA) or *heavy for dates* (HFD) is a birth weight above the 90th centile for that period of gestation.

The gestational age (GA) is estimated by determining the Ballard Score as illustrated in Figure 7.2.

The appropriate weight for the gestational age that is determined in this way is obtained from the Lubchenco chart (*see* Figure 7.3), which gives standards for size at birth. All those between the 10th and 90th percentile are appropriate-for-gestational-age (AGA) babies.

- Average weight: male 3 400 g, female 3 000 g
- Average length: 48 cm (range 46 to 52 cm)
- Average head circumference: 35 cm (range 33 to 37 cm)
- Respiratory rate: 40 to 60/min
- Heart rate: average 140 beats/min (range 120 to 160/min).

The full-term infant is fairly active, moves all four limbs, has a good tone, and a pink colour. The typical term infant's posture is that of the fetal position with flexion at hips, knees and elbows. For additional information on the details of examination, *see* Chapter 1, History-taking, physical examination, and evaluation of the sick child. Only those aspects unique to the newborn are dealt with here.

Skin of the normal newborn

The skin is covered with a thick, white substance, vernix caseosa. It is not necessary to wipe or rub this off.

Stork bites, or telangiectatic naevi (fine spider-like naevi), may be present over the nape of the neck, the glabella, and the upper eyelids. They are deep pink and flat, blanch easily and disappear during the first years of life.

The *mongolian spot* is an irregular area of blue-grey slate pigmentation distributed over the sacral and gluteal regions. It may, however, be so extensive that it involves much of the infant's back.

Milia are white pinpoint spots over the bridge of the nose, chin, or cheeks and are caused by retained sebum.

Erythema toxicum are small macules on a red base starting on the second or third day of life and disappearing within a few days. The cause is unknown.

Transient pustular melanosis is an eruption that may be present at birth as small non-erythematous vesiculopustules, which rapidly scale and form hyperpigmented macules that fade in a few weeks. These are sterile lesions and antibiotics are not indicated.

Head

Moulding of the head depends on the type of delivery, leading to overlapping of the sutures of the parietal, frontal, and occipital bones, and corrects itself. Asymmetrical moulding of the face occurs as a result of the intrauterine position of the baby during pregnancy.

Caput succedaneum is a soft, non-fluctuant swelling due to oedema of the presenting part of the scalp caused by pressure during delivery.

Mouth, tongue, palate, and teeth

Occasionally babies are born with one or two teeth, which should be removed. Epstein's pearls

Figure 7.2 Assessment of gestational age using the Ballard Score

Neuromuscular maturity

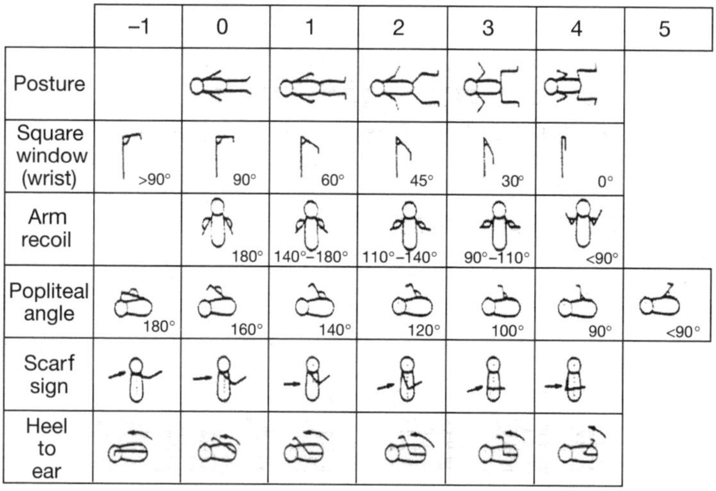

	−1	0	1	2	3	4	5
Posture							
Square window (wrist)	>90°	90°	60°	45°	30°	0°	
Arm recoil		180°	140°–180°	110°–140°	90°–110°	<90°	
Popliteal angle	180°	160°	140°	120°	100°	90°	<90°
Scarf sign							
Heel to ear							

Physical maturity

	−1	0	1	2	3	4	5
Skin	sticky friable transparent	gelatinous red, translucent	smooth pink, visible veins	superficial peeling &/ rash, few veins	cracking pale areas rare veins	parchment deep crackling veins	leathery cracked wrinkled
Lanugo	none	sparse	abudant	thinning	bald areas	mostly bald	
Plantar surface	heel – toe 40–50mm: −1 <40mm: −2	>50mm no crease	faint red marks	anterior transverse crease only	creases ant.2/3	creases over entire sole	
Breast	imperceptible	barely perceptible	flat areola no bud	stippled areola 1–2mm bud	raised areola 3–4mm bud	full areola 5–10mm bud	
Eye/Ear	lids fused loosely: −1 tightly: −2	lids open pinna flat stays folded	sl. curved pinna soft slow recoil	well-curved pinna, soft but ready recoil	formed & firm instant recoil	thick cartilage ear stiff	
Genitals male	scrotum flat, smooth	scrotum empty, faint rugae	testes in upper canal rare rugae	testes descending few rugae	testes down good rugae	testes pendulous deep rugae	
Genitals female	clitoris prominent labia flat	prominent clitoris small labia minora	prominent clitoris enlarging minora	majora & minora equally prominent	majora large minora small	majora cover clitoris & minora	

Maturity rating

score	weeks
−10	20
−5	22
0	24
5	26
10	28
15	30
20	32
25	34
30	36
35	38
40	40
45	42
50	44

Source: JL Ballard et al. Pediatrics 1991; 119:417–423. Copyright American Academy of Pediatrics.

Figure 7.3 Combined intra-uterine growth chart for height, weight and head circumference (OFC)

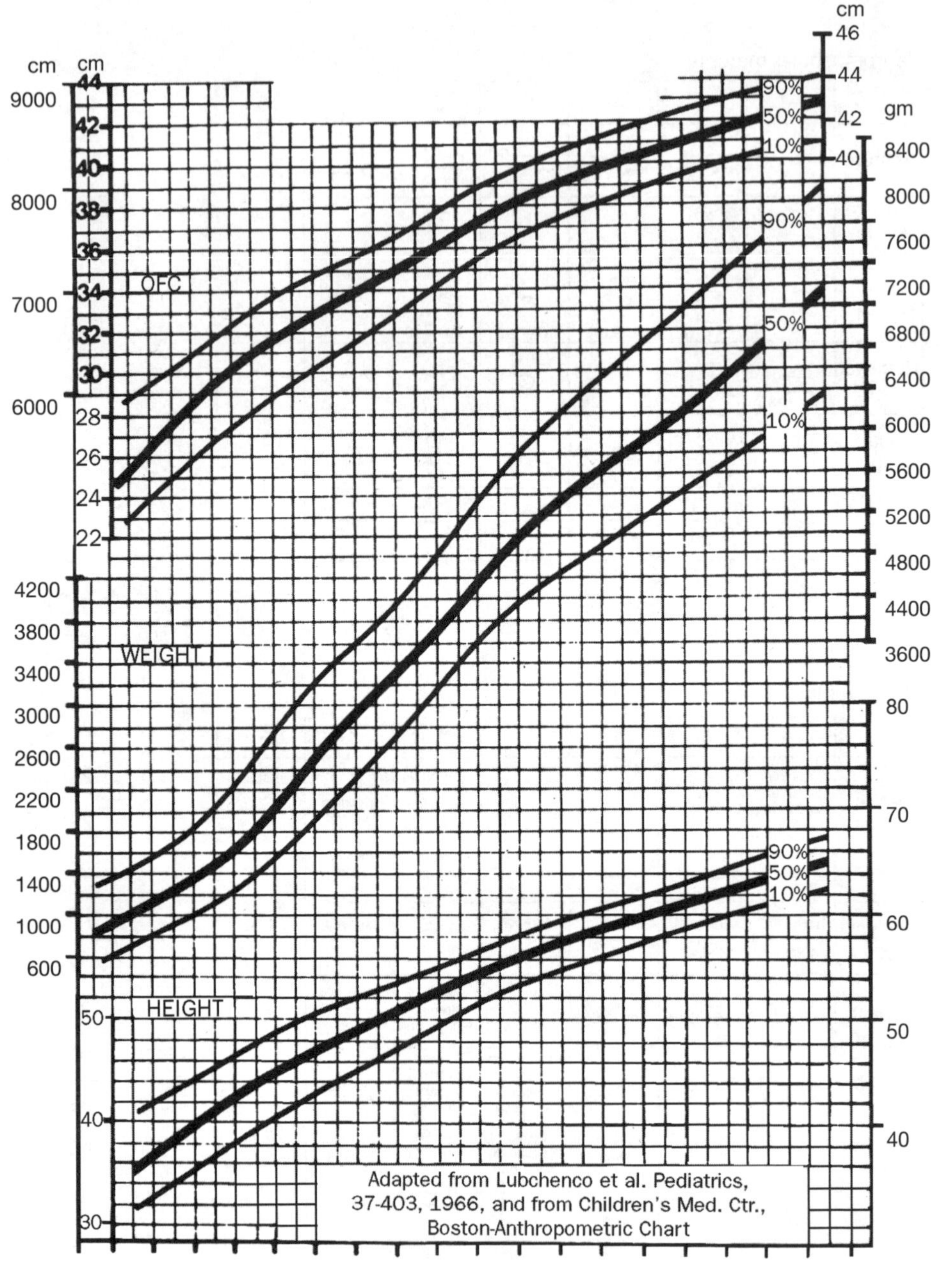

Adapted from Lubchenco et al. Pediatrics,
37-403, 1966, and from Children's Med. Ctr.,
Boston-Anthropometric Chart

Source: Lubchenco, L.O., 'Intrauterine growth charts', Pediatrics, vol. 37, no. 3, p. 403. Copyright American Academy of Pediatrics.

are small white nodules on the hard palate on either side of the midline. Retention cysts may occur on the gum margins. A partial cleft of the posterior soft palate has to be excluded by palpation.

Eyes

Redness of the conjunctiva and oedema of the eyelids due to chemical irritation are common and subconjunctival haemorrhages may be seen following a difficult delivery.

Neurological system

A number of primitive reflexes can be elicited in the newborn and young infant.

Abnormal responses include an absent or asymmetric response, or persistence of a reflex after the age at which it usually disappears.

The neurological examination is similar to that of older infants, but the plantar reflex always shows a Babinski (upgoing) response. The vision of a newborn infant is assessed by its ability to follow a face or a bright light, or by the

Table 7.5 Neonatal primitive reflexes			
Reflex	**Method of eliciting**	**Response**	**Disappearance**
Grasp reflex	Place finger in either the palm of the hand from the ulnar side or the sole of the foot	Reflex flexion and grasping of the finger from 26 weeks gestational age	4–6 months of age
Rooting reflex	Stroke the cheek with the finger or mother strokes with the nipple	Turning of the infant's head to the side of the stimulus and opening of the mouth for insertion of the nipple. It develops from 28 weeks' gestational age	4–6 months of age
Stepping/ placing reflexes	Stimulate the dorsum of the foot by bringing it in contact with the edge of a table or couch	The foot is raised and placed on the table or couch	4–6 months of age
Moro reflex	Sudden supported extension movement of the head in relation to the position of the spine	Extension and abduction of the arms and legs, followed by adduction of the arms and flexion of the elbows and fingers across the chest. It develops from 28 weeks gestational age	4–6 months of age
Sucking reflex	Place baby's hand in the mouth or offer mother's breast	Strong sucking response in the term infant, rather weaker in the preterm. Becomes well coordinated with swallowing. It develops from 34 to 35 weeks' gestational age	Becomes a voluntary response
Asymmetric tonic neck reflex	Infant spine and head should be aligned. The head is turned slowly to one side	Extensor tone occurs in the arm on the side to which the head is turned and flexor tone in the opposite arm. Reflex appears by 35 weeks	7 months of age

opticokinetic response. Response to a noise by a startle reaction suggests hearing ability.

Routine care of the healthy term newborn

Following delivery room procedures, the baby should be with the mother:
- To encourage breastfeeding, and
- To promote her observation and caring skills in keeping baby warm, dry and clean. The cord must be kept clean and dry by repeated application of an alcohol solution. Attention to drying the skin folds is essential, as moisture readily permits monilial infection.

Clothing should be changed daily, with meticulous washing, rinsing, and drying of garments.

The biggest danger of infection arises from the contaminated hands of hospital staff members, so routine hand-washing or spraying with a disinfectant before handling any baby is very important.

Urine should be passed within the first 24 hours and stool within 36 hours of birth. The latter is in the form of meconium for two to three days and is followed by a transitional stool, which is green to black with milk curds for several days; after one week the normal non-offensive soft, yellow, acid stools appear.

The normal infant loses up to 10 per cent of body weight in the first few days but usually regains this within 10 days. The rate of weight gain thereafter is in the range of 200–300 g per week. Breastfeeding difficulties must be anticipated and managed with expertise to foster the mother's confidence and success (*see* Chapter 9, Feeding of infants and young children).

Routine care of the healthy low birth weight baby

Ideally, all LBW infants should be assessed for special care. Some need intensive care, but these facilities are rarely freely available in developing countries. Apart from efficient primary health care, emphasis should be placed on meticulous routine nursing care, which in itself achieves a great deal for these special infants. Sophisticated monitoring and life-support systems make a negligible contribution to overall survival, while making crippling demands on personnel and the budget.

The management of the healthy preterm baby is relatively simple, requiring very basic facilities and careful nursing.
- Minimal handling is important, especially if ill. Minor procedures such as a nappy change may result in a sharp drop in oxygen saturation. Traumatic procedures should be kept to a minimum and in the event of apnoea, bradycardia, or hypoxaemia occurring the procedure should be terminated.
- Meticulous monitoring of the respiration rate, heart rate, colour, peripheral perfusion, and temperature with timely intervention in the case of abnormalities improves the overall prognosis for the small baby. The blood sugar level should be monitored regularly until feeding is established and maintained in the range 2–7.5 mmol/l.
- Maintenance of a normal body temperature is the first and most important step in the management. Day and night skin-to-skin contact with the mother has been shown to be very effective both in the prevention and management of hypothermia. More sophisticated equipment can be used where available.
- Early feeding, either orally or by gavage, is the next stage of management. Frequent small feeds or continuous nasogastric drip feeds are essential to avoid complications, starting with a total of 60 ml/kg/day and increasing by 25 ml daily to 200 ml/kg/day if tolerated.
- Intravenous feeding is advisable for the sick preterm baby, giving 60 ml/kg/day on day one, and gradually increasing the volume to 150 ml/kg/day. Factors that increase insensible water loss, such as tachypnoea and high ambient temperature (overhead warmer, phototherapy), need to be taken into account in calculating fluid requirements.

Healthy newborn babies should not be kept in hospital or separated from their mothers.

- The signs of respiratory distress must be noted and oxygen administered for cyanosis. The airway must be kept clear at all times by correct positioning. Apnoeic episodes must be recognized early for appropriate management.
- Particular attention must be paid to measures that prevent infection. Staff hand hygiene is crucial if cross-infection and hospital-acquired infection are to be controlled. Regular hand-washing before and after handling each baby, and spraying the hands with a 70% alcohol solution are essential.
- Even mild degrees of jaundice must receive consideration if bilirubin encephalopathy is to be avoided.
- Haemoglobin levels must be checked serially at weekly intervals, starting on the first day.

Once the clinical condition of the infant is stabilized, and life-threatening complications of the first few days of life adequately dealt with, the preterm baby is observed, while taking continued precautions against infection. Great patience and considerable time are required to support the mother in establishing breastfeeding. Monitoring weight gain will assist in evaluating the baby's wellbeing. The environmental temperature can be decreased gradually, bearing in mind that failure to gain weight is often an early sign of undue heat loss. Promoting mother and baby contact to establish bonding is an important aspect of preterm care. The multiplicity of procedures and apparatus in the nursery are often intimidating for the mother, who is at risk of withdrawing from involvement with her baby.

The process of bonding must be fostered carefully, as failure may result in maternal rejection and reluctance to breastfeed and cuddle the baby. Lack of maternal cooperation and interest in the baby are features suggestive of rejection. Any indication of this must be handled sensitively. Where facilities exist, professional counselling must be called for.

The baby is ready for discharge when:
- Breast feeding has been fully established.
- Temperature is maintained.
- Weight gain of about 1 per cent of body mass per day is occurring.

- The suitable weight for discharge should be determined individually, depending to some extent on available health services and conditions at the unit of delivery. Earlier discharge is possible with kangaroo mother care.
- The mother has been counselled on general care and hygiene, particularly with regard to washing hands, signs of illness, breastfeeding, preparation of the oral rehydration fluid, and fertility control.
- The mother has been familiarized with the most convenient primary health care facility for continued maternal and child care with the Road-to-Health-Card.
- Routine BCG and polio immunization have been given.

These aspects must receive particular emphasis in mothers who are at risk, such as:
- Adolescents
- Those with a poor obstetric history
- Those who have received counselling regarding antiretroviral therapy.

Wherever possible, home visits should be arranged. The mother and preterm baby must be seen by an experienced health worker within a week of discharge.

'Kangaroo mother care' of low birth weight babies

'Kangaroo mother care' or 'skin-to-skin contact' is a simple, cost-effective method of keeping clinically stable, small preterm infants warm. The mother places her baby on her chest under protective clothing. This technique reduces crying and promotes early breastfeeding by early initiation of non-nutritive sucking. Kangaroo mothercare units are being established worldwide to provide supervised environments where mothers can be supported in caring for their low birth weight babies before they are ready to be discharged home. Such babies tend to breastfeed for longer periods, gain weight more readily, and

> The prevalence of low-birth-weight (LBW) infants is a reflection of the health status of the community.

are ready to leave the hospital sooner. Of course, fathers may also give their babies kangaroo care.

In highly developed countries no more than 7 per cent of births fall into this category, whereas in some underprivileged communities more than 30 per cent of infants weigh less than 2 500 g at birth. The majority of infants in the former group are truly preterm, whereas intra-uterine growth restriction makes a considerable contribution to the latter. LBW constitutes up to 74 per cent of perinatal mortality, and the risk of dying during the first year of life is 20 times greater in LBW than in appropriately grown infants. They also tend to grow up to be malnourished, develop into short-statured adults, and in turn produce LBW infants. Major factors contributing to LBW infants are:

- Poor socio-economic circumstances
- Low maternal weight
- Adolescent pregnancy
- Short birth intervals
- Physical exertion late into pregnancy
- Low-grade amniotic fluid infection. This is more prevalent in undernourished mothers and those who practise unprotected coitus (without condom) during pregnancy.

In a large referral hospital one must anticipate 12–20 per cent of births to be LBW.

The high-risk neonate

Morbidity and mortality are appreciably reduced by identifying risk factors both during pregnancy and after birth. All babies born from a high-risk pregnancy or labour, as well as those outlined in Table 7.6, must be considered high-risk neonates. The next step is careful observation during the first few days or weeks and careful follow-up for long-term complications.

Transport of the high-risk patient

Once the high-risk mother or baby has been identified and the immediate needs assessed, the question of transfer to a referral centre arises. Transport of the fetus is preferable *in utero*, but delivery during transportation is hazardous. Active maternal haemorrhage and fetal distress are contra-indications to transporting the mother in labour until appropriately managed by maternal and fetal resuscitation.

Conditions requiring transfer of the mother before delivery include eclampsia, severe pregnancy-induced hypertension, abruptio placentae, multiple pregnancy, significant maternal disease, and poly- or oligohydramnios.

The referral centre should always be informed before transferring any patient. The escort must have adequate knowledge of the baby's condition and must be able to care for the baby during transit.

The infant must be in a reasonably stable condition to withstand the rigours of transport. Therefore hypothermia, hypoglycaemia, and hypotension should be corrected. A nasogastric tube should be passed. Monitoring equipment, such as a saturation monitor and infusion controller, are advisable. However, these may not be available and clinical monitoring will be necessary.

The following precautions must be taken in transit:

- Ensure a clear airway.
- Ensure that suction and oxygen are available.
- Prevent heat loss during transfer; skin-to-skin contact with the mother is most efficient, but at times a transport incubator is preferable.
- Monitor colour, respiration, and heart rate.
- Monitor the drip rate and volume control if an intravenous line has been established.
- Ensure that appropriate medical information accompanies the patient.

Table 7.4 Factors identifying the neonate at risk	
High risk	**Medium risk**
Pre-term or post-mature	Birth weight
Small for gestational age	1.5–2.49 kg
Large for gestational age	Clinically stable
Birth weight	after resuscitation
<1.5 kg or >4 kg	Birth trauma
Neurological depression	Abnormal CNS signs
after resuscitation	Cold exposure
Metabolic problems	Low blood sugar
after birth	Jaundice
Any congenital	Anaemia
abnormality	Multiple births

Table 7.7(a) Risks of immaturity

System	Risks of immaturity
Respiratory centre immaturity	Periodic pattern of respiration or apnoeic episodes (i.e. 20 seconds or more) More sensitive to effects of hypoxia and maternal sedation
Lung immaturity	Surfactant deficiency and hyaline membrane disease
Liver immaturity	Earlier development of neonatal jaundice and a tendency to bleed due to lack of vitamin K-dependent coagulation factors (II, VII, IX, and X)
Gastrointestinal and feeding	Before 35 weeks of gestation sucking and swallowing not yet well coordinated leading to significant feeding difficulties, with risk of regurgitation and aspiration. Stomach emptying and gut motility is slower. Abdominal distension due to a relatively atonic bowel aggravates feeding difficulties. Immaturity of digestive enzymes affects feed tolerance in some babies
Renal immaturity	A low glomerular filtration rate (GFR) and poor tubular function lead to the inability to excrete a water and solute load. The GFR is about 0.45 ml/min at 28 weeks and 5 ml/min at term. During the first week the plasma creatinine levels are a reflection of the mother's levels. The preterm infant suffers high sodium losses; under 33 weeks the fractional excretion of sodium is 3 to 5 per cent and between 33 and 37 weeks 1 per cent. The maximum urine osmolality is 500–700 mmol/l. Therefore oedema is frequently seen in the preterm infant
Neurological immaturity	Intraventricular haemorrhage is a constant hazard due to the rich network of unsupported capillaries in the germinal matrix. Fetal hypoxia, birth asphyxia, fluctuations in the blood pressure, and an unstable metabolic status render these delicate vessels prone to rupture with ensuing peri- or intraventricular haemorrhage
Immature immunity	Shorter duration of last trimester means that less maternal antibody protection has been transferred into baby. General immaturity increases risk of Gram-negative infections
Bone marrow immaturity	Anaemia is a common problem due to exaggerated physiological factors and sluggish erythropoietic response. Late anaemia occurs with rapid growth and depletion of relatively poor iron and folate stores. Vitamin E deficiency may contribute to the development of anaemia in a preterm baby

Table 7.7(b) Risks of small body size

Physiological parameter	Risks of small body size
Temperature control	Small stores of glycogen and fat predispose preterm and underweight-for-gestational-age (UGA) babies to poor temperature regulation. In addition, the large surface area, poor muscle tone, and inability to shiver compound the difficulty of temperature control. Maintenance of a neutral thermal environment is essential
Blood sugar control	Hypoglycaemia occurs with greater frequency in preterm babies due to inadequate stores of glycogen

The preterm infant

The clinical features consist of immaturity of external appearance and of neurological development, well described in the criteria for the assessment of the gestational age (*see* Figure 7.2). The markedly preterm infant shows very obvious clinical features. It is important, however, to consider intra-uterine growth restriction and wasting, which might make a greater contribution to the baby's low birth weight than prematurity alone. A rapid but superficial impression can be obtained by scrutinizing the breast, nipple development, the plantar creases, and muscle tone.

Risks and complications of prematurity

In the appropriate-for-gestational-age (AGA) preterm neonate, most organs are functionally and metabolically immature. Risks and complications arise because of immaturity and because of small body size (*see* Table 7.7). Additionally, there may be a reason for preterm labour such as maternal infection, which predisposes the baby to pneumonia at birth.

The underweight-for-gestational-age (UGA) baby

These babies can be classified as symmetrically growth-restricted or asymmetrically wasted. The former implies an early intra-uterine insult or other constitutional factors resulting in a small baby with weight, length, and head circumference below the 10th centile. (*See* Figure 7.3.)

Asymmetrical wasting is due to uteroplacental factors in the later stages of pregnancy; these cause failure to gain weight or even loss of

> Common causes of symmetrical intra-uterine growth restriction (IUGR) are low maternal weight, genetic abnormalities, chromosomal defects, chronic intra-uterine infection, and teratogenic agents such as alcohol.
>
> Asymmetrical wasting may be caused by pregnancy-induced hypertension, placental infarction, partial separation of the placenta, poor nutrition of the mother, severe physical exertion late into pregnancy, and smoking during pregnancy.

weight of the fetal trunk and limbs, while length and head circumference are relatively spared.

The essential clinical feature common to all these babies is a birth weight under the 10th centile for gestational age. The symmetrically growth-restricted infant may show features of the causative disease such as a chromosomal defect or intra-uterine infection. A high index of suspicion should be maintained for the features of the fetal alcohol syndrome (*see* Chapter 3, Medical genetics and birth defects).

Asymmetric wasting of late onset causes loss of subcutaneous fat and minimal or absent vernix caseosa. The facial appearance is one of alertness, with a wizened expression. The skin is thickened and desquamating with a parchment-like quality. The muscle tone is generally increased. As the liquor may well have been meconium-stained for some considerable period, the skin and umbilical cord may have a dirty green discoloration.

Risks and complications. Many problems are similar to those experienced by preterm babies and are related to the risks of small body size and low stores (*see* Table 7.7).

As the UGA infant may have been exposed to chronic oxygen and nutritional deprivation *in utero*, the acute stress of the birth process is not well tolerated. The infant is therefore additionally predisposed to a number of clinical problems.

- Fetal hypoxia is the most important, and can be detected by monitoring the fetal heart rate during labour and delivery.
- *There is a great risk of meconium aspiration* both *in utero* and at birth in the term growth-restricted baby, and pneumonia in the preterm baby. Hyaline membrane disease, in contrast, is relatively uncommon and less severe.
- Infections occur more readily in the UGA baby due to suppressed immunity.
- Chronic hypoxia stimulates erythropoietin production, resulting in polycythaemia and its complications.

Prognosis. The asymmetrically wasted baby is likely to do fairly well if adequately fed postnatally. Many UGA infants are not growth restricted but only wasted. Therefore intra-uterine growth restriction (IUGR) is not the same as UGA. The symmetrically small baby (IUGR) appears to have been programmed early *in utero* and in general remains small after birth. There is a slightly increased risk of cerebral palsy and mental retardation in term UGA infants, and they are at increased risk of manifesting minor neurological disorders. On the other hand, the preterm UGA infant appears to have a higher incidence of major handicap than the term UGA and the AGA preterm infant.

Management. The mother with the growth-restricted fetus must be regarded as having a high-risk pregnancy, which calls for the best attention available. Early delivery should be considered if there is continued evidence of fetal stress. During labour, careful monitoring of the fetal heart will give an indication of the need for oxygen and glucose infusion to the mother. Early intervention is called for if there is evidence of acute fetal distress.

During the delivery of a growth-restricted baby, one must anticipate and prevent meconium aspiration, and institute early management.

Subsequent observations must be geared to early detection of respiratory distress, of hypoglycaemia by frequent monitoring with reagent strips, and of hypothermia by frequent measurement of peripheral temperature.

The neonate with symmetrical growth restriction requires investigation for specific causative factors. Feeding is not so problematic in UGA babies – they are usually wide awake and take feeds avidly. Early feeding is essential. Every effort must be made to ensure adequate nutrition after discharge by making the mother aware of the deficit which must be made up and the risks to which the baby is predisposed.

In other respects, the management corresponds to that of the preterm baby.

The very-low-birth-weight (VLBW) baby

Babies weighing less than 1.5 kg at birth represent a small percentage of live births (1–2 per cent), but they contribute more than 50 per cent to the overall neonatal mortality. Survival rate with tertiary care is about 80 per cent. However, the cost of intensive and high care of this group of babies is enormous. Furthermore, the social background is an important consideration for the after-care; many of these VLBW babies are born to adolescent or other disadvantaged mothers. Often the pregnancy is unplanned and the babies are frequently rejected. The VLBW baby therefore places a considerable financial and social burden on the community in general.

Prevention. Education and fertility control of the teenager must receive serious consideration. Adequate antenatal care is essential so that early detection and appropriate management of preterm labour is effected to delay delivery where feasible. Women with threatened labour before 32 weeks of gestation need early transfer, so that optimal conditions for delivery and efficient after-care can be provided.

Immediate problems in the neonatal period. As the homeostatic balance of the VLBW baby is even more precarious than the larger LBW baby, meticulous attention is essential. Prompt, skilled resuscitation is the single most important determinant of a favourable outcome.

- Temperature regulation is critical because the thermo-neutral range in the smaller baby is narrow, with a marked tendency to hypothermia.
- Hypoxia and hyperoxia readily occur in recurrent and prolonged episodes, as tissue levels of oxygen fluctuate widely. Poor respiratory excursion and apnoea occur spontaneously and are often induced by handling. The most serious effect of hypoxia is on the delicate unsupported vessels of the periventricular area, resulting in haemorrhage. Hyperoxia occurs as a result of over-zealous treatment of apnoeic episodes or respiratory distress, risking injury to the retina (retinopathy) and lungs (broncho-pulmonary dysplasia).
- The incidence of hypoglycaemia is higher, particularly if feeding is delayed.
- Fluid and electrolyte balance may be difficult to achieve. The hazards of fluid restriction in these babies are well established. Hyponatraemia, acidosis, hypoglycaemia, and hyperbilirubinaemia are very real hazards unless close attention is paid to early feeding. Monitoring for clinical signs of dehydration and for biochemical disturbances is essential to maintain homeostasis.

In the long term there are several problems. General health in the first year of life is likely to be affected by frequent infections, particularly of the respiratory tract. The mortality rate is high due to brain damage or acute respiratory illness. The *sudden infant death syndrome* (SIDS) occurs more often in the VLBW than in the full term. Neonatal problems cause a delay in regaining the birth weight for two to three weeks, but following recovery, growth should proceed at the normal rate. Those who are appropriate for gestational age can be expected to grow at the same velocity as a full-term infant of the same conceptual age. Poor growth occurs in the UGA infant, and those with prolonged undernutrition in the early weeks of life. Visual, auditory, speech, and other neurological deficits must be expected.

Retinopathy of prematurity (retrolental fibroplasia) is emerging as one of the leading causes of childhood blindness in middle-income developing countries. It is an iatrogenic disease unknown in undeveloped countries and is caused by the hyperoxygenation of small preterm babies. Oxygen therapy in preterm babies should ideally be monitored by pulse oximetry and arterial oxygen saturation should be between 89–92 per cent. Where oximetry is not available, the least amount of oxygen required to keep the baby's tongue pink must be used with attempts to reduce the oxygen concentration every few hours. Immature babies requiring prolonged oxygen therapy should be transferred to specialized units where monitoring is available. All babies of birth weight less than 1 250 g and gestational age of 30 weeks or less require examination by an ophthalmologist six weeks post-natally. Treatment with cryotherapy or laser in the early stages of the disease prevents blindness.

The overweight-for-gestational-age (OGA) baby

The best-known association of OGA babies with a birth weight above the 90th centile for gestational age (4.0 kg at term) is maternal diabetes. Large mothers and those with excessive weight gain during pregnancy can expect to have OGA babies. The Beckwith syndrome is a much rarer cause and has associated macroglossia, macrosomia, and small genitalia.

The OGA infant is at risk of peripheral and intracranial birth trauma. As shoulder dystocia is a further possibility, Caesarean section is often indicated.

Management of the OGA baby delivered vaginally includes a careful search for cerebral birth trauma, fractured clavicle, or brachial plexus injury. There is a need to monitor the blood sugar level of the infant for the first 36 hours, and maternal diabetes must be excluded.

There appears to be an increased risk of mental subnormality in this group, which is thought to be related to cerebral complications. Delivery by Caesarean section and careful monitoring of the blood sugar level after birth to prevent hypoglycaemia decreases this risk substantially.

Signs of illness in the neonate

The neonate reveals illness by a limited number of non-specific physical signs. Knowledge of these and the ability to evaluate them are important.

Disorders of adaptation to extra-uterine life

Temperature instability

Temperature regulation in the neonate is very delicately balanced between heat loss (mainly by evaporation and radiation, and to a lesser extent by conduction to clothing and sheets and by convection) and heat production. Energy for heat production is obtained from glycogen stored in the liver and myocardium. In the absence of further intake, these stores are depleted within four to eight hours. Both hypo- and hyperthermia increase the metabolic rate. If there is associated hypoxia or hypoglycaemia, metabolic acidosis will complicate the picture and cause tissue damage. In the care of neonates a neutral thermal environment, which will allow a normal temperature to be maintained at a minimum metabolic rate, is essential. There are marked individual variations depending on the size, maturity, and state of health of the baby. It is important to achieve this environment so that insensible water loss is kept to a minimum and energy can be utilized optimally for growth.

Hypothermia

In LBW babies, hypothermia raises the mortality by at least 25 per cent. The most common cause of hypothermia is a low ambient temperature at birth. The asphyxiated, hypotonic

UGA baby requiring resuscitation is at greatest risk: hypoxia interferes with heat production, while hypotonia diminishes metabolism in the muscles and increases exposure from extended limbs. Furthermore, the LBW UGA baby has no brown fat stores on which to draw. Hypothermia is particularly likely to occur if there is a need for resuscitation and during transport. Associated sepsis further interferes with metabolism and hence heat production.

The metabolic rate and oxygen demand increase rapidly with cooling. Vasoconstriction occurs and apnoea may ensue. The adverse effects of hypothermia include metabolic acidosis, hypoglycaemia, decreased surfactant production, and a rise in free fatty acids. Slow or delayed weight gain may occur. The overall effects are reflected in an increased morbidity and mortality.

Management. Prevention of heat loss is essential: rewarming the neonate is difficult, time-consuming, and fraught with further complications. At birth every baby must be dried and wrapped in a prewarmed towel. The head must be included

Table 7.8 Signs of illness in the neonate

Sign	Causes and associations
Central cyanosis (tongue)	Most commonly indicates severe respiratory distress. May be due to congenital heart disease. May be a manifestation of a convulsion, sepsis or hypoglycaemia
Peripheral cyanosis	Indicates a temperature change or hypotension. The peripheral perfusion will be prolonged in both cases. Correction of hypotension is best achieved by infusing crystalloid solutions
Grunting	An expiratory sound made by the baby with inadequate oxygen uptake at alveolar level. Associated with pneumonia, hyaline membrane disease and pulmonary oedema, but not with airtrapping
Pallor	Of face or extremities suggests anaemia, haemorrhage, hypoxia, shock, sepsis, hypoglycaemia
Convulsions	Suggests CNS disorder such as asphyxia or meningitis. May occur as a non-specific sign of severe illness, hypoglycaemia, or hypocalcaemia
Apnoea	May be the first sign of a convulsion, severe respiratory disease, hypoglycaemia or hypothermia
Lethargy	Maternal sedation and analgesia, hypoglycaemia, asphyxia, infection
Failure to feed	Important sign of serious disease, particularly if feeding well before. Meningitis, other serious infections and moniliasis, metabolic disease. If poor feeding from birth in term infant consider asphyxia
Fever	Dehydration or, unusually, due to serious infection – note herpes
Hypothermia	Exposure, severe infection, CNS and circulatory disorders
Jaundice	A serious sign in the first 24 hours of life due to blood group incompatibility or infection
Vomiting	Bile-stained is significant, always exclude obstruction, consider infection
Diarrhoea	Acute gastroenteritis or a non-specific sign
Failure to move a limb	Fracture/dislocation, nerve injury, local infection, bone or joint infection

as it is the site of appreciable heat loss. Skin-to-skin contact with the mother provides warmth and prevents heat loss. When this is not possible and additional risk factors are present, warmers, cotton wool, aluminium swaddlers, and incubators can be used.

Rewarming of the cold baby is critical when hypothermia has been prolonged, and must be carried out as soon as possible. Again skin-to-skin contact with the mother is very effective and can be carried out in any situation. The skin temperature must be monitored and metabolic acidosis corrected. Complications such as infection, haemorrhage, and cerebral insults may develop.

Neonatal cold injury

Prolonged exposure to cold results in neonatal cold injury. Not infrequently the temperature is 32 °C or less. There is oedema, generalized redness, poor feeding, and lethargy. Sclerema, hypoglycaemia, shock, hypoxia, decreased surfactant production, convulsions, uraemia, and pulmonary haemorrhage may be encountered. There is an increased risk of sepsis and haemorrhage associated with cold injury. The mortality in this serious condition is very high. Treatment is symptomatic and as for hypothermia.

Overheating

When exposed to unnecessarily high environmental temperatures the baby becomes overheated. Term babies in incubators are particularly at risk. There is vasodilatation with increased insensible water loss, which results in dehydration and hypernatraemia. Apnoeic episodes may occur, and heat stroke and death may ensue.

Management is by lowering the environmental temperature, giving fluids either orally or by nasogastric tube, and correcting any serious metabolic disturbances.

Blood sugar control

Hypoglycaemia

Hypoglycaemia (i.e. a blood sugar level less than 2.0 mmol/l or a serum sugar level less than 2.5 mmol/l) is an important risk in UGA, preterm, and OGA babies. (For clinical features and causes *see* Chapter 10, Metabolic disorders.)

The blood sugar level (BSL) must be monitored within one hour of birth in infants at risk of hypoglycaemia, i.e. UGA and preterm neonates, those of diabetic mothers, and those that have been asphyxiated or hypothermic.

Hyperinsulinism is responsible for the hypoglycaemia of babies born to diabetic mothers and of those with severe erythroblastosis fetalis. An increased rate of consumption of blood glucose occurs in conditions such as hypothermia, hypoxia, respiratory distress, and infection. There is also a distinct possibility of rebound hypoglycaemia if a glucose infusion is interrupted.

Thereafter it must be determined two-hourly for the first eight hours and then six-hourly for the rest of the first 24 hours. Reagent strips can be used for screening, but biochemical analysis is advisable to confirm hypoglycaemia.

Management

- Commencing feeds within two hours of birth in the at-risk infants will usually prevent hypoglycaemia.
- A low blood sugar reading in an asymptomatic baby may be managed by an oral feed and monitoring of the BSL.
- A 10 per cent glucose solution must be infused intravenously as soon as possible in symptomatic infants or those with a BSL of <1.5 mmol/l. The infusion is started at 65 ml/kg per 24 hours (0.5 g/kg/hr).
- If the blood sugar does not reach normal levels, a 15% glucose infusion should be considered.
- If control is not achieved, glucagon 0.1 mg/kg per dose may be given repeatedly six- to twelve-hourly intramuscularly.
- Investigations must be considered to determine aetiology of prolonged hypoglycaemia (*see* Chapter 10, Metabolic disorders).
- Bolus infusions are generally not recommended as the intravascular consequences of a hyperosmolar solution and the effects on insulin levels cause unacceptable metabolic stress.

- The blood sugar is monitored hourly and small volume milk feeds (breastmilk) are commenced as soon as possible.
- When the patient is asymptomatic and the BSL has stabilized, the infusion is decreased slowly, while the milk feeds are slowly increased.

Infant of the diabetic mother

Good diabetic control during pregnancy decreases the risk of the majority of the problems which the infant of the diabetic mother (IDM) is likely to suffer. Congenital malformations vary from 5–13 per cent and include neural tube or vertebral defects, sacral agenesis, and cardiac malformations such as ventricular septal defect, transposition, and coarctation. (*See* Chapter 28, Cardiovascular disorders.) To prevent the latter it is critical to ensure preconceptual BSL control.

The other major risk is due to maternal hyperglycaemia, which places the developing baby in a state of continuous hyperinsulinism and accelerated growth. This causes an OGA baby with relative immaturity for gestational age.

The problems include:

- Birth injuries because of the large size: brachial plexus injury and fractures of the humerus following shoulder dystocia are the most common
- Hypoglycaemia, which may develop within the first one to two hours after birth. This complication implies poor maternal blood glucose control during pregnancy
- Poor feeding and sucking
- Jaundice
- Hypocalcaemia
- Respiratory distress syndrome
- Polycythaemia
- Cardiomyopathy, which may lead to cardiac failure
- Small left colon syndrome, presenting as transient intestinal obstruction, which resolves spontaneously
- Renal vein thrombosis, which presents as macroscopic haematuria.

Management includes three-hourly monitoring of the BSL from birth and early feeding.

Hyperglycaemia

Hyperglycaemia is defined as a blood sugar level (BSL) above 7.5 mmol/l with glycosuria.

It may occur as a consequence of severe stress, asphyxia, and sepsis, especially in the VLBW infant. Hyperosmolar solutions will induce an osmotic diuresis, which can result in significant dehydration.

Transient neonatal diabetes within the first six weeks of life occurs rarely in UGA babies. Usually there is failure to thrive with extreme hyperglycaemia and dehydration without acidosis. Insulin corrects the hyperglycaemia.

Management. The aim is to reduce the concentration of glucose in any infused fluid. The blood and urine sugar must be monitored carefully to detect the fall in the glucose levels. If these simple measures fail and the blood sugar remains above 15 mmol/l, insulin is infused at a dosage of 0.05–0.1 unit/kg/hr with very strict monitoring of the BSL to prevent hypoglycaemia. The very ill infant may be exquisitely sensitive to insulin and the BSL may fall within 15 to 20 minutes of the insulin injection.

Respiratory distress (RD)

Respiratory problems are a leading cause of neonatal deaths. It is important to recognize that disturbances of almost any system may manifest with respiratory signs and symptoms. Respiratory disturbances may present as:

- Respiratory distress
- Central cyanosis
- Inspiratory stridor
- Apnoea.

It is not uncommon for newborns soon after birth to have transient mild respiratory distress. This is an expression of adaptation from intrauterine to extra-uterine conditions; the distress settles within one to two hours and does not warrant investigation.

The causes commonly encountered are listed in Table 7.9

Respiratory distress (see Figure 7.4) is diagnosed when two or more of the following signs are present:
- Respiratory rate of 60/min or more (tachypnoea)
- Expiratory grunting
- Intercostal and/or sternal recession
- Central cyanosis while breathing air.

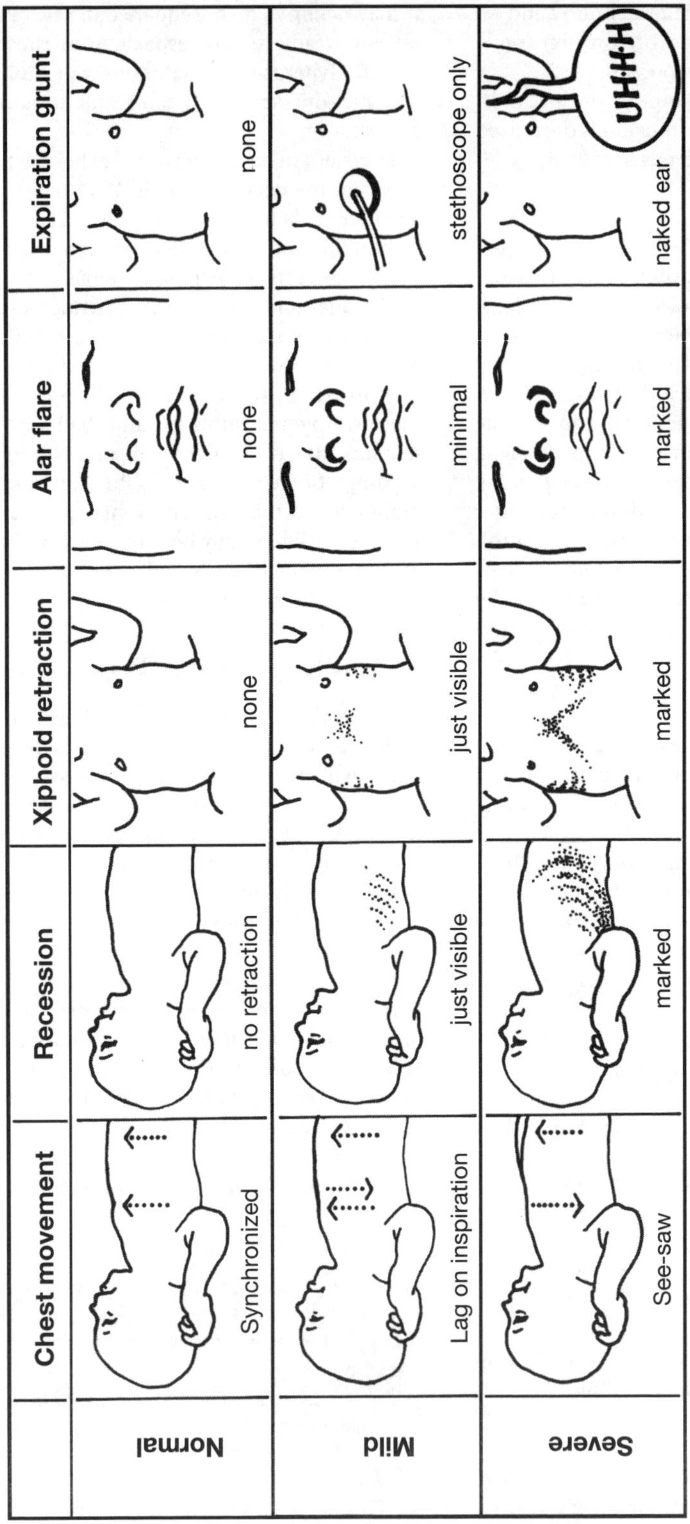

Figure 7.4 Clinical features of respiratory distress

	Chest movement	Recession	Xiphoid retraction	Alar flare	Expiration grunt
Normal	Synchronized	no retraction	none	none	none
Mild	Lag on inspiration	just visible	just visible	minimal	stethoscope only
Severe	See-saw	marked	marked	marked	naked ear

Central cyanosis is most commonly due to pathology of the respiratory tract. Although parenchymal lung disease is the most common cause of cyanosis, congenital heart disease must be suspected if the cyanosis is not relieved by oxygen. (*See* Chapter 28, Cardiovascular disorders.) Upper airway obstruction may simply be due to secretions or meconium and is readily relieved by suction. Rarely it is due to a structural abnormality such as choanal atresia.

Inspiratory stridor indicates an upper airway abnormality such as laryngeal webs or cysts or laryngomalacia. Mass lesions at the base of the tongue may present with intermittent or positional stridor.

Apnoea or poor respiratory effort may be caused by failure or depression of the respiratory centre or severe respiratory distress.

Immediate respiratory difficulties

Acute respiratory distress soon after birth requires careful clinical assessment to determine whether it is due to parenchymal lung disease, extra-pulmonary conditions, or congenital abnormalities. Early diagnosis of congenital abnormalities in particular reduces mortality and morbidity, as surgical intervention is often required.

Failure of the baby to breathe at birth suggests asphyxia or severe parenchymal lung disease.

Upper airway obstructive conditions that may present at the time of birth are choanal atresia and Pierre Robin syndrome. (*see* Chapter 34, Disorders of the ear, nose, and throat). A thick plug of mucus in the nostrils may present similar difficulties, but the obstruction is immediately relieved by nasal suction. The features of nasal obstruction are cyanosis and suprasternal recession when the mouth is closed, relieved by crying. Cyanosis and respiratory obstruction occurring in the supine position and relieved immediately on turning the baby are indicative of the tongue falling back and occluding the airway. These features, together with micrognathia, are found in the Pierre Robin syndrome.

Stridor may follow resuscitation either as a result of vigorous suctioning or intubation. Vocal cord paralysis or congenital abnormalities of the larynx such as webs, cysts, and laryngomalacia may also be diagnosed by direct laryngoscopy. An urgent tracheostomy may be necessary (*see* Chapter 34, Disorders of the ear, nose, and throat). Persistent extension of the neck with stridor may be associated with a retrosternal goitre or a vascular ring, which can be confirmed by an X-ray with a contrast swallow. The baby who has increased secretions from the time of birth and *chokes, coughs, or becomes cyanosed with feeding* must be regarded as having oesophageal atresia. This is easily confirmed by failure to pass a nasogastric tube into the stomach (*see* Chapter 8, Surgical conditions of the newborn). A chest radiograph with the tube *in situ* will confirm the presence of a pouch with the coiled tube visible.

Respiratory distress with *diminished breath sounds on one side of the chest*, suggests a pneumothorax, which is readily confirmed radiologically or by chest transillumination. Other signs include increasing respiratory difficulty, cyanosis, restlessness, and apparent malposition of the cardiac apex.

Ideally, all newborns who are at risk of developing respiratory problems should be delivered at centres with special care facilities.

Transfer of selected infants to such centres is warranted where there is moderate to severe respiratory distress or if there is deterioration; the latter is suggested by a need for increasing amounts of oxygen, a steady increase in the heart and respiratory rate or repeated apnoeic

Table 7.9 Causes of respiratory distress		
Pulmonary	**Extra-pulmonary**	**Congenital abnormalities**
Respiratory distress syndrome	Cold exposure	Pneumothorax
Meconium aspiration	Cardiac failure	Diaphragmatic hernia
Congenital pneumonia	Cerebral damage	Tracheo-oesophageal fistula
Transient tachypnoea	Metabolic disturbances	Lung cysts
Acute pulmonary haemorrhage	Acute blood loss	
	Septicaemia	

or cyanotic attacks. Often seriously ill neonates, such as those in haemorrhagic or septic shock, may benefit from respiratory support. Babies with severe asphyxia, convulsions, hypothermia, or hypoglycaemia should not be transferred immediately, but corrective management must be instituted first in consultation with the referral unit.

Principles of management of respiratory distress

From the list of causes of respiratory distress it can be seen that *it is imperative to have a chest radiograph.*

- Oxygen is administered in a concentration that abolishes cyanosis and keeps the oxygen saturation between 89–92 per cent.
- Blood gas analysis (if available) should be performed approximately one hour after clinical improvement and correction of any metabolic acidosis.
- A whole blood transfusion is indicated if the haemoglobin is below 12.0 g/dl (PCV below 35), giving 10–20 ml/kg over three hours.
- A plasma or crystalloid (normal saline, Ringer's lactate or haemacell) infusion should be given if the peripheral perfusion and pulse volume are poor.
- Circulation is assessed by the capillary filling time while the renal function is assessed by the urine output.
- Apart from the routine care, the blood sugar level must be monitored.
- Antibiotics are indicated in conditions such as respiratory distress syndrome and congenital pneumonia.

Principles of, and indications for, oxygen therapy

- Give as little oxygen as possible and as much as necessary to abolish central cyanosis and grunting.
- Oxygen administered indiscriminately, particularly to the preterm infant, may lead to retinopathy and blindness. (*See* Chapter 33, Disorders of the eye.) However, too little oxygen leads to hypoxic brain damage.
- If at all possible, the percentage oxygen given and the blood oxygen saturation must be monitored.

- Oxygen therapy without additional ventilatory support is sufficient if the respiratory effort is good and there is reasonable tone and cry. Blood gas analysis should show no carbon dioxide retention and a PaO_2 of 50–100 mmHg in an ambient oxygen concentration of up to 60%.
- Continuous positive airway pressure (CPAP) of 5 cm by nasal prongs or cannulae is indicated if cyanosis cannot be corrected with headbox oxygen.

The main indication for oxygen therapy is cyanosis or a change in colour, such as pale extremities and a central duskiness.

Oxygen should not be given for respiratory distress *per se*. If the baby is obviously cyanosed or has had a cardiac arrest, 100% oxygen must be given. This must be reduced once a clinical response occurs, which may take up to 20 minutes.

A baby with poor colour should be given 30–40% oxygen and once again reduced once clinical improvement is seen. This concentration of oxygen can be achieved by running 2–3 l/min into a headbox or incubator.

Cyanosis

Cyanosis of the skin and tongue is a guide to the state of oxygenation of the newborn. The degree of cyanosis depends on the arterial oxygen saturation, the haematocrit, the pH, the peripheral circulation, and the temperature of the baby. Intermittent cyanotic episodes may occur during vigorous crying; this is the result of right-to-left shunt through the ductus or foramen ovale. Vasomotor instability may cause generalized mottling of the skin.

Apparent cyanosis may be due to the blue phototherapy light or polycythaemia.

The causes of cyanosis include:
- Pulmonary pathology
- Congenital cardiac defects
- Hypothermia
- Metabolic disturbances, e.g. hypoglycaemia
- Infection, e.g. septicaemia, meningitis
- Severe intracranial disturbances, e.g. intra cranial haemorrhage, meningitis.

Management. With the infant supine, the head should be slightly extended, the airway kept clear by suctioning, and oxygen administered. The temperature and blood sugar levels are monitored and enteral feeds discontinued or withheld to avoid aspiration. Commence intravenous fluids to maintain hydration and electrolyte balance. As is the case with apnoea, further management depends on the cause of the cyanosis.

Hyaline membrane disease (HMD)

This condition is the clinical manifestation of lung immaturity. The lipoprotein, surfactant, which is necessary for normal alveolar expansion is deficient, either because of lack of production or failure of release from alveolar Type II cells. The air sacs collapse, the pulmonary capillary permeability is increased and protein-containing fluid and red cells ooze into the alveoli. The protein (fibrin) coagulates to form a membrane, which lines the alveolar sac; the sac itself contains oedema fluid and blood. This eosinophilic staining material seen on histology is a non-specific response of the lung to injury. Within a few days, the alveolar macrophages gradually remove the membranes and, as surfactant is produced, the normal physico-chemical properties of the gas–liquid interface in the air sacs are restored and the alveoli are able to maintain a spherical shape in expiration.

The assessment of lung maturity and of alveolar Type II cells is possible by measuring the ratio of lecithin to sphingomyelin (L-S ratio) in the amniotic fluid. The more mature the fetus, the closer the L-S ratio approaches 2:1.

The bubble or shake test is a simple bedside means of assessing lung maturity: 1 ml of amniotic fluid obtained by amniocentesis and 1 ml of absolute alcohol are shaken vigorously for 30 seconds in a clean 10 ml glass tube. After another 15 seconds the bubble score is read. The higher the score the more mature the lungs:

    0 = no bubbles
    1+ = a single ring of bubbles
    2+ = two rings of stable bubbles
    3+ = more than two rings of bubbles and a
         clear centre
    4+ = all of the miniscus covered in bubbles.

A score of 2+ can be considered 'safe' with regard to lung maturity. The shake test can also be performed on a sample of clear gastric aspirate collected within 30 minutes of delivery.

The pathophysiological effects of HMD on pulmonary function are as follows:

- Reduced lung compliance
- Ventilation perfusion imbalance
- Pulmonary vasoconstriction resulting in a large right-to-left shunt of blood
- Reduced alveolar ventilation and functional residual capacity
- Increased minute ventilation and work of breathing.

These changes result in hypoxaemia, hypercapnia and eventually metabolic acidosis. The classical radiological findings are an air-bronchogram, and reticulogranular pattern. However, this characteristic picture does not exclude infection.

The management is similar to that for respiratory distress and supportive care, and includes surfactant replacement therapy as discussed below.

Surfactant replacement therapy (SRT) is a major advance in the care of the preterm infant with respiratory distress syndrome. Mortality and the incidence of air leaks are reduced by this form of therapy. However, there has been no effect on the incidence of bronchopulmonary dysplasia (BPD), intraventricular haemorrhage, and patent ductus arteriosus.

Surfactant is commercially available as a natural or a synthetic preparation, with the natural version acting more rapidly than the synthetic preparation. Surfactant has to be administered with ventilatory support. Although large trials have shown no real differences between the two surfactants with regard to death or chronic lung disease, the natural surfactant of either bovine or porcine origin is preferred for the rapid clinical action. SRT is administered, via the endotracheal tube, prophylactically in the high-risk preterm infant or as 'rescue' therapy in those with established HMD. In South Africa the limited financial and physical resources for neonatal intensive care and the high cost of surfactant prohibits its prophylactic use. Ventilated infants with HMD are therefore selected to receive SRT if the FiO_2 exceeds 0.60 at three to four hours after birth and fails to maintain an arterial pO_2 of 55–75 mmHg.

Prevention of HMD includes the use of antenatal steroids. The effect of antenatal steroids is significant if delivery occurs 48 hours after or within seven days of the administration of the drug. A secondary benefit is the reduction in intraventricular haemorrhage and necrotizing enterocolitis. There appears to be no increased risk of infection to the mother or the baby. Administration of antenatal steroids will decrease or even prevent the incidence of HMD and thereby also the use of the costly SRT.

Massive pulmonary haemorrhage

This catastrophic situation most commonly arises in the low-birth-weight infant during the acute or recovery phase of an illness such as asphyxia, infection, or hypothermia. It occurs most frequently between the second and fourteenth day.

Treatment with transfusion and ventilation is unsatisfactory as the mortality rate is high. Probably of greater importance is the prevention of predisposing factors.

Meconium aspiration

This condition usually occurs in UGA, and term and post-term infants suffering from fetal distress before and during labour. The passing of grade 1 meconium *in utero* is of doubtful significance. Although grade 2 and 3 meconium do not mean inevitable aspiration, the risk is high. The monitoring of labour to detect fetal compromise and its management are the most important factors in the prevention of this condition. However, significant morbidity and mortality may be decreased by suction of the mouth and throat at delivery of the head, followed by direct pharyngeal and/or tracheal suction immediately after delivery if resuscitation is needed. The aspiration of meconium may have a number of effects on the lungs and heart:

- Small airways obstruction with areas of atelectasis and air trapping
- Acute pneumonitis presenting with various degrees of severity, shock, and acute pulmonary oedema or respiratory distress
- Pneumothorax
- Persistent pulmonary hypertension of the newborn.

If there has been severe hypoxia and hypotension, cerebral oedema and renal problems with fluid overload may readily occur. The natural history is one of full clinical and pulmonary recovery within weeks, unless of course severe hypoxia or pneumonitis causes death.

Management is as for respiratory distress (*see above*).

Chronic lung disease

Chronic lung disease is diagnosed if a baby is ventilated and/or oxygen dependent for 28 days or more and has characteristic features on chest X-ray. Chronic lung disorder (bronchopulmonary dysplasia) may be associated with patent ductus arteriosus, pulmonary haemorrhage, infection, and milk aspiration. The principles of management include prevention of nosocomial infection, adequate nutrition, treatment of cardiac failure if present, and maintaining the haemoglobin above 12 g/l, and the oxygen saturation between 85 and 92 per cent. The chest X-ray and electrocardiograph should be checked regularly for the development of right heart involvement. Theophylline may help to wean the baby from oxygen therapy or the ventilator; in addition it may improve lung compliance. Dexamethasone must be used with great caution and as a short course. Nebulization with ipratropium bromide or salbutamol may be of benefit.

In a population with a high prevalence of HIV infection, some babies with chronic lung disease of infancy may be expected to also suffer from vertically acquired HIV infection. Accordingly, a high index of suspicion should be maintained for additional HIV infection in any baby showing unusual features or responses.

Persistent pulmonary hypertension of the newborn (PPHN)

In this condition right-to-left shunting through the foramen ovale and ductus arteriosus occurs as a result of high pulmonary vascular resistance (persistent 'fetal circulation'). Profound hypoxia resulting in cyanosis occurs soon after birth. The heart is structurally normal, the chest X-ray may show pulmonary oligaemia, and the ECG is most often normal.

PPHN may present as a primary disorder (the lungs appear normal or oligaemic on chest X-ray) or with HMD, meconium aspiration, polycythaemia, and diaphragmatic hernia.

Mechanical ventilation with a high FiO_2 has little effect on severe hypoxia. Correction of the acidosis and systemic hypotension may be followed by improving oxygenation as pulmonary vascular resistance improves. Maintenance of a normal to high systemic blood pressure is important. The following options may be considered: $MgSO_4$ at a dose of 200 mg/kg body weight IVI over 20 to 30 minutes, followed by a continuous infusion of 20–50 mg/kg per hour, surfactant replacement therapy, sildenafil or nitric oxide, which may be available in some centres.

Wet lung syndrome or transient tachypnoea of the newborn (TTN)

This brief, self-limiting, relatively benign condition follows a normal full-term pregnancy. The infant usually has mild respiratory distress, which settles within a few days. Some may require oxygen. Radiological changes are those of perihilar streaking, fluid in the lung fissures, and a slightly enlarged cardiac silhouette.

Apnoeic and cyanotic episodes

Apnoeic episodes and periodic breathing in the preterm infant are considered to be one end of a spectrum of disturbed respiratory regulation. The heart rate and oxygenation remain normal with periodic breathing, but apnoeic spells result in bradycardia and cyanosis after 20 seconds. Should this persist, hypotonia and unresponsiveness may develop.

The following conditions may be associated with apnoeic episodes:

- Immaturity
- Respiratory distress, particularly due to obstructed airways
- Respiratory failure due to pulmonary pathology of any type
- Central nervous system pathology, e.g. convulsions, meningitis, raised intracranial pressure due to cerebral haemorrhage or oedema
- Septicaemia
- Metabolic disturbances, e.g. hypoglycaemia, hypocalcaemia, hyponatraemia, acidosis
- Hyperpyrexia
- Drugs given to the mother, particularly diazepam and magnesium sulphate.

It is important to emphasise that apnoea attacks may indicate convulsions, as the typical features of a seizure are rarely seen in a neonate.

Management. The respiration of patients at risk of apnoeic episodes must be monitored carefully. The basic management of an apnoeic or cyanotic episode is:

- Firstly gentle pharyngeal suction
- Oxygen is given per mask and
- The baby is stimulated by flicking the foot
- Intermittent positive pressure ventilation

has to be commenced if bradycardia persists
- If the pulse rate increases but remains of poor quality, then plasma 10 ml/kg may be infused over 20 minutes and respiratory support considered if a ventilator is available.

Once apnoea of immaturity is diagnosed by exclusion of other causes, oral theophylline 5 mg/kg is given, followed by 2 mg/kg 12-hourly.

Gastrointestinal disorders

Gastrointestinal disorders are common problems in the newborn. The major concern is to exclude surgical conditions (*see* Chapter 8, Surgical conditions of the newborn).

Vomiting

Vomiting is a very common sign in the first few hours of life. Regurgitation of the first few feeds may reflect irritation of the gastric mucosa by swallowed blood or meconium. A gastric lavage will confirm this diagnosis and is therapeutic.

Vomiting may be the first sign of serious organic disease, especially if it is persistent, bile-stained, or associated with abdominal distension or constipation. (*See* Chapter 24, Gastrointestinal disorders.)

Infections, both enteral and parenteral, are commonly associated with vomiting.and include meningitis, septicaemia, urinary tract infections, and necrotizing enterocolitis. Intestinal obstruction must be excluded (*see* Chapter 8, Surgical conditions of the newborn).

Intracranial injury and congenital abnormalities may cause persistent vomiting. Rarer causes include metabolic problems such as uraemia, congenital adrenal hyperplasia, and inherited metabolic disturbances.

Abdominal distension

This is a fairly common physical sign in the newborn. It may be a sign of serious illness. It should be established whether the distension is due to gas, fluid, or organ enlargement, and whether associated physical signs such as constipation and vomiting are present.

- *Gaseous distension* occurs as a result of the accumulation of air in the gut due to

139

obstruction or paralytic ileus. The causes of intestinal obstruction are congenital abnormalities of the gut, hernias, volvulus, and malrotation (*see* Chapter 8, Surgical conditions of the newborn). Meconium ileus is a pointer to cystic fibrosis and must be considered in babies of Caucasian origin who present with partial or complete obstruction. Paralytic ileus occurs as a result of hypoxia, shock, electrolyte imbalance, and infection, which may be systemic or confined to the gut.

+ *Abdominal masses* contributing to abdominal distension are most commonly due to organ enlargement such as hepatosplenomegaly, renal masses, dilated bladder, liver cysts, tumours, and ovarian masses. Rare causes include gut duplication, mesenteric cyst, and retroperitoneal tumours. Urogenital causes are not uncommon so that abdominal ultrasound and urological investigations may be required to detect these.

+ *Ascites* is a rare clinical finding in the newborn and most commonly occurs in babies with generalized oedema. This is seen in severe anaemia (as in Rh disease), cardiac failure, nephrotic syndrome, and chronic intra-uterine infections.

Management. Surgical conditions must be excluded first. An erect abdominal radiograph is obtained and an abdominal ultrasound performed in the case of an abdominal mass. A paediatric surgical opinion should be obtained.

Diarrhoea

The most common cause of loose stools in a neonate is dietary in origin. In the fully breastfed infant a loose stool with each feed is not uncommon and is due to a mild lactose maldigestion. This self-limiting condition clears within days or weeks and does not require a feed change if the baby is thriving.

Infective diarrhoea may occur and may be associated with parenteral infection (*see* Chapter 24, Gastrointestinal disorders).

It is extremely difficult to differentiate parenteral from enteral infection in the newborn. The clinical presentation may vary from mild disease to severe dehydrating disease with acidosis and electrolyte imbalance. Many babies are afebrile, yet others become hypothermic or pyrexial.

Necrotizing enterocolitis

The incidence varies in different centres, being rare in some and reaching epidemic proportions in others. It occurs more commonly in infants weighing less than 1 500 g.

The pathogenesis is poorly understood but ischaemia of the immature gut is a critical factor, followed by a combination of infection and release of inflammatory mediators. Perinatal hypoxia, prematurity, sepsis, artificial feeds, shock and exchange transfusions are contributing factors. Following the ischaemic insult, luminal gas enters the necrotic bowel wall to produce classical pneumatosis intestinalis. Organisms associated with this disease include *Escherichia coli*, klebsiella, acinetobacter, pseudomonas, and *Clostridium difficile*. Strict adherence to exclusive breastmilk feeding has reduced the incidence in some units.

Clinical features. Abdominal distension is the earliest sign. It may occur within a few hours of birth and as late as one month of age. A poor colour and shock may ensue with the full picture of septicaemia. Stools are usually scanty but blood-streaked in 20–25 per cent of cases. Perforation of the gut may occur.

Investigations. A low white count may be present; thrombocytopaenia, particularly a falling platelet count, is a poor prognostic sign and disseminated intravascular coagulation may be present. An X-ray of the abdomen shows intestinal distension with thickened bowel walls, intramural air, and sometimes gas in the intrahepatic portal venous system. Signs of pneumo-peritoneum will be present if the gut has perforated.

Management. The general principles of treatment of septic infants must be observed:

+ All feeds are stopped.
+ A nasogastric tube is passed and left open to drain to prevent accumulation of air and gastric content.
+ Intravenous alimentation is mandatory once the clinical condition is stable.
+ Monitor and correct electrolyte imbalance.
+ Correct low Hb, and low platelet count.
+ Broadspectrum antibiotics are commenced once appropriate cultures have been taken.
+ Regular consultation with a paediatric surgeon is essential as immediate

intervention is necessary for perforation, and strictures may develop later.

Prognosis. Prompt diagnosis, nasogastric drainage and intravenous alimentation have vastly improved the outlook in this serious disease. In the individual patient, however, the degree of prematurity and any associated conditions will affect the prognosis. In some centres mortality rates have decreased from 75 to less than 20 per cent.

Neonatal jaundice

Jaundice becomes apparent at 85–120 μmol/l (1mg/dl of bilirubin = 17 μmol/l). Jaundice is pathological if:
- It occurs within the first 24 hours of life.
- Total serum bilirubin exceeds 275 μmol/l or the upper limit of normal for the age in days.
- Bilirubin rises by more than 85 μmol/l per day.

Or:
- If the direct serum bilirubin exceeds 34 μmol/l.
- If jaundice persists for more than a week in the term and more than two weeks in the preterm baby.

The usual causes of jaundice in the first week of life are shown in Table 7.10.

Physiological jaundice
Up to 50 per cent of normal newborns and considerably more preterm infants become jaundiced in the first week of life. The normal newborn has a number of factors involving bilirubin metabolism and transport:
- Increased breakdown of fetal Hb red cells

- Immature uptake, conjugation, and excretion of bilirubin
- Increased enterohepatic circulation of bilirubin.

These result in raised unconjugated serum bilirubin levels in the first week of life. In physiological jaundice, the total serum bilirubin (TSB) level does not exceed the upper limit of normal for age in days. In the term neonate it usually peaks at 150 μmol/l on the third day, and in the preterm 170–200 μmol/l on the fifth to seventh day. The diagnosis of physiological jaundice is largely by exclusion.

Bilirubin encephalopathy
Bilirubin encephalopathy occurs when the fat-soluble unconjugated free bilirubin crosses the blood–brain barrier. Areas of the brain with high blood flow and high metabolic rates are susceptible to bilirubin toxicity. *Kernicterus* refers to the yellow staining of the basal ganglia and hippocampus seen at autopsy in infants dying of bilirubin toxicity.

Factors that interfere with albumin binding and allow a higher level of free bilirubin in the circulation, are:
- A low serum albumin (<30 g/l)
- Certain drugs such as sulphonamides, which compete with bilirubin for binding sites on albumin
- Non-esterified fatty acids (associated with starvation or total parenteral nutrition (TPN)
- Acidosis.

The preterm infant is at risk of encephalopathy at appreciably lower serum bilirubin levels than the term baby. Bilirubin encephalopathy is rarely seen in term infants with total serum

Table 7.10 Usual causes of neonatal jaundice in the first week of life	
Onset within the first 3 to 5 days	**Onset after day 5 to day 7**
Blood group incompatibility	Infections, e.g. UTI, hepatitis, Gram-negative sepsis
Blood collections, e.g. cephalhaematoma	Neonatal hepatitis syndrome
Physiological jaundice	Biliary atresia
Infection (intrauterine)	Metabolic disorders, e.g. galactosaemia
Immaturity	Endocrine, e.g. hypothyroidism
Maternal diabetes	Miscellaneous, e.g. Down's syndrome, pyloric stenosis

bilirubin levels below 400 μmol/l unless there is underlying pathology or factors that enhance the deposition of free bilirubin.

Hypoxia, sepsis, acidosis, hypoglycaemia and hyaline membrane disease predispose to kernicterus.

In general, unconjugated hyperbilirubinaemia originating from sources other than increased haemolysis does not commonly cause bilirubin encephalopathy.

Clinical features. The clinical picture of bilirubin toxicity may be transient or irreversible. The signs may not develop for several hours after toxic levels have been reached. Initially the signs are reluctance to take feeds, temperature instability, irritability, and cycling movements. An exchange transfusion at this stage may arrest the process. Progression of the disease shows up as generalized increase in extensor tone with opisthotonus and crossed extension of the legs. The cry is high-pitched and paralysis of the extraocular muscles causes a 'setting sun' sign. In the surviving infant hypotonia eventually occurs with developmental delay. Long-term manifestations include choreoathetosis or spastic cerebral palsy, clumsiness, intellectual impairment, and high tone deafness. Dental dysplasia may occur. In the preterm infant the initial physical signs may be quite different with fisting, an increase in tone, and apnoea.

Bilirubin encephalopathy should occur infrequently now to reflect an overall improved care of the newborn.

Haemolytic disease of the newborn

Rhesus haemolytic disease

Pathogenesis. There are five distinct Rhesus (Rh) antigens c, C, D, e, and E. Incompatibility to the D antigen is the most severe. About 85 per cent of Caucasians have the D antigen. Rh negativity denotes absence of the D antigen, indicated by d. When fetal cells carrying the D antigen leak across the placenta into the circulation of a Rh-negative mother, they stimulate antibody production in the mother to the specific fetal antigen. These antibodies, in turn, cross the placenta causing haemolysis of the fetal red cells.

Rhesus disease increases in incidence and severity if there has been prior sensitization due to feto-maternal bleeding at abortion, amniocentesis, external cephalic version, or delivery. Severity of the disease is also related to parity and to the stage of pregnancy during which the antibody crosses the placenta. The earlier the antibody crosses the placenta, the more severe the disease. Haemolytic disease commencing in the second trimester may result in severe anaemia, hepatosplenomegaly, liver damage (hypoproteinaemia, oedema), cardiac failure, and ascites (hydrops fetalis). When haemolysis occurs nearer to term the infant is born less anaemic but rapidly develops jaundice which may be severe.

Prevention. Antenatal investigation of Rh-negative women for the presence of Rhesus antibody will detect potentially affected fetuses. Amniocentesis with the measurement of bilirubin concentration and optical density has been the method of assessing severity. Recently tertiary centres have been performing cordocentesis to measure the haematocrit and analyse the blood groups. Direct fetal transfusion is performed if indicated.

All Rh-negative women must be given human Rh-hyperimmune gammaglobulin (100 to 200 mg IM) within 48 hours of birth or any procedure which could result in sensitization. The gammaglobulin binds to the fetal cells which are then rapidly removed from the maternal circulation. This procedure has resulted in a dramatic decline in the incidence of Rh-haemolytic disease.

Management of the infant. The jaundiced infant is managed as outlined below. Low-grade haemolysis may continue in the affected infant, resulting in anaemia at two to four weeks and may require a transfusion at that time. The early administration of iron and folate supplementation may reduce the severity of the late anaemia.

ABO incompatibility

The frequency of ABO blood group incompatibility is similar in tropical and non-tropical areas. As Rh disease has become uncommon, ABO incompatibility assumes greater importance. The latter rarely presents with as severe manifestations as Rh disease, e.g. hydrops fetalis, severe anaemia, and early onset of jaundice. Although the Coombs' test is often negative, sensitization may be suggested by the presence of immune anti-A or anti-B antibodies in the baby's serum or on the surface of the red cells. ABO incompatibility can occur where the mother has the blood group O and the baby either group A or B.

Management of hyperbilirubinaemia

Figure 7.5 gives guidelines for the management of hyperbilirubinaemia. The aim of therapy is to prevent bilirubin encephalopathy. Careful observation of the baby is important to detect and correct any of the above-mentioned predisposing factors.

Phototherapy. This should be regarded as both prophylactic and curative. Optimal results are obtained with blue light, but daylight is adequate. Nappies should be left untied so that the maximum surface is exposed. Phototherapy should be given to all LBW infants as soon as jaundice is noticed, to all infants with extensive bruising, to those with cephalhaematomas, as well as to full-term infants with total serum bilirubin (TSB) approaching exchange level.

Phototherapy should be discontinued as soon as there is a sustained fall in the unconjugated bilirubin level. Adequate hydration must be maintained throughout the therapy with frequent breastfeeds. The eyes must be covered throughout the procedure.

Side-effects include hyperthermia, loose stools, and skin rashes.

Intravenous immunoglobulin (IVIG) may be considered in haemolytic disease when the bilirubin level is rising. The IVIG is given at 1 gm/kg over eight hours on three consecutive days. IVIG binds the red cell antibodies, preventing further haemolysis. IVIG is not a substitute for an exchange transfusion.

Exchange transfusion. Although the TSB level gives an indication of the potential risk of bilirubin encephalopathy, each baby has to be assessed individually. An exchange transfusion may be required at a lower level of TSB if risk factors are present. (See Chapter 36, Procedures.)

The frequency of monitoring TSB levels depends on the severity of the jaundice, clinical condition, and available facilities. Mild to moderate jaundice may require daily assessment, whereas severe jaundice requires four- to six-hourly determinations. If a bilirubinometer is being used, the standards must be checked regularly.

Hydrops fetalis

Hydrops fetalis describes a grossly oedematous fetus, which is born anaemic, has hepatospleno-megaly, ascites, and pleural effusions. Besides Rh disease, congenital infections, most commonly syphilis, cytomegalovirus, and toxoplasmosis may cause hydrops fetalis. Cardiac failure, hypoproteinaemia due to hepatic and renal disease, twin-to-twin transfusion, thalassaemia, and a host of miscellaneous conditions may be responsible for this condition.

The management involves respiratory support, removal of the ascitic and pleural fluid (if they contribute to respiratory embarrassment) and slow correction of the anaemia by exchange transfusion.

Furosemide may be of assistance in controlling the cardiac failure. Haemorrhage may be prevented by the administration of vitamin K after birth and exchange transfusion with fresh whole blood. Hypoglycaemia may also occur in these infants.

Haematological problems

(*See also* Chapter 23, Disorders of the blood.)

Acute anaemia

Acute blood loss anaemia is a medical emergency. Pallor indicates hypoxia or, importantly, anaemia due to acute blood loss before, during, or after delivery.

The causes of acute anaemia may be related to the placenta, such as tearing of aberrant placental veins, and feto-maternal or twin-to-twin transfusion. Blood loss may occur during a traumatic delivery with intracranial or intra-abdominal haemorrhage. After birth, blood loss may occur if the cord is unclamped, and the infant is held above the level of the placenta. Cephalhaematoma, soft tissue bruising, and bleeding from the cord are other common causes. Rarely, coagulation defects or thrombocytopaenia may cause bleeding.

Initially the baby may be pale with normal heart rate and pulse volume. Some minutes or hours later peripheral vasoconstriction occurs with tachycardia, a thready pulse, and low blood pressure. During the second phase the baby becomes restless and finally lethargic and quiet. Without intervention death will ensue. When in doubt, serial haematocrit and haemoglobin estimations at hourly intervals will signify the need for transfusion.

Figure 7.5 Phototherapy and Total Serum Bilirubin (TSB) monitoring in the first week of life at primary care (South African Neonatal Academic Hospitals 2006)

- Refer/discuss all jaundiced infants who are: <2 kg or <35 weeks gestation.
- Refer all infants of mothers who have Rhesus antibodies on antenatal screening.
- Discuss ALL infants receiving phototherapy, daily, with MOU doctor (day) or referral hospital (night).
- Stop phototherapy when TSB >50 µmol/l below phototherapy line.
- If TSB continues to fall after phototherapy has been stopped, then no more TSB measurements are needed.

Figure 7.5a

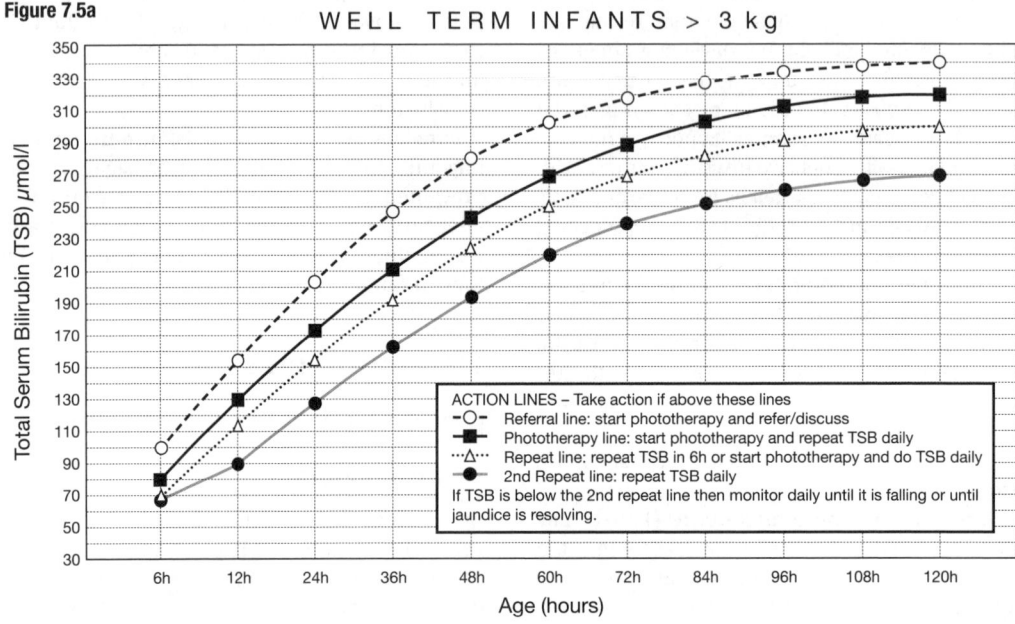

Figure 7.5b

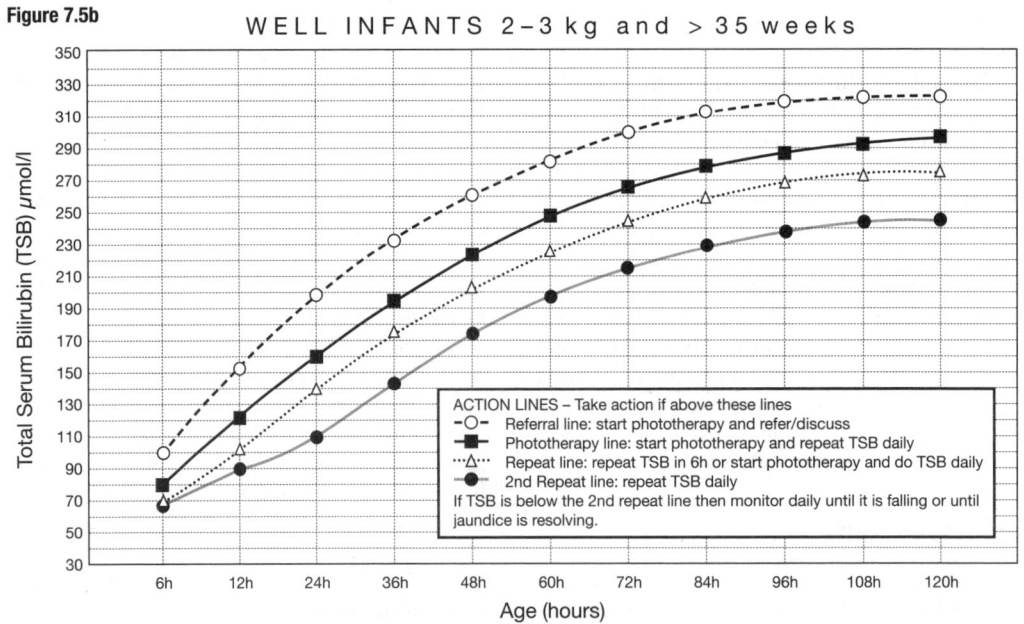

Figure 7.5a

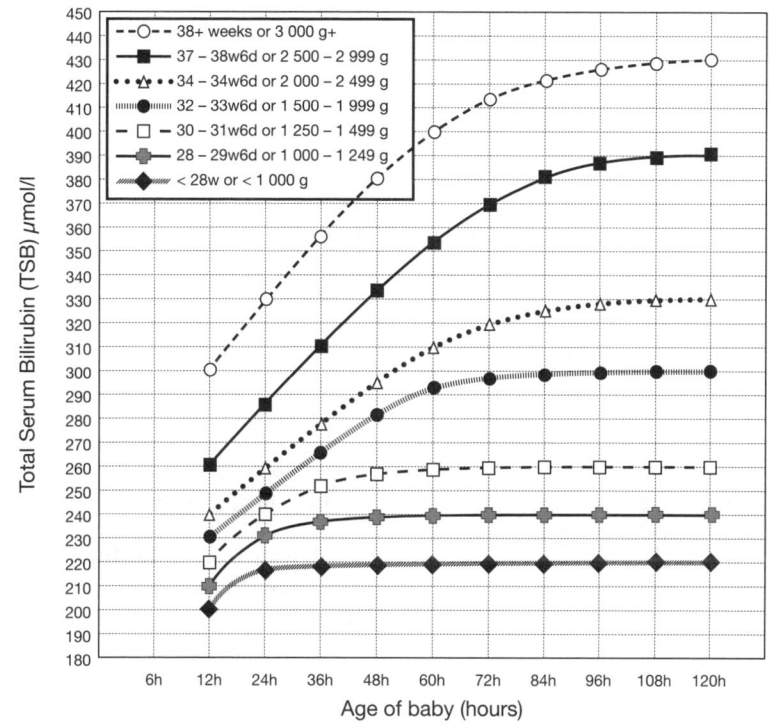

EXCHANGE TRANSFUSION
South African Neonatal Academic Hospital Guidelines: 2006
In presence of sepsis, haemolysis, acidosis, or asphyxia,
use one line lower (gestation below) until <1 000 g.
If gestational age is accurate, use gestational age (weeks) rather than body weight.

Note: 1. Infants who present with TSB above threshold should have exchange done if the TSB is not expected to be below the threshold after 6 hours of intensive phototherapy.
2. Immediate exchange is recommended if there are signs of bilirubin encephalopathy and usually also if TSB is >85 μmol/l above the threshold at presentation.
3. Exchange if TSB continues to rise above 17 μmol/l/hour with intensive phototherapy.

Management. This depends on clinical assessment of severity (see Table 7.11). Severely anaemic infants need oxygen and may need respiratory support. It is wise to check the prothrombin index to exclude haemorrhagic disease of the newborn. The blood sugar level must be monitored before and during an emergency transfusion.

Chronic anaemia

Chronic anaemia at birth is suggested by pallor and a well-compensated cardiovascular system, hepatosplenomegaly, and jaundice. Oedema may be present if the anaemia is very severe. Blood group incompatibility, particularly Rh disease, must be excluded. Chronic intra-uterine infections, mainly congenital syphilis, may present with anaemia.

Anaemia presenting late in the neonatal period may be due to frequent blood sampling or infection. The physiological anaemia of prematurity presents at four to six weeks. Ideally, a record should be kept of blood volumes removed at each venipuncture. Elemental iron 2 mg/kg is given daily once the baby is well. The VLBW infant should also receive 25 IU of vitamin E daily.

Polycythaemia

Polycythaemia is diagnosed when the haematocrit is over 65 per cent, and is associated with hyperviscosity which may have serious consequences, such as necrotizing enterocolitis. The infants at risk are those with hypovolaemia following twin-to-twin or materno-fetal transfusion, underweight for gestational age, wasted infants, and infants of diabetic mothers. Polycythaemia is to be excluded by checking the haemoglobin (Hb) and haematocrit levels in at-risk babies four to eight hours after birth.

Serious signs of hyperviscosity include central cyanosis, respiratory distress, apnoea, convulsions, abdominal distension, cardiac decompensation, and hypoglycaemia. Less ominous features include poor feeding, vomiting, irritability, lethargy, and hypotonia.

A partial exchange transfusion should be performed, using 20 to 30 ml/kg of fresh frozen plasma for any patient with a haematocrit over 70 per cent, or 65 per cent plus any of the serious signs. In view of the great risk of complications, such as cerebral infarcts, it is recommended that the plasma is infused into a peripheral vein, while blood is withdrawn in equal volumes from the umbilical vein.

Bleeding disorders

Bleeding disorders in the neonate include:
- Haemorrhagic disease of the newborn
- Consumption coagulopathy
- Platelet disorders
- Congenital deficiency of coagulation factors.

Haemorrhagic disease of the newborn

This disease is more common in developing countries with poor socio-economic conditions. Bleeding due to lack of vitamin K-dependent factors (II, VII, IX, X) classically occurs 48 hours after delivery. Bleeding commonly occurs from injection sites, cord stump, nose, and gastrointestinal tract, but there may be intracerebral haemorrhage. Multiple sites are commonly involved.

The diagnosis is confirmed by a prolonged prothrombin time (International Normalized Ratio or INR) which improves within two to four hours following the administration of vitamin K, 1 mg IV. Preterm infants respond with a slower rise in the INR or prothrombin index and may require fresh plasma or fresh whole blood in order to control bleeding

Using Apt's test (*see below*) one can distinguish fetal from maternal blood if the baby has haematemesis and melaena. Similarly, if haematemesis persists after a stomach wash-out, it is almost certainly not maternal blood.

It is essential that all babies, including those of low birth weight, receive vitamin K 1 mg IM at delivery in order to prevent this disease.

Consumption coagulopathy (DIC)

Neonates with infection or hypoxia are liable to develop this form of bleeding disorder (*see* Chapter 23, Disorders of the blood).

Consumption coagulopathy may be associated with systemic infection, asphyxia, hypothermia, severe acidosis, and macerated twin. It

Table 7.11 Management of blood loss according to severity

Colour	Pulse	BP	Hb	Haematocrit	Management
Good	Normal	Normal	>15	65%	Observe, check Hb/HCT 2 hours later
Good	Normal	Normal		30–35%	Transfuse – not urgent
Pale	Normal	Normal		Irrespective	Transfuse – urgent, cross-match
Pale	Thready	Low		Irrespective	Transfuse immediately. Use a plasma expander while awaiting blood

usually presents in a seriously ill neonate, with purpura, bruising and bleeding from many sites, including haematuria and intraventricular haemorrhage.

Diagnosis. Clinical features are highly suggestive. The full blood count reveals anaemia, thrombocytopaenia, and red cell fragmentation. Prothrombin, partial thromboplastin, and thrombin times may be prolonged. In severe cases fibrinogen levels are reduced and fibrin degradation products are elevated.

Management. The baby must be treated vigorously for the underlying condition and the clotting defects corrected with fresh plasma 10 ml/kg, platelet concentrates, and fresh whole blood.

Thrombocytopenia

The clinical expression of thrombocytopaenia in the neonate is very variable. The platelet count is usually less than 50 000/mm³. Common causes of thrombocytopaenia are overwhelming bacterial infections, chronic intra-uterine infections, consumption coagulopathy, maternal drugs, auto-immune disease, severe erythroblastosis fetalis, repeat exchange transfusions, and congenital leukaemia. Specific treatment for the underlying condition will reduce the bleeding tendency. Platelet transfusions may be considered if the count is less than 10 000/mm³. An exchange transfusion with whole blood is also recommended.

Thrombasthenia

A bleeding disorder with the features of thrombocytopaenia may occur in the presence of a normal platelet count and coagulation factors; but platelet function may be defective. Chronic ingestion of aspirin by the mother may give rise to this problem.

Congenital deficiency of coagulation factors

These are rare conditions. The usual presentation is one of prolonged bleeding from skin puncture sites in an otherwise well infant. Classical haemophilia (Factor VIII) and Christmas disease (Factor IX) are the most common deficiencies (*see* Chapter 23, Disorders of the blood). The diagnosis rests on family history and demonstration of the relevant deficiency.

Fluid and electrolyte homeostasis

(*see also* Chapter 10, Metabolic disorders).

Maintaining fluid and electrolyte homeostasis has revolutionized the care of the neonate at risk. As the baby adapts to the external environment and independent existence, immaturity of gut, liver and kidneys together with delay in onset of feeding can result in a number of biochemical derangements.

Water balance

Basal fluid requirements are approximately 60 to 150 ml/kg/day, increasing with age. The less mature the baby, the greater are the losses, in particular with the use of the open incubator, radiant heaters, and phototherapy lamps. Osmotic diuresis (e.g. due to glycosuria in the stressed infant receiving a 10 per cent dextrose infusion), excess fluid losses from the gut, and diuretic therapy are examples of increased fluid losses. Fluid retention occurs in severely ill infants with asphyxia, poor renal function, and 'leaky' capillaries. Inappropriate antidiuretic hormone (ADH) secretion may occur in those with neurological and pulmonary problems.

Infants therefore vary greatly in their water requirements and need an assessment of fluid balance six- to twelve-hourly, depending on the clinical state. The following are guidelines of normal urine values: urine volumes 50–100 ml/kg/day, osmolality 75–300 mOsmol/kg, and specific gravity 1005–1012.

The initial intravenous infusion should contain 30–50 mmol/l of sodium and 20 mmol/l potassium with adjustments according to the

In the following situations parenteral fluids should be considered in place of oral feeds:
- *At birth* – severe birth asphyxia, weight less than 1.5 kg, major surgical conditions, severe respiratory distress
- *Later* – respiratory distress, apnoea, cyanosis, intolerance of oral feeds.

electrolyte levels. The glucose requirement is adjusted to the blood sugar level. Most infants are commenced on a 10 per cent glucose infusion.

Oedema

Oedema is a common clinical problem. Accumulation of oedema fluid can be brought about by decreased plasma oncotic pressure or decreased tissue hydrostatic pressure. Immediately after birth the extracellular fluid mass is greater than the intracellular fluid compartment. During the first few days, however, the situation is reversed and weight loss occurs. Within a few days of birth the glomerular filtration rate rises with improved urinary concentration and no change in serum proteins. The body water may also be influenced by the amount of blood infused from the placenta and the mode of delivery: elective Caesarean section babies have a higher water content. The term baby tends to retain salt and may show oedema if challenged with a salt load.

The preterm infant may have moderate oedema, probably due to increased capillary permeability rather than hypoalbuminaemia. Factors such as poor perfusion, acidosis, shock, sepsis, severe respiratory distress, and hypothermia aggravate this situation.

Common causes of severe neonatal oedema are Rh disease and severe haemolytic states, chronic intra-uterine infection, and congenital nephrotic syndrome. In the VLBW baby with HMD, fluid retention causes fairly severe oedema. The syndrome of inappropriate ADH (SIADH) secretion is commonly responsible for oedema in hypoxic ischaemic encephalopathy and severe parenchymal lung disease. This is characterized by hyponatraemia.

Careful assessment of salt and water intake is important in the oedematous baby. Maintenance fluids, plasma, or bicarbonate infusions should be carefully administered. The weight, urine output, peripheral perfusion, blood pressure, and temperature must be carefully monitored. The known causes of oedema must be considered and appropriate treatment instituted.
- Fluid restriction is the first step in controlling oedema.
- A volume expander such as plasma and salt-poor albumin may be infused, followed by a diuretic such as furosemide.
- Underlying metabolic and temperature disturbances need to be corrected.
- Oedema due to SIADH secretion frequently clears with fluid restriction.

Hypocalcaemia

(*See* Chapter 10, Metabolic disorders.)

Approximately one-third of LBW babies and about 50 per cent of the infants born to mothers with diabetes develop hypocalcaemia, which may occur within the first three days of life. In infants fed unmodified milk hypocalcaemia may be seen after the end of the first week as a result of the high phosphate content of cow's milk.

In term infants a serum calcium level of less than 2 mmol/l and in preterm infants less than 1.8 mmol/l are regarded as hypocalcaemia.

Predisposing factors:
- Relative hypoparathyroidism
- Preterm infants are relatively calcium deficient, and factors such as asphyxia, correction of acidosis, and exchange transfusions may precipitate hypocalcaemia.

Treatment. In babies with the predisposing factors, 3 ml of 10% calcium gluconate may be added prophylactically to each 100 ml of glucose infusion from the first day of life, and the calcium level monitored.

Asymptomatic infants may be given oral calcium carbonate, gluconate or lactate as elemental calcium 30 mg/kg daily in divided doses, and the blood level is then monitored.

Symptomatic infants should receive 2 ml/kg of 10% calcium gluconate diluted in 5 ml of 5% glucose and infused very slowly. Calcium may have to be given intravenously or orally over days or even weeks, and the dose gradually decreased and stopped.

Hypomagnesaemia

This disturbance is very infrequent and diagnosed when the serum magnesium level is below 0.62 mmol/l. Signs are indistinguishable from hypocalcaemia and may occur in the UGA baby, the infant of the diabetic mother, or during exchange transfusion. Hypomagnesaemia is corrected by giving 0.1–0.3 ml/kg of 50% magnesium sulphate IV or IM 12-hourly, with a maximum of three doses.

Hypermagnesaemia

This uncommon disturbance occurs when eclamptic mothers are treated with excessive magnesium sulphate. Profound central nervous system depression with apnoea may occur, necessitating ventilation for a number of hours.

Hypernatraemia

(*See* Chapter 10, Metabolic disorders.)

Hypernatraemia is a serum sodium level above 150 mmol/l. Insufficient fluid administration, and dehydration from excessive insensible water loss are the main causes. Phototherapy lamps and radiant heaters tend to cause hyperthermia and diarrhoea. Excessive sodium bicarbonate administration during resuscitation is a further iatrogenic element.

Hyponatraemia

(*See* Chapter 10, Metabolic disorders.)

Hyponatraemia is a serum sodium level less than 125 mmol/l. VLBW infants under 32 weeks' gestation are unable to conserve sodium and may lose more than 3 mmol/kg/day in their urine. Severe asphyxia or respiratory distress may cause SIADH, with water intoxication. Diarrhoea may be a cause of excess sodium losses.

Hyperkalaemia

The causes are severe catabolism, acute renal failure, hypoxia, shock, acidosis, and congenital adrenal hyperplasia.

Birth trauma

Minor superficial injuries

Superficial abrasions on the infant's face, scalp, or other parts may be caused by blood sampling, rupture of the membrane by toothed forceps, or scalpel cuts during Caesarean section. Suturing may be necessary to prevent excessive blood loss. These lesions should be kept clean and dry.

Extensive bruising is often seen in the markedly preterm neonate. Oedema, bruising, and haematomas may involve the vulva, scrotum, and testes following breech delivery of the baby. These injuries settle in a few days. This extravasation of blood may contribute to hyperbilirubinaemia and anaemia.

Subconjunctival haemorrhage follows on difficult delivery. It usually clears spontaneously within a week, requiring no therapy other than reassurance to the mother.

Head injuries

Skull moulding denotes overriding of the cranial bones due to compression in the birth canal. It does not necessarily imply intracranial injury. The skull bones assume a normal position within a few days.

Swelling of the head is caused by caput succedaneum, vacuum extraction, cephalhaematoma, or subaponeurotic haemorrhage. (*See* Table 7.12 and Figure 7.6.).

Skull fractures may be linear, stellate, or depressed. Occasionally there is overlying soft tissue swelling, but rarely intracranial damage. Nevertheless, observations for 36 to 48 hours for signs of neuropathology are advisable. Depressed fractures resemble a ping-pong ball indentation and usually require elevation.

Limb fractures

Fractures of the clavicle, humerus, and femur may occur during difficult deliveries. Movements of the affected limb are restricted and very painful. Splinting is usually not needed for the upper limb, but femur fractures may require traction. In every case the mother must be warned that a large callus is likely to form.

Nerve injuries

Facial nerve paralysis, either due to forceps application or occurring spontaneously, is characterized by diminished movement of the affected
side of the face, with or without ability to close
the eye on the affected side. The baby may have
difficulty in sucking. Treatment consists of keeping the affected eye clean by periodic instillation of sterile saline solution. The baby should
be nursed on the unaffected side. The weakness
usually resolves in hours to days.

Brachial plexus injury is a serious injury, which
is usually caused by excessive traction in cases of
impacted shoulders or breech delivery. Upper
arm paralysis results from injury to cervical roots

Table 7.12 Swellings of the head

	Caput succedaneum	Vacuum extraction haematoma	Cephalhaematoma	Subaponeurotic haemorrhage
Site	Diffuse over presenting part	Localized at site of vacuum application. Skin and subcutaneous tissue involved	Localized, usually over parietal bones, under periosteum. Extension limited by periosteal adhesion of sutures	Diffuse over whole head underneath cranial aponeurosis
Cause	Oedema and bruising of presenting part	Oedema ± haemorrhage at vacuum site	Haemorrage often due to cephalo-pelvic disproportion	Diffuse haemorrhage; sometimes follows vacuum extraction or poorly applied forceps
Onset	Present at birth	Present at birth	Often only detected 6–12 hours after birth. Becomes progressively larger over 1–2 days	May be present at birth; swelling often increases during first 2 days
Distinguishing features	Diffuse. Petechiae over swelling	Usually well defined. Localized abrasions at periphery of swelling. Overlying skin may be purple	Well defined. Does not cross suture lines. May be bilateral, but then a groove is present between the two swellings. Skin normal	Diffuse and sometimes massive haemorrhage. Crosses suture lines. Bluish discoloration of upper eyelids or behind ears. Skin normal
Course	Disappears within 48 hours	Subsides within 5–7 days	Persists 6–8 weeks. Centre may become fluctuant	Gradual reabsorption of blood
Complications	Nil	Anaemia, infection, jaundice	Anaemia, jaundice, infection if aspirated. Rarely, underlying skull fracture	Severe anaemia, shock, jaundice
Treatment	Nil	Local antiseptic to abrasions. Treat complications	Usually nil. Observe complications	Vitamin K. May need urgent blood transfusion

5 and 6 (Erb-Duchenne paralysis). The arm is rotated internally and hangs limply at the shoulder, the elbow is extended, the forearm pronated, while the fingers are flexed in a 'waiter's tip' position. Wrist action and grasp reflex are normal.

Total arm paralysis (Klumpke paralysis) is due to injury to the 7th and 8th cervical nerves.

Complete rupture of nerve roots results in permanent lesions. If the paralyses are due to bruising of nerve roots, function returns within several months. Physiotherapy can be given to prevent contractures.

Spinal cord injury. This rare injury usually results from traction on the legs in breech delivery. There is flaccid paralysis with loss of sensation below the level of the lesion and bladder distension. The prognosis is poor.

Abdominal viscera

Occasionally a difficult delivery results in rupture of the liver and/or spleen. Large babies are particularly prone to this serious injury. The first sign is usually shock, followed by anaemia and some abdominal distension. An urgent blood transfusion and laparotomy are called for. An additional dose of vitamin K is advisable.

Intracranial haemorrhage

The extent of the injury and the outcome depend on the underlying pathogenic factors. There are four major categories of haemorrhage in the newborn: subdural, primary subarachnoid, periventricular-intraventricular, and intracerebellar. haemorrhage (*See* Figure 7.6.)

Figure 7.6 Caput succedaneum and intra- and extracranial haemorrhage

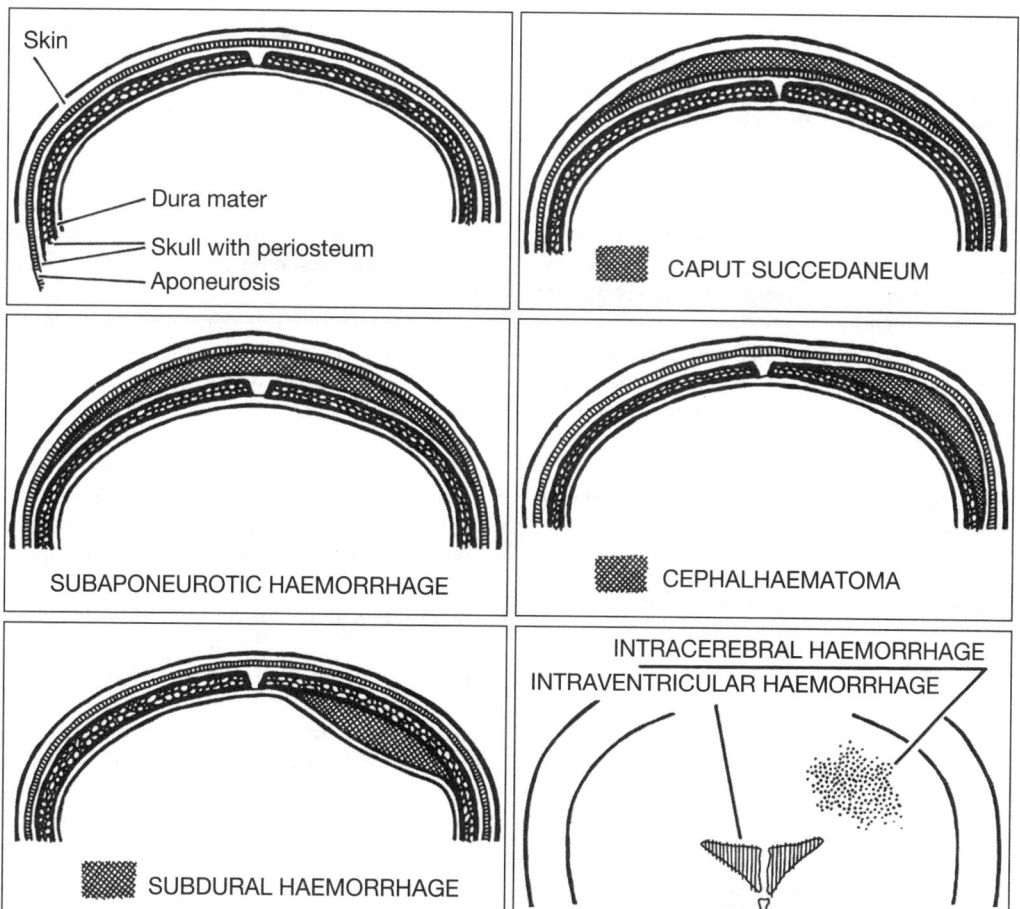

Subdural fluid collections

This is the second most common cause of abnormal head enlargement. The three main pathological types are haematoma, hygroma, and effusion and all are managed along similar lines.

Bleeding in the subdural space is due to disruption of bridging veins from the cerebral surface to the major venous sinuses (*see* Figure 7.6). Birth trauma accounts for the majority of cases. Major factors are cephalopelvic disproportion, the duration of labour, and the manner of delivery. Acute subdural haemorrhages in the neonatal period generally have a poor prognosis.

Less commonly, bleeding disorders and dehydration cause subdural bleeds. Hygromas result from laceration of the pia arachnoid and effusions as the result of infections. In an acute subdural bleed the lysing blood clot creates an osmotic gradient which draws fluid into the space, enlarging the lesion and thus promoting further bleeding.

Massive *infratentorial haemorrhage* manifests from the time of birth. The signs are due to brainstem compression, namely deviation of the eyes, unequal pupils, rapid respiration, and opisthotonus. If haemorrhage progresses coma ensues, the pupils become fixed and dilated, ocular bobbing appears, and finally respiratory arrest occurs. If the haemorrhage is less catastrophic the infant may survive with the late development of hydrocephalus.

Minor subdural haemorrhage over the cerebral convexities may be asymptomatic. Focal seizures may occur together with other focal cerebral signs.

Hygromas do not expand because the pia is less vascular and the effusions are absorbed with resolution of the infection.

Figure 7.7 The cerebral consequences of asphyxia

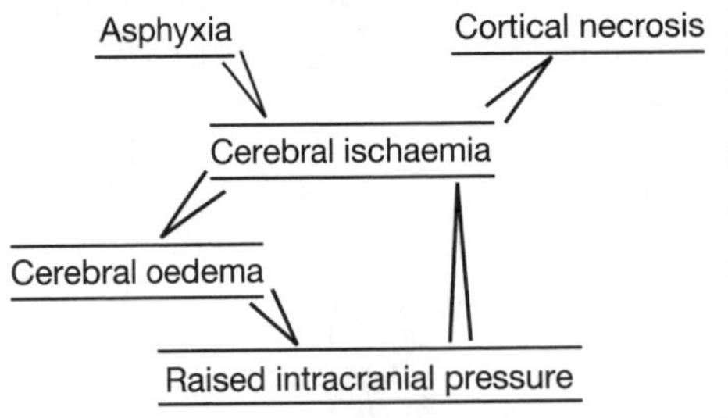

Diagnosis. In acute subdural bleeds, subhyaloid haemorrhage may be seen on fundoscopy. A computerized tomography (CT) scan is the investigation of choice.

Treatment. Subdural clotted blood may be difficult to drain by needling and require a burrhole. However, the chronic subdural collection is easily tapped (*see* Chapter 36, Procedures). Chronic collections may be tapped repeatedly over three to four weeks and if they do not subside, surgical intervention is indicated, possibly with a temporary subdural peritoneal shunt. In the acute variety the blood must be evacuated.

Hypoxic damage

Hypoxic ischaemic encephalopathy (HIE)

This results from significant hypoxia of the fetus or newborn. Hypoxia is due to the failure of gas exchange at placental level in the fetus and pulmonary level in the newborn. Perinatal hypoxia is predominantly an antenatal event, with no more than 10 per cent occurring postpartum. HIE is probably the major cause of cerebral palsy in the developing world. The pathogenesis of brain damage resulting from hypoxia is illustrated in Figure 7.7.

As fetal respiration is controlled by placental circulation, fetal hypoxia implies some degree of placental ischaemia. The systemic response to hypoxia, hypercarbia, and mixed acidosis is maintenance of cerebral blood flow at the expense of other organs. It follows that if an episode of hypoxia is sufficiently prolonged and severe, other organs such as the heart will be affected. With further decreased cardiac output, hypotension occurs and perfusion of the brain, kidney, lung, and gut is compromised. The clinical effects are those of ischaemia of these organs. The duration and severity of signs depend on the period of hypoxia and/or ischaemia.

Clinical features. These are caused by hypoxia and ischaemia occurring simultaneously or in sequence. Following severe intra-partum hypoxia and/or ischaemia, the infant goes into coma and has convulsions. Hypoxia during labour may be followed by a lucid interval of 12 to 18 hours, before convulsions occur, which at times are subtle and expressed as **apnoeic** or **cyanotic attacks**. The respiration is often irregular with a Cheyne-Stokes pattern suggesting diffuse bilateral hemisphere pathology. With a severe insult brain-stem signs occur, such as fixed, dilated pupils, and abnormal or absent eye movements. Motor weakness is the main clinical manifestation of primary ischaemia. The fontanelle may become full as a result of cerebral oedema.

The clinical grades of HIE are mild, moderate, or severe, depending on the severity and duration of neurological signs. Early improvement suggests a good prognosis.

Management. The most important aspect is prevention, by identifying the fetus at risk of hypoxia and taking the necessary steps to prepare for prompt resuscitation. Where a baby has been hypoxic, brain-oriented management is important and is directed at relieving factors that aggravate or contribute to hypoxia.

- Raise the head to 30 degrees above the plane of the body.
- Adequate control of seizures is essential. (*See below*). Some seizures are subtle.
- Keep the infant's core temperature at 35 °C for 48 hours. This reduces the risk of progressive brain damage.
- Avoid hypoglycaemia by maintaining the blood sugar level above 2.5 mmol/l.
- Monitor the blood pressure. Hypotension occurs frequently in severely hypoxic infants. If fluid replacement does not restore normotension, dopamine may be used. Dopamine is of value in the baby with poor urine output as well.
- Routine administration of alkali is not recommended. Acidosis corrects spontaneously if the infant is adequately and efficiently resuscitated at birth.

- Clotting disturbances may occur and are most often due to disseminated intravascular coagulation. Management is supportive, the infant should receive vitamin K, fresh frozen plasma, platelet transfusion, and fresh whole blood as the clinical condition demands.
- Feeding is by a nasogastric tube, the volume not exceeding 80 ml/kg/day for the first two to three days.
- Respiratory support for a limited period may be considered for the infant with severe HIE.
- Meningitis may be clinically indistinguishable from HIE. If in any doubt, a lumbar puncture and examination of the cerebrospinal fluid should be performed.

A number of drugs such as calcium channel blockers, magnesium sulphate, prostaglandins, and neurotransmitter inhibitors are under investigation but not yet recommended.

Complications such as pneumonia, hypoglycaemia, inappropriate antidiuretic hormone secretion, must be borne constantly in mind. Long-term follow-up of the child is essential to detect complications and developmental handicap. Appropriate rehabilitative measures must be introduced.

Fortunately an appreciable proportion of those who make rapid and early progress remain free of any deficit.

Convulsions

Neonatal seizures result from an insult to the brain. In themselves they are also injurious to the neurones. Furthermore, the concurrent res-

---

Mild HIE manifests neurological signs such as feeding and tone disturbances for 24 to 48 hours.
Moderate HIE includes convulsions and signs which last for four to five days.
Severe HIE is diagnosed if the physical signs are severe and persist for seven to 14 days or more.

The prognosis depends on the duration and severity of the cerebral insult. A neonate with prolonged loss of consciousness and generalized hypotonia with severe convulsions very rarely makes a complete recovery especially if the signs remain beyond seven days. Cerebral palsy, microcephaly, and lesser degrees of neurological impairment are the sequelae of profound cerebral hypoxia.

piratory disturbance causes hypoxia and hypercapnia (*see* Figure 7.8).

Subtle convulsions are very common. The physical signs include deviation of the eyes, repetitive blinking or fluttering of the eyelids, drooling, sucking, cycling movements of the lower limbs, rowing movements of the upper limbs, tonic posturing of a limb, apnoea attacks, cyanotic episodes, an abnormal cry, and stertorous respiration.

Tonic seizures indicate severe encephalopathy.
Clonic convulsions may be focal or multifocal. Lastly there are *myoclonic seizures*, which are single or multiple flexion jerks of groups of muscles.

Jitteriness must be distinguished from convulsions: it is not accompanied by loss of consciousness or abnormal eye movements and stops as soon as the limbs are held. However, it starts again easily with stimulation. Bradycardia, pallor or cyanosis do not occur.

The most common causes of neonatal convulsions are HIE, birth trauma, metabolic disturbances such as hypoglycaemia and hypocalcaemia, hypothermia, intracranial infections, electrolyte disturbances (particularly sodium imbalance), and narcotic and alcohol withdrawal.

Management

- Convulsions must be controlled as a matter of urgency. *See* Table 7.13
- Supportive care is provided as for any unconscious neonate.
- The airway must be kept clear with regular, gentle naso- and oropharyngeal suction.
- Oxygen is given for cyanosis
- The baby is nursed prone or on the side with regular changing of position to facilitate drainage of secretions.

Figure 7.8 The pathogenesis of brain damage in neonatal convulsions

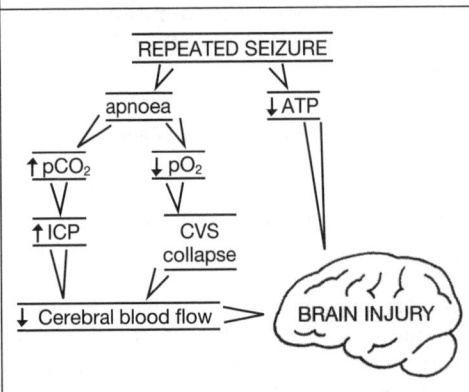

Table 7.13 Anticonvulsant drug use	
Drug	**Dose**
Seizure control	
Phenytoin intravenous and Phenobarbital oral	Loading dose 15 mg/kg in 3 ml 0.9% NaCl over 30 minutes slow IV infusion Loading dose 20–40 mg/kg via orogastric tube
or	
Clonazepam and Phenobarbital	Loading dose 0.1–0.15 mg/kg slow IV injection Loading dose 20–40 mg/kg via orogastric tube
Maintenance	
Phenytoin Phenobarbital	IVI/oral: 5–8 mg/kg/24 hours in 3 divided doses 5 mg/kg/day in 2 divided doses

- Monitor temperature, blood pressure, oxygen saturation, and blood sugar levels.
- The baby must be tube-fed, commencing with 80 to 100 ml/kg/day.

When seizures have ceased for 24–48 hours, the anticonvulsant dosage may be reduced gradually over days.

Prognosis. The nature of the underlying neurological disease will determine the eventual outcome in the individual baby with seizures. Generally:

- Babies with convulsions due to HIE have only a 50 per cent chance of normal development.
- Hypoglycaemia-associated convulsions have a similar outcome.
- Convulsions due to intracranial infection are associated with permanent damage in 20–50 per cent of cases.
- Severe intraventricular haemorrhage causes 65–100 per cent morbidity with a mortality of 50–65 per cent.

Follow-up. It is essential that all babies who have had convulsions are assessed neurologically at regular intervals in order to detect deficits, which usually manifest within nine to twelve months. Minor problems are often not detected during the pre-school period, but arise later as attention and learning difficulties. With expert counselling of the parents and correct management, many difficulties may be overcome at home. Infants with significant neurological deficits may require the assistance of a physiotherapist, occupational therapist, and clinical psychologist. Hearing, vision, and speech assessments may be necessary.

Subarachnoid haemorrhage

This haemorrhage is related to hypoxia in term infants. The development of the haemorrhage probably occurs as a result of vascular injury following hypoxia and ischaemia. Small bleeds occur commonly without clinical manifestations. Very few will have a structural lesion such as an aneurysm or a vascular malformation.

The clinical features are difficult to outline because of the associated manifestations of hypoxia. Convulsions may occur on the second day of life. Between seizures these babies appear very well and the prognosis is excellent. A massive haemorrhage runs a fatal course and is often associated with trauma. The cerebrospinal fluid is bloody, and later xanthochromic, with a high protein and an increased cell count.

Intraventricular haemorrhage (IVH)

This classical haemorrhage of the preterm infant occurs within the first 72 hours of life, often in association with respiratory distress. It starts as a haemorrhage into the germinal matrix and then may burst into the ventricles. The delicate vessels of the germinal matrix form a large unsupported network of capillaries, which ruptures easily. In 20–40 per cent of lesions the haemorrhage is confined to the brain tissue (germinal matrix) and does not rupture into the ventricles. As the fetus matures, the germinal matrix becomes less vascular. This form of haemorrhage is therefore rare in the term baby.

The **pathogenesis** has as yet not been fully clarified. However, hypoxia and ischaemia are major factors; in addition, raised cerebral venous pressure occurring during resuscitation contributes. Furthermore, there is marked fibrinolytic activity in the newborn, which promotes spread of the haemorrhage.

The **clinical presentation** is variable and depends on the size and rate of bleeding. Small haemorrhages may produce no signs. With large haemorrhages loss of consciousness, apnoea, convulsions, a full fontanelle, and anaemia may occur. Altered muscle tone, behaviour disturbances, and progressive head enlargement may be the only signs.

The classical clinical features make the diagnosis easy. Ultrasonography is used for confirmation; in difficult cases a CT scan may be indicated. These are also used for grading of the lesions.

> Grade I (bleed into the germinal matrix only) and Grade II (extension of the bleed into the ventricles) can be expected to achieve a full recovery. Grade III (ventricles dilated with blood) is associated with a risk of obstructive hydrocephalus. An associated periventricular venous infarct is also called a Grade IV intraventricular haemorrhage.

A unilateral Grade IV IVH may lead to a porencephalic cyst and hemiplegia; bilateral lesions are usually fatal. No definite guidelines for treatment have been established. Intervention is not indicated for those with severe haemorrhage, as the mortality is in the region of 90 per cent and the remaining patients have severe morbidity. Blood transfusions, anticonvulsants, and eventual shunting may be indicated. Approximately 35 per cent of babies with IVH develop posthaemorrhagic hydrocephalus.

Recent evidence indicates that the outcome in the milder cases does not depend on the extent of the haemorrhage but on the initiating events and circumstances. With steady improvement in the management of these small babies, the incidence and complications of IVH are decreasing.

Periventricular leucomalacia (PVL)

PVL occurs when ischaemia is prolonged or severe in a preterm infant. This degenerative process may resolve or progress to multiple small cysts; clinical features are determined by the site and extent of the injury. The diagnosis is made by intracranial ultrasonography after the first few days of life.

Parasagittal cerebral damage

This typical cerebral lesion occurs in the term infant. There is necrosis of the cerebral cortex and subcortical white matter with characteristic bilateral symmetrical distribution leading to leucomalacia of the parasagittal and superomedial aspects of the cerebral hemispheres. The 'watershed' infarct that follows cerebral hypoperfusion emphasizes the ischaemic nature of the lesion. In severe cases, necrosis extends to the lateral cerebral convexity. Clinically, spastic motor deficit, seizures, and intellectual impairment occur.

Focal ischaemic cerebral injury

Focal ischaemic lesions may also occur as a result of generalized cerebral hypoperfusion, with the middle cerebral arteries being most frequently involved. Infarction occurs with subsequent cystic development, which may or may not communicate with the lateral ventricles. The unilateral lesion results in hemiparesis and multiple lesions may cause quadriparesis.

Infection

Newborn babies may be infected before birth, at birth, or in the neonatal period.

Acquired neonatal infections

The reported prevalence of infection in neonatal units varies from 7–30 per cent. Certain predisposing factors increase the risk of infection in the neonate. These are:

- ◆ Maternal infection both acute and chronic
  - – Amniotic fluid infection syndrome (chorioamnionitis) is a common condition
- ◆ Newborn babies become colonized at the same time that they have to develop their own immunity
- ◆ Immature host defence mechanisms – both qualitative and quanitative
  - – Newborns do not have IgM and IgA antibodies; the latter protects the mucosal surfaces
- ◆ Low birth weight and prematurity – passive transfer of antibodies occurs late in gestation
- ◆ Obstetric or resuscitative procedures
- ◆ Anatomic: long cord stump, delicate or cracked skin
- ◆ Nursery environment: crowding, under-staffing, poor hand-washing facilities.

For these reasons, neonates become infected with Gram-negative bacteria as well as all the 'usual' infections, and if infected, they are particularly likely to develop septicaemic illness.

The prevention of infection is very important and prompt recognition is necessary for optimal management. It is equally important to stop antibiotic therapy when the investigations and subsequent clinical picture do not support the diagnosis of infection. Antibiotic therapy is not only a discomfort to the patient and a considerable expense, but also increases the risk of developing resistant organisms.

Common organisms

The common bacterial pathogens are the Gram-positive organisms, such as Group B streptococcus, *Streptococcus faecalis*, *Staphylococcus aureus*, and *Listeria monocytogenes*. Gram-negative organisms are *Escherichia coli* and *Klebsiella pneumoniae*. Infection due to herpes, enteroviruses, chlamydia, and *Pneumocystis jirovecii* may present in the same manner.

Superficial infections

Constant vigilance for infections is essential in the following areas: skin, umbilicus, eye, mouth, and perineum.

Systemic antibiotics are rarely indicated. Any pustules and abscesses of the skin should be opened and the pus collected for a Gram stain and culture. The lesions are cleaned with alcohol or chlorhexidine and left exposed to air. Strict hand-washing should be observed and the baby isolated if possible.

Conjunctivitis requires prompt treatment, preceded by a Gram stain and culture (*see* Chapter 33, Disorders of the eye). The eyes must be cleaned with saline and a broad-spectrum antibiotic instilled two- to four-hourly. If the eyelids are red and swollen (blepharitis), ceftriaxone 125 mg IM or IV is given in a single dose.

For *oral thrush*, nystatin suspension is instilled after each feed. Nystatin cream must be applied to the perineal area when this is involved. Monilial infection of the mother often calls for concomitant therapy.

An *umbilical flare* without induration may be regarded as a superficial infection. Shortening the stump and spraying the area frequently with alcohol is all that is required. Dressings should not be applied but the area should be observed for spread of infection.

Septicaemia

The diagnosis of infection may be very difficult in the newborn because of subtle and non-specific presentation. Certain clinical features, however, are highly *suggestive* of infection, while others indicate *obvious* sepsis.

Septicaemia should be suspected when three of the following are present:
♦ Predisposing factors as above
♦ Unstable temperature
♦ Lethargy
♦ Poor colour

♦ Apnoea
♦ Feeding difficulties
♦ Vomiting
♦ Abdominal distension
♦ Sclerema
♦ Superficial sepsis.

A combination of the following signs is strongly indicative of serious infection: purpura, anaemia, jaundice, hepatomegaly, splenomegaly, full fontanelle or a swollen joint.

Investigations. To confirm suspected infection a full blood count and smear and blood culture are performed and material from superficial lesions is examined by Gram stain. Cerebrospinal fluid (CSF) is examined and cultured if there is clinical suspicion of meningitis. Urinary tract infections generally occur after the first week of life and may be considered in late-onset infections. A C-reactive protein (CRP) estimation is very useful; in conjunction with the white cell count it gives support to a clinical diagnosis of sepsis. Both of these are also of value in assessing response to treatment. A chest radiograph should be considered even in the absence of signs of respiratory distress. A Gram stain of the gastric aspirate before the first feed is helpful if chorioamnionitis is suspected: the presence of organisms and pus cells is indicative of infection. In the tuberculosis-exposed infant chest radiograph, lumbar puncture for the tubercle bacillus and a baseline full blood count, tuberculosis blood culture and liver function tests are done (*see* Chapter 17, Tuberculosis).

Babies exposed to tuberculosis should receive prophylaxis with isoniazid and rifampicin for three months.

Management
♦ Penicillin and an aminoglycoside are started early once infection is suspected until culture reports are available, when antibiotics are either stopped or changed according to microbial sensitivity.
♦ The duration of antibiotic therapy depends on the nature of the organism and the clinical condition of the patient, but in general, proven septicaemia is treated for seven to ten days.
♦ Supportive care of the infected neonate in respect of metabolic derangements, hypothermia, abdominal distension,

hypoxia, poor perfusion, and so on is as important as the specific antibiotic.

Prevention

- All personnel handling neonates must be trained in the prevention of and the dangers of infection. Contamination from the hands of attendants is the most important source of infection. Hand-washing before and after handling an individual baby is recommended and attendants' hands must be sprayed with antiseptic before touching a baby.
- Careful attention to the umbilical cord and meticulous cleaning of the skin before venepuncture are mandatory. The use of prophylactic antibiotics in newborn infants should be discouraged.
- Exclusive breastfeeding and kangaroo mother care are most important aspects in the prevention of infection. Both colonize the infant with community bacteria of low pathogenicity and protect against harmful hospital bacteria.
- Overcrowding must be avoided and isolation facilities for highly infectious illnesses, such as acute infective diarrhoea, must be available in all units.

Pneumonia

Pneumonia is an important cause of morbidity and mortality in the neonatal period. Infection may be transmitted via the placenta, by aspiration during delivery, or acquired postnatally.

The clinical features include those of respiratory distress and the specific infection.

Aspiration pneumonia is acquired during the last days of pregnancy or at birth by aspirating infected material and can occur in the presence of intact membranes (chorioamnionitis) or ruptured membranes (if ruptured for more than 12 hours). Sometimes aspiration of maternal faecal material at the time of delivery may result in pneumonia. Clinically the liquor may be offensive and the onset of the illness occurs within minutes or hours of birth. Signs of respiratory distress may be mild or severe and delayed for a day or two. The microbes involved are group B beta-haemolytic streptococcus, pneumococcus, and coliforms.

In postnatally acquired pneumonia, the signs of respiratory distress usually appear after the first week of life. Common bacteria are coagulase positive staphylococci, streptococci, *Escherichia coli*, and *Klebsiella pneumoniae*. Respiratory syncytial virus, influenza A and B, adenovirus, and echoviruses have been associated with outbreaks of pneumonia in nurseries. *Chlamydia* and *Pneumocystis jirovecii* may be responsible for infection, particularly in premature babies.

Another form of nursery-acquired infection occurs in babies supported by respirators. This disastrous, often low-grade, chronic pneumonia from organisms such as *Klebsiella* and *Pseudomonas* contributes to mortality and chronic pulmonary disability. These organisms are harboured in equipment such as humidifiers and suction apparatus. Once established, these organisms are extremely difficult to eradicate.

Meningitis

This is perhaps the most difficult diagnosis to make on clinical grounds alone. *The classical signs occur very late* in the neonate. An added difficulty is the fact that a full fontanelle and convulsions are frequently not due to meningitis. Should these signs occur in the presence of meningitis, the prognosis is poor.

Meningitis is therefore diagnosed on clinical suspicion, and an examination of the CSF is recommended in any infant who is suspected of having sepsis. Ventriculitis is a characteristic feature of neonatal meningitis and is very resistant to treatment.

Osteitis and septic arthritis

There are two anatomical reasons why these conditions occur together so frequently. Firstly, the capsules of the hip and shoulder joint are attached below the metaphysis of the femur and humerus respectively. Infection of the epiphyseal cartilage will extend into the joint space, causing purulent arthritis. Secondly, during the first year of life capillaries perforate the epiphyseal plate of the long bones and provide a communication between metaphysis and joint space so that spread readily occurs. The most common organism is *Staphylococcus aureus* followed by Group B streptococcus and Gram-negative organisms. This disease may follow certain invasive procedures, such as femoral vein puncture and umbilical catheterization.

The most useful physical sign is decreased movement of the affected limb; redness and swelling are late signs. Of all the serious infections this is most often diagnosed late. Early X-rays may still be normal (*see* Chapter 31, Orthopaedic disorders).

Specific infections

Chlamydia trachomatis

The organism is acquired by the baby from the mother's birth canal and colonizes the nasopharynx in the majority of cases.

Conjunctivitis occurs within five to 14 days and may be mild or very severe with purulent discharge.

Pneumonia develops in about 25 per cent of babies with nasopharyngeal colonization. The onset is insidious about one to three months after birth. Cough and tachypnoea are present, but the absence of fever and significant wheezing serves to differentiate this infection from that caused by respiratory syncytial virus. The peripheral blood smear often shows significant eosinophilia.

Diagnosis is by culture or serology.

Treatment with erythromycin has to be prolonged for 14 days for a response.

Streptococcus agalactiae (Group B beta haemolytic streptococcus – GBS)

This common commensal of the genital and gastrointestinal tract of pregnant women may colonize their babies. The mothers are usually asymptomatic but may have urine infection or chorioamnionitis.

Early-onset infection (within 72 hours to seven days) is more common than late-onset disease. Many babies are symptomatic at birth, indicating exposure *in utero*, which often arises in amniotic infection. Immature, low-birth-weight babies are particularly prone. Clinically, babies suffer from pneumonia with respiratory distress which can mimic hyaline membrane disease. This is often complicated by pulmonary hypertension. Bacteraemia occurs frequently, and the patients may have disseminated disease, including meningitis and septic shock. The mortality rate is high.

Late-onset infection accounts for 20 per cent of cases. This can develop at any time, but after one month of age is usually associated with prematurity and immunodeficiency. This presents as bacteraemia or meningitis. Disseminated foci of infection can develop.

Diagnosis is by culture of blood, CSF or other fluids.

Treatment is with penicillin G.

Listeria monocytogenes

This facultative anaerobic Gram-positive bacillus may cause disease in a similar way to GBS. Infection during pregnancy may be associated with spontaneous abortion, stillbirth, or disseminated disease in a premature baby. This frequently presents with a diffuse pustular rash, hepatosplenomegaly and a very high mortality. This organism may present early or late in infection.

Treatment: Ampicillin and an aminoglycoside are used together. Listeria are not susceptible to the cephalosporins.

Chronic intra-uterine infection

Congenital infections are acquired *in utero* because of transplacental spread of infection within the mother's bloodstream, or because of direct spread from infected amniotic fluid. They affect the fetus in two ways:

♦ By inducing organ damage, which persists after the maternal infection has been treated or overcome. These are teratogenic influences for maldevelopment or permanent changes

♦ By blood-spread dissemination and persistence of the infection at the time of birth. Such babies show pathology and dysfunction of many organ systems at birth together with a septicaemic presentation.

The prenatally acquired infections should be diagnosed in the presence of a combination of hepatosplenomegaly, jaundice, anaemia, and purpura in the newborn baby. Apart from the above, HIV infection, tuberculosis, hepatitis B

A number of pathogens are involved in causing similar clinical manifestations, conveniently remembered by the word, TORCHES:

▪ **T** Toxoplasmosis
▪ **O** Other viruses
▪ **R** Rubella
▪ **C** Cytomegalovirus
▪ **He** Herpes virus
▪ **S** Syphilis.

and listeriosis should be considered. In syphilis, typical skin lesions and/or metaphysitis may occur in isolation or together with this constellation of signs.

HIV-exposed neonates suffer an additional burden of disease, especially in the small, wasted preterm infant. These babies may experience a number of co-infections, including tuberculosis, syphilis, cytomegalovirus, herpes simplex, fungal infections and recurrent acute bacterial infections. These babies present in the latter part of the second week or in the third week of postnatal life. The mode of presentation in infants infected with HIV during pregnancy is one of persistent or recurrent pneumonia, fungal or bacterial infections. These latter infections may be superficial or systemic.

Fetal varicella syndrome

This syndrome can occur in 10–13 per cent of fetuses whose mothers contract chickenpox in the first trimester of pregnancy, and in 5 per cent if the mother contracts chickenpox after the first trimester. The major features are skin lesions, cerebral atrophy, and eye abnormalities. Pregnant women in contact with varicella or who contract varicella should receive varicella zoster immunoglobulin (VZIG) within 96 hours of exposure.

Congenital rubella

The main importance of the disease is the transplacental transfer of the virus to the fetus when a pregnant woman contracts rubella. The virus may spread widely in the fetus, damaging differentiating cells in many organs, leading to abortion, stillbirth, or a malformed child. The risk of embryopathy is highest the earlier in pregnancy the mother is infected: in the first month >80 per cent of fetuses exhibit embryopathy; by the fourth month the risk has dropped to 5 per cent. Congenital rubella is rare in South Africa, since most women in the reproductive age group have protective antibodies.

Embryopathy consists of one or several of the following:

+ *Temporary damage.* Thrombocytopaenia, hepatitis, skeletal change, pneumonia, haemolysis, and small-for-gestational age
+ *Permanent damage.* Congenital heart disease, cataracts, microphthalmia, deafness, psychomotor retardation, microcephaly, and spastic quadriparesis.

Serological **diagnosis** is by IgM specific antibody.

Pregnant women who are exposed to rubella in the first trimester in pregnancy should be tested and if found to be infected, therapeutic abortion should be advised. Immunoglobulin therapy is of no value in such cases. Immunization with the live virus rubella vaccine is not advised in pregnancy.

Congenital cytomegalovirus (CMV) infections

The incidence of congenital infection ranges from 0.2–2 per cent. Currently CMV infection is the next commonest co-infection to tuberculosis in the newborn. The exact incidence in South Africa is not known. The majority are asymptomatic (only 5–10 per cent develop disease). Asymptomatic infants may subsequently develop deafness. In those with disease, hepatosplenomegaly, jaundice, purpura, microcephaly, cerebral calcifications, and chorioretinitis may occur together or singly. Neurological involvement, (e.g. deafness, visual loss, cerebral palsy) may not be evident for some time. Extraneural disease is usually reversible.

Confirmation of diagnosis is by detection of large, inclusion-bearing cells in urine, specific IgM antibody in cord serum, CMV PCR on secretions and by virus isolation. The differential diagnosis includes congenital toxoplasmosis, rubella and herpes simplex infection, as well as bacterial sepsis.

Congenital syphilis

Syphilis is most commonly acquired transplacentally, the fetus being infected by an infected mother. Rarely, infection may occur from contact with infectious lesions during passage through the birth canal.

The incidence is not known, but the number of cases of congenital syphilis correlates with the incidence of primary and secondary syphilis in women, and the adequacy of antenatal care. There appears to be a worldwide resurgence. Sero-surveys from Africa indicate that 2–25 per cent of pregnant mothers are infected. The spectrum of syphilis in childhood is outlined in Table 7.14.

Pathogenesis. It has been shown that infection may occur as early as the first trimester, even though histological evidence of syphilis is rarely seen until the second trimester. Clinico-pathological effects in syphilis are determined by host immune responses and therefore a possible explanation is that the fetus is able to exhibit an inflammatory response only in the second tri-mester. Syphilis is not a common cause of early abortion and adequate therapy of the mother during the first trimester prevents congenital syphilis in the fetus. Haematological spread from an infected mother involves the placenta

Table 7.14 Manifestations of congenital syphilis		
	Early	**Late**
Skin	Bullae Desquamation Red maculo-papules Condylomata	
Mucous membranes	Fissures Scars Rhinitis	Scars at corners of mouth (rhagades) Flat nasal bridge ('saddle nose')
Liver/spleen	Hepatosplenomegaly Jaundice Hepatitis	
Haematological	Anaemia 　Haemolytic 　Leuco-erythroblastic 　Normocytic, normochromic Leukaemoid reaction Thrombocytopaenia DIC	
Bones	Metaphysitis Diaphysitis Periostitis	Sabre tibia Bossing Deformities of maxilla
CNS	Meningo-encephalitis Convulsions Hydrocephalus	Chronic meningo-vascular disease Hydrocephalus Mental retardation Cranial nerve palsies Hemiplegia Paresis and tabes
Renal	Nephrotic syndrome	
Other	SGA Pseudoparalysis Oedema Pancreatitis Gastrointestinal disease Pneumonia alba Susceptibility to other infections Chorio-retinitis	Malnutrition Hutchinson's teeth Mulberry molars Caries Nerve deafness Painless synovitis Interstitial keratitis Argyll Robertson pupil Optic atrophy

and may lead to pathology in many organs in the fetus.

The placenta in congenital syphilis is large, pale, and greasy. Vasculitis may lead to infarction and intra-uterine death, premature delivery, or intra-uterine growth retardation.

Clinical manifestations. Prenatal infection may be obvious at birth or signs and symptoms may be delayed for weeks or months. The lesions correspond roughly to those seen in the secondary stage of syphilis. Those occurring during the first two years of life are referred to as early congenital syphilis and those manifesting after this time, late congenital syphilis. Overlapping may occur.

Early congenital syphilis

(*See also* Chapter 32, Skin disorders.)

The skin and mucous membranes are commonly involved. The earliest sign is often a transient bullous eruption containing many spirochaetes (syphilitic pemphigus). Characteristically involving the palms and soles, the bullae rapidly rupture, leading to desquamation and a glazed pink appearance to the palms and soles. Reddish maculo-papules, not confined to the soles and palms, which darken with age but which may also desquamate, appear later.

Condylomata lata — flat, wartlike, moist structures near the anal margin — are occasionally seen and are highly infectious. Mucous patches in the mouth may lead to fissuring and scarring at the angles of the mouth.

Rhinitis frequently occurs after the first week or two. The mucous discharge from the nose (snuffles) may become tinged with blood and is teeming with spirochaetes.

Hepatosplenomegaly is present in a very high percentage of affected infants. Jaundice may occur but is less common.

Haematological involvement manifesting with anaemia is very common. Erythroblastosis, with many nucleated red cells on a peripheral smear, together with hydrops fetalis and haemolytic anaemia, may produce a picture which has to be differentiated from iso-immunization. A leuco-erythroblastic picture with immature white and red cells may be seen on a peripheral blood smear. At autopsy extramedullary haemopoiesis involving the liver and spleen is a common finding.

Thrombocytopaenia and disseminated intra vascular coagulation may lead to purpura or bleeding from other sites.

Congenital syphilis is a rare cause of a leukaemoid reaction.

Bone involvement should be sought on radiographs of the long bones (*see* Figure 7.9) in any infant suspected of being syphilitic.

The long bones are most commonly involved but, rarely, the phalanges (syphilitic dactylitis) and metacarpals may also be affected. Involvement of the maxilla may lead to facial deformities and involvement of the skull to bossing. In the newborn only 40 per cent may have long bone involvement

Characteristically, multiple bones are involved, usually symmetrically, and the lower limbs tend to be more affected than the upper limbs. The metaphysis, diaphysis, and periosteum may be involved, but the epiphysis is spared.

Translucent bands in the juxta-epiphyseal areas are the earliest manifestations of syphilitic bone disease. Frank bone destruction at the metaphysis, appearing as 'rat bitten' or nibbled-out areas, tends to occur after the neonatal period. Wimberger's sign is this type of involvement of the upper medical aspects of the tibiae. Patchy, irregular 'moth eaten' lesions of the diaphysis, together with cortical thickening, are evidence of more extensive bone involvement and fractures may occur. Periostitis, appearing as an elevation of the periosteum, is a common finding, although a periosteal reaction may be a simple growth phenomenon or be caused by many other pathological states. Syphilitic periostitis may persist long after resolution of metaphyseal and diaphyseal lesions, and lead

Figure 7.9 Bone changes in syphilis

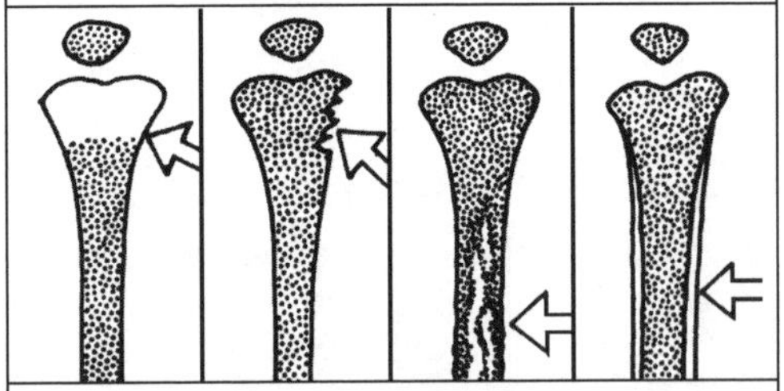

| 1 Metaphyseal translucent band |
| 2 Wimberger's sign |
| 3 Diaphysitis |
| 4 Periostitis |

to chronic thickening. Involvement of the tibiae leads to 'sabre' deformity of late congenital syphilis. Bone involvement causes pain which is responsible for the irritability commonly found in infants suffering from congenital syphilis. In some instances, pseudoparalysis of a limb occurs (Parrot's pseudoparalysis). The exact cause of this is not defined but may in part be due to bone disease.

Central nervous system (CNS) involvement,, when present, leads to convulsions and, if untreated, can cause mental retardation and hydrocephalus. Routine examination of the cerebrospinal fluid will reveal abnormalities in more than one-third of patients.

Renal involvement should always be sought in the presence of oedema. The nephrotic syndrome is a well-recognized complication of syphilis. The onset is usually within the first six months, but may occur later without other clinical evidence of congenital syphilis. Immune complex deposition leads to a membranous nephropathy. Adequate antisyphilitic therapy results in complete resolution of the condition. *Pretibial oedema* is a frequent finding in early infancy and may occur as a result of hypoproteinaemia unrelated to renal involvement.

Babies with congenital syphilis are not infrequently *small-for-gestational age* and many fail to thrive as a result of gastrointestinal involvement. The pancreas and intestines frequently reveal spirochaetes at autopsy, a *fibrous pancreatitis* being a common finding.

A *pericellular fibrosis* of the lungs may also be found at autopsy (pneumonia alba). *Pneumonia* complicating congenital syphilis is usually of intercurrent bacterial origin.

Patients with congenital syphilis have impaired cell-mediated immunity, and secondary bacterial infections, including septicaemia, occur frequently.

Diagnosis. Symptomatic congenital syphilis may be mimicked by any of the causes of intrauterine infection and by bacterial infections acquired after birth.

The only way to make a definitive diagnosis of syphilis is through microscopic identification of the *Treponema pallidum* in secretions, by dark ground illumination, or by examination of the pathological tissues. However, although not foolproof, serological tests are of great practical value in establishing the diagnosis. Treponemal

infection leads to production of both non-specific antibodies known as reagins and specific anti-treponemal antibodies. Examples of the non-specific serum antibody tests are the Wasserman, Kahn, and Venereal Disease Research Laboratory (VDRL) tests. The last-mentioned is one of the most commonly employed as a screening test for syphilis and as a quantitative serological method to assess the efficacy of treatment or activity of disease. A disadvantage is false positive reactions, which may be technical or due to other infections or connective tissue disorders.

Specific antibody tests have been devised in an attempt to overcome false positive reactions. Of these, the fluorescent treponemal antibody (absorbed) test (FTA Abs) has proved reliable in most instances. The FTA test detects both IgG and IgM antibodies. A baby born to a syphilitic mother may show a positive FTA IgG test merely as a result of passive transplacental transfer of maternal IgG, but a positive IgM test usually indicates infection of the infant. Biological false positive FTA tests may occur occasionally but, for practical purposes, a positive FTA IgM test in young infants is indicative of congenital syphilis infection which requires treatment. Unfortunately, when syphilis is acquired by a mother late in pregnancy, her baby may not produce IgM FTA antibody until three months of age. A cerebrospinal fluid examination should always be done to exclude meningeal involvement.

Treatment. An asymptomatic infant without meningeal involvement requires benzathine penicillin 50 000 units/kg/IM in a single dose. For a symptomatic infant without meningeal involvement, procaine penicillin G, 300 000 units IM daily for 10 days is essential. A symptomatic infant with meningeal involvement is given aqueous penicillin G, 50 000 units/kg/IV in two divided doses daily for 10 days.

Follow-up. Ideally, all infants with congenital syphilis should be seen at three-monthly intervals after completion of treatment, for quantitative VDRL tests and clinical examination to assess efficacy of treatment. Treatment should be repeated if the VDRL remains positive 12 months after therapy.

The mother and father of the infant should be investigated and treated if necessary.

Prevention. Adequate antenatal care of the mother should include serological testing and treatment, where necessary, during the second and third trimester of pregnancy.

Late congenital syphilis

Scars of early syphilitic lesions and subsequent developmental changes give rise to stigmata. These include rhagades (scarring at corners of the mouth), sabre tibiae, bossing of the skull, 'saddle nose' and other deformities of the maxilla, together with characteristic deformities involving permanent teeth. The upper central incisors tend to be peg- or barrel-shaped, with convergent lateral borders and thickened bodies. The cutting edge becomes notched with usage (Hutchinson's teeth). Moon's mulberry molars have multiple small cusps instead of the normal four. These deformities cause a predisposition to caries.

A wide variety of neurological sequelae may result from chronic meningovascular syphilis, including hydrocephalus, cranial nerve palsies, hemiplegia, juvenile paresis, and tabes.

Late hypersensitivity reactions include interstitial keratitis, nerve deafness, and painless synovitis (Clutton's joints) commonly involving the knees.

Congenital malformations of the central nervous system

The common disorders of the central nervous system (CNS) in the neonate fall into two major categories, namely developmental defects and perinatally acquired conditions (*see* Table 7.15).

A number of disorders of the CNS are preventable. The risk of neural tube defects may be reduced by the administration of folate preconceptually, the fetal alcohol syndrome by the avoidance of alcohol preconceptually and throughout pregnancy, and the screening of mothers over 35 years for chromosomal defects.

Only the commonly encountered conditions and those requiring urgent treatment will be discussed.

Meningomyelocele

This is the most common neonatal CNS disorder referred to neurosurgeons. This midline defect of the skin and vertebral arch containing both meninges and neural tissue occurs most commonly in the lumbosacral region. The aetiology

is poorly understood. The prevalence is 0.2–0.4 per 1 000 births with variation in different population groups. There is evidence that adequate folate supplementation preconceptually and during the first trimester will reduce the risk of this condition occurring. The risk of recurrence is increased in subsequent pregnancies. The Arnold Chiari malformation is the most common associated congenital abnormality and causes hydrocephalus.

Many cases are diagnosed by ultrasound in early pregnancy when termination can be offered. The diagnosis is usually quite obvious at birth, with motor and sensory impairment, and bladder and bowel incontinence depending on the level of the lesion. Cranial ultrasound is used to demonstrate the initial ventricular size and to monitor subsequent distension. Associated abnormalities can be excluded by CT scan. Careful neurological assessment of the lower limbs, bladder, and bowel function is important for prognostic purposes.

Management. (*See also* Chapter 8, Surgical conditions of the newborn.) Post-operatively the orthopaedic, renal, and general problems must be evaluated. The head circumference

---

Table 7.15 Lesions of the central nervous system

I. Developmental defects

1 Neural tube defects
   encephalocele, myelomeningocele, spina bifida occulta, anencephaly

2 Defects in growth and differentiation
   chromosomal defects, porencephaly, hydranencephaly, megalencephaly, holoprosencephaly

3 Defect in cerebrospinal fluid circulation
   hydrocephalus, Dandy-Walker malformation, aqueduct stenosis

II. Perinatally acquired conditions

1 Hypoxic ischaemic encephalopathy

2 Intracranial haemorrhage
   subdural, subarachnoid, intraventricular, intracerebral, and intracerebellar

3 Metabolic encephalopathy
   hypoglycaemia, kernicterus, hypothyroidism

4 Infections

must be closely monitored as *hydrocephalus is a common sequel* requiring ventricular shunting. The prenatal diagnosis of neural tube defects by means of serum alpha feto-protein determination and antenatal ultrasonography must be offered to the mother for her future pregnancies.

Spina bifida occulta

In this condition, which occurs most commonly at L5 and S1, there is a defect of the vertebral arch with failure of posterior fusion of the vertebral laminae, and frequently absent spinous processes. Associated vertebral body anomalies such as hemivertebrae may occur. The overlying skin may be quite normal or there may be a tuft of hair, telangiectasia, or subcutaneous lipoma. It is often an incidental finding. Less commonly there are neurological signs including those associated with meningomyelocele, e.g. unilateral leg and foot lesions or bladder dysfunction. Diagnosis is by X-ray of the spine, and further investigation is indicated only if there is progression of neurological signs. Associated tumours may be removed without neural tissue damage.

Anencephaly

Anencephaly is obvious at birth with absence of the vault of the skull and cerebral hemispheres. The brain stem and basal nuclei may be seen at the base of the skull. These infants are still-born or die within hours or days of birth. Most cases are now diagnosed with routine antenatal ultrasound.

Microcephaly

Isolated microcephaly is not associated with destructive disease and is a disorder of cell proliferation, therefore brain growth as a whole is defective and the resultant head size is below the 3rd centile. The condition may occur in males as an X-linked disorder. Developmental abnormalities affecting the fetus or the young infant may also lead to poor brain growth. Pathologically there is a decrease in total brain weight, a decrease in the number, size, and the complexity of the gyri. The frontal lobes are usually more severely affected; following perinatal insults there may be associated gliosis and neuronal loss in the cerebral cortex. Often the cerebellum

is relatively spared and appears disproportionately large. Clinically the head is small compared to the body and the circumference well below the 3rd centile. The forehead tends to recede and may appear relatively large. Initially, motor development appears reasonable but as the head fails to grow, motor and mental retardation become more apparent. The outcome is better if the baby with a small head demonstrates head growth along a particular centile without fall-off. Skull X-rays, serological tests, and a lumbar puncture assist in the diagnosis of microcephaly due to intra-uterine infection. Periventricular calcifications occur in congenital cytomegalovirus infection; diffuse cerebral calcifications occur in congenital toxoplasmosis.

The *fetal alcohol syndrome* is a very important cause of microcephaly and growth retardation. This condition must be suspected in a baby with the following features:

- Small palpebral fissures and apparent hypertelorism
- Smooth upper lip and absent philtrum
- Symmetrical growth retardation
- Abnormalities of heart, skeleton, and palmar creases.

(*See also* Chapter 3, Medical genetics and birth defects.)

Microcephaly must be distinguished from *cranial synostosis* affecting the sagittal and coronal sutures which results in a small head. The prematurely closed suture can usually be palpated clinically, and raised intracranial pressure is evident as papilloedema and on skull radiograph. This condition can be treated surgically.

Hydrocephalus

This term refers to an abnormally large head with an increase in CSF, which is or has been under increased pressure. Where the flow of CSF out of the ventricular system is obstructed, the pressure effect is from within the brain. In the communicating variety, on the other hand, there is interference with CSF flow or absorption outside the brain.

Aetiology. The aetiology is unknown in the majority of congenital varieties of hydrocephalus where there is a range of malfunctions. In a small proportion, congenital infections and genetic factors play a role. Meningitis, trauma, and intracranial haemorrhage are the common causes of acquired hydrocephalus.

Clinical features. The big head may be obvious at birth, or even diagnosed antenatally. At times the head enlargement develops gradually with very few signs early on, but subsequently anorexia, vomiting, irritability, and lethargy are seen. A bulging fontanelle and separation of the sutures are invariably present. Superficial venous engorgement is variable, and the classical sign of the 'setting sun' eyes appears late.

Benign enlargement of the head (or constitutional macrocephaly) must be differentiated from hydrocephalus. Once soft tissue swelling of the scalp has been excluded, serial head circumference measurements will demonstrate proportional growth in the former. There will also be no evidence of raised intracranial pressure.

Subdural fluid accumulation must also be considered in the differential diagnosis. Rarely intracranial cysts or tumours present a similar clinical picture.

Intervention. The prolonged pressure effect causes CSF to leak into the surrounding white matter with resultant atrophy. In the first instance it is important to record and plot serial head circumference measurements. Early referral for shunting is necessary as soon as excessive head enlargement is demonstrated. If cranial ultrasonography is available and shows progressive enlargement of the lateral ventricles, along with the development of a full fontanelle, referral for shunting is indicated.

The prognosis depends on the severity of associated malformations and the extent of subsequent brain damage.

Complications are not uncommon and often necessitate reinsertion of the shunt. Patients with arrested hydrocephalus require prolonged observation for low-grade pressure build-up.

Inherited errors of metabolism presenting in the neonatal period

(*See also* Chapter 10, Metabolic disorders.)

Inherited metabolic disorders may present in the neonatal period, when a previously healthy newborn baby may present severely ill and with deranged metabolism.

The following patterns are seen: severe illness with poor feeding, lethargy, vomiting, neonatal metabolic acidosis, recurrent or persistent hypoglycaemia, coma and convulsions. These features are indistinguishable from septicaemia or intracranial haemorrhage, but occur in infants with a normal prior course and with no evidence of infection on investigation. Severely dysmorphic infants should also be investigated for inborn errors of metabolism.

Prompt suspicion and laboratory diagnosis is essential as many conditions can now be treated and the family appropriately counselled.

A number of congenital endocrine and metabolic disorders may not present in the neonatal period. Screening of the newborn may detect some, allowing for the initiation of therapy and the prevention of damage. Congenital hypothyroidism is the most important of these (*see* screening programmes in Chapter 3, Medical genetics and birth defects; and hyperthyroidism in Chapter 19, Endocrine disorders).

Failure to thrive

(*See* Chapter 9, Feeding of infants and young children.)

Failure to thrive means that the baby fails to gain weight adequately. Following initial weight loss for a few days, the healthy term baby should regain its birth weight by the tenth day and the preterm baby by the fourteenth day. Thereafter the expected weight gain is a minimum of 150 g per week in a term infant or on average approximately one per cent of body weight per day; a baby who does not gain weight at this rate must be regarded as failing to thrive.

The most common cause is incorrect feeding practices: firstly, those related to breastfeeding such as difficulty with sucking, poor technique, and inadequate frequency of feeding; secondly, dilute or infrequent formula feeds.

In the preterm infant careful calculation of feed volumes is essential. Often insensible water loss is underestimated, particularly in VLBW infants and those nursed in incubators, under phototherapy units and radiant warmers.

Metabolic acidosis develops occasionally in some artificially fed healthy preterm babies, particularly during rapid growth when hydrogen ions are produced, which may not be excreted by the immature kidney. This build-up of acidosis will in turn result in poor weight gain, which is easily corrected by giving oral sodium bicarbonate 2–4 mmol/kg/24 hours for a short while. If acidosis persists, it should be investigated.

Anaemia and occult infections such as urinary tract and chronic intra-uterine infections including HIV and TB are not uncommon causes. Subclinical cold stress occurs when babies nursed in temperatures below thermoneutrality, use up energy in an attempt to maintain body temperature. Congenital heart defects, urinary and gastrointestinal tract malformations, chronic chest conditions, metabolic diseases, endocrine disorders, and brain damage may all cause failure to thrive.

The common causes must be excluded by taking a careful history, particularly in respect of feeds, vomiting, and stools, and doing a detailed relevant clinical examination. Special investigations must be selected with circumspection.

A very important aspect of thriving is the mother–child relationship. Some infants with growth failure and developmental lag have been shown to have suffered as a result of maternal psychosocial disturbances, such as maternal depression. On correction of these problems the babies improved both physically and developmentally. This form of failure to thrive is at one end of the spectrum of child abuse and neglect. Preterm babies and twins are at particular risk of this problem.

8

Surgical conditions of the newborn

Structural defects in the newborn baby may be life-threatening and require urgent surgical correction. Occasionally neonatal surgery is justified to preserve organ function, particularly renal function. However neonates are high-risk surgical patients and a careful assessment of the risk-benefit ratio is required before surgery is prescribed.

There are two varieties of congenital abnormalities; overt and covert. While the former are revealed by inspection of the patient, covert anomalies are manifested by abnormal function in the affected system in a neonate that appears to be outwardly normal. Both varieties will only be revealed with certainty if routine examination and observation are applied to all newborns.

The following overt anomalies require urgent intervention:

- Body wall defects
- Absent or misplaced orifices
- Neural axis defects
- Neonatal tumours
- Facial clefts
- Ambiguous genitalia.

These are frequently accompanied by premature birth where adaptive processes to extra-uterine life may be incomplete and reflexes immature.

Surgery should be one element of a continuum of care. Pre-operative preparation and post-operative care are essential components without which success is unlikely.

One element of post-operative care that is often neglected is pain relief. It must be appreciated that neonates experience pain, which makes a significant contribution to the stress of an operative procedure. Therefore, pain relief is an important component of postoperative care.

Surgical lesions cannot be treated in isolation. Success is based upon an accurate history and examination, and upon the orchestrated input of a team that includes the surgeon, paediatrician, anaesthetist, and nurse. Parents should also be involved.

Transportation

The centralization of neonatal intensive care and neonatal surgical services makes inter-hospital transfer of neonates inevitable. However the principles of neonatal transport are independent of distance and are as important when transporting a baby between the ward and the X-ray department as they are when the transfer is between hospitals.

Whenever a transfer is contemplated there must be direct communication between the sending and receiving staff and an appropriate level of care during transport must be arranged. *Speed is rarely, if ever, essential; care and planning is.*

The following factors are important determinants of successful surgical management:
- Blood glucose and temperature homeostasis
- Defence mechanisms against infection
- Hepatic maturity and clotting factor deficit
- Pulmonary maturity and control of breathing
- Circulatory stability.

> Surgically-ill babies need to be kept warm, have their stomach and small bowel decompressed by a well-managed nasogastric tube, and have their circulating blood volume restored by intravenous infusion of an appropriate fluid. Supplementary oxygen is advised.

All this is readily achieved without recourse to expensive technology and is within the ambit of any healthcare facility.

The mnemonic TWO SIDES is a useful aide memoire when considering inter-hospital transfer:

- **T**ube; A nasogastric tube is placed to drain gastric contents. This prevents vomiting and aspiration, decompresses the bowel maximizing intestinal mucosal blood flow, reduces abdominal distension thereby reducing resistance to diaphragmatic descent and making breathing easier. None of these advantages are seen if the tube is spigotted, knotted or blocked by blood or dried mucus. It requires constant supervision.
- **W**armth; Keeping a warm baby warm is simply a matter of wrapping him or her, including the head, in insulation. Aluminium foil from the kitchen is perfectly adequate. If the baby has exposed viscera, e.g. gastroschisis, these should be wrapped in non-adherent plastic such as Klingfilm®. An incubator is not essential.

  Wrapping a cold baby in insulation will, of course, keep him cold. Cold babies must be rewarmed as part of the stabilization prior to transfer.
- **O**xygenation; Supplementary oxygen improves oxygen delivery to the gut mucosa and is important in maintaining the integrity of the mucosal barrier.
- **S**tabilization; Ambulance journeys are not good for babies. Prior to transfer the sending physician must ensure that the baby is rewarmed, normovolaemic and normoglycaemic.
- **I**ntravenous fluids; Fluid loss is almost pathognomic of surgical pathology. The small circulating blood volume of the neonate means that fluid losses must be replaced on a continuing basis or

hypovolaemia will rapidly result. Surgical babies lose isotonic fluid and replacement with Ringer's Lactate is ideal.
- **D**ocumentation; All relevant X-rays and blood results, as well as a detailed referral letter must accompany all transfers. Failure to do this compromises care in the receiving institution.
- **E**scort; Care of a neonate during transport is the pinnacle of nursing achievement, and should be the domain of the most skilled and experienced personnel available. It is never appropriate to dispatch a baby in the care of his mother only.

Road or air?

In most parts of South Africa roads are adequate and transport by road is appropriate. In remote areas there may be a need for aero-med evacuation of sick babies. There are, however, difficulties with air transport, be it fixed wing, or helicopter, and thought must be given to patient selection.' Most importantly, in all aircraft gas expands. 'Pressurized' aircraft have a cabin pressure set usually to an altitude of around 3 600 m. Thus in any form of air transport, the air within an incarcerated hernia, pneumothorax, pneumoperitoneum, diaphragmatic hernia, or in a loop of intestine will expand to the detriment of the patient. The volume increase is related to the pressure according to Boyle's Law, and the pressure is related to the altitude. (*See* Table 8.1). There are also problems relating to turbulence and the displacement of tubes and lines. In helicopters lack of space and access make interventions difficult. Air transport is also weather dependent.

Table 8.1 Gas volume relative to altitude	
Altitude (m)	**Relative gas volume**
0	1.0
1 500	1.2
3 000	1.5
4 500	1.9
5 400	2.0
6 000	2.4

Discussion with the receiving unit will allow a decision on the correct transport vehicle as well as any additional requirements for a specific baby with a specific pathology.

Congenital abnormalities

The causes of some anomalies are well known (e.g. thalidomide – phocomelia) but in most patients the cause remains a mystery. However, it is well established that interference with fetal blood supply may result in major defects in the affected part, and this is well demonstrated in small-bowel atresia. Many other fetal insults – maternal alcohol, smoking, drugs, physical trauma, or infections – result in anatomical defects if they occur during the critical first trimester when organ development is proceeding rapidly. Any insult at such an embryologically busy time is likely to affect more than a single anatomical structure and result in non-random associations of defects (e.g. duodenal atresia in trisomy 21 or the VATER association, an acronym for **V**ertebral abnormality, **A**norectal malformation, **T**racheo-oesophageal fistula associated with o**E**sophageal atresia and **R**adial dysplasia; secondary associations include cardio **V**ascular defects and **R**enal anomalies). Such mnemonics serve to remind the clinician to look for further defects if one of these is discovered. Many anomalies are recognizable on antenatal investigations, particularly through ultrasound scanning. Antenatal diagnosis means that the patient can be delivered at a tertiary centre, but prior consultation with a specialist team is desirable so that the fetus may be appropriately managed. Combinations of defects, particularly when a chromosomal abnormality is included, present management and ethical difficulties that are cumulative.

Overt anomalies

Body wall defects

Babies may be born with anterior thoraco-abdominal defects allowing herniation of viscera, either covered by a membrane of amnio-peritoneum (exomphalos, syn. omphalocele) or unprotected, but with a thick fibrinous exudate over the herniated bowel (gastroschisis). Due to antenatal evisceration the abdominal cavity fails

to develop its full capacity. It may be impossible to return the evisceration safely to the patient. The sequelae of such defects are hypothermia, hypovolaemia, and peritonitis due to exposure. There may be associated intestinal malrotation and obstruction or hypoglycaemia (Wiedemann-Beckwith syndrome).

Primary management is directed towards excluding associated defects and maintaining body temperature. This can be achieved most readily by enclosing the herniated viscera or sac in a non-adhesive plastic (e.g. Klingfilm®) inside a covering of gamgee and aluminium foil. Gastric decompression by nasogastric tube, to prevent vomiting and postnatal herniation of previously enclosed bowel, is essential. The blood sugar level must be maintained within normal limits. Antibiotics should be commenced at the time of diagnosis.

Definitive management. Emergency surgery is necessary in all babies at risk of peritonitis. Where the abdomen cannot be stretched to accommodate the viscera, a temporary silastic tent must be manufactured to enclose it. Where an intact sac presents, surgery may still be desirable, particularly if the sac volume is small. Non-operative treatment with the daily application of silver sulphadiazine or an equivalent dressing will allow epithelialization over a period of weeks. The resultant ventral hernia can be electively repaired later.

Anorectal malformations

These anomalies are common, both singly or as part of a syndrome, particularly in association with oesophageal atresia and defects of the lower abdominal wall. The absence of an anus at the usual site is diagnostic. The diagnosis is rarely delayed in babies born at home as most mothers examine their newborn child thoroughly. Diagnostic delay is almost exclusively a phenomenon of institutional care. Anorectal malformations are classified as high or low, describing the relationship of the bowel end to the muscles of continence.

Low lesions

The bowel ends distal to the muscles of continence. In females an ectopic orifice often exists, which allows intestinal decompression. In males a fistula may run from an occluded anus along the median raphe of the scrotum to the penis. It is recognizable as beads of white desquamated cells, or meconium, along the line of the raphe. Such a fistula rarely allows adequate intestinal decompression. In some males, as there is no evidence of fistula or anal orifice, radiography is necessary to distinguish it from a high lesion. Where effective decompression exists there may be no signs of intestinal obstruction.

High lesions

In high lesions the bowel either ends blindly above the pelvic floor or more commonly ends as a fistula into the bladder or posterior urethra in males, and into the uterus or upper vagina in females. Diagnostic delay allows the signs of low intestinal obstruction to develop, with abdominal distension leading eventually to vomiting, respiratory embarrassment, caecal perforation, and death. Meconium may be evacuated in small quantities via the vagina or in the urine, and its presence in the nappy may mislead attendants. Diagnosis rests upon noting the absence of a patent anus.

Primary management. For both high and low lesions the child is in danger of intestinal obstruction. Following diagnosis, nasogastric decompression will minimize bowel distension and thus maximize diaphragmatic excursion. Intravenous replacement of loss through gastric aspirates or vomitus will be required. Careful examination must be carried out to exclude other defects or disorders.

Definitive management. In low lesions a perineal exploration and anoplasty are performed with a good prognosis for subsequent continence. In high lesions an initial colostomy is followed by definitive surgery at three to six months. The procedure can be performed laparoscopically if the fistula is above the prostate, as it is in most cases The prognosis for continence must be guarded, as several elements required for normality, e.g. internal sphincter, an anal canal lined with skin, will be absent, and the function of existing elements may be compromised by surgery or secondary defects, e.g. sacral abnormalities.

Neural axis defects

While these lesions are discussed in detail elsewhere it is appropriate to discuss indications for surgery here. There is clearly no place for surgery in anencephaly or severe microcephaly, which may be accompanied by a large meningo-encephalocele. In the more usual dilemma of the baby with a spinal meningomyelocele, it would be cruel to subject to surgery a baby for whom such surgery carries no prospect of any benefit. Congenital hydrocephalus, a large lesion on the back, a thoraco-lumbar situation, patulous anus, urinary dribbling, spastic diplegia, club feet, and kyphosis are all individually and collectively poor prognostic signs. Surgery may be indicated in any baby without hydrocephalus who can control the hips, but many babies fall into a grey area between two extremes. In referring such babies for specialist opinion it is important not to encourage unrealistic expectations in family members. Surgery never improves the existing neurological deficit.

Neonatal tumours

Tumours may appear virtually anywhere, and should always be investigated. The most common lesion is the sacrococcygeal teratoma. The features include a large swelling attached to the coccyx with anterior displacement of the anus and frequently intrapelvic extension, which is palpable rectally. The condition is rarely seen in males and commonly associated with prematurity. These tumours are often larger than the host, and bleeding into the tumour may cause anaemia or fetal death. Early complete removal along with the coccyx is essential to prevent recurrence and malignant transformation, and surgery in the neonatal period is appropriate.

Cleft lip and palate

These defects are quite obvious, except incomplete palatal clefts, which must be actively sought. While some units are achieving excellent results with neonatal surgery for cleft lip, conventional wisdom suggests that lips be repaired at 10 to 12 weeks and the palate at 10 to 12 months. Secondary surgery in later life may be needed as growth distorts the anatomy. Feeding problems can be overcome either by spoonfeeding, by special teats where clefts are partial, or by tube feeding as a last resort. A facial cleft does not always prevent sucking and a trial of breastfeeding is worthwhile.

Ambiguous genitalia

(*See also* Chapter 19, Endocrine disorders.)

Failure of sexual differentiation may not be an emergency in the usual meaning of the word. It is, however, important to recognize and investigate urgently in order to exclude adrenogenital syndrome with electrolyte abnormalities and to allow gender assignment for normal psychosocial development. It is important to realize that gender assignation depends not only on chromosomal sex but, perhaps more importantly, on phenotypic sex, and the latter depends upon normal gonadal development and end organ sensitivity to sex hormones. One can rarely tell the appropriate gender by looking at ambiguous genitalia. It is preferable to avoid assigning a gender until a definitive plan of management has been designed. Altering an inappropriately assigned gender can be difficult, traumatic, and in some instances impossible. Referral to a tertiary centre for investigation is thus imperative.

Covert anomalies

By their very nature, covert anomalies are not obvious to inspection, and their diagnosis depends upon the recognition of disordered function, which may be present at the time of birth, or delayed for hours, days, or in some cases months or years.

Ventilation

The causes of disordered breathing in the neonate are legion (*see* Figure 8.1).

Abdominal distension

The most common 'surgical' disorder presenting with breathing difficulty is abdominal distension. As the neonate is an obligate diaphragmatic breather, fatigue and respiratory distress will ensue if increased intra-abdominal pressure has to be overcome. Nasogastric decompression reduces intestinal distension. Occasionally paracentesis is justified with ascites or pneumoperitoneum to improve respiratory excursion.

> Functions commonly disturbed by covert anomalies include:
> - Ventilation (respiratory distress)
> - Feeding (vomiting)
> - Micturition (oliguria, anuria)
> - Defaecation (constipation)
> - Movement (paralysis).

Space-occupying lesion

Any space-occupying lesion within the chest will compromise ventilation. The most common such lesion is the congenital diaphragmatic hernia (*see below*). Pneumothorax behaves as a space-occupying lesion, and even without 'tension' may present as respiratory embarrassment.

Pneumonia/consolidation

Inhalation of vomitus, sometimes associated with intestinal obstruction, is the most common surgically related cause. Nursing patients prone or in the lateral position rather than supine will minimize the risk of aspiration in otherwise healthy individuals. Aspiration of saliva or gastric juice is a common presenting feature in oesophageal atresia, a lesion which must be excluded by being able to pass a nasogastric tube (*see below*).

Airway obstruction

Congenital obstruction occurs due to lesions such as choanal atresia, laryngeal webs or laryngomalacia.

Diaphragmatic hernia

Because intrathoracic pressure is lower than intra-abdominal pressure, any defect in the diaphragm will allow abdominal viscera to herniate into the chest.

The possible sites are:
- Posterolateral diaphragm (Bochdalek's hernia)
- Retrosternal (Morgagni's hernia)
- Oesophageal hiatus (hiatal hernia)
- Muscular diaphragm ('eventration').

Bochdalek's hernia

The posterolateral defect in the diaphragm represents persistence of the pleuro-peritoneal canal. As abdominal viscera, principally bowel and liver or spleen have been present in the chest throughout intra-uterine development, the abdominal cavity will be small, never having been stimulated to maximal development. It is likely that the primary event is failure of the lung to develop (pulmonary hypoplasia) and the bowel is simply occupying the space that the lung has failed to fill. The hernia itself is of secondary importance and treatment is directed to encouraging lung growth and avoiding pulmonary hypertension.

Pathology. Although the obvious defect is in the diaphragm, a secondary problem lies in the wall of the pulmonary arteries and arterioles where, in conjunction with pulmonary hypoplasia, there is hypertrophy of the muscle. This hypertrophied muscle responds to a variety of stimuli, e.g. cold, acidosis, hypoxia and pain, by constriction, thereby causing pulmonary hypertension. Although the ipsilateral lung is predominantly affected, in fact both lungs are abnormal. With acidosis and hypoxia, pulmonary hypertension ensues. This in turn results in persistent fetal circulation (*see* Chapter 7, Care of the newborn). Although closure of the diaphragmatic defect will contribute little to correction of the basic pathology, it will give the hypoplastic lung the opportunity to expand and grow.

Presentation. Patients present with dyspnoea and cyanosis at a variable time after birth. Early onset of symptoms of respiratory distress implies gross pulmonary inadequacy and hence a bad prognosis. Those babies in whom presentation is delayed for 24 hours or more have a good prognosis. Presentation may be accelerated if bowel within the chest cavity becomes filled with air, as may happen during ventilation by mask, crying, or swallowing; this compresses any ipsilateral lung tissue, displaces the mediastinum, and impedes the contralateral lung.

Diagnosis. In these babies respiratory distress is accompanied by a scaphoid abdomen and the mediastinum may be clinically deviated. Bowel sounds in the chest are an unreliable sign. A chest radiograph shows multiple loops of bowel, usually on the left side. Very rarely, staphylococcus pneumonia or congenital lobar emphysema may produce somewhat similar appearances.

Primary management. Surgery is not a 'fire-engine' emergency, but transfer to a paediatric surgeon is required.

Early postnatal presentation. Many patients with virtual pulmonary aplasia are unable to sustain postnatal life, and may die before diagnosis. When the diagnosis is made, a nasogastric tube

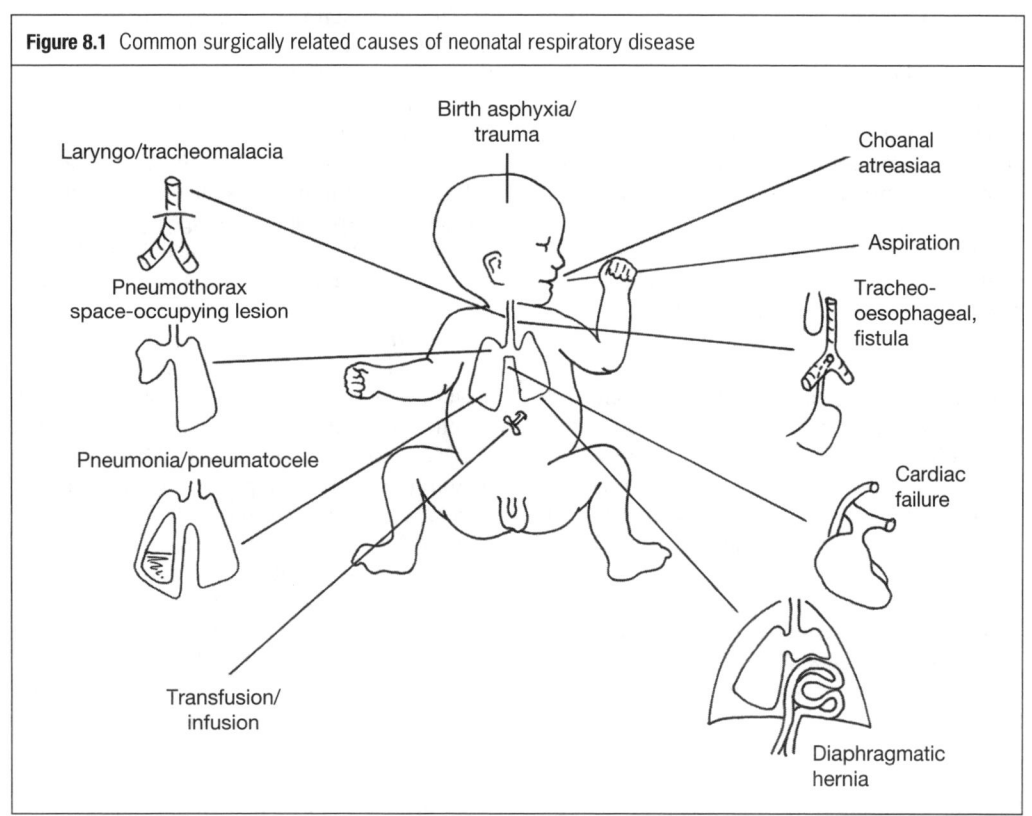

Figure 8.1 Common surgically related causes of neonatal respiratory disease

Laryngo/tracheomalacia

Birth asphyxia/ trauma

Choanal atreasiaa

Aspiration

Pneumothorax space-occupying lesion

Tracheo-oesophageal, fistula

Pneumonia/pneumatocele

Cardiac failure

Transfusion/ infusion

Diaphragmatic hernia

is passed and allowed to drain freely. The factors known to exacerbate pulmonary hypertension are avoided, particularly cold and hypoxia. Ventilation will require endotracheal intubation. No attempt should be made to 'expand' the compressed hypoplastic lung by increasing ventilation pressure, as this will simply cause contralateral pneumothorax. Transfer may be indicated if the patient's condition is stabilized. *Unpressurized air transport is not advised, as this may cause air in the bowel within the chest to expand, with potentially disastrous results.*

Delayed presentation. Where symptoms begin after 24 hours, pulmonary function is clearly adequate to sustain life and the prognosis is good. Similar primary care is instituted but endotracheal intubation is rarely necessary.

Definitive management. On arrival at a paediatric unit patients are reassessed and adverse factors (e.g. cold), which are frequently associated with transportation, are corrected. Surgery is delayed until the patient is stable. Intra- and postoperative epidural anaesthesia may be used in addition to general anaesthesia to obviate the effects of pain on pulmonary artery pressure. Trans-abdominal repair is performed and closure of the diaphragm is rarely problematic. Closure of the abdomen may be more difficult and stretching may be needed. Surgery in many patients is now performed using minimally invasive thoracoscopic techniques Postoperative care is directed to preventing pulmonary hypertension. The return of a fetal circulatory pattern, often after a 'honeymoon period' of satisfactory progress, represents treatment failure.

Morgagni's hernia
Retrosternal or Morgagni's hernias are rare and usually not large enough to compromise ventilation seriously. Bowel may occasionally incarcerate in such a defect. Diagnosis is made by lateral chest X-ray when the anterior disposition of mediastinal bowel shadows becomes clear.

Oesophageal hiatal hernia
This is further discussed under gastro-oesophageal reflux. Not all hiatal herniae result in reflux, however, and they may present with mass effect or incarceration.

Eventration
Massive eventration is pathologically identi-

cal to a Bochdalek's hernia, and is more properly described as a diaphragmatic hernia with a sac. Lesser degrees of eventration may result in recurrent or chronic chest infection or remain asymptomatic — these may be revealed as an irregular diaphragm on a routine chest X-ray. Most eventrations of any significance should be repaired.

Oesophageal atresia

Congenital obstruction of the oesophagus occurs in approximately 1 in 2 500 live births. While several patterns are seen (*see* Figure 8.2), in 90 per cent of cases the oesophagus ends blindly in the upper mediastinum while the lower oesophagus arises from the trachea. This tracheo-oesophageal fistula is usually at the level of the carina.

Pathophysiology. The effects of this anatomical derangement can be deduced from a study of Figure 8.2 (3). Firstly, at each breath a proportion of the tidal volume will be diverted into the oesophagus and thence the stomach. Gaseous distension results, with effective splinting of the diaphragm. Gastro-oesophageal reflux is promoted and gastric juice will reflux into the trachea and lungs. Pneumonitis and pneumonia rapidly result. Saliva, and any feeds that are offered, will accumulate in the upper blind pouch and then spill over into the trachea, aggravating the pneumonitis. As the baby is breathing through an oesophago-pharyngeal pool of saliva, bubbles and froth appear at the lips. Finally, any attempts at feeding will promote massive aspiration, often with cyanosis and bradycardia.

Clinical presentation. Oesophageal atresia may be seen as an isolated anomaly or as part of a syndrome, e.g. VATER association (*see above*). Given the dramatic nature of the abnormality it is surprisingly often missed. Maternal polyhydramnios is often reported and prematurity affects 50 per cent of patients. The babies usually look perfectly normal and have normal Apgar scores; however, a high index of suspicion should be raised by the presence of any other anomaly, particularly anorectal malformations.

The babies are typically 'bubbly' and choke on feeding. It is impossible to pass a stiff nasogastric tube beyond 11–12 cm. (It is possible to cause a soft tube to curl up in the upper pouch, giving a false impression of oesophageal continuity.)

An erect chest and abdominal radiograph is

taken with the tube in place confirming its arrest in the upper thorax. No other investigations are necessary, but an air contrast oesophagogram can be performed, if desired, outlining the upper pouch. Contrast media other than air are dangerous; a tracheobronchogram may result in deterioration of the respiratory status.

Progressive pneumonia occurs if the diagnosis and primary management are delayed. Starvation and depletion of energy stores further worsen the prognosis.

Primary management. A baby with oesophageal atresia can be made 'safe', allowing time for improvement of general condition, transportation or surgery. All feeding attempts are stopped immediately the diagnosis is suspected. A wide tube (preferably double lumen) is passed into the upper pouch, which is kept dry by fre-

quent aspiration or continuous suction. Gastrooesophageal reflux may be reduced by nursing the patient 'head up', and in the prone position, and its effects minimized by intravenous cimetidine or an equivalent. Pneumonitis or pneumonia is treated with antibiotics and oxygen supplementation, physiotherapy, or intubation and mechanical ventilation. Intravenous fluids are required, as no oral intake is possible.

Definitive management. At a paediatric surgical unit, associated abnormalities, if present, are evaluated. Surgery is performed as soon as possible but time can be spent pre-operatively to improve the condition of babies in whom pneumonia or other problems have arisen.

Treatment is surgical At thoracotomy the fistula is divided and the trachea repaired.

Oesophageal continuity is restored where

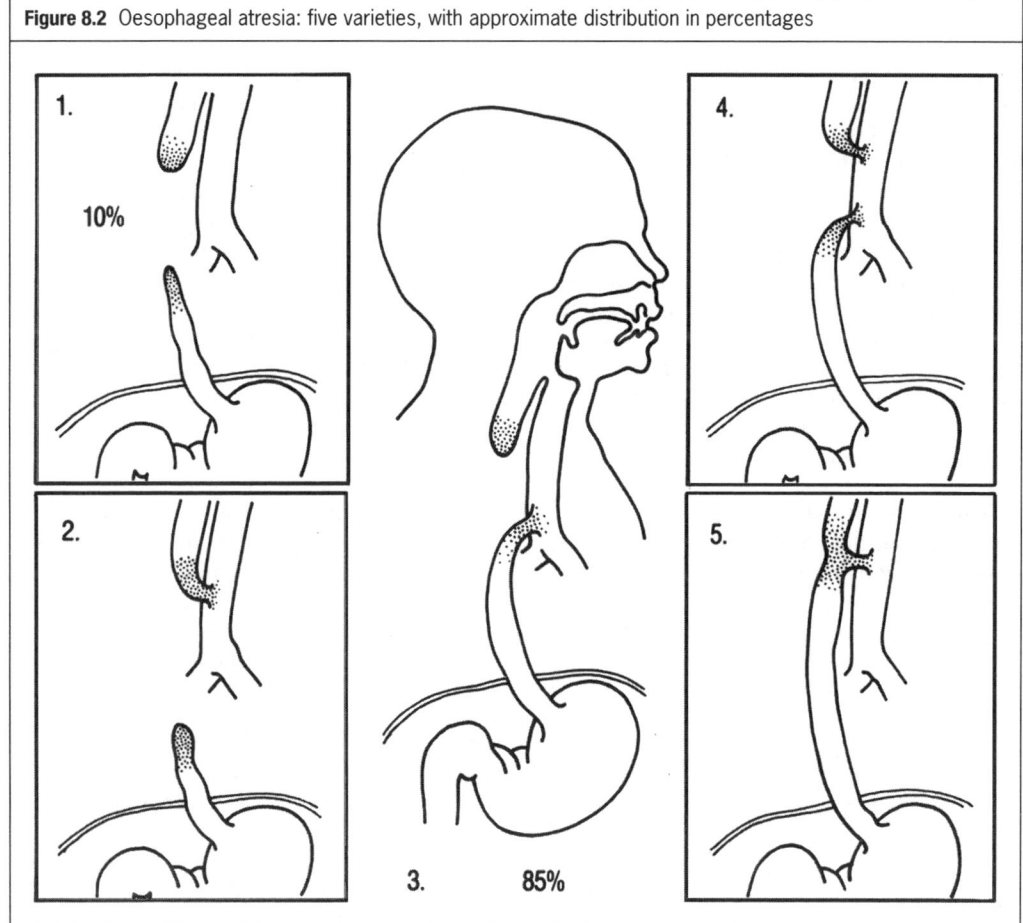

Figure 8.2 Oesophageal atresia: five varieties, with approximate distribution in percentages

1.

10%

2.

3.   85%

4.

5.

possible. A cervical oesophagostomy or salivary fistula may be necessary if the oesophageal ends cannot be brought together without unacceptable tension. In patients with oesophageal atresia without a fistula there is rarely sufficient distal oesophagus to allow an anastomosis.

Postoperative care consists of a continuation of pre-operative management. Gastrostomy or naso-gastric tube feeds are generally begun at 48 hours and are introduced at low pressure lest feeds reflux into the oesophagus. A contrast swallow is usually performed on the fifth to seventh day, and if satisfactory, graded oral fluids are commenced.

Prognosis. Low birth weight, other major anomalies, and pneumonia have an important bearing on survival. Large, well babies with no other anomalies have a 95 per cent chance of survival. If diagnosis is delayed and pneumonia allowed to develop, the survival drops to 75 per cent. In the presence of other anomalies the overall survival is 65 per cent, but major cardiac, neural axis, or pulmonary anomalies carry a much worse prognosis. Patients with recognizable chromosomal lesions which are of themselves life-limiting are offered no active treatment.

Vomiting

While some regurgitation of feed may be sufficiently common as to be regarded as normal, true vomiting is always pathological. Bile-stained vomitus is indicative of intestinal obstruction and always warrants the attention of the surgeon. Non-bilious vomiting is less commonly due to a 'surgical' cause, but if persistent requires investigation.

Intestinal obstruction

Obstruction of the bowel, whether mechanical or paralytic, at any age, is characterized by cessation of aboral progression of intestinal content and nutrient absorption, resulting in starvation. There is distension of bowel above the obstruc-tion due to secretions and swallowed air, resulting in abdominal distension to a degree dependent upon the level of obstruction. Fluid derived from the total body fluid accumulates within static bowel loops and dehydration results. Once the bowel distal to the obstruction has emptied, no further passage of faeces or flatus occurs, i.e. absolute constipation. Bacterial proliferation in the stagnant fluid above the obstruction may result in 'faeculent fluid' in the small bowel. Distension may be sufficient to compromise intestinal mucosal blood flow, thereby destroying the mucosal barrier to luminal organisms and toxins. Periodic decompression of the proximal bowel is provided by vomiting, which will be bilious or faeculent. In the rare case of pre-ampullary obstruction the vomitus will be bile-free. There will be additional features of toxaemia or peritonitis if a strangulating obstruction is present (*see* Table 8.2).

Features of respiratory distress may dominate the picture, due to aspirated vomitus, often aggravated by abdominal distension.

Primary management. Whatever the cause of intestinal obstruction the patient can best be served by:

- *Passage of a nasogastric tube*. Properly supervised this prevents vomiting, reduces abdominal distension (and thus improves respiratory function), and maximizes intestinal blood flow. Nasogastric tubes should never be closed but allowed to drain freely with frequent intermittent aspiration.
- Intravenous fluids. Except in unusual circumstances, isotonic fluid losses can be replaced by an isotonic fluid such as Ringer's lactate with added dextrose. The volume replaced is guided by signs of fluid deficit, particularly pulse rate, blood pressure, and urine output.
- General care. This includes maintenance of body temperature, relief of pain, and, where indicated, antibiotic therapy.

Table 8.2 Clinical features of intestinal obstruction			
Level of obstruction	**Vomiting**	**Distension**	**Constipation**
High	Early	Minimal	Late
Mid	Variable	Moderate	Variable
Low	Late	Marked	Early

Diagnosis of intestinal obstruction is clinical. Radiology may help to localize the site and occasionally the nature of the obstruction. Both supine and erect films are required and the hallmark of 'obstruction' is the presence of air-fluid levels within the bowel, and an absence of air shadows in the pelvis. Unfortunately, the presence of air-fluid levels is not pathognomonic of intestinal obstruction and they may be seen in inflammatory bowel disorders, particularly gastroenteritis and dysenteries. Clearly the clinical picture in such conditions precludes a diagnosis of obstruction, but the distinction can at times be taxing. Despite these reservations, the cardinal investigation of all neonates with bilious vomiting remains the erect chest and abdominal radiograph. Abnormal air-fluid levels or evidence of a large fluid-filled stomach should prompt surgical referral. Specific causes of intestinal obstruction in the neonate are discussed here. Pathology more characteristic of infants and children is discussed in Chapter 30, Paediatric surgical disorders.

Intestinal atresia

Congenital occlusion of the bowel lumen can affect any part of the gut but most commonly affects the duodenum or proximal jejunum. Most forms of congenital intestinal obstruction can be diagnosed antenatally by ultrasound. Polyhydramnios is invariably present. Antenatal diagnosis provides an opportunity to diagnose associated syndromes, e.g. Down's Syndrome and to counsel parents on the likely post-natal management.

Duodenal atresia

Duodenal atresia occurs at the level of the ampulla of Vater, and is thought to represent a failure of recanalization of the embryonic duodenum. There is a non-random association with Down's syndrome, which itself increases the risk of congenital heart lesions and other associated anomalies. Clinically, patients present with early onset of bilious vomiting with little, if any, epigastric distension. An erect chest and abdominal radiograph reveals the double-bubble caused by a large gastric air-fluid level on the left and a large air-fluid level in the duodenum on the right. There is no gas distally. These babies are often small and maintenance of body temperature is vital. A nasogastric tube is passed and the proximal bowel decompressed. This fluid is replaced in addition to the baby's maintenance requirements. Where multiple abnormalities do not preclude an acceptable prognosis, surgical bypass of the atretic area is performed at laparotomy. Postoperatively, gastroduodenal inertia may delay feeding, such that parenteral nutrition may be required.

Jejuno-ileal atresia

In a classic series of experiments in Cape Town, Louw and Barnard showed that atresia results from interference with the fetal blood supply to the bowel. Atresia is most common in the proximal jejunum. Bilious vomiting is the principal symptom. Abdominal distension will depend upon the site of obstruction. Babies with atresia may pass inspissated meconium on one or two occasions with consequent diagnostic delay. Radiographs will show air-fluid levels in proportion to the length of bowel above the most proximal obstruction. Management is as in duodenal atresia. Resection of atretic areas with intestinal anastomosis is usually required. The prognosis depends upon the nature of the defect and general state of the patient at presentation; however, as a rule the more distal the obstruction the more favourable the prognosis.

Meconium ileus

One method of presentation of patients with cystic fibrosis is neonatal intestinal obstruction. In this condition intraluminal obstruction of the distal ileum is caused by tacky meconium with the consistency and tenacity of chewing gum. The clinical features of ileal obstruction are present but radiologically the viscid intestinal content prevents the formation of air-fluid levels but gives a 'ground glass' appearance to the lower abdomen. Volvulus of the ileum may supervene. The cystic fibrosis gene is prevalent among whites. Many patients present with 'meconium ileus equivalent' but subsequent testing fails to confirm true cystic fibrosis. Gastrografin, which is hygroscopic, instilled per rectum, may enter the terminal ileum and relieve the obstruction. Sometimes operative clearance is required, which may involve intestinal resection. The ultimate prognosis depends upon the expression of other features of cystic fibrosis.

Intestinal malrotation

As the intestine outgrows the fetal abdominal cavity it herniates into the base of the umbilical cord. During its return, at approximately the tenth week of pregnancy, the midgut undergoes rotation about the axis of the superior mesenteric artery (*see* Figure 8.3).

The effect of this 270 degree counter-clockwise rotation is to provide the midgut loop with a long attachment to the posterior abdominal wall extending from the left upper quadrant to the right lower quadrant and minimizes the risk of volvulus (*see* Figure 8.4).

Any abnormality of rotation will result in a shorter posterior attachment of the midgut loop and a higher incidence of volvulus. Any such volvulus presents as a duodenal obstruction. It is doubtful whether peritoneal bands extending from a displaced caecum to the lateral abdominal wall (Ladd's bands) cause extrinsic duodenal obstruction, and any child presenting with symptomatic malrotation must be assumed to have volvulus neonatorum, syn midgut volvulus.

Clinical presentation. Midgut volvulus can present at any age with 80 per cent occurring below one year and 30 per cent below one month. The presentation is of a high intestinal obstruction with bilious vomiting. Bloody stools strongly suggest bowel infarction, which is usually associated with prostration and toxaemia. Volvulus can occur without bowel necrosis and may be intermittent, causing recurring symptoms over a long period.

Diagnosis. Duodenal obstruction, complete or incomplete, may be seen on plain abdominal films. Confirmation comes from a contrast meal that shows abnormal configuration of the duodenal loop and a duodeno-jejunal flexure to the right of the midline even when the radiological signs of obstruction are absent.

Treatment. Malrotation is a surgical emergency. Presentation with duodenal obstruction implies that volvulus has occurred. Should volvulus proceed to midgut necrosis, the bowel from duodenum to splenic flexure becomes gangrenous, an unsalvageable situation. The aim of surgery is to devise a stable arrangement and to recreate a long posterior midgut attachment to prevent future volvulus, obviously before necrosis occurs. This is achieved by derotating the bowel to the fetal position of non-rotation

Figure 8.3 Normal intestinal rotation occurring counter-clockwise around the axis of the superior mesenteric artery

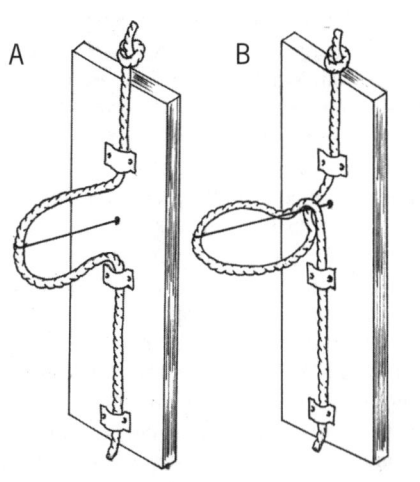

A. Prior to rotation
B. The proximal limb representing duodenum comes to lie posterior to the distal limb representing transverse colon

Figure 8.4 Normal rotation, demonstrating the long posterior attachment of the midgut loop

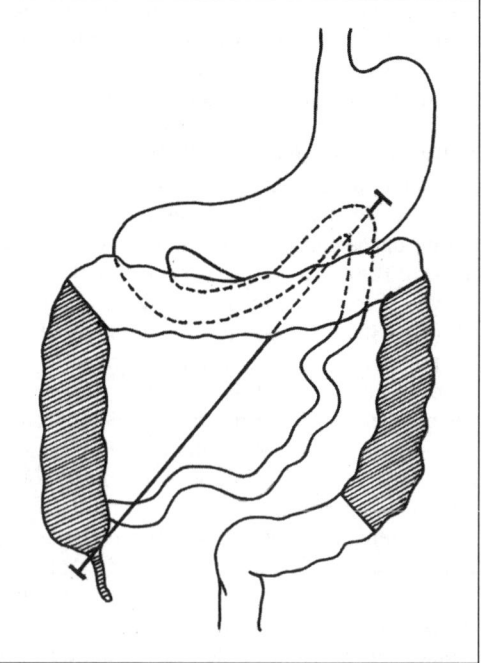

wherein the small bowel lies to the right of the abdomen, and the colon to the left.

Constipation

Most newborns pass meconium during the first 24 hours of life, and failure to do so requires investigation, particularly if there is accompanying abdominal distension. Causes include:
- Mechanical
  - Proximal atresia or other obstruction
  - Ectopic or stenotic anus
- Functional
  - Meconium plug
  - Aganglionosis/neuronal dysplasia
  - Small left colon syndrome.

Meconium plug

Where delay in passage of meconium is recognized, rectal examination or gentle saline enema may reveal an inspissated plug of pale meconium followed by the passage of apparently normal meconium associated with clinical decompression. However, a diagnosis of meconium plug obstruction can only be made with any confidence once colonic aganglionosis has been excluded. All patients with such histories require long-term follow-up.

Congenital intestinal aganglionosis (CIA) (Hirschsprung's disease)

This condition is underdiagnosed in neonates in a developing world environment and may still present only in infants and children. Rarely the condition presents for the first time in adulthood in a patient who has been unaware of his bowel habit being abnormal. In all patients a diligent interrogation will reveal that symptoms started in the neonatal period, the most consistent of which is delay in the passage of meconium.

Approximately one in three patients initially diagnosed as suffering from meconium plug obstruction will turn out to have intestinal aganglionosis.

An absence of ganglion cells in the neuronal plexi of the bowel wall results in a failure of transmission of the wave of relaxation which precedes peristaltic contraction. Embryonic ganglionic migration takes place from the region of the coeliac axis distally and may stop at any level but most commonly reaches the sigmoid or upper rectum. Total colonic or even total intestinal aganglionosis may occur.

Clinical presentation. In neonates delay in stooling is cardinal. Older patients may present with failure to thrive, abdominal distension secondary to megacolon, or simply with chronic constipation. Rectal examination in such patients may be followed by explosive decompression as the unrelaxing aganglionic internal sphincter is forced to dilate by the examining finger. Aganglionosis may result in perforation of the caecum due to increasing pressure within the colon secondary to distal obstruction, or to fulminating enterocolitis. In view of this, neonatal management is of some urgency. Where neonatal diagnosis can be established by rectal mucosal biopsy a primary transanal pull-through can be performed leaving the abdomen completely unscarred. In the developing world a more satisfactory solution is a colostomy placed in a ganglionic portion of the colon. Definitive surgery can be performed around the age of six months and normal bowel function thereafter can be anticipated.

Diagnosis. Following clinical suspicion, the diagnosis can be confirmed by plain X-ray films or contrast enema which will reveal a rectum and sigmoid of apparently normal calibre with dilated proximal bowel above. Pressure studies will show an absence of physiological internal sphincter relaxation in response to rectal distension. This investigation may be difficult to interpret in neonates, but is a useful screening test in older children. Rectal biopsy will show hypertrophied nerves and absence of ganglion cells in both Auerbach's and Meissner's plexi.

Small left colon syndrome

Infants of diabetic mothers, or of those taking certain psychotropic drugs, may present with a meconium plug-like syndrome. Contrast enema reveals an apparently unused colon from splenic flexure distally. A gastrografin enema is therapeutic and colonic function thereafter appears normal but there may be some difficulty distinguishing this condition from long segment aganglionosis. There is clearly a spectrum of neonatal colonic dysfunctional states with similar clinical and radiological appearances, and correct diagnosis may well involve manometry and biopsy.

Micturition

In the absence of hypovolaemia normal babies pass urine within four to six hours of delivery.

Failure to do so may be indicative of a urinary tract abnormality. Such abnormalities may reflect abnormalities of urine production or excretion. It is important that in all neonates the time of first micturition and, where possible, the nature of the urinary stream are noted. There is a clear association between abnormalities of fetal urine production/excretion and pulmonary development. Urine production starts at around the eighth to tenth intra-uterine week and is an important contribution to amniotic fluid volume. Hence urinary dysfunction will have been present for six months or more before presentation with consequent renal damage — the latter governs overall prognosis. Oligohydramnios is an important signal that urinary production has been inadequate *in utero*.

Urinary obstruction

Unilateral obstruction, such as pelvi-ureteric junction obstruction, causes no interference with micturition and overall renal function is protected by a contra-lateral normal kidney.

In females bilateral obstruction may rarely be due to bilateral ureteroceles obstructing the ureterovesical junction. In males, in whom lower urinary obstruction is many times more common, the most important cause is valvular urethral obstruction.

Posterior urethral valves

In the normal urethra small mucosal folds spread from the veru montanum to the side walls of the prostatic urethra. Exaggeration of these folds results in 'valves', which obstruct, partially or totally, the passage of urine. There is dilatation of the prostatic urethra proximal to the obstruction, hypertrophy and trabeculation of the bladder with diverticula, dilatation of both ureters, and bilateral hydronephrosis. By the time of birth this urinary obstruction is already long standing and the prognosis depends entirely upon the number of residual nephrons. Patients who present early have the most complete obstruction, most renal damage, and poorest prognosis. Patients who survive into childhood have a correspondingly good prognosis.

Clinical presentation. A neonate may have been noted to have failed to pass urine or to have passed a poor stream. Bilateral hydronephrosis may be palpable as may a hypertrophied thick-walled bladder. Abnormal renal function will be evidenced by raised blood urea and creatinine. A small proportion of patients will present with urinary ascites, and oedema of the abdominal wall and lower limbs.

Primary management. Valvular obstruction is truly valvular. There is no obstruction to passage of a catheter or feeding tube. This should be passed under sterile conditions as nephrons can equally be destroyed by infection as by persisting obstruction.

Radiology. Sonography is often diagnostic but a voiding cysto-urethrogram is more readily interpretable.

Definitive management. Disruption of the valves can be performed in the neonate if small calibre optics are available. In their absence urinary diversion, either cystostomy or ureterostomy, must be performed as a temporary measure. When the urethra is large enough to admit a cystoscope, the valves can be destroyed by diathermy or disrupted by a balloon catheter.

Neonatal GIT bleeding

Blood may be present in vomitus (haematemesis) or in the stool (haematochezia).

Haematemesis
(*See* Chapter 30, Paediatric surgical disorders.)

Haematochezia
Bleeding per rectum is most frequently a manifestation of haemorrhagic disease of the newborn (*see above*), particularly in an otherwise well baby. Bloody stools are, however, an important feature of intestinal mucosal necrosis secondary to necrotizing enterocolitis, volvulus neonatorum, and neonatal dysenteries.

Necrotizing enterocolitis (NEC)
The intestine bears the brunt of any hypoxic or hypovolaemic insult as blood is diverted from the splanchnic circulation to vital organs, especially the heart and brain. Within the bowel, blood is shunted away from the mucosa to perfuse the muscle layers. This compromises the mucosal barrier and allows luminal toxin and organisms access to the deeper layers of the bowel wall, giving rise to the clinical features of NEC. Bloody stools are a feature of this disease. Thus NEC represents the final common pathway of many primary pathologies. The clinical and radiological features are described elsewhere (*see*

Chapter 7, Care of the newborn) and treatment in the majority of patients is non-operative.

Surgery is required where there is evidence of full-thickness bowel necrosis, namely pneumoperitoneum, intra-abdominal mass (omentum and small-bowel loops), peritonitis (manifested often by abdominal wall oedema and erythema), and failure to respond to medical treatment. The latter is the most difficult indication to define but falling platelet and white cell counts are helpful indicators. Late surgery may be required to deal with strictures that result from the healing of circumferential ulceration. Patients who have perforated the bowel should have a drain inserted under local anaesthetic by the attending medical officer before transfer to a surgical unit.

Volvulus neonatorum

See Intestinal malrotation, *above*. It must be remembered as a cause of bloody stools in the neonate but such a presentation suggests that intestinal necrosis has already occurred and the prognosis is poor.

Other neonatal surgical problems

Labial fusion

Baby girls are often seen with a normal anus but with a covered vagina, giving rise to a misdiagnosis of vaginal atresia. These girls pass urine normally and are otherwise healthy. This appearance is due to midline fusion of the labia minora; the defect is painlessly corrected by gentle separation using an ear swab or blunt probe. Once separated a non-adherent dressing keeps the labia apart to prevent refusion.

Amniotic bands

Congenital constriction rings affecting ankles and wrists, and sometimes fingers and toes, are not uncommon. The aetiology remains unclear but fibrous bands within the amniotic fluid are held responsible. Often there is spontaneous amputation of the digit or limb distal to the constriction.

Surgery is required in the form of multiple Z-plasties. This can safely be performed in the neonatal period, with good results.

Circumcision

There are few, if any, indications for neonatal circumcision. There are some absolute contra-indications, however (*see below*).

The controversy surrounding circumcision stems from the incorrect use of terms such as 'phimosis' and 'pinhole meatus', as well as a lack of awareness of preputial physiology. It is unnecessary to retract the prepuce to wash the glans. It is also untrue that removal of the prepuce prevents masturbation and that circumcision is necessary to prevent penile cancer. The profession should adopt a stance of reassurance and re-education of both the laity and of professionals who perpetuate such myths.

The prepuce forms a protective cover for the glans penis and prevents excoriation of the glandular epithelium by nappies and urine.

In less than 5 per cent of newborns the prepuce is retractable but it should never be forcibly retracted. The prepuce and glans are joined by a viable cell layer which breaks down with time leaving epithelial debris in the coronal sulcus. This debris is not pus and is not associated with inflammation. Ballooning of the prepuce during micturition will occur in all boys until the urinary meatus can be exposed, and may in fact be the natural force causing separation.

Attempts to retract the prepuce will reveal the line of cell union which may appear 'pinhole'. However, if it allows the passage of urine at this age it is adequate. At four to six years the prepuce is retractable in 90 per cent of boys.

Mothers should be told to keep the genital area socially clean and not to retract the prepuce for hygiene or any other purpose. They should be reassured about 'ballooning' and that the 'pinhole meatus' will mature into a wide channel of communication. Social or traditional circumcision can be performed at or around the age of puberty with the understanding and consent of the individual.

Phimosis

Phimosis represents the end result of the healing of skin trauma caused by forced retraction. This manoeuvre produces longitudinal splits in the inner preputial layer which result in severe burning dysuria or 'crying on micturition', and ultimately fibrosis and stricturing of the preputial orifice. Circumcision may be indicated. The

Contra-indications to circumcision:
- *Hypospadias*. The prepuce provides useful and sometimes essential tissue for reconstruction and should never be discarded prematurely.
- *Buried penis/microphallus*. In this condition assessment of an appropriate resection is impossible, and inadequate skin may be available for future surgery.
- *Nappy (diaper)*. No matter how careful a mother may be, her infant will spend some time each day in a wet nappy. Glandular mucosa so exposed becomes ulcerated and scarred. Occasionally the meatal orifice is so affected that it leads to stenosis, requiring further surgery.
- *Systemic diseases* such as jaundice, infection, and heart disease, which require priority management and which increase the risks of surgery or anaesthesia.

condition is largely preventable by parental and professional education.

Inguinal hernia

In children, with rare exceptions, inguinal herniae are of the indirect variety representing persistence of the processus vaginalis. This outpouching of peritoneum extends as a sleeve to the upper pole of the testis and is thought to play an important role in testicular descent. Patency of this tube either wholly or in part will allow abdominal contents to descend into the scrotum.

The condition is more common in males. However, when present in girls, herniae are more often bilateral. Most commonly bowel or omentum is found as sac content, but ovaries, Fallopian tubes, and even free ascaris worms have been encountered.

Clinical presentation. Usually the mother notices an intermittent inguinal swelling, initially during crying. When examined, the inguino- scrotal region may appear quite normal. It may, however, be possible to appreciate a slight thickening of the cord on the affected side. Even when examination is unhelpful the maternal history is relied upon and elective surgery booked. In females an irreducible 'node' – in fact the ovary – may remain although the child is otherwise asymptomatic.

Complications. The presence of a hernia is of itself a benign condition but is the necessary precursor of potentially lethal complications — incarceration (irreducibility) and strangulation (gangrene of the hernial content). Herniae should be repaired to prevent these complications. The younger the patient, the higher the risk of complications, and therefore the earlier surgery should be prescribed.

Incarceration presents with a fixed inguino-scrotal swelling, usually in a patient with prior experience of a similar but reducible swelling. Intestinal obstruction follows any prolonged incarceration, and is associated with abdominal distension and vomiting. The increased intra-abdominal pressure tends to perpetuate and exacerbate the incarceration, which proceeds inexorably to intestinal gangrene if not treated. This may affect a whole bowel loop or just an arc of the bowel circumference. The final result of either is intestinal perforation, toxaemia, and death.

Strangulation is heralded clinically by local signs of inflammation, often to the point where an abscess is seriously considered. Intestinal obstruction, toxaemia, and dehydration are present to a variable degree.

Management. When incarceration is diagnosed, the aim is early reduction of the hernia followed by later elective repair. This is done because acute repair implies a greater anaesthetic risk and the oedematous friable tissues add to the surgical hazard. Thus a nasogastric tube is passed, IV fluid therapy initiated, and the child is given a sedative (e.g. Vallergan®). The foot of the cot is elevated and the child is watched for 60 minutes after falling asleep, whereafter gentle pressure is applied to reduce the hernia. Repair is arranged after a 48-hour period. The child should be kept under observation during this time lest incarceration recurs. Should reduction fail or if the initial impression is of strangulation, there is no alternative but to resuscitate the patient for emergency surgery. Bowel infarction requires intestinal resection but timeous surgery may allow ischaemic bowel to survive, hence surgery is urgent. It is important to remember that the blood supply to the testis also passes through this space and the testis is threatened in either incarceration or strangulation. This should be discussed with the parents before surgery as orchidectomy may be necessary.

Hydrocele

In children hydroceles usually 'communicate' with the peritoneal cavity. In other words, they are in fact herniae, but the communication is too narrow to allow bowel to descend to the scrotum. Peritoneal fluid tends to accumulate in the scrotum by day and flow back to the abdominal cavity at night. The child presents with a painless scrotal swelling, often worse in the evening. One can get above the swelling and perhaps appreciate thickening of the spermatic cord. Trans illumination cannot be relied upon in small children as even herniae containing bowel will allow the passage of light. The testis is often impalpable.

Hydroceles that persist after 12 months may be treated by herniotomy. Most hydroceles resolve spontaneously by 12 months of age.

Pyloric stenosis

Hypertrophic pyloric stenosis is a condition of unknown aetiology in which the thickened pyloric ring causes an incomplete gastric outlet obstruction. It is rare in the developing world and the diagnosis is often delayed due to the similarity of some of the clinical features to gastroenteritis.

Clinical presentation. Symptoms start at around three weeks of age. The cardinal symptom is bile-free vomiting which increases in frequency and forcefulness until it occurs after every meal and is truly projectile. Occasional flecks of blood in the vomitus are a reflection of underlying gastritis. In the developing world 30 per cent of patients will have diarrhoea at presentation, making differentiation from gastroenteritis particularly difficult. Associated features are weight loss due to failure of adequate intake, dehydration secondary to fluid loss in vomitus, and obvious hunger unless the patient is moribund. On examination, which ideally is performed while the baby is feeding, visible peristalsis crossing the epigastrium from left to right may be seen. A palpable pyloric mass may be felt, at the right edge of the rectus abdominis midway between the umbilicus and costal margin, when it is forced into prominence by an antral peristaltic contraction.

Biochemistry. Due to late presentation and diagnosis, severe nutritional and biochemical deficits are frequently seen. Pure loss of gastric juice results in a metabolic alkalosis with hyponatraemia, hypochloraemia, and hypokalaemia. There is usually a paradoxical aciduria. Recognition of the biochemical lesion and the importance of correcting it pre-operatively have reduced the mortality of pyloric stenosis to less than 1 per cent in most units.

Diagnosis. A clinical diagnosis may require no confirmation in experienced hands. However, the rarity of the disorder in the developing world, and the difficult differential diagnosis, means that confirmation will be required in many cases. Barium meal is the most accurate diagnostic tool, allowing visualization of a large stomach with vigorous peristalsis and a long, very narrow pyloric channel (string sign). Ultrasound scanning has a false negative rate of 10–20 per cent.

Treatment. The management of pyloric stenosis is surgical but it is not an emergency. Alkalosis is corrected by infusion of normal saline made up to a 10 per cent dextrose solution. When sufficient volume has been infused to stimulate a urinary output, potassium is added to the infusion. Serial checks of the electrolyte profile allow an optimal time to be selected for surgery, usually within 48 hours of admission. Gastric lavage to remove sour curds from the stomach may ameliorate gastritis. Ramstedt's pyloromyotomy, first performed in 1912, remains the ideal operation. The hypertrophied pyloric muscle is split, allowing the mucosa to pout out. If care is taken to avoid perforating the mucosa no further procedure is necessary.

Postoperative care. Patients may start taking small volume feeds as soon as they are fully awake following surgery, and well-nourished babies may be home by the second postoperative day. In patients with marked gastritis, postoperative vomiting may delay resumption of full feeds. The sequelae of malnutrition, particularly wound infection and dehiscence, and chest infections complicate recovery in up to 10 per cent of cases. Deaths, however, even in the developing world, should be rare.

Umbilical problems

Umbilical granuloma

A dull reddish polypoid lesion at the umbilicus appearing at the time of cord separation is likely to be an umbilical granuloma – exuberant granulation tissue representing healing of the umbilical cicatrix. Frequently there is a modest mucopurulent exudate. Less frequently, vitello-intestinal or urachal remnants may present, distinguishable by faeculent or urinary discharge.

Umbilical granulomata are satisfactorily treated by one or two applications of silver nitrate. It is important to protect surrounding normal skin with petroleum jelly or equivalent, and to cover the treated umbilicus with a dressing to prevent indelible staining of the baby's clothes.

Omphalitis

Umbilical infection, manifested locally by tenderness and erythema with or without a discharge, is a serious condition. Because infection may spread via the umbilical vein to the portal vein with resultant thrombosis, the lesion is of surgical interest. Aggressive antibiotic therapy is vital, and risk of tetanus must be remembered. Drainage, debridement with umbilical vein division, may be required.

Umbilical hernia

Contraction of the umbilical ring occurs as a normal postnatal event. Delay in closure of the ring results in a defect allowing herniation of abdominal viscera. Defects just above the umbilical ring – supra-umbilical hernia – have a different natural history. Umbilical hernia is common, affecting up to 50 per cent of black children and a lesser percentage of other ethnic groups. As the pathology is one of 'delay', spontaneous 'closure' of the hernia can be predicted. While these herniae, like any other, are subject to incarceration and strangulation, such events are rare and do not justify routine surgical repair. Umbilical herniae that persist after six years should be closed electively. Supra-umbilical herniae do not disappear spontaneously and require surgery at about two to three years of age.

The umbilical hernia provides a window into the abdomen and, where the size of the defect permits, palpation of the viscera through the hernia may be particularly rewarding. Similarly, as the hernia represents skin lined with peritoneum, the signs of peritonitis are readily elicited by gently 'tapping' the hernia.

9

Feeding of infants and young children

(Condensed, with permission, from '*WHO Infant and young child feeding. Model Chapter for textbooks for medical students and allied health professionals*'. 2009 (ISBN 978 92 4 159749 4) http://www.who.int/nutrition/publications/infant-feeding/9789241597494/en/)

The first two years of life provide a critical window of opportunity for ensuring children's appropriate growth and development through optimal feeding. Based on evidence of the effectiveness of interventions, achieving universal coverage of optimal breastfeeding could prevent 13 per cent of deaths occurring in children less than five years of age globally, while appropriate complementary feeding practices would result in an additional 6 per cent reduction in under-five mortality.

WHO and UNICEF's global recommendations for optimal infant feeding as set out in the Global Strategy are:
- exclusive breastfeeding for six months
- nutritionally adequate and safe complementary feeding starting from the age of six months with continued breastfeeding up to two years of age or beyond.

Exclusive breastfeeding means that an infant receives only breast milk from his or her mother or a wet nurse, or expressed breast milk, and no other liquids or solids, not even water, with the exception of oral rehydration solution, drops or syrups consisting of vitamins, mineral supplements or medicines.

Complementary feeding is defined as the process that starts when breastmilk is no longer sufficient to meet the nutritional requirements of infants, and therefore other foods and liquids are needed, along with breastmilk. The target range for complementary feeding is generally taken to be six to 23 months of age, even though breastfeeding may continue beyond two years.

These recommendations may be adapted according to the needs of infants and young children in exceptionally difficult circumstances, such as pre-term or low-birth-weight infants, severely malnourished children, and in emergency situations. Specific recommendations apply to infants born to HIV-infected mothers.

Disadvantages of not breastfeeding

Breastfeeding confers short-term and long-term benefits on both child and mother, including helping to protect children against a variety of acute and chronic disorders. The long-term disadvantages of not breastfeeding are increasingly recognized as important. Reviews of studies from developing countries show that infants who are not breastfed are 6–10 times more likely to die in the first months of life than infants who are breastfed. Diarrhoea and pneumonia are more common and more severe in children who are artificially fed, and are responsible for many of these deaths. Diarrhoeal illness is also more common in artificially-fed infants, even in situations with adequate hygiene. Other acute infections, including *Haemophilus influenza* meningitis, otitis media, and urinary tract infection, are less common and less severe in breastfed infants.

Artificially-fed children have an increased risk of long-term diseases with an immunological basis, including asthma and other atopic conditions, type 1 diabetes, coeliac disease, ulcerative colitis and Crohn's disease. Artificial feeding is also associated with a greater risk of childhood leukaemia. Several studies suggest that obesity in later childhood and adolescence is less common among breastfed children, and that there is a dose-dependent effect, with a longer duration of breastfeeding associated with a lower risk. The effect may be less clear in populations where some children are undernourished. A growing body of evidence links artificial feeding with risks to cardiovascular health, including increased blood pressure, altered blood cholesterol levels and atherosclerosis in later adulthood. Breastfeeding has been associated with greater intelligence in late childhood and adulthood, and the difference was greater among those children who were born with low birth weight. which may affect the individual's ability to contribute to society.

For the mother, breastfeeding also has both short- and long-term benefits. The risk of postpartum haemorrhage may be reduced by breastfeeding immediately after delivery, and there is increasing evidence that the risk of breast and ovarian cancer is less among women who breastfed.

Exclusive breastfeeding for six months

If the breastfeeding technique is satisfactory, exclusive breastfeeding for the first six months of life meets the energy and nutrient needs of the vast majority of infants. No other foods or fluids are necessary. Several studies have shown that healthy infants do not even need additional water during the first six months if they are exclusively breastfed, even in a hot climate. Breastmilk itself is 88 per cent water, and is enough to satisfy a baby's thirst.

Extra fluids displace breastmilk, and do not increase overall intake. However, water and teas are commonly given to infants, often starting in the first week of life. This practice has been associated with a two-fold increased risk of diarrhoea. The advantages of exclusive breastfeeding compared to partial breastfeeding were recognized when a review of available studies found that the risk of death from diarrhoea of partially breastfed infants 0–6 months of age was 8.6-times the risk for exclusively breastfed children. For those who received no breastmilk the risk was 25-times that of those who were exclusively breastfed. Exclusive breastfeeding for six months has been found to reduce the risk of diarrhoea and respiratory illness compared with exclusive breastfeeding for three and four months respectively.

For the mother, exclusive breastfeeding can delay the return of fertility, and accelerate recovery of pre-pregnancy weight. Mothers who breastfeed exclusively and frequently have less than a 2 per cent risk of becoming pregnant in the first six months postpartum, provided that they still have amenorrhoea.

From about six months, an infant's need for energy and nutrients starts to exceed what is provided by breastmilk, and complementary feeding becomes necessary to fill the energy and nutrient gap. If complementary foods are not introduced at this age or if they are given inappropriately, an infant's growth may falter. In many countries, the period of complementary feeding from 6–23 months is the time of peak incidence of growth faltering, micronutrient deficiencies and infectious illnesses. Even after complementary foods have been introduced, breastfeeding remains a critical source of nutrients for the young infant and child. It provides about one half of an infant's energy needs up to the age of one year, and up to one third during the second year of life. Breastmilk continues to supply higher quality nutrients than complementary foods, and also protective factors. It is therefore recommended that breastfeeding on demand continues with adequate complementary feeding up to two years or beyond. Complementary foods need to be nutritionally-adequate, safe, and appropriately fed in order to meet the young child's energy and nutrient needs. However, complementary feeding is often fraught with problems, with foods being too dilute, not fed often enough or in too small amounts, or replacing breastmilk while being of an inferior quality. Both food and feeding practices influence the quality of complementary feeding, and mothers and families need support to practise good complementary feeding.

Breastmilk composition

Breastmilk contains all the nutrients that an infant needs in the first six months of life, including fat, carbohydrates, proteins, vitamins, minerals and water. It is easily digested and efficiently used. Breastmilk also contains bioactive factors that augment the infant's immature immune system, providing protection against infection, and other factors that help digestion and absorption of nutrients.

Breastmilk contains about 3.5 g of fat per 100 ml of milk, which provides about one half of the energy content of the milk. The fat is secreted in small droplets, and the amount increases as the feed progresses. As a result, the *hindmilk* secreted towards the end of a feed is rich in fat and looks creamy white, while the *foremilk* at the beginning of a feed contains less fat and looks somewhat bluish-grey in colour. Breastmilk fat contains long chain polyunsaturated fatty acids (docosahexaenoic acid or DHA, and arachidonic acid or ARA) that are not available in other milks. These fatty acids are important for the neurological development of a child. DHA and ARA are added to some varieties of infant formula, but this does not confer any advantage over breastmilk, and may not be as effective as those in breastmilk.

The main carbohydrate is the milk sugar lactose, a disaccharide. Breastmilk contains about 7 g lactose per 100 ml, which is more than in most other milks, and is another important source of energy. A number of oligosaccharides (sugar chains) in breastmilk function as important prebiotics in the protection against infection.

Breastmilk protein differs in both quantity and quality from animal milks, and it contains a balance of amino acids which makes it much more suitable for a baby. The concentration of protein in breastmilk (0.9 g per 100 ml) is lower than in animal milks. The much higher protein in animal milks can overload the infant's immature kidneys with waste nitrogen products. Breastmilk contains less of the protein casein, and this casein in breastmilk has a different molecular structure. It forms much softer, more easily-digested curds than that in other milks. Among the whey, or soluble proteins, human milk contains more alpha-lactalbumin; cow milk contains beta-lactoglobulin, which is absent from human milk and to which infants can become intolerant.

Breastmilk normally contains sufficient vitamins for an infant, unless the mother herself is deficient. The exception is vitamin D. The infant needs exposure to sunlight to generate endog-

enous vitamin D – or, if this is not possible, a supplement (*see* chapter 12, Rickets and metabolic bone disorders). The minerals iron and zinc are present in relatively low concentration, but their bioavailability and absorption is high. Provided that maternal iron status is adequate, term infants are born with a store of iron to supply their needs; only infants born with low birth weight may need supplements before six months (*see* Chapter 23, Disorders of the blood).

Breastmilk contains many factors that help to protect an infant against infection including:

- Immunoglobulin, principally secretory immuno-globulin A (sIgA), which coats the intestinal mucosa and prevents bacteria from entering the cells
- Macrophages and colony-forming lymphocytes
- Whey proteins (lysozyme and lactoferrin) which can kill bacteria, viruses and fungi
- Prebiotic oligosacccharides, which prevent bacteria from attaching to mucosal surfaces.

The protection provided by these factors is uniquely valuable for an infant. Breastmilk sIgA contains antibodies formed in the mother's body against the bacteria in her gut, and against infections that she has encountered, so they protect against bacteria that are particularly likely to be in the baby's environment.

Other protective factors include *bile-salt stimulated lipase*, which facilitates the complete digestion of fat once the milk has reached the small intestine. Fat in artificial milks is less completely digested. *Epidermal growth factor* stimulates maturation of the intestinal mucosa, so that it is better able to digest and absorb nutrients, and is less easily infected or sensitised to foreign proteins.

Colostrum and mature milk

Colostrum is produced in the first days of life, about 40–50 ml on the first day, which is all that an infant normally needs at this time. Colostrum is rich in white cells and antibodies, especially sIgA, and it contains a larger percentage of protein, minerals and fat-soluble vitamins (A, E and K) than later milk. Vitamin A is important for protection of the eye and for the integrity of epithelial surfaces, and often makes the colostrum yellowish in colour. Colostrum provides important immune protection to an infant when he or she is first exposed to the microorganisms in the environment, and epidermal growth factor helps to prepare the lining of the gut to receive the nutrients in milk. It is important that infants receive colostrum, and not other feeds, at this time. Other feeds given before breastfeeding is established are called *prelacteal feeds*. Milk starts to be produced in larger amounts between two and four days after delivery, making the breasts feel full; the milk is then said to have 'come in'. On the third day, an infant is normally taking about 300–400 ml per 24 hours, and on the fifth day 500–800 ml. From day seven to 14, the milk is called *transitional*, and after two weeks it is called *mature milk*.

Animal milks and infant formula

Animal milks are very different from breastmilk in both the quantities of the various nutrients, and in their quality. For infants under six months of age, animal milks can be home-modified by the addition of water, sugar and micronutrients to make them usable strictly as short-term replacements for breastmilk in exceptionally difficult situations, but they can never be equivalent or have the same anti-infective properties as breastmilk. After six months, infants can receive full cream milk that has been briefly boiled. Infant formula is usually made from industrially-modified cow milk or soy products. During the manufacturing process the quantities of nutrients are adjusted to make them more comparable to breastmilk. However, the qualitative differences in the fat and protein cannot be altered, and the absence of anti-infective and bio-active factors remains. Powdered infant formula is not a sterile product, and may be unsafe in other ways. Life threatening infections in newborns have been traced to contamination with pathogenic bacteria, such as *Enterobacter sakazakii*.

Anatomy of the breast

The breast structure (*see* Figure 9.1) includes the nipple and areola, mammary tissue, supporting connective tissue and fat, blood and lymphatic vessels, and nerves. The mammary tissue includes the alveoli, which are small sacs made of milk-secreting cells, and the ducts that carry the milk to the outside. Between feeds, milk collects in the lumen of the alveoli and ducts. The alveoli are surrounded by a basket of *myoepithelial*, or muscle cells, which contract and make the milk flow along the ducts. The *nipple* has an average of nine milk ducts passing

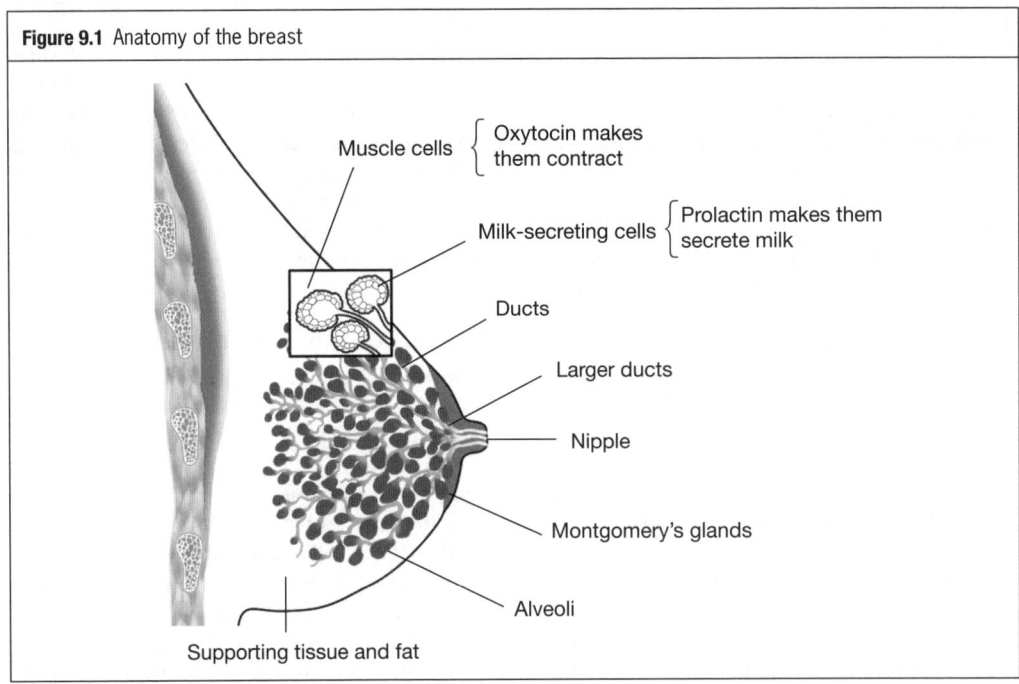

Figure 9.1 Anatomy of the breast

Muscle cells { Oxytocin makes them contract

Milk-secreting cells { Prolactin makes them secrete milk

Ducts

Larger ducts

Nipple

Montgomery's glands

Alveoli

Supporting tissue and fat

to the outside, and also muscle fibres and nerves. The nipple is surrounded by the circular pigmented *areola*, in which are located *Montgomery's glands*. These glands secrete an oily fluid that protects the skin of the nipple and areola during lactation, and produce the mother's individual scent that attracts her baby to the breast. The ducts beneath the areola fill with milk and become wider during a feed, when the oxytocin reflex is active.

Hormonal control of milk production

There are two hormones that directly affect breastfeeding: *prolactin* and *oxytocin*. A number of other hormones, such as oestrogen, are involved indirectly in lactation. When a baby suckles at the breast, sensory impulses pass from the nipple to the brain. In response, the anterior lobe of the pituitary gland secretes prolactin and the posterior lobe secretes oxytocin.

Prolactin is necessary for the secretion of milk by the cells of the alveoli. The level of prolactin in the blood increases markedly during pregnancy, and stimulates the growth and development of the mammary tissue, in preparation for the production of milk. However, milk is not secreted then, because progesterone and oestrogen, the hormones of pregnancy, block this action of prolactin. After delivery, levels of progesterone and oestrogen fall rapidly, prolactin is no longer blocked, and milk secretion begins. When a baby suckles, the level of prolactin in the blood increases, and stimulates production of milk by the alveoli (*see* Figure 9. 2).

The prolactin level is highest about 30 minutes after the beginning of the feed, so its most important effect is to make milk for the next feed. During the first few weeks, the more a baby suckles and stimulates the nipple, the more prolactin is produced, and the more milk is produced. This effect is particularly important at the time when lactation is becoming established. After a few weeks there is not a close relationship between the amount of prolactin and the amount of milk produced. However, if the mother stops breastfeeding, milk secretion may stop too – then the milk will dry up. More prolactin is produced at night, so breastfeeding at night is especially helpful for keeping up the milk supply. Prolactin seems to make a mother feel relaxed and sleepy, so she usually rests well even if she breastfeeds at night. Suckling affects the release of other pituitary hormones, including *gonadotrophin releasing hormone* (GnRH), *follicle stimulating hormone,* and *luteinising hormone*, which results in suppression of ovulation and menstruation. Therefore, frequent breastfeeding can help to delay a new pregnancy. Breastfeeding at night is important to ensure this effect.

Oxytocin makes the myoepithelial cells around the alveoli contract. The oxytocin reflex is also sometimes called the 'let-down reflex' or the 'milk ejection reflex'. Oxytocin is produced more quickly than prolactin. It makes the milk that is already in the alveoli flow along and fill the ducts for the current feed, and helps the baby to get the milk easily (*see* Figure 9.3). Sometimes the milk is ejected in fine streams. Oxytocin starts working when a mother expects a feed as well as when the baby is suckling. The reflex becomes conditioned to the mother's sensations and feelings, such as touching, smelling or seeing her baby, or hearing her baby cry, or thinking lovingly about him or her. If a mother is in severe pain or emotionally upset, the oxytocin reflex may become inhibited,

Table 9.1 Factors affecting lactation

	Favourable	Unfavourable
Environment	Calm, relaxed	Noisy, stressful
Frequency of feeds	Frequent	Infrequent
Breast contents	Empty	Engorged
Emotional state	Relaxed	Anxious
Physical state	Comfortable	Pain, tense
Drugs	Metoclopramide	Oestrogen
	Oxytocin (sub-lingual)	Testosterone
		Bromocriptine
		Sedatives (large doses)

Figure 9.2 Prolactin

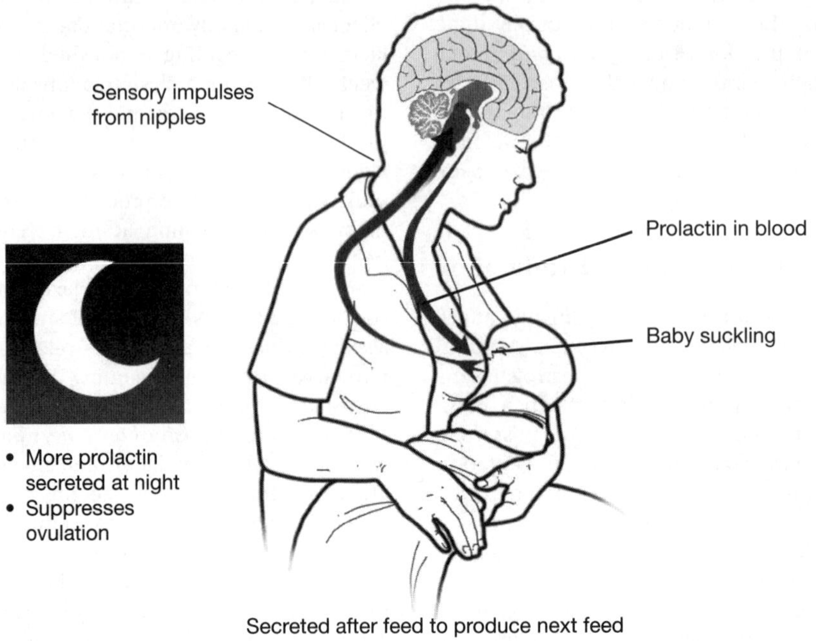

Sensory impulses from nipples

Prolactin in blood

Baby suckling

- More prolactin secreted at night
- Suppresses ovulation

Secreted after feed to produce next feed

Figure 9.3 Oxytocin

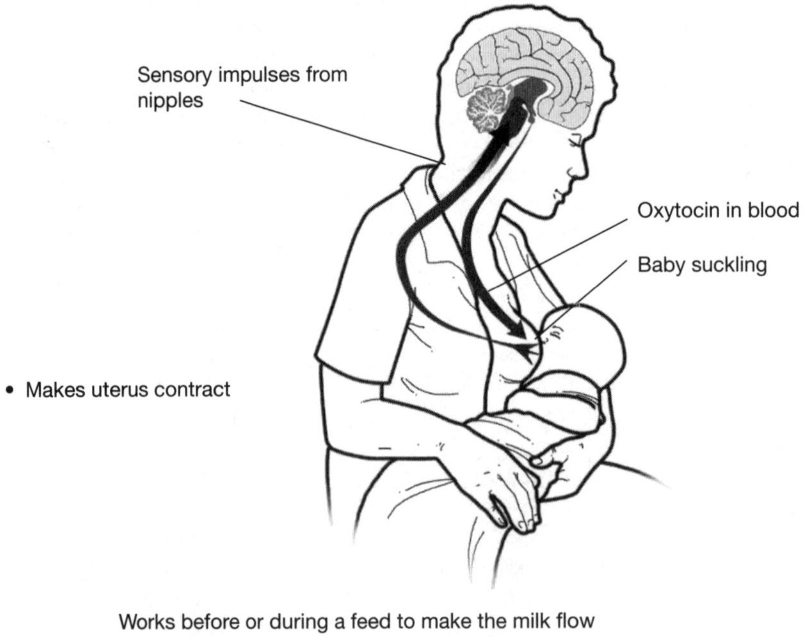

Sensory impulses from nipples

Oxytocin in blood

Baby suckling

- Makes uterus contract

Works before or during a feed to make the milk flow

and her milk may suddenly stop flowing well. If she receives support, is helped to feel comfortable and lets the baby continue to breastfeed, the milk will flow again. Understanding the oxytocin reflex is important in practice, because it explains why it is important to keep a mother and baby together and for them to have skin-to-skin contact, to help the flow of milk. Oxytocin makes a mother's uterus contract after delivery and helps to reduce bleeding. The contractions can cause severe uterine pain when the baby suckles during the first few days.

Mothers may notice signs that show that the oxytocin reflex is active:
- A tingling sensation in the breast before or during a feed
- Milk flowing from her breasts when she thinks of the baby or hears him crying
- Milk flowing from the other breast when the baby is suckling
- Milk flowing from the breast in streams if suckling is interrupted
- Slow deep sucks and swallowing by the baby, which show that milk is flowing into his mouth
- Uterine pain or a flow of blood from the uterus
- Thirst during a feed.

If one or more of these signs are present, the reflex is working. However, if they are not present, it does not mean that the reflex is not active. The signs may not be obvious, and the mother may not be aware of them.

Oxytocin also has important psychological effects, and is known to affect mothering behaviour in animals.

In humans, oxytocin induces a state of calm, and reduces stress. It may enhance feelings of affection between mother and child, and promote bonding. Pleasant forms of touch stimulate the secretion of oxytocin, and also prolactin, and skin-to-skin contact between mother and baby after delivery helps both breastfeeding and emotional bonding.

Feedback inhibitor of lactation (FIL)

Milk production is also controlled in the breast by a substance called the *feedback inhibitor of lactation*, or FIL (a polypeptide), which is present in breastmilk. This exerts local control of milk production independently within each breast and allows one breast to stop making milk while the other breast continues, for example if a baby suckles only on one side. If milk is not removed, the inhibitor collects and stops the cells from secreting any more, helping to protect the breast from the harmful effects of being too full. If breastmilk is removed the inhibitor is also removed, and secretion resumes. Therefore, if the baby cannot suckle for whatever reason, then milk must be removed by expression to prevent milk secretion from stopping. FIL enables the amount of milk produced to be determined by how much the baby takes, and therefore by how much the baby needs. This mechanism is particularly important for ongoing close regulation after lactation is established. At this stage, prolactin is needed to enable milk secretion to take place, but it does not control the amount of milk produced.

Reflexes in the baby

The baby's reflexes are important for appropriate breastfeeding. The main reflexes are *rooting, suckling* and *swallowing*. When something touches a baby's lips or cheek, the baby turns to find the stimulus, and opens his or her mouth, putting his or her tongue down and forward. This is the *rooting reflex* and is present from about the 32nd week of pregnancy. When something touches a baby's palate, he or she starts to suck it. This is the *suckling reflex*. When the baby's mouth fills with milk, he or she swallows. This is the *swallowing reflex*. Preterm infants can grasp the nipple from about 28 weeks gestational age, and they can suckle and remove some milk from about 31 weeks. Coordination of suckling, swallowing and breathing appears between 32 and 35 weeks of pregnancy. Infants can only suckle for a short time at that age, but they can take supplementary feeds by cup. A majority of infants can breastfeed fully at a gestational age of 36 weeks. When supporting a mother and baby to initiate and establish exclusive breastfeeding, it is important to know about these reflexes, as their level of maturation will guide whether an infant can breastfeed directly or temporarily requires another feeding method.

How a baby attaches and suckles at the breast

To stimulate the nipple and remove milk from the breast, and to ensure an adequate supply and a good flow of milk, a baby needs to be *well attached* so that he or she can *suckle effectively*. Difficulties often occur because a baby does not take the breast into his or her mouth properly, and so cannot suckle effectively.

Figure 9.4 shows how a baby takes the breast into his or her mouth to suckle effectively. This baby is well attached to the breast. The points to notice are:

- Much of the areola and the tissues underneath it, including the larger ducts, are in the baby's mouth.
- The breast is stretched out to form a long 'teat', but the nipple only forms about one third of the 'teat'.
- The baby's tongue is forward over the lower gums, beneath the milk ducts (the baby's tongue is in fact cupped around the sides of the 'teat', but a drawing cannot show this).
- The baby is suckling from the breast, not from the nipple.

As the baby suckles, a wave passes along the tongue from front to back, pressing the teat against the hard palate, and pressing milk out of the sinuses into the baby's mouth from where he or she swallows it. The baby uses suction mainly to stretch out the breast tissue and to hold it in his or her mouth. The oxytocin reflex makes the breastmilk flow along the ducts, and the action of the baby's tongue presses the milk from the ducts into the baby's mouth. When a baby is well attached his mouth and tongue do not rub or traumatise the skin of the nipple and areola. Suckling is comfortable and often pleasurable for the mother. She does not feel pain.

Figure 9.5 shows what happens in the mouth when a baby is not well attached at the breast. The points to notice are:

- Only the nipple is in the baby's mouth, not the underlying breast tissue or ducts.
- The baby's tongue is back inside his or her mouth, and cannot reach the ducts to press on them.

Suckling with poor attachment may be uncomfortable or painful for the mother, and may damage the skin of the nipple and areola, causing sore nipples and fissures (or 'cracks'). Poor attachment is the commonest and most important cause of sore nipples, and may result in inefficient removal of milk and apparent low supply.

Signs of good and poor attachment

Figure 9.6 shows the four most important signs of good and poor attachment from the outside. These signs can be used to decide if a mother and baby need help. The four signs of *good attachment* are:

- More of the areola is visible above the baby's top lip than below the lower lip.
- The baby's mouth is wide open.
- The baby's lower lip is curled outwards.
- The baby's chin is touching or almost touching the breast.

All four signs need to be present to show that a baby is well attached. In addition, suckling should be comfortable for the mother.

Figure 9.4 Good attachment

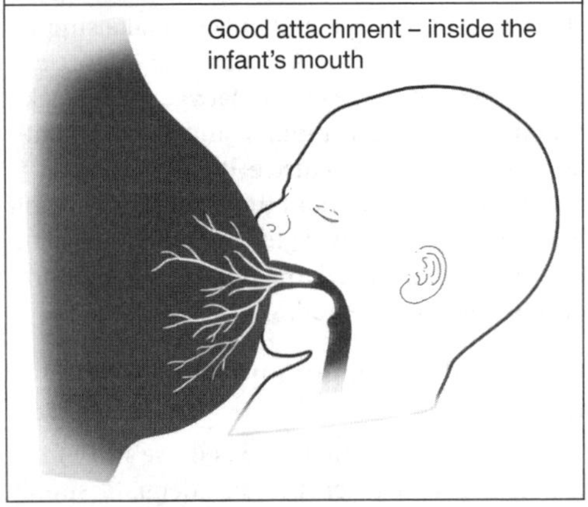

Good attachment – inside the infant's mouth

Figure 9.5 Poor attachment

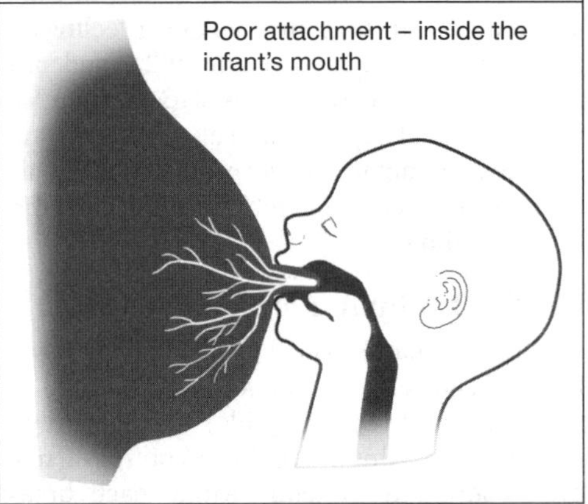

Poor attachment – inside the infant's mouth

The signs of *poor attachment* are:

- More of the areola is visible below the baby's bottom lip than above the top lip – or the amounts above and below are equal.
- The baby's mouth is not wide open.
- The baby's lower lip points forward or is turned inwards.
- The baby's chin is away from the breast.

If any one of these signs is present, or if suckling is painful or uncomfortable, attachment needs to be improved.

Effective suckling

If a baby is well attached at the breast, then he or she can suckle effectively. Signs of effective suckling indicate that milk is flowing into the baby's mouth. The baby takes slow, deep suckles followed by a visible or audible swallow about once per second. Sometimes the baby pauses for a few seconds, allowing the ducts to fill up with milk again. When the baby starts suckling again, he or she may suckle quickly a few times, stimulating milk flow, and then the slow deep suckles begin. The baby's cheeks remain rounded during the feed. Towards the end of a feed, suckling usually slows down, with fewer deep suckles and longer pauses between them. This is the time when the volume of milk is less, but as it is fat-rich hindmilk, it is important for the feed to continue. When the baby is satisfied, he or she usually releases the breast spontaneously. The nipple may look stretched out for a second or two, but it quickly returns to its resting form.

Signs of ineffective suckling

A baby who is poorly attached is likely to suckle ineffectively. He or she may suckle quickly all the time, without swallowing, and the cheeks may be drawn in as he or she suckles showing that milk is not flowing well into the baby's mouth. When the baby stops feeding, the nipple may stay stretched out, and look squashed from side to side, with a pressure line across the tip, showing that the nipple is being damaged by incorrect suction.

Consequences of ineffective suckling

When a baby suckles ineffectively, transfer of milk from mother to baby is inefficient. As a result:

- The breast may become engorged, or may develop a blocked duct or mastitis because not enough milk is removed.
- The baby's intake of breastmilk may be insufficient, resulting in poor weight gain.
- The baby may pull away from the breast out of frustration and refuse to feed.
- The baby may be very hungry and continue suckling for a long time, or feed very often.
- The breasts may be over-stimulated by too much suckling, resulting in oversupply of milk.

Causes of poor attachment

Use of a feeding bottle before breastfeeding is well established can cause poor attachment, because the mechanism of suckling with a bottle is different. Functional difficulties such as flat and inverted nipples, or a very small or weak infant, are also causes of poor attachment. However, the

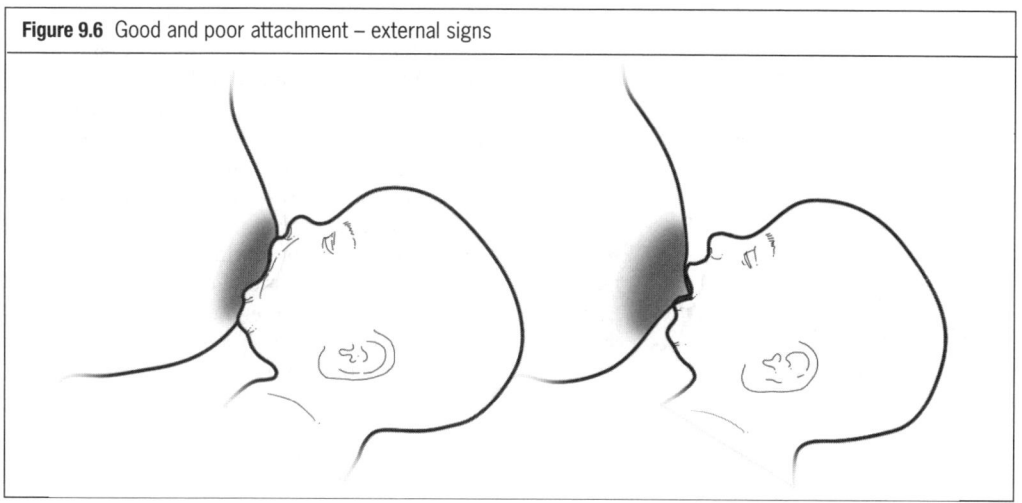

Figure 9.6 Good and poor attachment – external signs

most important causes are inexperience of the mother and lack of skilled help from the health workers who attend her. Many mothers need skilled help in the early days to ensure that the baby attaches well and can suckle effectively. Health workers need to have the necessary skills to give this help.

Positioning the mother and baby for good attachment

To be well attached at the breast, a baby and his or her mother need to be appropriately positioned.

The **mother** can be sitting or lying down (*see* Figure 9.7) or standing, if she wishes. However, she needs to be relaxed and comfortable, and without strain, particularly of her back. If she is sitting, her back needs to be supported, and she should be able to hold the baby at her breast without leaning forward.

The **baby** can breastfeed in several different positions in relation to the mother. Whatever the position of the mother, and the baby's general position in relation to her, there are four key points about the position of the baby's body that are important to observe.

Figure 9.7 Baby well positioned at the breast

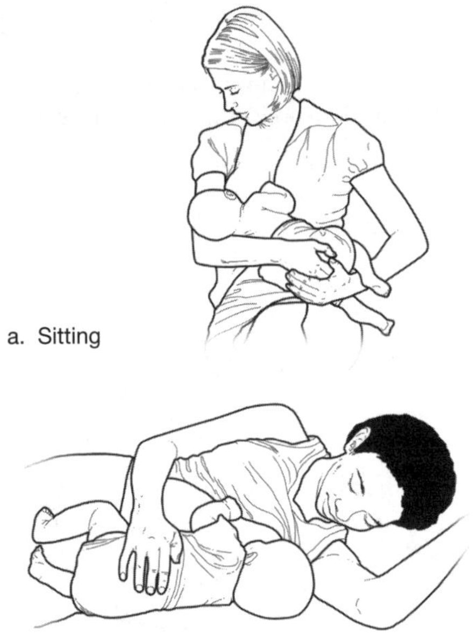

a. Sitting

b. Lying down

◆ The baby's body should be straight, not bent or twisted. The baby's head can be slightly extended at the neck, which helps his or her chin to be close in to the breast. He or she should be facing the breast. The nipples usually point slightly downwards, so the baby should not be flat against the mother's chest or abdomen, but turned slightly on his or her back and able to see the mother's face.

◆ The baby's body should be close to the mother, which enables the baby to be close to the breast, and to take a large mouthful.

◆ His or her whole body should be supported. The baby may be supported on the bed or a pillow, or the mother's lap or arm. She should not support only the baby's head and neck. She should not grasp the baby's bottom, as this can pull him or her too far out to the side, and make it difficult for the baby to get his or her chin and tongue under the areola.

These points about positioning are especially important for young infants during the first two months of life.

Demand feeding

To ensure adequate milk production and flow for six months of exclusive breastfeeding, a baby needs to feed as often and for as long as he or she wants, both day and night. This is called *demand feeding, unrestricted feeding*, or *baby-led feeding*. Babies feed with different frequencies and take different amounts of milk at each feed. The 24-hour intake of milk varies between mother-infant pairs from 440–1 220 ml, averaging about 800 ml per day throughout the first six months. Infants who are feeding on demand according to their appetite obtain what they need for satisfactory growth. They stop feeding because of satiety, not because the breast is empty. However, breasts seem to vary in their capacity for storing milk. Infants of women with low storage capacity may need to feed more often to remove the milk and ensure adequate daily intake and production. It is thus important not to restrict the duration or the frequency of feeds – provided the baby is well attached to the breast. Nipple damage is caused by poor attachment and not by prolonged feeds. The mother learns to respond to her baby's cues of hunger and readiness to feed, such as restlessness, rooting (searching) with his mouth, or sucking hands, before the baby starts to cry. The baby should be allowed to continue suckling on the breast until he or she spontaneously releases the nipple. After a short rest, the baby can be offered the other side, which he or she may or may not want.

If a baby stays on the breast for a very long time (more than one half hour for every feed) or if he or she wants to feed very often (more

---

Table 9.2 Medical reasons for use of breastmilk substitutes

Infant conditions

Infants who should not receive breast milk or any other milk except specialized formula:
- Infants with classic galactosaemia: a special galactose-free formula is needed
- Infants with maple syrup urine disease: a special formula free of leucine, isoleucine and valine is needed
- Infants with phenylketonuria: a special phenylalanine-free formula is needed

Infants for whom breast milk remains the best feeding option but who may need other food in addition to breast milk for a limited period:
- Infants born weighing less than 1 500 g (very low birth weight)
- Infants born at less than 32 weeks of gestation (very preterm)
- Newborn infants who are at risk of hypoglycaemia by virtue of impaired metabolic adaptation or increased glucose demand (such as those who are preterm, small for gestational age) or who have experienced significant intrapartum hypoxic/ischaemic stress, those who are ill and those whose mothers are diabetic if their blood sugar fails to respond to optimal breastfeeding or breast-milk feeding.

Maternal conditions

Maternal conditions that may justify permanent avoidance of breastfeeding:
- HIV infection: if replacement feeding is acceptable, feasible, affordable, sustainable and safe.

Maternal conditions that may justify temporary avoidance of breastfeeding:
- Severe illness that prevents a mother from caring for her infant, for example sepsis
- Herpes simplex virus type 1 (HSV-1): direct contact between lesions on the mother's breasts and the infant's mouth should be avoided until all active lesions have resolved

- Maternal medication:
  - sedating psychotherapeutic drugs, anti-epileptic drugs and opioids and their combinations may cause side effects such as drowsiness and respiratory depression and are better avoided if a safer alternative is available
  - radioactive iodine-131 is better avoided given that safer alternatives are available – a mother can resume breastfeeding about two months after receiving this substance
  - excessive use of topical iodine or iodophors (e.g. povidone-iodine), especially on open wounds or mucous membranes, can result in thyroid suppression or electrolyte abnormalities in the breastfed infant and should be avoided
  - cytotoxic chemotherapy requires that a mother stops breastfeeding during therapy.

Maternal conditions during which breastfeeding can still continue, although health problems may be of concern:
- Breast abscess: breastfeeding should continue on the unaffected breast; feeding from the affected breast can resume once treatment has started
- Hepatitis B: infants should be given hepatitis B vaccine, within the first 48 hours or as soon as possible thereafter
- Hepatitis C
- Mastitis: if breastfeeding is very painful, milk must be removed by expression to prevent progression of the condition
- Tuberculosis: mother and baby should be managed according to national tuberculosis guidelines
- Substance use:
  - maternal use of nicotine, alcohol, ecstasy, amphetamines, cocaine and related stimulants has been demonstrated to have harmful effects on breastfed babies
  - alcohol, opioids, benzodiazepines and cannabis can cause sedation in both the mother and the baby.
- Mothers should be encouraged not to use these substances, and given opportunities and support to abstain.

often than every 1–1½ hours each time) then the baby's attachment needs to be checked and improved. Prolonged, frequent feeds can be a sign of ineffective suckling and inefficient transfer of milk to the baby. This is usually due to poor attachment, which may also lead to sore nipples. If the attachment is improved, transfer of milk becomes more efficient, and the feeds may become shorter or less frequent. At the same time, the risk of nipple damage is reduced.

Acceptable medical reasons for use of breastmilk substitutes

A small number of health conditions of the infant or the mother may justify recommending that she does not breastfeed temporarily or permanently. These conditions, which concern very few mothers and their infants, are listed in the box together with some health conditions of the mother that, although serious, are not medical reasons for using breastmilk substitutes.

Monitoring of adequacy of feeding

There are two reliable signs that a baby is not getting enough milk:
- ◆ Poor weight gain
- ◆ Low urine output.

Passing meconium (sticky black stools) four days after delivery is also a sign of the baby not getting enough milk.

Poor weight gain

Babies' weight gain is variable, and each child follows his or her own pattern. You cannot tell from a single weighing if a baby is growing satisfactorily – it is necessary to weigh several times over a few days at least. Soon after birth a baby may lose weight for a few days. Most recover their birth weight by the end of the first week, if they are healthy and feeding well. All babies should recover their birth weight by two weeks of age. A baby who is below his or her birth weight at the end of the second week needs to be assessed.

From two weeks, babies who are breastfed may gain from about 500 g to 1 kg or more each month. All these weight gains are normal. The baby should be checked for illness or congenital abnormality and urine output. The technique and

pattern of breastfeeding, and the mother-baby interaction should also be assessed, to decide the cause of poor weight gain, as explained below.

Low urine output

An exclusively breastfed baby who is taking enough milk usually passes dilute urine 6–8 times or more in 24 hours. If a baby is passing urine less than six times a day, especially if the urine is dark yellow and strong smelling, then he or she is not getting enough fluid. This is a useful way to find out quickly if a baby is probably taking enough milk or not. However, it is not useful if the baby is having other drinks in addition to breastmilk.

Management and support of breast-feeding in maternity facilities

The Baby-Friendly Hospital Initiative

Many deliveries take place in hospitals or maternity facilities, and health care practices in these facilities have a major effect on infant feeding. To

---

The reasons for a low breastmilk supply are:

Breastfeeding factors:
- Delayed initiation of breastfeeding
- Poor attachment, so that the baby does not take the milk from the breast efficiently
- Short or infrequent feeds
- Using bottles or pacifiers which replace suckling at the breast, so the baby suckles less
- Giving other foods or drinks causes the baby to suckle less at the breast and take less milk.

Psychological factors of the mother:
A mother may be depressed, lacking in confidence, worried, or stressed; or she may reject the baby or dislike the idea of breastfeeding. These factors do not directly affect her milk production, but can interfere with the way in which she responds to her baby, so that she breastfeeds less.

Mother's physical condition:
A few mothers have low milk production for a pathological reason including endocrine problems (pituitary failure after severe haemorrhage, retained piece of placenta) or poor breast development. A few mothers have a physiological low breast-milk production, for no apparent reason.

encourage breastfeeding from the time of child-birth, to prevent difficulties from arising and to overcome difficulties should they occur, mothers need appropriate management and skilled help.

Support and counselling should be available routinely during antenatal care, to prepare mothers; at the time of birth to help them initiate breastfeeding; and in the postnatal period to ensure that breastfeeding is fully established.

Mothers and other caregivers who are not able to breastfeed need counselling and support for alternative methods of infant feeding. The Baby-friendly Hospital Initiative (BFHI) was launched in 1992 with the aim of transforming maternity facilities to provide this standard of care. Without the BFHI, practices often undermine breastfeeding, with damaging consequences for infant health. Hospitals become baby-friendly by implementing the *Ten Steps to Successful Breast-feeding*, summarized below, and complying with relevant sections of the International Code of Marketing of Breastmilk Substitutes and subsequent relevant Health Assembly resolutions. Facilities that are working to achieve baby-friendly accreditation are formally assessed on their policies, training, and full implementation of all of the Ten Steps including compliance with the Code.

South African Code of Ethics for the marketing of breastmilk substitutes

South Africa endorses the Code of Ethics accepted by the WHO Assembly in 1981, which applies to developed and developing countries. The aim of the code is to control the promotion of artificial feeds, not to ban the sale or use of infant feeds. Its essence is to protect children from the abuse or misuse of such products. All health personnel, especially those involved with infant nutrition, should be familiar with the Code.

The aim of the Code is to contribute to the provision of safe and adequate nutrition for infants by the protection and promotion of breastfeeding, and to ensure the proper use of artificial feeds.

The scope of the Code applies to infant formulae; other milk products, foods and beverages; feeding bottles and teats.

Principles of the Code:

 • There should be no advertising or other form of promotion to the general public of products within the scope of the Code.
 • Manufacturers and distributors should not provide free samples or gifts of products to the public.
 • There should not be any contact between the marketing personnel and mothers.
 • There should be no promotion to induce sales directly to the consumer at retail level, such as special displays, discount coupons, premiums, special sales, loss-leaders or tie-in sales for the products.
 • Neither the container nor the label should have pictures of infants or text which may idealize the use of infant formulae.
 • No health care facility should be used for the promotion or advertisement of infant formulae or other products within the Code.
 • Health workers should not accept nor give any gifts from manufacturers and distributors to the public.
 • No financial or material inducement should be offered to health workers or marketing personnel for the promotion of the products.

The ten steps to successful breastfeeding

1 Have a written breastfeeding policy that is routinely communicated to all health care staff.
2 Train all health care staff in skills necessary to implement this policy.
3 Inform all pregnant women about the benefits and management of breastfeeding.
4 Help mothers initiate breastfeeding within one half hour of birth.
5 Show mothers how to breastfeed and how to maintain lactation even if they should be separated from their infants.
6 Give newborn infants no food or drink other than breast milk, unless medically indicated.
7 Practice rooming-in – allow mothers and infants to remain together – 24 hours a day.
8 Encourage breastfeeding on demand.
9 Give no artificial teats or pacifiers (also called dummies or soothers) to breastfeeding infants.
10 Foster the establishment of breastfeeding support groups and refer mothers to them on discharge from the hospital or clinic.

Source: *Protecting, promoting and supporting breast-feeding: the special role of maternity services. A joint WHO/UNICEF statement, 1992*

Low-birth-weight babies

(*See* also chapter 7, Care of the Newborn)

Being born with low birth weight is a disadvantage for the infant. LBW directly or indirectly may contribute to 60 – 80 per cent of all neonatal deaths. Appropriate care of LBW infants, including their feeding, temperature maintenance, hygienic cord and skin care, and early detection and treatment of infections can substantially reduce excess mortality. This section deals with feeding low-birth-weight babies. It summarizes what, how, when and how much to feed to low-birth-weight babies.

What to feed?

A baby's own mother's milk is best for LBW infants of all gestational ages. Breastmilk is especially adapted to the nutritional needs of LBW infants, and strong and consistent evidence shows that feeding mother's own milk is associated with lower incidence of infections and better long-term outcomes. Not all LBW infants are able to feed from the breast in the first days of life. For infants who are not able to breastfeed effectively, feeds have to be given by an alternative, oral feeding method (cup/spoon/direct expression into mouth) or by intra-gastric tube feeding. In these situations, the options available for feeding the LBW infant are, in order of preference:

- Expressed breastmilk (EBM) (from his or her own mother)
- Donor breastmilk
- Infant formula: standard infant formula for infants with birth weight >1 500 g, and preterm formula for infants with birth weight <1 500 g.

A LBW baby who is not able to breastfeed usually needs care in a special newborn care unit. Every effort should be made to enable a mother to stay in or near this unit. Otherwise, she should spend as much time there as possible every day. When breastfeeding is established, care can continue at home with close follow-up. A baby should have as much skin-to-skin contact with his or her mother as possible, to help both bonding and breastfeeding. If a baby is too sick to move, the mother should at least be able to talk to him or her, and to have hand contact. A mother should be given skilled help to express her milk and to establish lactation starting, if possible, within six hours of birth. She should express at least eight times in 24 hours, expressing at home if she is not staying in the health facility. The EBM can be given every 1–3 hours according to the age and weight of the baby. Supplements of vitamin D and phosphate may be recommended as soon as enteral feeding commences for VLBW infants, and supplements of iron are recommended for all LBW infants from the age of 6–8 weeks.

How to feed?

Babies of 36 weeks gestational age or more can often suckle well enough at the breast to feed themselves fully. Help the mother to have skin-to-skin contact with the baby, and to let the baby try to suckle as soon as possible after delivery. Make sure that the baby is well attached at the breast. When a LBW baby first suckles, he or she may pause quite often and for long periods during a feed, and may need to continue feeding for an hour. It is important not to take the baby off the breast during these pauses. The baby should be allowed to suckle every three hours, or more frequently on demand. If a baby has difficulty suckling effectively, tires quickly at the breast or does not gain adequate weight, offer expressed milk by cup after the breastfeed, or give alternate breast and cup feeds.

Babies of 32 to 36 weeks gestational age need to be fed partly or fully on EBM by cup or spoon until full breastfeeding can be established. Feeds can start as soon as the baby is clinically stable, if possible within one hour of birth, and should be given 2–3 hourly. To stimulate breastfeeding, these babies should be allowed to suckle or lick the breast as much as they wish. Offer the full amount of feed by cup initially. If the baby has already had some milk from the breast, he or she may refuse to finish the cup feed. If the baby is suckling well and gaining weight, cup feeds can be reduced. If the baby is still having difficulties attaching correctly at the breast, encourage the mother to express her milk directly into her baby's mouth. Bottle feeding should be avoided, as it may interfere with the baby learning to breastfeed.

Babies less than 32 weeks gestational age usually need to be fed by gastric tube. They should not receive any enteral feeds in the first 12–24 hours. Table 9.2 shows the quantity of milk that a LBW baby fed by gastric tube needs each day and Table 9. 3 shows how much is needed at each feed.

Table 9.2 Recommended fluid intake for LBW babies

Day of life	Fluid requirements (ml/kg/day)		
	2 000–2 500 g	1 500–2 000 g	1 000–1 500 g
Day 1	60	60	60
Day 2	80	75	70
Day 3	100	90	80
Day 4	120	115	90
Day 5	140	130	110
Day 6	150	145	130
Day 7	160+	160	150*

*If the infant is on intravenous fluids, do not incease above 140 ml/kg/day

Table 9.3 Recommended feed volumes for LBW infants

Day of life	Feed volumes (ml)		
	2 000–2 500 g (3-hourly)	1 500–2 000 g (3-hourly)	1 000–1 500 g (every 2 hors)*
Day 1	17	12	6
Day 2	22	16	7
Day 3	27	20	8
Day 4	32	24	9
Day 5	37	28	11
Day 6	40	32	13
Day 7	42	35	16

If the baby is cup feeding, add 5 ml per feed to allow for spillage and variability of infant's appetite.
*For infants with birth weight <1 250 g who do not show signs of feeding readiness, start with small 1–2 ml feeds every 1–2 hours and give the rest of the fluid requirement as intravenous fluids.

The quantity needs to be exact. However, babies less than <1 500g may need to receive some of these requirements as intravenous fluids, as they may not tolerate full enteral feeds. The quantities in the table are calculated according to the baby's need for:

- 60 ml/kg on day 1, increasing by 10 or 20 ml per day over seven days up to 160 ml/kg/day.
- Eight feeds in 24 hours. If a baby has more than eight feeds in 24 hours, the amount

per feed must be reduced accordingly, to achieve the same total volume in 24 hours.

A baby who is cup fed needs to be offered 5 ml extra at each feed. This slightly larger amount allows for spillage with cup feeding. Also, a baby having cup feeds may take more or less than is recommended. Adding 5 ml allows for different amounts to be taken at each feed. It is important to keep a record of the 24-hour total and ensure that it meets the required total ml/kg per day for the baby's weight.

Quantities after seven days

If a baby is still having EBM by cup or gastric tube after seven days, increase the quantity given by 20 ml/kg each day until the baby is receiving 180 ml/kg per day. The baby's weight needs to be monitored. Satisfactory weight gain should be more than 15 g/kg each day. If the weight gain is less than 15 g/kg each day over three days, the quantity of milk should be increased by 20 ml/kg each day until 200 ml/kg is reached. As the baby begins to breastfeed more frequently, the amount of EBM given by gastric tube or cup may be gradually reduced.

Discharge

A LBW baby can be discharged from hospital when he or she is:

* Breastfeeding effectively or the mother is confident using an alternative feeding method
* Maintaining his or her own temperature between 36.5 °C and 37.5 °C for at least three consecutive days
* Gaining weight, at least 15 g/kg for three consecutive days
* The mother is confident in her ability to care for her baby.

Before discharging a mother and her LBW baby from hospital, a discussion should take place with her on how she can be supported at home and in the community.

If a mother lives a long distance from the hospital and it is difficult for her to return for a follow-up visit, her baby should not be discharged until he or she fully meets the criteria. If possible, the mother should stay with her baby to establish breastfeeding before discharge. She should be given the name and contact details of any local breastfeeding support groups, whether health facility or community based.

Follow up of LBW babies

The baby should have follow-up visits at least once 2–5 days after discharge, and at least weekly until fully breastfeeding and weighing more than 2.5 kg. Ideally these should be home visits by a community breastfeeding counsellor, or visits by the mother to a nearby health facility. Further follow-up can then continue monthly as for a term baby.

Kangaroo mother care (KMC)

KMC is a way in which a mother can give her LBW or small baby benefits similar to those provided by an incubator. The mother has more involvement in the baby's care; and she has extended skin-to-skin contact, which helps both breastfeeding and bonding, probably because it stimulates the release of prolactin and oxytocin from her pituitary gland. KMC helps a mother to develop a close relationship with her baby, and increases her confidence.

Management. The mother keeps her baby in prolonged skin-to-skin contact day and night, in an upright position between her breasts. The baby is supported in this position by the mother's clothes, or by cloths tied around her chest. The baby's head is left free so that he or she can breathe, and the face can be seen. The baby wears a nappy for cleanliness and a cap to keep the head warm. KMC has been shown to keep the baby warm, to stabilize his or her breathing and heart rate, and to reduce the risk of infection. It helps the mother to initiate breastfeeding earlier, and the baby to gain weight faster. Most routine care can be carried out while the baby remains in skin-to-skin contact. When the mother has to attend to her own needs, skin-to-skin contact can be continued by someone else, for example by the father or a grandparent, or the baby can be wrapped and put into a cot or on a bed until KMC can be continued. It is not essential for a baby to be able to coordinate sucking and swallowing to be eligible for KMC. Other methods of feeding can be used until the baby is able to breastfeed. Close contact with the mother means that the baby is kept very near to her breasts, and can easily smell and lick milk expressed onto her nipple. He or she can be given breastmilk by direct expression into his mouth until able to attach well.

KMC should be continued for as long as necessary, which is usually until the baby is able to maintain his or her temperature, is breathing without difficulty and can breastfeed without the need for alternative methods of feeding. It is usually the baby who indicates that he or she is ready and 'wants to get out'. If the mother lives near the hospital or health facility the baby may be discharged breastfeeding and/or using an alternative feeding method, such as cup feeding with the mother's EBM. The mother and her baby should be monitored regularly.

In the first week after discharge, the baby should be weighed daily, if possible, and a health-care worker should discuss any difficulties with the mother, providing her with support and encouragement. Monitoring should continue until the baby weighs more than 2.5 kg. When the baby becomes less tolerant of the position, the mother may reduce the time in KMC and then stop altogether over about a week. Once the baby has stopped KMC, monthly follow-up should be continued to monitor feeding, growth and development until the baby is several months old.

Relactation

The re-establishment of breastfeeding is an important management option in emergency situations, and for infants who are malnourished or ill. Most women can relactate even years after their last child, but it is easier for women who stopped breastfeeding recently, or if the infant still suckles sometimes. A woman needs to be highly motivated, and well supported by health care workers. Continuing support can be provided by community health workers, mother support groups, women friends, older women and traditional birth attendants.

Stimulation of the breasts is essential, preferably by the infant suckling as often and for as long as possible. Many infants who have breastfed before are willing to suckle, even if there is not much milk being produced currently. Suckling causes release of prolactin, which stimulates growth of alveoli in the breast and the production of breastmilk. The mother and infant must stay together all the time. Skin-to-skin contact, or kangaroo mother care are helpful. If the infant is willing to suckle, the mother should put him or her to the breast frequently, at least 8–12 times every 24 hours, ensuring that attachment is good. If the infant is not willing to suckle, she can start the relactation process by stimulating her breasts with gentle breast massage and then with 20–30 minutes of hand expression 8–12 times a day.

Supplementary feeds for the infant. The infant needs a temporary supplement, which can be expressed milk, artificial milk or therapeutic formula. The full amount of supplement should be given initially, in a way that encourages the infant to resume breastfeeding. Avoid using feeding bottles or pacifiers. Whenever the baby wants to suckle, he or she should do so from the breast. For infants who are not willing to suckle at the breast, the supplementary suckling technique is useful.

The supplementary suckling technique usually needs to be practised under supervision at a health facility. A breastfeeding supplementer consists of a tube which leads from a cup of supplement to the breast, and which goes along the nipple and into the infant's mouth. The infant suckles and stimulates the breast at the same time drawing the supplement through the tube, and is thereby nourished and satisfied. Encourage the mother to let the infant suckle on the breast at any time that he or she is willing – not just when she is giving the supplement. When the infant is willing to suckle at the breast without the supplement, then she can start giving breastmilk by cup instead. This should be more feasible in home conditions.

Quantity of supplement to give. The full amount of milk normally required by a term baby is 150 ml/kg body weight per day. To start relactation, give the full amount of supplement each day. Divide this into six to twelve feeds depending on the infant's age and condition. Young, weak or sick infants will need more frequent, smaller, feeds. Monitor the infant's weight and urine production. When the infant is gaining weight, and there are signs of breastmilk production, the supplement can be reduced, by 50 ml per day every few days.

Signs that breastmilk is being produced

These include:

- *Breast changes*: The breasts feel fuller or firmer, or milk leaks or can be expressed.
- *Less supplement consumed*: The infant takes less supplement while continuing to gain weight.
- *Stool changes*: The infant's stools become softer, more like those of a breastfed infant.

Lactogogues

Drugs are sometimes used to stimulate increased lactation, if the above measures are not effective by themselves. Drugs used are metoclopramide (given 10 mg three times a day for 7–14 days) or domperidone (given 20–40 mg three times a day for 7–10 days). However, drugs help only if the woman also receives adequate help and her breasts are fully stimulated by the infant suckling.

Follow-up. When relactation is well under way, the mother-baby pair can be discharged for daily community-level follow-up and support

Complementary feeding

By the age of six months, a baby has usually at least doubled his or her birth weight, and is becoming more active. Exclusive breastfeeding is no longer sufficient to meet all energy and nutrient needs by itself, and complementary foods should be introduced to make up the difference. At about six months of age, an infant is also developmentally ready for other foods. The digestive system is mature enough to digest the starch, protein and fat in a non-milk diet. Very young infants push foods out with their tongue, but by between six and nine months infants can receive and hold semi-solid food in their mouths more easily.

Thus, approximately six months is the recommended appropriate age at which to introduce complementary foods. During the period of complementary feeding, children are at high risk of undernutrition. Complementary foods are often of inadequate nutritional quality, or they are given too early or too late, in too small amounts, or not frequently enough. Premature cessation or low frequency of breastfeeding also contributes to insufficient nutrient and energy intake in infants beyond six months of age. The *Guiding principles for complementary feeding of the breastfed child*, summarized in the box, set standards for developing locally appropriate feeding recommendations. They provide guidance on desired feeding behaviours as well as on the amount, consistency, frequency, energy density and nutrient content of foods. The guiding principles are explained in more detail in the paragraphs below.

Breastfeeding should continue with complementary feeding up to two years of age or beyond, and it should be on demand, as often as the child wants. Breastmilk can provide one half or more of a child's energy needs between 6–12 months of age, and one third of energy needs and other high quality nutrients between 12–24 months. Breastmilk continues to provide higher quality nutrients than complementary foods, and also

protective factors. Breastmilk is a critical source of energy and nutrients during illness. Children tend to breastfeed less often when complementary foods are introduced, so breastfeeding needs to be actively encouraged to sustain breastmilk intake.

Optimal complementary feeding depends not only on what is fed but also on how, when, where and by whom a child is fed. Behavioural studies have revealed that a more active style of feeding can improve dietary intake. The term *'responsive feeding'* is used to describe caregiving that applies the principles of psychosocial care. A child should have his or her own plate or bowl so that the caregiver knows if the child is getting enough food. A utensil such as a spoon, or just a clean hand, may be used to feed a child, depending on the culture. The utensil needs to be appropriate for the child's age. Many communities use a small

---

Guiding principles for complementary feeding of the breastfed child

1 Practise exclusive breastfeeding from birth to six months of age, and introduce complementary foods at six months of age while continuing to breastfeed. Continue frequent, on-demand breastfeeding until two years of age or beyond.
2 Practise responsive feeding, applying the principles of psychosocial care.
3 Practise good hygiene and proper food handling.
4 Start at six months of age with small amounts of food and increase the quantity as the child gets older, while maintaining frequent breastfeeding.
5 Gradually increase food consistency and variety as the infant grows older, adapting to the infant's requirements and abilities.
6 Increase the number of times that the child is fed complementary foods as the child gets older.
7 Feed a variety of nutrient-rich foods to ensure that all nutrient needs are met.
8 Use fortified complementary foods or vitamin-mineral supplements for the infant, as needed
9 Increase fluid intake during illness, including more frequent breastfeeding, and encourage the child to eat soft, favourite foods.
10 After illness, give food more often than usual and encourage the child to eat more.

Responsive feeding

- Feed infants directly and assist older children when they feed themselves. Feed slowly and patiently, and encourage children to eat, but do not force them.
- If children refuse many foods, experiment with different food combinations, tastes, textures and methods of encouragement.
- Minimize distractions during meals if the child loses interest easily.
- Remember that feeding times are periods of learning and love – talk to children during feeding, with eye-to-eye contact.

spoon when a child starts taking solids. Later a larger spoon or a fork may be used. Whether breastfeeds or complementary foods are given first at any meal has not been shown to matter. A mother can decide according to her convenience, and the child's demands.

Microbial contamination of complementary foods is a major cause of diarrhoeal disease, which is particularly common in children 6–12 months old. Safe preparation and storage of complementary foods can prevent contamination and reduce the risk of diarrhoea. The use of bottles with teats to feed liquids is more likely to result in transmission of infection than the use of cups, and should be avoided. All utensils, such as cups, bowls and spoons, used for an infant or young child's food should be washed thoroughly. Eating by hand is common in many cultures, and children may be given solid pieces of food to hold and chew on, sometimes called 'finger foods'. It is important for both the caregiver's and the child's hands to be washed thoroughly before eating. Bacteria multiply rapidly in hot weather, and more slowly if food is refrigerated. When food cannot be refrigerated it should be eaten soon after it has been prepared (no more than two

Five keys to safer food:
- Keep clean
- Separate raw and cooked
- Cook thoroughly
- Keep food at safe temperatures
- Use safe water and raw materials.

hours), before bacteria have time to multiply. Basic recommendations for the preparation of safe foods are summarized in the box.

The overall quantity of food is usually measured for convenience according to the amount of energy – that is, the number of kilocalories (kcal) – that a child needs. Other nutrients are equally important, and are either part of, or must be added to, the staple food.

Figure 9.8 shows the energy needs of infants and young children up to two years of age, and how much can be provided by breastmilk. It shows that breastmilk covers all needs up to six months, but after six months there is an energy gap that needs to be covered by complementary foods. The energy needed in addition to breastmilk is about 200 kcal per day in infants 6–8 months, 300 kcal per day in infants 9–11 months, and 550 kcal per day in children 12–23 months of age. The amount of food required to cover the gap increases as the child gets older, and as the intake of breastmilk decreases.

Table 9.4 summarizes the amount of food required at different ages, the average number of kilocalories that a breastfed infant or young child needs from complementary foods at different ages, and the approximate quantity of food that will provide this amount of energy per day. The quantity increases gradually month by month, as the child grows and develops, and the table shows the average for each age range.

The actual amount (weight or volume) of food required depends on the *energy density* of the food offered. This means the number of kilocalories per ml, or per gram. Breastmilk contains about 0.7 kcal per ml. Complementary foods are more variable, and usually contain between 0.6 and 1.0 kcal per gram. Foods that are watery and dilute may contain only about 0.3 kcal per gram. For complementary foods to have 1.0 kcal per gram, it is necessary for them to be quite thick and to contain fat or oil, which are the most energy-rich foods. Complementary foods should have a greater energy density than breastmilk, that is, at least 0.8 kcal per gram. The quantities of food recommended in Table 9.4 assume that the complementary food will contain 0.8–1.0 kcal per gram. If a complementary food is more energy dense, then a smaller amount is needed to cover the energy gap. A complementary food that is more energy-dilute needs a larger volume to cover the energy gap.

Table 9.4 Practical guide on weaning food

Practical guidance on the quality, frequency and amount of food to offer children 6–23 months of age who are breastfed on demand

Age	Energy needed per day in addition to breast milk	Texture	Frequency	Amount of food an average child will usually eat at each meal
6–8 months	200 kcal per day	Start with thick porridge, well mashed foods Continue with mashed family foods	2–3 meals per day Depending on the child's appetite, 1–2 snacks may be offered	Start with 2–3 table-spoonfuls per feed. increasing gradually to $\frac{1}{2}$ of a 250 ml cup
9–11 months	300 kcal per day	Finely chopped or mashed foods, and foods that baby can pick up	3–4 meals per day Depending on the child's appetite, 1–2 snacks may be offered	$\frac{1}{2}$ of a 250 ml cup/bowl
12–23 months	550 kcal per day	Family foods, chopped or mashed if necessary	3–4 meals per day Depending on the child's appetite, 1–2 snacks may be offered	$\frac{3}{4}$ to full 250 ml cup/bowl

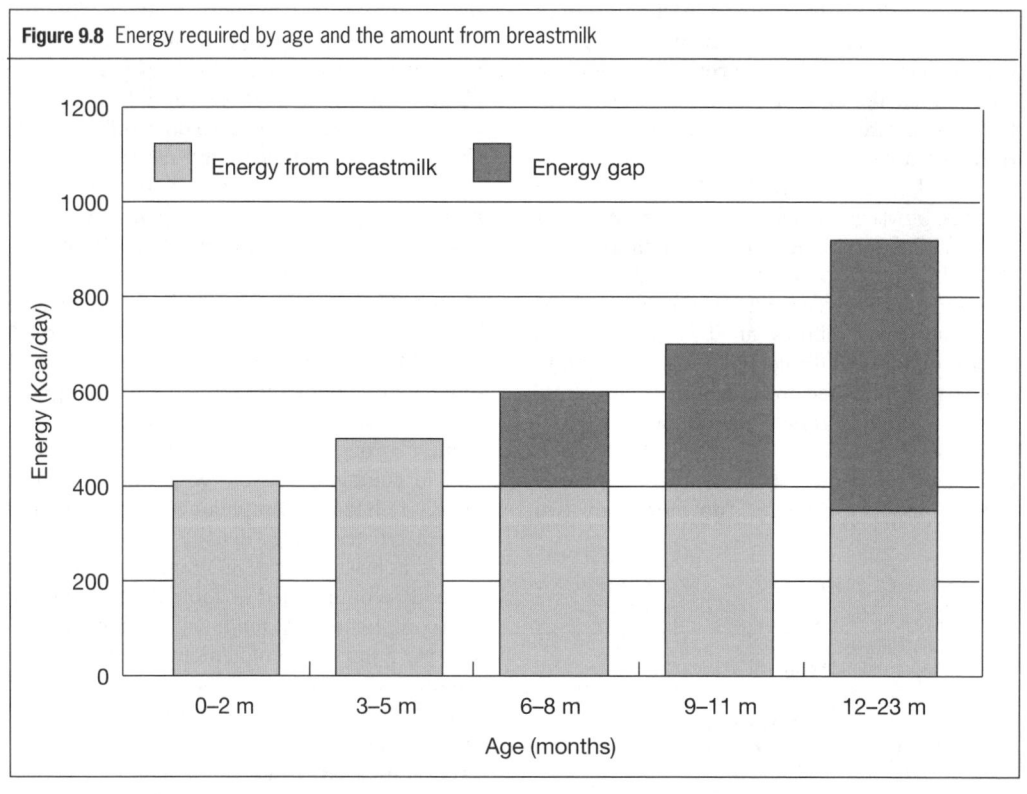

Figure 9.8 Energy required by age and the amount from breastmilk

When complementary food is introduced, a child tends to breastfeed less often, and his or her intake of breastmilk decreases, so the food effectively displaces breastmilk. If complementary food is more energy-dilute than breastmilk, the child's total energy intake may be less than it was with exclusive breastfeeding, an important cause of malnutrition. A young child's appetite usually serves as a guide to the amount of food that should be offered. However, illness and malnutrition reduce appetite, so that a sick child may take less than he or she needs. A child recovering from illness or malnutrition may require extra assistance with feeding to ensure adequate intake. If the child's appetite increases with recovery, then extra food should be offered.

The most suitable consistency for an infant's or young child's food depends on age and neuromuscular development. Beginning at six months, an infant can eat pureed, mashed or semi-solid foods. By eight months most infants can also eat finger foods. By 12 months, most children can eat the same types of foods as are consumed by the rest of the family. However, they need nutrient-rich food, and foods that can cause choking, such as whole peanuts, should be avoided. A complementary food should be thick enough so that it stays on a spoon and does not drip off. Generally, foods that are thicker or more solid are more energy- and nutrient-dense than thin, watery or soft foods. When a child eats thick, solid foods, it is easier to give more kcal and to include a variety of nutrient-rich ingredients including animal-source foods. There is evidence of a critical window for introducing 'lumpy' foods: if these are delayed beyond 10 months of age, it may increase the risk of feeding difficulties later on. Although it may save time to continue feeding semi-solid foods, for optimal child development it is important to gradually increase the solidity of food with age.

As a child gets older and needs a larger total quantity of food each day, the food needs to be divided into a larger number of meals. The number of meals that an infant or young child needs in a day depends on:

- *How much energy the child needs to cover the energy gap.* The more food a child needs each day, the more meals are needed to ensure that he or she gets enough.
- *The amount that a child can eat at one meal.* This depends on the capacity or size of the

child's stomach, which is usually 30 ml per kg of the child's body weight. A child who weighs 8 kg will have a stomach capacity of 240 ml, about one large cupful, and cannot be expected to eat more than that at one meal.

- *The energy density of the food offered.* The energy density of complementary foods should be more than breastmilk, that is, at least 0.8 kcal per gram.

If the energy density of food is lower, a larger volume of food is needed to fill the gap, which may need to be divided into more meals. As shown in Table 9.4, a breastfed infant 6-8 months old needs 2-3 meals a day, and a breastfed infant 9-23 months needs 3-4 meals a day. Depending on the child's appetite, 1-2 nutritious snacks may be offered. Snacks are defined as foods eaten between meals, often self-fed finger foods, which are convenient and easy to prepare. If they are fried, they may have a high energy density. The transition from two to three meals, and from smaller to larger meals, happens gradually between those ages, depending on the child's appetite and how he or she is developing. If a child eats too few meals, then he or she will not receive enough food to cover energy needs. If a child eats too many meals, he or she may breastfeed less, or may even stop breastfeeding altogether. In the first year of life, displacement of breastmilk may reduce the quality and amount of the child's total nutrient intake.

Complementary foods should provide sufficient energy, protein and micronutrients to cover a child's energy and nutrient gaps, so that together with breastmilk, they meet all his or her needs.

Figure 9.9 shows the energy, protein, iron and vitamin A gaps that need to be filled by complementary foods for a breastfed child 12-23

Good complementary foods are:
- Rich in energy, protein and micronutrients (particularly iron, zinc, calcium, vitamin A, vitamin C and folate)
- Not spicy or salty
- Easy for the child to eat
- Liked by the child
- Locally available and affordable.

months of age. The filled part of each bar shows the percentage of the child's daily needs that can be provided by an average intake of 550 ml of breastmilk. The empty part of the bar shows the gap that needs to be filled by complementary foods. The largest gap is for iron, so it is especially important that complementary foods contain iron, if possible from animal-source foods such as meat, organs, poultry or fish. Pulses (peas, beans, lentils, nuts) fed with vitamin C-rich foods to aid absorption provide an alternative, but they cannot replace animal-source foods completely.

The basic ingredient of complementary foods is usually the local staple. Staples are cereals, roots and starchy fruits that consist mainly of carbohydrate and provide energy. Cereals also contain some protein; but roots such as cassava and sweet potato, and starchy fruits such as banana and breadfruit, contain very little protein. A variety of other foods should be added to the staple every day to provide other nutrients. These include:

- *Foods from animals or fish* are good sources of protein, iron and zinc. Liver also provides vitamin A and folate. Egg yolk is a good source of protein and vitamin A, but not of iron. A child needs the solid part of these foods, not just the watery sauce.
- *Dairy products*, such as milk, cheese and yoghurt, are useful sources of calcium, protein, energy and B vitamins.
- *Pulses – peas, beans, lentils, peanuts, and soybeans* are good sources of protein, and some iron. Eating sources of vitamin C (for example, tomatoes, citrus and other fruits, and green leafy vegetables) at the same time helps iron absorption.
- *Orange-coloured fruits and vegetables* such as carrot, pumpkin, mango and papaya, and dark-green leaves such as spinach, are rich in carotene, from which vitamin A is made, and also vitamin C.
- *Fats and oils* are concentrated sources of energy, and of certain essential fats that children need to grow.

Vegetarian (plant-based) complementary foods do not by themselves provide enough iron and zinc to meet all the needs of an infant or young child aged 6–23 months. Animal-source foods that contain enough iron and zinc are needed in addition. Alternatively, fortified foods or

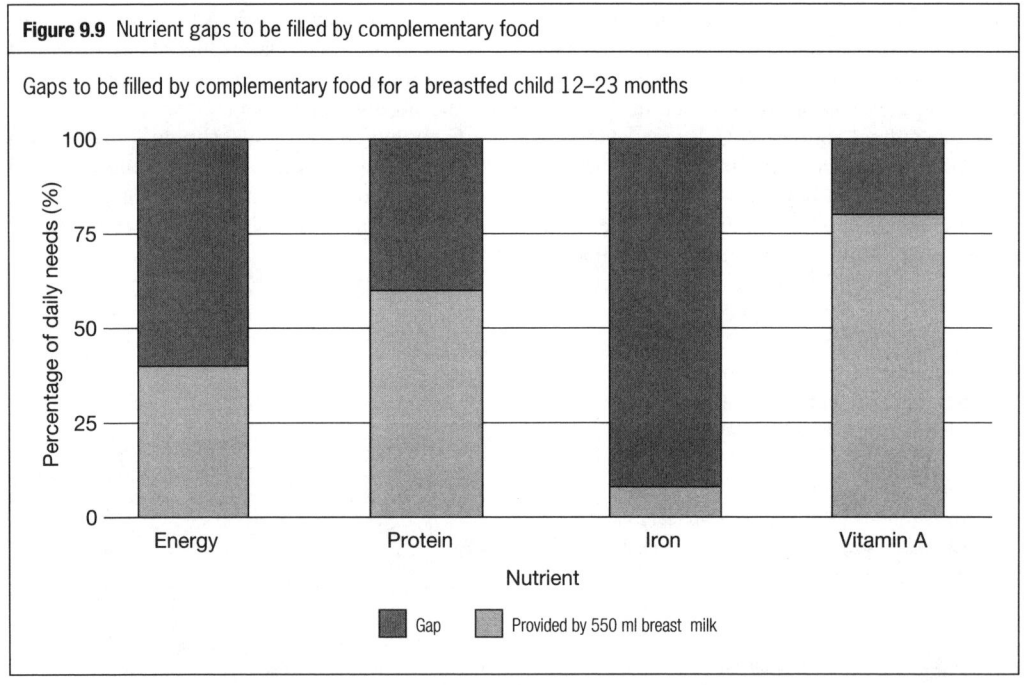

Figure 9.9 Nutrient gaps to be filled by complementary food

Gaps to be filled by complementary food for a breastfed child 12–23 months

Percentage of daily needs (%)

Nutrient: Energy, Protein, Iron, Vitamin A

■ Gap   ■ Provided by 550 ml breast milk

micronutrient supplements can fill some of the critical nutrient gaps.

Fats, including oils, are important because they increase the energy density of foods, and make them taste better. Fat also helps the absorption of vitamin A and other fat-soluble vitamins. Some fats, especially soy and rapeseed oil, also provide essential fatty acids. Fat should comprise 30–45 per cent of the total energy provided by breast-milk and complementary foods together. Fat should not provide more than this proportion, or the child will not eat enough of the foods that contain protein and other important nutrients, such as iron and zinc.

Sugar is a concentrated source of energy, but it has no other nutrients. It can damage children's teeth, and lead to overweight and obesity. Sugar and sugary drinks, such as sodas, should be avoided because they decrease the child's appetite for more nutritious foods. Tea and coffee contain compounds that can interfere with iron absorption and are not recommended for young children.

Concerns about potential allergic effects are a common reason for families to restrict certain foods in the diets of infants and young children. However, there are no controlled studies that show that restrictive diets have an allergy-preventing effect. Therefore, young children can consume a variety of foods from the age of six months, including cow milk, eggs, peanuts, fish and shellfish.

Unfortified complementary foods that are predominantly plant-based generally provide insufficient amounts of certain key nutrients (particularly iron, zinc and vitamin B6) to meet recommended nutrient intakes during comple-mentary feeding. Inclusion of animal-source foods can meet the gap in some cases, but this increases cost and may not be practical for the lowest-income groups. Furthermore, the amounts of animal-source foods that can feasibly be consumed by infants (e.g. at 6–12 months) are generally insufficient to meet the gap in iron. The

difficulty in meeting the needs for these nutrients is not unique to developing countries. Average iron intakes in infants in industrialized countries would fall well short of recommended intake if iron-fortified products were not widely available. Therefore, in settings where little or no animal-source foods are available to many families, iron-fortified complementary foods or foods fortified at the point of consumption with a multinutrient powder or lipid-based nutrient supplement may be necessary.

During an illness, the need for fluid often in-creases, so a child should be offered and encour-aged to take more, and breastfeeding on demand should continue. A child's appetite for food often decreases, while the desire to breastfeed increases, and breastmilk may become the main source of both fluid and nutrients. A child should also be encouraged to eat some complementary food to maintain nutrient intake and enhance recovery. Intake is usually better if the child is offered his or her favourite foods, and if the foods are soft and appetizing. The amount eaten at any one time is likely to be less than usual, so the caregiver may need to give more frequent, smaller meals. When the infant or young child is recovering, and his or her appetite improves, the caregiver should offer an extra portion at each meal or add an extra meal or snack each day.

Recommendations for micronutrient supplementation

Micronutrients are essential for growth, dev-elopment and prevention of illness in young children. As discussed earlier, micronutrient supplementation can be an effective interven-tion in some situations. Recommendations are summarized below.

Vitamin A

WHO and UNICEF recommend universal sup-plementation with vitamin A as a priority in chil-dren aged 6–59 months in countries with a high

Table 9.5 Prevention of vitamin A deficiency

High-dose universal distribution schedule for prevention of vitamin A deficiency	
Infants 6–12 months of age	100 000 IU orally, every 4–6 months
Children >12 months of age	200 000 IU orally, every 4–6 months

risk of deficiency. In these countries, a high dose of vitamin A should also be given to children with measles, diarrhoea, respiratory disease, chicken-pox, other severe infections or severe protein-energy malnutrition, or who live in the vicinity of children with vitamin A deficiency.

Iron

As a rule, fortified foods should be preferred to iron supplements for children during the complementary feeding period. Caution should be exercised with iron supplementation in settings where the prevalence of malaria and other infectious diseases is high. In malaria-endemic areas, universal iron supplementation is not recommended. If iron supplements are used, they should not be given to children who have sufficient iron stores as the risks of severe adverse events appear to be greater in those children. Prevention and management of anaemia in such areas requires a screening system to identify iron-deficient children, and the availability of and accessibility to appropriate anti-malarial and other anti-infective treatments.

Iodine

Universal salt iodization (USI) has been introduced in South Africa as a safe, cost-effective and sustainable strategy to ensure sufficient intake of iodine by all individuals. However, in areas with severe iodine deficiency, vulnerable groups – pregnant and lactating women and children less than two years – may not be adequately covered when USI is not fully implemented, and iodine supplementation may be necessary.

Zinc

Zinc supplementation is recommended as adjunct therapy in the management of diarrhoea. Zinc (20 mg/day) should be given to all children with diarrhoea for 10–14 days. In infants below six months of age the dose should be 10 mg/day.

Local adaptation of complementary feeding recommendations

Develop a list of locally available foods and find out the nutrient content of the local foods from food tables. Calculate the amount of various foods that would provide a child with his or her daily needs of the various nutrients. Assess which foods and quantities of foods caregivers

---

Remember

Foods rich in iron:
- Liver (any type), organ meat, flesh of animals (especially red meat), flesh of birds (especially dark meat), foods fortified with iron

Foods rich in Vitamin A
- Liver (any type), red palm oil, egg yolk, orange coloured fruits and vegetables, dark green vegetables

Foods rich in zinc
- Liver (any type), organ meat, food prepared with blood, flesh of animals, birds and fish, shell fish, egg yolk

Foods rich in calcium
- Milk or milk products, small fish with bones
- Foods rich in Vitamin C
- Fresh fruits, tomatoes, peppers (green, red, yellow), green leaves and vegetables

---

and families accept as suitable for children, and identify their feeding practices and preferences.

Whether or not vitamin-mineral supplements should be included in the recommendations depends on the micronutrient content of locally-available foods, and whether children can eat enough suitable foods.

Monitoring the adequacy of feeding

(*See* Figure 9.10)

The most important parameter to consider is the child's rate of growth. If there are concerns, a useful guide and approach is presented in Figure 9.10.

Appropriate feeding in exceptionally difficult circumstances

These circumstances include babies who are low birth weight (see above), and infants and young children who are malnourished (*see* Chapter 13, Nutritional disorders), who are living in emergency situations, or who are born to mothers living with HIV.

Infants and young children living in emergency situations

In emergencies infants and young children are more likely than older children or adults to become ill and die from malnutrition and disease. Optimal feeding is often disrupted because of lack of basic resources such as shelter and water, and physical and mental stress on families. Breastfeeding may stop because mothers are ill, traumatised, or separated from their babies, and yet it is particularly valuable in emergency situations. Artificial feeding is more dangerous because of poor hygiene, lack of clean water and fuel, and unreliability of supplies. There may be no food suitable for complementary feeding, nor facilities for preparing feeds and storing food safely. Breastmilk substitutes including infant formula and feeding bottles may be sent to emergency situations in inappropriate amounts

by donors who believe that they are urgently required, but who are poorly informed about the real needs. Without proper controls, stocks run out before more arrive for those who might have a genuine need. The result is inappropriate and unsafe use of breastmilk substitutes, and a dangerous and unnecessary increase in early cessation of breastfeeding. Babies may be given unsuitable foods, such as dried skimmed milk, because nothing else is available.

Management in emergencies

For the majority, the emphasis should be on protecting, promoting and supporting breastfeeding, and ensuring timely, safe and appropriate complementary feeding. Most malnourished mothers can continue to breastfeed while they are being fed and treated themselves. A minority of infants will need to be fed on breastmilk substitutes, short term or long term. This may be

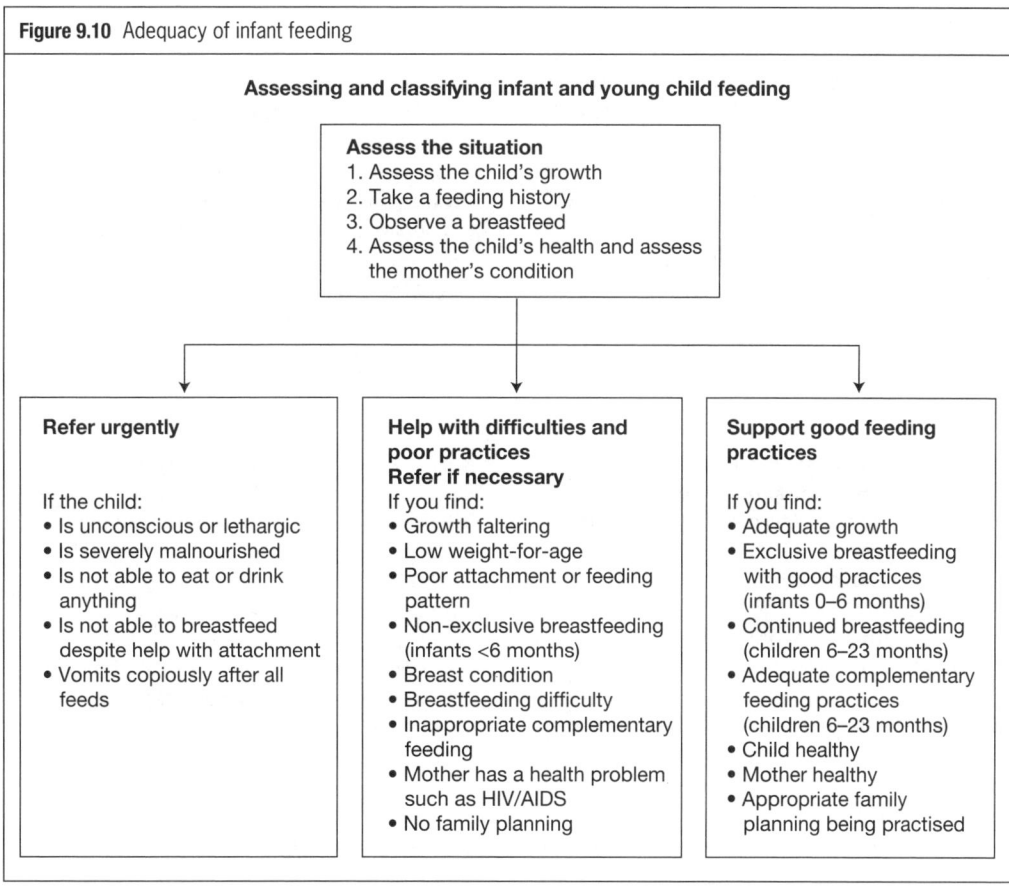

Figure 9.10 Adequacy of infant feeding

Assessing and classifying infant and young child feeding

Assess the situation
1. Assess the child's growth
2. Take a feeding history
3. Observe a breastfeed
4. Assess the child's health and assess the mother's condition

Refer urgently	**Help with difficulties and poor practices** **Refer if necessary**	**Support good feeding practices**
If the child: • Is unconscious or lethargic • Is severely malnourished • Is not able to eat or drink anything • Is not able to breastfeed despite help with attachment • Vomits copiously after all feeds	If you find: • Growth faltering • Low weight-for-age • Poor attachment or feeding pattern • Non-exclusive breastfeeding (infants <6 months) • Breast condition • Breastfeeding difficulty • Inappropriate complementary feeding • Mother has a health problem such as HIV/AIDS • No family planning	If you find: • Adequate growth • Exclusive breastfeeding with good practices (infants 0–6 months) • Continued breastfeeding (children 6–23 months) • Adequate complementary feeding practices (children 6–23 months) • Child healthy • Mother healthy • Appropriate family planning being practised

necessary if their mothers are dead or absent, or too ill or traumatised to breastfeed, and no wet-nurses are available; or for infants who have been artificially fed prior to the emergency or whose HIV-positive mothers choose not to breastfeed.

Infants of HIV-positive mothers

Feeding infants of HIV-positive mothers is a major concern of governments and agencies concerned with infant feeding. The aim of preventing mother-to-child transmission of HIV (MTCT) through breastfeeding needs to be balanced with the need to support optimal nutrition of all infants through exclusive and continued breast-feeding and adequate complementary feeding.

Mother-to-child transmission of HIV

(*See* Chapter18, HIV infection)

Without intervention, an estimated 5–20 per cent of infants born to HIV-infected women acquire the infection through breastfeeding. Transmission can occur at any time while a child is breastfeeding, and continuing to breastfeed until the child is older increases the overall risk. Exclusive breastfeeding in the first few months of life carries a lower risk of HIV transmission than mixed feeding. The main factors which increase the risk of HIV transmission through breastfeeding include:

- Acquiring HIV infection during breastfeeding, because of high initial viral load
- The severity of the disease (as indicated by a low CD4+ count or high RNA viral load in the mother's blood, or severe clinical symptoms)
- Poor breast health (e.g. mastitis, sub-clinical mastitis, fissured nipples)
- Possibly, oral infection in the infant (thrush and herpes)
- Non-exclusive breastfeeding (mixed feeding)
- Longer duration of breastfeeding
- Possibly, nutritional status of the mother.

Women and their partners should be encouraged to accept HIV testing and counselling during pregnancy, so that they know their status, and so that they can take advantage of help that is available and make appropriate decisions before the baby is born. All women should be made aware of the risk of MTCT in general, and that there is an increased risk of transmission if they become infected during breastfeeding.

Current feeding recommendations

The United Nations recommendations for feeding of infants by mothers who are HIV-infected include:

- The most appropriate infant feeding option for an HIV-infected mother depends on her individual circumstances, including her health status and the local situation, but should take consideration of the health services available and the counselling and support she is likely to receive.
- Exclusive breastfeeding is recommended for HIV-infected mothers for the first six months of life unless replacement feeding is acceptable, feasible, affordable, sustainable and safe for them and their infants before that time (see box for definitions).
- When replacement feeding is acceptable, feasible, affordable, sustainable and safe,

---

Definitions of Acceptable, Feasible, Affordable, Sustainable and Safe (AFASS)

Acceptable: The mother perceives no significant barrier to choosing a feeding option for cultural or social reasons or for fear of stigma and discrimination.

Feasible: The mother (or other family member) has adequate time, knowledge, skills and other resources to prepare feeds and to feed the infant, as well as the support to cope with family, community and social pressures.

Affordable: The mother and family, with available community and/or health system support, can pay for the costs of replacement feeds – including all ingredients, fuel and clean water – without compromising the family's health and nutrition budget.

Sustainable: The mother has access to a continuous and uninterrupted supply of all ingredients and commodities needed to implement the feeding option safely for as long as the infant needs it.

Safe: Replacement foods are correctly and hygienically prepared and stored, and fed in nutritionally adequate quantities, with clean hands and using clean utensils, preferably by cup.

avoidance of all breastfeeding by HIV-infected mothers is recommended.

- All HIV-exposed infants should receive regular follow-up care and periodic re-assessment of infant feeding choices, particularly at the time of infant diagnosis and at six months.
- At six months, if adequate feeding from other sources cannot be ensured, HIV-infected women should continue to breastfeed their infants and give complementary foods in addition, and return for regular follow-up assessments. All breastfeeding should stop once an adequate diet without breastmilk can be provided.
- Breastfed infants and young children who are HIV-infected should continue to breastfeed according to recommendations for the general population.

Every effort should be made to ensure that HIV-infected women who fulfil the eligibility criteria for lifelong antiretroviral therapy for their own health should receive antiretroviral drugs, as they are the women most likely to transmit HIV through breastfeeding. Comparative studies in women who do not yet require treatment on the safety and efficacy of antiretroviral drugs taken during breastfeeding solely to reduce transmission are ongoing. There is increasing evidence from observational studies that in women who are taking lifelong antiretroviral drugs for their own health, the risk of transmission through breastfeeding is low. Additional evidence suggests that giving infants antiretroviral prophylaxis such as daily nevirapine while breastfeeding, also significantly reduces transmission from breastmilk. These interventions, in addition to exclusive breastfeeding, offer HIV-infected women the prospect of being able to breastfeed their infants and avoid the risks of HIV transmission while still gaining all the benefits of breastmilk.

Counselling about feeding options

Counselling about feeding options for HIV-positive women needs to start during pregnancy. HIV-positive women and their partners should be informed about:

- The risks of mother-to-child transmission of the virus
- Feeding options that are appropriate and feasible in the local context, considering national policies
- The advantages and disadvantages of each feeding option
- The risk of breastfeeding transmission is significantly reduced if the mother is on antiretroviral treatment or if the infant receives daily antiretroviral prophylaxis such as daily nevirapine.

They should also be made aware that:

- Replacement feeding carries an increased risk for the child of morbidity and mortality associated with malnutrition and infectious diseases other than HIV, when compared with breastfeeding.
- Mixed feeding carries both the risk of transmission of HIV and the risk of other infections and is the worst option.
- It is important for the mother to take care of her own health and nutrition, but that breastfeeding will not affect her health adversely.
- It is particularly important to practise safer sex when the baby is breastfeeding, because of the greater risk of transmission of HIV to the infant should the mother be infected at this time.

HIV-positive women should be given guidance to help them decide what is the best infant feeding method for their own situation, and they should be taught how to carry out their chosen method safely.

Usually, only the two main feeding options (replacement feeding and exclusive breastfeeding) need to be discussed during counselling, but others may be explained if the woman appears interested.

Support for the chosen feeding method

If an HIV-positive mother chooses to give replacement feeding, she will need to be taught how to measure ingredients and how to prepare breastmilk substitutes hygienically. Programmes should try to improve conditions that make replacement feeding safer for HIV-infected mothers and families. If an HIV-positive mother chooses to breastfeed her baby herself, she should be given support to help her to breastfeed exclusively, with a good technique to ensure a plentiful supply of milk and to prevent mastitis and sore nipples; and guidance about treating these conditions early should they occur.

If an HIV-positive mother chooses to stop breastfeeding early, she will need help to change to replacement feeding and to stop breastfeeding completely over a time period of a few days to 2–3 weeks. She will need support to:

- Express her breastmilk and accustom the baby to cup feeding of heat-treated EBM
- Gradually reduce breastfeeds, and replace them with heat-treated EBM
- Change from EBM to replacement feeds given by cup; if the baby is receiving replacement feeds and EBM at the same time, then the EBM should be heat treated
- Comfort the baby by cuddling, rubbing and rocking, and by giving him or her a finger or forearm to suck on
- Keep her breasts healthy, by expressing enough milk to prevent engorgement until milk production stops.

The milk should be discarded, or if used to feed the infant, it should be heat treated. HIV-positive women who choose to express and heat treat their milk, need guidance on expression, heat treatment, cup feeding and quantities of EBM to give. If a family decides on a wet-nurse, she will need all the support that a breastfeeding mother needs, and counselling about avoiding any risk of HIV infection while she is feeding the baby. All mothers and caregivers should receive follow-up care for at least two years to ensure that the child is adequately fed and growing and that other foods are introduced when the child is six months old

The document *HIV and Infant Feeding: Framework for Priority Action* has been endorsed by United Nations agencies. In the context of the Global Strategy, five priority areas for national governments are proposed to

1 Develop or revise (as appropriate) a comprehensive national infant and young child feeding policy, which includes HIV and infant feeding.
2 Implement and enforce the International Code of Marketing of Breastmilk Substitutes and subsequent relevant World Health Assembly resolutions.
3 Intensify efforts to protect, promote and support appropriate infant and young child feeding practices in general, while recognizing HIV as one of a number of exceptionally difficult circumstances.
4 Provide adequate support to HIV-positive women to enable them to select the best feeding option for themselves and their babies and to successfully carry out their infant feeding decisions.
5 Support research on HIV and infant feeding, including operations research, learning, monitoring and evaluation at all levels, and disseminate findings.

Replacement feeding

Replacement feeding is the process of feeding a child who is not breastfeeding with a diet that provides all the nutrients the child needs, until the child is fully fed on family food. Replacement feeding includes replacement of breastmilk with a suitable breastmilk substitute in the first six months of life, and ensuring adequate complementary food and replacement of breastmilk from six months to two years. This is the period during which a child is at greatest risk from malnutrition. To replace breastmilk, a child needs a breastmilk substitute of suitable composition, and of which the supply is reliable and uninterrupted. Heat-treated expressed breastmilk can also be used (though not strictly a replacement feed, it needs hygienic preparation and measuring so is included here). To prepare feeds, a mother or caretaker needs water, soap, fuel and utensils, time to make the feeds, and knowledge of how to prepare them accurately and hygienically. She needs detailed guidance on how to measure milk, water and other ingredients and how to clean utensils.

Commercial infant formula must be prepared carefully according to the instructions on the label, and given in quantities appropriate for the child's weight and age. Information about the volume of feeds is also included on the label.

Heat-treated breastmilk. The mother expresses enough milk for one or two feeds, heats it to boiling in a small pan or in a small metal container standing in a pan of water, leaves the milk to cool in a clean, covered container, and feeds it by cup.

Volume of milk required: Give 150 ml of prepared milk per kg of the child's body weight per day, divided into eight feeds in 24 hours:

- For the first few days of life, start with 60 ml/kg per day on the first day, and increase the total by 20 ml/kg per day, dividing into eight feeds in 24 hours.
- After complementary foods are introduced, milk feeds continue at approximately the same amount as is given to the child at six months of age, but may vary according to availability of milk and other foods and the child's demands.

Home-modified cows milk is no longer recommended as a safe replacement feed for infants less than six months of age. (Note that it can be used for a short period in emergency circumstances).

PART 4

Metabolic and nutritional disorders

10

Metabolic disorders

The body's homeostatic mechanisms concerned with acid-base balance, blood glucose control, electrolytes, and clearance of metabolic waste products may be disturbed by numerous acquired disease processes and are frequently deranged in congenital and inherited disorders of metabolism. The metabolic disturbance itself may aggravate the clinical condition and may require correction additional to the management of an underlying disorder.

The following clinical circumstances call for biochemical tests assessing metabolic function:

- Acute neurological symptoms, including a disturbed level of consciousness and convulsions
- Any severe illness
- Severe dehydration
- Malnutrition with additional symptoms and signs of illness
- Disturbances of neuromuscular function and tone
- Failure to thrive
- Persistent or recurrent symptoms, such as vomiting and/or diarrhoea, breathing disturbances, and urine abnormalities.

There is clinical overlap between the symptoms of acquired and congenital metabolic disturbances. Frequently, it is only the recurrent or persistent nature of the symptoms, together with a suspicious history, which will lead the health professional to the clinical suspicion of an inherited metabolic disorder.

Acute acquired metabolic disturbances

Disorders of acid-base regulation

The pH of the body fluids is normally maintained within a fairly narrow range. Acidosis indicates a disturbance which can lead to a body pH below normal (7.4 ± 0.02). Conversely, alkalosis indicates a condition in which the pH may become higher than normal. A large number of hydrogen ions are produced daily from metabolic sources; these are mopped up by the body's buffer systems. While haemoglobin and the plasma proteins have the biggest buffering capacity, the bicarbonate/carbonic acid system is the most important buffer because of the body's ability to excrete carbon dioxide through the lungs and thus rapidly adjust the hydrogen ion concentration:

$$H^+ + HCO_3^- \longleftrightarrow H_2CO_3 \longleftrightarrow CO_2 + H_2O$$

If the primary disturbance lies in an altered pCO_2 through either alveolar hypo- or hyperventilation, it is classified as respiratory acidosis or alkalosis. If the defect primarily effects the $[H^+]$ or $[HCO_3^-]$, it is classified as a metabolic disturbance. Compensatory respiratory or metabolic mechanisms come into play in all disturbances to oppose the effect of the primary problem in order to maintain a constant pH level.

Assessment

The clinical circumstances indicate the possibility of a disturbance in acid-base regulation (*see* Table 10.1).

Clinical examination is performed for evidence of dehydration or shock, respiratory disease and cyanosis, ketosis, rickets, or other abnormalities.

In metabolic acidosis, respiratory compensation results in deep, rapid respiration with pursed lips, but with no signs of pulmonary disease. In severe acidosis, peripheral vasoconstriction and poor capillary filling is often present even without other signs of shock. In neonates, sig-

nificant acidosis may be unaccompanied by the usual physical signs. In severe metabolic alkalosis, the breathing pattern becomes shallow and infrequent.

The acid-base status is measured by means of a blood gas analysis. The pH is the most important measurement, indicating the severity and need for treatment. The pCO_2 and HCO_3^- levels indicate the respiratory and metabolic components respectively.

Often ancillary investigations help to elucidate the problem. The '**anion gap**' refers to the difference between the sum of cation concentrations

Table 10.1 Acid-base disturbances		
Disorder	**Mechanism**	**Common associated conditions**
Metabolic acidosis	Anaerobic glycolysis	Tissue anoxia
	Lactic acidosis	Shock
	Keto-acidosis	Starvation
		Diabetes mellitus
		Glycogen storage disease
	Organic acidaemia	Branch chain amino-aciduria, e.g. maple syrup urine disease
	Administration of acidifying agents	NH_4Cl administration
	Reduced renal excretion of H^+	Renal tubular acidosis
		Renal failure
		Renal immaturity
	Gastrointestinal: loss of HCO_3^-	Acute diarrhoea
	Renal loss of HCO_3^-	Chronic renal failure
		Renal tubular acidosis
		Acetazolamide treatment
Respiratory acidosis	Retention of CO_2 by the lung	Pulmonary disease
		Muscle paralysis or spasm
Metabolic alkalosis	Loss of H^+ from gut	Excess vomiting, e.g. pyloric stenosis, gastric drainage
	Loss of H^+ through kidneys	Diuretic: furosemide
	Excess renal HCO_3^- retention	Hypochloraemia
	Administration of alkali	Hyperaldosteronism
		Hypokalaemia
		Bicarbonate administration
		Citrate administration
		Lactate administration
Respiratory alkalosis	Hyperventilation with exhalation of CO_2	Voluntary hyperventilation – emotional
		Central respiratory stimulation
		– drugs, e.g. salicylates
		– brain-stem involvement

Na^+, K^+, Mg^{++}, Ca^{++} and the sum of the anion concentration Cl^-, HCO_3^-, SO_4^-, PO_4^-. This difference normally reflects the anionic contribution of plasma proteins and other organic acids. An anion gap larger than 16 mmol/l indicates abnormal acid accumulation, such as:

- Lactic acid, found in shock, hypoxia, circumstances of anaerobic metabolism and disturbances of glucose production
- Ketoacids, found in starvation and diabetic ketoacidosis
- Endogenous organic acid, found in inherited organic acid disorders and uraemia
- Exogenous acids, such as salicylates in salicylate intoxication.

The serum electrolytes may show hypokalaemia or hypochloraemia, while a high Cl^- out of keeping with the serum sodium is often a clue to a long-standing low plasma bicarbonate level.

Management

Appropriate treatment must be directed at the underlying disorder, e.g. fluid and/or glucose deficit, shock, vomiting, hypoxia, or respiratory failure. That is all that is required in the majority of instances. The pH must be corrected if outside the range 7.2 to 7.5, as this is important for cellular function.

Clinical signs of metabolic acidosis suggest a base deficit of 10 or more and if it is not possible to measure the pH, $NaHCO_3$ may be given as a slow bolus intravenously (8.4% bicarbonate, 2 ml/kg). One should generally only half correct the acidosis, as treatment of the predisposing

---

In **metabolic acidosis**, $NaHCO_3$ is given IV according to the formula:
Base deficit × 0.3 body mass (kg) = mmol HCO_3^- required
(8.4% bicarbonate = 1 mmol/ml;
4.2% bicarbonate = 0.5 mmol/ml)

In **severe metabolic alkalosis**, NH_4Cl (5% solution = 1 mmol/ml) can be given according to the formula: Base excess × 0.3 body mass (kg) = mmol NH_4Cl required

---

condition allows the normal compensatory mechanisms to come into play.

Complications of acid-base disturbance treatment. Rapid administration of bicarbonate for correction of pH may result in fluid overload and a drop in serum-ionized calcium level, causing tetany, as well as hypokalaemia and hypernatraemia, especially if more than 8 mmol/kg is given per day (1 mmol bicarbonate = 1 mmol Na^+).

It is well-documented in neonates that the administration of bicarbonate is associated with intraventricular haemorrhage.

Hypoglycaemia

The blood glucose level reflects the balance between glucose production and utilization. In the fasting state, glucose is produced by the processes of glycogenolysis and gluconeogenesis. Intake of glucose from dietary sources or intravenous administration contributes to the blood glucose level. Glucose utilization occurs obligatorily by red blood cells, brain, and kidney as their major source of energy, and by other tissues primarily under the influence of insulin.

In neonates, even asymptomatic hypoglycaemia may impair normal brain development. A whole blood glucose level less than 2.2 mmol/l constitutes hypoglycaemia (*see* Chapter 7, Care of the newborn). Symptomatic hypoglycaemia is an important risk factor for brain damage, particularly in low-birth-weight babies.

Symptoms and signs due to hypoglycaemia result from deranged cerebral metabolism:

- In neonates the symptoms are non-specific and include lethargy, hypotonia, poor feeding, apnoea attacks, jitteriness, or convulsions.
- An acute fall of blood sugar in older children may trigger sympathetic effects including a feeling of hunger and weakness; pallor, tachycardia, and sweating. Headaches, visual disturbances, drowsiness and coma, or convulsions may follow.
- A slow, gradual drop of blood sugar may occur, especially in malnourished patients and only present with no or limited warning signs before the patient becomes comatose or convulses due to neuroglycopaenia.

Thus, *seriously ill infants, especially while on restricted intake, need to have blood glucose levels monitored regularly*, e.g. with glucose test strips. This is especially true for malnourished patients who have decreased glycogen stores. In kwashiorkor, the development of hypoglycaemia is regarded as a serious clinical sign, signalling severe substrate deficiency and inability to maintain serum glucose through gluconeogenesis. (*See* Chapter 13, Nutritional disorders.)

Symptomatic hypoglycaemia calls for urgent treatment. Where an IV line is not available, oral glucose 10 to 25% solution should be given by nasogastric tube in a dose of 1 g/kg body mass. Otherwise 1 g/kg or 2 ml/kg of a 50% solution should be diluted to 10–20 per cent and given IV. The symptoms should be rapidly relieved unless hypoglycaemia has been of long duration, or there are other complications, e.g. liver failure. After this initial management, it is important to confirm that the blood sugar has risen and is maintained within normal levels.

Once hypoglycaemia has been identified and treated, the cause must be determined, as only then can appropriate preventive therapy be instituted. The approach to investigation of a patient with hypoglycaemia depends on the history and examination.

In recurrent, unexplained episodes of hypoglycaemia, blood samples should be obtained for glucose, urea and electrolytes, blood gas analyses, liver function tests, including ammonia, insulin, lactate, ketones, and cortisol, prior to giving intravenous glucose. Always remember to test the urine for the presence of ketones and to store a urine specimen in the freezer compartment of the fridge. It might be useful for further investigations later if required.

Blood sugar disturbances are summarized in Table 10.2.

Electrolyte disturbances

Electrolyte disturbances are summarized in Table 10.3.

Sodium is the principal extracellular cation. Major changes in serum sodium cause alterations in the osmolality of the extracellular fluid in relation to the intracellular compartment; hence water moves along the concentration gradient. The serum sodium level is thus inversely proportional to the intracellular fluid volume.

Hyponatraemia

In hyponatraemia, water moves into the intracellular compartment with reduction of the extracellular volume and early development of circulatory insufficiency with any extra fluid losses.

Symptoms occur if there is an acute drop in the level of serum sodium. As the sodium level falls below 125 mmol/l, nausea, vomiting, muscle twitching, and lethargy may appear. Below 115 mmol/l, seizures and coma may occur. If the sodium level gradually decreases, the patients may be relatively asymptomatic.

Severe hyponatraemia of less than 120 mmol/l requires correction. If the patient is dehydrated, the replacement fluid should have a sodium concentration equal to that of normal saline (e.g. Ringer's lactate, normal saline). In the absence of dehydration, the formula employed for acute correction is as follows:

{130 minus serum Na^+ level} $\times$ 0.6 $\times$ wt (kg)
= mmol Na^+ required for the correction of hyponatraemia
(0.9% NaCl = 0.15 mmol/ml; 3% NaCl = 0.5 mmol/ml; 5% NaCl = 0.87 mmol/ml)

This is in addition to the daily requirement of 1–3 mmol/kg body mass and may be administered as saline or hypertonic saline, and could be added to intravenous rehydration fluids.

Hypernatraemia

In *hypernatraemia with dehydration*, the osmotic gradient ensures water movement from the intracellular into the extracellular and intravascular compartments. This means that clinical signs of dehydration are masked. Therefore the signs and symptoms of hypernatraemic dehydration are predominantly those of intracellular water loss from brain cells, with depressed sensorium, irritability, and even convulsions. The severity of neurological symptoms depends on the degree and the rate of rise of plasma osmolality. Therapy of hypernatraemic dehydration is directed at two goals: rapid restoration of intravascular volume by means of plasma expanders such as Ringer's lactate if circulatory insufficiency is present; and secondly, a more gradual correction of the water deficit over 48 hours. Rapid downward correction of hypernatraemia at a rate faster than

1 mmol/l/hr carries the risk of water movement into brain cells down the osmotic gradient with resultant cerebral oedema and convulsions. The rate of fall in the serum sodium depends on the speed of administration as well as on the sodium concentration of the infused fluid. For patients with a serum sodium above 160 mmol/l, the sodium concentration of the infused fluid is therefore initially raised to between 90 and 105 mmol/l by adding sodium bicarbonate 8.4%, 15–20 ml to the first 500 ml of half-strength Darrows/dextrose for about six hours in acidotic patients. Thereafter half-strength Darrows in 5% dextrose can be used. The fluid is given at a steady rate of 10 ml/kg/hr, unless the patient has large continuing stool losses, in which case the speed of administration must be adjusted.

The treatment of the *hypernatraemic patient without dehydration* consists of an adequate oral water supply and salt restriction. This occurs occasionally due to inadvertent excessive salt administration. If fluid overload is severe, peritoneal dialysis may remove a large amount of sodium.

Hypokalaemia

(*See also* Chapter 24, Gastrointestinal disorders.)

The symptoms associated with hypokalaemia,

Table 10.2 Blood sugar disturbances		
Disturbance	**Mechanism**	**Common conditions**
Hyperglycaemia	Insulin deficiency	Diabetes mellitus
	Defective glucose uptake	Sick-cell syndrome
		Hypokalaemia
	Increased gluconeogenesis	Steroid therapy or excess
	Increased glycogenolysis	Stress-mediated catecholamine release
	Iatrogenic	High-concentration glucose administration
Hypoglycaemia Decreased availability or production of glucose	Substrate deficiency	Small for gestational age
		Protein-energy malnutrition
		Chronic diarrhoea
		Starvation
		'Ketotic' hypoglycaemia
	Defects of glycogenolysis	Glycogen storage disease
	Defects of gluconeogenesis	Endocrine deficiencies
		Enzyme deficiencies
	Mixed hepatic damage	Liver disease and failure
	Hepatotoxins	'Impila' poisoning
		Jamaican vomiting sickness
		Salicylates
		Alcohol
	Idiopathic	
Increased utilization of glucose	Hyperinsulinism	Infant of diabetic mother
		Beckwith syndrome
		Erythroblastosis fetalis
		Leucine sensitivity
		Insulin treatment
		Oral hypoglycaemic agents
		Islet cell adenoma
		Nesidioblastosis
		Tumours of mesothelial origin

Table 10.3 Electrolyte disturbances

Disturbance	Mechanism	Common conditions
Hyponatraemia <130 mmol/l	Na⁺ deficiency in excess of fluid losses	Diarrhoea Burns Water enema Sweat losses Low solute feeding Malnutrition Hot climate Adrenal insufficiency
	Water retention	Renal tubular dysfunction Congestive cardiac failure Cirrhosis Nephrotic syndrome Syndrome of inappropriate ADH secretion
Hypernatraemia >150 mmol/l	With dehydration water loss >Na loss Without dehydration	Diarrhoea Diabetes insipidus Osmotic diuresis Defective thirst sensation Concentrated feeds
Hypokalaemia	Deficient intake Gut losses Renal wasting	Protein-energy malnutrition Diarrhoea Enemas Congenital Cl⁻ losing diarrhoea Renal tubular disease Alkalosis Diuretic treatment Muscle wasting Endocrine disease
Hyperkalaemia	Alteration in cell metabolism Decreased renal excretion	Acidosis Hypoxia Oliguria Acidosis Hypoaldosteronism
Hypocalcaemia	Lack of intake, lack of absorption, hyperphosphataemia	Neonatal hypocalcaemia Hypoparathyroidism Pseudohypoparathyroidism Rickets Renal disease
Hypomagnesaemia	Decreased intake Gut losses Urine losses	Decreased intake Chronic diarrhoea Chronic diuretic therapy
Hyperphosphataemia	Decreased renal excretion	Renal failure Parathyroid hormone deficiency
Hypophosphataemia	Inadequate intake Renal losses	Premature neonate Hyperparathyroidism Renal tubular disorder

to a certain extent, depend on the rate of change in the serum potassium level. Heart, skeletal and smooth muscle, kidney, and brain are affected. Weakness, and hypotonia with paralysis and areflexia, occurs. This may resemble poliomyelitis with respiratory muscle depression. Cardiac arrhythmias and ECG changes may occur. Ileus may develop. Prolonged hypokalaemia leads to renal tubular changes, with reduced concentrating ability and subsequently interstitial nephritis.

It is advised that 3–6 mEq/kg/24 hours potassium chloride is administered orally to treat hypokalaemia. In conditions with severe renal losses, e.g. Bartter's syndrome, high dosages up to 10 mEq/kg/24 hours may be required to correct the deficit and maintain a stable serum potassium concentration. The concentration of potassium in intravenous fluids should not exceed 40 mmol/l (1 mEq = 1 mmol; 1g KCl = 13 mEq, 1 ml 15% KCl = 2 mmol.)

Hyperkalaemia

This is a life-threatening complication and must be considered an emergency.

A substantial increase in total body potassium is incompatible with life. A moderate elevation of serum potassium is quite normal in the neonatal period, but thereafter a rise above 6.5 mmol/l is associated with altered myocardial function with a risk of ventricular fibrillation and death. The ECG will show peaked T waves, flattening of the P wave, prolongation of the PR interval and progressive widening of the QRS complex.

Treatment for hyperkalaemia
- Eliminate all potassium intake.
- Administer sodium bicarbonate to correct underlying metabolic acidosis.
- Salbutamol nebulisation (Dilute 5 mg of salbutamol in 2–4 ml 0.9% saline and allow nebulisation over 20 minutes).
- Inject 10 % calcium gluconate, 0.5–1.0 ml/kg IV slowly.
- Give IV glucose, 1–3 g/kg over 1 hour. Soluble insulin, 1 unit/3 g glucose, may be added to this infusion.
- Sodium polystyrene sulphonate: 1 g/kg orally or per rectum.
- Furosemide, 1 mg/kg IV.
- Consider peritoneal dialysis if there is no improvement.

As haemolysis of a blood specimen may cause an erroneously high potassium level, the decision to treat a patient for hyperkalaemia should be taken when a level of 6.5 mmol/l or above is associated with these specific ECG changes.

Hypomagnesaemia

Magnesium is an essential co-factor for many enzyme systems in oxidative phosphorylation, glucose utilization, and muscle contraction. It is the second most important intracellular cation after potassium. It is required for the normal release of parathyroid hormone in response to hypocalcaemia. Deficiency is common in conditions of protein energy malnutrition and chronic diarrhoea, or with prolonged diuretic therapy. A dose of 250–500 mg $MgSO_4$ (0.5–1.0 ml 50% $MgSO_4$) given IM or IV daily for three to five days will usually correct the deficit.

Hypocalcaemia

Symptoms occur when there is a decrease in the ionized fraction of serum calcium, which accounts for about 50 per cent of the total serum calcium if the serum albumin level is normal. The measured total serum calcium may be reduced by as much as 0.2 mmol/l for every 10 g/l decrease in serum albumin, without any clinical features of hypocalcaemia.

The proportion of ionized calcium is increased in the presence of metabolic acidosis, but reduced in alkalosis, and may result in symptoms despite near-normal calcium levels. Hypokalaemia can mask symptoms of hypocalcaemia. Sustained hypocalcaemia with onset in, or persistence beyond, the neonatal period is due to deficiency or resistance to parathyroid hormone; vitamin D deficiency or resistance; chronic lack of calcium intake or absorption; and conditions leading to hyperphosphataemia such as chronic renal disease.

The clinical features of hypocalcaemia are those of increased neuromuscular irritability, jitteriness, seizures, and signs of raised intracranial pressure, eye and skin changes, and cardiac manifestations. Tetany is the occurrence of spontaneous spasms of motor muscles with sensory disturbances or central nervous excitability. The characteristic carpopedal spasm consists of flexion and adduction at the wrist and metacarpophalangeal joints, with similar muscle spasms around the ankles. Laryngeal spasm (*laryngis-*

mus stridulus) results in a stridulous, interrupted type of crowing inspiratory noise or it may lead to apnoea. Sensory disturbances consist of tingling or numbness of the extremities. Latent tetany may be detected by positive **Chvostek** or **Trousseau** signs. The former is elicited by tapping over the facial nerve anterior to the ear, and results in a twitching of the muscle of the ipsilateral side of the face. The latter consists of carpal spasm when a blood pressure cuff on the arm is kept inflated to just above the systolic blood pressure for three minutes.

The symptoms of neonatal hypocalcaemia include tremor or cyanotic attacks and may resemble symptoms of septicaemia, intracranial pathology, or other metabolic disturbances. *Chronic hypocalcaemia* leads to dystrophic manifestations, which include lenticular cataracts, dry and scaling skin, coarse hair, brittle nails, and enamel hypoplasia of teeth.

The **management** involves attention to rapid reversal of the underlying conditions. A slow intravenous injection of 2 ml/kg of calcium gluconate 10% is given with monitoring of the heart rate during injection to detect and avoid bradycardia. Thereafter, oral calcium supplements may be prescribed, but this depends on the underlying or associated disorder.

Hyperphosphataemia

This occurs under the following main sets of circumstances:

- Decreased glomerular filtration rate as in acute or chronic renal failure
- Increased load due to a large intake, e.g. cow's milk in young infants or phosphate-containing enemas
- Increased load from endogenous tissue destruction, e.g. cytotoxic therapy
- Increased tubular reabsorption of phosphate due to deficiency of or resistance to parathyroid hormone.

Hyperphosphataemia depresses the serum calcium level and this may lead to secondary hyperparathyroidism. A major clinical sequel of hyperphosphataemia is soft tissue calcification due to an increased $[Ca] \times [P]$ product.

Treatment involves identification of the predisposing cause. When the cause is reduction of renal phosphate excretion, intestinal phosphate-binding compounds such as magnesium trisilicate and aluminium hydroxide, are used. The intake of dietary phosphate should also be reduced.

Hypophosphataemia

In view of the important role of phosphate on intracellular processes (ATP; cAMP; 2,3-DPG), as well as in mineralization of bone, phosphate deficiency can have a variety of effects. These include neurological manifestations ranging from irritability and paraesthesiae to convulsions and coma, as well as diminished tissue oxygenation and impaired leukocyte function.

Hypophosphataemia is caused by excessive renal losses, e.g. familial hypophosphataemic rickets, renal tubular acidosis, or hyperparathyroidism, inadequate intake, e.g. premature infants, prolonged parenteral nutrition, malabsorption or severe malnutrition, and rapid flux from extracellular to intracellular compartments, that may occur during correction of diabetic ketoacidosis.

The **treatment** involves the correction of precipitating factors, as well as phosphate supplementation. This should be given several times a day to maintain adequate phosphate levels.

Hyperammonaemia

The accumulation of ammonia is responsible for some of the features of hepatic encephalopathy, such as vomiting, drowsiness, confusion, coma, and seizures. Apart from being found in conditions associated with liver failure, it is also seen in hepatic immaturity of neonates exposed to excessive protein intakes. It is also a prominent feature of some inherited disorders of metabolism. The management depends on the degree of hyperammonaemia and the underlying cause, and requires dietary protein restriction to limit ammonia production and, in symptomatic cases, intravenous sodium benzoate. Sodium benzoate 250 mg/kg/day serves to decrease the serum ammonia level and should be advised in severe hyperammonaemia even if the case is not definitely due to an inborn error of metabolism.

Inherited metabolic disorders

Incidence

Although individual inherited metabolic disorders are rare, there are more than 600 well described conditions. There is a wide variation in the regional incidences due to factors such as genetic drift, founder effect, consanguineous marriages and environmental influences.

The rarity of inherited metabolic diseases in developing countries may be more apparent than real due to the lack of facilities and expertise. In addition, the true incidence may be masked by a high prevalence of nutritional and infective disorders, and a high infant mortality rate.

Pathogenesis

A genetically determined deficiency of enzymes, or co-factors lead to the manifestations of disease in several ways (*see* Figure 10.1).

In classification, three different groups of disorders can be identified.

Group 1 comprises the disorders where there is a problem with the synthesis or catabolism of large molecules. It includes lysosomal storage disorders, peroxisomal disorders, congenital defects of glycosylation and disorders of abnormal cholesterol synthesis. These disorders present with permanent and progressive symptoms independent of food intake and intercurrent events.

Group 2 includes all the inborn errors of intermediate metabolism and they present episodically with accumulation of toxic compounds proximal to the metabolic block. The symptoms are due to intoxication, and progressive damage occurs although they may have symptom free intervals. These conditions typically have recurrent episodes of ketosis, acidosis and hyperammonaemia, lethargy, coma, liver failure, vomiting and thromboembolic complications. The group includes aminoacidopathies, organic acidurias, sugar intolerance and congenital urea cycle defects.

Group 3 are the disorders with predominant deficient energy production. The clinical symptoms are due to accumulation of toxic products and lack of energy. These patients present with hypoglycaemia, hyperlactacidaemia, severe hypotonia, failure to thrive, cardiomyopathy, SIDS and sometimes malformations. The specific disorders are the glycogenoses, defects in gluconeogenesis, congenital lactacidaemias, fatty acid oxidation defects and mitochondrial disorders.

Diagnosis

Neonates and young infants have a limited range of non-specific responses to severe illness, including irritability, poor feeding, lethargy, vomiting, and failure to thrive. These symptoms and signs tend to occur much more frequently in conditions that are not primarily inherited metabolic disorders. The picture is often that of an infant in deep coma or with vascular collapse, and the first impression is that of a septicaemia or cerebral haemorrhage.

However, the circumstances in which the symptoms develop are usually more characteristic than the symptoms themselves, and include:

- Onset after several hours or days of good health
- Occurrence in a full-term baby, following a non-traumatic delivery
- A relentless recurrence and progression of symptoms once they do appear
- A family history of consanguinity or unexplained early neonatal loss
- A suspicious association of symptoms and biochemical abnormalities.

An inborn error ought to be seriously considered at an early stage if no obvious cause of the illness can be established. The laboratory tools available

---

Figure 10.1 Genetically determined origins of disease

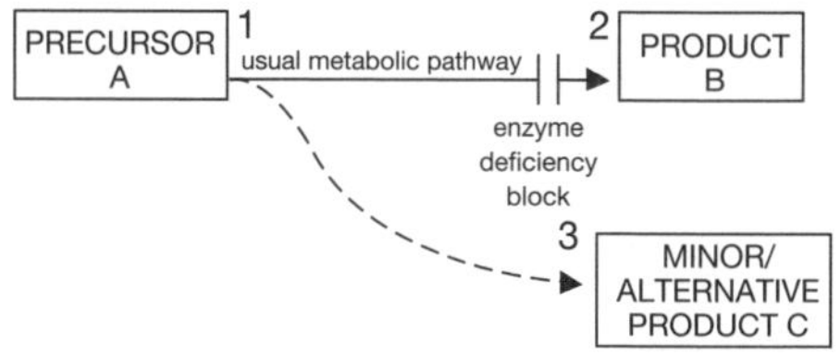

1 Substrate and precursor accumulation
  Intracellular storage
  Blood accumulation
  Loss through gut or urine

2 Product deficit

3 Utilization of minor or alternative pathways
  Abnormal product accumulation

Any child presenting with *unexplained* hypoglycaemia, acidosis, recurrent vomiting, impaired consciousness, apnoea attacks or seizures must be suspected of having an inherited metabolic disorder.

to investigate these conditions vary greatly in their complexity, but the screening methods for detecting them are few in number:

+ Hypoglycaemia
+ Electrolyte imbalance
+ Metabolic acidosis with raised anion gap (serum chloride needs to be measured)
+ Ketonuria
+ Ketonaemia
+ Raised ammonia and
+ Raised lactate.

Many late-onset **presentations**, usually occurring after six months of age, are preceded by insidious or intermittent warning symptoms which are commonly misdiagnosed or overlooked:

+ Gastrointestinal associated features: failure to thrive, recurrent vomiting, hepatomegaly and jaundice
+ Neurological manifestations: developmental delay, progressive retardation, long-tract signs, lethargy, seizures
+ Musculoskeletal findings: floppiness, rickets
+ General: abnormal odour, dysmorphic appearance, failure to grow normally
+ Specific entities: anaemia, cirrhosis, cardiomyopathy, tubulopathy, cataracts.

Screening and initial management

To facilitate the clinician's task, simple screening procedures to be carried out in the ward or in a simple laboratory are recommended to confirm or refute a suspicion of 'metabolic' diagnosis (*see* Table 10.4). Correct technique instructions and the freshness of the reagents must be assured. If recurrent hypoglycaemia is the main problem, sampling at the critical time may avoid the performance of hazardous diagnostic procedures. Thus, clinical and laboratory data can be assembled in a few hours, precluding long waiting periods for sophisticated results or inappropriate referrals.

Table 10.4 Screening procedures in the newborn nursery

Blood	Glucose
	Electrolytes
	Acid-base
	Ca, P, Mg
Urine	Colour
	Smell
	Reducing substances
	Ferric chloride and
	Phenistix®
	Acetest or Ketotest®
	2.4-DNP-hydrazine

Table 10.5 Plan for preliminary management of infant with suspected metabolic disorder

Total protein restriction where patient presents with acute metabolic crisis
Maintain high urine output, especially for lactic acidosis
Intake 150 ml/kg/day with added bicarbonate to achieve alkaline urine
Sustain anabolism and energy intake with dextrose especially
Provide minerals and vitamins according to requirements
Consider megavitamin cocktail (as available)
   Thiamine 50–100 mg
   Riboflavin 20–50 mg
   Pyridoxine 200–500 mg
   Folic acid 10–25 mg
   Ascorbic acid 250–500 mg
   Biotin 100 mg
   Carnitine 100 mg/kg/day
Sodium benzoate 250 mg/kg/day for hyperammonaemia
Lactulose and neomycin for symptoms of liver failure
Re-introduction of minimum protein intake

Once suspicion has been aroused, supportive measures are undertaken, an expert in a tertiary centre is consulted and a few laboratory investigations are sent off. While awaiting a definitive diagnosis, confirmatory or otherwise, a common plan of management needs to be instituted, even if only one positive element is available. What may seem like shot-gun therapy may increase the infant's chances of survival without major neurologic damage (*see* Table 10.5).

Definitive diagnosis entails sophisticated biochemical investigations on blood, urine or skin biopsy samples and is an essential prerequisite for possible effective management and especially for genetic counselling. Every effort – usually no more than arranging transport of a few specimens to a distant laboratory – should be made to ensure that a young couple are offered future prenatal diagnosis.

Access to special milks, substrates, and megavitamins will undoubtedly be problematic in remote areas but early contact with a tertiary centre may help the coordination of the treatment plan. Close dietary supervision and frequent biochemical monitoring may also be impractical, but expert advice can be obtained by telephone.

Despite the rarity of these disorders and the perceived lack of relevance in the context of more pressing health needs of many communities, real benefit may be derived from a raised index of suspicion and the use of preliminary inexpensive screening tests with early access to experts.

11 Poisoning

Children are natural explorers. Infants and young children are likely to experiment and over 60 per cent of cases of accidental poisoning occur in children under five years of age. Serious poisonings are rare after five years. In many instances the family is immediately aware that the child has been in contact with a potentially toxic substance, but in other instances, no such information is available. Poisoning should then be considered whenever there is sudden unexplained illness in a child previously thought to be perfectly healthy.

The following situations related to poisoning will occur:

Allegedly known toxin exposure – the child is brought with an observed or suspected exposure:

- ◆ Symptoms and signs match the known properties of the alleged substance
- ◆ Symptoms and signs do not match the known properties: manage as for an unknown poison.

Sudden onset of symptoms in a previously healthy child not known to have been exposed to a toxin:

- ◆ Coma and convulsions: exclude hypoglycaemia and neurological disease
- ◆ Recognizable syndromes of poisoning:
  - Paraffin and volatile hydrocarbons: respiratory distress, hypoxia
  - Organophosphates: salivation, miosis, bradycardia, muscle symptoms, convulsions
  - Atropine-like effects: mydriasis, flushing, tachycardia, excitability, dry mouth
  - Sedatives, anticonvulsants: coma, hypotension, respiratory depression
  - Salicylates: acidosis, sweating, fever, coma
  - Corrosive substances: local erythema, oedema, erosions
- ◆ Unrecognizable syndrome of symptoms and signs: manage as for unknown poison.

The majority of accidental poisonings involve medicines and drugs. They have usually been left inadvertently accessible to the child by the carelessness of an adult. Household cleaning products, paraffin for cooking, and alkali cleaning fluids are other hazards that children may experiment with, especially if the products have been decanted into drink bottles or food containers.

Children are sometimes tempted to taste brightly coloured berries, mushrooms, or other garden plants that may be potentially poisonous. However, accidents associated with rat and insect poisons are more common.

In many communities of developing countries, local medicines dispensed by traditional healers are often the first line of treatment. Most such medicines contain a cocktail of ingredients that are not standardized for infants or young children, or which may be contaminated by toxic compounds. Accidental poisoning may then complicate the illness of an already sick child.

Most poisonings in childhood are accidental. However, the miseries of adolescence may precipitate a suicide attempt. Some adolescents, through peer group pressure, may experiment with alcohol, glue sniffing, and drugs. This may lead to severe and dangerous intoxication. Rarer still is deliberate poisoning of a child by a parent or guardian to fabricate illness: Munchhausen-by-proxy syndrome.

Chronic poisoning may sometimes occur in children living in polluted slum environments that are often sited near industrial and petro-chemical complexes. Certain heavy metals such as lead and mercury have been implicated.

Management of acute poisoning

The management of acute poisoning in the child depends on when and where the child is first seen. Specific issues are of concern at the site of the suspected poisoning, the health centre, and in the hospital.

Most acute poisonings occur in or around the home. The child should receive immediate first aid attention. The specific measures will depend on the type of poisoning.

Diagnosis

The diagnosis of a specific poisoning depends on an understanding of the epidemiology, a careful history and examination. It is useful to assess the level of consciousness on first encounter (coma score, *see* Chapter 26, Neurological and muscular disorders). This will indicate the severity, the line of action to be taken and the possible prognosis.

Table 11.1 Immediate management of acute poisoning		
Environment	**What are the concerns**	**Action**
Home	Immediate reaction What poison is it? Identify by container, specimen of poison, or vomitus Assess child's condition. If child is convulsing, consider hypoglycaemia	**Possible gas, fumes or smoke**: Carry into the fresh air and administer 100% oxygen, if available, through a face-mask. **Contact poisons** include herbicides and pesticides such as chlorinated hydrocarbons and organophosphates. All contaminated clothing should be removed and the skin, hair, and nails washed first with water and then with soap. The child must then be rinsed thoroughly and dried. **Poisons in the eye**: Irrigate gently with lukewarm water for up to 10 minutes. **Ingested poisons**: If a household product, detergent, and corrosive alkali or acid has been swallowed, a glass of milk or water can be given. No attempt at neutralizing an acid or alkali should be made, as it will cause more severe tissue damage through a thermal reaction. **Unless the suspected poison is known to be innocuous, urgently take to hospital**
Clinic/ health centre	First aid management Assess condition Reduce or prevent continuing absorption of the poison Refer to hospital	If child is unconscious, maintain airway and ventilate with bag and mask Assess circulation: Blood pressure, pulse If child is convulsing, consider hypoglycaemia Give activated charcoal
Hospital	Assess clinical state Identify specific measures	Maintain airway and ventilation Correct shock and circulation Contact poison centre for specific complications and antidotes Consider forced diuresis, peritoneal or haemodialysis as may be required

Table 11.2   Signs and symptoms of some common acute poisons

Symptoms and Signs		
General	Flushing	Atropine, belladonna alkaloids, anticholinergic drugs, tricyclic antidepressants, quinine
	Sweating	Organophosphates, salicylates, nitrates, muscarinic mushrooms
	Fever and hyperthermia	Atropine, antihistamines, salicylates, tricyclic antidepressants
	Hypothermia	Barbiturates, alcohol, phenothiazines
	Burns/stomatitis	Corrosive acids and alkalis
	Smell	Alcohol, acetone, salicylates and camphor
	Salivation	Organophosphates, muscarinic mushrooms
	Dry mouth	Atropine, antihistamines
	Cyanosis without respiratory distress	Aniline, antimalarials, methaemoglobinaemia, sulphaemoglobinaemia (nitrates)
	Jaundice	Paracetamol, mushrooms
The eyes	Lacrimation	Organophosphates, irritants
	Blurred vision	Organophosphates, atropine, alcohol
	Miosis (constricted pupils)	Organophosphates, opiates, phenothiazines, muscarinic mushrooms
	Mydriasis (dilated pupils)	Atropine, antihistamines, tricyclic antidepressants, alcohol, cocaine
	Nystagmus	Organophosphates, alcohol, barbiturates, phenytoin
Cardiovascular System	Tachycardia	Atropine, tricyclic antidepressants, theophylline, caffeine
	Bradycardia	Digoxin, organophosphates, opiates, nitrites
	Hypotension	Organophosphates, barbiturates, benzodiazepines, phenothiazines
	Hypertension	Antihistamines, tricyclic antidepressants
	Arrhythmias	Digoxin, tricyclic antidepressants, theophylline, antimalarials (quinine, halofantrine)
Respiratory System	Dyspnoea	Paraffin, hydrocarbons, petroleum products
	Tachypnoea	Salicylates, carbon monoxide
	Respiratory depression	All tranquillizers and sedatives, opiates, antidepressants, organophosphates
Central nervous system	Coma	All tranquillizers, barbiturates, phenothiazines, alcohol, carbon monoxide, salicylates, narcotics
	Ataxia	Organophosphates, alcohol, antihistamines, barbiturates, tricyclic antidepressants
	Delirium/hyperexcitability	Atropine, tricyclic antidepressants, phenothiazines, theophylline
	Convulsions	Organophosphates, tricyclic antidepressants, atropine, theophylline, alcohol, camphor, hypoglycaemia
	Dystonic movements	Phenothiazines, metoclopramide, tricyclic antidepressants, phenytoin
	Muscle fasciculations	Organophosphates
	Muscle weakness	Organophosphates, carbamates, herbicides

Any child who presents with unexplained altered mental status, respiratory or haemodynamic compromise, seizures or metabolic derangement should be considered for a toxic ingestion. A thorough examination should include special attention to vital signs, mental and neurological status, pupillary size and reactivity, skin colour and hydration, respiratory effort, pulses and perfusion. If a child is convulsing, hypoglycaemia can be confirmed with a glucostix and treated immediately with 5 ml of 50% dextrose given intravenously.

Poisoning should also be considered when there is sudden unexplained illness in a previously healthy child with the signs and symptoms listed below. Many poisons can be suspected on the basis of specific clinical features, so-called 'toxidromes' (see Table 11.2). Laboratory investigations can be helpful. Toxicological screening for some drugs may be useful for monitoring and management. Blood glucose, electrolytes, and blood gases are important for monitoring progress. ECG monitoring is useful to detect arrhythmias or gross electrolyte imbalance. There is no substitute for regular clinical assessment and examination of the patient.

Management of the conscious child

Although most accidental paediatric poisonings cause minor or no effects, a few substances can lead to severe toxicity or even death, even when ingested in small amounts. Identifying those high-risk patients allows clinicians to decide whether any decontamination techniques would be of benefit or if any specific antidotes or special interventions are required. Patients who present with serious signs and symptoms or have potentially life-threatening toxic exposures should be admitted to PICU for close monitoring and management.

Prevention of absorption

Emesis

Emesis is of value up to six hours after ingestion and even after 12 hours, for children who have taken salicylates or tricyclic antidepressants which delay gastric emptying.

Ipecacuanha is the only antiemetic that is recommended. It is given as a syrup at a dose of 10–15 ml followed by a glass of water. If vomiting has not occurred within 20–30 minutes, a repeat dose may be given.

Contra-indications to inducing emesis include:

- Depressed consciousness with the slightest danger of absent or diminished cough and swallowing reflexes
- Convulsions and coma
- Poisoning with all petroleum products, paraffin and hydrocarbons such as benzene and turpentine
- Poisoning with corrosive products, acids and alkalis.

Gastric lavage

Gastric lavage should only be performed in children who are conscious or who have an endotracheal tube to protect their airway. The widest bore tube should be inserted orally. The child should be positioned on the left side with the head slightly lower than the body to minimize the potential for aspiration. Half-strength tepid

Management plan for poisoning	
Consider	**Action**
State of child and careful monitoring	Supportive management, circulation, level of consciousness
Parental anxiety and panic	Allay anxiety, take detailed history
Type of poison or drug taken	Obtain specimen and container
Prevention of absorption	Consider emesis, activated charcoal, whole bowel irrigation
Specific antidotes	Involve poison information centre

saline is then instilled, 50 ml at time, and then drained. This may be repeated until 500 ml has been used or until the fluid returned is clear.

Contra-indications to gastric lavage:

◆ Petroleum products and volatile hydrocarbons. There is a danger of aspiration pneumonitis with these substances.

◆ Corrosive alkalis and acids. Insertion of the gastric tube may cause trauma and even perforation.

Activated charcoal

This can be taken orally or instilled by gastric tube. The aim is to avert toxicity by adsorbing the poison within the gastrointestinal tract, thereby preventing systemic absorption. Efficacy is greatest when charcoal is given as soon as possible after the ingestion. Thirty grams of charcoal are mixed with about 150 ml of water and swallowed. If instilled by naso-gastric tube it may take time to drain because of its consistency.

Activated charcoal is recommended for the following poisonings:

◆ Aspirin (salicylates)
◆ Phenobarbitone
◆ Carbamazapine (Tegretol®)
◆ Phenothiazines
◆ Tricyclic antidepressants
◆ Phenytoin
◆ Dapsone
◆ Quinine
◆ Digoxin
◆ Theophylline/aminophylline.

Whole bowel irrigation

Polyethylene glycol electrolyte solution is administered orally or via a nasogastric tube. The recommended dosing schedule is 500 ml/hr for children nine months to six years, 1 000 ml/hr for children 6–12 years and 1 500–2 000 ml/hr for adolescents. It is best to start at a lower rate and slowly advance to the desired dose. The patient is placed upright, sitting on a commode and the solution is continued until the rectal effluent is clear.

Whole bowel irrigation has its greatest potential benefit in substances that are slowly absorbed from the gastrointestinal tract and for potentially toxic ingestions of sustained-release or enterically coated drugs.

Polyethylene glycol is not absorbed and does not produce fluid and electrolyte imbalance.

Contraindications to whole bowel irrigation:

◆ Impaired airway reflexes or intractable vomiting
◆ Obstructed bowel, ileus and gastrointestinal haemorrhage.

Table 11.3 Specific antidotes for common poisons

Poison	Antidote
Alcohol (ethyl alcohol)	Glucose (to prevent hypoglycaemia)
Methyl alcohol and ethylene glycol	Ethyl alcohol (competitive inhibition)
Aniline; nitrobenzene dyes	Methylene blue
Atropine (belladonna alkaloids)	Physostigmine
Carbon monoxide	100% oxygen or hyperbaric oxygen
Coumarins (warfarin)	Vitamin K (10–15 mg)
Cyanide	Sodium nitrite 3% (10 mg/kg)
	Sodium thiocyanate 50%
	Dicobalt edetate
Iron	Desferrioxamine: Oral 50 mg in 5 ml water, IV 15 mg/kg by continuous infusion
Isoniazide	Pyridoxine
Opiates (morphine, pethidine, diphenoxylate hydrochloride)	Naloxone 0.01 mg/kg IM or IV
Organophosphates, carbamates	Atropine 0.02–0.05 mg/kg (repeat as indicated)
	Pralidoxime 25 mg/kg (cholinesterase reactivator)

Specific antidotes

Specific antidotes may be administered to neutralize drugs. An antidote is no substitute for careful monitoring and good clinical and nursing support of the child.

Common specific poisons

There are hundreds of different drugs, medicines, chemicals, herbicides, insecticides or industrial and domestic products that are potential poisons. Only those that are common in childhood have been selected. Before assuming that any compound or product is innocuous, the local poison centre should be contacted for information.

Acute poisoning

Paracetamol® (acetaminophen)

Accidental poisoning is uncommon in infants and children. Adolescents may take an overdose in a suicide attempt.

Pathogenesis Centrilobular necrosis of the liver occurs when glutathione levels fall below 70 per cent and reactive metabolites of acetaminophen combine with hepatic macromolecules.

Clinical features Usually delayed for 48 to 72 hours when vomiting, jaundice, and signs of liver failure occur.

Treatment A specific antidote, N-acetylcysteine, is given by oral and intravenous route in the event of a severe overdose. Toxic levels and prognosis can be estimated from plasma paracetamol levels relative to the time elapsed since ingestion.

Salicylates (Aspirin®)

Some preparations taste pleasant and children may consider them as sweets.

Pathophysiology. There is an initial stimulation of the respiratory centre, which causes a transitory respiratory alkalosis with alkaluria. This is followed by a metabolic acidosis due to uncoupling of oxidative phosphorylation. Glucose metabolism is disturbed which may cause hypo- or hyperglycaemia. Hepatotoxicity occurs in severe cases leading to increased prothrombin time and bleeding.

Clinical features Initially there may be tachypnoea, fever, tachycardia, and sweating followed by signs of acidosis, dehydration, vomiting, hypoglycaemia, convulsions, coma, and liver or renal failure.

Treatment Take a serum sample for salicylate level, blood gas, and electrolyte analysis. Dehydration is present in all severe cases and should be managed with intravenous fluids. Acidosis and electrolyte imbalance should be corrected and a forced alkaline diuresis may be necessary. Dialysis may be indicated in severe toxicity.

Tricyclic antidepressants

Young children who ingest even quite small amounts of tricyclic antidepressants may become seriously ill because the therapeutic/toxic ratio is low.

Pathogenesis. Tricyclic antidepressants act by blocking acetylcholine, nor-adrenaline, and alpha-adrenergic receptor uptake by neurons. They also block the uptake of serotonin, 5-hydroxytryptamine, and dopamine. In excess this causes an anticholinergic syndrome.

Clinical features. Initially there may be drowsiness but this is followed by dry mouth, tachycardia, cardiac arrhythmias, pupillary dilatation, excitability, and hallucinations. There may be a progression to convulsions and coma. Urinary retention and constipation are also features.

Treatment. Induce emesis, do gastric lavage and administer activated charcoal. The child should be monitored in an intensive care unit so that cardiac arrhythmias can be detected early and treated. Sodium bicarbonate is given to raise the pH to between 7.45 and 7.55. The particular anti-arrhythmic drug given will depend upon the type of arrhythmia induced.

Antimalarials

Children may be tempted to experiment, although antimalarial tablets are bitter.

Pathogenesis. Quinine can cause hypoglycaemia in children especially if given parenterally. It stimulates the pancreatic beta cells, causing increased insulin levels. Quinine, mefloquine and halofantrine can all cause arrhythmias by interfering with myocardial conduction.

Treatment. Admit for cardiac monitoring. Any arrhythmia is treated as indicated.

Alkalis and acids

Alkalis and acids are found in many domestic

and kitchen cleaning products. Children may come into contact through exploring the kitchen or toilet cupboards.

Pathogenesis. Alkalis tend to cause more serious tissue damage than acids. They bind to fats and oils in the tissues and cause necrosis. The mucous membranes of the mouth and oesophagus are most commonly involved.

Clinical features. Acute inflammation and ulceration of the mouth, oesophagus, and eyes occurs. Local tissue necrosis can cause stricture formation in the oesophagus.

Treatment. No attempt at emesis or lavage should be made. Nasogastric intubation can lead to perforation of the oesophagus. Oesophagoscopy may be performed 48 hours after ingestion to assess the extent of tissue damage and anticipate whether future stricture formation or surgery is indicated.

Tranquillizers, sedatives and hypnotics

Most tranquillizers and sedatives act directly on the central nervous system (CNS).

Benzodiazepines

They act by depressing the CNS, causing drowsiness, ataxia, loss of consciousness, coma, and respiratory depression.

Phenothiazines

They cause depression of the CNS, extrapyramidal signs and symptoms that mimic a psychotic episode.

Barbiturates

Barbiturates depress the CNS and in excess cause respiratory failure. Initial symptoms of confusion, ataxia, hypotension and miosis may present before loss of consciousness.

Antihistamines

Some long-acting preparations are particularly dangerous. Many antihistamines directly depress CNS activity although children may react with initial symptoms of hyperexcitability. Antihistamines also have an anticholinergic effect causing a dry mouth, fever and dilated pupils.

Treatment. Because tranquillizers and sedatives affect consciousness and many have an anti-emetic action, the induction of vomiting with ipecacuanha syrup is best avoided. Respiratory depression will follow CNS depression, and

ventilation must be maintained by oxygen and artificial ventilation if necessary. Physostigmine at a dose of 0.5–2 mg will reverse the anticholinergic actions of antihistamines.

Alcohol (ethyl alcohol)

Alcohol (ethyl alcohol) has a social function in many cultures and children may easily gain access to it. Other alcohols include methyl alcohols (methylated spirits, meths), isopropyl alcohol, and ethylene glycol, which may be found in industrial solvents, cleaners, and as antifreeze.

Pathophysiology. Alcohol depresses the central nervous system. In children, alcohol interferes with glucose metabolism and can cause hypoglycaemia. Cerebral oedema may occur in severe acute alcohol poisoning.

Clinical features. Sedation, ataxia, and slurring of speech are initial signs followed by progressive incoordination, stupor, coma, and respiratory failure. Hypoglycaemia may be profound, causing sweating, tachycardia, and convulsions.

Treatment. Emesis is dangerous where consciousness is impaired but activated charcoal will reduce absorption. Intravenous glucose will prevent hypoglycaemia and also rehydrate the child. In cases of methanol or ethylene glycol poisoning, ethyl alcohol can be given to competitively inhibit damage to the liver and brain.

Insecticides

Insecticides that include **organophosphates and carbamates** are widely used in rural and farming communities. Children may become poisoned through direct contact and ingestion.

Pathophysiology. Organophosphates act by inhibiting the enzyme cholinesterase which breaks down the neurotransmitter acetylcholine. Accumulation of acetylcholine leads to symptoms of toxicity. Red cell cholinesterase levels give an indication of severity of poisoning.

Clinical features. Sweating, excess salivation, increased bronchial secretions, muscle fasciculations, muscle weakness, constriction of pupils, bradycardia, diarrhoea, convulsions, and coma are all features of a cholinergic crisis.

Treatment. If the child is conscious, emesis may be induced or gastric lavage performed. If the skin is contaminated the clothes must be removed and the child should be washed thoroughly. Specific treatment is atropine in an initial dose of 0.05 mg/kg intravenously as an initial dose followed by a dose of 0.02 mg/kg every 15 minutes until salivation stops and the pupils begin to dilate.

Hydrocarbons and petroleum products (paraffin, turpentine, white spirit, benzene)

Hydrocarbons are used in a wide variety of domestic and industrial products. They cause toxicity by direct contact, ingestion and inhalation. The more volatile the substance, the more toxic it is. Children may ingest paraffin when it is stored in unlabelled soft drink bottles.

Pathogenesis. Local toxicity is caused by leaching out of oils and fat from the skin and causing local irritation to mucous membranes. Aspiration or inhalation of even a small amount causes a severe necrotizing and haemorrhagic pneumonitis. Systemic toxicity is caused by CNS depression and sensitization of heart muscle. Liver and kidney damage may occur.

Clinical features. Coughing, tachypnoea and dyspnoea may be the first signs of aspiration or inhalation pneumonitis. Signs and symptoms may continue for over a week. CNS toxicity will cause loss of consciousness, coma and convulsions.

Treatment. No attempt should be made to induce emesis or perform gastric lavage. Treatment is usually supportive with maintenance of hydration and ventilation where necessary.

Iron

Children usually become poisoned with iron after taking their mother's antenatal iron pills. The pills may resemble sweets because some preparations are coloured and taste pleasant.

Pathogenesis. Excess elemental iron causes direct irritation and necrosis of the gastric and intestinal mucosa, producing vasodilatation, inflammation and bleeding. Once absorbed, the iron accumulates in the mitochondria. It interferes with electron transport across mitochondrial membranes, causing damage to organs, in particular the liver. Bleeding and hypoglycaemia may result.

Clinical features. Due to local irritation, gastrointestinal symptoms of vomiting, diarrhoea, abdominal pain, and haematemesis may be the initial symptoms. After 12 to 24 hours signs of clinical shock may develop with metabolic acidosis, fever, and hypotension. Liver damage may cause a bleeding tendency and hypoglycaemia. A late complication may be pyloric stenosis caused by fibrosis due to the local corrosive effect of iron.

Treatment. The amount of iron ingested can be assessed by measuring plasma serum iron levels. Emesis should be induced as soon as possible. This may be followed by gastric lavage and the instillation of a specific antidote desferrioxamine in the stomach as 1 g diluted in 1 l of water to which sodium bicarbonate has been added. Desferrioxamine chelates iron. It may be given by slow continuous intravenous infusion at 15 mg/kg/hr. In severe cases peritoneal or haemodialysis may be considered.

Carbon monoxide

Carbon monoxide poisoning can occur in children who sleep in a room or hut with inadequate ventilation and in which there is a coal or charcoal fire. Inhalation of smoke, car exhaust fumes, and fumes from blocked chimneys in confined and poorly ventilated spaces can also cause carbon monoxide poisoning.

Pathogenesis. Toxicity is due to hypoxia. Carbon monoxide binds tenaciously to haemoglobin, forming carboxyhaemoglobin, thereby preventing the carriage of oxygen. The half-life of carboxyhaemoglobin is about 200 minutes in air but 40 minutes in 100% oxygen. Hypoxia causes cerebral oedema and damage to cardiac muscle and other organs.

Clinical features. Headache and dizziness with gradual loss of consciousness are the first signs. Tachypnoea and tachycardia occur as hypoxia increases. Ultimately convulsions, coma, respiratory and circulatory failure supervene.

Treatment. Immediate, 100% oxygen therapy should be started and, if available, hyperbaric oxygen, which is also beneficial. To prevent cerebral oedema, an infusion of mannitol and intravenous dexamethasone 1 mg/kg every six hours should be started. After recovery the child should be monitored closely for a week because delayed pulmonary oedema, cardiac failure, and myoglobinuria can complicate convalescence.

Botanical poisons

There are hundreds of species of berries, plants and mushrooms that look alluring but are potentially toxic. Fortunately many of the berries are bitter and will be spat out before much is ingested.

Mushrooms

Accidental mushroom poisoning can occur when poisonous mushrooms are mistaken for edible ones. Cooking will inactivate many of the toxins but not all. There are many variable factors which determine the degree of toxicity; these include the stage of maturity, the species, and the method of cooking.

Gastrointestinal upset is common with mushroom poisoning. Vomiting, diarrhoea, and abdominal cramps help to expel some of the offending plant. Mushrooms of the species *Inocybe* contain muscarine which can cause a cholinergic crisis. Symptoms of lacrimation, salivation, bronchospasm, miosis and urinary and faecal incontinence can be reversed by giving atropine – 0.05 mg/kg.

The most dangerous types of poisonous mushrooms are the *Amanita* and *Galerina* species. Their toxins cause cell necrosis in the liver, kidneys, and gut. Supportive management is indicated as complications arise.

Belladonna and atropine poisoning

Deadly nightshade (belladonna) and plants that contain the belladonna alkaloids such as stramonium, Jimsonweed and green and sprouting potatoes (solanine) cause atropine poisoning. The symptoms are dry mouth, dilated pupils, fever, decreased sweating, and tachycardia. Fortunately the symptoms tend to last only four to six hours. Physostigmine 0.5–2 mg may be given to reverse the effects of atropine.

'Impila' poisoning

The tuber *Callilepsis laureola*, which is also known as 'impila' is contained in some herbal medicines. One of its constituents, atractyloside, causes hypoglycaemia, renal damage, and centrilobular necrosis of the liver. Patients presenting with impila poisoning are predominantly young African children of variable nutritional status, with a short history of diminishing level of consciousness, convulsions and gastrointestinal symptoms. They are usually tachypnoeic and have acidotic-type breathing, and are often profoundly hypotonic and hyporeflexic, but there is no jaundice, hepatic foetor, focal neurological signs or meningeal irritation. Hypoglycaemia is invariable and is very frequently accompanied by signs of renal impairment, with hyperkalaemia, uraemia and acidosis. There are always biochemical indices of hepatic failure, with liver function tests showing elevated serum enzyme levels, prolonged prothrombin time and a raised blood ammonia level. Evidence of renal failure may accompany and sometimes precede the development of hepatic failure. Management is for the hypoglycaemia, hepatic failure and renal failure.

Chronic poisoning

Over-the-counter (OTC) cough and cold medication

These medications are widely marketed for relief of common cold symptoms despite little evidence demonstrating their efficacy in young children. Most children will eventually improve on their own with no intervention. In addition, these medications can be associated with significant morbidity and even mortality in both acute overdoses and when administered in correct doses for chronic periods of time.

The potential toxicities of cough and cold medicines vary with their composition. Many products contain multiple substances including a decongestant, cough suppressant, antihistamine, and/or antipyretic, and/or analgesic.

Pseudoephedrine and phenylpropanolamine (PPA) are sympathomimetics that reduce nasal congestion by stimulating the alpha-adrenergic receptors on vascular smooth muscle. Both drugs have a low therapeutic index with toxic complications evident at 3–4 times the therapeutic dose.

Clinical toxicity presents with central nervous system (CNS) stimulation, hypertension and tachycardia with pseudoephedrine ingestion, and bradycardia with PPA ingestion. CNS stimulation can manifest as extreme agitation, restlessness, insomnia, psychosis and seizures. Serious complications after decongestant ingestions and/or overdoses include hypertension, tachycardia, bradycardia, seizures, stroke and cerebral haemorrhage.

Antihistamines, namely H_1 blockers, are structurally similar to histamine and prevent its effects at receptor level. They also possess antimuscarinic, antispasmodic, antiemetic, sedative and anticholinergic effects. Chlorpheniramine and brompheniramine are commonly used. Adverse effects and clinical toxicity are characterized by a spectrum of anticholinergic symptoms and CNS depression. Tachycardia, blurred vision, agitation, hyperactivity, toxic psychoses and seizures may be evident.

Dextrometomorphan, an antitussive, (at dosages 10 mg/kg and greater), has also been associated with toxic side effects such as lethargy, stupor, hyperexcitability, ataxia, abnormal limb movements and coma.

Cough and cold medicines, therefore, are not administered without risk. Often physicians fail to ask specifically about over-the-counter medication use in the evaluation process, presuming that when asked about medicine use parents will include all medication. However, most parents perceive questions about medications as pertaining to prescription medication only and not over-the-counter preparations.

Traditional/ herbal medication

The use of herbal medication is a regular practice in many communities. The reasons for this are multiple and include the following:

- Ill health in children with the aim of alleviating disease
- As an alternative medicine in sick children when there is no improvement on prescription medication
- Inability to tolerate the side effects of prescribed drugs
- A belief that these agents repel or protect against evil spirits
- Prophylactically to promote good health
- A belief that natural products are harmless, and
- As a family tradition, as many parents have learnt the use of herbal medicines from their parents, even in the absence of ill health.

Some herbal medications as well as OTC medications have known side effects. *Ginkgo biloba*, evening primrose, arnica flower, devils claw, licorice, horse chestnut, quassia, red clover and sunflower seeds are known to increase bleeding potential.

There is also the potential for drug-to-drug and drug-to-herb interaction and the possibility of contamination with heavy metals during processing cannot be excluded.

Parents should understand that herbal or natural products are not inherently safer than prescribed drugs just because they are derived from plant sources and sold without a prescription.

There is a need for research to evaluate the safety and efficacy of alternative paediatric therapies.

Prevention

Prevention of accidental poisoning is the ideal for what is clearly a misadventure. However, the natural curiosity of children, carelessness of adults and hazards of the environment, mean that not all incidents can be avoided. Parents and adults should be made aware that it is their responsibility to ensure that children are not exposed to potential poisons. Sensible steps to minimize the risk of exposure can be taken in the home and surroundings.

Measures to help prevent poisoning include the following:
- Safe and lockable cupboards to store dangerous substances out of reach of children and the keys kept separately
- Household cleaning solutions, garden poisons and garage products, pesticides and insecticides should all be kept out of sight and reach of children
- Food and cleaning products must never be stored together
- Medicines and drugs should be stored separately in their original child-proof containers
- Children are great imitators and so medicines should not be taken by an adult in the presence of children
- Children should never be induced to take medicines by describing them as sweets or as anything other than medicine
- Potentially poisonous substances should never be kept in unlabelled bottles. Paraffin, industrial spirits and petroleum products are often kept in soft drink bottles, which is a particularly dangerous situation.

These are precautions that can be applied in any household. It is easier to control the situation in one's own home than elsewhere. Many accidental poisonings occur when children are visiting relatives, particularly grandparents and the elderly, who arrange their household to suit themselves without normally having to consider young children.

Fortunately most cases of accidental poisoning in children have a favourable outcome. Every year new household products, herbicides and medicines become available as old ones are discarded. Where available, a poison information centre will be able to identify and advise on appropriate management of such potentially new poisonous products.

12

Rickets and metabolic bone disorders

Metabolic bone diseases in children may present with an array of symptoms and signs. The following are common presenting features:

- Bony deformities
- Short stature
- Delayed development
- Hypotonia
- Convulsions
- Acidosis
- Recurrent lower respiratory tract infections in an infant.

Bony deformities

These result from pathological fractures (in rickets, osteoporosis, and osteopetrosis), or from disturbances at the growth plate (in rickets). The latter result in:

- Widening of the metaphyses of the long bones, which may be clinically palpable at the wrists, knees and ankles
- Progressive bow-legs, knock-knees, or windswept deformities
- Frontal and parietal bossing of the skull in the young infant and craniotabes
- Harrison's sulcus (which may also occur in children with cardiac or chronic pulmonary problems)
- Rickety rosary
- Kyphoscoliosis may occur as a compensatory abnormality
- Spinal deformities due to vertebral fractures in osteoporosis.

A degree of bow-legs occurs normally in infants and young children, and disappears with age;

but, if progressive, should be investigated. Blount's disease (*see* Chapter 31, Orthopaedic disorders) may give rise to severe bow-legs in the young black child.

Short stature

This is a feature in children with long-standing rickets, in particular those due to renal phosphate loss. These children may be classified as having disproportionate short stature, as may children with severe osteogenesis imperfecta or bone dysplasias (*see also* Chapter 19, Endocrine disorders).

Developmental delay

A delay in gross motor milestones (*see* Chapter 2, Growth and development) is due to the hypotonia and muscle weakness characteristic of vitamin D deficiency. Motor milestones are generally normal in children with X-linked hypophosphataemic rickets and dietary calcium deficiency.

Developmental milestones such as the closure of cranial fontanelles and the eruption of primary and secondary teeth, may also be delayed in privational rickets.

Hypotonia

Hypotonia and proximal muscle weakness are characteristic features of rickets associated with vitamin D deficiency or with abnormalities of vitamin D metabolism. The presence of hypotonia/muscle weakness helps to differentiate vitamin D deficiency from X-linked hypo-phosphataemic rickets. Unlike the hypotonia and muscle weakness associated with other conditions (*see* Chapter 26, Neurological and muscular disorders), deep-tendon reflexes are often brisk in children with rickets.

Convulsions

Generalized seizures and/or apnoeic attacks may occur in association with hypocalcaemia and may also be associated with other clinical features of low plasma ionized calcium values, such as *tetany* (carpopedal spasm), tingling of the fingers, a positive Chvostek's sign, or Trousseau's sign (*see* Chapter 10, Metabolic disorders) and laryngospasm. Generally, hypocalcaemia of sufficient degree to cause seizures only occurs in the early stages of vitamin D deficiency in young infants (usually less than one year of age) or in severe rickets. In the former, there may be no clinical signs of vitamin D deficiency and hypocalcaemia will only be diagnosed if serum calcium measurements are made in any young infant with convulsions.

Metabolic bone disease in children may present clinically in one of several ways:

- **Osteomalacia and rickets**, in which there is failure of, or delay in, mineralization of uncalcified osteoid or bone matrix. Thus the ratio of uncalcified osteoid to calcified bone is increased. Rickets manifests as a delay in mineralization at the growth plate and thus only occurs in children whose epiphyses have not yet fused. Osteomalacia refers to a delay in mineralization at the endosteal bone surface and thus occurs in both children and adults. In children, rickets and osteomalacia occur concomitantly.
- **Osteoporosis**, in which the total amount of bone per unit volume is decreased. The ratio of uncalcified osteoid to calcified bone is normal. The pathogenesis is related to either inadequate formation of bone matrix or to increased resorption of preformed bone.
- **Osteosclerosis**, in which there is an increase in calcified bone per unit volume, generally due to a failure of normal bone resorption or an increase in bone formation.

Acidosis

The presence of rapid breathing in a child should draw attention to the possibility of a metabolic acidosis or associated with soft ribs and thoracic cage abnormalities.

Recurrent lower respiratory tract infections in an infant

These may indicate underlying pulmonary complications due to soft pliable ribs and ineffective ventilation secondary to rickets or osteogenesis imperfecta (Lethal type – OI type II).

It should be noted that osteomalacia and osteoporosis frequently may be found together in the same patient, and that in renal failure all forms of bone disease may occur together.

Rickets

Rickets is the only form of metabolic bone disease occurring commonly in children. Important points to remember:

- There are a number of different causes of rickets. It presents typically with progressive bone deformities and with a delay in motor milestones.
- In infants, vitamin D deficiency is the most common cause. It occurs most frequently in those who were born prematurely, who are breastfed, and who live in overcrowded urban communities, where exposure to sunlight does not occur.
- In older children, dietary calcium deficiency and the inherited forms of hypophosphataemic rickets are more common.
- In the young infant, the prevention of vitamin D deficiency is important. This may be achieved by encouraging mothers to expose their infants to sunlight for short periods every day.

The diagnosis of rickets in a primary health care situation

Figure 12.1 provides a schematic approach to the management of a child with suspected rickets in a primary health care situation.

Clinically, mild rickets is extremely difficult

to diagnose accurately, as the signs are often difficult to assess, and are not pathognomonic of active rickets. In the child with gross bone deformities, other diseases such as osteogenesis imperfecta should also be considered. Craniotabes, although a sign that should alert the health professional to the possibility of rickets, is frequently a normal finding in young infants (especially in those who were born prematurely). Rachitic rosary and widening of the wrists are difficult signs to interpret, especially in the thin child. It is therefore advisable that a child should not be treated for rickets without radiological confirmation of the disease. Further, if the child is walking (i.e. older than a year to 18 months), biochemical support should be obtained to help elucidate the aetiology of the rickets, as vitamin D deficiency is less likely in the child who can walk and therefore get out into the sun. In the infant, vitamin D deficiency is likely to be the cause, and a trial of therapy with vitamin D can be initiated without biochemical confirmation; it

is important that the infant returns for radiological confirmation of healing of the rickets approximately eight weeks after initiating therapy. If healing is not evident on the radiographs or the child is outside the infant age group, then biochemical investigations are helpful in differentiating the various causes (*see below*).

A urine dipstick to detect the presence or absence of glycosuria, proteinuria, and alkaline pH is a useful screening test to exclude Fanconi's syndrome and renal tubular acidosis.

The patient who does not respond to vitamin D therapy, or who has features consistent with other causes of rickets, should be referred to a centre for further investigation and initiation of therapy.

Vitamin D-deficiency rickets as a public health problem

During the 19th and early 20th centuries, rickets was a major public health problem in industrial-

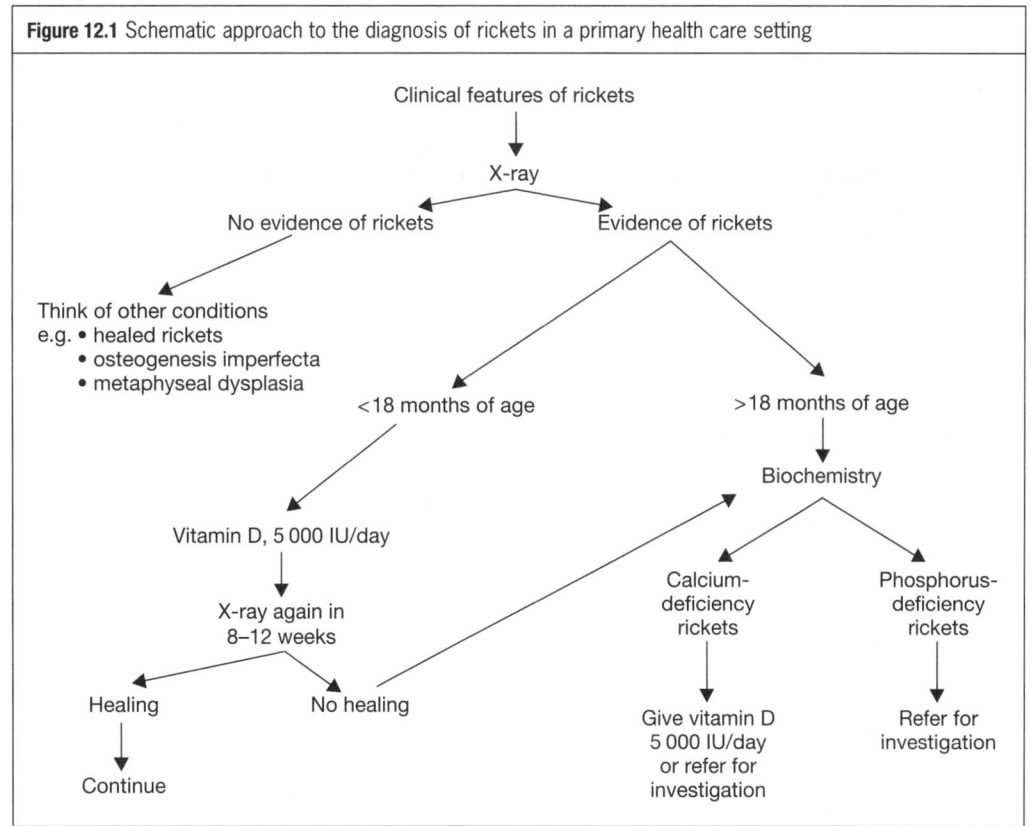

Figure 12.1 Schematic approach to the diagnosis of rickets in a primary health care setting

ized countries. Effective public health measures, such as the provision of vitamin D drops and the vitamin D supplementation of milk and certain other foods, had almost completely eradicated vitamin D deficiency from Europe and America by the middle of the last century. However, in Britain rickets is still seen in Asian children due in part to the high melanin content of the skin decreasing the amount of vitamin D formed by suboptimal ultraviolet light exposure, the lack of skin exposed to sunlight due to clothing, the lack of vitamin D in the diet, and the low calcium and high phytate content of the typical vegetarian diet. Furthermore, in the USA the prevalence of rickets is once again increasing in breastfed infants born to African American mothers who themselves are often vitamin D deficient during pregnancy, and in Europe among children of immigrant communities from Africa, the Asian subcontinent and the Middle East.

In developing countries, the problem of rickets has perhaps been largely neglected because attention is concentrated on more serious conditions, such as malnutrition, gastroenteritis, and infectious diseases. In southern Africa, accurate figures of the prevalence of rickets are not available; it appears, however, that the prevalence of vitamin D deficiency has decreased dramatically over the last three decades, although it is still seen in infants living in high rise buildings in the inner city areas of Johannesburg.

Globally, several factors predispose infants to rickets, the most important of which are:

• A lack of sunlight exposure, especially in an urban environment where air pollution is marked, and particularly in communities living in the extremes of latitude
• Increased skin pigmentation which prevents adequate conversion of 7-dehydrocholesterol to vitamin D, especially during the winter months in countries at high latitude.
• Cultural traditions, which prevent adequate sunlight exposure of the skin, for example wearing clothes that completely cover the skin, or customs that keep the pregnant mother or infant indoors away from sunlight
• Vegetarian diets
• Prolonged breastfeeding without vitamin D supplementation
• Infants delivered to mothers who are vitamin D deficient.

Vitamin D deficiency is not of short-term interest only, but can lead to considerable morbidity and mortality if not prevented or detected early. Growth failure and limb deformities are well recognized, but pelvic deformities leading to obstructed labour in later life, apnoeic attacks and convulsions in the young infant, and severe chest deformities leading to recurrent pneumonia and respiratory failure are perhaps less often considered as complications of rickets. Furthermore, epidemiological studies are suggesting that vitamin D deficiency might also alter immune function and increase the risk of asthma and type 1 diabetes and predispose subjects to an increased risk of certain cancers.

With the disappearance of vitamin D-deficiency rickets as a major public health problem, the rarer and more complex causes of rickets have become more apparent, although probably not more common.

Metabolism of vitamin D

In order to understand the pathogenesis of rickets, a knowledge of the role of vitamin D and its metabolites in the control of calcium homeostasis is necessary (see Figure 12.2).

Vitamin D, the generic parent compound, may be in the form of either vitamin D_3 (cholecalciferol), which is obtained from skin synthesis, or vitamin D_2 (ergocalciferol), which is obtained from irradiated plant material.

People acquire vitamin D either through the absorption of ingested vitamin D or by the conversion of 7-dehydrocholesterol to vitamin D_3 in the skin under the influence of ultraviolet irradiation (sunlight). Most diets are deficient in vitamin D and thus people rely on that formed in the skin to prevent the occurrence of vitamin D deficiency.

Once absorbed from the gastrointestinal tract or formed in the skin, vitamin D is either stored in muscle and fat, or transported to the liver where it is hydroxylated to 25-hydroxyvitamin D (i.e. 25-OHD), the major circulating form of the vitamin. Both these compounds are inactive in people at physiological concentrations. When 25-OHD is transported to the kidney, it undergoes further metabolism. Under the influence of parathyroid hormone (PTH) or hypophosphataemia, 25-OHD is hydroxylated to 1,25-dihydroxyvitamin D (i.e. 1,25-$(OH)_2$D), the active metabolite. Thus 1,25-$(OH)_2D$ plays a central role in calcium homeostasis. Its principal sites of action are the gut, where it promotes calcium, and to a lesser extent phosphorus, absorption, and bone, where it acts synergistically with parathyroid hormone to increase bone resorption. Both of these actions increase the serum concentrations of calcium and phosphorus. 1,25-$(OH)_2D$ also appears to have important paracrine actions on a vast array of tissues in the human body influencing cell differentiation and function.

Figure 12.2 The metabolism of vitamin D. Vitamin D is converted to 25-OHD_3 in the liver, while both 1,25-$(OH)_2D_3$ and 24,25-$(OH)_2D_3$ are formed in the kidney

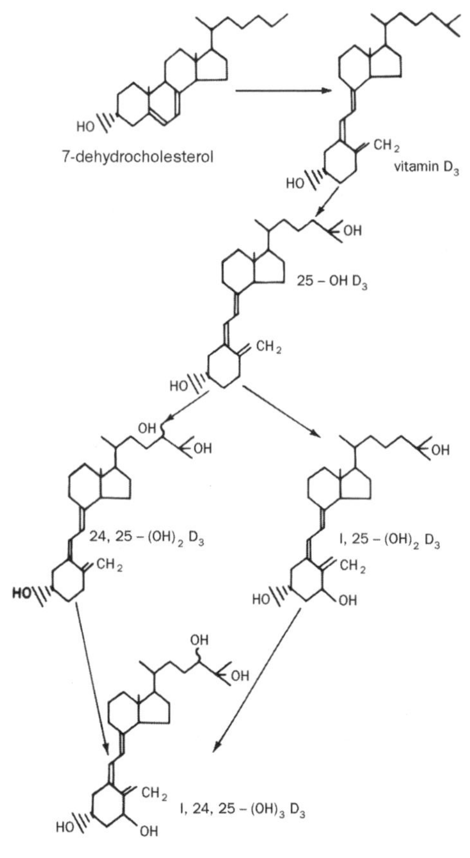

Causes of rickets

The causes of rickets may be divided into:

- Those primarily resulting in an inadequate supply of calcium (calcium-deficiency rickets)
- Those primarily producing hypophosphataemia (phosphorus-deficiency rickets).

Table 12.1 lists the common causes of rickets.

Table 12.1 The causes of rickets/osteomalacia in children

Calcium-deficiency rickets

a. Abnormalities in vitamin D metabolism

Nutritional rickets
- dietary deficiency of vitamin D; inadequate exposure to sunlight

Impaired absorption of vitamin D
- steatorrhea, e.g. coeliac disease
- biliary obstruction, e.g. biliary atresia impaired hydroxylation of vitamin D to 25-hydroxyvitamin D
- liver immaturity
- prematurity

Increased metabolism of vitamin D
- anticonvulsant drugs, e.g. phenobarbitone

Decreased renal synthesis of 1,25-dihydroxy-vitamin D
- renal failure
- vitamin D-dependency rickets

End-organ resistance to 1,25-dihydroxyvitamin D

b. Dietary deficiency of calcium
- diets deficient In dairy products

Phosphorus-deficiency rickets

Decreased intake of phosphate
- prematurity

Decreased intestinal absorption of phosphate
- ingestion of large amounts of aluminium hydroxide

Increased renal losses of phosphate
- hypophosphataemic vitamin D-resistant rickets: X-linked sporadic
- Fanconi's syndrome
- mesenchymal tumours

Calcium-deficiency rickets

The causes of calcium-deficiency rickets are those that are associated with a lack of vitamin D, with abnormalities in its metabolism to 1,25-(OH)$_2$D, with end-organ resistance to 1,25-(OH)$_2$D or with a dietary lack of calcium. (See Figure 12.3.)

Lack of vitamin D or abnormalities of vitamin D metabolism

Nutritional vitamin D deficiency

Aetiology. The aetiology is an inadequate vitamin D intake, coupled with a lack of exposure to sunlight. Once the infant is walking (one to two years of age) vitamin D deficiency is rarely seen in South Africa because of the abundant sunshine.

Breast milk contains only very small quantities of vitamin D or its metabolites. Their concentrations are normally insufficient to meet the daily requirements of the breastfed infant, who is thus dependent on sun exposure or vitamin D supplementation to maintain an adequate vitamin

D status. Cow's milk contains almost no vitamin D. Thus, all infant milk formulae in South Africa are supplemented with vitamin D (400 IU/l) to prevent vitamin deficiency in infancy. Except in the rare case where the mother is vitamin D deficient, rickets does not manifest in the first few months of life. The reason for this is that 25-OHD$_3$ crosses the placenta, and at birth the neonate's levels correlate well with maternal concentrations.

Clinical features. (See Table 12.2.) In the early stages of vitamin D deficiency, bone deformities are not present. The infant may pass through this phase with no symptoms whatsoever and present later with bone deformities; or may present early with apnoeic spells or convulsions due to hypocalcaemia. Laryngismus stridulus, a peculiar tremulous crowing inspiratory noise due to tetany of the vocal cords, is a rare clinical sign of hypocalcaemia due to vitamin D deficiency. This is found particularly in the young infant. Craniotabes, the sign elicited by being able to depress the skull bones above and behind the ears, is often present in young infants presenting with rickets, but is not pathognomonic of the

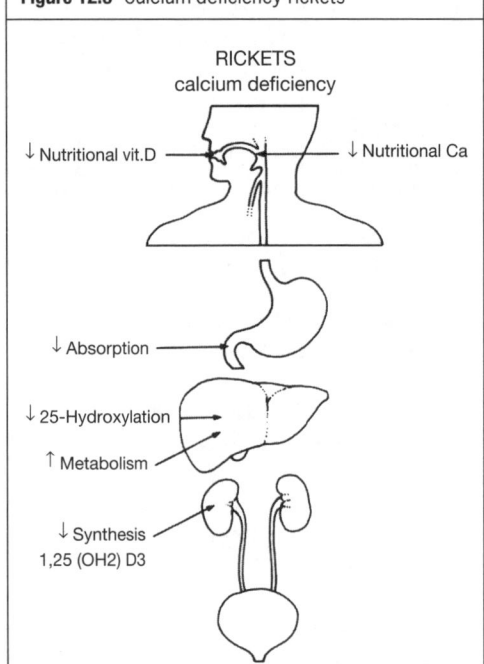

Figure 12.3 Calcium-deficiency rickets

RICKETS
calcium deficiency

↓ Nutritional vit.D

↓ Nutritional Ca

↓ Absorption

↓ 25-Hydroxylation

↑ Metabolism

↓ Synthesis
1,25 (OH2) D3

Table 12.2 The clinical features of vitamin D-deficiency rickets
Signs of hypocalcaemia
– convulsions
– apnoeic attacks
– tetany
– laryngospasm
Signs of muscle weakness
– hypotonia
– delayed motor milestones
– prominent abdomen
Signs of delayed mineralization
– widened metaphyses (especially wrists and knees)
– craniotabes in the young infant
– delayed closure of fontanelles
– enlarged costochondral junctions (rickety rosary)
– Harrison's sulcus
– deformities of the long bones (bowing, knock-knees, windswept)

disease. Muscle weakness may be a prominent feature of vitamin D deficiency; the weakness being more apparent in the proximal muscles. Delayed motor milestones are frequently found.

Rickets in the infant presents in its severest form with bone deformities, particularly involving the wrists, legs, chest-cage, and skull. The severely affected infant has a protuberant abdomen and sweats excessively. Such infants commonly suffer from recurrent chest infections and bronchopneumonia.

Chest deformities such as Harrison's sulcus involving the lower ribs, and the violin case deformity of the upper ribs are due to the effects of the diaphragm and intercostal muscles acting on abnormally pliable and soft ribs. The metaphyses of the wrists, ankles, and knees may become palpably enlarged. Enlargement of the costo-chondral junctions produces the rickety rosary. The child who lies with his head frequently turned to one side may develop an asymmetric skull. The fontanelles are often large and closure is delayed. Frontal and parietal bossing may give the typical hot-cross bun appearance. Dentition may also be affected, with a delay in the eruption of primary dentition and, if rickets has been present for a prolonged period of time, enamel hypoplasia may occur. The extent and site of the deformities are determined largely by pressure effects such as those occurring during crawling. Leg deformities include knock-knees or bow-

The radiological features consist of:
- Delay in epiphyseal development
- Widening of the growth plate (>1mm distance between the epiphysis and metaphysis)
- Splaying and cupping of the metaphysis
- Irregularity and fraying of the end of the metaphysis
- The bones are osteopenic with thin cortices and a coarse trabecular pattern
- Signs of hyperparathyroidism such as subperiosteal erosions may be present.

legs. In the young infant anterior bowing of the distal tibia may occur. Signs of hypocalcaemia may also be present.

Radiological features. (*see* Figure 12.4) The radiological features of early rickets are difficult to detect as they consist only of a decrease in the bony density due to inadequate calcification. This demineralization is most easily seen on lateral skull radiographs. Some blurring of the metaphyseal plates may be seen on radiographs of the wrists.

On the other hand, the radiological features of severe rickets are diagnostic. The best sites to assess the presence of rickets are those of rapid bone growth, i.e. the wrists and knees.

In addition to the features listed above, pathological fractures and bone deformities

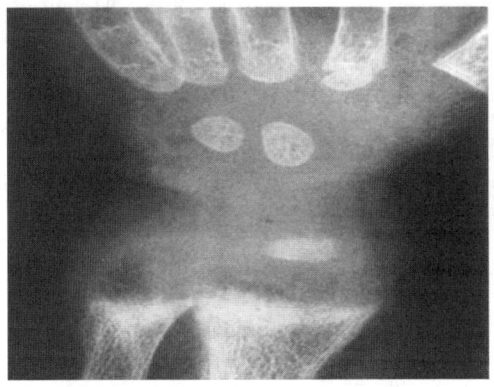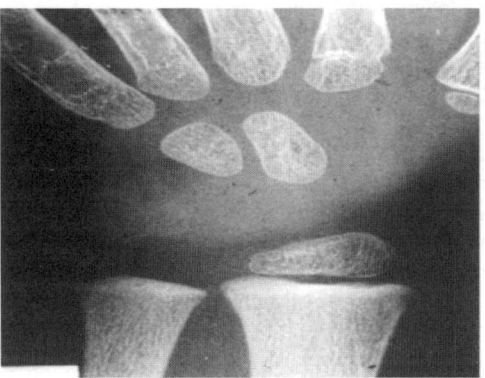

Figure 12.4 Nutritional rickets in a young child. Note the widening of the growth plate and the splaying, fraying and loss of the distinct zone of provisional calcification at the distal end of the metaphysis. The radiograph on the right is of the same wrist taken several months after the commencement of treatment with vitamin D 5 000 IU/d.

may be seen, corresponding to the clinical abnormalities identified. The radiographic bone deformities may persist even after healing has occurred. Healing of rickets can be observed radiographically by demonstrating an increasing density at the zone of provisional calcification of the metaphyseal plate. The metaphyseal cupping becomes progressively less evident and there is less fraying and irregularity. Then the growth plate narrows and remodelling occurs.

Biochemical features. The biochemical features depend on the degree and duration of vitamin D deficiency and the effect of compensatory physiological mechanisms. The typical biochemical features of vitamin D deficiency are hypocalcaemia, hypophosphataemia, elevated serum alkaline phosphatase concentrations, elevated parathyroid hormone levels, and low 25-OHD values. The urinary excretion of calcium is decreased (less than 2 mg/kg/24 hours), while phosphate and cyclic AMP excretion is increased. A generalized amino aciduria occurs and in some cases, glycosuria has been noted. These urinary changes are probably due to the effects of hyperparathyroidism on the renal tubule.

Prior to the development of severe bone deformities, hypocalcaemia may be the only abnormal biochemical finding. However, with the development of secondary hyperparathyroidism, serum phosphorus values fall and alkaline phosphatase concentrations rise.

The normal values of certain parameters used to detect and classify the various types of rickets are age dependent. Serum phosphorus concentrations are highest in the immediate neonatal period (1.8–2.6 mmol/l), falling rapidly over the next six months to a plateau (1.3–2.0 mmol/l) which persists until puberty, when values gradually fall to adult levels (<1.3 mmol/l). In infancy, concentrations of alkaline phosphatase may be slightly higher than throughout childhood (100–300 IU/l). During the adolescent growth spurt, values rise (often up to 500 IU/l) and then fall rapidly to adult levels (<100 IU/l). Serum calcium values (normal 2.25–2.75 mmol/l) change little throughout life, although there is a slight fall from childhood to old age. Total serum calcium values are dependent on albumin concentrations, thus hypocalcaemia could be due to an actual decrease in ionized calcium levels or to hypoalbuminaemia (of particular relevance in the malnourished child).

Treatment. Vitamin D deficiency is easily corrected by oral administration of vitamin D (1 000–5 000 IU/day) for a period of six weeks to three months. Within a month biochemical improvements will be observed and early evidence of radiological healing will be noted. If hypocalcaemia is a prominent feature, calcium supplements may be necessary in the early stages of treatment. If convulsions or apnoeic attacks occur, calcium gluconate (10%, 1–2 ml/kg) may be given slowly as an intravenous infusion, while the heart rate is closely monitored. In the young child, bone deformities may correct spontaneously over a period of months, thus orthopaedic correction of any deformities should be delayed as long as possible.

Prevention is as important as the curative treatment of vitamin D deficiency. Even in South Africa with its abundant sunshine, an adequate vitamin D intake should be ensured, particularly during the first year of life. The average diet contains little vitamin D, and cow's milk is almost devoid of vitamin D. It is thus recommended that all infants should be supplemented with vitamin D (400 IU/day) from birth, unless they are on a fortified milk formula, or adequate exposure to sunlight is ensured.

Impaired absorption of vitamin D

Dietary vitamin D, being fat-soluble, is absorbed by a mechanism similar to that of dietary fats. Thus any condition causing steatorrhoea may impair vitamin D absorption. If adequate exposure to sunlight occurs, the reduction in intestinal vitamin D absorption may be compensated for and not produce any deleterious effects. However, in infants or sick children not exposed to ultraviolet light, vitamin D deficiency may develop. Large doses of vitamin D (10 000–50 000 IU/day) may be necessary to overcome the malabsorption. The problem is further compounded by a concomitant calcium malabsorption due to the formation of insoluble calcium soaps with the malabsorbed fatty acids. In infants, neonatal hepatitis and biliary atresia might lead to severe rickets through this mechanism.

Impaired hydroxylation of vitamin D to 25-hydroxyvitamin D

Impaired formation of 25-OHD in the liver may occur in severe liver disease, and it has been suggested as a cause of rickets in premature infants who have an immature hepatic enzyme system. This latter possibility has not yet been adequately documented.

Increased metabolism of vitamin D

Anticonvulsants, especially phenobarbitone, increase hepatic hydroxylation and excretion of vitamin D. Further, diphenylhydantoin directly blocks calcium absorption from the intestine and may also impair bone mineralization. Thus, anticonvulsants may predispose children to a higher prevalence of rickets by several mechanisms. This is particularly so in institutionalized children, whose vitamin D intakes may be sub-optimal. The problem can be overcome by supplementing the diet with vitamin D (1 000 IU/day).

The biochemical features of anticonvulsant rickets are similar to those described in vitamin D deficiency. However, the serum alkaline phosphatase concentration is a poor indicator of the presence of rickets, as alkaline phosphatase levels may be elevated due to an increase in the serum concentrations of the hepatic iso-enzyme. The latter rise is a manifestation of the hepatic effects of phenobarbitone rather than an indicator of bone disease.

Decreased renal synthesis of 1,25-dihydroxyvitamin D

Vitamin D-dependency rickets is a rare, autosomal recessive condition which presents in infancy with a picture similar to that seen in vitamin D deficiency. However, the bone disease only responds to large doses of vitamin D (25 000–50 000 IU/day). Unlike vitamin D deficiency, vitamin D-dependency rickets is associated with normal serum levels of 25-OHD, but low to very low $1,25\text{-}(OH)_2D$ concentrations. The disease responds dramatically to physiological doses of $1,25\text{-}(OH)_2D_3$ (0.5 µg/day). Studies have found mutations in the gene encoding for the $1\text{-}\alpha\text{-}$hydroxylase enzyme, which converts 25-OHD to $1,25\text{-}(OH)_2D$ in the kidney. This form of rickets is very rare in South Africa.

Renal failure is associated with decreased levels of $1,25\text{-}(OH)_2D$ and may present with rickets and osteomalacia, but the bone disease of renal failure (renal osteodystrophy) has a complicated pathogenesis. Early on in the development of renal failure, decreased renal excretion of phosphorus leads to hyperphosphataemia, secondary hypocalcaemia, and concomitant hyperpara-

thyroidism. Long-standing hyperparathyroidism leads to osteoporosis, osteitis fibrosa cystica, and osteosclerosis. The secondary hyperparathyroidism can be partially controlled by the administration of an oral phosphate-binding agent such as calcium carbonate, which decreases serum phosphorus concentrations. Besides secondary hyperparathyroidism and $1,25\text{-}(OH)_2D$ deficiency, chronic acidosis may aggravate bone loss in chronic renal failure. Aluminium hydroxide should not be used as a phosphate binding agent in renal failure as the absorbed aluminium has toxic side-effects on bone.

Radiologically, the features of renal osteodystrophy are variable, with signs of either secondary hyperparathyroidism or rickets and osteomalacia predominating. Epiphyseal slipping and epiphysiolysis may occur and lead to severe deformities of the limbs.

The biochemical abnormalities of renal osteodystrophy can be distinguished from other forms of rickets, because of the elevated serum creatinine and urea levels characteristic of renal failure. Further, although hypocalcaemia is a feature of other forms of vitamin D-related rickets, hyperphosphataemia is usually found only in renal osteodystrophy.

Treatment requires careful monitoring. Serum calcium and phosphorus concentrations should be maintained within the normal range by means of calcium supplementation and phosphate-binding agents. Vitamin D therapy may be required, particularly if osteomalacia is a prominent feature, but the dose needed varies widely from patient to patient, and therefore should only be increased slowly. More recently, $1,25\text{-}(OH)_2D_3$ (Rocaltrol®) or 1α-cholecalciferol (One Alpha®) has been used in place of vitamin D with good results. In some instances, partial parathyroidectomy may be required to control the hyperparathyroid bone disease.

End-organ resistance to 1,25-dihydroxy vitamin D

A rare syndrome of peripheral resistance to $1,25\text{-}(OH)_2D$ has been described (vitamin D-dependency rickets type II). These children present with features of calcium-deficiency rickets, do not respond to the usual therapeutic doses of vitamin D, and have markedly elevated serum concentrations of $1,25\text{-}(OH)_2D$. This syndrome is not a single disease entity, as several different mutations in the gene coding for the intracellular vitamin D receptor have been described. The net effect of these receptor defects is a failure of response of the target organs to normal circulating concentrations of 1,25-$(OH)_2$D. One apparently homogeneous disease entity within this syndrome is associated with total alopecia. Treatment of this condition is unsatisfactory as the patients respond only partially to massive doses of 1,25-$(OH)_2D_3$ or to large oral calcium supplements.

Dietary deficiency of calcium

Low dietary calcium intakes are a recognized cause of osteoporosis in animals and have been implicated in the pathogenesis of involutional osteoporosis in humans. However, only recently has this deficiency been shown to lead to rickets and osteomalacia in vitamin D-replete children. Several cases of rickets in rapidly growing infants on very low calcium diets have been reported.

Studies conducted in South Africa, Nigeria and Bangladesh suggest that children in these countries may suffer from a similar problem, due to the low calcium content of their diets, if milk or other dairy products are not consumed on a regular basis. Patients with this condition generally present between three and 16 years of age with leg deformities characteristic of rickets, hypocalcaemia, variable serum phosphorus concentrations, elevated alkaline phosphatase values, and normal serum 25-OHD levels. Radiographs reveal the presence of osteopenia and active rickets at the metaphyses of the long bones. The features of rickets on X-ray may be so mild as to be missed at a cursory glance, but all have histological evidence of osteomalacia on bone biopsy. The biochemical and radiological abnormalities respond to calcium supplementation without the addition of vitamin D. Dietary calcium intakes are estimated to be between 100 and 300 mg/day in these children (recommended dietary intake: 800–1 200 mg/day).

It is apparent that vitamin D deficiency and dietary calcium deficiency are at two ends of the spectrum of causes of privational rickets. It is becoming clearer that many infants and children with privational rickets have a combination of both vitamin D insufficiency and low dietary calcium intakes which combine to exacerbate the onset of rickets.

Phosphorus-deficiency rickets

Phosphorus depletion, despite an adequate vitamin D intake, may lead to the development of rickets. Unlike calcium or vitamin D deficiency, the disease is not accompanied by secondary hyperparathyroidism. Thus, low urinary calcium excretion and a generalized amino-aciduria are generally not features of the disease. Furthermore, phosphorus depletion can be differentiated from vitamin D or calcium deficiency, because phosphorus depletion is characteristically normocalcaemic.

The causes of phosphorus-deficiency rickets may be grouped into two large categories:
- those associated with inadequate intake or impaired absorption
- and those associated with a failure of renal conservation of phosphorus (increased renal excretion).

Decreased intake of phosphorus

The average diet usually contains more than enough phosphorus to meet requirements. However, premature infants fed on soya-bean milk preparations have been reported to develop rickets, which has responded to phosphorus supplementation. Soya-beans, like cereals, contain a portion of their phosphorus in the form of phytates, a complex phosphate molecule from which phosphorus is thought to be poorly absorbed. Furthermore, in breastfed very low-birth-weight neonates (<1 500 g) the low phosphorus intakes are thought to be responsible for the elevated alkaline phosphatase values, osteopenia, and rickets in these infants which become manifest at about 12 weeks of age. Although breast-milk contains sufficient mineral to sustain the growth of healthy full-term infants, the phosphorus content is insufficient to meet the requirements of the rapidly growing VLBW infant. Thus it is now recommended that if very low-birth-weight infants are fed breast milk, the feed should be supplemented with calcium and phosphorus.

Decreased intestinal absorption of phosphorus

Unlike calcium, phosphorus absorption by the intestine is only partially controlled by body needs and is generally very efficient. Although $1,25\text{-}(OH)_2D_3$ does increase phosphate absorption, it is little impaired in vitamin D-deficiency states. Phosphorus absorption can be inhibited, however, by the ingestion of a phosphate-binding agent such as aluminium hydroxide, which is frequently used as an antacid in the treatment of peptic ulceration. If phosphate absorption is impaired sufficiently to induce hypophosphataemia, rickets and osteomalacia may occur.

Increased renal excretion of phosphate

Phosphate excretion by the kidney is controlled mainly in the proximal tubule. Although the mechanisms are not fully understood, two separate mechanisms have been described, one sensitive to parathyroid hormone and the other sensitive to calcium.

Hypophosphataemic vitamin D-resistant rickets

The classic example of this syndrome is X-linked hypophosphataemic rickets (XLH). The disease has been linked to mutations in the PHEX gene (Phosphate-regulating gene with homology to endopeptidases on the X chromosome). Clinically, it is characterized by early growth failure, bone deformities, and excess renal phosphate loss. Biochemically, normocalcaemia and normal concentrations of parathyroid hormone distinguish it from the vitamin D-related causes of rickets. Further, unlike Fanconi's syndrome, there is no amino-aciduria, and glycosuria is uncommon. In countries where vitamin D fortification of all milks is routine (e.g. the USA), it has become the most common form of rickets seen in hospital. In South Africa, it occurs in all racial groups, but the prevalence is unknown.

Although generally inherited as an X-linked condition, some 30 per cent of cases appear to be the result of sporadic mutations. Affected males and females appear to have similar phenotypes, which vary considerable from one child to another. Muscle weakness, a feature of vitamin D-related causes of rickets, is absent in this condition. The diagnosis is made by confirming a low tubular reabsorption of phosphorus in the absence of hyperparathyroidism.

Radiologically, the picture is that of rickets, although signs of secondary hyperparathyroidism are absent. Osteopaenia is also generally not seen.

Treatment is aimed at correcting the persistent hypophosphataemia. This is achieved by increasing the oral intake of phosphorus (Joulies solution: 1.5–3 g phosphorus/24 hours in five divided doses). As the increased phosphate load impairs calcium absorption and induces hypocalcaemia and secondary hyperparathyroidism, $1,25\text{-}(OH)_2D$ or 1-alpha cholecalciferol at a dose of 0.5–1 µg/d is also given. If treatment is adequate, growth rates usually increase and the bone disease heals. At present, treatment is recommended until late adolescence when growth has stopped and the epiphyses have fused. Treatment may be needed again in later life, when symptomatic osteomalacia may occur.

Fanconi's syndrome

Fanconi's syndrome does not constitute a single disease entity, but all are associated with proximal renal tubular dysfunction. In the severest form, the syndrome consists of phosphaturia, hypokalaemia, amino-aciduria, glycosuria, proximal renal tubular acidosis, and an absence of renal concentrating ability. Rickets and short stature are but two of the presenting signs, other features being more prominent depending on the aetiology.

Cystinosis, an autosomal recessive disease characterized by the deposition of cystine crystals in many tissues, is associated with progressive renal failure, hepatomegaly, acidosis, and hypo kalaemia.

Lowe's syndrome (oculocerebrorenal syndrome) is characterized by mental retardation, cataracts, and glaucoma, together with Fanconi's syndrome.

Other causes of Fanconi's syndrome include tyrosinaemia, galactosaemia, hereditary fructose intolerance, Wilson's disease, and toxicity due to heavy metals such as cadmium and lead. An idiopathic form of the disease also exists. Treatment is mainly symptomatic, with $1,25\text{-}(OH)_2D$ and phosphate supplements being used to treat the phosphaturia and rickets. Potassium and citrate or bicarbonate supplements may be needed if potassium wasting and renal tubular acidosis are present. Despite vigorous therapy, growth and development may remain poor.

Distal renal tubular acidosis

Distal renal tubular acidosis should be considered in any child with failure to thrive, unexplained acidosis and rickets. Typically the children present with hypophosphataemia, phosphaturia and hypercalciuria and an alkaline urine in the face of a metabolic acidosis. Children generally respond rapidly to alkali therapy (Shohl's solution or bicarbonate at a dose of 2–3 mmol/kg/day in 3–4 divided doses).

Tumour-induced rickets/osteomalacia

Rarely, children may present with hypophosphataemic rickets due to phosphaturia produced by phosphatonins (fibroblast growth factor 23 (FGF-23) and matrix extracellular phosphoglycopotein (MEPE)), that are secreted by mesenchymal tumours. Unlike X-linked hypophosphataemic rickets, tumour-induced osteomalacia presents more commonly with marked osteopaenia, muscle weakness, fatigue and fractures. Removal of the tumour corrects the biochemical abnormalities and heals the bone disease.

Osteoporosis

Osteoporosis usually manifests clinically with fractures after minimal or no trauma, rather than bone deformities as occurs in rickets. The diagnosis of osteoporosis is difficult as the facilities for the accurate assessment of bone mineral content are not available in most hospitals (the technique required is dual energy X-ray absorptiometry (DXA)). Thus the diagnosis is dependent on the subjective impression of thin cortices and decreased bone density on routine X-rays. The picture is further complicated in older children, in whom growth has ceased, because osteomalacia may present with a similar radiological pattern to that of osteoporosis. However, the two syndromes can usually be differentiated biochemically, as osteoporosis is generally associated with normal serum calcium, phosphorus and alkaline phosphatase concentrations.

Osteoporosis is an unusual problem in clinical paediatric practice, although a number of chromosomal abnormalities, such as Down's syndrome, have decreased bone density. Table 12.3 lists the more frequent causes of osteoporosis in paediatrics.

The paediatrician or general practitioner is much more likely to be consulted by parents who are worried that their apparently normal child might have osteoporosis, as he/she had fractured his/her forearm while playing. It should be remembered that approximately 50 per cent of boys and 30 per cent of girls will have fractured one or more bones sometime during their childhood (it appears that the fracture rate may be lower in black than white children in South Africa). The peak fracture rate is during the adolescent growth spurt. There is some evidence that children who fracture have slightly lower bone mass than children who do not, however there is no indication for the active treatment of these children, rather the parents and children should be reassured once the child has been examined to exclude other causes of osteoporosis.

Table 12.3 Causes of osteoporosis
Decreased bone matrix formation: • osteogenesis imperfecta • corticosteroid excess or steroid-induced (osteoporosis) • protein-energy malnutrition • vitamin C deficiency • copper deficiency
Increased bone resorption: • immobilization • marrow hyperplasia, e.g. thalassaemia • juvenile osteoporosis • hyperparathyroidism, e.g. renal failure

Decreased bone matrix formation

Osteogenesis imperfecta

(*See* Figure 12.5)

Osteogenesis imperfecta is an inherited disorder characterized by decreased bone formation due to abnormalities in collagen synthesis. It is not a single disease entity, the majority of cases being inherited as autosomal dominant traits with several different clinical presentations. Mutations in the genes coding for the collagen molecules have been documented at a number of different sites in patients with osteogenesis imperfecta. Because of the numerous different genetic defects possible, the diagnosis of osteogenesis imperfecta by means of gene probes is not widely available.

Osteogenesis imperfecta is typically divided into four clinical subgroups, although another three rare subgroups (Types V-VII) have been recently added to the classification:

♦ **OI I**, which is usually a mild disease associated with blue sclera and deafness in adulthood. Fractures of the long bones may occur, but are relatively infrequent, and become less frequent once adolescence is reached. This form is inherited as an autosomal dominant condition. Teeth defects (dentinogenesis imperfecta) may also be seen (25 per cent). Stature is generally normal or only mildly affected.

♦ **OI II** is the lethal form of osteogenesis imperfecta. It is inherited as an autosomal dominant condition (although many cases are new mutations) and usually presents with multiple intra-uterine fractures, severe bone deformities at birth and death in the neonatal period.

♦ **OI III** is also inherited as an autosomal dominant trait, but is less severe than OI II: fractures are frequent in this group of children and bone deformities may develop. The sclera are often blue. The children are typically short statured with shortened limbs and have a triangular facies. Dentinogenesis imperfecta occurs in 80 per cent.

♦ **OI IV** is inherited as an autosomal dominant, but tends to be more severe than OI I; the sclera in this form of the disease are normal. Short stature is variable, and dentinogenesis imperfecta occurs in approximately 60 per cent.

Hydrocephalus may be a complication of osteogenesis imperfecta. Dentinogenesis imperfecta is a dental defect that may or may not be present in patients with osteogenesis imperfecta due to the lack of dentin, which contains collagen Type I. The teeth appear stained and translucent, and are subject to early development of caries. Other common clinical manifestations are those of joint hyperlaxity and hypermetabolism (increased sweating, heart rate and temperature).

The radiographs in osteogenesis imperfecta may vary from a picture of mild to severe osteoporosis with fractures, extremely thin cortices, and narrowing of the total width of the bone. The skull may show multiple wormian bones with platybasia.

Until recently, no specific therapy was available for the treatment of osteogenesis imperfecta. However, over the past few years the use of bisphosphonates in the management of severe OI has shown considerable promise. Fractures heal well with adequate callus formation, but care must be taken

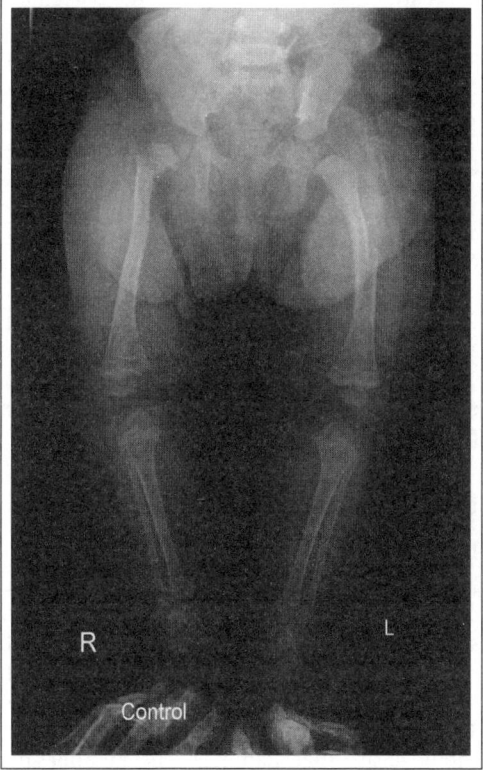

Figure 12.5 Osteogenesis imperfecta in a 10-month old child. Note the thin cortices, mid-shaft fracture of the left femur, shepherd-crook deformity of the femoral necks, and dense metaphyseal transverse line as a result of a single intravenous dose of bisphosphonates given some months previously.

to prevent deformities and limb shortening. Bisphosphonate therapy has been shown to increase bone mass, reduce bone pain, improve mobility and probably reduce fracture Incidence.

A multidisciplinary approach in the form of physiotherapy, corrective surgery for deformities and counselling is mandatory in the management of these children in order to improve their quality of life.

Corticosteroid excess or steroid-induced osteoporosis

Cushing's disease, due to adrenal tumours or excess ACTH secretion, is relatively rare in children but is associated with osteoporosis secondary to endogenous hypercortisolism. However, corticosteroid therapy is used fairly frequently in a number of paediatric disorders such as juvenile rheumatoid arthritis, juvenile dermatomyositis, Duchenne muscular dystrophy and nephrotic syndrome. Steroid-induced osteoporosis is generally more severe in children who receive corticosteroids daily, as compared with those who receive therapy on alternate days.

The pathogenesis is, firstly, a failure of adequate matrix formation due to a direct effect of the steroids on the osteoblast, and, secondly, a block in calcium absorption from the gastrointestinal tract. Osteoporosis is further aggravated by the development of secondary hyperparathyroidism due to decreased calcium absorption, and by immobilization, which often results from the primary illness that is being treated with corticosteroids.

Treatment of the osteoporosis is difficult once bone loss is far advanced. However, the block in calcium absorption can be overcome by the administration of large doses of vitamin D and calcium supplements. To be effective, this form of therapy should be started early in the course of the disease.

Protein-energy malnutrition (PEM)

Although fractures are rarely a problem, most children admitted to hospital with protein-energy malnutrition have radiological evidence of osteoporosis. The aetiology of this is multifactorial, but protein deficiency probably plays a major role. Many of these infants are also on low calcium diets. Treatment should be aimed at correcting the primary nutritional deficiency.

Vitamin C deficiency

In paediatric practice, scurvy is now a rare disease, but most cases of scurvy occur in the second half of the first year in infants fed almost exclusively on cow's milk.

Clinically, scurvy presents in the infant with irritability, loss of appetite, and tenderness of the long bones. This may be associated with a refusal to sit or stand. Eventually the child refuses to move, lying with the arms and legs semi-flexed. Movement of the limbs elicits acute pain. Swelling and ecchymoses around the joints may also be noted.

The radiographic changes are usually characteristic: the bones are generally osteopenic, with a ground-glass appearance of the shaft. The cortices are thin but well defined. The zone of provisional calcification at the growing ends of the bones is well demarcated, but beneath this line is an area of rarefaction.

Subperiosteal haemorrhages, which produce the severe bone pain, are generally not visualized on admission; however, when healing occurs, the elevated periosteum calcifies, and the extent of the haemorrhages can be seen.

Treatment should be aimed at the prevention of vitamin C deficiency; thus, vitamin C supplementation of the diet should be recommended during the first year of life. Scurvy responds to vitamin C therapy (250 mg/day).

Copper deficiency

With the advent of prolonged intravenous alimentation for various gastrointestinal disorders, particularly chronic diarrhoea, cases of copper deficiency are now being reported. Copper deficiency leads to anaemia, neutropenia, and severe osteoporosis. Metaphyseal lesions may also be noted, but these can usually be differentiated from those produced by vitamin D deficiency.

Increased bone resorption

Immobilization

Immobilization of any limb may produce marked osteopenia. In paediatrics this is most commonly seen in children with myelomeningoceles, with resulting paralysis of the legs. It is also seen in the affected limbs following poliomyelitis. Therapeutically, there is little to offer, but carers should ensure that vitamin D deficiency does not aggravate the problem as many of these children do not spend time in the sun.

Hyperplasia of the bone marrow

Chronic haemolytic anaemias, especially thalassaemia major, may be complicated by osteoporosis, with marked thinning of the cortices and extreme fragility of the long bones. Specific therapy is not available to correct the osteoporosis.

Hyperparathyroidism

Primary hyperparathyroidism is a rare disease in children; however, secondary hyperparathyroidism complicates a number of conditions, such as vitamin D deficiency and renal failure.

Hyperparathyroidism may present with osteoporosis or osteitis fibrosa cystica (where resorbed bone is replaced by fibroblasts and connective tissue). The characteristic radiological features of hyperparathyroidism are localized areas of subperiosteal resorption of bone, seen particularly along the metacarpals or phalanges. The lateral ends of the clavicles may also be severely demineralized. The lamina dura, a dense line of bone around the teeth, disappears due to resorption. Metaphyses may become ragged and frayed, so as to resemble the abnormalities seen in rickets.

The treatment of hyperparathyroid bone disease depends on whether the aetiology is primary or secondary. Treatment of primary disease requires the removal of the parathyroid glands, while the treatment of secondary hyperparathyroidism is directed towards treatment of the primary cause, such as renal failure.

Juvenile osteoporosis

Juvenile osteoporosis is a disease of unknown aetiology, which presents in late childhood with symptomatic osteoporosis. The disease may be difficult to differentiate from mild cases of osteogenesis imperfecta, but the absence of any family history may be helpful. Symptoms usually subside once the patient reaches puberty, and at present there is no specific therapy, but bisphosphonates may be helpful.

Osteosclerosis

Osteosclerosis is characterized by increased density of bone, secondary to an abnormality in bone resorption and remodelling. Although dense, the bones may be abnormally brittle. Except for the patchy increase in bone density that may occur in renal osteodystrophy, osteosclerosis is uncommon; thus, only two of the causes will be discussed.

Osteopetrosis

Osteopetrosis may be inherited as either an autosomal dominant or recessive trait. The pathogenesis of osteopetrosis is typically a failure of production of osteoclasts or a lack of function of the formed osteoclasts, resulting in a failure of bone remodeling and modeling with accumulation of bone.

The autosomal recessive condition is invariably fatal unless therapy is undertaken. It is associated with anaemia, neutropenia, thrombocytopenia, increased susceptibility to infections, extra medullary erythropoiesis and complications due to nerve compression. Deafness and blindness occur due to the entrapment of the

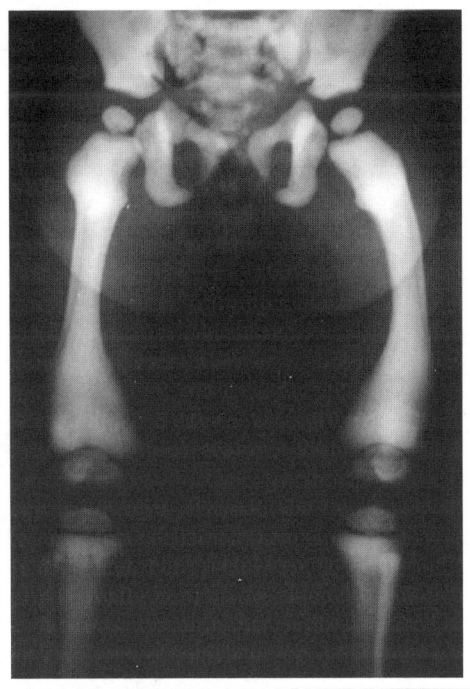

Figure 12.6 Osteopetrosis. Note the very dense bones with no medullary cavity and the abnormal modelling.

cranial nerves as they pass through the skull, and hydrocephalus may develop. Dental sepsis is frequent, with osteomyelitis of the jaw occurring as a complication.

Radiologically, all the bones are excessively dense, with tubular bones having no marrow-cavity (*see* Figure 12.6).

Hand radiographs may reveal the classic 'bone within a bone appearance'. Recently, bone marrow transplants have had some success in reversing this condition.

The autosomal dominant variety of osteopetrosis is a milder disease, symptoms only becoming apparent in adolescence or adulthood. Skeletal X-rays show alternate zones of osteopetrosis and relatively normal bone, while unlike the recessive condition, the medullary cavity is maintained. Anaemia is unusual in the dominant form, but nerve compression, with deafness and blindness, still occurs.

Diaphyseal dysplasia

This disease usually presents in early childhood with tender swollen legs and muscle weakness. The diaphyseal portions of long bones are markedly thickened and hyperostosis of the skull may occur. Anaemia and elevated erythrocyte sedimentation rates have been reported. No specific therapy is available; however, corticosteroids may help to relieve bone pain and improve muscle power.

13

Nutritional disorders

A steady supply of nutrients is required for the maintenance of biological function and, in childhood, for normal growth and development. In the absence of a regular supply of nutrients in the quantities required by the child, there is a biological cost. This expresses itself in a variety of ways, from subtle alteration only, through to obvious and major disorders of structure and function that inhibit normal interaction with, and response to, the child's internal and external environment.

A normal nutritional state is therefore vitally important for normal health. The body adapts to undernutrition initially to maintain vital functions as far as possible; this usually involves slowing down of cell growth and differentiation, as well as decreasing the metabolic rate. Disease occurs when adaptation fails or when additional metabolic demands result from infective stress. Accordingly, nutritional disorders evolve through stages depending on the duration, degree, and pattern of deficiency, as well as the presence of complicating and precipitating factors.

Nutritional disorders are very rarely manifestations of a pure, single-component deficiency. Usually there is multifactorial deficiency, and the clinical features depend on the interplay and relative proportions of nutrient imbalances.

Factors that predispose to undernutrition

Certain children have an increased risk of suffering from nutritional deficiencies. Clinical disorders of nutrition must be expected and specifically looked for in a child who has a history of one or more of the following:

- Was born prematurely or with low birth weight
- Is not being, or has not been, breastfed in poor social circumstances
- Is a twin
- Has diarrhoea, pneumonia, infectious disease, or tuberculosis
- Is affected or infected by HIV
- Has cancer or chronic disease
- Has a mother who is in poor social circumstances, in poor health, incompetent, or who already has many children
- Has a father who is an alcoholic or out of work
- Has lost a parent by death or desertion
- Has a working mother and there is inadequate child-minding
- Is in a home without piped water supply or other source of clean water.

Most patients suffer from several coexisting deficiencies. However, the most important determinant is the quantity and type of protein (as a source of essential amino acids) and energy available; accordingly the most important global nutritional disorder is protein-energy malnutrition (PEM).

> By far the most common nutritional disorder is undernutrition due to a lack of sufficient food intake, associated with poverty.

Assessment of the nutritional state

Clinical nutritional assessment

This is a vital component of every complete physical examination. It is performed as follows:

- **Dietary history**, to determine the amount and quality of nutrient intake and to indicate the possibility of deficiency. This must be obtained in a very sensitive and tactful way, as mothers may feel threatened by detailed questions regarding the way they feed their children.
- **Clinical nutritional assessment** is the clinical evaluation of parameters that may be affected by nutrient deficiencies. This is the simplest and most reproducible method, which is satisfactory in most instances.
- **Laboratory evaluation** of the nutritional state must complement clinical judgement. There is no definitive laboratory test which is entirely satisfactory for the assessment of protein-energy status.

The classical biochemical finding in PEM is a reduced serum albumin concentration. It is relatively insensitive as an index compared with the earlier manifestations of PEM, e.g. early growth failure.

Hypo-albuminaemia is caused by a variety of conditions (*see* Table 13.1).

Once serum albumin concentration is persistently below 30 g/l, it has been shown that there is a drop in serum insulin, a rise in human growth hormone, diminished serum valine and alanine, a drop in serum beta-lipoprotein and cholesterol, and a drop in serum colloid osmotic pressure.

Many other biochemical tests for PEM including measurements of transferrin, blood urea (which is always low), serum amino acid patterns, urinary hydroxyproline secretion, urinary creatinine-height index, 3-methylhistidine excretion, have been evaluated but have not proved to be useful in practice. Abnormalities of serum electrolyte concentrations such as hypokalaemia, hypocalcaemia, hypomagnesaemia, and low plasma zinc are frequently found, but are not diagnostic of PEM *per se*, but rather of its complications.

Clinical nutritional examination

This is done as follows:

- Anthropometry: measure and record weight-for-age, length-for-age, and weight-for-height
- Skin changes are seen in undernutrition:
  - desquamating, pigmented dermatosis (PEM, pellagra)
  - follicular hyperkeratosis and perifollicular haemorrhages (vitamins A and C)
  - peri-oral and peri-anal erythematous maculopapular rashes (zinc)
- Skin appendages:
  - brittle, discoloured hair (PEM, copper deficiency)
  - finger and toe nails (thinning, brittleness: PEM, calcium; koilonychia: iron deficiency)

Table 13.1 Mechanisms and conditions associated with hypoalbuminaemia

Mechanisms	Conditions associated with hypoalbuminaemia
Insufficient intake or absorption of dietary protein	Protein energy malnutrition (e.g. kwashiorkor, marasmus, intestinal malabsorption)
Reduced protein synthesis	Chronic liver disease (e.g. cirrhosis, liver failure)
Increased losses	Renal losses (e.g. nephrotic syndrome) Gut losses (e.g. protein losing enteropathy Surface losses (e.g. burns, bullous skin conditions, exudative conditions)
Catabolic states	Acute phase response (e.g. sepsis)

♦ Eyes:
- xerophthalmia, Bitot's spots, keratomalacia: vitamin A deficiency
- pale mucosa of haematinic deficiency

♦ Mouth and tongue:
- angular stomatitis (PEM, riboflavin)
- atrophic glossitis and mucosa (PEM, riboflavin, niacin)
- tongue colour changes (magenta in riboflavin deficiency; scarlet in niacin deficiency)

♦ Subcutaneous oedema (hypoalbuminaemia, sodium, and potassium disturbances)

♦ Subcutaneous tissue and fat: skinfold thickness (mainly energy balance)

♦ Muscle bulk (mid-upper arm circumference: PEM)

♦ Bones (rickets: vitamin D, calcium)

♦ Organomegaly:
- liver (fatty infiltration)
- thyroid (iodine)

♦ Mental state: iron, PEM, niacin.

Symptoms and signs of nutritional disorders

The following symptoms and signs are seen in nutritional disorders:
- Abnormally low or high body mass for age
- Growth faltering (nutritional dwarfing)
- Failure to thrive
- Oedema
- Frequent infections and delayed recovery
- Changes in body appearance.

Protein-energy malnutrition (PEM)

Epidemiology

PEM characteristically occurs among pre-school children in the age group six months to five years. However, no age group is immune, and juvenile and adult cases of PEM can occur under certain environmental, nutritional, and diseased (e.g. intestinal malabsorption) circumstances. Manifestations in older individuals are usually less frequent and clinically less obvious, because protein and energy requirements per kilogram mass are not as great as in childhood.

PEM is found where food is scarce and is particularly prevalent in the so-called developing world. There is a high prevalence in all countries of Africa, in India, South-East Asia, the Middle East, the Caribbean, and South and Central America.

In urban areas, PEM occurs in families of low socio-economic status and in broken homes. Here poverty, large numbers of children, lack of sophistication and education preclude the purchase of sufficient food and particularly sufficient high-protein foods. Cheap or refined carbohydrate foods tend to form the basis of the diet. Early cessation of breastfeeding compounds the problem. The worldwide migration of people from rural to urban areas is aggravating the PEM problem enormously and large numbers of children in squatter communities at the periphery of cities suffer from it.

In *rural* areas in poor countries PEM is endemic and increases in prevalence are seen during periods of drought, famine, or disaster. Cereal staples are often the only foods available under these conditions. When breastfeeding was universally practised well into the second year of life, children still obtained some high class protein from this source; in its absence, protein energy malnutrition is an inevitable consequence. Lack of water or contaminated water promotes intestinal and other infection, and this in turn worsens nutritional status.

Particularly in urban areas, the sociological phenomenon of the *working mother* has implications for the pre-school and primary school child. Many of these children have only two meals per day and on this they are unable to grow adequately and are at risk of PEM. Child-care facilities are often not available, inadequate, or episodic.

The prevalence of the individual syndromes of malnutrition varies in different communities and parts of the world. In a poor community, *severe* forms may make up 2–3 per cent of the child population, with 10–60 per cent of the same population suffering from *milder* forms. Age of weaning, availability of food, local or individual prejudices and customs, environmental and economic circumstances, and family stress are some of the more common factors that will collectively or individually determine prevalence and clinical picture.

Individual cases of PEM can occur where intake, absorption, or utilization of nutrients is interfered with by disease or dysfunction of most organ systems, but occur most notably in the presence of paediatric HIV, chronic diarrhoea and malabsorption.

The clinical syndromes of malnutrition are usually precipitated by an intercurrent stress such as an acute infection. In well-nourished communities, morbidity and mortality from gastroenteritis, measles, or tuberculosis is negligible, but this may be 20 to 50 times higher in poor communities due to the underlying malnourished state.

Causes of PEM

Intake of protein and/or energy below minimal requirements for growth and health is the basic underlying cause of PEM.

In children with borderline nutrition, infection precipitates PEM through its effect on reducing intake of and increasing requirements for nutrients because of the infection-mediated catabolic state.

The high worldwide prevalence is aggravated by food production and distribution failing to keep pace with population growth. It is to be noted that the intake requirements for children, particularly in the pre-school age group, are relatively greater per kilogram mass than those for adults. This is because of the demands for growth, and the younger a child, the faster his growth. It should also be appreciated that the quality of a food protein depends on the pattern and quantity of essential and non-essential amino acids that it contains. Requirements will therefore vary immensely with quality, e.g. when calculating protein requirements for a toddler in a sophisticated country, the doctor works on a considerably lower figure, e.g. 1–1.5 g/kg/day of egg, meat, milk, or fish protein, than his colleague in a developing country, where the basic diet is mixed vegetable or plain vegetable protein, 1.5–2.0 g/kg/day (*see* Table 13.2).

An illustration of the practical implications of the relationships between quality and quantity of protein and the nitrogen uptake in the tissues is shown in Figure 13.1.

It can be seen from this diagram that if milk is the source of protein, the nitrogen uptake at an intake of 200 mg/kg/day (protein 1.2 g/kg/day) is greater at that level than the uptake from a vegetable-based protein. At higher intakes, the milk and the vegetable-mix protein are equally effective. A poor quality protein, such as maize, has a very unsatisfactory nitrogen uptake at all levels. It can therefore never meet growth and health requirements, if fed without supplementation.

Figure 13.1 Relationship of source of protein to nitrogen retention. At low levels of absorption (intake), nitrogen from a vegetable mixture is not as well retained as it is from a mixture that contains a small amount of animal protein. At higher levels of absorption, nitrogen retention of a vegetable mixture equals that of milk. Therefore, when appetite is poor, animal protein or milk should be included in the diet.

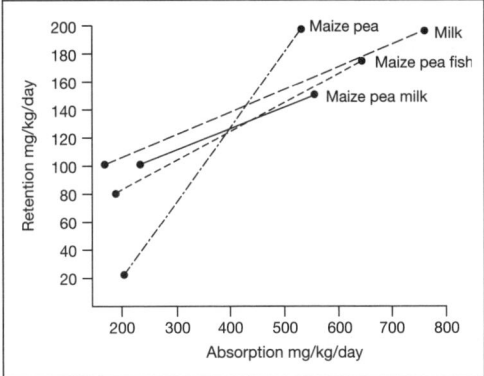

Table 13.2 Protein requirement			
Reference protein	**Milk, egg protein**	**Mixed veg. protein**	**Single veg. protein**
Chemical score	100	70	60
FAO/WHO requirement (g/kg/day)	1.19	1.70	2.08

All food contains energy or calories so there is no difference in energy requirement between vegetarian or animal protein diets; but an adequate energy intake is essential for proper utilization of protein. Energy requirement is made up of three components – maintenance, growth, and physical activity, as illustrated for a one-year-old child in Table 13.3.

The energy intake of children in developing countries is commonly 320 kJ/kg/day. This is only just enough for maintenance, with the result that there is no margin for growth and physical activity. Studies have shown that an energy intake of 30 per cent below normal results in marked reduction of physical activity. It is not surprising, therefore, that children with PEM have growth retardation and are apathetic and inactive, and this may affect the children's capacity for responding to their environment, and consequently the response to them by their caregivers, resulting in lack of stimulation and educability.

Protein quality, total protein, and energy intake are thus all equally important for optimal growth and development. If these are not supplied, for whatever reason, PEM will result. It will also occur where there is excessive loss of nutrients in diarrhoea, vomiting, intestinal fistulae, and malabsorption syndromes. The increased metabolic demands of infection, e.g. septicaemia, tropical disease, HIV disease and tuberculosis, will also precipitate PEM in instances where dietary therapy is neglected. Children hospitalized with these problems must be assessed regularly with regard to nutritional status.

Pathogenesis of clinical disease in PEM

The pathogenesis of clinical disease in PEM relates to failure of adaptation.

Table 13.3 Energy requirement		
		kJ/kg/day
Maintenance	1.5 BMR (220 kJ/kg)	330
Growth		20
Physical activity		80
	Total	430

Free radical damage occurs when infection-mediated free oxygen radicals are not removed or neutralized by the body's defence mechanisms, e.g. in conditions of deficiency of vitamins A and E, zinc, and of decreased activity of glutathione peroxidase. This results in cell membrane damage. Many of the clinical features of kwashiorkor, such as oedema, fatty liver, and excess mortality, can be ascribed to such free radical excess in circumstances of nutritional deficiency.

Aflatoxin or other environmental toxins can be shown to be accumulated in the liver of many patients with kwashiorkor. Such hepatotoxins have been postulated to be involved in the pathogenesis of the clinical features of kwashiorkor. On the other hand, the fatty liver of malnourished patients does not clear environmental toxins successfully, leading to tissue accumulation. In dry climates, there is little evidence of aflatoxin, but kwashiorkor certainly exists.

Classification of PEM

There is a spectrum of clinical syndromes that fall under the umbrella term of protein-energy malnutrition, ranging from kwashiorkor to marasmus and including pellagra. The criteria for distinguishing between them remain essentially clinical. Essentially, the clinical recognition of visible severe wasting and of the presence of bipedal oedema is important to identify severe malnutrition. A variety of classifications has been proposed to help interpret the anthropometric measurements of such children, but the use of Z-scores (standard deviation scores) of weight-for-age (WAZ) and weight-for-height (WHZ) is considered to be more useful in defining severity of malnutrition. Even though Z scores are not strictly comparable to percentile graphs, a Z score of 0 corresponds to the median (or 50th centile), and a Z score of –2 to approximately 80% of the median (or approximately the 3rd centile on a weight-for-age graph).

Pellagra, which has very similar clinical features to kwashiorkor, but which usually occurs above the age of six years, can also be regarded as a form of PEM. Although pellagra is specifically associated with deficiency of niacin, it must be appreciated that the precursor of niacin is the amino acid tryptophan, an essential amino acid.

Pathophysiology of PEM

Body composition

In PEM, there is a profound change of body composition. This involves the amount and distribution of body water, body fat, minerals, trace elements, and total body protein, particularly muscle wasting.

Total body water (TBW). With cessation or slowing of growth, there is a gradual increase of TBW as a percentage of body weight. This is mainly due to the disappearance of fat stores, and wasting of muscle and other tissues. There is an inverse relationship between being underweight and the total body water content. Thus children with marasmus who exhibit the most tissue wasting have the highest TBW. The high body water content of children with PEM resembles that of newborn infants. The children are therefore not only small for age, but have the body water composition of much younger children. Associated with an increase of TBW is a proportionate rise in extra-cellular fluid (ECF). Children with oedema have more water in the extra-cellular space than those without oedema. On recovery, some of the excess ECF is taken up into the cells and some is lost by diuresis, causing an initial loss of weight.

Potassium. Total body potassium is severely reduced in PEM. The loss is due to wasting of lean tissue and loss in diarrhoeal stools. The metabolic effects are promotion of oedema because of reciprocal sodium retention, hypotonia of muscles, diminished insulin secretion, and renal function disturbance. Serum potassium concentration correlates poorly with the overall potassium deficiency.

Other minerals. There is some evidence of a magnesium deficiency in PEM and autopsy studies have shown diminished total body calcium and phosphorus. Iron deficiency can occur as in any other condition.

Trace elements. Zinc deficiency occurs in PEM and aggravates ulcerative skin lesions. Zinc supplementation improves these and leads to better retention of nitrogen during recovery. Vanadium is considered to be an essential trace element affecting reproductive performance.

Total body protein. This is severely reduced in PEM. In particular, non-collagen protein is affected. Collagen protein is affected to a very limited extent.

Plasma proteins. In PEM, total albumin mass is reduced by about 50 per cent, the extravascular pool being more depleted than the intravascular pool. A striking feature of PEM is hypoalbuminaemia, which is more marked in kwashiorkor, but is also present to a lesser degree in many cases of marasmus.

On a low protein diet, both synthesis and catabolism of albumin are decreased and there is increased re-utilization of ammonia from endogenous urea. Muscle mass is greatly diminished and may be only 30 per cent of normal mass for age. This supports the concept that muscle acts as a buffer in the adjustment of protein metabolism to deficiency in the diet. The synthesis rate is reduced when dietary deficiency occurs and rises immediately when the diet is corrected. It appears to be controlled by the rate of amino acid supply, particularly the branched-chain amino acids. Rates of protein breakdown and synthesis are higher in marasmus than in kwashiorkor.

The metabolism of the gamma globulins and immunoglobulins is quite different. Serum immunoglobulins are normal or elevated. Synthesis and turnover are unaffected and may even be increased in the presence of infection.

Nitrogen balance. Protein is adequately digested, even though pancreatic enzyme function is reduced. Absorption of nitrogen may be reduced from a normal of 90 per cent to between 70 and 80 per cent of the intake. However, nitrogen retention is much more efficient in the child with PEM than in the well-nourished child, and again, full utilization is made of whatever protein is offered to a child with PEM.

Body fat. In marasmus, body fat may drop to as low as 5 per cent of body weight (normally 19 per cent). In contrast to marasmus, the child who develops kwashiorkor on a low protein but relatively high carbohydrate diet may have subcutaneous and other fat stores preserved to a remarkable degree.

Endocrine system

The endocrine glands show atrophy, affecting particularly the pituitary and adrenal glands, although there is little correlation between endocrine function and the macroscopic appearance of the glands.

Pituitary. Human growth hormone levels are normal or supranormal in both marasmus and kwashiorkor. Serum IGF-1 levels are, however, decreased by undernutrition. This appears to be an adaptive response which allows available substrate to maintain homeostasis rather than be used up for growth. Thyroid stimulating hormone (TSH) is elevated and TSH response to synthetic thyrotropin-releasing hormone is prompt, exaggerated and sustained with a normal reserve.

Thyroid. No evidence of thyroid deficiency or abnormality has been described in PEM. Once enough protein and energy are supplied in the diet, intense metabolism and growth occurs, and 'catch-up' growth is dramatic.

Adrenals. Plasma cortisol levels in kwashiorkor and marasmus are elevated. There is a prompt response to corticotrophin, suggesting reasonable functional reserve. Because of hypoalbuminaemia, there is decreased binding of cortisol and a higher 'free' content in the plasma. This may contribute to the clinical features of the 'moon facies', abnormal glucose tolerance, and oedema. Aldosterone secretion rates and plasma levels are also normal or elevated in PEM.

Clinical features of PEM

The clinical presentation of PEM depends very much on the degree and duration of protein and/or energy deficiency, the age of the individual, the previous nutritional status and modifications produced by disease, and by possible associated vitamin, mineral and trace element deficiencies.

> The mechanism of growth retardation in PEM is therefore not related to pituitary, adrenal, or thyroid dysfunction, but rather to the lack of energy and/or protein intake.

Table 13.4 summarizes the clinical features of the common PEM syndromes.

Growth faltering (nutritional dwarfing)

The first effect of protein-energy malnutrition (PEM) is on growth, as manifest by:

- Slowing or cessation in linear growth
- Slowing or cessation of weight gain, or weight loss
- Decrease in mid-upper arm circumference (MUAC)
- Delayed bone maturation
- Normal or diminished weight/height ratio
- Normal or diminished skinfold thickness.

The most useful indicators are weight and height. International reference levels derived from populations in optimal, stable nutritional environments should be used in the assessment of growth performance. The body mass can fluctuate acutely depending on acute changes in food intake, acute illness or starvation. Accordingly, body mass for age is an indirect measure of the total food energy recently available to the individual. A child with a body mass for age outside

Table 13.4 Clinical features of PEM

	Underweight	Marasmus	Kwashiorkor	Marasmic kwashiorkor
Weight	↓	↓↓	↓	↓↓
Height	↓	↓	↓	↓
Dermatosis	o	o	+	+
Oedema	o	o	++	+
Apathy, irritability	o	+	++	++
Muscle wasting	+	++	++	++
Enlarged liver	+/−	+/−	++	+
Anaemia	+/−	+	++	+
Infections	+/−	+	++	++

Key:	↓ = decreased	o = not present	++ = severe
	↓↓ = marked decrease	+ = mild	+/− = presence variable

the normal range (<3rd centile or >97th centile) has only a 3 per cent chance of being normal.

In areas where marasmus and kwashiorkor are found, there are many children whose dietary deficiency has not been sufficiently severe to produce clinical disease or symptoms. These children are underweight and stunted, while at the same time they have relatively normal body proportions, e.g. weight-to-height ratios. Because of the latter the diagnosis of PEM is frequently missed unless weight and height for age are charted. There are no specific physical stigmata and the only biochemical abnormality may be a slightly reduced serum albumin concentration. Children with this type of mild PEM are very susceptible to the effects of infections such as gastroenteritis, respiratory disease, or infectious fevers, e.g. measles and tuberculosis.

Patterns of growth failure vary considerably. There may be *acute weight loss or wasting* due to recent restriction of energy or due to underlying infection or malabsorption. Here there will be a diminished weight-to-height ratio. At the other extreme, *chronic shortage* of protein and/or energy leads to failure of weight and height gain or *stunting*, with a normal or little changed weight-to-height ratio. Other parameters, such as mid-upper arm circumference (MUAC), skinfold thickness, and bone age maturation, are useful to assess growth where age is not known. Eruption of deciduous teeth may be delayed slightly in PEM, but there is much less effect than that occurring on height, weight, and bone age.

It is essential that all health workers recognize underweight or growth-retarded children by ensuring regular growth and weight monitoring. Any child who is below the 3rd percentile weight or height for age must be suspected of suffering from PEM (<80 per cent expected weight or <90 per cent expected height). Failure to appreciate the underlying presence of PEM in patients who present with a variety of ailments will lead to

> - Low weight-for-age in a normally grown individual reflects mainly energy deficit
> - Low height-for-age reflects the totality of long-term nutrition, endocrines, and health
> - Weight-for-height deficit indicates recent weight loss or wasting.

ineffective therapy, repeated hospital visits, and frequently a fatal outcome.

Kwashiorkor

This is a severe and characteristic form of PEM. It occurs mostly after weaning from the breast or bottle, its maximum prevalence being between nine months and two years, but no age group is immune. The diet is commonly devoid of milk or other high protein food, and consists principally of refined carbohydrate, cereal and/or vegetable foods. Presenting symptoms are mainly those of failure to thrive, oedema, anorexia, diarrhoea, skin and mucous membrane lesions, and misery or apathy.

On clinical examination the important features are the following:
- **Growth failure**, as manifested by low body weight and decreased length for age. Oedema and excess subcutaneous fat from a high carbohydrate diet may give a deceptively chubby appearance.
- **Muscle wasting**. This causes increasing weakness resulting in an inability to run, walk, sit or hold the head up.
- **Oedema** first appears on the dorsum of the feet or over the lower tibia. It can be slight, or generalized and gross, depending on the state of hydration, and the availability of salt and water in the diet. Ascites rarely occurs and this is a distinguishing point in the differential diagnosis of renal, hepatic, and cardiac oedema. The presence of oedema is a striking physical sign in kwashiorkor as opposed to marasmus. It is also a fact that a child with 'marasmus' can become oedematous overnight and thus becomes a 'marasmic kwashiorkor'.

  The pathogenesis of the oedema is complex but closely related to total body potassium depletion (from diarrhoea), and reciprocal retention of sodium and water. Hypersecretion of antidiuretic hormone (ADH) and aldosterone does not appear to be important in this respect. Certainly, potassium supplements early in treatment speed up the resolution of oedema. It is aggravated by the low colloidal osmotic pressure of the plasma (hypoalbuminaemia), decreased cardiac output and lowered glomerular filtration rate, infection, and anaemia. Deficiency of vanadium has been postulated to stimulate the sodium pump and so promote oedema.

- **Dermatoses**. These are pellagroid in type and characterized by dryness, scaling and pigmentation ('crazy paving') and depigmentation where skin has flaked off ('flaking enamel paint'), pseudo-purpura or even bullous desquamation. The skin changes may extend over the whole body or be localized. Sometimes they develop acutely. In gross cases their appearance is similar to a burn. The lesions are distributed in exposed and unexposed areas of skin like groin or flexures, in contrast to pellagra where lesions occur in exposed areas only. In toddlers the perineum and buttock areas are particularly affected. The mouth often shows reddening with atrophied tongue papillae and fissuring at the corners (angular stomatitis). The hair is sparse, thin, easily pulled out and in tropical regions, changes its colour to red or grey. The eyes may reveal xerophthalmia as there is frequently an associated vitamin A deficiency.

- **Immune suppression**. Malnutrition and infection are very closely interlinked. The child who is malnourished is often infected, while infection in the sub-optimally nourished child may precipitate frank marasmus or kwashiorkor. Infections in such children tend to be more severe, are more frequently associated with complications and account for a higher mortality. There is a three-way relationship between malnutrition, immunodeficiency, and infection: PEM leads to immuno-deficiency, which predisposes to infection, which further aggravates the nutritional state. This condition has been termed the **Nutritionally Acquired Immune Deficiency Syndrome (NAIDS)**. The combination of NAIDS and common childhood infections is considered to be the leading cause of human mortality, accounting for up to 10 million childhood deaths per year.

The frequency and severity of infections in PEM is explained by the observed defects in the immune response. This is supported by the

Immunodeficiency

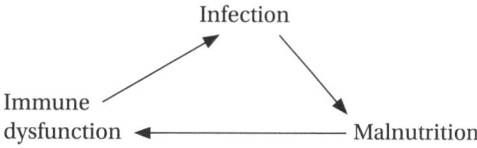

clinical finding of anergy. While this results in a lower incidence of clinical allergy, it also causes a decreased ability to deal with and recover from infection. Even serious infection can be silent and unaccompanied by fever. Hidden infections must always be suspected in any child presenting with malnutrition.

Deficiencies of vitamins A and C, nutrients such as iron and folate, and trace elements such as zinc may also cause a predisposition to infection.

- **Infections** Depression of CMI may encourage severe infection, in particular measles and Herpes simplex infection, tuberculosis, moniliasis, and gastro-enteritis. Malnutrition is one of few circumstances (the others being the neonate, HIV disease, malignancy, and measles) in which herpes virus tends to disseminate and cause convulsions, hepatomegaly, purpura, pox-like herpes skin lesions, collapse, and death. Tuberculosis is common and debilitating, and as the tuberculin test is often negative despite the presence of active tuberculosis, a routine chest X-ray is indicated. In poor environmental conditions malnourished children are particularly susceptible to respiratory and gastro-intestinal infections, and to septicaemia. The risk of Gram-negative septicaemia is serious enough to

> Immune deficiency manifests as predominantly decreased cell-mediated immunity (CMI), but abnormalities occur in all limbs of the immune response: inverted T-helper/suppressor cell ratios, diminished eosinophil and natural killer-cell numbers, diminished responses to T-cell dependent antigens, decreased secretory IgA responses, decreased complement, transferrin, lysozyme and interferon.

warrant aggressive therapy. *Pneumocystis jirovecii* may cause a progressive pneumonia which is difficult to diagnose. *Giardia lamblia* infestation of the bowel is common and aggravates the nutritional deficiencies. Intestinal parasites such as roundworms and hookworms are almost invariably present.

- **Mental and neurological changes**. Apathy and irritability are always present. The children are constantly unhappy and there is no play activity. A few children develop Parkinsonian-like tremors ('kwashi shakes', Kahn's syndrome) which disappear after two to three weeks of treatment.
- **Liver enlargement**. A large fatty liver is characteristic of PEM, especially kwashiorkor. Microscopically the fat appears first in the periportal area and then spreads to the central vein area. With recovery, the fat disappears from the liver in about three weeks and follow-up biopsies have failed to reveal any damage. The lipid that accumulates is triglyceride and has a similar fatty acid pattern to adipose tissue. Plasma lipids, particularly cholesterol, triglycerides, and phospho-lipids, are usually low in kwashiorkor and low to normal in cases of marasmus. Free fatty acids (FFA) are raised in both conditions. On refeeding, plasma triglycerides and cholesterol rise dramatically.
- **Other features** frequently associated with kwashiorkor include abdominal distension (pot belly) with small-bowel dilatation, glucose intolerance and hypoglycaemia, possibly related to deficiency of glucagon or diminished lean tissue, e.g. muscle, which in turn means lessened stores of glycogen, hypokalaemia that may cause ileus, and anaemia due to protein and iron or folic acid deficiency. A less frequent finding is purpura due to low platelets and bleeding due to low prothrombin.
- **Diarrhoea** is a major problem in PEM, so it is not surprising that there are profound structural and functional changes in the gut. Macroscopically, the bowel is atrophic throughout its length. The mucosal changes range from almost normal to severe villous atrophy, with only convolutions or ridges being seen. On light microscopy, the brush border of the mucosal cells may be abnormal and there is a lymphocyte and plasma cell infiltrate in the mucosa and submucosa. On electron microscopy, there are gross epithelial cell changes, with a sparse brush border and shortened microvilli. The nuclei are irregular and there is disorganization of the mitochondria and cytoplasmic organelles. The disaccharidase enzymes are frequently diminished, especially lactase, and this may be related to the mucosal atrophy. Marked improvement of the mucosal histology and of the enzyme levels occurs with dietary therapy, though in some children, lactase deficiency may become permanent as a consequence of an anticipation of the genetically determined primary adult hypolactasia. The functional effects of the above changes are manifested by lactose intolerance and in some cases, sucrose and glucose intolerance. With regard to protein absorption, there is little effect, except in cases with severe diarrhoea. Fat malabsorption does, however, occur and lasts for a short while after treatment has commenced. It is due to low pancreatic lipase levels, reduced transit time, impaired micellar solubilization of lipids, and decreased conjugated bile acids. Infection, e.g. with *Giardia lamblia*, may be important in producing malabsorption. (*See also* Chapter 24, Gastrointestinal disorders.)

The pathogenesis of the diarrhoea of PEM has, therefore, several factors of which the following seem important:

- Enteric infection with pathogens (e.g. salmonellae, shigellae, *Escherichia coli, Entamoeba histolytica, Giardia lamblia*) viruses (e.g. rotavirus), and intestinal moniliasis, have all been identified to

Clinical features of severe kwashiorkor include:
- Drowsiness or stupor
- Poor capillary filling
- Temperature <35 °C
- Significant infection (e.g. pneumonia)
- Persistent diarrhoea
- Obvious anaemia
- Jaundice
- Failure to respond to out-patient therapy.

a greater or lesser degree in different geographical situations. Contamination of the upper small bowel with bacteria is also thought to contribute.

◆ The grossly atrophied bowel mucosa with abnormalities of digestion and absorption.

The prognosis is poor in kwashiorkor patients with severe infection, hypothermia, hypoglycaemia, jaundice, and collapse due to dehydration.

Marasmus

This is the childhood equivalent of starvation and occurs when the diet is grossly deficient in energy. Such a diet also necessarily fails to meet protein requirements. Marasmus is mostly commonly seen during the first year of life. It occurs most frequently after early weaning onto dilute or low energy (density) bottle feeds or cereal paps, or due to prolonged severe diarrhoea with severe malabsorption or other infections. In the age group one to five years, marasmus occurs when grossly too little food of any kind is available, such as under conditions of war, civil unrest, famine, and extreme poverty, or if there is a lack of care.

The presenting symptoms are failure to thrive, irritable crying, or, alternatively, apathy. Diarrhoea is frequent and vomiting is sometimes a complaint. The children are usually ravenously hungry, but some are anorexic.

On examination, the child has a shrunken, wizened, stark appearance due to the absence of subcutaneous fat. The degree of underweight for age is extreme, the children being less than 60 per cent of their weight for age. Voluntary muscles are weak and atrophic. The dermatosis, hair changes, mucous membrane lesions, and oedema characteristic of kwashiorkor are not features of pure marasmus. A mixed picture, however, often occurs (*see* marasmic kwashiorkor). Where marasmus complicates chronic diarrhoea, patients may have a distended abdomen with visible peristaltic loops, the stool pH is low and shows reducing sugars on Clinitest® or even glucose on dipstick examination.

In the differential diagnosis, nutritional marasmus due to deficient intake must always be distinguished from the severe weight loss resulting from persistent diarrhoea, chronic infections such as tuberculosis, AIDS, and tropical infestations. Such patients demonstrate obvious wast-

ing by a much reduced weight for height ratio. Psychological factors, especially maternal deprivation, can be severe enough to bring about marasmus through depression of appetite or through rumination.

Marasmic kwashiorkor

The pure syndromes of marasmus and kwashiorkor are probably not so common as the many borderline cases and intermediate conditions which have some clinical signs of both. This is because, in practice, diets vary enormously and sometimes from season to season. Local conditions determine the availability and intake of carbohydrates, water, minerals and vitamins.

In addition, infection and diarrhoea modify presenting symptoms and signs. The term marasmic kwashiorkor is used to describe the wasted intermediate forms of PEM which have a variety of clinical dematoses and/or oedema characteristic of kwashiorkor. Confusion sometimes arises when a child who appears to be marasmic is admitted to hospital and becomes, by definition, a case of kwashiorkor overnight because oedema and skin lesions are more apparent when hydration has improved.

Ambulatory treatment of mild to moderate PEM

The early identification and management of preclinical malnutrition is the greatest challenge for the primary health care worker who can prevent many infections and other morbidity by simple nutritional intervention. In a child who has been attending a clinic for healthcare, the occurrence of clinical malnutrition represents a failure of the healthcare system.

Many different forms of supplementation have been introduced in various parts of the world, making use of locally produced foods. The aim of these is to improve the biological value of the protein, and increase the protein and energy content of the staple foods.

In Africa, staples such as maize, bread, or rice can be supplemented by milk, egg, or fish, but these, if indeed they are available, are expensive. Vegetable protein supplements such as beans, peas, lentils and nuts (peanuts) are excellent substitutes for animal protein.

If milk is available, it remains the best form of

The most important aspects regarding the provision of nutritional supplementation to an ambulatory patient are as follows:

- As much as possible use should be made of available staple foods. Advice on increasing the usual diet by introducing an extra one or two meals a day will frequently suffice. Even if the diet is of poor quality, giving more will supply more protein and energy. No small child can grow on less than three meals per day and usually requires five meals just to be able physically to eat adequate quantities. Increasing the energy density of weaning foods by the addition of oil or margarine will also assist in supplying basic requirements.
- Specific supplements, whether of energy or protein, should be cheap and easily available. Skim milk powder, 2 teaspoons/kg/day added to the food, will supply an extra 1.5 g/kg/day of protein.
- Changes in diet should be acceptable to the patient, the mother, the family, and the traditions of the community.
- The child must be followed up to confirm an improvement in weight gain.

protein supplement for a basic cereal diet. There is 1 g of protein in each 30 ml whole or skimmed milk. This means that 30–60 ml milk/kg of body mass will supply 1–2 g protein/kg which is sufficient, together with the basic diet, to cover any child's protein requirement. Even 15 ml milk/kg/day added to a cereal diet will be sufficient to promote recovery and prevent malnutrition. From a practical point of view, 600 ml milk added to the pot of porridge daily would be sufficient for four children.

Clinics usually have dried milk powder or other sources of high-protein foods to issue to patients who need protein supplementation in treatment over the short term. Ready-to-use therapeutic foods (RTUF) are increasingly being made available. Here it is important to appreciate that it takes much time and patience on the part of doctors, nurses, and nutritional advisors to obtain the understanding and cooperation of the mother.

Follow-up is essential for every case and the best measure of efficacy of dietary treatment is weight gain, which should be monitored at least until the child has reached the normal centile range in the Road-to-Health Chart (*see* Chapter 4, Community paediatrics, child health and survival).

Any child presenting with mild PEM should be checked and treated for infection including intestinal parasites, the social and economic circumstances assessed, and advice and assistance given where possible.

Hospital treatment of severe PEM

These children should be hospitalized because of the danger of death from dehydration, electrolyte disturbances, hypoglycaemia, and infection. Treatment can be divided into the phases described below:

Table 13.5 Guide to outpatient or inpatient management of malnutrition

Outpatient supplementary feeding	Hospital care
For uncomplicated malnutrition: all the criteria below:	For severe/complicated malnutrition:
Weight for height >70% of expected (WHZ >−3)	Marasmus or kwashiorkor PLUS any of the following:
No oedema	Anorexia
Clinically well	Dehydration
Eating well	Lethargic or unwell
Not lethargic	Fever ≥38.5 °C Pneumonia Severe anaemia Severe diarrhoea

Resuscitation and stabilisation (First day) Dehydration, severe anaemia (Hb less than 6 g per decilitre), hypoglycaemia, and electrolyte imbalances must be managed appropriately in the first instance. A dehydrated child with a satisfactory peripheral circulation (i.e. not in shock) receives oral rehydration fluid (Sorol® or equivalent), 10 ml/kg/hour until he passes urine and his hydration has improved. (*See also* Chapter 24, Gastrointestinal disorders.) In the presence of shock or severe anaemia, Ringer's lactate with 5% dextrose, plasma or blood should be given initially at a dose of 15 ml/kg within one hour. If the child's status starts to improve, a further 15 ml/kg should be given over the next hour and then fluid therapy is switched to oral rehydration with Sorol®. This therapy will assist in correcting dehydration and acidosis. During the period of resuscitation, no food or milk should be given. This precaution lessens the complication of vomiting and gastric distension that frequently occurs if feeding is started before adequate circulatory stabilization; however, feeding should be resumed as soon as possible thereafter.

Metabolic management. Mineral supplements in the form of potassium, (3–4 mmol/kg/day) and magnesium (0.4–0.6 mmol/kg/day), have been found helpful in correcting gross deficiencies. Zinc sulphate or acetate in a dose of 2 mg/kg/day, and copper (0.3 mg Cu/kg/day) assist in correcting possible deficiencies of these trace elements.

Hypoglycaemia. Routine blood glucose screening is mandatory because patients may be too ill to mount a sympathetic response to hypoglycaemia (blood glucose <3 mmol/l), which may then go undetected. Mild asymptomatic hypoglycaemia should be treated with 10 per cent dextrose water, 50 ml orally, and be followed with the first feed as soon as possible.

Hypothermia. A low body temperature is associated with increased mortality in malnourished children. This often accompanies hypoglycaemia. Whenever the axillary temperature reaches below 35 °C, monitor for hypoglycaemia, and ensure regular two hourly feeds. Hypothermia is also a frequent warning sign of septicaemia. The child should be clothed and adequately covered with a warmed blanket, including the head. Beware of potential burns if heaters or hot water bottles are brought into direct contact with skin.

Infection. If the child has open skin lesions, overt infection, or is critically ill, antibiotics should be given immediately, preferably after blood cultures and other bacteriological specimens have been obtained. Initially antibiotics should be given intravenously where possible. Infection is very commonly due to Gram-negative organisms, therefore a broad-spectrum antibiotic should be given according to local bacterial sensitivity patterns and antibiotic availability. A second generation cephalosporin, amoxycillin/ampicillin or co-trimoxazole may be used successfully. If a broader spectrum is needed, the third generation cephalosporins or the aminoglycosides kanamycin, gentamycin, or amikacin are valuable. Suspicion or proof of pseudomonas infection informs the choice of piperacillin in addition to an aminoglycoside.

Where parasitic infections such as malaria, amoebiasis, giardiasis, ancylostomiasis, and ascariasis are endemic or present, these should be dealt with as soon as possible.

Underlying tuberculosis is a frequent concern and must be treated immediately if there is any suspicion of this infection. The possibility of HIV infection or AIDS must be considered when there is failure of response to therapy.

Measles is fatal to children with severe PEM. Accordingly, this disease must be prevented by administration of immunoglobulin if there is any risk of hospital-acquired infection.

Herpes virus infection may become disseminated in patients with severe PEM. Oral acyclovir is used if there is evidence of oral herpes.

Due to the depressed cell-mediated immunity of patients, oral candida should be treated actively with local nystatin to avoid dissemination.

No specific therapy is needed for skin lesions, apart from protecting ulcerated areas from moisture and contamination. Barrier creams are applied to raw areas. Local nystatin is used for candida superinfection.

Diet and supplements after resuscitation

After initial resuscitation measures, it is usually possible to commence feeds on the same day. Small, frequent milk feeds, orally or by nasogastric tube should be started in two- to three-hourly feeds around the clock to supply a volume of 130 ml/kg/day, followed by extra oral rehydration solution if rehydration is still necessary. The World Health Organization recommends a starter milk formula called F-75 (75 kcal/100 ml, protein 0.9 g/100 ml, low lactose) for initial feeding, to achieve an energy intake of about 100 kCal/kg/day. The milk feeds are gradually increased by 10–20 ml/kg/day to a total of 150 ml/kg/day. Too rapid an increase in food intake can lead to gastric distension and vomiting. When diarrhoea is a problem, a lactose-free formula is usually started, and if diarrhoea has not started to improve within 48 hours, further diet modification may be undertaken to avoid maldigestion and malabsorption-induced aggravation of the diarrhoea. (*See also* Chapter 24, Gastrointestinal disorders.) If milk is not available or poorly tolerated because of lactose intolerance, milk substitutes, such as soya milk, egg added to porridge, or other lactose-free food or formula (usually expensive) may be given.

Cereal and other foods are introduced after about three or four days and gradually increased. By the end of a week, a higher protein and energy intake should be provided (F-100 catch-up formula: 2.9 g/100ml and 400 kJ/100ml). It is essential to maintain frequent feeds also at night in order to achieve the high energy and protein intakes needed for catch-up growth. Supplements of potassium, zinc, and magnesium should be maintained for at least five days after admission.

Studies have shown that the use of ready-to-use therapeutic foods (RTUF) prepared with groundnut paste to obtain a much higher energy density than the presently suggested F-100 or milk-oil-formula, can achieve more rapid nutritional rehabilitation. An ideal RTUF could be based on locally available produce and should have the following attributes: low cost, good nutritional quality in respect of protein, energy and micronutrient composition, long shelf-life, be palatable and have a consistency suitable for feeding infants, should not support bacterial growth and should require no processing prior to feeding.

Vitamin supplementation. It is wise to add vitamin A because of the danger of xerophthalmia and because it has been shown that vitamin A therapy decreases the morbidity and mortality of infections. All children should have an oral dose of vitamin A (<6 months: 50 000 IU, 6–12 months: 100 000 IU, >12 months : 200 000 IU) on day one. In addition, all children should receive a multivitamin supplement and folic acid, 5 mg daily, for at least two weeks. Vitamin D should be given even though most children with PEM

do not show signs of rickets. As patients with kwashiorkor and hepatomegaly usually have a reduced prothrombin activity, vitamin K 5 mg is given as a single dose.

Iron supplements are commenced when oedema has settled after 10–14 days' therapy, when transferrin levels can be assumed to have returned to normal.

Usually there is an obvious improvement in the child within the first two to three days of treatment. Appetite returns and apathy and irritability lessen. Many children with marasmus may become temporarily oedematous and oedema may increase in kwashiorkor. This is not a bad sign and represents sodium retention while the child is still potassium-depleted. Diuresis and loss of oedema (and weight) will occur by the eighth to tenth day. By two or three weeks, the child is smiling once more, gaining weight, and is ready to go home.

Course of the disease

Most deaths occur in the first three days from uncontrollable infection, diarrhoea, or electrolyte imbalance. The mortality rate with good treatment and care should not exceed 10 per cent. Those who recover may gain weight (because of water retention) for the first three to four days, then have a massive diuresis, with loss of oedema and weight reduction from the fifth day. Thereafter a steady gain in weight of about 10 g/kg/day should be achieved. Poor weight gain or persistent oedema suggests infection, inadequate refeeding or other complication. A smiling child is a welcome sign of improvement and hospitalization is rarely necessary for more than two to three weeks, depending on conditions at home.

Rehabilitation

Play therapy and tender loving care during the hospital stay will restore the child's natural interest and learning abilities more quickly.

It is important to ensure that before discharge from hospital, the parents understand the reasons for the child's illness and know what to do for follow-up care and prevention. As far as possible, post-discharge planning should include arrangements for completing any outstanding immunisations and follow-up.

During recovery from severe PEM (marasmus or kwashiorkor) catch-up weight gain precedes catch-up in length. Convalescent cases therefore may go through a period of apparent obesity. In these instances, measurement of length at monthly intervals will reveal the growth spurt and the weight/height discrepancy will disappear with time.

Follow-up

Every case of PEM should be followed up at regular monthly intervals after discharge to check on weight gain. It is desirable that the child should catch up to at least the third percentile on the weight chart, or growth rate should parallel the percentile lines. Mothers are particularly interested in this aspect and if properly instructed will aid the doctor or clinic nurse in achieving this goal. There are relatively few cases that relapse. Care must be taken to ensure that other members of the family, e.g. the father and grandmother, also understand the causes of and preventive measures for PEM. It is important that the relevant social services are mobilized to assist these families. There are various schemes, governmental and voluntary, in most countries, whereby subsidized milk or food can be obtained at welfare clinics for children recovering from or at risk of malnutrition. Full use should be made of these schemes by all health workers.

Prevention

PEM is essentially a problem of poverty, whether this is brought about by famine, social or family disorganization, unemployment, or migrant labour. The eradication of PEM is therefore an extremely complex challenge and is one that faces two-thirds of the world population. The World Bank and numerous international agencies have struggled with variable success to improve the lot of the poor people of the world. It has been shown that even countries with a low GNP per capita can successfully provide social security.

The following macro-economic measures have been found to be effective in alleviating malnutrition in developing countries:

- Economic growth which includes participation of the poor; this is an investment for future wellbeing.
- Social security for the poor; this includes easy access to food ('food security'). Such interventions meet the immediate needs for food consumption.

Preventive measures applicable at a clinic or community level

- Identification of risk. This is an essential component of the IMCI strategy. All children at high risk for malnutrition should have regular follow-up and growth monitoring. The recognition that the child's growth is deviating from its centile line should alert the health workers to improve nutritional intake and support the social circumstances prior to the development of clinical malnutrition.
- Nutritional assessment at all contact opportunities. Doctors, nurses, and all members of the health team working in infant welfare clinics, health centres, hospital out-patient departments, or in the community, should include nutritional assessment in the clinical examination of every child. This applies in particular to children who present with gastroenteritis, pneumonia, or other infections. Attention to dietary needs is an essential part of treatment of these conditions, to avoid poor results, relapse and constant re-attendance for minor and major illnesses.

Measures applicable at local authority or national level

- Promotion of adequate wage structure for unskilled workers.
- Encouragement of production of protective foods. These include meat, milk, eggs, fish, and high-protein vegetables. This should be done with due regard to agricultural possibilities of the area and social and cultural factors. Agricultural and technical services should work hand in hand with health authorities to produce, market, and distribute food equitably to the population.
- Food subsidies. These can significantly lower the price of basic and essential protective food for the poor.
- Health education. Use of mass media for propagation of sound advice on nutrition should be widely employed.
- Notification of nutritional diseases. This aids identification of families at risk so that some form of assistance can be given to these families.

Long-term effects of PEM

Growth retardation. Follow-up of cases of kwashiorkor occurring within the first two years of life has revealed that growth retardation is reversible provided malnutrition is corrected and social circumstances and subsequent food intake are adequate.

Malnutrition and cognitive performance. Malnutrition and poverty are so closely interwoven that the effects on development of one cannot be distinguished from the other. Therefore the consequences of malnutrition on intellectual function must be seen as being inseparable from those of a poor socio-economic environment. It follows that therapeutic interventions should include not only food, but improvements in other essential components of life, such as the residential environment, employment, and education.

Where malnutrition is endemic, children who have had PEM in earlier years enrol late in school, drop out early, and have impaired aptitudes. Children with stunting (i.e. chronic PEM) do less well in school than their peers. Nutritional rehabilitation, and health and educational inputs can improve aptitude and school performance.

In a 15-year follow-up a Cape Town group found no difference in scholastic attainment or social adjustment between PEM survivors and the children of the socio-economic environment from which they came. With respect to intellectual development, the survivors could not be distinguished from their siblings at the age of 10 years, on intelligence testing.

The effects of PEM on the intellectual development of children are reversible if adequate treatment and sustained improvement of dietary intake, stimulation and social circumstances occur. Environmental and nutritional enrichment in the first two years of life reduce the chance of intellectual impairment in the long term. This has highlighted the problem of separating the effects of malnutrition on brain growth

per se (the physical aspect) from the effects of poor stimulation. The two often go together. With malnutrition in early years (pre-school), a child's capacity for exploring, learning, and gaining experience is reduced because of apathy and weakness. It is probably through this mechanism, rather than biochemical or structural change to the brain, that malnutrition exerts its main effect. Most of the alterations in the brain structures found during malnutrition eventually recover with refeeding, but more recent neuropharmacological research reveals long-lasting changes in brain neural receptor function which are more concerned with behaviour, adaptability, and emotional responses to stressful events than to cognitive defects *per se*. However, *extended* deprivation of food throughout the growing period (up to 18 years of age) is likely to lead to adult stunting and diminished intellectual potential.

Therefore, in a poor social and emotional environment, PEM lasting throughout childhood results in small adult stature, apathy, and lack of initiative.

Vitamins, minerals, and trace elements

Deficiencies and toxicities

In contrast to protein and energy, requirements for vitamins do not differ significantly throughout the age range. Some daily requirements are listed in Table 13.6.

Vitamins and minerals are present in most mixed diets, but under certain circumstances pure deficiencies do occur. In children in South Africa, iron and vitamin A and D deficiency are common; pellagra occurs in maize-eating populations but scurvy is uncommon.

Mineral deficiencies

In addressing the nutritional status of infants and

Table 13.6 Daily requirements of vitamins and minerals				
Vitamin A µg	Vitamin C mg	Vitamin D IU	Calcium mg	Iron mg
300–750 (2 000–5 000 IU)	40	400	500	5–10 (Female adolescents 12–24)

children, it is important to decide whether the following mineral deficiencies are relevant in a particular case.

Iron deficiency. This is common in the first year of life because milk, the basic diet, is low in iron content. However, iron-deficiency anaemia must be considered at all ages.

In South African children, one in ten was found to be iron-deficient or iron-depleted, and 5 per cent had iron-deficiency anaemia. The effects of a lack of iron on tissues other than red cells are given in Table 13.7 (*see also* Chapter 23, Disorders of the blood).

Sodium, potassium, and magnesium deficiency. Diarrhoea, vomiting, or loss of fluid from the gastrointestinal tract from suction, fistulae, ileostomy, and colostomy may give rise to acute or chronic deficiencies of the minerals sodium, potassium, and magnesium. They form part of most therapeutic supplements in treatment of these conditions and must never be omitted in serious cases.

Calcium deficiency. This occurs in some areas (*see* Chapter 12, Rickets and metabolic bone diseases) where milk is in short supply. Infants, school-age children, and the elderly may be affected.

Trace element deficiencies

Fluoride. The chief source is drinking water, which, if it contains 1 part per million (ppm) or 1 mg/l, supplies 1–2 mg per day. Soft waters contain less and deficiency leading to dental caries may occur. (*See* Chapter 35, Oral and dental disorders.)

Iodine deficiency. This occurs in certain areas and gives rise to goitre and hypothyroidism (*see* Chapter 19, Endocrine disorders). In community surveys, the prevalence of visible goitre can be taken to reflect the iodine status of that community. In a South African survey, children under the age of six were found to have a 1 per cent prevalence of goitre. Iodine deficiency is successfully prevented by iodination of table salt.

Zinc deficiency. There is currently much interest in this trace element. Deficiency of zinc is a feature of the rare disease acrodermatitis enteropathica, in which erythematous peri-oral and peri-anal rashes are found. Zinc supplements improve the lesions dramatically.

Zinc has a role in numerous metabolic pathways including lymphocyte function and immunity, scavenging of free radicals, integrity of epithelial surfaces, and growth. Zinc deficiency occurs in prolonged parenteral nutrition, malabsorptive states, and chronic diarrhoea. Deficiency is associated with PEM, small for dates, and low birth weight babies. It has also been shown that serum zinc levels can be very low in cases of kwashiorkor with ulcerative skin lesions and in small-for-date infants. In treatment, zinc sulphate or acetate is given in a dose of 2 mg/kg/day for a week. Excess zinc therapy has been shown to precipitate evidence of copper deficiency.

Vitamin deficiencies and toxicities

Vitamin A (retinol) deficiency

This fat-soluble vitamin is found in milk (butter), egg yolk, fish oils, etc. Its provitamin, beta carotene, is responsible for the yellow/red colour of vegetables and some fruits. Dark green leaves are a good source of beta carotene, and carrots

Table 13.7 Non-erythroid effects of iron deficiency	
Immune system:	Immunodeficiency
	Increased incidence of infections
Gastrointestinal system:	Histological changes
	Variable duodenal and jejunal atrophy
	Hypochlorhydria
	Impaired absorption of food, D-xylose, vitamins
Thermoregulation:	Impaired homeostatic response to hypothermia
Physical work:	Reduced efficiency
Cognition and behaviour:	Impaired or abnormal

Vitamin deficiencies	
Vitamin A:	xerophthalmia, increased morbidity and mortality from infections
Vitamin B complex:	pellagra, macrocytic anaemia, failure to thrive, skin and mouth changes
Vitamin C:	scurvy; anaemia, poor iron absorption
Vitamin D:	rickets
Vitamin E:	haemolytic anaemia (newborns); neuropathy, ataxia
Vitamin K:	haemorrhagic disease (newborns).

are an excellent source. Where animal foods are seldom eaten, all vitamin A intake comes from such sources. Beta carotene is transformed by intestinal mucosa to retinol. This and dietary vitamin A are absorbed in chylomicrons, transported to the liver, and stored as retinyl palmitate. From there it is released into the circulation as retinol bound to retinol-binding protein (RBP). One international unit of vitamin A is equivalent to 0.3 µg of retinol.

Retinol is essential for vision in dim light and for integrity of tissues, particularly the epithelial tissue of the eye and the skin. Daily requirement of vitamin A is 300 µg in infants to 750 µg in adolescents.

Pathogenesis of deficiency. The human infant is dependent on milk for her supply of the vitamin. Later carotene-containing vegetables and fruit are an additional source, but in many rural districts the supply is inadequate, especially in the dry season, and in urban areas, these foods may be too expensive. The diets of children with vitamin A deficiency are almost invariably deficient in other nutrients, especially in protein and energy content. In Africa vitamin A deficiency tends to occur together with PEM, particularly in severe kwashiorkor and marasmus, whereas in the East, where the staple diet is rice, it may occur in a more specific and endemic form. In the development of eye lesions, precipitating factors such as gastro-enteritis, measles, and tuberculosis are important, in addition to a hot, dusty climate.

Epidemiology. Night blindness and xerophthalmia are found in the Middle East, Africa,

India, South and East Asia, and Latin America. The peak incidence is between two and five years of age. The exact incidence worldwide is unknown, but one estimate is that keratomalacia causes 20 000 children per annum to become permanently blind.

The reported frequency of vitamin A deficiency in severe PEM varies from 74 per cent in Indonesia, to 1–2 per cent in Lebanon, Uganda, and South Africa. These differences are explicable on the basis of the vitamin A content of the basic diet. In a large survey, it was found that 33 per cent of South African children under the age of six had a marginal vitamin A status as indicated by a serum vitamin A level of less than 20 µg/dL. This indicates vitamin A deficiency to be a serious public health problem in South Africa.

Studies in developing countries have shown a strong association between vitamin A deficiency and increased incidence of respiratory and diarrhoeal infections. In addition infections have been shown to reduce serum concentrations of vitamin A. This vicious circle can be broken by vitamin A supplementation, as has been shown in trials in Indonesia, India, and Nepal, where vitamin A supplementation resulted in significant reduction in morbidity and mortality from common childhood infections. There is now adequate evidence that vitamin A supplementation during complicated measles shortens the duration of complications, lowers the incidence of new infections, and reduces the mortality rate and should therefore be included as part of the routine of primary health care. One of the pathways by which vitamin A is thought to have its effect in reducing severity and incidence of infection is by repairing and maintaining the integrity of the epithelial tissue of the respiratory and gastro-intestinal tract and thus providing an effective barrier against infectious agents.

Cancer. Currently much research is in progress over the possible role of vitamin A deficiency in the aetiology of various types of cancer.

Clinical features. *Eyes*. Although night blindness is the classical clinical feature of vitamin A deficiency in older children or adults, xerophthalmia is characteristic of the deficiency in infants and younger children. The earliest sign is dryness of the conjunctivae (xerosis conjunctivae). There is a loss of transparency and thickened vertical folds of conjunctivae appear. Often a small plaque of silvery-grey hue, Bitot's spot, is raised above the surface of the conjunctiva (*see* Figure 13.2).

The next stage is corneal xerosis, characterized by unwettability and loss of transparency, which leads to haziness of the cornea. This is reversible, but irreversible corneal ulceration can be the next stage. Perforation and iris prolapse may occur.

Keratomalacia, a passive softening of the cornea, is another manifestation that can occur suddenly, even during therapy. Here again there may be perforation and panophthalmitis as a complication.

Xerophthalmia is seen particularly in association with severe PEM and should always be looked for in these children, as well as in severe measles cases. A retinol plasma concentration of less than 15–20 µg/100 ml (normal 20–50 µg/100 ml) suggests deficiency. The plasma RBP is also low.

Differential diagnosis. Xerophthalmia may also be due to disease of the lacrimal glands, e.g. pemphigus or trachoma, or it may result from overexposure of the conjunctiva or cornea.

Skin. Perifollicular keratosis (phrynoderma, 'toad skin') is thought to be due to vitamin A deficiency. It has also been associated with exposure to dry, cold atmosphere, deficiency of fatty acids and the vitamin B complex group. So it is in general difficult to ascribe the condition solely to vitamin A deficiency. Sunbathing enthusiasts believe that vitamin A oil protects or relieves the skin from sunburn. The scientific evidence for such claims is uncertain. Acne in adolescents is currently being treated with concentrated vitamin A preparations. The results vary with the enthusiasm of the investigators.

Treatment. Where clinical vitamin A deficiency is suspected, a dose of 30 mg of retinol

(100 000 IU) daily for three days should be started as soon as the diagnosis is suspected. Half of the dose should be given orally and half intramuscularly as a water-miscible retinyl palmitate. All cases of PEM should receive vitamin A prophylactically as a vitamin supplement containing vitamin A. Antibiotics help in the prevention and treatment of secondary infection. Local treatment of the eye will only be required if disorganization is already present, in which case an ophthalmologist should be consulted.

Prevention of vitamin A deficiency. In countries with large-scale vitamin A deficiency, high dose vitamin A capsules should be distributed once or twice a year to all children aged six to seven months in areas of high risk. A national vitamin A policy has been introduced in South Africa. Infants aged 6–12 months receive 100 000 IU, and children older than 12 months receive 200 000 IU. In addition, diets containing green leafy vegetables, squash, pumpkin, carrots, or yellow and orange fruits, which are locally available or cheap should be encouraged as good sources of beta carotene.

Where blindness from keratomalacia is a major public health problem, single large prophylactic doses of 60 mg (200 000 IU) of retinol in oily solution should be given orally at four- to six-monthly intervals to all children, if personnel and facilities are available. Other means of fortification of local food, e.g. sugar, are being investigated.

Vitamin A toxicity

Acute poisoning following overdose of sunburn tablets or vitamin preparations or excessive ingestion of fish or shark liver has been described. The symptoms are restlessness, headache, and vomiting, sometimes with signs of raised intracranial pressure. Recovery occurs without residual damage on removal of the vitamin A source.

Chronic poisoning from extended excessive dosing occurs occasionally. In its mildest form, carotenaemia or yellow staining of skin occurs, particularly in children who have had over-enthusiastic dosing with carrots or vitamin preparations. In more severe forms, the clinical picture can include coarse sparse hair, cracked lips, and dry skin. Arthralgia, headache, and weakness can occur and in the long bones, thickening of shafts and widened metaphysis have been reported.

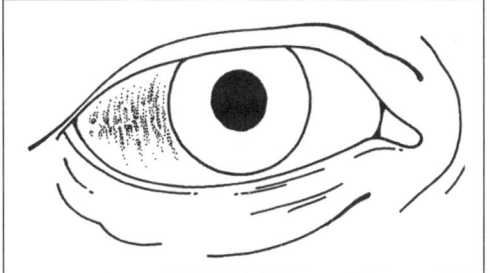

Figure 13.2 Bitot's spots resulting from vitamin A deficiency

A fasting serum retinol value of more than 250 µg/100 ml is diagnostic. Recovery occurs with withdrawal of the vitamin.

Vitamin E

The actions of vitamin E (α-tocopherol) are mainly anti-oxidant. It is present in human tissues and widely distributed in foods, so primary deficiency of the vitamin is unlikely. However, a deficiency of vitamin E could aggravate oxidant stresses on cell membranes.

In paediatrics at present, it is accepted that deficiency in premature and small-for-date infants results in haemolytic anaemia. Prophylactic vitamin E to prevent or treat this is given routinely in some neonatal units.

A form of vitamin E-deficiency peripheral neuropathy has been described in patients with biliary atresia or other types of congenital cholestatic liver disease. A feature of this condition is a paralysis of conjugate deviation of the eyes. In addition there is patchy loss of peripheral sensation and loss of tendon reflexes.

Apart from small infants, vitamin E deficiency is sometimes considered in cystic fibrosis patients with severe malabsorption.

Vitamin B complex

Initially considered to be substances each protecting against a specific disease, it is now known that the water-soluble B complex vitamins are essential co-factors in many metabolic processes. Specific deficiencies of single vitamins are quite rare.

Thiamine (vitamin B₁) deficiency

Thiamine is the least labile portion of the B complex, and deficiency leads to beriberi. In children in Africa, clinical beriberi is very rare, as the basic diet, maize or wheat, contains B_1. It does occur in the Far East in those populations that exist solely on polished rice or highly refined wheat flour. Infants breastfed from a mother on such a diet may develop beriberi at two to five months. In southern Africa, infants with recurrent attacks of diarrhoea have been found to have biochemical evidence of B_1 deficiency, but no specific clinical features were noted. Beriberi occurs in adult alcoholics in most countries.

The clinical features of beriberi in infants are those of acute cardiac failure, occurring suddenly with cyanosis and/or oedema, aphonia because of laryngeal paralysis, and pseudomeningeal signs, with drowsiness and head retraction. A lowered erythrocyte transketolase activity is suggestive of beriberi.

Treatment. Emergency administration of 50–100 mg of thiamine hydrochloride, IM or IV, should be followed by oral maintenance of 5–10mg daily for several days. Recovery is rapid.

Nicotinic acid deficiency: pellagra

Nicotinic acid is biosynthesized from the essential amino acid tryptophan. Diets low in nicotinic acid or tryptophan lead to the deficiency disease pellagra. Africa appears to be the only continent where pellagra is an important public health problem. In parts of southern Africa it remains endemic, with outbreaks in the spring and summer months. The reason for this is that the basic diet of a great proportion of the population is maize.

Maize protein is deficient in tryptophan and although maize contains nicotinic acid, it is present in a bound form unavailable to the consumer. People on unsupplemented maize porridge diets are thus predisposed to developing pellagra. Pellagra can be regarded both as a vitamin deficiency disease or one of the syndromes of PEM, because of its association with nicotinic acid and its percursor tryptophan, an essential amino acid.

Clinical features. Traditionally pellagra has been known as the disease of the three Ds: dermatitis, diarrhoea, and dementia. In children dementia is rare and pellagra is characterized by the skin lesions and features akin to protein deficiency.

The disease affects children from the age of five years. The skin lesions of pellagra are almost identical to those of kwashiorkor. In fact, before kwashiorkor became established as a term for severe protein malnutrition, it used to be labelled as 'infantile pellagra'.

The lesions consist of erythema or pigmentation over areas exposed to ultraviolet radiation of sunlight or other irritants. In children with pellagra, the lesions are on the neck (Casal's necklace), forehead, face, back of hands, wrists, forearms and legs; covered areas are spared, while the perineum, buttock, and flexural areas are affected in infants with kwashiorkor.

A red beefy tongue, angular stomatitis, and cheilosis are frequently present. The more severe features of kwashiorkor, e.g. gross oedema, diarrhoea, apathy, or infection, are not so prominent in pellagra, because in older children protein requirement is not as critical as in the rapidly growing infant or toddler. It is advantageous to regard pellagra in children as a manifestation of kwashiorkor in an older child. In affected families, children under three years will have kwashiorkor and the older children, pellagra.

Diagnosis. This is made on clinical appearance and history. A reduced N-methylnicotinamide excretion in the urine is helpful academic confirmation. Fasting plasma tryptophan ranges from 1.0–4.5 mg/l in pellagra and 6.5–8.8 mg/l in healthy adults. As in PEM, there may be a degree of hypoalbuminaemia.

Treatment. Nicotinamide or nicotinic acid, 100 mg orally every four hours, will give relief, but it is more important to improve the diet with sources of animal protein, such as milk, meat, cheese, fish, eggs, or with legumes such as beans, peas, and lentils. Recovery is complete and rapid.

Prevention. A mixed diet or maize enrichment with nicotinic acid will assist in preventing pellagra. Commercial maize enrichment is now becoming more universal in southern Africa and pellagra is less common than it used to be.

Riboflavin (vitamin B₂) deficiency

Deficiency of this vitamin rarely occurs alone and is usually associated with kwashiorkor or pellagra. The skin lesions of riboflavin deficiency cannot be distinguished from these conditions.

Pyridoxine (vitamin B₆) deficiency

Most foodstuffs contain this vitamin and isolated deficiency is very rare. Convulsions have been described in established deficiency due to heat-processing of commercial milks, malabsorption or drug antagonism (isoniazid). In addition, some newborn infants of mothers who had been on large doses of pyridoxine as anti-nausea medication for a long time present with jitteriness and convulsions, which respond to the intramuscular administration of pyridoxine.

In addition to convulsions in infants, pyridoxine deficiency in older persons has been described to cause peripheral neuritis, dermatitis with cheilosis, glossitis, and seborrhoea.

Folic acid and B₁₂ deficiency

Megaloblastic anaemia is associated with these deficiencies. (*See* Chapter 23, Disorders of the blood.) Where there is a poor diet, diarrhoea, or malabsorption associated with intestinal parasites and megaloblastic anaemia, deficiency of folic acid should be considered. Apart from the anaemia, affected patients have a smooth red tongue, are irritable, and fail to thrive. Folic acid supplementation before and during the early part of pregnancy has recently been shown to reduce the incidence of congenital malformations, including neural tube defects in the newborn, e.g. myelomeningocele.

Vitamin B₁₂ deficiency tends to occur in vegans (those who are true vegetarians and who eat no source of animal protein, as compared with the lacto-ovo vegetarians who do allow eggs and milk in their diet). Dietary B₁₂ deficiency from a pure vegetable diet may take months or even years to develop and is thus hardly ever seen in children. However, B₁₂ deficiency may occur very rarely due to a specific malabsorption or due to resection of large parts of the ileum. The neurological features seen in adults with this deficiency are very rarely seen in children.

Vitamin C (ascorbic-acid) deficiency – scurvy

The minimum requirement of vitamin C is 40 mg/day throughout all age groups. Vitamin C is found in fresh vegetables and fruit.

In infancy, requirements are met by breastmilk, which is rich in vitamin C, or by fruit juices or artificial supplements when feeding is by bottle. It is important to appreciate that cow's milk is low in vitamin C and that boiling or processing destroys the vitamin. Infants fed solely on unsupplemented processed milks are thus prone to develop scurvy at four to six months of age.

Vitamin C promotes the release of free folic acid from conjugates in food and, most importantly, facilitates the absorption of iron. In the tissues, vitamin C deficiency results in defective function of intercellular ground substance. In skin, bone and blood vessels, the deficiency leads to defective collagen, resulting in poor wound healing, rupture of capillaries, and haemorrhage.

Clinical features. Scurvy in paediatrics is a disease of infancy, usually at the age of four to ten months. The presenting symptom is irritability, made worse by picking up or by moving limbs. This is due to the tenderness and pain of subperiosteal and other haemorrhages. For this reason patients are often referred to surgeons with a provisional diagnosis of osteitis. The pseudo-paralysis induced by pain leads to a characteristic frog-like position of the legs.

Haemorrhage may occur in any tissue but is commonly seen in skin and muscle in response to minor trauma. Gum bleeding is rare in infants before tooth eruption. There is beading of the ribs at the costochondral junction. X-rays of long bones show diagnostic changes of periosteal elevation because of haemorrhage, especially well seen in recovery when it becomes calcified. There is a ground glass appearance in the shaft, thinning of the cortex, and broadening of the zone of provisional calcification. In the epiphyses, the ground glass appearance within the centre of ossification, and the surrounding dense epiphyseal line, give the appearance known as 'ringing' of the epiphyses.

On recovery there is return to normality without deformity.

Scurvy has to be differentiated from other bleeding disorders and causes of purpura. Herpes virus stomatitis is occasionally mistaken for scurvy.

Osteitis, septic arthritis, and non-accidental injuries have to be excluded and the radiological changes of rickets and congenital syphilis must be distinguished from those of scurvy.

Treatment. This must be immediate because of the danger of further bleeding. Ascorbic acid 250 mg four times a day causes prompt improvement and initiates healing.

Prevention. Scurvy tends to occur only in the first year of life. A source of vitamin C (fruit juice or vitamin preparation with 40 mg vitamin C) must be given daily from birth to infants on artificial (bottle) feeding.

Vitamin K (phytomenadione) deficiency

This fat-soluble vitamin occurs in plants and is also produced by bacteria in the gut. Vitamin K is a co-factor for the synthesis of prothrombin in the liver. Primary deficiency of this vitamin occurs in the neonate because the gut is sterile and there is very little vitamin K in breastmilk and cow's milk. Infants in the first week of life therefore have low prothrombin in their blood. There is spontaneous improvement in a few days, but haemorrhagic disease of the newborn may supervene in the interim. Bleeding from the second to fifth day of life can occur from any internal or external site and may be fatal. The condition can be completely avoided by administration of 1 mg of vitamin K_1 IM at birth. This should be a routine at every delivery.

Vitamin K deficiency after the newborn period tends to occur with hyperalimentation regimes, liver disease, biliary obstruction and fistulae, PEM and intestinal malabsorption syndromes, and as a result of long-continued antibiotic therapy. Prophylactic administration of vitamin K_1 by mouth or by injection will prevent bleeding in these circumstances.

Diseases of overnutrition

Obesity

Definition

Obesity is overweight due to excess fat. In childhood, obesity may be defined as the infant or child who is too heavy for his length or height. Obesity is obvious on inspection; however, in order to determine obesity objectively, weight and length must be charted on standard growth reference curves. In practice, this means a child who is 10 to 20 percentiles or more in weight than his percentile length or height. This excess weight for height may also be expressed in terms of a Body Mass Index (BMI) at or above the 90th percentile for age, calculated as follows:

$$\frac{\text{weight in kg}}{\text{height in metres}^2}$$

BMI varies with age in childhood. Sex-specific BMI charts are available and must be used for accurate identification of obesity. In general, if the BMI exceeds 19 at age five years, 20 at age 10 years and 25 at age 18 years, a diagnosis of obesity is likely. Skinfold measurements can be used as additional evidence and charts are now available for these in childhood. In adults, men should be considered obese if the triceps skin fold exceeds 15 mm and women if it exceeds 25 mm.

Prevalence of obesity

In many developed countries more than 10–15 per cent of school-going children are obese. Societies in demographic transition may have particularly steep increases in the prevalence of obesity. It is more common in girls than in boys, particularly during adolescence. While moderate obesity is a disorder of affluence and therefore more frequent in rich countries, pathological obesity is found independent of socio-economic status.

Pathogenesis

The immediate cause of simple obesity is a positive energy balance. Excess fat is laid down if energy intake chronically exceeds energy expenditure. Every person has a genetically pro-grammed, physiologically maintained, homeo-static body mass set point. This prevents large swings in body mass over short periods of time despite large variations in intake. Lifestyle changes and a *persistently* increased intake of energy above that which is required for homeo-stasis can alter body weight.

Epidemiological evidence is accumulating to indicate that low birth weight due to fetal under-nutrition (especially thinness at birth, i.e. low weight for length) is associated with a significant risk of subsequent adult obesity, hypertension, type 2 diabetes mellitus, and coronary artery disease (metabolic syndrome). This appears to be due to metabolic programming, whereby an insult at a critical, sensitive period of organ mat-uration results in long-term changes in physiol-ogy or metabolism.

A number of genes are associated with obesity, predominantly through their influence on bio-chemical pathways involved in the complex neu-roendocrine control of hunger and food intake. Hormones, neurotransmitters and autonomic nerve signals are involved in complex feedback loops centred in the hypothalamus. While at least seven genes are known to cause obesity, most obesity is due to the interaction of multiple genes and environmental factors.

Whether there is an abnormality of metabolism or not, obesity in infants tends to occur with artificial as opposed to breastfeeding in the first year of life. In pre-school and school years, obesity is propagated by the eating habits of families that favour the excess consumption of refined (sugar, cold drinks, white bread, cakes, sweets) as opposed to unrefined (fruit, potatoes, brown bread, vegetables) carbohydrate sources. Also, an excess of fat, e.g. butter, fried foods, fatty meat, will promote obesity. These children tend to have obese parents and other family members as well.

Genetic factors predisposing to obesity appear to be less important. Although obesity is more common in the children of fat parents, pseudo-hereditary influences, e.g. family eating patterns and environment, appear to be the operative factors. Lack of exercise through excessive time spent TV viewing rather than on the playing field, and psychological causes of overeating, e.g. boredom, insecurity, poor family relationships, or mental and physical handicaps, are important in modern-day society.

Clinical assessment

Obesity as defined above should be recorded at all ages at well-baby follow-up at clinics, at pre-school assessments, at school, and during adolescence. The doctor or primary health care worker should include the presence of obesity in the diagnostic assessment, so that appropriate advice can be given before the condition becomes chronic and complications occur. While fat infants do not necessarily go on to become obese adults, obesity in childhood and adolescence is definitely associated with a higher risk of adult obesity.

Complications

Obesity is now considered to be a disease. The risks of obesity are found in social and psycho-logical stress, physical and metabolic disorders, and in complications in adulthood.

Infancy and pre-school. Fat infants and chil-dren are prone to repeated respiratory infections, hypoventilation, and airways disease. The most severe cases may lead to carbon dioxide reten-tion (Pickwick syndrome). During gastroenteri-tis, dehydration is more difficult to assess in a fat child and this may result in inadequate fluid therapy. Impaired glucose tolerance is a problem that may eventually lead to diabetes.

School age and adolescence. The psycho-logical effects of obesity in this age group may be profound, leading to feelings of rejection and poor self-image that in themselves propagate the overeating habit or, alternatively, could pre-cipitate anorexia nervosa. Orthopaedic com-plications include slipped capital femoral epiphyses, flat feet, and an association with Blount disease.

Long term. Increased mortality and morbidity from hypertension, diabetes, heart disease, or joint problems are increasingly recognised.

In addition to the factors dicussed above, the pattern of nutrition during childhood may be an important determinant of degenerative arterial disease in adulthood. An elevated serum cholesterol is now an established cardiovascular risk factor and intervention is indicated when it is above 4.2 mmol/l in children and adolescents. This takes the form of appropriate advice on lifestyle, e.g. a 'prudent' diet (fat intake limited to between 20 and 30 per cent of total energy intake), daily exercise, and control of stress. This is particularly important when there is a family history of cardiovascular disease, diabetes, and familial hyperlipidaemia. In the latter instance, screening of children above the age of two years is indicated.

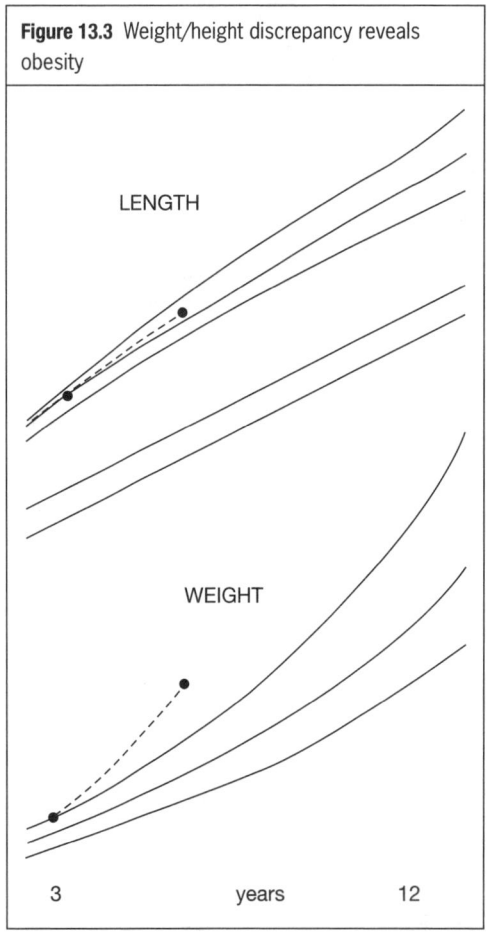

Figure 13.3 Weight/height discrepancy reveals obesity

LENGTH

WEIGHT

3   years   12

Differential diagnosis

Large infants. During the first year of life large infants are frequently confused with obese infants. During the first six to twelve months, an infant tends to put on more fat than muscle and looks chubby. The distinction between the two is made clear by charting weight and length (*see* Figure 13.3). The large, as opposed to obese, infant will have a length corresponding to the weight on the percentile lines.

Endocrine disorders. Hypothyroidism, Cushing's syndrome, and hypothalamic disorders (craniopharyngioma) may present with apparent obesity and weight-for-height will be increased. However, the height-for-age in these cases is usually reduced, whereas in simple obesity height is also increased. (*See* Chapter 19, Endocrine disorders.)

Rare congenital disorders associated with mental deficiency and dwarfism, e.g. Prader Willi syndrome, have to be considered in cases where the clinical picture does not fit with simple obesity.

Treatment

A well-motivated parent and patient are essential if treatment is to be attempted. Obesity runs in families and it is usually impossible to distinguish what is genetic and what is environmental. However, the paediatrician should watch the weight gain of children so that parents can be advised at the earliest sign of obesity. A dietician can be of great assistance in all age groups.

In infancy. Excessive gain of weight compared with height can be detected on weight charts. Here, simple advice is to cut down feeds to requirements, e.g. after six months 500 ml of milk per day is enough on a weaning diet. Avoid adding sugar to feeds and use it sparingly on porridge to cut energy intake. In practice, skim milk in place of whole milk effectively cuts energy intake without need for further dieting. The aim should always be to keep weight static rather than to try to promote loss of weight. This will enable the infant to continue growing and so 'grow into his weight.'

The best time for treatment is at *primary school entry*, since a modest reduction in the normal rate of fat storage between the ages of five and twelve will convert the obese five-year-old into a child of normal weight at entry to secondary school.

In adolescence. This is a more complicated age for treatment, but emphasis should be on:

- Increased activity: many obese adolescents are extremely inactive.
- Sensible dieting: Concentrate on foods with high fibre and low fat, e.g. salads. Avoid refined carbohydrates (cold drinks, cakes, sweets, white bread). Porridge, brown bread, potatoes, and rice can be eaten in moderation. The diet should be adapted as closely as possible to family and cultural eating habits.
- Psychological support: Frequent counselling and follow-up visits boost self-discipline.

Group therapy is often helpful.
Organizations such as Weigh-Less may be helpful.

Prevention

The detection of obesity in infancy and childhood and its treatment will prevent multiple complications in later life. Health education, during and after pregnancy, at infant welfare centres and the school medical service is therefore mandatory if prevention is to be effective. Proper use of growth and weight charts will detect early predisposition to obesity and should be available in all doctors' rooms and clinics.

PART 5

Infections

14

Principles of infection in children

Infections are the most common reason for consultation at all levels of the health service. In developing countries two-thirds of the 10 million annual deaths in children under the age of five years are due to infections.

Predisposition to infection

Mild infections are common in all children and raise only normal anxiety. However, frequently recurrent, severe, or unusual infections with delayed recovery should alert the clinician to underlying predisposing factors to infection.

Frequent infections occur under the following circumstances:

- Frequent exposure in overcrowded environments. This includes children who attend day-care centres. An otherwise healthy pre-school child may suffer from six to eight attacks of acute respiratory infection per year, most of which are self-limiting and are followed by an uncomplicated recovery.
- Anatomical or structural abnormality of organs may predispose to recurrent local infection, e.g. obstruction to a bronchus may cause recurrent pneumonia in the same region of the lung, an obstruction of the ureter may cause recurrent urinary tract infections.
- Acquired immunodeficiency, which is most commonly due to HIV infection, malnutrition (NAIDS, *see* Chapter 13, Nutritional disorders), post-measles infection and during treatment with cytotoxic therapy or long-term steroids.

- Primary or inherited immunodeficiency involving isolated or combined limbs of the immune system, e.g X-linked agammaglobulinaemia, Di George syndrome, complement deficiencies, and neutrophil disorders. Such conditions are rare, but some specific therapies are available (e.g. immunoglobulin treatment), and information about the course and prognosis can assist parents in dealing with the problem. Some clinical features associated with these immunodeficiency disorders include petechiae, eczema, mucocutaneous candidiasis, ataxia, chronic diarrhoea, facial abnormalities, multifocal infections, or lack of lymphadenopathy. Basic investigations which should be done include a full blood count with differential white cell count, serum immunoglobulins and complement, CD_4 and CD_8 counts, and tests measuring antibody responses to recall-antigens; e.g. those used in routine immunization of children such as tetanus toxoid (*see* chapter 21, Immune and connective tissue disorder).

Pathogenesis of disease in infection

The mode of infection to cause disease differs between the organ sites that are involved. The most common forms of severe infections include lower respiratory tract infections and gastroenteritis. Less common forms of severe disease include sepsis, which may also be associated with diarrhoea and pneumonia, as well as meningitis.

There is a close link between preceding respiratory virus infection and superimposed bacterial infections with *Streptococcus pneumoniae* and *Staphylococcus aureus*.

Respiratory viruses may be transmitted through airborne spread as well as through fomite and self-inoculation, as occurs with respiratory syncytial virus. Similarly, transmission of *S. pneumoniae* may occur through small-droplet particle transmission or through self-inoculation. The nasopharynx of children under six years of age is commonly colonized by a multitude of potentially pathogenic bacteria, including *S. pneumoniae*, which these children may transmit to other susceptible close-contacts. Although the majority of these nasopharyngeal colonizing episodes in children and adults are asymptomatic events, underlying risk factors may result in disease, especially due to newly-acquired colonizing bacteria.

The transmission of enteric viruses and bacteria causing gastroenteritis is generally through oral-faecal transmission. Whereas poor sanitation is especially associated with a heightened susceptibility to pathogenic bacteria including *Escherichia coli*, *Salmonella* sp., *Vibrio cholera* and *Shigella* sp., enteric viruses are less reliant upon poor sanitation for transmission. The most common enteric-viral cause of diarrhoeal disease is rotavirus, to which all children are exposed to at least one infection episode by two years. The severity of rotavirus infection may however be greater in settings where infections occur during the first year of life, outside of the neonatal period, as well as where the risk of concurrent enteric pathogenic bacterial infections is greater. Despite a number of strains of rotavirus which may differ annually, disease following infection by the virus is most severe after the first episode of infection.

Presenting features of infection

The hallmark of infection is the presence of fever; however, many newborn, malnourished, anergic or severely ill children do not respond to infection with fever, some localized infections (e.g. on the skin) do not elicit fever, while there are also a number of non-infectious causes of fever.

In general, the effects of an infection are due to the pathology caused by the infectious agent and the body's responses to it. The following groups of symptoms and signs may be indicative of infection:

- Fever alone
- Haemodynamic instability and shock in the absence of evident fluid or blood losses
- Fever and rash
- Purpuric rash
- Fever plus specific organ-based symptoms or signs.

Fever

Fever is a common presenting symptom of infectious and non-infectious disease in children and may be the sole reason for a consultation in about 20 per cent of cases. It is important to know the mechanisms maintaining normal temperature in order to understand fever.

In healthy individuals, body temperature is strictly maintained within a narrow range of 36.5–37.2 °C. The body requires three levels of control to achieve such fine temperature regulation:

- Receptors to detect thermal changes in the skin, spinal cord, and hypothalamus
- A reference mechanism situated in the hypothalamus which maintains temperature at a set point (compare with thermostat)
- Effector channels to retain or release heat in order to keep temperature at the set point.

Temperature regulation is achieved through the metabolic rate (heat production), vasoconstriction or vasodilatation, sweating and behavioural responses (e.g. putting on warm clothing).

Changes in environmental temperature. In cold weather, heat is retained in the body by vasoconstriction, increased heat production (by brown fat in neonates, by shivering in children), and lack of sweating. In hot weather there is increased loss of heat from the body through vasodilatation (by conduction and convection), and sweating (by evaporation). These responses to changes in environmental conditions keep internal body temperature at the set point.

Changes to the set point in the hypothalamus. At the onset of sleep the set point is reduced, thereby lowering the internal body temperature through the appropriate thermoregulatory mechanisms. The opposite happens in febrile states: the hypothalamic set point is displaced upward, and therefore the internal body temperature is higher than normal. This higher temperature is maintained by decreasing heat loss (through vasoconstriction) and increasing heat production (by increasing metabolism and shivering). The threshold for the set point is raised in infections by the following process: exogenic pyrogens, e.g. bacterial products such as endotoxins, viruses, yeasts, spirochetes, protozoa and immune reactions stimulate mononuclear phagocytes to release endogenous pyrogens, such as interleukin I, interleukin 6 and TNF-α (cachectin) which increases synthesis of prostaglandins in the hypothalamus. It is not known how prostaglandins, especially PGE, reset the hypothalamic thermostat. This results in an increase in the production of heat and a reduction in the loss of heat, until the body's temperature reaches the new set-point. Acetyl-salicylic acid acts by reducing synthesis of prostaglandins. Thermoregulatory mechanisms are not fully developed in neonates, especially preterm babies, and hence they do not adjust adequately to changes in ambient temperatures and may not produce fever in response to infection.

Clinical considerations

Certain signs which relate to the appearance and behaviour of the child suggest a potentially serious infection; these observations include changes in the child's reactions to stimuli (smiling, anxiety, crying), level of consciousness, skin colour, and hydration. High temperatures in excess of 38 °C are more often due to bacterial infections than are lower temperatures. In infancy, bacterial infections are accompanied by fever in the majority of cases. However, newborns and malnourished children often do not manifest a high temperature, despite severe underlying infection. About 97 per cent of premature babies with bacterial infections do not have fever. The reason for this paradoxical situation is the relative immune anergy of these babies to exogenous antigens.

The common causes of mild to moderate fever in well-nourished children are non-specific viral disease, upper respiratory tract infections, and some of the common exanthems. However, an apparently benign fever may reflect the early stage of severe infections, such as meningitis, septicaemia, or pneumonia. Of particular concern are children who present with acute pyrexia without an obvious focus, or with pyrexia of unknown origin.

Pyrexia without a focus

Acute pyrexia without an obvious cause is a common problem in infants and young children and frequently poses a diagnostic and therapeutic dilemma. In infants, especially those aged less than three months, always consider bacterial infections. There are no definitive guidelines for the management of such children and the approach is usually individualized.

Well-looking infant over three months of age. If the rectal temperature is less than 39 °C, observe the child and advise the mother to return if any other signs or symptoms develop. If the rectal temperature is more than 39 °C, investigate as indicated below and consider empiric treatment with antibiotics as an out-patient.

Well-looking infant less than three months of age. If the infant looks well, do a blood count and urine examination. If the white cell count is normal and there is no evidence of urinary tract infection, observe the patient and advise the mother to return immediately if any other abnormality occurs.

Children who are ill and toxic. Refer urgently for admission to hospital and perform the appropriate investigations, which must include a blood and urine culture and full blood count. A cerebrospinal fluid (CSF) examination would be recommended in most infants and in older children if meningitis is suspected. Treatment depends on associated findings, but will usually include antibiotic therapy.

Pyrexia of unknown origin (PUO)

Although there is no standard definition for PUO, a working definition may include a temperature greater than 38.3 °C in whom no specific diagnosis has been made following investigation after two outpatient visits or three days in hospital. Additional categories include:.

- ◆ Nosocomial PUO in hospital patients with fever of 38.3 °C on several occasions caused by a process not present or incubating on admission, where initial cultures are negative and diagnosis still unknown after three days investigation.
- ◆ Neutropaenic PUO includes patients with

fever as above with $<1 \times 10^9$ neutrophils with initial negative cultures and diagnosis uncertain after three days
- HIV-associated PUO includes HIV-positive patients with fever as above for four weeks as outpatients or three days as inpatient, with an uncertain diagnosis after three days investigation where at least two days have been allowed for cultures to incubate.

The causes of PUO vary according to the age of the child:
- Infections, especially tuberculosis, HIV, occult abscesses: 30–50%
- Collagen vascular diseases: 10–20%
- Malignancies: 5–10%
- Miscellaneous causes (drug fever, metabolic causes): 5%
- No cause found: 30%

In addition, the spectrum of causes varies by geographic area. In developing countries infections are more common (*see* Table 14.1), while in developed countries the relative contribution of the other causes would be greater. The approach to a patient with PUO should be individualized. Nevertheless, some basic, generic guidelines must be followed.

History-taking must be comprehensive and include details about symptoms from all major systems and general complains, e.g. weight loss, headaches, rashes. Fever pattern, geographic

Table 14.1 Common infectious illnesses to be suspected and investigated for when considering a diagnosis of 'Pyrexia of Unknown Origin' in developing countries

Disease	Clinical features and relevant diagnostic tests
Bacteria	
Tuberculosis	Fever, anorexia, loss of weight , history of contact, tuberculin skin test and/or interferon gamma release assay, CXR
Abscesses	Toxic, repeat positive blood or site specific cultures, abdominal symptoms. Sonar kidney, liver, spleen
Typhoid	Toxic, swinging temperature, splenomegaly – leucopaenia, Widal test, blood and stool culture
Malaria	Febrile episodes, anaemia, jaundice, splenomegaly – blood film
Amoebiasis	Bloody stools, pain in right hypochondrium, anaemia – leucocytosis, serology, stool examination
UTI	Fever – urine examination, sonar kidney (perinephric abscess may have a normal urine analysis)
Osteitis	Fever, bone pain – blood culture
Endocarditis	Fever, changing murmurs, splenomegaly, petechiae – leucocytosis, blood culture, echocardiography
Viruses	
HIV infection	Failure to thrive, generalised adenopathy, recurrent diarrhoea, recurrent pneumonia, chronic respiratory disease. 75% of unexplained fever may be infection related, 20–25% are due to malignancies and a small fraction (5%) are due to HIV itself. Test involves HIV-PCR if <18 months of age or HIV ELISA in older children.
AIDS-related	CMV, cryptosporidium, tuberculosis, opportunistic infections
Herpes viruses	Cytomegalovirus, EBV. Constitutional symptoms with localization. EBV serology, p65Ag CMV.
Other	Rickettsia, exposure to animals and ticks, eschar formation (check on scalp), maculopapular or purpuric rash, splenomegaly – serology.

location, and environmental conditions (water and sanitation), travel to areas of endemic tropical diseases (malaria), exposure to a known case of tuberculosis, exposure to domestic or wild animals (leptospirosis, toxoplasmosis), ingestion of unpasteurized milk (brucellosis), and pica (toxocara). Enquire about any underlying medical condition that may predispose to a specific infection (*see* Table 14.2). Additionally, drug history should be recorded, to include over-the-counter medications, prescription medications and any illicit substances. Immunization status and timing should be documented. Also enquire about family history of illnesses.

The clinical examination must be detailed. Look for any clinical signs that may indicate a specific diagnosis of infection. In addition, the presenting clinical features may suggest a specific

organism. It is important to examine the child on a number of occasions, as the emergence of new clinical findings may be an important clue to diagnosis. Rectal examination should be done to detect pelvic abscesses.

Where there is multisystem involvement and infection has been excluded, collagen diseases must always be considered. Malignancies such as lymphoma may also produce fever, and therefore bone tenderness, lymphadenopathy, anaemia, and splenomegaly should be specifically sought.

Special investigations are important aids to diagnosis. The choice of tests is dependent upon their availability, the epidemiology of local diseases, the presence of underlying disorders, the age of the patient, and the detection of physical signs.

Table 14.2 Causes of fever in children with underlying disease

Disease	Likely infection
Malnutrition	Septicaemia, herpes, adenovirus, fungal infections
Post-measles	Septicaemia due to *S. pneumoniae*, *Staphylococcus aureus*, herpes, adenovirus, tuberculosis, candida
Rheumatic fever and congenital heart disease	Endocarditis, brain abscess
Nephrotic syndrome	Pneumococcal infections
Schistosomiasis	Typhoid fever, hepatitis B
Renal tract abnormalities	Gram-negative infections
Head injury	Pneumococcal meningitis
Hydrocephalus	Ventriculitis (staph infection)
Malignancies	Septicaemia, fungal infections
Sickle-cell anaemia	Pneumococcal infections
HIV infection	TB, CMV, *Pneumocystis jirovecii*, bacterial and viral infection, cryptosporidium

Treatment of fever

Therapy should obviously be directed at the cause of the fever. However, in many cases the aetiology is not immediately clear, and the clinician has to treat on the basis of probability. If there is a strong suspicion of tuberculosis it is better to start specific therapy immediately, and to discontinue treatment if investigations do not support the diagnosis. Basic side room techniques (urine, CSF, stools, white cell count) must be done immediately in order to facilitate a rational choice of antibiotics.

Although there is no agreement on whether antipyretics are required or not, in practice most clinicians would administer them.

A Cochrane review of clinical trials reported that paracetamol was not superior in its antipyretic effect when compared to placebo. Children tolerate temperatures between 38 and 40 °C fairly well, but above 41 °C problems arise; these include anorexia, irritability, discomfort, and the likelihood of convulsions in those who are susceptible. The disadvantages of reducing the temperature are the risks of side-effects of the drugs, and masking the underlying cause. Fever also appears to benefit immune responsiveness by its effect on increased phagocytosis, enhanced leucocyte mobility, lymphocytic activation, interferon production, and decreased iron mobilization. The final decision to treat rests on an assessment of risks and benefit, also to anxious parents and attendants.

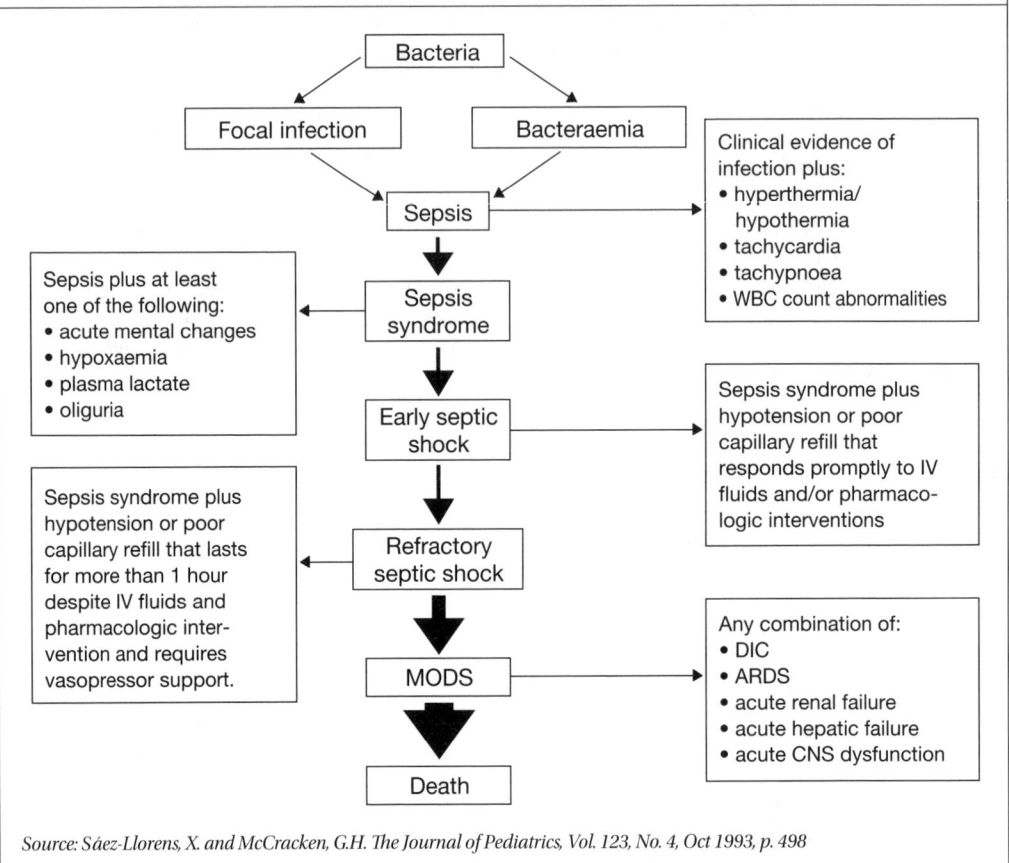

Figure 14.1 Proposed terminology of the septic process (systemic response syndrome) in children. In general, the risk of dying increases as one moves down the spectrum from sepsis to multi-organ dysfunction syndrome (MODS) (risk is indicated by width of arrows). WBC, white blood cell; IV, intravenous; DIC, disseminated intravascular caogulation; ARDS, adult respiratory distress syndrome; CNS, central nervous system

Source: Sáez-Llorens, X. and McCracken, G.H. *The Journal of Pediatrics, Vol. 123, No. 4, Oct 1993, p. 498*

Symptomatic treatment of a child with fever is as follows:

* **Physical methods**. Tepid baths, sponging, removal of excess clothing, maintaining hydration.
* **Drugs**. Paracetamol 10–20 mg/kg six-hourly. Ibuprofen 5–10 mg/kg six-hourly. Aspirin should be avoided in the treatment of febrile children because of the risk of Reye's syndrome.

Septicaemia and septic shock

Septicaemia is defined as the presence of organisms in the bloodstream associated with additional clinical features. If untreated, sepsis can lead to shock, multiple organ failure, and death (*see* Figure 14.1). The pathogenesis of sepsis and septic shock is outlined in Figure 14.2.

Septicaemia should be considered in any child with an acute, severe illness, haemodynamic instability and pyrexia, in whom no cause for the fever can be found.

Causes

Staphylococcus aureus and *Streptococcus pneumoniae* are the most frequent Gram-positive infections. Common Gram-negative infections causing sepsis and shock in children include *Escherichia coli*, *Klebsiella* spp., *Salmonella* spp, *Haemophilus influenzae* and *Neisseria meningitidis*. In infants, group B streptococcal and *E. coli* infections predominate. Immunocompromised individuals are at high risk for sepsis from the above-mentioned infections, as well as the more unusual ones such as *Acinetobacter* sp. and *Serratia* sp.

Clinical features

Septicaemic children present acutely with non-specific signs and symptoms, fever or hypothermia. There may be no obvious focus of infection, but they have a peculiarly 'sick' appearance with alternating apathy/drowsiness and irritability. Tachypnoea, tachycardia, hypotension and alterations in level of consciousness may be present. In some cases a focus of infection such as meningitis, osteitis, or pneumonia may be evident. If untreated, shock, coma, and multiple organ failure may occur, leading to death. Cutaneous manifestation such as petechiae, ecchymosis, and peripheral gangrene may be present.

Diagnosis

Laboratory evidence of septicaemia may include a positive blood culture, bacteria in urine, CSF or plasma, or visualization of organisms in skin scrapings. Other frequent laboratory abnormali-

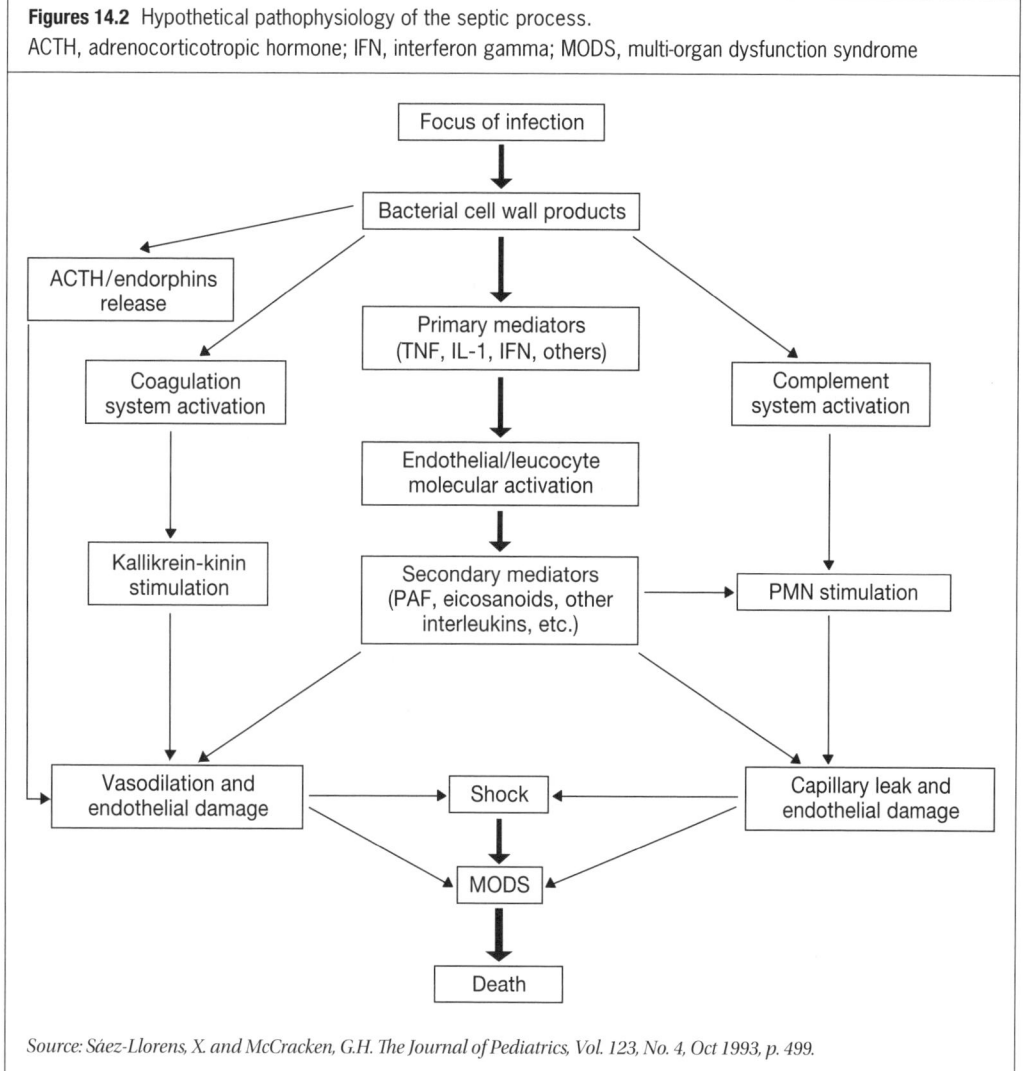

Figures 14.2 Hypothetical pathophysiology of the septic process.
ACTH, adrenocorticotropic hormone; IFN, interferon gamma; MODS, multi-organ dysfunction syndrome

Source: Sáez-Llorens, X. and McCracken, G.H. The Journal of Pediatrics, Vol. 123, No. 4, Oct 1993, p. 499.

ties include evidence for disseminated intravascular coagulation (DIC), metabolic acidosis, anaemia, elevated neutrophil count, or neutropaenia and hypoglycaemia.

Treatment

Children with septicaemia should be treated with broad-spectrum antibiotics; either ampicillin and gentamicin or a third-generation cephalosporin while waiting for laboratory confirmation of the offending organism and sensitivity. If staphylococcal infection is suspected, add cloxacillin. Cases of septic shock should ideally be managed in an intensive care unit. Hypoxia should be treated with oxygen. If hypoventilation is present, consider artificial ventilation. Provide adequate fluid intake. Children in septic shock are usually intravascular volume depleted, due to capillary leakages and require high resuscitation volumes of fluids (20–40 ml/kg *ad lib*), even if no clinical signs of dehydration are present. If normal blood pressure cannot be maintained with fluid therapy, treat with sympathomimetic agents such as dopamine. If hypotension remains refractory, adrenaline or nor-epinephrine may be tried. If DIC with bleeding is present, treat with fresh frozen plasma and platelet infusions. The role of steroids in treatment of septic shock is controversial, but may improve sensitization to inotropes. Mortality rates for septic shock, especially in the presence of DIC, remain high despite the improvements in intensive care therapy. Therapy with monoclonal antibodies against endotoxins and cytokines have not been found to be useful.

Fever and rash

In most instances fever and rash are a consequence of a viral or rickettsial infection, but may also be the result of a bacterial infection, or of a non-infectious disease. The diagnosis is usually made on the basis of history and examination. Frequently a definite clinical diagnosis cannot be made and special investigations are required. The following are medical emergencies:

  ◆ A child presenting with a haemorrhagic rash.
  ◆ Any rash associated with toxaemia, bleeding tendency, depressed level of consciousness, or other signs of neurological disturbance.

Such cases should be urgently treated with intravenous antibiotics and referred to hospital.

History-taking. This should include enquiring about the onset of rash in relation to illness, duration, progression and distribution of rash, prodromal illness, and other associated symptoms. Ask about recent contact with another similar case, travel history, insect bites, exposure to animals, prior immunizations, and antibiotic usage.

Examination. Do a comprehensive examination. Measure the temperature and look for lymphadenopathy, hepatosplenomegaly, characteristic mucosal involvement (enanthem), arthritis, and other systemic manifestations.

The characteristics of the rash should be documented and are conveniently classified as maculopapular, blistering, crusting or desquamating, or haemorrhagic. Often, a maculopapular rash becomes petechial or haemorrhagic in severe expression of disease. Tables 14.3, 14.4 and 14.5 summarize the important infections associated with such rashes.

Special investigations. If a clinical diagnosis is not possible, perform the relevant investigations, which should include a full blood count, differential count, blood culture, serology, and viral culture.

Diseases associated with erythematous rashes

(*See* Table 14.3.)

Measles (rubeola)

Epidemiology

Measles is an acute, highly contagious disease caused by an RNA paramyxovirus. Up to the age of three to four months, infants are protected by passively acquired maternal antibodies. Large families living in crowded conditions predispose to the disease being introduced into a household by an older sibling, and thus infants in developing countries can acquire measles very early in life.

In many countries the epidemiology of measles is changing following increased immunization coverage and mass immunization campaigns. Together with routine immunization, mass campaigns have resulted in a 90 per cent reduction in measles mortality in a few African countries during the past decade. Nevertheless, in disadvantaged, marginalized communities, measles

Table 14.3 Erythematous maculopapular rashes

Disease	Description of rash	Prodrome	Other features	Complications	Cause
Measles	Generalized maculopapular starting behind ears and face, spreading to trunk and limbs, becomes confluent	Fever, cough, conjunctivitis, Koplik spots	Post-measles staining	Pneumonia, croup, eye complications, diarrhoea, suppression of immunity	Morbillivirus
Rubella	Fine generalized discrete maculopapular rash	Mild fever	Suboccipital adenopathy, arthralgia	Rarely encephalitis, thrombocytopaenia	Rubivirus
Non-polio enterovirus	Measles-like, may be petechial	Abrupt onset	Common under 5 years. Associated herpangina often	Many including meningo-encephalitis, gastoenteristis, myopericarditis, others	Coxsackie and Echo viruses
Infectious mononucleosis	Generalized maculopapular, usually precipitated by ampicillin treatment, may become purpuric	Malaise, headache, fever, sore throat, adenopathy, splenomegaly	Few clinical features under 4 years. Lifelong latent infection established	Heamolytic anaemia, thrombocytopaenia, hepatitis, oncogenesis	Epstein-Barr virus (HHV 5)
Erythema infectiosum	'Slapped cheek' flushed appearance, then lace-like macular rash on trunk and limbs	Unusual	Afebrile, generally well. Palms and soles are spared	Arthritis, arthralgia, transient aplastic crisis, chronic hypoplastic anaemia	Parvovirus B19
Roseola infantum	Rose-coloured discrete lesions spread from trunk to face and proximal extremities	Upper respiratory signs, then high fever, irritability, some with febrile convulsions	Rash appears as fever subsides	Rare encephalitis	Herpesvirus 6 and 7
Scarlet fever	Punctate erythema on face or generalized circumoral pallor	Fever and sore throat	'Strawberry' tongue	Nephritis, rheumatic fever	Group A beta-haemolytic streptococcus
Toxic shock syndrome	Diffuse macular erythroderma with subsequent desquamation on hands and feet	Unusual	High fever, hypotension, myalgia, 'strawberry' tongue, diarrhoea	Renal failure, ARDS, circulatory failure	Toxin–producing *Staphylococcus aureus*
Kawasaki disease	Diffuse maculopapular, scarlatiniform or erythema multiforme	Fever	Bulbar conjunctival injection, mucosal erythema and strawberry tongue, cervical adenopathy, desquamation of fingers, palms and soles	Coronary aneurysms	Unknown
Drug reactions	Usually morbilliform	Antibiotic exposure often for febrile illness	Rash unrelated to fever, pruritus, improves on drug withdrawal	Unusual	Antibiotic exposure often for febrile illness

remains an important cause of infant and child-hood morbidity and mortality. Sporadic disease in young children is declining, but outbreaks affecting predominantly 5–14-year-old children are common. In developed countries, the disease affects mainly older children and adolescents as a consequence of waning immunity or incomplete immunization.

The disease is transmitted by droplet spread and is communicable for about seven days from the onset of the prodrome. However, prolonged excretion of the virus may occur for up to a few weeks in severe disease of poorly nourished and immunocompromised children. HIV infected children may be susceptible to measles infection at an earlier age, due to reduced maternal-derived antibody.

Severe measles occurs in:
- Infants <1 year
- Malnourished children
- The immunocompromised (including HIV infection)
- Vitamin A-deficient children
- Patients from crowded homes.

The disease must be considered to be serious when complicated by:
- Pneumonia
- Encephalitis
- Diarrhoea
- Laryngotracheobronchitis (LTB).

Measles commonly causes:
- Malnutrition
- Secondary bacterial infection, identified in 50 per cent of measles-associated deaths
- Immune depression
- Recurrent infections, including chronic pulmonary disease.

Measles can be prevented by vaccination.

Pathophysiological factors

The clinical expression of infection and complications is influenced by the extent of virus-induced epithelial damage, by the degree of immune suppression, and by the patient's vitamin A status. The pathological effects of measles virus infection and vitamin A deficiency are remarkably similar, in that both are responsible for epithelial damage and immune suppression. In addition, measles induces a rapid drop in vitamin A levels, which may manifest itself biochemically or in the development of xerophthalmia.

The clinical significance of measles virus immunosuppression is well recognized. Lymphopenia due to lower T and B lymphocyte levels, impaired antibody response, and reduced C3 levels are predictors of the clinical severity of measles.

Low vitamin A status has been associated with a higher rate of complications and a higher death rate. Even in the USA, where clinical vitamin A deficiency is virtually unheard of, low serum vitamin A levels have also been associated with an increased risk of hospitalization and severe disease.

Clinical features

After an incubation period of 10–11 days, a prodrome or catarrhal phase occurs with fever, cough, coryza, and conjunctivitis. On the fourth day the rash appears. Koplik's spots appear two days before the rash and are usually present for four days. This **enanthem**, which is pathognomonic of measles, consists of small red spots on the buccal and labial mucous membrane, each with a minute white centre, not unlike salt grains.

The **exanthem** is an erythematous maculo-papular (morbilliform) eruption, which spreads from the face to the trunk and arms, and continues on to the legs on the third day. It begins to fade by the third day in order of appearance. After the second or third day of the rash, the temperature falls rapidly and convalescence ensues. If the child is feverish beyond the third day of rash, a complication should be suspected. A brown staining of the skin follows and lasts for one to two months, while fine desquamation, sparing the hands and feet, may occur as the rash fades.

Complications

Complications that tend to occur early during the clinical course (within a week of the appearance of the rash) such as croup, diarrhoea, and pneumonia, may be due to the effects of the measles virus itself and even though they may be severe, they are not usually life threatening. Later complications are usually due to secondary viral or bacterial infections. Post-measles pneumonia, croup, and diarrhoea are the most common life-threatening complications. Corneal ulceration may result in blindness. Other common complications include malnutrition, otitis media, and herpes gingivo-stomatitis. The frequency of complications varies in different parts of the world. In the USA, complications were reported in 20 per cent of cases, and these included diarrhoea, otitis media, pneumonia, and encephalitis. In developing countries, hospital-based surveys have shown that the three major problems which are associated with a significantly higher mortality than others are pneumonia, diarrhoea, and croup, occurring in up to 75, 80 and 25 per cent of hospitalized cases respectively.

Recovery following acute measles may be delayed for many weeks and even months and is characterized by failure to thrive, recurrent infections, persistent pneumonia, and diarrhoea. It is probably due to viral persistence with immune suppression. If present, vitamin A deficiency will aggravate these problems. The survival rate of children during this phase is also significantly reduced. These problems underscore the importance of long-term follow-up once the child with measles recovers from the acute illness.

Uncommon complications include acute encephalitis, nephritis, pneumomediastinum, myocarditis, pericarditis, hepatitis, ileocolitis, appendicitis, and subacute sclerosing panencephalitis (SSPE).

Pulmonary complications. These are common and are the main cause of death from measles.

Pneumonia following measles may be due to bacterial superinfection (50 per cent of cases), often by a combination of Gram-positive and Gram-negative organisms. Just as frequently the cause is viral: the measles virus itself or superinfection by adenovirus and herpesvirus leads to bronchiolar and interstitial necrosis. Healing may be slow and incomplete, leading to obliterative bronchiolitis or bronchiectasis. Concomitant infection with measles and adenovirus produces the most severe symptoms, most prolonged course and highest mortality rate.

Laryngotracheo-bronchitis (LTB). Mild laryngitis is a common feature of measles. More significant inflammation of the upper airway may occur, and obstruction of airflow results in stridor and retractions. LTB occurs during the period of the rash, but also in the post-measles state, when the cause is sometimes due to secondary infection by viruses such as adenovirus, para-influenza, or herpes simplex.

Encephalitis, acute. This occurs in about 0.1 per cent of cases, with onset usually during the rash, but it can occur before the rash appears or in the post-measles period. The CSF displays a typical viral picture, although in rare instances it may be normal.

The course is variable, but in general, 60 per cent recover, 15 per cent die, and the remainder have neurological sequelae.

Immunosuppressive measles encephalopathy. Children with defective cellular immunity under cytotoxic therapy may have mild or atypical measles infection, followed by encephalitis one to six months later. The prognosis is poor, with survivors having severe neurological damage.

Subacute sclerosing panencephalitis (SSPE). In about 1 in 100 000 cases of measles, SSPE occurs some years after the initial disease (mean six years). This slowly progressive encephalitis almost always ends fatally. It has followed most often where measles occurred in the very young. Despite this, the prevalence is no higher in communities where the disease is rife at an early age.

Diarrhoea is a common complication, reducing food intake and contributing to a negative nitrogen balance. Florid malnutrition may be precipitated by measles in children with suboptimal nutrition. Cellular damage of the absorptive surface of the bowel leads to diarrhoea, protein-losing enteropathy, and lactose intolerance.

Otitis media, a common complication in measles, almost pales into insignificance in measles cases in developing communities, because of the high incidence of pneumonia, diarrhoea, and LTB. It should nevertheless be sought in all patients during convalescence, as it may not resolve, resulting in chronic infection and hearing loss.

Corneal ulceration following conjunctivitis is especially likely to occur in malnourished children.

Herpes simplex gingivo-stomatitis. There is an increased susceptibility to this condition in children with measles. Dissemination of the virus can occur, particularly in children with kwashiorkor.

Prognosis

The prognosis for measles has improved as living conditions for children have become better. Universally high morbidity and mortality occurs among children who are malnourished, immunosuppressed, and under one year of age, and where an increased viral load occurs due to overcrowding of children in a home. Case fatality rates in hospitalized children are high and frequently exceed 5 per cent. Most of these deaths follow complications such as pneumonia, croup, and diarrhoea, and are also frequently associated with malnutrition. Lymphopaenia of less than $2\,000/mm^3$ in the first two days of the rash also carries a poor prognosis and indicates slow recovery from complications. This lymphopaenia is due to a decrease in numbers of both B- and T-lymphocyte cells and is significantly associated with the histocompatibility leucocyte antigen (HLA) AW32.

Treatment

Measles is usually an uncomplicated self-limiting disease in well-nourished children and requires supportive management, which consists of an antipyretic and a cough mixture.

In less favoured communities, where the course is often complicated, more intensive therapy is required. Admission to hospital is warranted if a complication other than otitis media is present.

The nutritional status is compromised as a result of the catabolic effects of the disease and the fever, associated diarrhoea and vomiting, refusal to take food because of mouth ulcers, or anorexia. Maintain and encourage breastfeeding. If not breastfed – continue feeding even if diarrhoea is present. Provide additional vitamins and minerals and increase the energy content of the food. Nasogastric tube-feeding may be necessary. Along with oral or intravenous rehydration fluids if required for diarrhoea, continuation of milk feeds is recommended. A low lactose or semi- elemental feed may need to be substituted for cow's milk if diarrhoea becomes prolonged. (See Chapter 24, Gastrointestinal disorders.)

Cleansing of the eyes with warm saline prevents superinfection with viral conjunctivitis. Antibiotic eye ointment may also be necessary, especially if there is secondary bacterial infection. Do not use steroid ointments. If there are signs of xerophthalmia, make sure that the child has been given vitamin A. Apply a protective eye pad to prevent other infections.

Mouth ulcers are frequently due to secondary herpes infections and may be complicated by anaerobic sepsis. Clean the mouth with clean water or saline. Metronidazole should be prescribed if anaerobic infection is present.

Antibiotics should only be given if there is a specific indication such as pneumonia, otitis media, or dysentery. Indiscriminate use of antibiotics may result in unnecessary complications, such as antibiotic-associated diarrhoea, drug reactions, and emergence of drug-resistant organisms, at present a problem in many parts of the world. The role of prophylactic antibiotics to prevent the bacterial complications of measles is unclear. Nevertheless, broad-spectrum antibiotics (ampicillin or co-trimoxazole) are recommended for children at risk for secondary bacterial infections. This includes children with severe malnutrition, AIDS, and xerophthalmia.

Vitamin A therapy has been shown to reduce significantly the risk of complications (particularly pneumonia, diarrhoea, and corneal ulceration) as well as the death rate. The dose of vitamin A recommended by the WHO is indicated in the next column.

Prevention

Measles-attenuated live virus vaccine. This vaccine may cause a fever or a mild measles-like illness seven to 10 days after administration. The incidence of reactions is higher in the poorly nourished, but even those with kwashiorkor show seroconversion, although this is delayed. Because vaccine virus, like the wild virus, causes temporary immunoparesis, use of the vaccine in the malnourished should be restricted to those at home (as opposed to those at increased risk for superinfection, e.g. in a hospital), or to those whose nutritional rehabilitation has been initi-

Vitamin A for measles schedule:

Age	Dose at diagnosis	Dose next day
Infants		
<6 months	50 000 IU	50 000 IU
Infants		
6–11 months	100 000 IU	100 000 IU
Children		
>12 months	200 000 IU	200 000 IU

Note: Repeat dose at four to six months in children with ophthalmic evidence of Vitamin A deficiency.

ated. Interim protection if needed is achieved by giving human measles immunoglobulin or pooled gammaglobulin, followed in six weeks by active immunization. Failures of seroconversion may be due to improper handling and storage of the vaccine, but also to the presence of maternal antibody in those under one year of age.

In developing communities the risk of measles in the first year is high and carries increased mortality and morbidity. The Schwartz strain of vaccine virus (grown on chick embryo fibroblasts) is recommended at nine months of age with a booster dose of vaccine at 15–18 months of age. In low-risk communities with satisfactory socio-economic conditions, measles vaccine (Schwartz) is given at 15 months, when it can be administered with rubella and mumps vaccines. Repeat vaccination at four to six years of age.

Measles vaccine can be given at the same time as the first DTP and OPV if the primary immunizing course is started after one year of age.

Rubella (German measles)

Rubella is a common childhood exanthem and is caused by an RNA virus belonging to the toga virus family. In susceptible pregnant women it may cause congenital infection of the fetus. Rubella is a worldwide endemic disease, with irregularly occurring epidemics, and is usually seen in older children and young adults. The disease is preventable by means of vaccination. It is droplet spread, with an incubation period of 14–21 days. Children are infectious for seven days before and after the onset of the rash. Newborns with congenital infection may excrete the virus for six months or longer.

Clinical features

Many cases are asymptomatic. There is a prodrome of malaise, coryza, conjunctivitis, and tender lymphadenopathy, usually of suboccipital, post-auricular, and cervical nodes. The pink-red, maculopapular rash appears on the face, spreads rapidly to the trunk and limbs, and lasts for three days. Disease without the exanthem occurs and the rash is difficult to see on pigmented skin.

Serological diagnosis. The haemagglutination-inhibition antibody level rises within 24 to 48 hours of the rash, peaks at 12 days and persists. Complications, which are rare in childhood, are arthralgia, encephalitis, and purpura. The

disease is generally benign in children and life-long immunity is usual. Rubella must be differentiated from other childhood exanthems (*see* Table 14.3).

Prevention

The live-attenuated vaccine RA 27/3 has a high seroconversion rate (95 per cent) and virtually no untoward reactions when given to children. As with other live virus vaccines, it should not be given to pregnant women or to those who may become pregnant within three months of receiving vaccine. Reinfections with rubella can occur: in epidemics there is a much higher incidence of reinfection in vaccinated people (80 per cent) compared with those with natural immunity (40 per cent).

Infectious mononucleosis (IM)

The disease is caused by the Epstein-Barr virus (EBV), which is a member of the herpes virus group. It infects B lymphocytes of humans and primates and is transferred in saliva, from where it can be isolated for at least three months after the acute infection and for much longer in 30 per cent of cases.

EBV infection occurs early in life in underdeveloped communities, where 70 to 90 per cent of the population becomes serologically positive by six years of age. In children, IM is seldom recognized as a clinical entity; seroconversion follows subclinical or non-specific illness.

In developed communities over 50 per cent remain uninfected during childhood and classical IM occurs in adolescents and young adults. But even in this population, subclinical infections are two or three times more common than manifest disease. Infection is transmitted from person to person through contact with salivary secretions. The incubation period is usually 30 to 50 days.

Clinical features

Classical IM syndrome, seen mainly in young adults, has an insidious onset of malaise, headache, and nausea. After about two weeks, fever and pharyngitis occur, with or without tonsillar exudates and petechiae on the soft palate. In the majority of cases there is also lymphadenopathy (mainly posterior cervical and epitrochlear) and hepatosplenomegaly. Occasionally there is oedema of the eyelids and a maculopapular rash.

IM in infants and young children is rarely classical. The majority of seroconversions are subclinical or follow mild upper respiratory symptoms. Occasionally EBV infection is associated with hepatitis, Guillain-Barré syndrome, thrombocytopaenia, haemolytic anaemia, transverse myelitis, and meningo-encephalitis.

Like other herpes virus infections, EBV exhibits latency.

Reactivation may occur, especially in immuno-compromised individuals. It has been implicated as a cause of Burkitt's lymphoma, nasopharyngeal carcinoma, other B cell lymphomas, and lymphoid interstitial pneumonitis in children with AIDS.

Diagnosis

Leucocytosis with 20 to 40 per cent atypical lymphocytes is characteristic of IM.

EBV-specific tests. These immunofluorescent techniques, using different antigens, detect specific viral antibodies:

- IgG antibody to viral capsid antigen (VCA): titre peaks at two to three weeks, then declines, but persists for life.
- IgM antibody to VCA: this titre also rises early, but disappears within two to three months.
- IgG antibody to early antigen appears shortly after VCA appears, and disappears within six months of illness.
- Antibodies to EBV nuclear antigen: titre rises late, but persists for life.

Using a combination of these tests, diagnosis of recent or past infection can be made in all cases of EBV infection.

Differential diagnosis

Infections with cytomegalovirus, toxoplasmosis, and hepatitis virus must be considered. Streptococcal sore throat and diphtheria must be excluded when the pharyngeal signs are prominent. The rash and lymphadenopathy may be confused with those of rubella.

Treatment

Management is supportive and antibiotics should be avoided. Ampicillin in particular has been shown to cause a skin eruption.

Prognosis

The prognosis is good. Very rarely death has occurred from splenic rupture, Guillain-Barré syndrome, or haemolytic anaemia.

Cytomegalovirus (CMV) infections

CMV has the characteristics of herpes virus and causes a mononucleosis-like illness. Of worldwide distribution, both congenital and acquired infection is generally higher in those with a low standard of living. Virus is excreted in the urine, faeces, milk, saliva, and upper respiratory tract, and there is cervical shedding in pregnant women. The virus may be transmitted from any of these sources. Infection may also be transmitted via blood or through transplanted organs. Congenital infection follows infection via trans-placental blood spread. Acquired infection in the newborn is a consequence of contamination with cervical secretions.

Acquired CMV infections

In immunocompetent individuals infection is usually inapparent and the majority of children in developing countries would be infected with CMV by two to three years of age. Occasionally, CMV can be associated in infants with pneumonia, paroxysmal cough, petechial rash, hepatosplenomegaly, and polyneuritis. Older children exhibit an infectious mononucleosis-like syndrome. The prognosis is usually good.

In the immunocompromised (children with AIDS, transplants, and malignancies) the disease may manifest with pneumonia, colitis, hepatitis, and chorioretinitis. It is frequently severe and can be fatal.

Diagnosis is by virus isolation. Antibody titres are less reliable as cross-reactions with other herpes viruses occur. The serum pp65 antigen detection is a useful diagnostic test and strongly associated with active disease, especially in immunocompromised persons. CMV infections need to be differentiated from infectious mononucleosis and hepatitis due to A or B viruses.

Treatment

Ganciclovir, an acyclic nucleoside analogue, may be of use, but its efficacy has mainly been established in treatment of CMV chorioretinitis.

Treatment is usually given for two to four weeks. HIV infected immunocompromised individuals surviving treatment with ganciclovir for CMV pneumonitis may require ongoing prophylaxis after four to six weeks of treatment.

Diseases associated with vesicular/blistering rashes

(*See* Table 14.4.)

Chickenpox (varicella)

Primary infection with varicella zoster virus (VZV) causes chickenpox. VZV is identical to herpes virus hominis on electron microscopy. Chickenpox occurs at any age, with a peak age incidence at five to ten years. It is a highly communicable disease spread by droplets or by direct contact with vesicular fluid. Infectivity lasts from 24 hours before the rash appears until all lesions have scabbed, usually a period of six to seven days.

Clinical features

After a 13- to 17-day incubation, a mild pro-dromal illness (fever, headache, and malaise) lasting 24–48 hours occurs, followed by a crop of red papules, which rapidly develop into clear vesicles. Within 24 hours these become cloudy, then umbilicate, and dry to scabs. Crops of vesicles erupt for three to four days, starting from the trunk and spreading to the face, scalp, conjunctivae, and mucous membranes. At the height of the disease the eruption consists of all stages of the rash. Systemic reaction is usually minor.

Complications

Secondary bacterial sepsis caused by staphylo-cocci or streptococci is common. Rare complica-tions include thrombocytopaenia, pneumonia, myocarditis, hepatitis, glomerulonephritis, en-cephalitis, and Guillain-Barré syndrome. Cere-bellar ataxia is another well-recognized but rare complication. Recovery is usually complete. Adults tend to develop encephalitis character-ized by convulsions, depressed level of con-sciousness, and focal signs. About 10 per cent of Reye's syndrome cases are associated with varicella virus infection. Children with AIDS or malignancy, or on cytotoxic drugs and steroids are at risk of developing severe, disseminated, and fatal disease, which may manifest as a severe necrotizing pneumonia.

Differential diagnosis

Papular urticaria, bullous impetigo, scabies, mol-luscum contagiosum.

Perinatal varicella infection. Infants born to mothers in whom varicella occurs within seven days before or after delivery are at high risk of severe neonatal disease. Varicella develops in 33 per cent of these neonates, often with a severe course and 30–50 per cent mortality rate. Newborns born to mothers developing varicella during the first and second trimesters may develop severe congenital abnormalities.

Herpes zoster (shingles)

Zoster is thought to be a reactivation of latent infection with VZV. Following acute infection the virus may remain dormant in the dorsal nerve roots and reactivation at a later stage due to some stress factor results in herpes zoster or shingles. It is uncommon in normal children. There is an increased incidence of zoster in those immunosuppressed by malignancy, drugs, or in AIDS sufferers. The reactivated virus spreads from sensory ganglia along nerves to the skin and produces a vesicular eruption. The virus may be shed from skin lesions, producing varicella in susceptible subjects.

Clinical features

Pain and paraesthesiae occur over a sensory dermatome (spinal or cranial), followed in two to four days by a localized vesicular eruption. The disease may be complicated by meningitis, encephalitis, hepatitis, and post-herpetic neural-gia (uncommon in children).

Therapy of VZV infections

Prophylaxis. Zoster immune globulin (ZIG) is indicated for:

- Susceptible contacts if given within 72 hours of exposure. Prevention of disease is less effective in immunosuppressed contacts.

Table 14.4 Blistering and vesicular skin rashes

Disease	Description of rash	Other features and complications	Cause
Chickenpox	Crops of vesicles develop on red papules, spread from trunk, become turbid and umbilicate	Mild fever, secondary infection of ruptured vesicles. Ataxia, encephalitis, pneumonia	Varicella zoster virus
Herpes zoster (shingles)	Vesicles develop in the distribution of dermatomes	Uncommonly localized pain. In immunocompromised patients may disseminate	Varicella zoster virus
Herpes simplex gingivostomatitis	Thin-walled superficial blisters rupture early, inside of mouth and lips, extend to skin around mouth, may spread	Fever and irritability	Herpes simplex virus
Eczema herpeticum	Thin-walled superficial blisters clustering in areas of eczematous skin	Fever, Risk of dissemination and secondary infection	Herpes simplex virus
Hand, foot and mouth disease	Ulcers on tongue and buccal mucosa, vesicles on dorsal surfaces, palms and soles of hands and feet	Fever. Rarely aseptic meningitis, encephalitis	Coxsackie A 16 and Enterovirus 71
Impetigo	Vesicle on traumatized skin develops into honey-coloured, crusted plaque; oozes	No fever or constitutional symptoms. Regional adenopathy	Streptococci or staphylococci
Staphylococcal scalded skin syndrome	Localized bullous impetigo or generalized erythematous tender skin which closely resembles severe burn	Fever, irritability, skin tenderness. Secondary sepsis	Staphylococcus aureus
Papular urticaria	Various stages between erythematous wheals and oedematous redbrown papules	Pruritus. Secondary infection (impetigo)	Flea or insect bites Hypersensitivity reaction
Stevens Johnson syndrome	Macules, vesicles, bullae, desquamation, haemorrhagic crusting on face, trunk, extremities. Erythema multiforme, target lesions. Involvement of two or more mucosal surfaces	Corneal ulceration, scarring and strictures, pneumonia, myocarditis, hepatitis, renal failure	Mycoplasma pneumoniae Drugs (sulphonamides, NSAIDS, anticonvulsants)
Toxic epidermal necrolysis	Skin erythema and inflammation leads to full thickness skin loss in flaccid bullae. No target lesions. Conjunctivae and mouth often involved	Worst end of spectrum of erythema multiforme. Fever and constitutional symptoms	Infection and drugs Hypersentivity phenomenon

- Pregnant mothers
- Exposed premature newborns
- Infants born to mothers who develop chickenpox a week before or after delivery.

Zoster immune plasma (ZIP) is derived from convalescent zoster cases; 10 ml/kg IV is also effective in protecting susceptible contacts.

Management. The following should be considered:

- Drying lotions and antipruritics can be prescribed for the rash.
- In complicated cases and in immuno-suppressed subjects, ZIP is often effective.
- Radiotherapy or cytotoxic drugs must be stopped, but steroids should be continued.
- Never prescribe aspirin therapy (increased risk of Reye's syndrome).
- Acyclovir intravenously is indicated for children with severe disease, HIV/AIDS, malignancies, immune deficiency, and for neonatal varicella. Some authorities would recommend oral acyclovir 20 mg/kg six-hourly for all infants with chickenpox, since morbidity and mortality are usually highest in the first year of life.
- Antibiotics should be prescribed for those with secondary infections. Give cloxacillin if staphylococcal infection is suspected.

Prevention

A live-attenuated varicella vaccine has been developed, which is safe with a high protective efficacy in healthy children. Children should be vaccinated in the second year of life and the vaccine has been shown to be safe for HIV-infected children who are immunocompetent (CD4 ≥25 per cent). Following varicella vaccination, immunity may wane during early childhood and a booster dose may be required during adolescence. When given to leukaemic children in remission seroconversion and protection are slightly reduced and reactions more frequent. The vaccine may be useful in susceptible children as post-exposure prophylaxis provided it is given within 36 hours of exposure.

Herpes simplex virus type 1 (HSV1)

Infants are usually protected for a few months by maternal antibody to HSV1. Primary infection usually occurs between one and five years of age, but in an affluent society may be delayed to adulthood.

The virus spreads by close personal contact or by contamination with infected saliva. Primary infection is usually subclinical in childhood, with about 10 to 20 per cent developing clinical disease. Lesions in the form of vesicles are localized in skin or mucous membrane. Viraemia and dissemination of the infection may occur in the immunosuppressed (measles, malnutrition, malignancy). High-risk or very ill patients should receive acyclovir intravenously.

Clinical syndromes

Gingivostomatitis. HSV1 is the commonest cause of stomatitis in children under five years. The onset is abrupt or insidious, with fever, salivation, and refusal to eat. Vesicles develop on the lips, gums, tongue, and buccal membrane and rapidly rupture to leave shallow, painful coalescing ulcers with a thin red margin, covered with a yellow-grey membrane. The ulcers may extend into the nasopharynx and may be found also in the anterior nares, causing a clear discharge, which may be the cause of further herpetic vesicles around the nostrils and on the cheeks and chin. The acute phase, which is self-limiting, lasts between four and nine days. Primary infection of fingers and abrasions occur in adults at risk, e.g. health workers. In stomatitis, oral hygiene is most easily achieved by giving small, frequent fluid feeds. Local application of analgesic cream is useful and in severe cases, admission to hospital for tube feeding may be necessary.

Eczema herpeticum. Widespread primary infection of eczematous skin can occur with HSV1. The vesicles develop in crops for seven to ten days, after which scabs form and healing occurs. Systemic reaction with high fever is common.

Meningo-encephalitis is seen in all ages. HSV2 (*see below*) is the usual cause in neonates and HSV1 in older patients. It can occur during primary or recurrent infection, carries a high mortality rate, and frequently produces permanent neurological sequelae in survivors. There is some evidence of improved prognosis with acyclovir. (*See also* Chapter 26, Neurological and muscular disorders.)

Conjunctivitis and kerato-conjunctivitis are also manifestations of primary or recurrent infections. The diagnosis is suggested by herpetic vesicles of the eyelids (*see* Chapter 33, Disorders of the eyes).

Recurrent disease. The virus becomes latent in sensory ganglia. Recurrent attacks occur in 30 per cent of cases, despite adequate serum antibody levels. The virus spreads to the skin along cutaneous nerves, and vesicles occur in mucocutaneous areas such as the lips. Recurrences (so-called 'fever blisters') are associated with pneumonia, meningitis, malaria, exposure to cold or sun, menstruation, viral respiratory infections, and emotional stress.

Disseminated herpes. In children with secondary immunodeficiency (usually measles or malnutrition) who have herpes simplex infection, dissemination of virus is to be suspected in the presence of neurological signs, increasing hepatomegaly, signs of liver failure or DIC, worsening pneumonia, or pyrexia. These patients are usually anaemic and septicaemic, and require vigorous therapy with intravenous acyclovir.

Herpes virus type 2 (HSV2)

Infections are usually post-pubertal and transmitted venereally. The usual clinical expression is genital herpes, although cervical involvement is often subclinical. Sixty per cent of adults in lower socio-economic groups and 10 per cent in higher groups have antibodies to HSV2; 5 to 10 per cent of cases are due to HSV1.

Neonates may contract HSV2 from maternal genital herpes. The resultant disease is usually disseminated and often fatal.

Impetigo and other staphylococcal and streptococcal skin conditions

Staphylococci and streptococci commonly cause primary and secondary skin infections in children, particularly if they are malnourished and live in overcrowded, unhygienic conditions.

Impetigo is a very common, superficial, contagious skin infection, which may be caused by either staphylococci or streptococci from the patient's nose or from other children, but usually both. Infection often starts in the nostrils and the face is most commonly affected, but any part of the skin may be involved. The lesions, which may be single or multiple and confluent, start as superficial blisters and spread to form round, moist, eroded, or crusted areas, at the periphery of which the remains of the blister are usually visible (*see* Chapter 32, Skin disorders). Treatment consists of antibiotic ointments such as Polysporin® or Terramycin®, which should also be applied to the anterior nares because many patients carry the organism in their noses. Where lesions are widespread, an antibiotic should be given by mouth in addition. Erythromycin and cloxacillin are usually safe and effective where sensitivity tests are not available.

Impetigo neonatorum. Neonates are particularly susceptible to *Staphylococcus aureus* and easily develop generalized infections. In the newborn, staphylococcal impetigo may spread rapidly to form large superficial blisters, often containing pus. Swabs for culture should be taken from an unbroken blister and antibiotic treatment started immediately. Epidermolysis bullosa and bullous congenital syphilis should be excluded by biopsy and serology if necessary.

Staphylococcal scalded skin syndrome

The clinical picture resembles that of very superficial burns and is due to a toxin which causes erythema and desquamation. The site of the staphylococcal infection may be the nose, eyes, or skin. Staphylococci may be isolated from the primary infection, but are not found in the distant skin lesions due to the toxin (*see* Chapter 32, Skin disorders).

Skin eruptions secondary to streptococcal tonsillitis

Desquamation of the skin, particularly the palms and soles, may be the only complaint in a patient who is otherwise well and has not had scarlet fever. It is thought to be due to a previous asymptomatic infection with streptococci which produce an erythrogenic toxin. A fine rash, consisting of very small, diffuse, superficial papules, occurring in children with a fever, may be due to streptococcal tonsillitis (*see* Chapter 32, Skin disorders). The rash and fever respond rapidly to an oral antibiotic. Streptococcal tonsillitis may precipitate an attack of guttate psoriasis or seborrhoeic dermatitis and streptococcal infection is probably the most common cause of urticaria in children.

In any unusual rash in children, the possibility of streptococcal infection should be considered first.

Diseases associated with petechial/purpuric rashes

(*See* Table 14.5.)

Meningococcal disease

Meningococcal disease is caused by *Neisseria meningitidis,* a Gram-negative diplococcus transmitted from person to person by droplet spread. Risk factors for disease include overcrowding, creche attendance, and immune deficiency, particularly Complement 5–8 deficiency. The disease is endemic in many developed countries and sporadic outbreaks occur. Annual incidence rates vary between 0.5–5/100 000 population. In developing countries incidence rates vary from 5–50/100 000, with the higher incidence in African countries closer to the equator (meningitis belt region). During epidemics, which occur cyclically, disease incidence rates may exceed 300. In South Africa the average annual notifications number about 1 000 per year with an incidence rate of 3–6/100 000. Attack rates are highest in children younger than five years. There are five major serotypes (A, B, C, W135, Y) of *N. meningitides,* with serotype A being the most common cause of meningitis outbreaks in the meningitis-belt countries. In South Africa, while meningococcal meningitis occurs sporadically in most of the country, serotype B is the dominant serotype in the Western Cape and serotype W135 elsewhere. The dominant serotype may fluctuate over time.

Clinical features

After an incubation period of usually two to four days, approximately 35 per cent of cases present with meningitis, 15 per cent with septicaemia, and 50 per cent with both. Rare presentations include chronic meningococcaemia, pneumonia, and endophthalmitis.

The onset of the septicaemic illness is usually abrupt, with fever, chills and prostration. The rash is typically petechial or purpuric and evolves rapidly. It may be widespread and involve mucosal surfaces as well. Occasionally a maculopapular eruption may occur. In severe cases extensive purpura, DIC, and shock may be followed by coma and death within a few hours. Case fatality rates vary from 8–25 per cent. Factors predictive of a poor prognosis include rapid onset of disease, shock, coma, acidosis, seizures, DIC, and absence of meningitis.

Meningococcal meningitis is clinically indistinguishable from other causes of meningitis. Severe cases may present with convulsions, focal neurological signs, and depressed level of consciousness, but these features are less common in the acute phase than with *Haemophilus influenzae* type b or pneumococcal meningitis. Case fatality rates are generally less than 5 per cent.

Diagnosis

Non-blanching purpura in a sick and febrile child is virtually diagnostic of meningococcaemia. Other causes of purpura include Henoch-Schönlein purpura, occasionally bacterial infections, viral haemorrhagic disease, and idiopathic thrombocytopaenic purpura (ITP). The diagnosis is confirmed by blood culture. Organisms may also be seen in skin scrapings or biopsy. CSF examination should only be done if no signs of raised intracranial pressure are present.

Diagnosis of meningitis is confirmed by isolation of the organism in the CSF.

Antigen detection in CSF, urine, or serum by counter-immuno-electrophoresis or latex agglutination may be useful in situations where prior antibiotics have been used and when cultures may be negative.

Treatment

Meningococcal disease is a medical emergency. If a case is suspected administer the first dose of antibiotics, provide supportive care and refer urgently to hospital.

Treat meningococcal disease with parenteral penicillin or a cephalosporin for seven days. Penicillin-resistant isolates have been reported, but are rare. Management of septicaemic shock is outlined earlier.

Prevention

Primary prevention. Capsular polysaccharide vaccines are available against groups A, C, Y and W135. Immune response to group A antigen is satisfactory from the age of three months, protective titre of antibodies develop in one week and

Table 13.5 Petechial or purpuric rashes

Disease	Description of rash	Associated features and complications	Cause
Meningococcal septicaemia	Maculopapular, petechial or purpuric with ecchymoses, occasionally vesicular	Fever, pharyngitis, weakness and headache. Rapid progression to shock, DIC, coma. May develop pneumonia, myocarditis, arthritis, meningitis	*Neisseria meningitidis*
Disseminated intravascular coagulation	Petechiae and ecchymoses, also areas of skin necrosis can develop	Severe predisposing systemic disease process, bleeding from puncture sites, haemolytic and blood loss anaemia	Excessive activation of clotting in sepsis, shock, acidosis, snakebite, rickettsial infections, incompatible blood transfusions
Rickettsial diseases	Discrete pale red blanching maculopapular rash on limbs, palms and soles spread to whole body, may become purpuric	Fever, headache, myalgia, can develop DIC, meningoencephalitis, myocarditis, pneumonia	Rickettsiae
Viral haemorrhagic fevers	Maculopapular rashes on face and trunk become petechial, associated red enanthem on palate common	Prior fever, headache, myalgia, vomiting. DIC universal, leads to haemorrhagic tendency	Several viruses: Ebola, Marburg, Lassa, Dengue, Rift Valley, Congo
Acquired cytomegalovirus infection	Petechial rash occasionally	Subclinical in most, some with fever, pneumonitis, hepatitis, hepatosplenomegaly, adenopathy. Severe in immunocompromised	Cytomegalovirus
Henoch Schönlein purpura	Pink maculopapules blanching on pressure progress to palpable purpura on dependent areas (buttocks, legs, arms)	Mild fever, arthritis, abdominal pain, proteinuria	IgA-mediated vasculitis of small vessels
Idiopathic thrombocytopaenic purpura	Petechia and purpura (non-palpable), also in conjunctivae and mouth	Preceding viral infection, otherwise well Risk of intracerebral haemorrhage low	Platelet auto-antibodies triggered by virus infection

last for one to three years. The other groups of antigens are poor immunogens for those under two years of age. The vaccine is indicated to control outbreaks of meningococcal disease, for travellers to epidemic areas, and for household contacts of a patient. Quadrivalent (serotype A, C, Y, W135) polysaccharide-protein conjugate vaccines have been established to be immunogenic and efficacious in infants vaccinated as early as two, three and four months of age. Although there has been some progress in developing vaccines against serogroup B, the available vaccines are not efficacious against all subtypes of serogroup B, and consequently there is no available vaccine against serogroup B in Africa.

Secondary prevention. Since contacts of cases are at increased risk for disease, chemoprophylaxis is recommended for exposed household and day-care-centre contacts, but for hospital staff only if intensive and intimate exposure has occurred, such as following mouth-to-mouth resuscitation.

The drug of choice is rifampicin (adults 600 mg, infants 5 mg/kg and children 10 mg/kg twice daily for two days). Alternatives are ceftriaxone or, in adults, minocycline or ciprofloxacin. Sulphonamides are no longer recommended because of high resistance rates. Other antimicrobial agents are ineffective.

Rickettsial infections

Rickettsiae are obligate intracellular bacteria appearing as pleomorphic coccobacilli on light microscopy, with a diameter of 0.3–0.5 microns. The organism is transmitted to humans from an animal reservoir by arthropod vectors such as the tick, louse, flea and mite. Small vessel endothelium is invaded and subsequent proliferation of cells may result in thrombosis and/or plasma leakage. These changes occur principally in skin, meninges, brain, myocardium, kidneys, and lungs and are responsible for the characteristic symptomatology.

Rickettsial infections in childhood can be grouped according to a number of different criteria into the following:

- Typhus
- Scrub typhus
- Spotted fevers, e.g. tick-bite fever, Rocky Mountain spotted fever
- Q fever.

The main epidemiological and clinical features of these are summarized in Table 14.6.

Clinical features

Generally rickettsial infections are mild in children and often escape diagnosis.

Tickbite fever (tick typhus) is seen predominantly in Caucasian children. Early exposure causing mild illness and producing long-lasting immunity might account for the infrequent occurrence of this disease in other groups.

The dominant features are pyrexia and headache, which rapidly reach peak intensity and respond poorly to symptomatic treatment. A small eschar at the site of the bite is found in most patients with regional lymphadenopathy. The typical maculopapular or non-blanching purpuric rash of vasculitis appears on the second or third day in less than 50 per cent of patients. A moderate splenomegaly is sometimes encountered. Significant cardiovascular, respiratory, or neurological features are usually absent, but in rare cases severe meningo-encephalitis may be seen. The disease is self-limiting, with symptoms settling after a week.

Table 14.6 Rickettsial infections

Disease group	Causative agent	Vector	Animal host	Incubation period (days)	Rash (day of onset)
Typhus	R. prowazeki	Louse	Humans	14	4–7
Scrub typhus	R. tsutsugamushi	Mite	Rodents	6–11	5–8
Tick-bite fever	R. conori, australis, etc.	Tick	Mammals, rodents	5–8	2–3

Epidemic typhus occurs at times of war and during population shifts when facilities for hygiene are inadequate and there is general dislocation. It is the most severe of the rickettsioses in children, although not as serious as it is in adults. The disease is spread by contaminated faeces of an infected body louse. The faeces gain entry through abraded skin or the upper respiratory tract. After an incubation period of up to 14 days there is a sudden onset of severe pyrexia, headache, and malaise. The rash, which appears four to seven days after onset, blanches on pressure initially but in severe cases is haemorrhagic. In some cases the rash may be transient or not appear at all.

Stupor, delirium, circulatory collapse, and renal insufficiency suggest severe pathology and these features may be accompanied by pneumonia. The untreated patient improves during the third week and recovers completely thereafter.

Q fever, which rarely affects children, differs markedly from the others in that the mode of spread is by inhalation of infected animal material, with subsequent pulmonary symptomatology and varying degrees of systemic illness.

Diagnosis

Rickettsiosis must be considered in any patient with pyrexia of unknown origin. Meningococcaemia, typhoid, measles, meningitis, and encephalitis must be considered in the differential diagnosis. Typical features, i.e. rash and/or eschar, facilitate an early diagnosis.

Laboratory confirmation is achieved by indirect fluorescent antibody assay, but early diagnosis is not always possible. Treatment should not be withheld pending laboratory confirmation in clinically suspect cases.

Treatment

Chloramphenicol and tetracyclines both suppress but do not kill rickettsiae. Nevertheless, they have made a considerable difference to the severity of this disease complex.

Dosage (of either drug). 50–100 mg/kg/24 hours by mouth in four divided doses, or 30–40 mg/kg/24 hours IV in eight-hourly doses. Drug treatment should be continued until the child has been apyrexial for 48 hours. Doxycycline 2–4 mg/kg in one to two doses is a better alternative to tetracycline as the risk of dental staining is less.

Supportive measures, such as maintenance of hydration and nutrition are of utmost importance. Plasma or plasma expanders are used for circulatory collapse.

Prevention

Appropriate control measures must be instituted where conditions are conducive to epidemics. Rickettsiosis spread by ticks can usually be prevented by early search for and removal of ticks, as two or three days elapse before infection occurs.

Viral haemorrhagic disease

This group of diseases occurs in Africa, Asia, and North America. Only those that have occurred in southern Africa will be outlined here. They share the clinical features as indicated below.

Haemorrhagic fevers must be suspected in the presence of combinations of:
+ Fever and chills
+ Rash, often biphasic, may be haemorrhagic
+ Haemorrhagic diathesis
+ Headaches and/or encephalopathy
+ Hepatitis
+ Conjunctivitis
+ Myalgia and/or arthralgia
+ Vomiting and diarrhoea.

Differential diagnosis of acute haemorrhagic fever

The approach to a case of suspected acute haemorrhagic fever is to assume the worst: isolate and barrier nurse the patient, and take every precaution to prevent nosocomial spread; keep all contacts under close surveillance. Immediate notification of public health personnel and appropriate virus laboratory is mandatory. Management is supportive only.

Meningococcaemia, staphylococcal and streptococcal septicaemia, malaria, and trypanosomiasis are conditions to be considered in addition to the viral haemorrhagic fevers

Dengue fever

Four antigenic types of dengue virus and three other arthropod-borne viruses (chikungunya, o'nyong-nyong, and West Nile fever) cause similar or identical disease. The dengue viruses are transmitted by mosquitoes of the Stegomyia family and the reservoirs are monkeys, birds, and other wild animals. Because of the limited flying range of mosquitoes, spread of an urban epidemic is mainly through movement of viraemic humans. Where dengue viruses are endemic, children and susceptible foreigners acquire overt disease, indigenous adults having become immune.

Epidemics of dengue fever have not occurred in southern Africa in the past 50 years. Chikungunya fever is prevalent in the Limpopo Valley and adjacent areas.

Clinical features

After an incubation period of two to seven days, a biphasic feverish illness develops with headache, vomiting, myalgia, a transient, macular generalized rash, and lymphadenopathy. A secondary rise in temperature is accompanied by a generalized morbilliform, maculopapular rash, which spares the palms and soles. This lasts between one and five days. Prolonged malaise and bradycardia during convalescence are seen in adults, but seldom in children. The platelet count and coagulation factors are normal. Diagnosis is confirmed by serology and virus isolation. Treatment is supportive and the outcome is usually favourable.

Control of disease depends on measures against mosquito bites and mosquito breeding sites in stagnant water.

Dengue haemorrhagic fever (DHF)

DHF occurs where the different types of dengue virus are sequentially transmitted. Second infections with heterologous types are common. DHF is a disease almost exclusively of children and usually due to secondary infections. If it occurs during primary dengue infections, it affects infants whose mothers are immune. DHF is a biphasic illness similar to dengue fever, but

hepatomegaly and a haemorrhagic diathesis occur, sometimes with circulatory shock. Thrombocytopaenia, disseminated intravascular coagulation (DIC) and a rapid secondary-type rise in antibodies are the laboratory findings. Mortality rates vary from 5–40 per cent depending on the effectiveness of management.

Treatment consists of correction of shock and DIC.

Rift Valley fever (RVF)

Epizootics of RVF, affecting sheep and cattle, have occurred in southern Africa since 1951. The disease is acquired by humans when handling carcasses and tissues of affected animals and possibly from mosquito bites. RVF is spread among animals by mosquitoes. Person-to-person spread has not been noted.

After an incubation period of four to six days, a biphasic illness occurs with fever, painful eyes, myalgia, diarrhoea, and vomiting. During recrudescence of fever, encephalitis, hepatitis, and haemorrhagic diathesis are the main features. Management is supportive and fatalities do occur.

Marburg-Ebola fever

Marburg and Ebola viruses, while immunologically distinct, cause a similar disease. Epidemics have occurred in Uganda, Kenya, Sudan, Zaire, and South Africa. The viruses also cause infection in monkeys (*Cercopithecus aethiops*). The natural reservoir is unknown, as is the vector. Mosquitoes can be infected experimentally, but it is uncertain whether they can transmit the disease.

The incubation period is seven to fourteen days, after which sudden fever, headache, malaise, arthralgia, diarrhoea, vomiting, and conjunctivitis develop. On the fifth to the seventh day an erythematous macular rash appears, most marked on the upper arms and legs, followed by hepatic and renal damage and DIC.

Since secondary person-to-person infection has occurred, strict isolation of the patient is necessary. Attendants must take meticulous care with barrier nursing. Treatment is symptomatic. The mortality rate is considerable.

Lassa fever

The reservoir for this virus, the rodent *Mastomys nataliensis*, is widespread in Africa, but the disease in humans has so far been limited to West Africa. Subclinical disease can occur, but high mortality rates of 35–65 per cent among hospitalized cases have been reported. The modes of spread between humans, and rodent and human, have not been established, but virus has been isolated from the pharynx and urine. Rodents may contaminate the air, food, or water through their urine and saliva.

The incubation period is three to sixteen days, followed by fever, chills, headache, pharyngitis, and myalgia. The febrile stage lasts seven to twenty-one days. Hepatic and renal damage may occur with haemorrhage into the bowel and lungs.

Crimean-Congo haemorrhagic fever (CCHF)

Hyalomma ticks, which are the vectors of the disease, occur widely in Africa, eastern Europe, and Asia. Antibodies to CCHF are found in cattle all over South Africa, suggesting that the virus has occurred widely for years. Ticks are infected when feeding on viraemic small mammals (e.g. hares), and transmit the infection to livestock. While cattle and sheep do not become ill, they are briefly viraemic and can be a source of infection for humans. People are infected from a tick-bite, from squashing ticks, or from contact with livestock tissue or with patients. Such nosocomial infection involves direct contact with infective blood. Mild and inapparent infections occur. Case fatalities occur in 15–70 per cent of cases, the latter being in nosocomial outbreaks.

The incubation is about one week, followed by sudden onset of severe headache, fever, and chills. Frequently dizziness, amnesia, confusion, and changed behaviour supervene, accompanied by myalgia, diarrhoea, nausea, anorexia, and vomiting. Fever is often biphasic, and hyperaemia of the face and chest occurs with conjunctivitis, pharyngitis, bradycardia, and hypotension. Haemorrhagic diathesis appears in severe cases on the third to sixth day.

Special investigations may show anaemia, leucopaenia, thrombocytopaenia, abnormal coagu-

lation factors, and raised liver enzymes. Management is supportive.

Diagnosis of infection

At a primary care level investigations should be done only if there is suspicion of a specific disease, or if the fever does not settle within three to four days. The following investigations are frequently undertaken if the need arises to probe the cause of pyrexia: urine tests, full blood count, blood film for malaria, chest radiograph, tuberculin skin test, blood culture, lumbar puncture, stools and serological tests such as a Widal. Acute and convalescent serum should be taken for other serological tests as indicated.

Principles of treatment of infection

Supportive care, including ensuring haemodynamic stability is critical in addition to targeted therapy against pathogenic organisms. Treatment of infections should be targeted against the pathogens most likely to be causing the disease being managed, as well as in relation to the local antibiotic susceptibility patterns and patient-specific risk factors. Initial antibiotic regimens may however require broad-spectrum activity in order to optimize clinical outcomes, especially in severely sick individuals. This should be followed by modification of the regimen with a de-escalation strategy based on the patient's clinical response and the results of microbiological testing. Modification of the initial antibiotic regimen should include:
  ◆ Decreasing the number and/or spectrum of antibiotics, perhaps on the basis of culture and sensitivity results
  ◆ Shortening the duration of therapy in patients with uncomplicated infections who are demonstrating signs of clinical improvement
  ◆ Discontinuing antibiotics in patients who have a noninfectious aetiology identified for their signs and symptoms.

The injudicious use of broad-spectrum antibiotics should be avoided, unless absolutely required. The use of broad-spectrum antibiotics may select for the emergence of multi-resistant bacteria. Additionally, special attention needs to be applied to dosage and dosing regimens to optimise the pharmacokinetic/pharmacodynamic properties of antibiotics, especially in children.

Failure of fever to settle within 48 hours of initiating antibiotic therapy should lead to a review of the subject with the following in mind:

- Is there an alternative cause for the fever and has the correct diagnosis been made?
- Is there any indwelling catheter that may be causing the ongoing infection?
- Is the antibiotic being used adequately dosed?
- Is the antibiotic being used appropriate based upon available antibiotic susceptibility patterns of the targeted pathogen?
- Does the subject possibly have a collection of pus (abdominal organ abscess, osteomyelitis) that requires surgical drainage to optimise antibiotic therapy?
- Could the ongoing fever be related to the drug being used (usually resolves within 24 hours of stopping the drug)?

Nosocomial infections

A nosocomial infection can be defined as an infection that develops 48 hours after admission or following a visit to an outpatient department and which was not present or incubating before that admission/outpatient visit.

Nosocomial infections contribute significantly to patient morbidity and mortality. It is estimated that approximately 5 per cent of patients develop nosocomial infections. Rates tend to increase three- to four-fold in patients admitted to intensive care as well as during respiratory viral epidemics.

Other factors that contribute to the occurrence of nosocomial infections include:

- Impaired patient host defences, including HIV infection
- Prolonged hospitalization
- Overcrowding in wards and clinics
- Contamination of hospital supplies and equipment
- Exposure to invasive devices and procedures such as urinary catheters and intravenous cannulas

- Inappropriate use of broad-spectrum antibiotics
- Emergence of drug-resistant organisms
- Extremes of age
- Infection among staff members.

The spectrum of infections varies widely. In adults, urinary tract infections and wound sepsis are common. In children, respiratory, gastrointestinal and bacteraemic infections are common. While bacterial infections are most prevalent, outbreaks of viral infections, including respiratory syncytial virus (RSV), rotavirus and adenovirus infections may account for a substantial proportion of cases in children. Of particular concern is the proportion of nosocomial bacterial infections, in some cases in excess of 50 per cent, that are resistant to one or more antibiotic.

New, emerging and re-emerging infections

The last recorded naturally occurring case of smallpox was observed in Somalia in 1977, and in 1980 the World Health Organization (WHO) certified smallpox to be absent worldwide. The WHO has now targeted poliomyelitis and measles for eradication. Although many industrialized countries have been certified as being polio free, sporadic cases of polio continue to occur in Africa and polio remains endemic in parts of populous countries such as Nigeria, India and Indonesia. The last case of polio in South Africa occurred

---

Nosocomial infections can be prevented by adhering to policies that have been shown to reduce transmission of infection. These include:

- Hand-washing, which is the single most cost-effective strategy to prevent infection from person to person
- Minimizing the use of catheter devices
- Ensuring strict antiseptic procedures
- Sterilization of hospital equipment
- Isolation of patients where necessary
- Appropriate use of prophylactic and therapeutic antibiotics
- Education of staff.

almost two decades ago. Substantial progress has been made in reducing childhood mortality from measles, especially on the African continent Measles nevertheless is still estimated to cause 190 000 deaths in children under five years of age globally. Civil strife and population migration, especially in Africa, however makes it necessary to continue vaccinating and be vigilant for breakthrough cases caused by these pathogens. In addition to these diseases a number of other infectious diseases have been controlled as a consequence of widespread use of vaccines and socio-economic development.

Despite these tremendous advances in medical science, a number of new infections have emerged and, in the last 30 years, a number of old diseases have re-emerged. The most dramatic of the new infectious diseases is HIV infection, first recognized in the late 1970s and early 1980s. HIV related infections and other morbidity are now the leading cause of mortality in many sub-Saharan African countries. The HIV epidemic has also contributed significantly to the escalation and the re-emergence of other opportunistic infections, including tuberculosis. More recent examples of new emerging diseases include a variant of Creutzfeldt-Jakob disease, which was first described in 1996 in England, avian influenza, which is a well-known infection in birds but was first isolated in humans in Hong Kong in 1997, and SARS (severe acute respiratory syndrome) due to a hitherto unrecognized coronavirus, described in East Asia in 2003.

Recent examples of re-emerging infections include the diphtheria outbreak in the ex-Soviet Union in the mid-nineties, which occurred as a consequence of the collapse of the immunization services, and the reappearance of dengue in the Americas in the 1990s following breakdown in mosquito control programmes.

Factors contributing to emerging and re-emerging infections include:

- Erosion of public health infrastructure
- Social instability, war and famine
- Changes in human behaviour
- Globalization of travel and trade
- Migration of people
- Environmental changes
- Microbial adaptation and change.

Of particular concern to clinicians has been the emergence of multi-drug resistant organisms as a consequence of the inappropriate, widespread use of antibiotics. This has made the treatment of common conditions such as meningitis, dysentery, and tuberculosis difficult.

The WHO, through the Communicable Diseases Surveillance and Response Division, has developed a strategy to respond appropriately to the threats of emerging and re-emerging infections. For developing countries it provides technical advice and training to enhance skills in epidemiology, laboratory diagnosis, and public health interventions.

Prevention of infection

The principles of infection control apply. These consist of the following:

- Identify the infectious case: accurate diagnosis and notification
- Isolate the infectious case where appropriate
- Prevent person-to-person spread by barrier nursing where appropriate
- Safely dispose of fomites
- Use antibiotic prophylaxis where appropriate
- Provide passive immunization of susceptible contacts where appropriate
- Provide active immunization of the susceptible population.

Immunization

Immunization against infectious diseases has had a significant impact on reducing the burden of disease. Since the WHO's Expanded Programme on Immunization (EPI) began, the overall immunization coverage for measles, tuberculosis, pertussis, diphtheria, poliomyelitis, and tetanus has risen from 5 per cent to over 70 per cent in developing countries. This has resulted in a decline in deaths from these diseases during this period from over 10 million

---

Every contact by a health professional with a child must be seen as an opportunity to bring the immunization schedule up to date.

to about 1.5 million. The potential for reduction in infection-related morbidity and mortality has been further strengthened by the development of new vaccines targeting the most common bacterial cause of pneumonia (pneumococcal conjugate vaccine) and viral cause of diarrhoea (rotavirus vaccine).

While every effort is made to complete an immunization schedule in the optimum time, in developing countries this is often not possible; however, perseverance is necessary.

Immunization programmes have failed for the following reasons:
- Lack of political commitment by national decision-makers
- Inadequate funding, staff, supplies, and equipment
- Failure to implement comprehensive primary health care.

Immunization schedules

The schedule and availability of vaccines vary from country to country. The immunization schedule planned for South Africa from 2009 is as follows:
- Birth: OPV (oral polio vaccine), BCG (bacillus Calmette Guerain)
- 6 weeks: OPV, DaPT-IPV-HibCV, HBV, PCV, Rotavirus vaccine
- 10 weeks: DaPT-IPV-HibCV, HBV,
- 14 weeks: OPV, DaPT-IPV-HibCV, HBV, PCV Rotavirus vaccine
- 9 months: Measles, PCV
- 18 months: Measles, DaPT-HibCV
- 5 years: DT

OPV: trivalent oral polio vaccine
DaPT-IPV-HibCV: diptheria, acellular pertussis, tetanus toxoid, trivalent inactivated polio and Haemophilus influenzae type b conjugate vaccine combination vaccine
HBV: Hepatitis B Virus vaccine
PCV: pneumococcal conjugate vaccine

Missed opportunities

Opportunities to immunize are missed when they are not offered at every contact, are denied because of inappropriate contra-indications, or when only one vaccine is given when the child is eligible for more than one. Every opportunity should be taken to immunize children, even those attending health facilities that are not designated as immunization centres. A lapse in the immunization schedule does not necessitate restarting the whole schedule. The remaining dose or doses should be given as if the prolonged period had not occurred.

Immunization of older children not immunized in infancy

Give three primary doses of DaPT-IPV-HibCV and HBV spaced at least four to six weeks apart. Measles vaccine is given at the first visit. Booster DaPT-IPV-HibCV is given about a year following the last primary dose. BCG may be given if the tuberculin test is negative and there is no immunosuppression. PCV is given as a single dose if the child is 12–60 months of age.

Immunization of children with HIV/AIDS

The WHO recommends that children with HIV infection be immunized according to the normal schedule. Where resources permit, they should also be given influenza vaccines before the onset of symptomatic HIV disease. BCG should not, however, be given to children with AIDS or who are known to be HIV infected because of the risk of causing disseminated disease.

Contra-indications to immunization

Egg allergy. Children with a history of significant egg sensitivity (manifested by generalized urticaria, shock, wheezing, upper airway obstruction) should not receive vaccines against diseases such as measles, mumps, and yellow fever, nor influenzae vaccines which are produced in eggs or chick embryos. Refer for expert advice.

Immunosuppression. Children with malignant disease, or those who are receiving cytotoxic, high-dose prolonged steroid or irradiation therapy, should not be given live vaccines, i.e. BCG, measles, MMR, TOPV. Vaccination should be deferred for at least three months following cessation of immunosuppressive therapy. Low-dose or inhaled steroids are not contra-indications.

Pertussis vaccine. Do not give whole-cell pertussis containing vaccine if a child has a progressive CNS disease or if there was a severe reaction to a previous dose (e.g. shock, collapse, or anaphylaxis, persistent screaming for more than three hours, fever above 40.5 °C, convulsions within three days, or encephalopathy within seven days).

Polio vaccine. Immunosuppressed children and their household contacts should receive inactivated polio vaccine. The WHO does, however, recommend live TOPV for children with HIV or AIDS.

Administration of plasma or immunoglobulin. Measles, mumps, and rubella vaccines should be deferred for three months following such administration. Other vaccines need not be deferred.

Conditions that are not contra-indications to immunization

- Minor illness with low-grade fever (less than 38.5 °C), diarrhoea, and respiratory infections
- Malnutrition
- Breastfeeding
- Prematurity – immunization should commence at the same chronological age recommended for term infants
- Family history of convulsions
- History of non-specific allergies, asthma, hayfever, or rhinitis
- Dermatoses, eczema, or localized skin infections
- Allergy to antibiotics, except anaphylactic reactions to neomycin or streptomycin (they are contained in some vaccines)
- Soreness, redness, or temperature of less than 40 °C following a previous DPT vaccine
- Treatment with antibiotics
- Children treated with topical, inhaled, short-term (less than two weeks) or low-dose maintenance steroid therapy for a condition that is not immunosuppressive
- Chronic diseases of the heart, lung, kidney, or liver
- Static neurological disorders, such as cerebral palsy and Down's syndrome.

Pregnant mother

Live vaccines, including rubella, should not be administered during pregnancy. Susceptible pregnant mothers, particularly in areas of high risk for neonatal tetanus, must be given tetanus toxoid (in the context of NNT elimination). Other inactivated vaccines such as diphtheria, HBV, *Haemophilus influenzae*, and pneumococcal vaccine can be given to at-risk pregnant women. The pregnant mother is not at risk if children are vaccinated.

Practical points

Vaccination of preterm infants. Immunize at the recommended age with a full dose.

Missed opportunities. Avoid missed opportunities by offering immunizations at every contact, except if there is a true contra-indication to vaccinate.

Site of injection. Intramuscular: In infants (<12 months), inject into mid antero-lateral aspect of thigh using a 22 to 25 gauge needle with a minimum length of 25 mm. In older children, inject into deltoid (if muscle bulk is adequate), or mid antero-lateral aspect of thigh using a 22–25 gauge needle with a minimum length of 32 mm. Subcutaneous injections are given in the thigh in infants and deltoid in older children. Intradermal vaccines are administered on the volar aspect of the forearm.

Simultaneous administration. Most vaccines can be administered simultaneously. The exception (but not absolute) is yellow fever and cholera – give three weeks apart. Preferably space vaccines that are reactogenic, e.g. cholera and typhoid. Do not mix vaccines in the same syringe unless so licensed.

Interchangeability of vaccines from different manufacturers: Not a problem, however yet to be established for rotavirus vaccine and PCV.

Antimalarials and vaccination. Mefloquine (Lariam®) could affect immune responses to Ty21a typhoid vaccine. Chloroquine may interfere with rabies vaccine.

Blood transfusion or immunoglobulin therapy. Defer MMR for at least four to six weeks, unless absolutely essential.

Regurgitation of oral vaccines. Repeat once and if regurgitation persists, defer until next visit.

Steroid therapy. Live vaccines are not contra-indicated if therapy <2 weeks, low dose, alternate day, topical or aerosol. Immunosuppressive dose – prednisone 2 mg/kg daily or >20 mg daily.

Diphtheria-Tetanus-Pertussis Vaccine (DTP-whole cell). Common adverse reactions within 48 hours of vaccination are pyrexia 38.5 °C and local induration and tenderness.

Reactions that constitute absolute contra-indications to continuing DTP are convulsions, encephalitis, focal neurological signs, and collapse with shock.

Probable contra-indications to continuing DTP

are excessive somnolence, screaming attacks of more than three hours' duration, and a fever above 40 °C.

DTP is not embarked upon if the infant has progressive neurological disease, a history of fits, or has a significant febrile illness. Babies with a mild upper respiratory infection, low-grade fever, or diarrhoea can receive DTP.

The side-effects are largely due to the pertussis component of the triple vaccine. Thus, children who have any contra-indications to continuing or starting DTP, as well as those commencing the programme after the age of three years, are given DT and not DTP.

A booster of DT at school entry is needed to ensure a protective level of diphtheria antibody into adulthood, but tetanus antibody levels are usually adequate without this. Tetanus toxoid boosters are recommended every 10 years.

Acellular pertussis vaccine is to be introduced into the South African EPI program and in combination with tetanus and diphtheria can be used in children for whom whole cell vaccine is contra-indicated.

Storage and handling of vaccines (cold chain). Failure to adhere to recommended specifications will render vaccines impotent. Heat-sensitive vaccines include OPV, rotavirus vaccine, yellow fever, and measles. Vaccines that are sensitive to freezing include DPT, HBV, HiB, pneumococcal, and influenza vaccines. Keep fridge at 2–8 °C; do not place vaccines in the freezer or in the door of the refrigerator.

Passive immunization

Measles. Give exposed susceptible children immunoglobulin 0.25 ml/kg (for immunocompromised children give 0.5 ml/kg) with a maximum of 15 ml within six days of exposure.

Hepatitis A. Household or day-care centre contacts may be given immunoglobulin 0.02 ml/kg within two weeks after exposure. Although its efficacy has not been established, immunoglobulin may be given to infants of mothers who are jaundiced.

Hepatitis B immunoglobulin (HBIG). Newborns of mothers with acute or chronic hepatitis should be given HBIG within 12 hours of delivery; post-exposure prophylaxis.

Rabies immunoglobulin (RIG). 20 IU/kg – post-exposure.

Tetanus immunoglobulin (TIG). HTIG 500 IU for newborns; 2 000 IU for children as treatment; 75–250 IU prophylactically for severe wounds in incompletely immunized children.

Varicella zoster immunoglobulin (VZIG). 0.15 ml/kg for susceptible children within 96 hours, and for newborns of mothers who contracted chickenpox between five days before delivery to two days after delivery.

15 Systemic infections

Staphylococcal infections

Staphylococci are Gram-positive organisms. Strains are classified as *S. aureus* if they are coagulase positive. Coagulase negative strains include *S. epidermidis*.

Epidemiology

Staphylococci are colonizers of the skin and the nasal mucosa. Approximately 30 per cent of individuals carry *S. aureus* with a higher prevalence among older children, whereas *S.epidermidis* is part of the normal skin flora. Transmission of staphylococci is from person to person by direct contact, particularly via the hands. Coagulase-negative infections are common in immuno-compromised persons and those with indwelling catheters and CSF shunts. *S. aureus* is the second most common bacterial cause of pneumonia and a common secondary infection following measles. Community-acquired *S. aureus* is increasingly emerging as an important cause of serious soft-tissue infections. The strains of *S. aureus* responsible for community-acquired methicillin-resistant *Staphylococcus aureus* (MRSA) differ from those associated with hospital-associated MRSA infections, and phenotypically are more susceptible to a variety of non-beta lactam classes of antibiotics. Hospital- and community-acquired MRSA strains can be distinguished genotypically, with antibiogram susceptibility patterns, which also provide some cues as to the likely origin of the MRSA strain. Not all cases of *S. aureus* occurring in the community are, however, of the classical community-acquired MRSA strains. Hospital-associated MRSA may result in nasal colonization during hospitalizations and other health-care facility utilization. These strains may subsequently circulate in the community or cause illness in colonized individuals many months after health-care facility utilization. Hospital-associated MRSA strains causing disease in the general community are more correctly referred to as community-onset MRSA.

Clinical features

The clinical manifestations of *S. aureus* vary with the location of the infection. Superficial skin infection usually manifests as impetigo or carbuncles. Localized staphylococcal sepsis may manifest as myositis, acute bacterial endocarditis, septic arthritis, osteomyelitis, bacterial tracheitis, pneumonia, necrotising pneumonia and lung abscess. Community-acquired MRSA infection in the USA mainly manifests as soft-tissue infections, however there are reported cases of necrotising pneumonia with these MRSA strains.

Toxin-producing *S. aureus* cause **scalded skin syndrome** (due to an exfoliative toxin) or **food poisoning**, which usually presents two to six hours after ingestion of food containing pre-formed enterotoxin. Vomiting and watery diarrhoea are prominent features and usually resolve within 24 hours.

Diagnosis and treatment

Isolation of the organism from a septic focus or blood confirms the diagnosis.

The choice and duration of antimicrobial therapy depend upon the nature of the disease. Cloxacillin is the drug of choice even for severe methicillin-sensitive *S. aureus* infections.

Although rifampicin is active against most methicillin-susceptible *S. aureus,* it should not be used alone because of the risk of emergence of resistance. Fusidic acid, vancomycin and linezolid telithromycin are alternatives for drug-resistant infections. Deep-seated infections such as arthritis and endocarditis require at least six weeks of therapy. Depending on the local epidemiology, prevalence of healthcare-associated risk factors and severity of disease, consideration should be given to treating empirically for methicillin-resistant *S. aureus* in cases of severe disease in areas with a high prevalence of MRSA.

Toxic shock syndrome (TSS)

TSS is an acute multisystem disease characterized by high fever, hypotension, abdominal pain, vomiting, diarrhoea, and an erythematous rash caused by an exotoxin (TSS Toxin-1) produced by *S. aureus* and occasionally by exotoxin-producing streptococci.

TSS was initially described in females who use tampons, but has also been found to occur in males and in children. It may occur in association with bacteraemia or focal staphylococcal sepsis.

The **diagnosis** of TSS is based upon specific clinical and laboratory findings:
- Fever
- A diffuse macular erythematous rash which desquamates one to two weeks later
- Hypotension.

Plus involvement of three of the following systems:
- Gastrointestinal – diarrhoea and vomiting
- Muscular – severe myalgia or elevated creatine kinase
- Renal – elevated urea and creatinine
- Liver – elevated AST, ALT, or bilirubin
- Haematologic – thrombocytopaenia ($<100\,000 \times 10^9$)
- CNS – alteration in level of consciousness
- Negative serologic tests for measles, leptospirosis, and Rocky Mountain spotted fever.

The differential diagnosis includes scarlet fever, severe measles, leptospirosis, Kawasaki syndrome, and Rocky Mountain spotted fever. Treatment with beta lactamase-resistant anti-staphylococcal agents is recommended for about 10 days, or at least until antibiotic susceptibility profiles become available. Drainage of focal septic lesions, if present, should be done. Shock should be managed aggressively with adequate fluid therapy and inotropic support as required. It is essential to investigate for all possible sources of abscess collections, inlcuding undertaking ultrasound of the abdominal viscera and bone scans to exclude pyogenic arthritis and osteomyelitis. Failure to respond to appropriate antibiotic therapy, usually suggests the presence of an abscess that may require drainage.

Ecthyma

This is a deep form of impetigo in which the infection extends into the dermis, resulting in the formation of crusted ulcers, followed by depressed scars. It usually occurs on the legs following trauma or insect bites. Antibiotic or antiseptic ointments or wet antiseptic dressings such as diluted eusol or potassium permanganate solutions will remove the crusts and disinfect the ulcer. An antibiotic should always be given by mouth in addition, as the infection is too deep to respond to topical treatment only.

Boils (furunculosis)

Boils are due to a staphylococcal infection in and around hair follicles. They present as painful, raised, red nodules in which the centre is hard at first, but later softens and discharges pus. Isolated boils heal spontaneously and do not require treatment. However, in some children they are recurrent and may be associated with styes. These children and other members of the family are usually nasal carriers of staphylococci. Treatment of numerous and recurrent boils consists of systemic and topical antibiotics, which should be given for at least two or three weeks. Where sensitivity tests are not available, cloxacillin is preferred. Nasal carriers should be treated with an antibiotic ointment such as mupirocin, applied in both nostrils for at least two weeks. Systemic cotrimoxazole has been used additionally to reduce colonization with different rates of success. Occasionally, appropriate drainage, especially of closed-space abscess and deep seated soft-tissue abscess is required as an important adjunct to antibiotic therapy. Superficial abscesses typically resolve with drainage and debridement alone.

Streptococcal infections

Streptococci are Gram-positive cocci in chains. They are classified on the basis of their ability to lyse red cells into alpha haemolytic and beta haemolytic strains. Group A beta haemolytic streptococci (GAS) are further subdivided according to differences in the outer wall M protein (Lancefield groups).

Epidemiology

GAS or *Streptococcus pyogenes* is probably the most common bacterial infection worldwide. It is a normal inhabitant of the nasopharynx and is transmitted from person to person by droplet spread. Group B haemolytic streptococci (GBS) are normal inhabitants of the maternal genitourinary and gastrointestinal tract. Newborns acquire infection through vertical transmission from the mother.

Clinical features

GAS infections result in acute tonsillitis or pharyngitis with associated cervical adenopathy, impetigo, cellulitis, scarlet fever, and occasionally toxic shock syndrome.

Scarlet fever presents acutely with fever, pharyngitis, headache, a diffuse punctate erythematous rash which desquamates after a few days, circumoral pallor, and what is commonly referred to as a 'strawberry' tongue.

Acute glomerulonephritis and rheumatic fever are significant consequences of streptococcal infections.

GBS infections are associated with neonatal meningitis, arthritis, and septicaemia (*see* Chapter 7, Care of the newborn).

Cellulitis is an infection of the dermis and subcutaneous tissues. The affected skin is red, tender, swollen, and warm, and regional lymph glands may be enlarged and tender. Cellulitis requires treatment with systemic antibiotics and local topical antiseptic care if required. It is important to exclude underlying local bone involvement.

Erysipelas is a superficial form of cellulitis caused by streptococci. A raised, red, advancing margin is seen on the skin and sometimes blisters form on the surface.

Peri-anal cellulitis which is due to group A β-haemolytic streptococci is a cause of erythema and pain in the perineal area in young children.

Diagnosis and treatment

Streptococcal tonsillitis cannot be distinguished clinically from other causes of tonsillitis. Throat swabs should ideally be done. Scarlet fever should be differentiated from other erythematous exanthems (*see* Table 14.3 in Chapter 14, Principles of infection in children).

Treatment of streptococcal infections is with penicillin or amoxycillin. Treatment is recommended for at least 10–14 days. If children are allergic to penicillins then erythromycin or a cephalosporin is recommended. Cases of cellulitis, scarlet fever, and toxic shock syndrome (TSS) should be given parenteral antibiotics initially.

Haemophilus influenzae infections

H. influenzae is a Gram-negative pleomorphic rod. Six serotypes (a to f) are identifiable on the basis of the capsular polysaccharide. Other isolates are non-encapsulated and thus non-typeable.

Epidemiology

Transmission is from person to person by droplet spread. However spread of Hib is interrupted with the introduction of Hib conjugate vaccine, resulting in indirect protection of unvaccinated susceptible members of the community. Overcrowding is a major risk factor. The case fatality rate varies between 5 and 20 per cent. The burden of *Haemophilus influenzae* type b (Hib) infection, previously a major cause of severe invasive bacterial disease in children worldwide, has been reduced with the widespread use of *Haemophilus influenzae* type b conjugate vaccine in the childhood immunization programme. Rates in infancy have been reduced from >100/100 000 to <5 per 100 000. There does, however, remain a residual burden of disease, especially in HIV-infected children, who present mainly with bacteremia and pneumonia and less frequently with meningitis. Other rare manifestations of Hib disease include arthritis, septicaemia, cellulitis and epiglottitis, which is extremely rare in Africa. Unvaccinated, children aged less than two years are at greatest risk. With the introduction of Hib conjugate vaccine, there is an age shift to older immuno-compromised children developing Hib disease as a consequence of a decline in the immunity following vaccination during early childhood.

Clinical features

Clinical syndromes include asymptomatic bacteraemia, septic shock, meningitis, septicaemia, arthritis, cellulitis, and epiglottitis. They are clinically indistinguishable from other causes. Rare manifestations include pericarditis, endocarditis, peritonitis, endophthalmitis, neonatal sepsis, and primary lung abscess. Hib is also responsible for a small proportion of milder non-invasive (non-bacteraemic) diseases such as bronchitis, sinusitis, conjunctivitis, and otitis media.

Diagnosis

A definitive diagnosis of invasive Hib infection is made by isolation of the organism from the CSF, blood, pleural fluid, or aspirate from a joint or skin.

Antigen detection in CSF, urine, serum, joint, or pleural fluid by counter-immuno-electrophoresis or latex agglutination may be useful in situations where prior antibiotics have been used and where cultures may be negative. A positive culture from the nasopharynx is not diagnostic, since approximately 5–10 per cent of unvaccinated children may be carriers.

Management

Treat suspected invasive Hib infections with a third generation cephalosporin, especially if suspecting meningitis. Ampicillin alone is not recommended as resistance varies between 5 and 30 per cent. Once antimicrobial sensitivities are obtained, therapy with the appropriate single drug is recommended. Therapy should continue for 10 days for all cases except in cases of septic arthritis, where at least 14 days are required. Be aware that multiple foci of infection may occur, e.g. meningitis and pneumonia. Management of shock, meningitis, pneumonia, epiglottitis, and arthritis is carried out according to standard protocols.

Primary prevention

The Hib conjugate vaccines, using tetanus toxoid, outer membrane protein of *Neisseria meningitidis* or CRM_{197} (mutant diptheria toxoid like protein) as the carrier protein for an antigenic component of the polysaccharide of Hib, have been highly effective. In countries where these vaccines have been introduced invasive haemophilus disease has been virtually eliminated. The Hib conjugate vaccines are administered in conjunction with DTP and hepatitis B, and are available in combination formulations with DTP with/without Hepatitis B and inactivated polio virus vaccine. Children aged less than six months require three primary doses, those aged seven to eleven months two doses, and those aged 12 to 14 months one dose. A booster dose is given at age greater than 15 months. Doses should be spaced six to eight weeks apart. Children over the age of 15 months require a single dose only.

Streptococcus pneumoniae

Epidemiology

Of the 91 different pneumococcal serotypes, a select few (7–13) cause between 70–95 per cent of all invasive pneumococcal disease In children. Most children acquire asymptomatic infection of the nasopharynx by the age of five years and the prevalence of colonization in young children in developing countries ranges between 30–75 per cent. The prevalence of colonization is also especially high in children living in over-crowded settings, as well as in day-care centres, where mini-epidemics of pneumococcal infection may occur. Transmission is from person to person by droplet spread and children under six years of age are considered as being the most important sources of transmission within the community, including to older susceptible individuals such as the elderly. Pneumococcus is the leading cause of bacterial pneumonia and otitis media in most countries and the commonest cause of bacterial meningitis in children, outside of meningococcal meningitis epidemics. It is a common opportunistic infection in children with AIDS, sickle-cell disease, asplenia, and malignancies. The major serotypes causing disease vary between developed and developing countries and may change over time with the emergence of new dominant serotypes. Drug resistance is particularly related to serotypes 6, 9, 14, 19 and 23.

Clinical features

Pneumococci are a common cause of otitis media, sinusitis, pneumonia, bacteraemia, and meningitis. Mastoiditis, empyema, pericarditis, peritonitis, arthritis, and osteomyelitis may also occur.

Diagnosis

Isolation of pneumococci from the blood or a septic focus confirms the diagnosis, however only 5–15 per cent of children with pneumococcal pneumonia may have a positive blood culture. Antigen detection in CSF, serum, joint, or pleural fluid by latex agglutination may be useful in situations where prior antibiotics have been used and when cultures may be negative. Isolation of pneumococci from the nasopharynx in children with pneumonia is not diagnostic as asymptomatic colonization is highly prevalent.

Treatment

The major problem in the treatment of pneumococcal infections has been the emergence of drug resistance in many parts of the world. Treatment options must therefore be based upon knowledge of local antimicrobial susceptibility patterns. The emergence of drug-resistance demonstrated *in vitro* may, however, be overcome by the appropriate dosing of antibiotics. The favorable pharmacokinetic/pharmacodynamic (PK/PD) profile of beta-lactams in the treatment of pneumococcal pneumonia allows for successful treatment with penicillin derivatives, even in the presence of in-vitro resistance of MICs of <4 µg/ml. It is uncommon for pneumococcal strains to have an MIC of ≥4 µg/ml. Management of pneumococcal meningitis and acute otitis media associated with reduced antibiotic susceptibility strains is, however, more complex due to the differing PK/PD profile of antibiotics in managing these infections in compartments into which penetration of antibiotics is less than that which occurs in the blood stream or lung compartment. Antibiotic therapy of acute otitis media requires amoxicillin at 90 mg/kg/day (divided into 2–3 doses) and possibly the use of amoxicillin-clavulanic acid, if a beta-lactamase organism (e.g. *Haemophilus influenzae* non-typable or *Moraxella catarrhalis*) is suspected. Pneumococcal meningitis needs to be treated with a 3rd generation cephalosporin (cefotaxime or ceftriaxone), and infrequently may require vancomycin if there is resistance to the 3rd generation cephalosporin. Duration of therapy is usually about 5–7 days for acute otitis media and pneumonia, but 14 days for severe infections such as meningitis.

Prevention

The 23-valent polysaccharide vaccine is not immunogenic for many of the serotypes, nor efficacious in young children. In recipients older than two years, protective antibody levels are achieved in two weeks and last for five to eight years. The vaccine is indicated in high-risk patients, e.g. post splenectomy, sickle-cell anaemia, nephrotic syndrome, Hodgkin's lymphoma and still indicated for use in these children, after being adequately immunized with pneumococcal conjugate vaccine if under nine years of age.

A polysaccharide-protein conjugate vaccine including seven serotypes is currently available for vaccination of very young children. This formulation will be enhanced with the inclusion of additional serotypes (including 1, 5 and 7F in a 10-valent formulation). This vaccine has been shown to prevent invasive pneumococcal disease, pneumococcal pneumonia and recurrent acute otitis media in children immunized during early infancy. Although less immunogenic and efficacious in HIV infected children, the vaccine nevertheless prevents a high burden of pneumococcal disease in these children, although there is a possible need for booster doses of vaccine in later life.

Although the pneumococcal conjugate vaccine is highly effective in preventing invasive disease due to the serotypes included in the vaccine, there remains a significant residual burden of pneumococcal disease. This is in part attributable to 'replacement' disease occurring due to serotypes not included in the vaccine.

The recommended dosing schedule of the pneumococcal conjugate vaccine includes three doses during early infancy together with the other childhood vaccines and a booster dose in the second year of life. Children 6–12 months old are given two doses spaced one month apart, and a booster dose in the second year of life. Older children are given a single dose of vaccine.

In addition to conferring direct protection to immunized children, the pneumococcal conjugate vaccine has also been shown to reduce nasopharyngeal acquisition of vaccine-serotype pneumococci in vaccinated children. Consequently, mass immunization has been associated with reduced transmission of these specific serotypes in the community, resulting in indirect protection against invasive pneumococcal disease in unvaccinated sections of the population, including the very young and the elderly.

The high cost of the pneumococcal conjugate vaccine is likely to result in a lag before the vaccine becomes available to the majority of children in developing countries, where the burden of pneumococcal disease is the greatest.

Salmonellae

These are Gram-negative, motile, non-lactose fermenting, aerobic rods. The majority of the more than 1 700 serotypes known primarily infect animals, but may cause gastroenteritis, septicaemia ('enteric fever') or typhoid in humans. Transmission is by ingestion of dairy products, undercooked or cold meat, or contaminated food and water. Human carriers play a role in their spread. Enteric fever is a more inclusive term for typhoid fever and paratyphoid fever and is caused by *Salmonella enterica*, including *S. enterica* serotype Typhi (*S. typhi*) and serotype Paratyphi (*S. paratyphi* A, B and C). Eighty percent of cases in endemic areas are due to *S. typhi*, however *S. paratyphi* may be more common among travellers because of vaccination against *S. typhi*. A further emerging problem in Africa, especially in malnourished and HIV infected children is septicaemia and meningitis caused by *Salmonella non-typhi*.

Typhoid fever

Typhoid fever is endemic in Africa, the Middle and Far East, south-eastern Europe, and Central and South America. Sporadic cases have a worldwide distribution and occasional epidemics occur even in countries which, under normal circumstances, have a very low incidence of the disease. In the majority of instances, the infection is acquired while holidaying in countries where typhoid is endemic.

Salmonella typhi and *S. paratyphi* differ from other salmonellae in that they are primarily human pathogens. Humans are the only known reservoirs of these bacteria and transmission occurs through contaminated food, inadequate sanitation and faecal contamination of water by acutely ill or chronic carriers. Areas in southern Africa with the highest incidence have summer rains, with the peak incidence in the hottest

months, i.e. January to March. However, cases occur throughout the year and drought also leads to an increased number of cases. No age group is exempt, but schoolchildren and young adults have the highest incidence. Transplacental infection may lead to neonatal typhoid. Both sexes are equally affected.

Pathogenesis

Swallowed organisms multiply in the reticulo-endothelial tissues of the small intestine and, after an incubation period of 7–14 days (range 3–60 days), invade the bloodstream resulting in symptoms and signs initially presenting with influenza-like symptoms including fever, headache, malaise but few physical signs. Dissemination of organisms may lead to focal involvement of many organs. Focal necrosis of the liver and inflammation of the biliary passages and gall bladder are usually present. Reinvasion of the small intestine via the biliary tract leads to the characteristic hyperplasia, necrosis, and ulceration of Peyer's patches, which may progress to perforation or haemorrhage.

Lipo-polysaccharide endotoxins in the cell wall of the bacteria may also affect many organs and give rise to symptoms, signs, and complications.

Clinical features

As typhoid is both a septicaemia and a toxaemia, practically any organ or tissue in the body may be involved. A wide variety of symptoms and signs occur, and their severity and duration vary greatly from patient to patient. Ninety percent of typhoid fever cases in endemic areas occur in young children aged 3–19 years. Children admitted to hospital are frequently severely ill. Fever is the most constant of all clinical manifestations, is commonly high (39–40 °C), and may be sustained or intermittent (maximum during the afternoon) and may develop incrementally in a step-wise fashion over 5–7 days. This is followed by a period of 10–14 days of sustained fever of 39–41 °C. Severely anaemic children and those presenting in congestive cardiac failure may become pyrexial only when the anaemia has been corrected or the cardiac failure controlled. The temperature response to successful antibiotic therapy varies but often takes as long as seven to eight days. Rigors may be seen at the height of fever.

Anorexia and abdominal pain are common in children old enough to complain and constipation may be an early feature in the older child. In those under five years of age, diarrhoea and vomiting often dominate the clinical picture and mask the diagnosis, which may be missed unless the accompanying high fever alerts the clinician to the possibility of typhoid.

A tender, tumid abdomen together with hepatosplenomegaly in a febrile child in an endemic area is highly suggestive of typhoid. The incidence of splenomegaly varies in different childhood series from 30–100 per cent and may be dependent upon the timing of accessing health care. Symptoms and signs of respiratory tract involvement are present in many patients, cough being a complaint in almost half and signs of bronchitis in one-third. Headache is a frequent presenting complaint in the older child. Delirium and signs of meningeal irritation are common. Myalgia, arthralgia, and sore throat sometimes head the list of complaints, but epistaxis is uncommon in children. Rose spots (2–4 mm blanching erythematous maculopapular lesions), regarded as a diagnostic sign, are invisible or absent in pigmented skins, and mainly occur on the abdomen and chest in 5–30 per cent of cases. Anaemia is present in up to 40 per cent of patients in admission. When present, leucopaenia is of help in establishing the diagnosis, but is relatively uncommon. A moderate leucocytosis is often found when focal involvement gives rise to complications. Thrombocytopaenia, unre-

lated to drug therapy, may be present in one-fifth of patients, but is seldom severe. Complications of typhoid occur in 10–15 per cent of cases and are shown in Table 15.1 Case fatality rates in endemic countries are as high as 30 per cent. Chronic biliary carriage (shedding for more than a year) occurs in 2–5 per cent of cases, even after treatment. Clinical disease with S. paratyphi A is indistinguishable from that of S. typhi.

Diagnosis

The diagnosis is most often missed or delayed in the very young or when children present with symptoms and signs of focal complications. Confirmation of diagnosis is by culture of blood, stool, or urine. Rarely, S. typhi may be isolated from cerebrospinal fluid or pus. Blood cultures are positive in the majority of cases at presentation, however may be negative if antibiotics have been started, in which case bone marrow culture provides a better chance of isolating the organism. Samples should be collected at the height of fever and repeated whenever fever remains unexplained or occurs inappropriately in such clinical conditions as acute glomerulonephritis, hepatitis, cardiac failure, or profound anaemia.

Less commonly, cultures of stool and urine yield S. typhi, particularly in the first week of illness and the organism may also be cultured from rose spots. Leucopaenia, thrombocytopaenia and moderately elevated liver enzymes are common.

The Widal test is of limited value because it is neither sensitive nor specific and may be positive in those who had received the typhoid vaccine. A rising titre is supportive evidence for the diagnosis when the clinical picture suggests typhoid.

Treatment

The first line treatment of enteric fever is ceftriaxone (80 mg/kg IM or IV once a day) and alternately quinolones can be given if the local epidemiology suggest susceptibility to fluoroquinolones. Resistance of S. typhi (and more recently emergence thereof in S. paratyphi A) to previously used antibiotics including chloramphenicol (50–100 mg/kg/day) , ampicillin and co-trimoxazole limits the use of these antibiotics. Multi-drug resistance organisms may occur in 50–90 per cent of isolates in some areas in Asia.

Therapy with short course (five days) of ceftriaxone is as effective as three weeks of chloramphenicol. Ceftriaxone therapy is cost-

Table 15.1 Complications in 1 400 children with typhoid fever

Complications	%
Respiratory:	
Bronchopneumonia (radiological)	34
Lobar pneumonia (radiological)	2
Neurological	16
Hepatitis	5
Nephritis	4
Cardiovascular	4
Gastrointestinal:	
Intestinal haemorrhage	2
Perforation	2
Haemolytic anaemia	1

Source: South African Journal of Hospital Medicine, Vol. 2, No. 10, 1976

effective since it greatly reduces the length of hospital stay. Therapy with quinolones, such as ciprofloxacin for 5–7 days, has also been shown to be effective in the treatment of typhoid, however there is an emerging trend of resistance to this class of antibiotics as well, requiring higher doses and more prolonged therapy with the quinolones. Azithromycin appears to be a promising option and comparable to intravenous ceftriaxone in uncomplicated typhoid in children and adolescence.

Correction and maintenance of fluid balance and electrolytes and the provision of a nutritious diet are essential components of the treatment. Haemorrhage and shock require immediate and often life-saving blood transfusions.

Corticosteroids are believed to be antitoxigenic and have been recommended in severely ill obtunded patients. They apparently cause no increase in the incidence of perforation or haemorrhage. Perforation requires prompt surgical intervention if recognized reasonably early. Intravenous fluid therapy is recommended in advanced peritonitis and in the presence of ileus without perforation (*see* Chapter 30, Paediatic surgical disorders).

Relapses

Clinical relapse may occur within days or weeks of completion of therapy. In Durban, experience with amoxicillin and chloramphenicol therapy over many years has shown that 21 days of therapy reduces the rate to 1 per cent in patients treated with amoxycillin and to 5 per cent in patients treated with chloramphenicol. Relapse rate with ceftriaxone is similar to that with chloramphenicol.

Carriers

Convalescent carriage is relatively common. Most cases clear spontaneously without treatment. In Durban, convalescent carriers occur more commonly after chloramphenicol (6 per cent) than amoxycillin (less than 1 per cent). Permanent carriers are said to occur in 2–5 per cent of all patients, but are very rare in children.

Prevention

The whole-cell killed vaccines typhoid and paratyphoid A & B (TAB), although shown to be effective, are no longer used because of substantial adverse events.

Two new vaccines are licensed for prevention which include parenteral vaccines that take advantage of circulating antibody responses, and live attenuated oral vaccines which rely upon secretory IgA responses. Both vaccines are safe and well tolerated:

◆ Ty21a is the attenuated live *S. typhi* oral vaccine, which lacks the virulence (Vi) antigen, and is thus avirulent but contains immunogenic cell wall polysaccharide. Primary vaccination consists of one enteric-coated formulation or lyophilised sachet on alternate days for 3–4 doses. This vaccine provides 71 per cent protection in 5–9 year old children and 63 per cent efficacy in 10–14 year old children and does not cause adverse reactions. Vaccine efficacy among travellers may however be less (23 per cent). The live-attenuated vaccine is contraindicated in those with cell mediated immunodeficiency, children under six years of age and the concurrent use of antibiotics and anti-malarials may interfere with antibody response.

◆ A capsular polysaccharide Vi antigen vaccine given in a single parenteral dose results in 65–75 per cent protection for two years. It can be safety administered without any interference with other vaccines and anti-malarials. The vaccine is not recommended in children under two years. A new vaccine formulation is a Vi antigen conjugated to nontoxic recombinant *Pseudomonas aeruginosa* exotoxin A (Vi-rEPA). It has enhanced immunogenicity in children following a two dose schedule and has been shown to confer 89 per cent protection in 2–5 year olds up to 46 months of age.

None of the currently available vaccines protect against *S. paratyphi*.

Diphtheria

Diphtheria is characterized by fever, toxaemia, nasopharyngitis, and/or obstructive laryngotracheitis following infection by *Corynebacterium diphtheriae*. It occurs throughout the world. In well-immunized communities the disease is rare and tends to occur in adults, but where immunization is deficient, children of the poorer sector are mainly affected. In developing countries outbreaks have occurred in both children and adults.

Virulent diphtheria bacilli lodge in the nasopharynx following droplet spread from a case or carrier. The toxin produced by the multiplying organisms causes local tissue necrosis which, along with the inflammatory and exudative reaction, combines to form a membrane. Toxin is then absorbed into the bloodstream and can affect all tissues, but has a predilection for myocardium and nerve tissue. Once fixed in cells the toxin cannot be neutralized: antitoxin is only effective against circulating toxin. Occasionally disease may result from diphtheritic infection of skin lesions, e.g. a leg ulcer.

Clinical features

The disease is characterized by three stages:

- The patient presents with a sore throat and fever, which progresses rapidly to toxaemia. A white to grey membrane is seen in the nose or oropharynx, which ranges in size from a small patch to massive involvement of tonsils, palate, pharynx, and glottis. Attempts at removing the membrane results in bleeding. Laryngeal involvement results in hoarseness and stridor, and may lead to suffocation. Swelling of the neck due to cervical adenopathy and periadenitis ('bull neck') is often present.
- Myocarditis usually manifests in the second week of the illness and is characterized by a rapid, thready pulse, indistinct heart sounds and cardiac failure.
- Neuritis commences in the third to sixth week following onset of symptoms and usually follows a specific pattern. Palatal and pharyngeal involvement results in difficulty in swallowing, nasal-type speech, and regurgitation. Involvement of the ocular muscles causes strabismus and diplopia.

Paralysis of the intercostal muscles and diaphragm leads to difficulty with respiration. An early sign is a weak cough or cry. Involvement of peripheral nerves causes weakness or paralysis of the muscles of the limbs.

Pneumonia is a common complication and is usually secondary to laryngeal involvement, regurgitation, inability to cough up secretions, or weakness of the muscles of respiration.

Thrombocytopaenia and disseminated intravascular coagulation are seen in severe cases.

Renal failure occurs from direct toxic effect on the kidneys and from disseminated intravascular coagulation or is pre-renal following the low-output cardiac failure of myocarditis.

Diagnosis

Clinical clues to the aetiology of the pharyngeal membrane are a serosanguinous nasal discharge, cervical adenopathy with periadenitis ('bull neck'), and toxaemia. Culture of nose and throat swab is essential. Any unimmunized child with severe tonsillitis and a membrane must be suspected of having diphtheria.

Management

Treat with procaine penicillin (50 000 IU/kg/d in two doses) IM for 10 days. Alternative therapy is oral erythromycin 50 mg/kg/d in four doses for 10 days. Children with stridor should be intubated or have a tracheostomy. Extubation is usually possible in four to five days.

Antitoxin (ADS) is the most important therapy and is given if the diagnosis is strongly suspected as it is unwise to delay therapy until laboratory confirmation is received. The dose of antitoxin is determined by the extent of disease, ranging from 20 000 units for cases presenting with nasal diphtheria or a small pharyngeal membrane to 100 000 units IM or IV for cases of laryngeal diphtheria or those with a large membrane. Be extremely careful when administering the antitoxin, since this is a horse serum product and there is a risk of hypersensitivity (anaphylaxis). Before administering the antitoxin, give an intradermal test dose of a small amount as described in the product instructions. Make sure that adrenaline and steroids are on hand to immediately treat any adverse reactions.

If myocarditis occurs, strict bed rest is essential. If cardiac failure is present, restrict fluid intake, try to avoid parenteral fluids, and treat with diuretics and digoxin if available.

Avoid regurgitation by thickening feeds and by giving it via a nasogastric tube. Patients with a weak cough should be given physiotherapy and encouraged to cough up secretions to prevent the development of pneumonia. Those with respiratory muscle paralysis must be referred to a centre capable of providing mechanical ventilation. This is usually necessary for about two weeks.

Prevention

The patient must be isolated.

After an attack of diphtheria, immunity may not be permanent and active immunization with toxoid should be started in convalescence. Immunity may be acquired by inapparent infection or with mild symptoms and immune persons may become nasopharyngeal carriers.

Contacts should be isolated until the results of their nose and throat cultures are known. Those with negative cultures can be released from isolation. Those with positive cultures require antibiotic treatment for 10 days followed by a repeat culture.

Active immunization is recommended for contacts who have previously received a course of diphtheria toxoid or who are uncertain of their past immunization history. Diphtheria is readily preventable by means of vaccination. Booster doses of low-dose diptheria (dT) toxoid vaccine is recommended at school entry in addition to the primary series of vaccines provided during infancy and the booster dose of vaccine in the second year of life.

Prognosis

Prognosis is affected by several factors:
- The virulence of the organism
- The larger the membrane, the greater the amount of toxin produced
- Delay in receiving ADS therapy.

These all increase the likelihood of myocarditis, neuritis, and renal failure occurring.

If an immunized child contracts disease it is usually mild. In those who are non-immunized or who develop large membranes and receive specific treatment late or not at all, mortality rates go up to 50 per cent.

Pertussis (whooping cough)

Pertussis is an acute infectious disease of the respiratory tract typified by severe bronchitis. The disease is caused by the organism *Bordetella pertussis*. It shares minor antigenic components with *Bordetella parapertussis* and *Bordetella bronchiseptica*, both of which give rise to respiratory infections resembling pertussis. It is characterized by a forceful staccato-like cough which ends with a high-pitched inspiratory whoop and may be associated with vomiting, apnoea, cyanosis, and convulsions. Coughing paroxysms usually last for about two to four weeks.

Epidemiology

Pertussis occurs worldwide. It is spread by droplets, and since attack rates are highest following household exposure, it is likely that prolonged exposure is important in the spread of the disease. Disease incidence, morbidity, and mortality are greatest in infancy (no transplacental immunity is conferred to newborns), and decrease with increasing age. Approximately 40–50 per cent of cases are younger than one year, with a peak incidence between the ages of one to two months. Of the reported cases about 70 per cent of those younger than one year are hospitalized, compared with only 5 per cent of those older than five years; the case fatality rates (CFRs) range from 1–6 per cent in South Africa.

Pathogenesis

The organism does not invade tissues or blood, but it does cause necrosis of ciliated epithelium in the respiratory tract. Sticky mucus and sloughed cells which accumulate in bronchi result in obstruction, leading to patchy atelectasis and emphysema. The neurological and haematological effects probably result from haemagglutinins present in the organism.

Clinical features

The incubation period is seven days and the course of the disease is divided into three stages. The *catarrhal stage* lasts for one to two weeks. The symptoms are of an upper respiratory infection with a short, dry, nocturnal cough.

The *paroxysmal stage* lasts for two to four weeks. The cough becomes paroxysmal; it is followed by a forceful inspiration usually associated with a whoop. At the end of a paroxysm the child often vomits up mucus or feeds. Haemoptysis may occur. The cough is most common at night and is precipitated by eating, drinking, or crying. In the young infant the cough is often atypical: the whoop may be absent and paroxysms may be less frequent. Instead of a paroxysm, the baby may suffer apnoea attacks and cyanosis.

The *convalescent phase* lasts two to four weeks,

and is marked by a decrease in the severity and frequency of paroxysmal coughing, which finally ceases. Symptoms often recur for up to one year after the disease whenever the child contracts an upper respiratory infection.

Diagnosis

The diagnosis is usually made on the distinctive clinical features of the cough. A leucocytosis in excess of 10 000/mm³ (sometimes rising to 100 000/mm³) with a relative lymphocytosis, occurs from the second to fifth week of disease. Special techniques of nasopharyngeal culture using charcoal media or serology using the enzyme-linked immunosorbent assay (ELISA) method are available to confirm the diagnosis, but are not usually needed.

Differential diagnosis of the cough

A cough suggestive of pertussis may occur in infants with bronchiolitis, chlamydial pneumonitis, or cystic fibrosis. In older children a similar cough may accompany interstitial pneumonia, inhalation of a foreign body, or pressure on the trachea by enlarged tuberculous tracheobronchial glands.

Management

Severe cases, especially infants, are best managed in hospital where close nursing supervision is available. Administer oxygen to children during severe coughing paroxysms, if apnoeic or cyanotic spells occur or if severe pneumonia is present. Severe episodes may require intubation and mechanical ventilation to allow for paralysing of the child.

The child should be placed head down during a severe coughing paroxysm to avoid aspiration of gastric contents and to encourage expectoration of secretions, which can be cleared from the nose and pharynx by the use of brief and gentle suction.

Cough suppressants, sedatives, mucolytics, and antihistamines should not be given. There is no evidence that they control or prevent the cough. The best way to control the cough is to minimize stimuli that would trigger paroxysms, such as unnecessary suctioning, throat examinations, and insertion of nasogastric tubes. There is evidence that salbutamol (0.15 mg/kg/six-hourly) or steroids (prednisone 5–20 mg/kg/d for one week) are effective in reducing the paroxysms and shortening the course of the disease in infants with severe disease.

Erythromycin 50 mg/kg/d in four divided doses for 10–14 days is recommended to eradicate infection and prevent relapse. If given in the catarrhal phase, the clinical course may be shortened. Alternatives include cotrimoxazole and chloramphenicol.

Complications

Pneumonia is the most common complication and is due to secondary bacterial or viral infections, or aspiration of gastric contents during vomiting and is characterized by a rapid onset of fever and signs of respiratory distress. The choice of antibiotic will be dictated by the severity of pneumonia and prior antibiotic usage.

Atelectasis is due to obstruction of the airways by thick tenacious secretions and manifests by respiratory distress, but may only be detected by chest radiograph. Bronchiectasis may occur in persistent atelectatic segments, a complication now rarely seen in the developed world, but still a problem in poor communities. Gentle chest physiotherapy is recommended.

Encephalopathy may be due to anoxic brain damage, intracranial haemorrhage, or toxin mediated effects. Irritability, convulsions, and alterations in level of consciousness may occur. Administer oxygen therapy during the apnoeic or cyanotic attack and terminate convulsions with anticonvulsants.

Children frequently fail to thrive and become malnourished as a result of the persistent vomiting. Pay particular attention to providing adequate nutrition during the acute and convalescent stages of the illness. It may be useful to give the child smaller and more frequent feeds to minimize vomiting and aspiration of feeds which are frequently associated with the coughing paroxysm.

Subconjunctival haemorrhage and epistaxis are common. Treat symptomatically. Umbilical or inguinal hernias may be precipitated by the violent coughing spasms. Treat conservatively unless there is evidence of bowel obstruction. Refer for surgical consultation once recovered.

Congestive cardiac failure may occur in a few cases with severe pneumonia. Myocarditis due to the exotoxin of the bacterium may also be a factor. Treatment consists of oxygen, digitalis, and diuretics.

Prognosis

The case fatality rate has declined with reduction in severity of disease due to immunization and improved case management. Complications worsen the prognosis, and these occur most frequently in infancy. Most deaths occur in the first year of life.

Prevention

A patient is infectious from seven days after exposure to three weeks after the onset of paroxysms if untreated. Erythromycin therapy reduces communicability to about three to five days. Young infants who have been exposed to infection should ideally be given a five- to seven-day course of prophylactic erythromycin.

An acellular pertussis vaccine containing two or more purified and detoxified antigens has been shown to be protective against whooping cough, and to cause fewer adverse reactions than the whole-cell vaccine. This vaccine is recommended for use in children in whom the whole cell vaccine is contra-indicated and is increasingly replacing whole cell pertussis vaccines as part of routine immunization.

Leprosy

Leprosy is a chronic infectious disease caused by *Mycobacterium leprae,* which usually involves peripheral nerves and skin, and occasionally other tissues (*see* Figure 15.1).

Transmission occurs between humans through inhalation or across abraded skin and children usually acquire the disease from affected parents. As there is a prolonged incubation period of between three to seven years, leprosy in paediatric practice is a disease of older children. (*See* Table 15.2 for further details.)

Clinical features

The clinical features of the disease are influenced by two factors:

◆ The character of the immune response: a powerful cell-mediated immune reaction to *M. leprae* results in tuberculoid leprosy, while a deficient response is associated with a lepromatous picture.

◆ The preferred sites of the infection are nerves and skin; presentation is therefore determined by nerve damage or skin lesions.

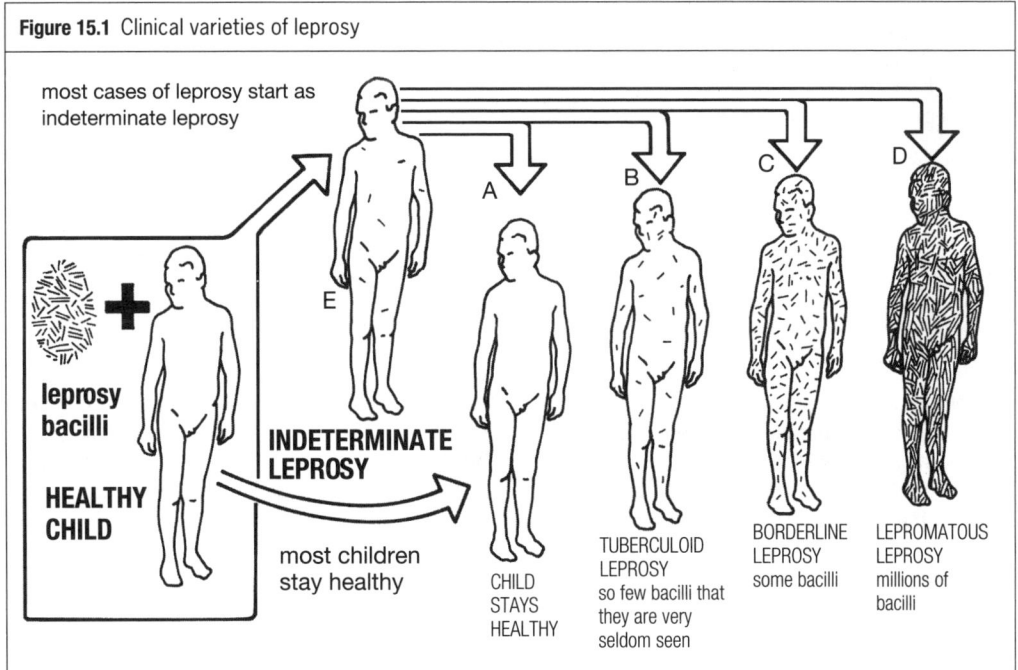

Figure 15.1 Clinical varieties of leprosy

most cases of leprosy start as indeterminate leprosy

A   B   C   D

E

leprosy bacilli

HEALTHY CHILD

INDETERMINATE LEPROSY

most children stay healthy

CHILD STAYS HEALTHY

TUBERCULOID LEPROSY
so few bacilli that they are very seldom seen

BORDERLINE LEPROSY
some bacilli

LEPROMATOUS LEPROSY
millions of bacilli

Table 15.2 Leprosy

	Tuberculoid	Lepromatous
Frequency in childhood	Common	Uncommon
Skin lesions	Few Well-defined edge Macule, raised erythematous edge, hypopigmented, anaesthetic, hairless	Numerous, bilateral, symmetrical Poorly defined edge Macule, erythematous or hypopigmented, no obvious progress to form plaques and nodules, and there is loss of eyelashes and eyebrows
Nerve lesions	Thickened cutaneous nerve at site of or away from skin lesions	Little nerve involvement in early stages. In late stages peripheral nerves thicken and cause anaesthesia and muscle weakness
Disseminated lesions	—	Rhinitis; conjunctivitis; keratitis, iritis; nodules in nose, palate, ear lobes; lymphoedema; lymphadenopathy; hepatosplenomegaly; testicular atrophy; deformities due to infection and injury
Complications	Rare	'Lepra' reactions occur spontaneously or during therapy, i.e. exacerbation of skin and nerve lesions. 'Erythema nodosum leprosum' (ENL), i.e. painful erythematous nodules
Cell-mediated immunity	Marked	Deficient
Lepromin test (delayed hypersensitivity to *M. leprae*)	+	–
Pathology	Non-caseating tuberculoid granuloma (epithelioid cells, giant cells, lymphocytes), nerves destroyed, few AFB	Macrophages containing many AFB, scanty lymphocytes, nerves intact during early stages

The earliest clinical evidence is an ill-defined, hypopigmented macule which usually retains sensation, has a diameter of about 5 cm, and occurs at any site. This lesion heals spontaneously in most instances and has been classified as an indeterminate form of the disease. A minority of children progress to the more serious manifestations of leprosy.

A comparison is drawn between the tuberculoid and lepromatous patterns of leprosy in Table 15.2. Various intermediate forms occur with accompanying shifts in immunological status. The most common are borderline tuberculoid (most common in Africans) and borderline lepromatous (most common in Asians and Europeans) leprosy.

Diagnosis

The clinical features of anaesthetic skin lesions and thickened nerves are pathognomonic. Skin smears for acid-fast bacilli or biopsy of skin or nerve tissue will confirm the diagnosis.

Management

Initial treatment for all varieties is dapsone (1 mg/kg/d), rifampicin (10 mg/kg/d), and clofazimine (adult dose 100 mg tds; paediatric dose not established) for six weeks.

Maintenance therapy:
Tuberculoid and borderline tuberculoid
* Dapsone daily until no signs of activity for three years.

Lepromatous and borderline lepromatous
* Continue dapsone, rifampicin, and clofazimine for six months; thereafter dapsone indefinitely.
* Severe ENL and lepra reactions (*see* Table 15.2): prednisone 2 mg/kg.

Provide education to minimize complications, appropriate physiotherapy, and surgery where indicated.

Prevention

BCG is used in some countries. Case-finding and prompt treatment limit spread.

Tetanus

Tetanus is a spastic paralytic illness caused by a potent neurotoxin, tetanospasmin, produced by *Clostridium tetani*, spores of which are found in soil and excreta of animals. Tetanus occurs world-wide and is endemic in developing countries. The most common form, neonatal tetanus, is an important cause of infant mortality. The WHO estimates that approximately 180 000 deaths occur annually as a result of neonatal tetanus. In developed countries the non-immunized elderly are usually affected.

Pathogenesis

Following contamination of the umbilicus in the newborn or wounds in older children and adults, spores multiply in anaerobic conditions and produce tetanospasmin. The toxin is released into the bloodstream, is picked up by the motor nerve endings, and travels in the perineural spaces to reach the anterior horn cells where it accentuates the reflex arc markedly. This results in muscular hypertonia and usually intermittent muscle spasms. It is also transmitted along the neurons from the site of infection, aided by muscular contraction. The short, seventh cranial nerve and the powerful contraction of the masseter make trismus an early and constant sign. Muscles in the region of the site of infection are also likely to be more severely affected and the last to lose their hypertonicity.

All wounds, no matter how trivial, should be regarded as tetanus-prone.

The incubation period is seldom less than five days. The disease is more likely to be severe if the incubation is shorter than eight days and the onset period from the first symptom to the first generalized spasm is less than 48 hours.

Clinical features

These include the following:
* **Generalized tetanus**. This is characterized by diffuse muscle rigidity and intermittent reflex muscle spasms. Trismus (lockjaw), which is due to rigidity of the muscles of mastication, is an early sign. Facial muscle rigidity with trismus results in risus sardonicus (sardonic smile) – raised eyebrows, tightly closed eyes, and clenched teeth. Painful dysphagia follows the spasms of the pharyngeal muscles. Reflex spasms are the result of sudden increase in muscle rigidity, occur spontaneously or following external stimuli, and last for a variable time period. Laryngeal spasms may result in asphyxia. The generalized tetanic seizure activity results in the adoption of a classic posture with opisthotonus, abduction, and flexion at the shoulders, flexion of elbows and wrists with clenched fists, and extension of the legs. The patients are extremely anxious but alert and conscious.
* **Neonatal tetanus**. This usually presents three to ten days after birth. It presents with poor sucking, difficulty in swallowing, and signs of generalized tetanus.
* **Local tetanus**. This is an uncommon and mild form of tetanus and tends to occur in incompletely immunized individuals. Rigidity and spasms are confined to the muscles around the injury and may persist for weeks. Local tetanus may develop into generalized disease.
* **Cephalic tetanus**. This is rare and follows wounds of the head, neck, face, and eye, and middle ear infections. It involves the motor cranial nerves, particularly the

seventh. It can progress to generalized tetanus and prognosis is poor.

Autonomic nervous system disturbances, characterized by excessive catecholamine release, occur in about 60 per cent of cases, usually in the second week of the illness. Features include labile hypertension, tachycardia, arrythmias, peripheral vasoconstriction, sweating, and in some cases episodes of hypotension.

Diagnosis

The diagnosis is essentially a clinical one. A positive culture of *C. tetani* is obtained in less than 30 per cent of cases. Serodiagnosis is of limited value. The cerebrospinal fluid is usually normal, but the protein level may be elevated.

Management

Patients should be nursed in a quiet environment as any external stimuli can provoke spasms. Control of the spasms frequently requires prolonged paralysis and supportive mechanical ventilation. Attention should be paid to control of fluid and electrolyte balance and adequate nutritional support must be provided. Anticoagulation therapy is necessary to prevent thrombosis and pulmonary embolism. Sucralfate, H_2 blockers, or antacids are recommended to prevent stress ulcers.

Treatment of neonates

The vast majority have severe tetanus and therefore require full intermittent positive pressure ventilation under muscle relaxation and sedation (IPPV).

- Human anti-tetanus immunoglobulin is given 500 units IM. Since few neonates are seen before the onset of reflex spasms, intrathecal therapy is less effective. The dose is 250 units given as a single dose.
- Sedation: chlorpromazine, 12.5 mg IM four- to six-hourly and phenobarbitone 5 mg/kg/dose IM once or twice daily as necessary OR diazepam, 15–30 mg/d, IV or by nasogastric infusion.
- Phenobarbitone may be added to the chlorpromazine regimen if required to gain extra control of spasms. Diazepam may be given alone in the dosage recommended above, or combined with chlorpromazine, when the lower dosage range is suggested.

If spontaneous spasms are still frequent or prolonged despite very heavy sedation, IPPV is indicated.

- A nasogastric tube is passed 30 minutes after sedation; laryngospasm if provoked, can be overcome by positive pressure ventilation with well-fitting face mask and oxygen.
- Fluids: expressed breastmilk – small feeds are given to lessen danger of regurgitation and aspiration. Fluid intake may need augmentation by IV fluids.
- Mouth suction and turning of infant 30 minutes after each dose of sedative if IPPV is not available.
- Penicillin is given for pneumonia and antiseptic measures to umbilicus.
- Monitor and maintain body temperature.

Prognosis

With the introduction of intensive care in developed and in some developing countries the mortality rate has declined to between 10 and 20 per cent. Sudden unexplained cardiac arrest (probably due to autonomic disturbances) accounts for between 40 and 60 per cent of all fatalities and is the leading cause of death even with optimal intensive care. Respiratory complications and sepsis are other important causes of death, especially in developing countries.

Poor prognostic features include severe disease at presentation, short incubation period, rapidly progressing disease, delay in seeking medical care, and cephalic or neonatal tetanus. In children who have had neonatal tetanus, mental retardation, cerebral palsy, growth retardation, and enuresis are common findings. In adults muscle weakness and atrophy, peripheral paresis, nervousness, decreased mental capacity, and difficulties in speech, balance, and memory have been noted.

Prevention

Tetanus can be prevented if certain guidelines are followed:

- Immunization of pregnant women with toxoid protects their infants for the first four to six months of age.
- Administer triple vaccine in infancy with a booster a year later and tetanus toxoid every 10 years thereafter.

- Wound care: cleanse and debride if necessary.
- Toxoid is also given if fully immunized but with booster more than five years previously. If the patient is non-immunized or the status unknown, a complete course of toxoid is given.
- If the wound is penetrating, contains a foreign body or soil, and/or is more than six hours old, human anti-tetanus immunoglobulin 250 units is given IM (in opposite limb to toxoid).
- An antibiotic (penicillin, metronidazole, erythromycin, cephalosporin) is given for five days or until the wound is healed.

Anterior poliomyelitis

Poliomyelitis has been targeted by the WHO for eradication. Strategies for eradication include maintaining the highest level of immunization coverage, implementing mass national or sub-national vaccination campaigns for all children under five years of age, conducting outbreak response immunization, providing mop-up immunization efforts to groups at high risk in situations where wild polio virus transmission may persist, and improving disease surveillance of acute flaccid paralysis to detect and investigate every suspected polio case.

Since 1988 the global initiative has made significant progress. Worldwide immunization coverage has increased from about 60 to 85 per cent and the reported cases of polio have declined from over 35 000 to a few thousand cases in select parts of Asia and Africa. In 1994 a significant milestone was achieved when the Western Hemisphere was declared polio-free. No cases of clinical poliomyelitis have been reported in South Africa since 1991, but eradication can only be certified once acute flaccid paralysis surveillance is able to identify all cases. This is measured by the ability to report all expected cases of acute flaccid paralysis, mainly due to Guillain-Barré syndrome with an expected incidence of 1 per 100 000.

Epidemiology

Poliovirus types 1, 2, and 3 are usually spread by faecal–oral contamination but also by droplets in epidemics. Humans are the sole natural reservoir.

The incubation period is about 10 days and the latter part of the incubation period and first week of disease are the most infectious.

Pathogenesis

The virus multiplies in the intestinal tract and its lymph nodes, with production of antibody. If the antibody response is rapid, the virus is neutralized, but sometimes the virus proliferates and becomes invasive. Access to the central nervous system occurs either across blood vessels into the cerebellum or by spreading along the nerve pathways from the gut.

The virus affects the anterior horn cells of the cord and several areas of the brain. Damage may be reversible, with recovery; but may go on to irreversible nuclear destruction, when muscle paralysis results.

Clinical features

- **Inapparent infection**. About 95 per cent of infections are subclinical, giving lasting immunity.
- **Abortive disease**. A minor illness of a few days occurs, with fever, sore throat, headache, abdominal pain, nausea, and vomiting. Lumbar puncture at this stage shows a normal CSF.
- **Non-paralytic poliomyelitis** resembles the abortive disease with meningism and pain in the back and legs. The CSF here usually shows pleocytosis and a slightly raised protein level.
- **Paralytic disease**. Weakness of skeletal or cranial muscle groups may follow closely upon the non-paralytic form or occur after a symptom-free period of some days.
- **Spinal form**. Involvement of muscles of neck, trunk, abdomen, thorax, diaphragm, and limbs.
- **Bulbar form**. Motor weakness of cranial nerves and/or dysfunction of medullary vital centres of respiration and circulation.
- **Bulbospinal form**. The above two forms frequently occur together.
- **Encephalitic form**. Irritability, disorientation, drowsiness, tremors.

There is flaccid muscle paralysis with reduced or absent superficial and deep tendon jerks and intact sensation. Improvement of muscle power following paralysis occurs for up to 12 weeks after onset. Muscle wasting is due to denervation of muscle, as well as disuse.

Diagnosis

The diagnosis is made on the clinical picture. The CSF is abnormal for about 10 days after onset of meningism. A rising serum antibody titre and culture of the virus from stool and urine is confirmatory evidence.

Poliomyelitis should be considered in the differential diagnosis of any case of acute flaccid paralysis such as Guillain-Barré syndrome, transverse myelitis, and traumatic neuritis. The essential differences are outlined in Table 15.3.

Complications

Superficial gut erosions with haemorrhage, hypertension, myocarditis, and transitory bladder paralysis are encountered at times. In the severely incapacitated, hypercalciuria may occur later, with urinary calculi.

Management procedures depend on whether the patient is in the acute, recovery or residual phase and usually require a multi-disciplinary approach involving physiotherapist, speech therapist and occupational therapist. In bulbar and bulbospinal disease care is taken to avoid aspiration while respiratory muscle paralysis requires a period of assisted ventilation. Isolation of the subject is essential during the acute phase. Most recovery of muscle power will occur in the first three months. Surgery may be required in selected case during the residual phase to overcome soft-tissue contractures and to improve function, and/or prevent deformity by tendon transfer, or by stabilization of flail joints. Legs that are unequal in length may need correction.

Prevention

OPV (Sabin) vaccine has the advantage of ease of administration and the induction of local gut immunity, which prevents the survival of wild polio virus. Recipients also shed vaccine virus, which can spread to and protect those that have not been vaccinated.

In the USA, the risk of paralytic vaccine poliomyelitis was found to be one in 2.5 million doses. The major disadvantage of OPV in developing communities is that serological failures are sometimes unacceptably high after three or four OPV doses. Many are due to widespread interference in the gut by other enteroviruses. To counter this, an extra (fifth) dose in the first year is suggested. Most of the residual polio cases are of serotype 1 and targeted immunization against this serotype has shown some success in those areas where polio remains uncontrolled. A return to the inactivated Salk vaccine (IPV) has been advocated. This vaccine, given by injection with boosters, gives a high seroconversion rate, and has no complications. From 2009, South Africa plans to use a combination of OPV (at birth and six weeks) and IPV at 6, 10, 14 weeks with a booster at 15–18 months of age.

Rabies (hydrophobia)

Rabies is a viral infection of the central nervous system (CNS), transmitted usually by contamination of a wound with saliva from a rabid animal.

Epidemiology and pathogenesis

Rabies is widespread in warm-blooded animals. The principal vectors vary in different countries. In Africa, meerkat, fruit bats, and stray dogs are the main transmitters of the disease to humans.

After entry through the skin, the virus possibly multiplies first in striated muscle, where antibody, interferon, and other host factors may retard nerve invasion. Ascent through sensory nerves follows and once in the CNS, neuronal destruction occurs maximally in the brain stem, pyramid cells, cranial nerves, and posterior horns of the spinal cord. The virus then moves out along nerves to mucous-secreting and salivary glands, where the amount of virus is variable, which may explain why only 50 per cent of bites by proven rabid dogs result in rabies. Since animals lick their claws, scratches by rabid animals can also transmit disease.

Bats cause disease by bites and individuals have been infected by the inhalation of virus-containing excreta in infested caves. In general, if a biting animal does not die within 10 days, it is unlikely to be rabid, although bats are often infected for long periods without symptoms.

Clinical features

The clinical features of rabies can be summarized as follows:

Table 15.3 Criteria for the differential diagnosis of poliomyelitis, Guillain-Barré syndrome, transverse myelitis, and traumatic neuritis

	Polio	Guillain-Barré syndrome	Traumatic neuritis	Transverse myelitis
Installation of paralysis	24 to 48 hours onset to full paralysis	from hours to 10 days	from hours to 4 days	from hours to 4 days
Fever at onset	high, always present at onset of flaccid paralysis, gone the following day	not common	commonly present before, during, and after flaccid paralysis	rarely present
Flaccid paralysis	acute usually, asymmetrical, principally proximal	generally acute, symmetrical, and distal	asymmetrical, acute, and affecting only one limb	acute, lower limbs, symmetrical
Muscle tone	reduced or absent in affected limb	global hypotonia	reduced or absent in affected limb	hypotonia in lower limbs
Deep-tendon reflexes	decreased to absent	globally absent	decreased to absent	absent in lower limbs early on
Sensation	severe myalgia, backache, no sensory changes	cramps, tingling, hypo-aesthesia of palms and soles	pain in gluteus, hypothermia	anaesthesia of lower limbs with sensory level
Cranial nerve involvement	only when bulbar involvement is present	often present, affecting nerves VII, IX, X, XI, XII	absent	absent
Respiratory	only when bulbar involvement is present	in severe cases, enhanced	absent	sometimes
Autonomic signs and symptoms	rare	frequent blood pressure alterations, sweating, blushing, and body temperature fluctuations	hypothermia in affected limb	present
Cerebro-spinal fluid	inflammatory	albumino-cytologic dissociation	normal	normal or mild increase in cells
Bladder dysfunction	absent	transient	never	present
Nerve conduction velocity: third week	abnormal: anterior horn cell disease (normal during the first two weeks)	abnormal: slowed conduction decreased motor amplitudes	abnormal: axonal damage	normal or abnormal, no diagnostic value

continued

Table 15.3 *continued*				
EMG at three weeks	abnormal	normal	normal	normal
Sequelae at three months	severe, asymmetrical atrophy, skeletal deformities	symmetrical atrophy of distal muscles	moderate atrophy, only in affected lower limb	flaccid diplegia atrophy after years

Source: 'The Diagnosis of Polio and Other Acute Flaccid Paralysis: A Neurological Approach'; Alcala, H., Olive, J-M. and de Quadros, C.; No. EPI/TAG/91/10. Document presented at the Ninth Meeting of the Technical Advisory Group on Vaccine-Preventable Diseases, held in Guatemala City, Guatemala, from 12 to 15 March, 1991.

- **Incubation**: Two weeks to one year; usually one to two months.
- **Prodrome of a few days**: Fever, malaise, headache, anorexia, vomiting, and paraesthesia at the site of the wound.
- **Acute neurological phase**: *Furious rabies.* This is characterized by hydrophobia and/or aerophobia, which lead to spasms of the larynx and pharynx with aspiration into the trachea. Hyperactivity and bizarre aggressive behaviour alternate with periods of lucidity. This is followed by ascending symmetrical paralysis, areflexia, and coma. Respiratory muscle paralysis or arrhythmias are the usual cause of death.
  Dumb rabies. In about 20 per cent of cases there is an ascending symmetrical paralysis without a furious phase. The cerebrospinal fluid (CSF) may be normal or show pleocytosis and elevated protein. No survivors have been reported in unimmunized cases.

Laboratory confirmation

Fluorescent antibody test on brain and a rise in serum antibody titre are diagnostic.

Control of disease in endemic area

Domestic animals must be kept immunized with live-attenuated virus vaccine. Measures against growth of vector population, e.g. meerkat, are a parallel approach.
Measures during an epidemic:
- Re-vaccinate domestic animals, and keep them fenced in or tied up.
- Restrict movement of domestic animals between rabies and rabies-free areas.

- Eliminate stray animals.
- Vaccinate high-risk humans (veterinarians, health inspectors, etc.).

The human diploid cell vaccine is given to at-risk individuals. The pre-exposure schedule is 1 ml IMI on days 0, 7, and 28 with boosters every one to three years depending on the level of exposure.

Biting animal	Condition of animal at time of attack	Treatment of humans with RIG* or V**
Wild	Regard as	RIG + V
Domestic	rabid	None
	Healthy***	RIG + V
	Unknown, escaped	RIG + V
	Suspected rabid	

*   RIG: Rabies immunoglobulin
**   V: Human diploid cell vaccine
*** Isolate for 10 days if bite was apparently unprovoked.

The **management** of a patient when bitten by a 'suspect' animal is as follows:
- Clean wound with soap and water, then apply a virucidal solution, e.g. 10% povidone iodine.
- Administer rabies immunoglobulin (RIG).
- Administer human diploid cell vaccine on days 0, 3, 7, 14, 30, and 90.

Note: Confirmation of rabies is possible by autopsy on the biting animal. Don't wait for this before giving RIG.

Mumps (epidemic parotitis)

Mumps is an acute viral illness, characterized by enlargement of the parotid and other salivary glands, caused by a paramyxovirus. Endemic in most urban communities, the mumps virus is spread by droplet infection and by infectious saliva from the human reservoir. Eighty-five per cent of infections occur under the age of 15 years. Infants are protected for about six months by passive placental transfer of antibodies. Immunity is lifelong after one attack.

The period of infectivity is from about six days before onset of symptoms to subsidence of salivary gland swelling: a period of seven to fourteen days in the average case. Inapparent infections occur in 30–40 per cent of persons; these remain infectious for a period similar to that of overt cases.

Clinical features

The incubation period is 14–21 days. Parotitis is unilateral in 30 per cent of patients. Submandibular and, rarely, sublingual gland infection is encountered. There is tender swelling which reaches a maximum during the first day but the opposite gland may be affected some days later. Opening the mouth may be difficult. There is oedema of the surrounding tissue with ear lobe displaced upwards and backwards. Stensen's duct may be inflamed. Headache, malaise, and anorexia are common symptoms. Sour food elicits pain along the duct and in the gland. Symptoms usually subside within a week. **Complications** could include the following:

* **Epididymo-orchitis** occurs in about 25 per cent of post-pubertal males.
* **Meningo-encephalitis**. Clinical features are seen in about 10 per cent of patients. The disease is usually benign but high fever and marked meningeal signs do occur. The CSF shows a mildly raised protein content and pleocytosis, with lymphocytes predominating.
* **Pancreatitis** occurs in about 7 per cent of patients, presenting with epigastric pain, fever, and vomiting.

* **Oophoritis, thyroiditis,** and **mastitis** are rare complications.

All complications may precede or occur in the absence of parotitis.

Deafness, post-infectious encephalomyelitis, facial nerve neuritis, myocarditis, arthritis, thrombocytopaenia, and haemolytic anaemia are further rare complications which have been described.

Diagnosis and treatment

The diagnosis is usually based upon the clinical findings. Virus can be isolated from the throat, saliva, and CSF. Serological tests usually require paired sera or determination of specific IgM.

Parotid enlargement may rarely be caused by other acute viral infections such as para-influenzae and coxsackie, or a bacterial infection. Chronic parotid enlargement is common with AIDS.

Treatment is entirely symptomatic.

Prevention

The mumps-attenuated virus vaccine has no untoward reactions and produces antibody titres which are protective in 95 per cent of cases, but are lower than titres following natural disease. While the use of this vaccine should not take priority over more essential community health needs, some complications of mumps are serious enough for the use of a safe vaccine, which is usually given as a combination vaccine with measles and rubella (MMR vaccine).

Influenza

The influenza virus genus belongs to the family orthomyxoviridae, classified into three types, A, B and C. Influenza A virus is subject to major shifts as well as minor drift in its antigenic components. Major shifts can be associated with large-scale severe pandemics. These occur regularly every 30–40 years, with the last pandemic strain having occurred in the mid-1970s. The major antigenic determinants of the influenza virus are the haemagglutinin (HA) and neuraminidase (N) antigens. The haemaglutinin (HA) protein is the outermost protein responsible for attachment to the host receptor and is critical in determining the host's immune response to the virus. Changes in the antigenic epitopes of HA therefore allow the virus to escape the host's specific immune response. Type A is further divided into subtypes on the basis of the antigenic epitopes of the HA and NA proteins. Each of the human subtypes H1N1, H2N2 and H3N2 are further subdivided into strains on the basis of more subtle antigenic properties of the HA protein. The predominant influenza epidemic strains since the mid-1970s are the H1N1 and H3N2 subtypes. Vaccines are updated annually based on recommendation by the World Health Organisation as to which influenza virus strains should be included in the vaccine based upon anticipated circulating strains. Influenza B virus undergoes only minor antigenic changes, with resultant major outbreaks at more variable intervals. In such epidemics, the attack rates with the new subtype are higher in children than in adults.

Clinical presentation

The manifestation of infection in older children is fairly typical of influenza, with abrupt onset (distinguishing it from the common-cold) of fever, headache, myalgia, sore throat, rhinitis, vomiting and respiratory signs. Severe complications such as coryza, croup, bronchitis, bronchiolitis, and pneumonia occur at a higher rate in younger children (20–30 per cent) than in adults. Influenza virus is also frequently associated with febrile seizures during influenza epidemics in young children. The rate of hospitalisation and death are increased in children under two years of age and especially in those under six months of age. Reye's syndrome, encephalitis, pericariditis and myocarditis have also rarely been reported in children as complications of influenza infection. Bacterial super-infection from S. pneumoniae and S. aureus is a common complication in children with influenza virus associated otitis media and pneumonia. Animal-model studies and epidemiological data indicate that the influenza virus enhances the host susceptibility to developing a superimposed pneumococcal infection, which contributes to severe pneumonia. Myocarditis, encephalitis, and Reye's syndrome are rare complications. Influenza C is a sporadic cause of upper respiratory tract infections.

Prevention

Influenza vaccine is the mainstay of influenza prevention strategies. The most widely available vaccine is a sub-unit or split-product (inactivated) vaccine that is administered intra-muscularly. Vaccination with the sub-unit vaccines is recommended for persons who are at high risk for influenza and its complications because of underlying medical conditions or who are receiving regular medical care for chronic conditions.

Some countries recommend routine immunisation of all young healthy children between 6–59 months of age. Children less than three years of age should receive 0.25 ml (or the paediatric formulation) on two occasions separated by one month, when vaccinated for the first time. Children 3–9 years who have never been vaccinated should receive two doses one month apart. Dosing in children between 9–12 years is the same as for in adults which is a single dose.

Newer vaccine formulations, not yet available in Africa, include live-attenuated influenza vaccines, which are administered intranasally. The live-attenuated vaccines have also been shown to provide some cross-protection against strains that are not matched for in the vaccine, and possibly provide protection into the second year after vaccination as well.

Treatment

The antiviral agents currently available for use include the M1 inhibitors (adamantanes) and the neuraminidase inhibitors. Widespread resistance has been documented to adamantanes and resistance to neuraminidase inhibitors is also emerging, including in South Africa. Neuraminidase inhibitors are nevertheless an important adjunct to influenza vaccination, in both the prevention and treatment of influenza. Because of concerns about the possibility of the development of viral resistance with overuse of these

Recommendations for influenza vaccination in South Africa include those with chronic pulmonary, cardiac, renal, hepatic, endocrine, neurologic, metabolic or immunological disease that increases the risk of severe influenza; children on current or chronic aspirin therapy; children who are family contacts of young children or contacts of high risk people. Vaccines should be given from at least two months prior to the onset of winter (March) in South Africa, but can be administered at any time thereafter at least until July-August.

agents, it is recommended that neuraminidase inhibitors should be reserved for sicker influenza patients. Two neuraminidase inhibitors are currently available for clinical use, namely oseltamivir (Tamiflu®) and zanamivir (Relenza®). The former is given orally as a prodrug and is distributed systemically to all potential infection sites. The latter is administered via inhalation and is deposited primarily in the respiratory tract. The current approved indications for oseltamivir are for the treatment of uncomplicated acute illness due to influenza infection in patients ≥ 1 year of age or older who have been symptomatic for 48 hours or less. Oseltamivir significantly reduces the complication rate from influenza in children by up to 40 per cent, reduces the need for hospitalisation, the length of hospitalisation in children already hospitalised and the length of illness. Oseltamivir is indicated for treatment of influenza in children older than one year of age to reduce the risk of complications and severity of illness and especially in children with risk factors for severe disease.

The mainstay of treatment available for severe illness is however supportive and symptomatic therapy. For those requiring hospitalisation, oxygen is a mainstay of treatment in hypoxic children. Children with suspected secondary bacterial infection or who are severely ill with pneumonia requiring hospitalisation should also be treated with an antibiotic for community acquired pneumonia.

Diagnosis

While most cases of influenza are diagnosed clinically, rapid tests (Binax Now Influenza A&B®, Directigen EZ Flu A+B®, Denka Seiken Quick Ex-Flu®, Fujirebio Espline Influenza A&B-N®, and Quidel QuickVue Influenza A+B Test®) are available in South Africa. Conventional testing of respiratory secretions by immunofluorescence or real-time RT-PCR is offered by most laboratories. Cell culture is used for epidemiological purposes. Diagnostic assays, especially culture and immunofluorescence, are more sensitive among children, in whom shedding of influenza virus is more prolonged (7–14 days) compared to adults.

Major antigenic shifts causing pandemics

Major antigenic shifts in influenza virus may

result in pandemics. It is forecast that the next major influenza pandemic may cause between 51 million and 81 million deaths, the majority (>90 per cent) of which would occur in the developing world.

Recently (2009), a new reassortant H1N1 ('swine flu') virus originating in Mexico has spread to many countries, including South Africa. Fortunately, it has so far not caused high case fatality rates. Nevertheless, public health authorities have been placed on high alert.

Prevention

In the event of a pandemic, control by means of case tracing and isolation will be impossible as virus is shed prior to the development of symptoms. Infection control specialists and virologists will be valuable primarily to inform clinicians of the arrival of the new strain and that patients should thereafter be treated presumptively.

The most important intervention during a pandemic would be an effective, widely available and cheaply produced vaccine.

Antiviral medications would represent the second most important intervention. This would, however, require early diagnosis to be effective and there is no way of predicting the effectiveness thereof during a pandemic.

Additional preparations should also include the stock-piling of antibiotics, as a large proportion of deaths occurring during recent, past influenza pandemics were attributable to superimposed pneumococcal and *S. aureus* infection.

Additionally, adequate vaccination of the population, including pneumococcal conjugate vaccination in children, may abrogate some of the influenza-associated morbidity and mortality. Pneumococcal conjugate vaccines have been shown to reduce hospitalization for influenza-virus associated pneumonia by 40 per cent during influenza epidemics. Additionally measures that would need to be planned for in a future pandemic include adequate health-care worker vaccination and education regarding infection control and disease management, as well as minimizing human to human contact.

Avian influenza (H5N1 subtype virus)

Another influenza strain currently posing a threat as a future pandemic strain of the virus is the avian H5N1 subtype virus. Sporadic cases, initially mainly occurring in South-East Asia, have been documented in Europe, North America and Africa. Case fatality rates due to H5N1 virus are 50–60 per cent, however children appear to be less often affected and have had a better outcome. Nevertheless, changes in the virulence factor of the virus following mutation to a strain able to transmit between humans makes it difficult to predict the outcome of individuals should this strain of virus contribute to the next influenza pandemic.

H5N1 influenza virus strain vaccines are currently under development.

Infections presenting mainly with lymphadenopathy

Local infections commonly present with tender draining lymphadenopathy. In patients in whom a local lesion is not immediately identifiable to explain lymphadenopathy, a number of other conditions have to be borne in mind:

- Specific infections, e.g. tuberculosis (Chapter 17, Tuberculosis), actinomycosis, *Bartonella henselae (LGV)*, viral infections such as E-B virus, cytomegalovirus (CMV), and HIV
- Lymphoreticular malignancy, e.g. lymphoma
- Generalized reticulo-endothelial activation, e.g. auto-immune disorders and Kawasaki disease.

Actinomycosis

The anaerobic causative organism *Actinomyces israeli* can be found on the teeth, pharynx, and tonsils of many healthy individuals. Trauma from a tooth extraction, pyogenic infection or possibly hypersensitivity to the organism is believed to precipitate the abscess formation, with multiple draining sinuses characteristic of the disease. Cervico-facial actinomycosis presenting as a gradually enlarging, painless swelling of the neck and jaw is the most common clinical form. Multiple sinuses form in the overlying skin and pus contains typical 'sulphur granules'. Infection may spread to involve bone or meninges.

Abdominal actinomycosis with the primary lesion in the caecum, appendix, or pelvic organs, presents as a hard, irregular, lower abdominal mass which may drain to the outside or progress to involve other abdominal organs.

Lung involvement leads to a chronic pulmonary infection commonly of the lower lobes which may extend to the ribs, pleura and subcutaneous tissues.

Treatment

Penicillin in massive doses (1–6 million units daily) are required for several months.

Surgical excision or drainage may be necessary adjuncts.

Cat scratch disease

Cutaneous inoculation with the Gram-negative bacillus *Bartonella henselae* results in regional adenitis which may suppurate and form a 'cold abscess'. Commonly, superficial scratch marks are associated. It must be differentiated from suppurative adenitis, tuberculous adenitis and other forms of lymphadenopathy. Diagnosis usually rests on serological tests and direct stains of histological specimens. Antibiotic therapy is not of proven benefit.

16

Parasitic and fungal diseases

Protozoal infections

Malaria

This is endemic in parts of tropical and subtropical regions of Africa, Asia, and America. Sporadic cases of malaria occur in non-malarious areas, often in individuals returning from visits to endemic areas. Freak transmission may occur when an infected mosquito is conveyed to a non-malarious area by car or aeroplane.

In southern Africa, malaria is endemic in Mozambique, Malawi, northern Namibia, the lowveld of Zimbabwe, and northern Botswana. Epidemic outbreaks occur in the Limpopo Province, Mpumalanga, northern KwaZulu-Natal, Zimbabwe and Swaziland, and in pockets in the Northern Cape Province.

Aetiology and pathogenesis

A vector-borne parasitic infection, malaria is caused by parasites of the genus *Plasmodium*. Four species, *P. falciparum, P. vivax, P. ovale,* and *P. malariae* infect humans and cause malignant tertian, tertian, ovale, and quartan malaria respectively. All four species occur in southern Africa. *P. falciparum* is the most prevalent and causes the most severe infection.

The life cycle is passed in two hosts, the asexual phase (schizogony) in humans, and the sexual (sporogony) in the Anopheles mosquito. After the female Anopheles mosquito injects sporozoites into the human bloodstream, development of the parasite occurs in the parenchymal cells of the liver (pre-erythrocytic phase). Invasion of circulating red cells by the parasite follows. Multiplication and maturation in the red cell leads to red cell rupture. Reinvasion of red cells occurs and the cycle is repeated many times (erythrocytic phase).

After schizogony has been repeated many times, sexual forms (gametocytes) appear and are sucked up by a feeding mosquito to start the sexual cycle in the insect host.

In *P. vivax, P. ovale,* and *P. malariae* infections, parasites may re-enter liver cells where they continue to multiply long after the initial bloodstream invasion has ceased (exo-erythrocytic cycles). Later reinvasion of the bloodstream results in a relapse of malaria. This may occur many years after the initial attack, especially in *P. malariae* infections, which have been known to relapse as long as 40 years after the initial infection. *P. falciparum* does not have an exo-erythrocytic cycle.

Although the bite of a mosquito is the usual mode of transmission, humans may acquire the infection by means of a blood transfusion from an asymptomatic infected donor. Rarely, an infected mother may transmit the parasite to her fetus.

The ability of the malarial parasites to proliferate and produce clinical manifestations depends on their virulence, the size of the infecting dose, and the immune status of the host.

An attack of malaria is followed by a rise in immunoglobulin levels. Initially the IgM fraction rises steeply, but in chronic malaria the increase is predominantly in the IgG fraction. Transplacental passive immunity from mother to fetus probably explains the rarity of congenital malaria and the relative freedom from infection

Figure 16.1 The life cycle of the malaria parasite

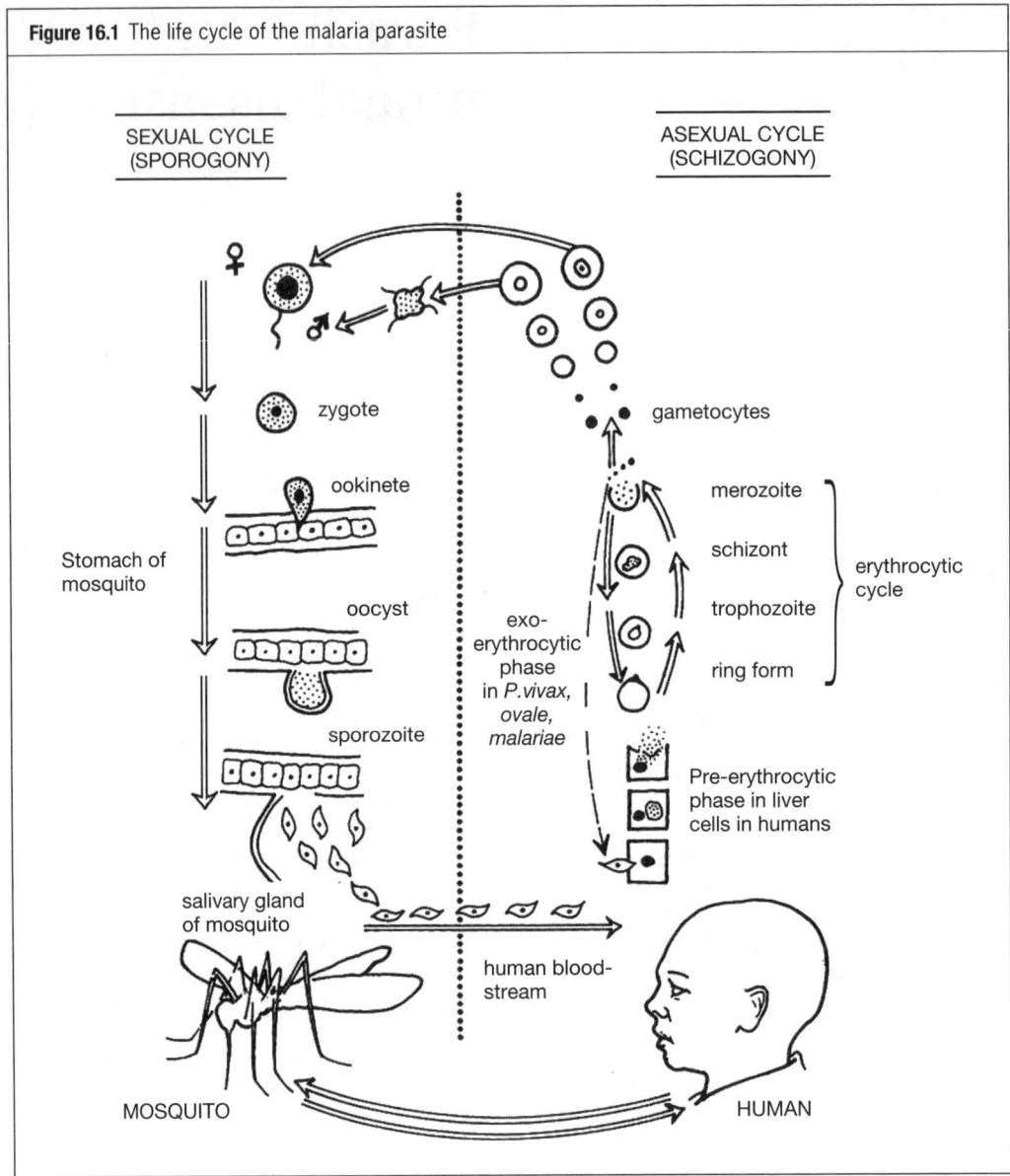

SEXUAL CYCLE
(SPOROGONY)

ASEXUAL CYCLE
(SCHIZOGONY)

zygote

gametocytes

ookinete

merozoite

schizont

Stomach of
mosquito

erythrocytic
cycle

oocyst

exo-
erythrocytic
phase
in *P. vivax,
ovale,
malariae*

trophozoite

ring form

sporozoite

Pre-erythrocytic
phase in liver
cells in humans

salivary gland
of mosquito

human blood-
stream

MOSQUITO

HUMAN

Transplacental passive immunity explains the
rarity of disease among young infants in endemic
areas.

Premunity represents a state of tolerance
between the host and parasite after repeated
exposures.

Innate immunity occurs in patients with G6PD
deficiency or the sickle cell trait.

in young infants in endemic areas. As passive
immunity wanes, clinical manifestations occur,
but repeated exposures to infection lead to a
tolerance between the host and the parasite.
Clinical manifestations thereafter no longer
occur, provided the host continues to be exposed
to infection. This state is known as premunity
and it is lost after a few years if the host leaves
a malarious area. Re-exposure after this time

results in a return of symptoms, but some degree of protection persists because fatalities rarely occur, unlike in a primary attack in a fully susceptible individual.

In certain hyperendemic areas an innate immunity to malaria may be present in addition to acquired immunity. G6PD deficiency and the sickle-cell trait appear to partially protect against *P. falciparum* infection and the absence of the Duffy antigen in red cells in certain inhabitants of tropical Africa is believed to protect them against *P. vivax* infections.

An attack of malaria results in marked activity and hyperplasia of the reticulo-endothelial system with subsequent hepatosplenomegaly. Malarial pigment, released when parasitized red cells rupture, is phagocytosed by cells of the reticulo-endothelial system, giving rise to pigmentation of the skin and internal organs.

Destruction of red cells leads to anaemia with reticulocytosis and to jaundice.

In *P. falciparum* disease, infected red cells tend to adhere to each other and to the vascular endothelium. Interference with circulation and resulting tissue damage may affect many organs in the body, leading to a variety of complications.

Clinical manifestations

Uncomplicated malaria

The incubation period is shortest in *P. falciparum* infections. Symptoms usually develop within seven to twelve days after exposure, while in *P. vivax*, *P. ovale*, and *P. malariae* infections, 10–30 days may elapse after infection before clinical manifestations occur. Incomplete prophylaxis or partial immunity may suppress symptoms and signs for longer periods after infection has occurred. The onset is usually abrupt.

Fever is the most common presenting sign and initially tends to be remittent, but after some days typical periodicity may be established.

In a classical attack, headache and muscle and joint pains rapidly progress to shivering and rigors. This is followed by flushing and complaints of feeling hot. Nausea and vomiting may occur, and severe headache and delirium may be present. Finally there is profuse sweating with relief of symptoms.

Cold, hot, and sweating stages are unusual in infants and children. Convulsions may occur during the height of the fever in the very young. The spleen tends to be enlarged and some degree of anaemia, together with a mild leucopaenia and thrombocytopaenia, is usually present.

Infections due to *P. vivax*, *P. ovale*, and *P. malariae* commonly present in this manner, but *P. falciparum* malaria frequently presents atypically. Periods of fever may be irregular, and an undramatic picture of fever and constitutional symptoms may suddenly deteriorate when complications occur.

Complicated malaria

Cerebral malaria is the most dangerous complication. It is due to *P. falciparum* and may be fatal Symptoms range from apathy to coma, disorientation to psychotic behaviour, focal or even extra-pyramidal signs and, convulsions. Hypoglycaemia must be excluded in all children with seizures or altered conscious state.

Gastrointestinal involvement leads to severe vomiting, abdominal pain and distension with profuse watery diarrhoea or even dysentery, with the passage of blood-stained stools. Occasionally an acute abdomen may be simulated.

Hepatic necrosis with marked jaundice and disturbed liver function tests may dominate the clinical picture.

Attacks of fever are believed to correspond with the end of each erythrocytic cycle, occurring at 48-hour intervals in *P. falciparum*, *P. vivax*, and *P. ovale* infections, and at 72-hour intervals in *P. malariae* infections.

If any of the following is present, diagnose severe malaria and treat as a medical emergency:

- Cerebral malaria (unrousable coma)
- Severe anaemia (haemoglobin <5 g/dl)
- Parasitaemia >10 000/µl
- Renal failure
- Pulmonary oedema
- Circulatory collapse
- Hypoglycaemia
- Spontaneous bleeding or DIC
- Repeated generalized convulsions
- Severe metabolic acidosis
- Malarial haemoglobinuria.

Acute renal failure with oliguria or anuria as a consequence of dehydration, hypotension, or intravascular coagulopathy may necessitate dialysis.

Massive intravascular haemolysis leading to haemoglobinuria and oliguria constitutes blackwater fever. This complication is believed to result from a hypersensitivity reaction of the host to the red cells, made auto-antigenic by repeated quinine therapy and malarial infection. Pamaquine or primaquine therapy in the presence of G6PD deficiency may also cause blackwater fever. Rarely, it may be seen in a first attack of malaria before treatment is given.

Haematological involvement, as shown by the presence of anaemia, is invariable. Anaemia, if severe, may lead to cardiac failure. Even non-parasitized cells have an increased osmotic fragility. Rarely, a positive Coombs' test suggests autosensitization. Purpura and bleeding from mucosal surfaces are consequences of disseminated intravascular coagulation.

Pulmonary complications are common in cerebral malaria. Oedema, congested capillaries, haemorrhages, and hyaline membrane formation may be found at autopsy and present clinically with severe refractory hypoxaemia. Bacterial pneumonia may also occur.

Algid malaria is a term given to a syndrome which resembles Gram-negative shock.

Severe complications are unusual in *P. vivax* or *P. ovale* malaria. Even in *P. falciparum* infections in the partially immune, mild fever with general malaise lasting for a few days may be the only manifestation, and symptomless parasitaemia is not uncommon. Exceptions occur in pregnant women who are liable to develop very severe attacks, as are splenectomized and immunosuppressed individuals.

Chronic malaria is seen in patients who have had inadequate or no treatment. As immunity develops, acute attacks gradually lessen. *P. falciparum* infections usually disappear within a year and *P. vivax* infections within two years. Splenic enlargement, which may be massive and lead to hypersplenism, or rupture in response to trauma, is a feature of chronic *P. malariae* infections. Malarial nephrosis is a further important complication of quartan malaria. It is a common cause of death from renal failure in children in West Africa, unless the condition is diagnosed and treatment is instituted early.

Diagnosis

The symptoms and signs are rarely sufficiently specific to make a clinical diagnosis and the only certain proof of malaria infection is the finding of the parasites in the peripheral blood. A single negative finding does not exclude malaria. Repeated blood films may be required and those taken during the height of fever are most likely to reveal parasites. These may be more easily seen in thick films, but thin films may be necessary to identify the species of the infecting plasmodium. Small doses of antimalarial drugs or other drugs such as sulphonamides may result in negative films. The finding of malarial pigment in neutrophils or monocytes is strongly suggestive of malaria, even in the absence of parasites.In cerebral malaria typical retinal changes are found on indirect and direct fundoscopy. These changes include retinal vessel whitening, haemorrhages and exudates.

Bone-marrow examination for detection of parasites may rarely be of value, particularly in chronic malaria. When the diagnosis is strongly suspected but not proven, antimalarial therapy may be prescribed. Provided drug resistance can be excluded, failure of response to therapy makes the diagnosis unlikely.

Serodiagnostic tests. A dipstick antigen-capture assay based upon the qualitative detection of *P. falciparum* histidine-rich protein 2 in peripheral blood has been developed. The test is quick and easy to use, but cannot detect low levels of parasitaemia. It would be of use in situations where there is no access to laboratory services. Other ELISA kits for the detection of malarial antigens have been shown to be of use in diagnosing acute malaria. Immunofluorescence or ELISA for detecting antibodies may also be of help in the diagnosis of chronic malaria.

Treatment

The choice of antimalarial therapy to be used should be determined by the species responsible for the infection, the severity of infection, the area where infection was acquired, and the pattern of drug resistance in the area.

Uncomplicated attack. Chloroquine is the drug of choice for rapid elimination of the asexual forms in all non *P. falciparum* species. Unfortunately, widespread resistance has developed to chloroquine making it unsafe for first line use in *P. falciparum* infections and all forms of severe or complicated malaria.

Chloroquine doses are: 10 mg base/kg orally immediately, then 5 mg base/kg six to eight hours later, and 5 mg base/kg daily for three days. (Commercial names of chloroquine = Aralan®, Nivaquine®; standard tablet = 150 mg base).

Primaquine should be given in addition to chloroquine in *P. vivax, P. ovale,* and *P. malariae* infections for the hepatic or exo-erythrocytic phase of the parasite. Dose: 0.3 mg/kg orally, daily for 14 days. Primaquine is also effective against gametocytes of all four species.

P. falciparum infections: Monotherapy other than quinine, should be avoided as it leads to rapid resistance. For oral therapy a combination of an artemesinin and another antimalarial drug is recommended by WHO:

CoArtem® (Artemether20/lumefantrine120) is a fixed dose combination tablet and is prescribed by body weight. The dose for children is as follows:

Weight	Dose of CoArtem
5–14.9 kg	1 tablet bd for 3 days
15–24.9 kg	2 tablets bd for 3 days
25–34.9 kg	3 tablets bd for 3 days
Adult	4 tablets bd for 3 days

The second dose should, ideally be taken eight hours after the first dose; all others are at 12 hour intervals. Lumefantrine is absorbed better if taken with fatty food.

Artesunate can be given in combination with amodiaquine. These drugs are taken once daily for three days.

Complicated malaria. For *specific therapy,* intravenous quinine is the drug of choice. Give a loading dose of 20 mg salt/kg in 5% dextrose or dextrose saline over four hours, followed by 10 mg/kg every eight hours until the patient can take oral quinine and is not vomiting or shocked. Complete seven days of treatment. If intravenous therapy is impossible, give by intramuscular injection (10 mg/kg IM at 0 and 4 hours and then 12 hourly). If a patient has received quinine or mefloquine before presentation, omit the loading dose of quinine.

Supportive therapy is as important as chemotherapy in severely ill patients and includes maintenance of fluid and electrolyte balance. Accurate diagnosis of the cause of oliguria and azotaemia, and careful monitoring are necessary to prevent iatrogenic pulmonary oedema. Blood transfusion may be necessary.

In cerebral malaria, convulsions are managed with diazepam and phenobarbitone or paraldehyde. Hyperpyrexia must be controlled. Hypoglycaemia is common in severe malaria and may be exacerbated by quinine therapy. It must be excluded or treated in all children with seizures or altered consciousness.

Hypotension and acidosis may occur and need to be treated with adequate fluid therapy

Prophylaxis

The choice of prophylaxis depends upon the level of drug resistance in the area to be visited.

Chloroquine 5 mg/kg once a week is recommended for protection against *P. vivax* and for *P. falciparum* in areas of low chloroquine resistance. This is usually given with proguanil (under two years – 50 mg/day; two to ten years – 100 mg/day and over ten years – 200 mg/day).

For protection where chloroquine-resistant *P. falciparum* is present, mefloquine or doxycycline can be used but only in children over the age of eight years. Fansidar is no longer recommended because of the high risk of significant side-effects. Likewise, pyrimethamine in combination with dapsone (Maloprim®) or chloroquine (Darachlor®) is no longer recommended. Mefloquine has been associated with significant neurological and psychiatric side-effects especially in those with pre existing depression or psychological disorders.

Malarone (atovoquine 250/proguanil hydrochloride100) is taken once daily with food as a prophylaxis. It should be started two days before travel and continued for seven days on return. A paediatric dose of atovoquine 62.5 mg/proguanil hydrochloride 25 mg is also available.

Side effects are few but it should be avoided in severe renal disease and will be less effective when taken with tetracycline, metoclopramide or rifampicin. It can be used for the treatment of non-severe *P. falciparum* malaria. Travellers should carry with them, and take if necessary, a course of antimalarial treatment for use as an emergency treatment.

Advise non-immune pregnant and lactating women and young children against entering malarious areas. Mefloquine and doxycycline are contra-indicated in pregnancy and in children under eight years. Chloroquine with proguanil is recommended if necessary.

Non-chemotherapeutic preventive measures include:

- Visiting malarious areas only during the dry season
- Applying insect repellent to exposed skin and clothes
- Using mosquito nets, screens or coils at night
- Wearing long sleeves and trousers if outside between dusk and dawn.

Toxoplasmosis

The protozoal parasite *Toxoplasma gondii* has a worldwide distribution and infects a wide range of animals, including domestic cats and birds. Infection is acquired by swallowing oocysts which contaminate soil, by close association with cats, or by eating undercooked meat. Humans are relatively resistant to infection and in the majority of cases infection is asymptomatic. *T. gondii* is an intracellular parasite and may cause depression of cell-mediated and humoral immunity. Latent infections may become active during immunosuppression or primary infections may occur in immunocompromised individuals, especially those with lymphatic or haematological cancer or HIV infection. Toxoplasmosis acquired during pregnancy is often symptomless in the mother or may only cause mild fever and malaise. Parasites form local lesions in the placenta and are released into the fetal bloodstream. It is generally believed that the earlier the infection occurs in pregnancy, the more severe the damage to the fetus. Abortion, stillbirth, or premature birth may result. The baby may show obvious neurological and visceral involvement at birth or be apparently normal and develop clinical manifestations after a latent period of months or longer. More than half of babies born to mothers who acquire toxoplasmosis during pregnancy are uninfected.

Clinical manifestations

Acquired toxoplasmosis. Most infections are asymptomatic. Lymphadenopathy, especially of the cervical nodes, is the most common manifestation and there is a predominance of mononuclear cells in the peripheral blood. Infectious mononucleosis is a common misdiagnosis.

Fever, myalgia, a transient maculopapular rash, hepatomegaly and rarely pneumonia, myocarditis, and glomerulonephritis have been described.

Meningo-encephalitis is the usual manifestation in immunocompromised individuals. Eye involvement in the form of necrotizing retinitis may be seen.

Congenital toxoplasmosis. Severely infected infants show features common to most intrauterine infections, such as jaundice, hepatosplenomegaly, anaemia, and skin haemorrhages. Microphthalmia, retinitis and hydrocephalus may occur.

Intracranial calcification, seen on skull radiographs, is usually not present at birth, but is a characteristic feature later. Microcephaly, mental retardation, and convulsions may be later manifestations.

Diagnosis

Demonstration of the parasite in cerebrospinal fluid (CSF) or in sections from fresh tissue may be possible in early symptomatic congenital toxoplasmosis, but serological tests are more commonly used to establish the diagnosis.

The indirect fluorescent antibody test is the most reliable. Both IgM and IgG antibodies may be measured. Failure to demonstrate IgM antibodies immediately after birth, in infants suspected of having toxoplasmosis, does not exclude the diagnosis. Repeat tests may be necessary to show a rising titre. Antibody levels may take months or years to decline after infection. Enzyme-linked immunosorbent assay (ELISA) tests for IgM are also available and useful.

Treatment

A combination of pyrimethamine 1 mg/kg/day and sulphadiazine 100 mg/kg/day in divided doses for 21 days is recommended for treatment of congenital toxoplasmosis. This treatment will prevent further harm from the infection, but has little effect on damage already present. Even asymptomatic infants with serological evidence of infection should be treated to prevent possible intellectual impairment at a later stage. Some authorities recommend alternative courses of pyrimethamine with sulfadiazine and spiramycin (not freely available) for one year.

Corticosteroids are recommended if there is chorioretinitis.

Both pyrimethamine and sulphadiazine may produce haematological complications and blood counts should be monitored during treatment.

Acquired toxoplasmosis is usually a self-limiting disease and does not require treatment.

Prevention

Women should avoid handling cat litter and eating undercooked meat during pregnancy. Those who have antibodies prior to pregnancy are safe from infecting their fetuses.

Trypanosomiasis

African trypanosomiasis is transmitted by the tsetse fly (genus *Glossina*) and American trypanosomiasis (Chagas' disease) by bugs.

African trypanosomiasis occurs between the latitudes 14°N and 29°S and has a focal distribution within this area. Two varieties are recognized. The East African form (due to *Trypanosoma rhodesiense*) is transmitted by *Glossina morsitans*, a tsetse fly which inhabits savannah country, while West African trypanosomiasis (caused by *T. gambiense*) is transmitted by *G. palpalis* flies, which prefer riverine areas. Geographical overlapping of the two forms may occur. *T. rhodesiense* and *T. gambiense* are morphologically identical, but show differences in biological behaviour.

East African trypanosomiasis

Animal hosts, usually ungulates, and the tsetse fly harbour the trypanosome and humans only become infected when they visit an affected area. Children are rarely infected.

The disease in those who live in endemic areas differs from that which occurs in non-immune people from non-endemic areas. In the latter, symptoms usually start abruptly eight to ten days after being bitten by a tsetse fly and features closely resemble those of malaria. Paroxysmal bouts of fever, headache, debility, dizziness, and anaemia are common symptoms. A trypanosomal chancre at the site of the bite is helpful in establishing the diagnosis, but is rarely present. CNS signs such as tremor, dullness, gait changes, slurred speech, and coma are more important clues for the diagnosis of sleeping sickness, but are late manifestations. The prognosis is poor if treatment is delayed until the onset of semi-coma. Lymphadenopathy and splenomegaly may be present. Myocarditis and oedema may occur. The duration of illness is usually four to nine months.

West African sleeping sickness

This tends to have a more acute onset in Caucasians than in Africans. Recurrent fever, blotchy erythematous rash, lymphadenopathy, and hepatosplenomegaly, together with the appearance of the trypanosomal chancre, are helpful pointers to the diagnosis in Caucasians. Insomnia and personality changes may be noted early in the disease. Later, cardiac failure and central nervous symptoms dominate the clinical picture. The course of the disease in Africans is more protracted. Children are more commonly infected than is the case in East African sleeping sickness.

Diagnosis. Identification of the parasite in thick blood films, lymph node aspirations, or on bone-marrow aspiration is necessary to establish the diagnosis. Repeated examinations may be necessary. Late in the disease trypanosomes may be seen in the CSF which also shows a pleocytosis and elevated protein level.

Treatment. In early cases, suramin 20 mg/kg is given IV at seven-day intervals for five doses. Suramin is nephrotoxic and should not be given to anyone with renal disease. Urine examination should be performed after each injection and therapy stopped if casts or haematuria are found. Pentamidine 3 to 4 mg/kg on alternate days for 10 days is an alternative. However, it is less effective for the East African form.

Once CNS involvement is present, IV melarsoprol is given: 0.4 mg/kg on three successive days at weekly intervals over four weeks. Anaemia should be corrected and parasites should be eliminated from the blood and lymphatic system by giving suramin before commencing this therapy.

American trypanosomiasis (Chagas' disease)

Trypanosoma cruzi, the causative protozoan, is transmitted by contamination of the mucous membranes of the eye, mouth, and nose by an infected bug or through skin abrasions. The infection is widespread in Central and South America.

The initial manifestation is a painful swelling in the eye or skin (the chagoma) together with enlargement of regional nodes. Fever follows and may persist for several weeks. In the young child, increasing debility progresses to cardiac failure, signs of meningeal irritation or encephalitis and death after many weeks. The disease may become chronic, especially in older children, with features of myocarditis persisting for variable periods of up to ten years or more. Involvement of the alimentary tract, with dilatation and loss of muscle tone in the oesophagus and colon, may lead to dysphagia or constipation. Mental deficiency, speech disturbances, and involuntary movements indicate either ongoing CNS pathology or partial recovery after encephalitis in the acute phase.

Diagnosis. Diagnosis depends on identifying the trypanosome in peripheral blood. Serological tests are not useful in endemic areas.

Treatment. If given in the acute stage, drug treatment may cure the disease.

Nifurtimox (a nitrofurazone) 25 mg/kg/d orally in three divided doses for the first week, then 10 to 15 mg/kg/d for two months plus metronidazole 20 mg/kg/d for one month.

Benznidazole (an imidazole) 5–7 mg/kg/d given orally for two months is an alternative therapy.

Preventative measures, which include improved housing and eradication of the vector, should be employed where possible.

Leishmaniasis

Caused by several different species of the protozoan leishmania, leishmaniasis is a collection of diseases that may involve the skin (cutaneous), skin and mucous membranes (mucocutaneous), and viscera (kala azar). Phlebotomine sandflies are the vectors responsible for the spread of the infection, but this may also occur by direct contact through abraded skin, by blood transfusion, and even transplacentally from mother to fetus. Reservoir hosts such as rodents, dogs, and humans with inapparent infection also play a role in spreading infection.

There is a wide range of reactions to infection, which usually leads to a T-lymphocyte-mediated response similar to that seen in tuberculosis and leprosy, demonstrated by the leishmanin skin test. The majority of infections are not apparent. In others, absence of T-cell-mediated immunity leads to diffuse cutaneous disease. Exaggerated delayed hypersensitivity is found in mucocutaneous forms, while depressed T-cell response and an abnormal humoral immunity are present in visceral leishmaniasis.

Leishmania tropica causes infection confined to the skin. Predominantly a disease of children, it is endemic in large areas of south-west Asia, in southern Europe, and North Africa. It also occurs in certain areas of southern Africa such as Namibia.

The typical lesion is an indolent granuloma. The sores develop on exposed areas of the body, and may be single or multiple. Initially presenting as irritating papules surrounded by erythema, they enlarge and are soon covered by brown scales or crusts which, when shed, reveal indolent ulcers with an offensive purulent discharge. Satellite lesions may occur in the immediate vicinity of the sore. Secondary bacterial infection often occurs and healing leads to scarring. There are no constitutional symptoms. Diagnosis is confirmed by demonstrating the parasite in smears or in biopsies of the ulcer.

Leishmaniasis recidiva. The delayed hypersensitivity response is exaggerated, but the infection is not eradicated. A chronic spreading lesion involves the face and resembles lupus vulgaris. A strongly positive leishmanin test establishes the diagnosis, but response to treatment is poor.

Diffuse cutaneous leishmaniasis. Little or no T-cell response and very limited cellular reaction allow for widespread dissemination of the parasite in the skin. Chronic lesions about the nose continue to spread for many years. Large numbers of amastigotes are seen in macrophages, but the leishmanin skin test is negative.

Kala azar, caused by *Leishmania donovani,* affects all age groups with a wide distribution in areas in Asia, central Africa, southern Europe, and Central and South America. The incubation period is usually two to six months and the onset insidious. Occasionally there is an abrupt onset with high fever which later becomes undulant. Splenomegaly is almost invariably present. In certain areas, lymphadenopathy is a prominent manifestation and simulates tuberculosis, leukaemia, and lymphoma. Anaemia, leucopaenia, and thrombocytopaenia occur later. In some, hepatomegaly and jaundice appear. Gastrointestinal symptoms are said to be common in India. A picture similar to mucocutaneous leishmaniasis with or without visceral involvement may be seen in Africa. If untreated, progressive debility leads to intercurrent infection and death. During or after treatment a depigmented macular rash or a papular lesion resembling leprosy may appear on the face and trunk. Typically, large amounts of gammaglobulin are produced but are nonprotective against widespread dissemination of the parasite in liver sinusoids, spleen, bone marrow, and lymph nodes.

The **diagnosis** is established by identifying parasites in aspirates from these organs.

Treatment. Therapy is not indicated for oriental sores, which are self-healing. When they involve the face, are extensive or diffuse, chemotherapy should be given.

Pentavalent antimony compounds, preferably given intravenously, are the drugs of choice. In children aged four to twelve years, the dose is 15 mg/kg/d for 30 days (maximum dose 400 mg and minimum dose 200 mg).

Amoebiasis

Amoebiasis is caused by a protozoan parasite *Entamoeba histolytica*. Pathogenic strains can be distinguished from non-pathogenic strains on the basis of isoenzymes (zymodenes). It has been estimated that 10 per cent of the world's population is infected, but in the majority of infections, *E. histolytica* is a harmless commensal. Amoebic dysentery occurs in about 5–20 per cent of infected persons and a smaller proportion develop extra-intestinal disease. The incidence of infection and disease is highest in subtropical and tropical areas, but lack of sanitation and personal hygiene are more important factors than are climatic conditions. The parasite is harboured in the large intestine and is spread by faecal contamination of food and water. No age group is exempt from infection. Dysentery and hepatic amoebiasis may occur in infants as young as three weeks of age, when the source of infection may be from the mother's perineum.

Aetiology and pathology

(See Figure 16.2.) Infection is acquired by swallowing cysts, which are 10–20 μ in size and contain up to four nuclei. Motile trophozoites emerge from the cysts and travel to the large bowel, the largest number tending to collect in areas of greatest faecal stasis such as the caecum, lower ascending colon, sigmoid colon, and rectum. Trophozoites are not usually passed in the stool, but any cause of diarrhoea may lead to

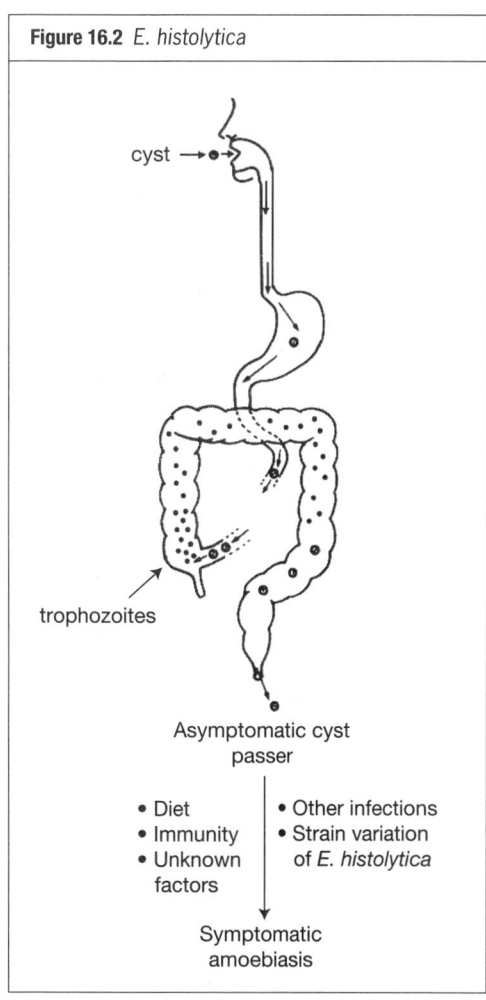

Figure 16.2 *E. histolytica*

cyst

trophozoites

Asymptomatic cyst passer

- Diet
- Immunity
- Unknown factors

- Other infections
- Strain variation of *E. histolytica*

Symptomatic amoebiasis

their rapid passage down the colon. The finding of trophozoites in a diarrhoeic stool does not necessarily indicate that the amoebae are causing the diarrhoea. There is some evidence that certain strains of E. histolytica may be more pathogenic than others. Invasion is accomplished by lytic enzymes secreted by trophozoites, which damage the bowel wall and capillaries. Trophozoites ingest red cells and produce ulcers varying in extent from pinhead-sized lesions confined to the caecum, to extensive, deep, confluent ulceration throughout the bowel. Studies have shown that in severe cases, trophozoites invade colonic blood vessels and cause well-demarcated areas of infarction. Extension through the bowel wall leads to peritonitis. Rarely, the extension occurs to the skin of the perineum. Access to the liver is via the portal vein. Here tissue necrosis leads to abscess formation. Rupture of the abscess may involve adjacent spaces or tissue. Blood-borne embolic spread to remote sites such as the lung or brain is encountered occasionally.

Clinical manifestations

Intestinal amoebiasis may be asymptomatic. Non-invasive parasites produce no symptoms and even mild colonic invasion evidenced by the passage of haematophagous trophozoites may not produce symptoms.

Abdominal discomfort and colonic tenderness may be found and liver tenderness elicited in the absence of hepatitis. Fever is usually absent or slight and the appetite unaffected. Proctoscopy or sigmoidoscopy frequently reveals undermining ulcers, varying in size and covered with a yellow exudate. The intervening bowel is normal. Transmural colitis temporarily sealed by omentum leads to abdominal distension with tenderness on palpation. In severe cases, dehydration and symptoms and signs of electrolyte imbalance develop rapidly. Generalized abdominal tenderness and distension suggest impending peritonitis even in the presence of bowel sounds.

> Symptomatic intestinal amoebiasis varies in severity from mild intermittent diarrhoea which may last for weeks or months, to severe fulminating dysentery, with the passage of many blood-stained mucoid stools which contain little or no faecal matter.

Local complications

Perforation and peritonitis are the common sequelae of severe amoebic colitis, usually the result of slow leakage from perforations. The onset is often insidious, with the development of relatively painless, increasing abdominal distension. Vomiting and signs of ileus follow. Rarely, a single ulcer may perforate and produce the more dramatic clinical picture of an acute abdomen. Generalized peritonitis is the usual sequel in children, but a localized abscess may occur. (See Figure 16.3.)

Although an uncommon complication, intussusception should be suspected if colicky abdominal pain develops during an attack of amoebic dysentery. Careful palpation may reveal a sausage-shaped mass.

Amoeboma, a granuloma of the bowel, presents as a tender mass, most commonly in the right iliac fossa. Strictures may follow at sites of severe ulceration. Erosion of a blood vessel in the bowel wall may lead to profuse haemorrhage with shock and collapse.

Post-dysenteric colitis leads to severe debility and emaciation, requiring weeks or months of supportive therapy. Repeated stool examination should be made to exclude a relapse of amoebic dysentery.

Systemic complications

Hepatic amoebiasis is the most common extra-intestinal complication. Amoebic liver abscess is the only pathologically proven form.

In childhood, the majority of liver abscesses present in the first three years of life. A history of previous or concomitant dysentery can be obtained in more than 50 per cent and swelling of the abdomen is a common complaint. Fever, tender hepatomegaly, and anaemia are almost invariable findings.

Hepatic amoebiasis should be considered in the differential diagnosis whenever there is unexplained fever, and in all instances of tender liver enlargement, especially when associated with anaemia.

Palpation often reveals a mass in the liver, which may be visible. A single abscess most often involves the right lobe, resulting in elevation of the diaphragm and signs at the right lung base. Multiple abscesses are more common in infancy and early childhood, but jaundice is

---

Figure 16.3 Complications caused by *E. histolytica* infection

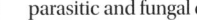

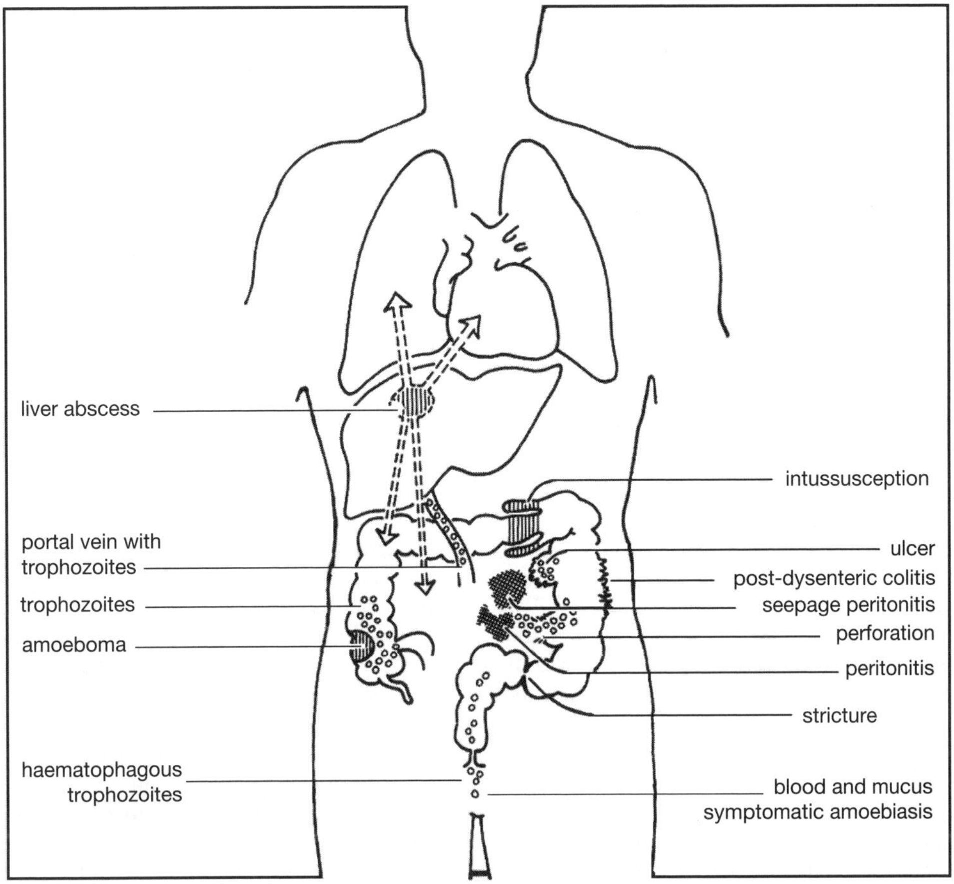

liver abscess

intussusception

portal vein with trophozoites

ulcer
post-dysenteric colitis
seepage peritonitis

trophozoites

amoeboma

perforation

peritonitis

stricture

haematophagous trophozoites

blood and mucus
symptomatic amoebiasis

---

rare. Extension or rupture of a liver abscess is a serious complication. In children rupture into the peritoneal cavity occurs more commonly than into the pleural space. A left-lobe abscess may cause an effusion in or rupture into the pericardium, resulting in sudden, severe distress and signs of cardiac tamponade. An effusion of the adjacent pleural space may complicate abscesses situated near the superior surface of the right lobe of the liver, while rupture of the abscess through the diaphragm leads to an amoebic empyema.

Bacterial contamination of the liver abscess may cause persistent fever and failure of the abscess to resolve, despite adequate anti-amoebic therapy.

Other very rare extra-intestinal complications are cutaneous amoebiasis involving the peri-anal area and perineum or blood-borne amoebic abscesses of the brain or lungs.

Diagnosis

Identification of haematophagous *E. histolytica* trophozoites in bowel contents or liver pus establishes the diagnosis of invasive amoebiasis. These motile trophozoites are most readily seen in freshly passed specimens or scrapings obtained from ulcers at sigmoidoscopy, or freshly aspirated pus. Repeated stool examinations may be needed before the parasite is identified. Amoebic cysts are less fragile and retain their characteristic features for hours after being passed, but as the number of cysts fluctuates a single negative finding does not exclude the diagnosis.

Aspiration of bacteriologically sterile pus is strongly suggestive of amoebic liver abscess. The typical pink or reddish-brown colour (anchovy pus) may not always be seen, being yellowish grey on first aspiration.

A full blood count very commonly reveals anaemia and neutrophil leucocytosis in amoebic liver abscess, while a chest radiograph may show elevation of the right diaphragm. Ultrasound examination of the liver is helpful in diagnosing the presence and number of abscesses. Radioisotope liver scanning provides similar information.

Serology. The gel diffusion test is an invaluable clinical tool and is positive in almost all children with invasive disease. Repeat tests in those who are negative will show seroconversion. A number of other serological tests are available but the advantage of a fluorescent antibody test based on whole amoeba is that it can be used to monitor IgG and IgM response.

Treatment

Metronidazole (Flagyl®) 50 mg/ kg/d for 5–7 days, or tinidazole (Fasigyn®) for three days, are highly effective in the vast majority of cases. In uncomplicated amoebic dysentery these preparations are given by mouth and symptoms subside rapidly. If they persist after 48 hours the diagnosis should be questioned. Asymptomatic carriage (intraluminal infection) is treated with diloxanide or iodoquinol.

In severe amoebic colitis with impending or established peritonitis, metronidazole should be given intravenously until such time as oral therapy becomes possible. Fluid and electrolyte losses should be corrected and gastric suction employed until signs of ileus subside. Profound anaemia indicates the need for blood transfusion. Gram-negative septicaemia and chest infection, which are often present, are indications for broad-spectrum antibiotic therapy. Steroid therapy is contra-indicated.

Amoebic liver abscesses may respond to metronidazole alone, but large abscesses with palpable masses and elevation of the diaphragm should be aspirated with a wide-bore needle. Persistence of symptoms despite adequate amoebicidal therapy is also an indication for aspiration. Repeated aspirations may be necessary. On rare occasions, posteriorly situated abscesses may require aspiration under direct vision at laparotomy.

Surgical repair is required in those rare instances where a single ulcer perforates to produce an acute peritonitis. Surgery is not indicated in the management of amoebomas and remains controversial in seepage peritonitis.

Asymptomatic individuals with amoebic cysts or trophozoites in the stool should be treated, as disease may occur at a later date. Metronidazole should be given by mouth.

Giardiasis

The flagellated protozoan *Giardia lamblia* has a worldwide distribution, but is more prevalent in tropical and subtropical areas and particularly in economically depressed communities. Children are infected more commonly than adults. Infection is acquired by transmission from person to person due to swallowing of cysts which may also contaminate food or water. The parasite lives in the duodenum and upper jejunum.

The parasites do not appear to enter mucosal cells, nor have they been convincingly shown to cause any morphological change in these cells. The majority of infections are asymptomatic and may persist for years or disappear spontaneously. The pathogenicity is unpredictable and the severity of symptoms is not related to the density of infection. Under certain circumstances diarrhoea occurs.

Clinical manifestations

Giardiasis is a common cause of traveller's diarrhoea and, in this instance, there is usually an explosive onset with foul-smelling stools accompanied by abdominal distension and flatulence. This diarrhoea characteristically has a longer incubation period and persists for longer than traveller's diarrhoea from other causes.

Giardiasis is also a well-recognized cause of outbreaks of diarrhoea in young children's nurseries. The diarrhoea is associated with loose, green stools and varies in severity. In some children, vomiting and dehydration are early complications. In others the diarrhoea is less severe but persists or relapses intermittently. Abdominal pain and tenderness may be features. Certain children become anorexic and fail to thrive.

Chronic giardiasis may be associated with evidence of malabsorption. Whether it is the sole cause of malabsorption in such cases is unclear. No consistent or characteristic mucosal bowel pattern has been shown to be associated with giardiasis. Normal jejunal mucosa is present in some, while in others, changes indistinguishable from coeliac disease or other causes of malabsorption may be found.

Giardiasis often coexists with protein energy malnutrition and congenital hypogammaglobulinaemia. In such cases it must be actively excluded and treated.

Diagnosis

Stools tend to be greasy and contain no blood or mucus. Trophozoites may be seen in the stool, but are often extraordinarily difficult to detect. Cysts usually only appear when symptoms have been present for a week or more. Repeated stool examination may be necessary to verify the diagnosis. As examination of duodenal aspirates may be needed to identify trophozoites, empiric treatment is justified when clinical suspicion is strong.

Treatment

Metronidazole given as a single daily dose for three days eradicates the infection in 90 per cent of cases. Children under four years require 50 mg daily and those between four and eight years 100 mg daily. Tinidazole in a similar dose is equally effective and may be better tolerated by some children.

Prevention

Travellers to endemic areas should refrain from drinking or using unboiled water. Fresh salads are also best avoided when travelling.

Cryptosporidiosis

The coccidian protozoan cryptosporidium is related to other coccidia infecting humans, such as *Plasmodium, Isospora*, and *Toxoplasma*. It is found in the intestinal and respiratory epithelium of mammals, birds, and reptiles. Since 1976 it has been recognized as an important human pathogen, causing severe resistant diarrhoea in immuno-compromised individuals, such as persons with AIDS, and is also associated with acute watery diarrhoea in otherwise healthy individuals. It has a worldwide distribution, but is more common in Africa than in the developed world, where several series have shown it to be one of the top three or four enteric pathogens associated with acute watery diarrhoea. Human to human transmission occurs and cryptosporidium is a common pathogen in traveller's diarrhoea, or in group outbreaks such as in day-care centres. Infection is more common during summer and autumn.

Clinical features

The small oocysts each release four flat sporozoites, which are immediately infective. In the small intestine, the trophozoites encyst in the microvillous brush border, where an enterotoxic mechanism results in severe watery diarrhoea without an inflammatory response. In immunocompetent individuals, this is associated with mild to moderate fever, significant cramp-like upper abdominal pain, nausea, anorexia, and weight loss. In severe infections, there is mucosal damage with malabsorption. Symptoms often last for up to three weeks even in well-nourished children. Auto-infection is common, and parasite clearance from the stools lags behind resolution of clinical symptoms by several weeks. In patients with severe malnutrition or immunodeficiency, the disease is often very prolonged and associated with severe mal absorption.

The diagnosis is made by finding the oocysts in the stools. As the parasite is small (2–5 μm), special stains and sometimes stool concentration techniques are required.

Treatment and prevention

There is no uniformly successful therapy, although treatment with the macrolide antibiotic spiramycin in high doses for 10 days has been described to reduce the duration of illness in immunocompetent patients. Nitazoxanide, a broad-spectrum anti-protozoal agent, has been recently licensed in the USA for the treatment of cryptosporidiosis in normal children. The mainstay of therapy is supportive, consisting of fluid and electrolyte replacement, and nutritional management of maldigestion and malabsorption as identified. Antidiarrhoeal medication has not been shown to be of benefit.

Balantidiasis

The large ciliated protozoan *Balantidium coli* is usually a harmless commensal in the large bowel of humans but, under rare circumstances, may invade the terminal ileum and colon to cause ulcers or abscesses of the mucosa and submucosa. Chronic recurrent diarrhoea, alternating with constipation, may be a complaint and, occasionally, severe dysentery with bloody mucoid stools, tenesmus, and colic may develop. Fatal cases have been described. Metronidazole is the treatment of choice.

Microsporidia

This intestinal parasite causes non-bloody chronic diarrhoea and occasionally an ascending cholangitis in the immunosuppressed patient. It is more common in adults than children. It is best identified in stool specimens using special stains – modified trichrome stain or calcuflour white. Treatment is four weeks of albendazole which is only effective against the encephalitozoon species of microsporidium.

Parasitic helminths: Trematodes (flukes)

Parasitic worms have a worldwide distribution, but are most prevalent in the tropics and subtropics where climatic conditions favour their spread. They multiply by laying eggs from which larvae hatch and mature to adult males and females. Most live in harmony with their human hosts and they are seldom the only cause of poor nutrition in a child. They may cause disease when they are present in large numbers, when infestations are repeated, and when the host defence mechanism is depressed. Helminths are divided into nematodes (roundworms), cestodes (tapeworms), and trematodes or flukes.

Schistosomiasis (bilharzia)

Three major species of the genus schistosoma commonly infect man, *S. haematobium* being largely responsible for genito-urinary disease, while *S. mansoni* and *S. japonicum* cause intestinal schistosomiasis.

Epidemiology

It has been calculated that 200 million people are infected world-wide. In South Africa, 2 million are thought to harbour the parasite. The popular belief that bilharzia only occurs in rivers flowing into the Indian Ocean in southern Africa is not correct, as the Vaal catchment area is not free from infection.

In southern Africa, the infection rate of schoolchildren with *S. haematobium* may be as high as 90 per cent in certain rural endemic areas such as northern KwaZulu-Natal. *S. mansoni* is considerably less common. *S. japonicum* infections occur in certain areas of the Far East.

The distribution of infection is dependent on the presence of the intermediate snail host. These snails are found in permanent fresh water in streams, pools, canals and, particularly, in storage dams and cement reservoirs. Snails multiply rapidly by laying eggs which hatch after 10–14 days, the young snail being susceptible to bilharzia at one day old and capable of reproduction by six weeks. Snails or their eggs are readily transported by insects, or on the feet of birds and animals, to a new habitat. They survive passage through water pumps and drying in sand or mud for months. Their most important habitats are collections of water near human habitation.

Wild animals have been infected with *S. mansoni* and, rarely, with *S. haematobium*, but it is doubtful whether animals play a role in the spread of schistosomiasis in southern Africa.

Urinary bilharzia is mainly a disease of children and young adults. Their fondness for swimming and their habit of urinating into the water in which they swim, play major roles in the spread and prevalence of *S. haematobium*. *S. mansoni* disease occurs in a wider age range and is the result of increasing faecal pollution of water due to rising population density and inadequate sanitation.

Life cycle

The life cycle of the species is similar. Miracidia hatch from eggs in water and enter the snail where cercariae develop in sporocysts. Cercariae pass from the snail and swim in water until they penetrate the skin of their human host. They lose their tails, become schistosomules, and migrate to the portal vessels of humans where maturation to adulthood occurs. After mating,

S. haematobium migrates to the vesical plexus and *S. mansoni* to the tributaries of the inferior mesenteric vessels. Eggs pass through the tissues and enter the bladder or large intestine. The degree of reaction of tissues through which the ova pass varies greatly and has resulted in a wide variety of opinions about the severity and clinical importance of bilharzia.

Pathology

This may be divided into three stages: the first coinciding with invasion by cercariae, the second with the onset of egg laying, and the third or chronic stage with the consequences of the host's response to eggs in various organs. In *S. haematobium* infection, the urogenital tract and lower bowel are the principal sites of pathology. *S. mansoni* and *S. japonicum* disease affects mainly the gut and the liver.

Eggs may reach the lungs through collateral circulation and may also get to the central nervous system. Multinucleated giant cells, histiocytes, and eosinophils surrounding eggs constitute the bilharzial granuloma.

A heavy parasite load, which is indicated by a high egg count in the stool or urine, is generally associated with more severe disease than a light load and a smaller egg count. The host response plays an important role in pathogenesis and accounts for differences in severity of disease in various race and population groups, even when exposure and egg loads are similar. The hypersensitivity reactions characteristic of the first and second stages are very rarely seen in African children in coastal KwaZulu-Natal, but occur in white children in the same area. A similar racial difference has been described in Zimbabwe.

Clinical features

An irritating erythematous papular rash referred to as 'swimmer's itch' may occur at the time and site of entry of cercaria.

> Immediate and delayed hypersensitivity reactions and immune complexes are responsible for the clinical findings of the first and second stages. Destruction of tissue and scarring is due to a granulomatous response to the eggs, which is also a form of delayed hypersensitivity.

Four to six weeks later a high fever, urticarial rashes, oedema, lymphadenopathy, and hepatosplenomegaly may be found. Complaints include severe headache, bronchospasm, and rigors. Symptoms and signs of encephalitis and cardiac involvement are also described in this syndrome, which is most severe in *S. japonicum* infections (Katayama's syndrome).

Urogenital bilharzia *S. haematobium* infection is often asymptomatic, or terminal haematuria may be the only symptom. Dysuria and suprapubic pain are less common and, rarely, precipitancy or dribbling incontinence occurs.

Obstruction of ureteric orifices or ureteric strictures may cause hydronephrosis or vesicoureteric reflux, and obstructive uropathy may lead to renal failure. Bladder calcification follows heavy and repeated infections. Ureteric and bladder lesions, demonstrated radiographically, frequently regress after treatment and may do so spontaneously. Chronic renal failure, which is the consequence of chronic bacterial pyelone-phritis, may supervene. In Egypt, salmonella infections are often responsible for this complication. Cancer of the bladder is a rare complication.

The vagina, cervix, and uterus may be involved in females and the urethra and prostate in males.

Bilharzial nephrotic syndrome

Advanced *S. mansoni* infection has been associated with the nephrotic syndrome in Brazil and Egypt. There is evidence that soluble immune complexes are formed and deposited on the glomeruli of these patients.

Gastrointestinal bilharzia.

S. mansoni infection may cause abdominal pain and diarrhoea with dysenteric stools in the early stages. More chronic infection leads to nodular thickening, ulceration, and polyp formation which are most marked at the rectosigmoid junction and in the lower colon. Blood and protein loss occurs and anaemia, oedema, and ascites may be the consequences of these bowel lesions.

Lateral-spined eggs found in stools or histologically in rectal biopsy specimens confirm the diagnosis.

Hepatic and hepatosplenic bilharzia. Massive or repeated infections encourage carriage of eggs to the liver via the portal vein. Granuloma formation followed by portal fibrosis results in pre-sinusoidal portal hypertension, with passive congestion of the spleen, portosystemic collaterals, and oesophageal varices. Hypersplenism, ascites, and oedema follow. Liver function tests usually remain normal. Patients with markedly abnormal liver function are often HBs Ag positive and it is thought that this associated infection is responsible for the cirrhosis which has been described in bilharzia.

S. mansoni and *S. japonicum* infections commonly involve the liver, but *S. haematobium* may also do so.

Pulmonary schistosomiasis. Eggs in the pulmonary circulation obstruct small arterioles and may cause necrosis of their walls, followed by thickening or fibrosis and obliteration of their lumens. If widespread and diffuse, this obliterative endarteritis leads to pulmonary hypertension and eventually to aneurysmal dilatation of the pulmonary artery. Right ventricular hypertrophy and failure follow, but respond to rest, digitalis, and diuretics. Patients with bilharzial cor pulmonale may survive for many years. Heart failure in bilharzia may also occur as a result of rare myocardial granulomatous involvement.

Granulomas situated near bronchioles and alveoli may cause parenchymatous lung disease, fibrosis, and scarring, giving rise to chronic bronchitis, bronchiectasis, and emphysema.

Pulmonary complications are rare in southern Africa. Most reported cases have been from South America and Egypt.

Central nervous system schistosomiasis. Eggs reach the nervous system via anastomatic vessels in the pelvis and vertebral venous plexuses. Spinal cord involvement is commonly due to *S. haematobium* and *S. mansoni*, whereas *S. japonicum* is more liable to cause encephalitis.

A bilharzial aetiology should be suspected when neurological symptoms and signs are associated with a marked eosinophilia. Cerebrospinal fluid shows a pleocytosis, raised protein level, and normal sugar level.

Focal epilepsy, mental changes, visual defects, and upper motor neurone palsies have been described in bilharzial encephalitis; the presentation may be that of an intracranial space-occupying lesion.

Cord involvement often presents as an acute transverse myelitis or radiculitis. A granuloma of the cord may lead to paraplegia or weakness, together with sensory changes. Treatment consists of antibilharzial therapy and corticosteroids. Surgery is indicated in certain instances and the diagnosis is confirmed by surgical biopsy specimens.

Diagnosis

The presence of viable eggs in urine, stool, or biopsy specimen is proof of infection. The diagnosis of *S. haematobium* infection is confirmed by finding terminal-spined ova in urine specimens. Maximum excretion of ova occurs at midday and specimens collected at this time give the highest yield of ova. Bladder calcification revealed on plain abdominal radiographs may be the first indication of urinary bilharzia. Excretory urograms are indicated to exclude obstructive lesions when renal function is impaired. Rarely, cystoscopy and even biopsy may be needed to establish the diagnosis.

Bilharzia is a common cause of eosinophilia and should be excluded whenever this is found in patients in endemic areas or in visitors to such areas.

The finding of granulomatous lesions, black pigment, and portal fibrosis of liver biopsies is suggestive evidence of hepatic bilharzia – even in the absence of ova.

Advances in serological tests have increased their usefulness in diagnosis. The most helpful are an ELISA based on schistosomal egg antigen, and fluorescent antibody test based on cercaria antigen.

Treatment

Praziquantel is the drug of choice and is effective in all species in a single oral dose (30 to 45 mg/kg) which may be repeated after one month. Side effects are uncommon but include abdominal colic for which antispasmodics may be necessary. Cure rates and reduction of schistosomal load are excellent.

Alternative drugs (e.g. niridazole, metriphonate, and oxamniquine) are available in some countries, but have a number of contra-indications and side-effects.

Prevention

Health education aimed at the avoidance of infection and the provision of clean water and adequate sanitation are important public health measures.

Eradication of the snail host may be achieved by the use of molluscicides, in addition to improved irrigation practices.

Mass treatment with praziquantel in areas of high endemicity should be considered. The cost of mass treatment must be weighed against the cost of morbidity and mortality of bilharzia in the target community.

Hydatid disease

Sheep and cattle are the intermediate hosts of the fluke *Echinococcus granulosus* and humans become accidentally involved by ingesting dog faeces containing eggs. Infections are most prevalent in sheep-farming areas.

Oncospheres penetrate mesenteric vessels and are carried to many organs, but the right lobe of the liver and the lung are most commonly involved. Hydatid cysts enlarge gradually and compress surrounding structures to produce symptoms and signs. Cysts usually remain intact for many years. If they rupture, they will spread to many other organs.

The presence of an eosinophilia and a tumour mass should alert the clinician to the possible diagnosis. Serological tests, including the indirect haemagglutination and latex agglutination, may be of help in establishing the diagnosis. Aspiration of the cyst is contra-indicated because of the danger of spread. Ultrasonography of the cyst will demonstrate smaller daughter cysts inside it.

Treatment. Initial treatment should be with albendazole 10–20 mg/kg/day for six weeks or longer, or mebendazole 20–40 mg/kg/day for at least eight weeks. If a cyst causes serious pressure effects or involves the eye, surgery is indicated and drugs should also be given to prevent relapse or recurrence.

Parasitic helminths: Nematodes (round worms)

Table 16.1 lists some of the common roundworm infections in humans and their usual modes of spread.

Ascaris lumbricoides

The ascaris is a soil-transmitted helminth which is a public health problem in regions with temperate and moist conditions. In some areas

> The ova or larvae of most roundworms require an incubation period in warm, moist soil before they become infective. Children are very commonly infected because of their playing habits.

Table 16.1 Common nematode helminths and their usual mode of spread

Worms	Sources of infection	Mode of entry into human host
Ascaris	Faecal contamination of soil + vegetable	Eggs swallowed
Trichuris	Faecal contamination of soil + vegetable	Eggs swallowed
Enterobius	Person to person. Contamination of families. Hands to anus to mouth	Eggs swallowed
Trichinella	Meat, especially pork	Encapsulated larvae swallowed
Hookworm	Damp ground, skin contact	Filariform larvae penetrate skin
Strongyloides	Damp ground, skin contact	Filariform larvae penetrate skin
Filaria	Blood-sucking insects	Filariform larvae deposited through insect bites

in the Pacific up to 94 per cent of the population were found to be infested. The distribution is largely determined by the local habits of disposal of human excreta. The intensity of infestation in the individual corresponds roughly to the prevalence of the worm in the community.

The worm and its life cycle

Ascaris is the largest roundworm infesting humans, with the adult female reaching up to 400 mm in length. The worm is white-pink in colour, and tapers at both ends with the posterior end of the male being curved. The 200 000 ova which can be put out daily by the adult female are ovoid in shape and measure approximately $60 \times 40\ \mu m$. In a favourable environment, e.g. moist clay soil, the ova can survive for up to two years.

The ovum matures and becomes infective within 10–15 days of being passed. Children playing in contaminated soil or eating vegetables treated with night-soil may become infected. The larvae hatch rapidly in the duodenum, penetrate the bowel wall, and enter the portal or lymphatic circulation. On reaching the lung they burrow into the alveoli and make their way up the air passages into the pharynx, and are then swallowed and finally come to rest and mature in the gut. The cycle takes approximately 65 days and the adult worm lives for one to two years.

Clinical features

Migration of the larvae through the lung is known to cause severe pulmonary eosinophilia (Loeffler syndrome) and may be accompanied by bronchospasm and pneumonitis. (*see* Chapter 25, Respiratory tract disorders). The pulmonary phase is associated with an appreciable eosinophilia in the peripheral blood, and a subsequent rise in the IgE. Some authors claim that pre-existing asthma is aggravated by ascariasis.

Intestinal symptoms occur as a result of the sheer numbers of worms in the lumen of the gut, such as worm boluses leading to colic, intestinal obstruction or volvulus, and as a result of worms migrating into the orifices of the appendix, bile and pancreatic ducts and causing obstruction (*see* Chapter 30, Paediatric surgical disorders).

> In tropical coastal countries, up to 40 per cent of patients presenting with surgical abdominal complaints suffer from ascariasis.

Large numbers of worms interfere with appetite and the digestion and/or absorption of carbohydrates, proteins, fats, and vitamins, thus contributing to malnutrition of the host.

Diagnosis and investigations

Stool microscopy confirms the diagnosis of ascaris infestation. Plain X-rays of the abdomen will show worms and/or demonstrate signs of partial or complete intestinal obstruction. The 'whirl-pool' or 'target' sign is produced by an intestinal volvulus. The vast majority of worms in the biliary tract can be demonstrated by intravenous cholangiography or ultrasound scanning. Barium meal examination may demonstrate worms in the duodenum, and those entering the bile duct are sometimes identified. Occasionally endoscopic cholangiography is used. Diagnosis of pancreatic involvement is also made by the above investigations and serum amylase estimations.

Prevention

As ascaris infestation depends on contamination of the soil by human faeces, public health measures must be directed towards providing adequate sanitation. The use of sewerage sludge as fertilizer is inadvisable as it almost certainly carries viable ova. Chemical treatment of contaminated vegetables is singularly unhelpful.

It has been recommended that older infants and children living in an environment where ascariasis is endemic should be given a vermifuge regularly every three to six months to reduce the worm load.

Treatment

Ascaris can be treated with piperazine citrate in syrup form 3–4 g, repeated after two days, or with broad-spectrum drugs such as:

- mebendazole 100 mg bd for three days
- pyrantel pamoate 10 mg/kg in one dose
- albendazole at age two to five years: 200 mg in one dose; over five years: 400 mg in one dose.

There is no specific treatment that is effective against the larval stage in the lungs.

Trichuris trichiura

Also known as *Tricocephalus trichiura* or whipworm because of its whip-like anterior portion, this parasite is very common in children in southern Africa and in most warm, moist areas of the world. Eggs mature within three weeks of being deposited in soil. After ingestion, larvae hatch in the terminal ileum and caecum and full maturation occurs in about three months. In heavy infestations, the ascending colon, sigmoid, and rectum are involved. Adult worms live for three to five years. Unlike most other intestinal parasites, visceral invasion does not occur.

Clinical picture

Most infections are mild and asymptomatic. Symptoms attributed to trichuris are often due to coexisting bacterial or other parasitic infections. Heavy infestations cause chronic diarrhoea with mucoid stools which may contain blood. Tenesmus is a common complaint. Rectal prolapse and iron-deficiency anaemia are complications and are frequently the presenting features. Anaemia may be severe and lead to cardiac failure. Oedema, as a result of hypoproteinaemia, is also seen. Some children with heavy infestations fail to thrive and hence become marasmic.

Blockage of the appendiceal lumen can lead to acute appendicitis.

Diagnosis

In heavy infestations, inspection of a prolapsed rectum or sigmoidoscopy will reveal multiple, flesh-coloured, fine, whip-like structures attached to the mucous membrane. The characteristic barrel-shaped eggs with bi-polar prominences are found in the stool.

Treatment

Mebendazole 100 mg bd for four days by mouth. Albendazole 400 mg daily for three days by mouth.

Hookworm

Ancylostoma duodenale and *Necator americanus* are widely distributed throughout the tropics and subtropics. Seventy per cent of schoolchildren have been found to harbour hookworm in some localities in northern KwaZulu-Natal, but infection is negligible in many other areas of southern Africa and when present, is often light and asymptomatic. It is more common in rural than urban communities.

Life cycle

Eggs deposited in the soil hatch within 24 hours. After maturation from rhabditiform to the infective filariform larvae, the latter penetrate the human host's skin (often the soles of bare feet) and are conveyed to the heart and lungs, from whence they migrate up the respiratory passages to the pharynx and are swallowed. Maturation to adult worms occurs in the upper small intestine. Worms attach themselves to the mucosa with perioral hooks and cause the loss of minute amounts of blood. Seven to ten weeks elapse from larval invasion to deposition of eggs in the stool.

Clinical findings

Most infections are asymptomatic. Larval invasion may cause an irritating papulovesicular dermatitis, commonly localized to the feet, and larval migration through the lungs may lead to bronchospasm and pneumonitis. Epigastric pain and tenderness suggestive of peptic ulceration are described and believed to be caused by the attachment of the worm to the upper intestinal mucosa. A ravenous appetite and pica may occur. The development of anaemia is dependent on the worm load and dietary iron intake. Symptoms and signs of anaemia develop slowly and patients may be in congestive cardiac failure when they first seek medical advice. Very heavy parasite loads also lead to diarrhoea with blood and mucus and hypoproteinaemia, which may be aggravated by oedema.

Diagnosis

Hookworm ova in the stool indicate infection, but unless the load is in the order of 20 000 eggs/gram of faeces or more, there is no proof that these worms are the cause of the patient's symptoms and signs.

Treatment

Pyrantel pamoate 10 mg/kg is effective as a single dose. Mebendazole 100 mg bd for three days, or albendazole 400 mg as a single dose (200 mg for children under two years) in mixed helminth infections.

Prevention

Wearing of shoes or protective clothing and improved sanitation may help to reduce the incidence in highly endemic areas.

Ancylostoma braziliense, a hookwom infesting cats and dogs in the tropics, is the cause of **cutaneous larva migrans** (creeping eruption) and rarely, if ever, occurs as an adult worm in humans. It is treated with oral mebendazole,or albendazole. Ivermectin 200 µg/kg (>5yrs of age) as a single dose is also effective. Topical thiabendazole (15 per cent) applied as a paste (made from a 500 mg tablet dissolved in water) is sometimes effective. Many worms disappear spontaneously after 1–2 months.

Strongyloides stercoralis

This roundworm has a worldwide distribution and is most prevalent in tropical areas where high humidity favours transmission.

Life cycle
Filariform larvae penetrate the skin and are conveyed to the lungs. They mature, migrate to the pharynx via the airways and are swallowed. Adult worms settle in the upper small intestine. Eggs containing rhabditiform larvae may be passed in the stool to commence a free-living cycle in soil or undergo maturation in the intestine before reinvading their host's circulation. This auto-infection explains the persistence of the parasite in humans for long periods after having left endemic areas. The severity of infection appears to depend on the host's resistance and the parasite load. Immunosuppression which occurs in malnutrition, malignant disease, or during cytotoxic therapy, predisposes to severe infections. Conditions such as megacolon or chronic constipation are thought to favour auto-infection.

Clinical picture
The majority of strongyloides infections are asymptomatic. Larvae found in various organs at necropsy are not necessarily responsible for the patient's death nor for symptoms and signs.

A creeping eruption which is red and irritating and often found in the buttock or peri-anal area may occur within a week of exposure. Oedema and urticaria may also be seen. Skin lesions tend to recur for many years. Bronchitis or pneumonitis may follow skin lesions and become chronic.

Intermittent attacks of abdominal distension, diarrhoea, or malabsorption are described.

Shock, intercurrent bacterial infections, and acute respiratory failure may follow the use of steroids or immunosuppressive therapy in the presence of strongyloides infection, and can lead to a fatal outcome.

Strongyloides larvae have been blamed for conveying pathogenic bacteria from the bowel to the biliary tract and bloodstream.

Diagnosis
Larvae rather than eggs are present in fresh stool specimens. Aspiration of duodenal juice may be necessary to establish the diagnosis.

Treatment
Thiabendazole 25 mg/kg/d divided into two doses orally for three days. High doses of mebendazole or albendazole are successful in 80 per cent of cases.

Preventative measures are similar to those for hookworm.

Enterobius vermicularis

Synonyms: oxyuris, threadworm, pinworm.

Transmission is favoured by lack of bathing, wearing excess clothing and overcrowding. Preschool and schoolchildren are very commonly infected and the infection rapidly spreads to the whole family. Eggs contaminate bed linen, clothes, toilet seats, toys, the fur of domestic pets, and remain viable in dust for long periods if the atmosphere is cool, moist, and poorly ventilated. Reinfestation from anus-to-hand-to-mouth is very common.

Life cycle
Embryonated eggs are swallowed, larvae hatch and mature in the small intestine, and gravid females migrate to the peri-anal area at night to deposit their eggs. Embryonated eggs may hatch in the peri-anal area and crawl back into the anus before migrating higher up into the bowel. This is known as retro-infection.

Clinical findings
Pruritus ani results from the gravid female's noctural wanderings and egg laying in the peri-

Unlike most other helminths, *Enterobius vermicularis* is more prevalent in temperate climates.

anal area. The irritation leads to scratching, secondary infection, and may interfere with sleep. Enuresis has been attributed to pinworm infection. Vaginitis, endometritis, and, very rarely, salpingitis may be complications.

Diagnosis

Transparent adhesive tape applied to the perianal skin is the most satisfactory method of obtaining ova for identification. Ova are rarely found in stools but the 10 mm enterobius female worm may occasionally be seen.

Treatment

Piperazine compounds, 75 mg/kg/ body weight daily for one week, or mebendazole, 100 mg as a single oral dose repeated in one week, are effective. High infestation rates often require repeated treatment. The whole family should be investigated and treated accordingly.

Prevention

Frequent bathing and changing underclothes help to control spread. Finger-nails should be kept short.

Trichinosis

The genus has four species the best known of which is *Trichinella spiralis*. This is found in poorly cooked pork, which contains encapsulated larvae. These larvae develop into adulthood in the upper small intestine. They penetrate the bowel wall and, having gained entry into the circulation, are deposited in muscle. Encapsulation of these larvae gives rise to acute inflammation. After ingestion the person is symptomless or develops diarrhoea,and abdominal pains. Two to three weeks later fever, muscle pain, facial oedema, lymphadenopathy and a marked eosinophilia occur. Encystment is found in voluntary muscles. Invasion of the brain and myocardium has been described but is rarely seen in children. Death may occur in widespread infestation. The diagnosis is confirmed by identifying larvae on biopsy or by intracutaneous immunofluorescent antibody test. Treatment is with albendazole 400 mg for three days if >10kg body weight, 200 mg if <10 kg body weight. Mebendazole and thiabendazole are also effective. The latter drug kills the larval stage of the infection.

Toxocariasis (visceral larva migrans)

This is a zoonotic infection caused by the dog and cat nematodes, *Toxocara canis* and *T. cati,* which resemble human roundworms but do not develop beyond the second larval stage in humans. Children in intimate contact with dogs, cats, or contaminated soil are infected when eggs are ingested.

Toxocara larvae produce eosinophilic granulomata in various organs. A tender hepatomegaly, marked hypergamma-globulinaemia and hyper-eosinophilia, in which up to 80 per cent of the differential count consists of eosinophils, are the most characteristic findings; symptoms may be predominantly respiratory with cough and wheezing. A perihilar pneumonitis is often demonstrated radiographically. Splenomegaly and lymphadenopathy may also occur. Anorexia, lassitude, failure to thrive, and intermittent fever may be the only manifestations. Rarely, encephalopathy with convulsions and coma, myalgia, or even myocarditis are seen.

In older children with no evidence of generalized disease, an ocular lesion involving only one eye may lead to visual deterioration, strabismus, and a central field visual loss. Retinal detachment and occasionally chronic endophthalmitis with secondary glaucoma may follow. Eye involvement mimics retinoblastoma and the diagnosis must be excluded if enucleation is being considered. (*See* Chapter 33, Disorders of the eye.)

Diagnosis

Eosinophilic leucocytosis is almost invariable in visceral larva migrans and persists for months and up to one year. A marked increase in serum IgM and IgE is also a usual finding, but is rarely present in ocular toxocariasis.

Serological tests tend to be unreliable because of cross-reactions with antibodies of other nematodes, but high or rising titres of ELISA and fluorescent antibody tests are suggestive of the infection.

Needle biopsy of the liver may demonstrate eosinophilic granulomas surrounding larvae, but failure to identify these granulomas does not exclude the diagnosis.

Management

Normally a self-limiting infection, the illness may last for weeks or months. Spontaneous improvement is usual.

Diethylcarbamazine is the most effective remedy (1 mg/kg body weight day one; 1 mg/kg weight tds day two; 2 mg/kg body weight tds day three; then 3 mg/kg body weight tds for 21 days). Or it can be given as 6 mg/kg bd for 3 weeks, or 2 mg/kg tds for 7–10 days. In ocular toxocariasis and seriously ill patients, prednisone should be given in addition. Mebendazole 100 mg bd for three days, or thiabendazole 25 mg/kg body weight bd for three days may be effective.

Prevention

Deworming puppies at two weeks of age and redosing twice at two-weekly intervals, and yearly deworming of adult dogs and all newly acquired puppies, will help to control the incidence of visceral larva migrans. Cats are less infective to children. Handwashing after handling animals should be encouraged.

Filariasis

Five distinct species of filarial worms are important causes of disease in humans. They are listed in Table 16.2. All are confined to the tropics and subtropics.

Acute manifestations are seen in children, but the chronic effects are usually confined to adults.

Clinical syndromes

Lymphatic filariasis. Immunological responses to adult worms in lymphatics lead to acute lymphangitis. In *Wuchereria bancrofti* infections, the lower limbs and spermatic cord are commonly involved, leading to funiculitis, epididymitis, or orchitis. In chronic cases, hydrocoele and elephantiasis occur. *Brugia malayi* and *B. timori* infestations tend to involve the upper limbs and cause more severe acute infections, with high fever and abscess formations.

Pulmonary eosinophilia syndrome. This syndrome is commonly caused by a hyperimmune response to *W. bancrofti* and *W. brugia* microfilariae and is characterized by chronic cough, wheezing, and persistent eosinophilia.

Onchocerciasis. This is transmitted by the bite of the black fly (*Simulium*) which breeds in fast flowing water. Adult worms become encapsulated to produce subcutaneous nodules which are found mainly on the hips and buttocks in Africa, but the microfilariae are responsible for more serious disease. Skin involvement initially causes an irritating eruption which may become secondarily infected with scratching. In chronic cases, loss of skin elasticity and atrophy leads to the appearance of premature ageing. Blindness as the result of a sclerosing keratitis is the most serious sequel to prolonged infection in hyperendemic areas.

Loiasis. Allergic reactions to the adult worms migrating through subcutaneous tissue causes recurrent calabar swellings. Adult worms may be seen migrating across the eyeball under the conjunctiva.

Treatment

Diethylcarbamazine, 75 mg/kg body weight, is effective in acute lymphatic filariasis. Heavily infected patients with *Onchocerca volvulus* and

Table 16.2 Common filarial infections which cause disease in humans			
Filarial worm	**Insect ventor**	**Geographical distribution**	**Disease produced**
Wuchereria bancrofti	Mosquito	Indian and other Asian countries, East Africa, Central and South America	Lymphatic filariasis
Brugia malayi	Mosquito	Indonesia, Far East	Lymphatic filariasis
Brugia timori	Mosquito	Indonesia	Lymphatic filariasis
Onchocerca volvulus	Simulium flies	West Africa, Central America, Yemen	Skin lesions, ocular lesions and blindness
Loa loa	Chrysops flies	West and Central Africa	Calabar swellings

Loa loa infections should be given test doses of 25 mg/kg to avoid side-effects. In heavy infestations, steroids are recommended before commencement of this therapy. Onchocericisis can be treated with ivermectin 150–200 µg/kg as a single dose. This kills microfilaria and not adult worms and so the dose should be repeated after 3–6 months. The addition of doxycycline reduces the female worm fertility.

Prevention

Wearing protective clothing and vector control help to reduce the incidence of infections.

Parasitic helminths: Cestodes (tape worms)

Tapeworms that cause disease in humans are listed in Table 16.3

These segmented flat worms consist of a head or scolex which becomes attached to the small bowel of the definitive vertebrate host, and segments or proglottids, whose chief function is that of reproduction. Both male and female reproductive organs are present in proglottids. These and fertilized eggs may be found in the host's stools. Eggs are ingested by susceptible intermediate hosts. After hatching, larvae or oncospheres develop.

Variations occur in the oncospheres of different tapeworms. They penetrate the tissues of the intermediate host which are eaten by the definitive host. Maturation of the larval stage to the adult worm in the definitive host completes the cycle.

Treatment of intestinal cestodes. Niclosamide 2 g by mouth on an empty stomach; small children should be given half this dose. Praziquantel 40 mg/kg in one dose, or mebendazole 100 mg bd for six days are also effective.

Taeniasis

Taenia saginata is common in the Middle East and Africa but is found worldwide. Humans are the only definitive hosts of the adult worm *Taenia solium*. Eggs are occasionally passed in the stools of the host into soil and vegetation which is eaten by pigs, the intermediate host. The ova develop into the larval form in the pig's gut and penetrate the mucosal lining of the intestine to be disseminated to the pig's muscles, brain and other tissues by the bloodstream. The larval stage or oncosphere consists of a small fluid-filled sac containing a single scolex which is called a cysticercus and which, when present in numbers in the tissues of the intermediate host, gives rise to measly beef (*T. saginata*), or pork (*T. solium*). To complete the cycle, man consumes undercooked or raw infected 'measly' pork containing the cysticerci which develop into adult worms in the upper part of the small intestine. Human faecal contamination of grazing lands and the eating of rare beef or undercooked pork favours spread. *T. solium* is less common, but has a similar distribution to *T. saginata*.

Clinical findings

Infestation with adult worms may cause

Table 16.3 Tapeworms which may infect humans			
Worm	**Definitive host**	**Intermediate host**	**Disease in humans**
Taenia saginata	Humans	Cattle	Gastrointestinal
Taenia solium	Humans	Pigs, humans	Cysticerosis
Diphyllobothrium latum	Humans, fish-eating animals	Fish	Megaloblastic anaemia
Hymenolepis nana	Humans	Humans	Gastrointestinal
Echinococcus granulosus	Dogs	Humans, sheep, cattle	Hydatid disease
Multiceps multiceps	Dogs	Herbivorous animals, humans	Central nervous system

abdominal pain, but the passage of segments in the stool is the presenting complaint of most patients.

Diagnosis

The eggs of the two species are identical and examination of proglottids is necessary to differentiate them.

Cysticercosis

Humans may also become the intermediate hosts of *Taenia solium* by ingesting tapeworm ova or auto-infecting themselves via the faecal–oral route. These hatch into the larval form, penetrate the intestinal mucosa into the circulation and eventually lodge in various parts of the body as cysticerci – small cysts which excite an inflammatory reaction and tend to become calcified. These are sometimes seen in muscles on plain X-ray. The most important site for pathology is the brain, where the condition presents as neurocysticercosis which is difficult to manage (*see* Chapter 26, Neurological and muscular disorders). Drugs used in treatment are albendazole, niclosamide or praziquantel.

Diphyllobothriasis

This tapeworm occurs in cold regions of the world such as the Scandinavian lakes regions, but is also found in certain parts of Africa. It has the ability to split the vitamin B_{12} intrinsic factor complex in the lumen of the host's bowel, thus preventing vitamin B_{12} absorption. Megaloblastic anaemia and neurological complications result.

Treatment is with praziquantel or niclosamide and vitamin B12 may be needed to treat the anaemia.

Hymenolepiasis

Hymenolepis nana or the dwarf tapeworm commonly infects children in institutions, especially when overcrowding and unsanitary conditions prevail. Humans act as both the definitive and intermediate host; the complete life cycle takes place in the bowel lumen and wall. This auto-infection leads to an increasing population of adult worms. Irritation of the bowel wall causes abdominal pain and diarrhoea. The finding

of typical double membrane eggs in the stool establishes the diagnosis.

Multiceps multiceps

This is another dog tapeworm which has herbivorous animals as intermediate hosts, but the larval stage, known as a coenurus, may infect humans. Symptoms are neurological and similar to those seen in cysticercosis.

Fungal infections

Of the thousands of known species of fungi, relatively few cause disease in man. Pathogenic fungi are divided into those causing superficial chronic disease of skin and nails, and the deep or systemic mycoses. These may involve viscera such as lung, kidney, gastrointestinal tract, or meninges, but in some instances may also involve skin and mucous membranes.

Certain systemic fungal infections have a world-wide distribution but only cause serious infection in immunosuppressed hosts. Candidiasis and cryptococcal meningitis are common opportunistic infections in AIDS. Others have a limited geographic distribution, often infect many individuals in these areas, but cause disease only in a minority of those infected. (*See* Table 16.4.)

Therapy of systemic fungal infections

The major therapeutic agents used in the treatment of fungal infections are:

Amphotericin B, the drug of choice for most severe mycoses.

Flucytosine is frequently used in combination with amphotericin B.

Table 16.4 Systemic fungal infections

Worldwide distribution	Limited distribution
Actinomycosis	Blastomycosis
Aspergillosis	Coccidioidomycosis
Candidiasis	Histoplasmosis
Crytococcosis	Mucormycosis
Nocardiosis	
Sporotrichosis	

Azole derivatives. They are useful alternatives to the above ones especially for less severe infections. Miconazole is mainly used topically, but can be used systemically. Fluconazole is useful in the immunocompromised patients, particularly those with AIDS who have cryptococcal meningitis or oropharyngeal candidiasis. Ketoconazole is a useful oral agent to use for non-life threatening mycoses and for oropharyngeal candidiasis not responsive to topical therapy.

Candidiasis

Candida albicans is a normal commensal on the mucous membranes in the respiratory, gastrointestinal and female genital tracts. It causes symptoms at the time of first colonization after birth, and subsequently when the local 'ecological balance' is disturbed by intercurrent infection or antibiotic therapy, and when there is interference with the normal cell-mediated immune suppression of fungal overgrowth.

An oval budding fungus which produces a pseudomycelium in tissues and exudates, it may cause lesions confined to mucous membranes as in thrush or monilial vaginitis, or be restricted to the skin and nails. Both skin and nails may be affected in mucocutaneous candidiasis. Rarely, invasion of the bloodstream gives rise to a candidaemia when multiple organs may be involved, or focal involvement of meninges, kidney, or endocardium may occur. Invasion is commonly via the gastro-intestinal tract, but may be via the skin or renal tract.

Thrush has long been recognized as a common disease of early infancy, especially in preterm neonates. The mother's vagina is thought to be the source of infection in most instances, but bottle teats and attendants' fingers may also spread infection. Trauma to the oral mucosa will increase the likelihood of thrush infection and the use of broad-spectrum antibiotics has caused an increased incidence. Thrush causes characteristic greyish-white or cream patches on the oral mucosa which leave a raw, bleeding area when scraped. Pain in the mouth or extension of the lesions into the oesophagus leads to feeding problems. Thrush oesophagitis has been shown to produce incoordination of swallowing and an aspiration pneumonia as a sequel. Blood-stained vomiting may be a symptom. Monilial

dermatitis of the peri-anal or buttock region is commonly present.

Pulmonary candidiasis in infants is a rare finding at autopsy. The diagnosis is difficult to make during life because there are no specific clinical or radiological features to distinguish the pneumonia as being of candidal origin. The isolation of candida in the mouth or pharynx is no proof of pulmonary candidiasis, but finding candida on blood culture in an infant with bronchopneumonia is strong presumptive evidence.

Disseminated candidiasis. Candidaemia is found in certain postoperative or immunosuppressed patients. A fluctuating fever is usual. Removal of intravenous catheters may abort the infection, but deep organ invasion such as endocarditis, urinary tract involvement, or meningitis may develop. Predisposing factors for dissemination include broad-spectrum antibiotic, AIDS or immunosuppressive therapy, diabetes mellitus, malignant disease, and surgery to the heart, brain or gastrointestinal tract.

Candida endocarditis usually involves mitral and aortic valves and may follow valve replacement or arise *de novo* in patients suffering from leukaemia. It should be considered in the presence of major arterial emboli and the finding of soft, white retinal plaques.

Diagnosis

Candida may be cultured on Sabouraud's glucose agar. Repeated attempts to isolate the organism may be necessary. A variety of serological tests are available, but normal individuals show the presence of antibodies in low titre and antibody formation is often defective in the immunosuppressed. A rising antibody titre is helpful in establishing the diagnosis.

Treatment

Thrush. Topical nystatin or clotrimazole. Azole derivatives can be used if topical therapy fails. *Systemic candidiasis.* Amphotericin B or flucytosine given IV.

Mucormycosis

Mucormycosis is caused by the organisms of the genera *Mucor*, *Rhizopus*, and *Absidia*, which are widely distributed as bread moulds. It is characterized by the penetration of hyphae into the walls of blood vessels, leading to thrombosis, infarction, and necrosis. The gastrointestinal tract is a common site for serious infection in preterm neonates and severely malnourished infants and children. The skin may be involved as a complication of burns. Diabetics are susceptible to infection, a characteristic site being the paranasal sinuses from whence spread to the meninges may occur.

In leukaemia the lungs are often involved or the infection disseminates. Any severe debilitating illness such as chronic diarrhoea or uraemia and prolonged corticosteroid or chemotherapy predispose to the development of mucormycosis.

The diagnosis is frequently made only at autopsy, but should be suspected when an infection is associated with infarction. Culture or histology of a biopsy specimen confirms the diagnosis.

Treatment. Local excision or debridement is combined with amphotericin B given IV and as local irrigation (1 mg/ml). Ketoconazole is also effective and can be given orally.

Blastomycosis

A systemic infection caused by *Blastomyces dermatitidis*, this disease is found in scattered areas of North America and Africa. Dogs and horses may be infected, but the organism is seldom isolated from the environment. It is found in soil and thought to be inhaled. Infection gives rise to micro-abscesses resembling miliary tuberculosis. Dissemination may occur to any organ, but bone and skin are most commonly involved. Culture of the organism confirms the diagnosis. Serological tests are less reliable, being negative in half the cases.

Treatment. Prolonged courses of Amphotericin B. More recently oral ketoconazole and especially itraconozale have been found to be equally effective.

Pneumocystis jirovecii

Most humans become infected with this extracellular parasite before the age of four years, but in healthy hosts the infection is asymptomatic. Suppression of disease occurs via cell-mediated immune mechanisms, and therefore patients with congenital or acquired defective cell-mediated immunity such as AIDS, or who are on cytotoxic treatment for malignancy or organ transplantation, are at risk. The disease is a progressive pneumonitis with fever, cough, tachypnoea, recession and prominent hypoxia. The severity of clinical disease is worse than expected by the findings on clinical examination. Without treatment, this is a progressive, fatal condition. Treatment is with high doses of cotrimoxazole and steroids.

Aspergillosis

Aspergillus fumigatus, flavus, niger and other aspergillus species (there are over 90 species 19 of which are associated with human disease) may produce a variety of diseases in debilitated children and, rarely, in previously apparently healthy individuals.

Pulmonary aspergillosis usually complicates pre-existing chronic pulmonary disease. It may take the form of a hypersensitivity reaction with bronchospasm. Eosinophilia, elevated levels of serum IgE, and the recovery of aspergillus organisms in secretions from the respiratory tract suggest the diagnosis.

Colonization of pre-existing lung cavities with the formation of fungal balls, or aspergillomata, may also occur. The lesion often causes no symptoms and may only be found at necropsy. Recurrent haemoptyses and the finding of a cavitated lesion with a solid centre on chest radiograph are suggestive of the condition during life.

Rarely, diffuse pulmonary infiltration and the picture of a severe pneumonia unresponsive to antibiotics may occur. Lung biopsy may be the only means of establishing the diagnosis.

Any debilitating disease or immunosuppression may lead to dissemination of the fungus to lungs, kidneys, the brain, or endocardium.

Treatment consists of Amphotericin B. Addition of 5 flucytosine may be of benefit. Itraconazole may be required long term. Surgical removal of an aspergilloma may be possible.

Histoplasmosis

This is common in the eastern-central USA, but sporadic cases occur in South America, Africa, Australia, and the Far East.

The causative organism, *Histoplasma capsulatum*, is found in soil contaminated by the excreta of birds and bats. Infection is by inhalation and the majority of infections are asymptomatic, but massive infection leads to an acute febrile illness with cough, dyspnoea, and chest pain. Marked radiological changes are often present despite minimal clinical signs.

Arthralgia and erythema nodosum or multi-forme may occur. Most cases resolve with rest but, rarely, chronic pulmonary histoplasmosis supervenes and mimics pulmonary tuberculosis. Acute disseminated disease may occur in infants or the immunosuppressed. The organisms multiply in the reticulo-endothelial system, giving rise to weight loss, hepatosplenomegaly, and thrombocytopenic purpura and death unless treated.

Culture of infected sites, histology, or serology establishes the diagnosis.

Treatment consists of Amphotericin B or itraconazole and fluconazole.

Sporotrichosis

Sporotrichum schenkii, a fungus of worldwide distribution in soil, on plants and on timber, is a problem for florists, farmers and gardeners. It gains entry through an abrasion and commonly causes a characteristic skin lesion. A localized ulcerating granuloma at the site of infection is followed by thickening of draining lymphatic channels and the development of subcutaneous nodules, which may also ulcerate along the thickened lymphatic cord. Dissemination of the infection may occur in debilitated individuals and, rarely, the primary infection may be in the lung. Chronic inflammation and necrotic granulomas result.

Treatment. Potassium iodide 10 drops in juice tds by mouth is effective but poorly tolerated in skin lesions. Amphotericin B, or oral itraconazole for 3–12 months may be indicated if systemic involvement occurs.

17

Tuberculosis

Poverty, HIV and increasing drug resistance drive the tuberculosis (TB) epidemic. Rigorous attention to case finding, identification of contacts, adherence to therapy and monitoring for drug sensitivity are sufficient to control the pandemic. TB is the most common opportunistic infection in HIV-infected individuals and the fact that these two diseases exacerbate each other has been referred to as the 'cursed duet'. However, the majority of children with TB remain HIV-uninfected, and both HIV-infected and uninfected children suffer a huge burden of disease in endemic areas. Although it should be on the differential diagnosis list for disease affecting virtually any organ in the body, it frequently presents with fairly well-defined chronic symptoms.

Aetiology

TB is caused by *Mycobacterium tuberculosis* (*M.tb*), an aerobic bacillus, ranging in length from 1–10 μm. The genus mycobacterium includes a diverse group of organisms, with various animal and environmental reservoirs. Due to the high mycolic acid (lipid) content of the cell wall, mycobacteria stain poorly with Gram stain, however, they retain specific dyes (such as carbolfuchsin) very strongly, despite attempted decolouration with acid or alcohol, and are therefore referred to as acid-fast bacilli (AFB). The bacillus is tough and able to evade destruction in the human body because of special characteristics: it multiplies slowly (about once a day) and is resistant to many antibiotics. It remains viable in macrophages by subverting macrophage-killing, while its waxy coat and many component substances depress immune responses against it.

Epidemiology

TB is an ancient disease, which has affected humankind for a very long time. Evidence of mycobacterial disease has been found in human remains from Africa and South America dating back more than 3 000 years, with proof that spinal TB occurred in ancient Egypt when the great pyramids were constructed. Although *M.tb* is uniquely adapted to survive in relatively small nomadic communities, urbanization and industrialization with close contact between large numbers of previously uninfected individuals in overcrowded conditions and subjected to the stress of poverty and malnutrition provided the ideal soil in which the bacterium could flourish. Poor living conditions, linked to urbanization, provided the impetus for epidemic waves of TB. In England this wave probably peaked in the mid-nineteenth century when mortality reached 1 000/100 000 population. By 1950 this had fallen to 50/100 000 and it is currently 5/100 000 or less in most developed countries.

In South Africa, TB was virtually unknown before European colonization. However, from the early nineteenth century the occurrence of rapidly fatal TB among the indigenous peoples of southern Africa was noted. By 1920, 70 per cent of adult populations and 25–60 per cent of 10-year-old children were tuberculin skin test (TST) positive. TB remains one of South Africa's major health problems with an incidence of up to

1 500/100 000 in some areas, which is three times higher than the limit set by the World Health Organization (WHO) to identify the worst affected nations. In sub-Saharan Africa the situation is greatly exacerbated by HIV/AIDS, where some countries reported a 300–400 per cent increase in the number of TB cases, and more than 70 per cent of adult patients are HIV-infected.

In developed countries children make up 5 per cent or less of the case-load. In high incidence countries, such as South Africa, children comprise 15–20 per cent of the TB case-load, with an estimated TB incidence of roughly 50 per cent that experienced by the adult population. However, certain groups such as the very young and/or immune compromised children are at far greater risk of developing active TB and require particular attention.

Pathogenesis

Clinical disease resulting from *M.tb* infection is determined by microbial and host factors. *M.tb* does not secrete exotoxins or possess endotoxins; its harmful effects result from direct tissue damage and the immune response it evokes. Many disease manifestations contain an element of immune-mediated pathology.

As with any infection, active disease can be viewed as the end result of two separate processes:

- Transmission of infection to an individual
- Failure by the individual to control the infection.

Transmission of infection

M.tb infection results from the inhalation of minute infectious droplets (<5 μm in diameter) that are deposited in the periphery of the lung. Adults with lung cavities whose sputum contains visible bacilli (microscopy smear-positive) produce the greatest number of infectious droplets. Approximately 60–70 per cent of children living in close household contact with such a case will become infected. Cramped, overcrowded, poorly ventilated living conditions increase the opportunity for the transmission of *M.tb* infection, which is exacerbated by tobacco smoke exposure and indoor combustion. The risk of infection following contact with sputum smear-negative, but culture-positive tuberculosis patients is less, but cumulatively

important, especially if the primary caregiver of the child is infected. Children can transmit tuberculosis, although this is uncommon as they rarely develop lung cavities. However, adolescent children (>10 years of age) frequently develop adult-type lung disease that is sputum smear-positive, making them as infectious as an adult case.

Development of disease

The risk of developing active disease following *M.tb* infection follows a fairly predictable course, referred to as the time table of tuberculosis (*see* Figure 17.1).

The balance between the multiplication and spread of bacilli versus the body's defense mechanisms ultimately determines the clinical outcome. The primary lesion in the periphery of the lung is characterized by the exudation of polymorphonuclear leucocytes followed by monocytes and is called the primary or Ghon focus. Tissue destruction rarely occurs and there are minimal clinical symptoms or signs, although bacilli multiply and spread via the lymphatics to regional lymph nodes. The primary focus in the lung (often with some overlying pleural reaction), together with the inflamed connecting lymph ducts and enlarged regional lymph nodes, are known as the primary or Ghon complex (also called Ranke's complex).

Formation of the Ghon complex is frequently followed by silent (occult) bacteraemia and establishment of minute metastatic foci in places like the apices of the lungs, anterior parts of vertebrae, the ends of long bones, meninges, and kidneys. Small metastatic foci, referred to as Simon's foci, contain low numbers of *M.tb* and may calcify. The Simon's foci are also visible on chest radiograph and are often the site of disease reactivation. During this phase, the sites for potential later disease are established.

Within four to eight weeks, the situation is radically altered by the establishment of cellular immunity, which is clinically manifested by a positive tuberculin skin test (TST) as a result of delayed-type hypersensitivity. T-cells are sensitized to specific antigens of the tubercle bacillus displayed on the macrophage surface; these sensitized T-cells liberate a number of lymphokines that activate macrophages in an attempt to control intracellular bacilli.

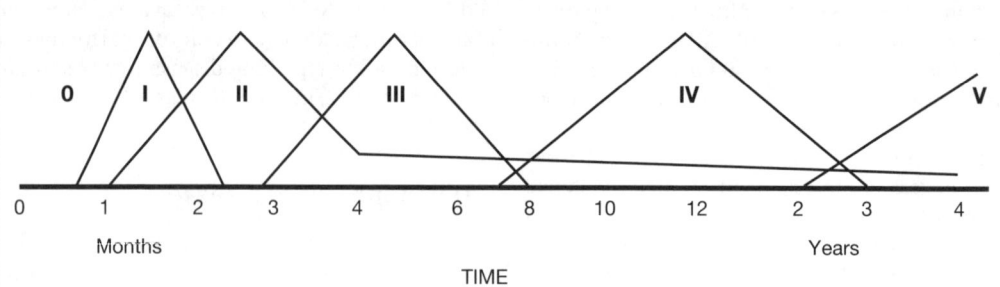

Figure 17.1 Schematic timeline, illustrating periods of greatest risk for particular disease manifestations following primary infection with *M. tuberculosis* in children

Phase of disease – adapted from the time-table of tuberculosis described by Wallgren[3]

0   Incubation phase
I   Hypersensitivity manifestations
II   Miliary tuberculosis and tuberculous meningitis
III   Lymph node and lymphobronchial disease in children <5 years; pleural effusion in those >5 years
IV   Osteo-articular tuberculosis in children <5 years and adult-type disease in those >10 years
V   Late manifestations such as urogenital disease and pulmonary re-activation

Not all these disease manifestations are equally common and while hypersensitivity is a nearly universal phenomenon following primary infection, the late manifestations are extremely rare. The vast majority of complications occur in the first 3–12 months following primary infection.

The host immune response results in the formation of granulomas with necrotic (caseating) centres, within which the acidic and hypoxic conditions are unfavourable for the multiplication of tubercle bacilli. However, *M.tb* is uniquely adapted to survive in an intermittently metabolizing (dormant, or 'latent') form within macrophages.

In children the greatest risk of disease progression occurs within the first year following primary infection and this risk is highest in the very young (<2–3 years of age) with immature immune responses. T-cells establish long-term memory following initial contact with *M.tb*, providing some protection against future re-infection events. Re-infection events are common in endemic areas with a high infection pressure (huge numbers of patients spreading the organism) and each re-infection event is associated with a new risk of disease development. Thus, although the risk of developing disease is greatest following initial infection, future disease may develop as a result of 'reactivation' of latent bacilli following immune compromise, or from re-infection.

This may explain why the disease manifestations seen in very young (immune immature) children are similar to those in immune compromised individuals. In these patients, extra-pulmonary and disseminated disease is more common, while immune competent adults are more likely to develop the typical lung cavities associated with pulmonary tuberculosis.

The reasons for the paradoxical destructive immune response experienced by some immune competent adults (and adolescent children) remain poorly understood. Some immune pro-

'Latent' bacilli are unlikely to cause disease as long as the immune response remains strong, but may cause future 'reactivation disease' if circumstances change.

Disease may result from an inadequate immune response or via immune mediated pathology.

cesses are essential to control bacillary multiplication and systemic spread, while others are decidedly harmful and are associated with tissue necrosis and the development of cavities in the lungs. It may be that different subsets of T-cells are responsible for the good and the bad effects. Like everything in the human body, an effective immune response represents a finely tuned balance; any disruption in this balance can lead to pathology. Antibodies are produced but B-cell mediated responses correlate poorly with protection.

As the initial immune response reaches its peak, it may be accompanied by fever, referred to as 'fever of initiation', enlargement of regional lymph nodes and/or hypersensitivity phenomena such as erythema nodosum and phlyctenular conjunctivitis. By this stage, the TST is usually highly reactive (>15 mm induration) and the immune response can control bacilli distributed throughout the body. In most TST-positive children the process goes no further and the infection is controlled. In a minority, however, the process continues and may lead to a wide spectrum of disease. The lifetime risk of disease following primary infection of an immune competent individual is estimated at approximately 10 per cent, but this is highly variable with the greatest risk occurring in the very young and within the first few years after infection. In immune competent children more than 95 per cent of disease manifestations occur within the first year after primary infection. In the timetable of tuberculosis (*see* Figure 17.1) it is evident that the first three to nine months following infection is the period of greatest danger, as the majority of cases with disseminated (miliary) tuberculosis, tuberculous meningitis (TBM), lymphobronchial tuberculosis, and pleural effusions will occur during this period. Unusual disease manifestations such as osteoarticular lesions may develop later, usually within two to three years after infection and rare urogenital tuberculosis usually occurs more than five years after infection.

Infants (less than one year of age) have a particularly high morbidity and mortality following infection. This risk stays high throughout the first two to three years of life while the immune system matures. Studies done before effective tuberculosis treatment became available (in the early 1950s) carefully documented the natural history of disease following infection with *M.tb*. The age-related risk of developing disease following primary infection is summarized in Table 17.1.

The age group 5–10 years old experiences the lowest risk and this is often referred to as the safe primary school age, when protection following primary infection seems optimal. Apart from very young age (<2–3 years) primary infection during adolescence (>10 years) represents a second danger period. Adolescent disease most often has the characteristic features of adult-type tuberculosis with cavitation in the lung apices. Large pleural effusions are often a sign of recent primary infection and may precede lung cavities. Adult-type tuberculosis first emerges during adolescence and tends to affect females earlier than males, probably reflecting a shift in the immune response occurring around the onset of puberty.

It has been estimated that in tuberculosis endemic settings approximately 10 per cent of HIV-infected individuals will develop active tuberculosis, either from reactivation or from recent infection (either primary or re-infection). The risk seems even higher in HIV-infected children where it has been recorded that up to 25 per cent, living in an endemic area and with limited access to antiretroviral therapy, develop active tuberculosis per year.

Tuberculosis presents with a wide range of clinical manifestations that represent different pathological mechanisms. Patterns are not as clear-cut as in leprosy (another mycobacterial disease), but the same variability in host responses is observed. In the optimal scenario effective cellular immunity quickly restricts and/or eliminates bacilli within granulomas, causing little damage to surrounding tissues. With immune compromise or immaturity, inefficient cellular immunity fails to control bacillary multiplication, resulting in regional and/or disseminated disease. At the other extreme an over-aggressive immune response may damage surrounding tissues in a failed attempt to contain

Apart from young age (immune immaturity) the likelihood that disease will develop is strongly influenced by immune compromise. HIV infection is the most powerful predisposing factor yet described.

Table 17.1 Age-specific risk of progressing to disease following primary infection with *M. tuberculosis* in immune competent children*

Age at primary infection	Risk to progress to active disease
<1 year	No disease 50% Lung disease 30–40% Disseminated (miliary) disease or TBM 10–20%
1–2 years	No disease 75–80% Lung disease 10–20% Disseminated (miliary) disease or TBM 2–5%
3–4 years	No disease 95% Lung disease 5% Disseminated (miliary) disease or TBM 0.5%
5–9 years	No disease 98% Lung disease 2% Disseminated (miliary) disease or TBM <0.5%
10–14 years	No disease 80–90% Lung disease 10–20% Disseminated (miliary) disease or TBM <0.5%
TBM–tuberculous meningitis	

the infection, leading to lung cavity formation. Conditions within these cavities support rapid multiplication of bacilli. Free communication with the airway then facilitates airborne transmission to those in contact with the patient. In the absence of lung cavities or extensive parenchymal involvement the organism load remains fairly low and the individual is unlikely to be infectious, as in most children. However, children with cavitary lung disease are likely to be as infectious as adult patients.

IRIS was previously referred to as paradoxical reaction. It has been documented after initiation of tuberculosis treatment and after nutritional rehabilitation, but is most commonly seen in HIV-infected children in the first few weeks/months after initiating antiretroviral therapy where there is successful viral suppression and immune recovery (increase in CD4 count). In HIV-infected children, IRIS frequently manifests as right sided axillary adenitis due to live *M. bovis* BCG vaccination given at birth.

Clinical manifestations

Due to the occult dissemination of *M.tb* following

> The immune reconstitution inflammatory syndrome (IRIS) represents pathology in sites of antigen exposure that results from increased inflammation following the reconstitution of a previously compromised immune response.

primary infection, virtually any organ or system may be affected. Nonetheless, it is helpful to discuss the clinical manifestations of tuberculosis in children under the headings of intra-thoracic and extra-thoracic disease, acknowledging that more than one organ or system may be involved in the same individual. The spectrum of disease observed in children treated for tuberculosis in a high prevalence area is reflected in Table 17.2.

Intra-thoracic tuberculosis

Infection without disease

These children have a positive TST, confirming that infection has taken place, but are asymptomatic with a normal chest radiograph. Although not yet diseased, very young and/or immune compromised children are at a considerable risk of developing disease and should therefore

Table 17.2 Disease spectrum documented in a prospective community-based survey of all children <13 years of age, treated for tuberculosis in a high prevalence area (N=439)	
Tuberculosis disease manifestation	**Total (%)**
Not tuberculosis	**85 (19.4)**
Intra- thoracic tuberculosis	**307 (69.9)**
Primary (Ghon) focus	
Uncomplicated (with/without hilar adenopathy)	16/307 (5.2)
Complicated	3/307 (1.0)
Lymph node disease	
Uncomplicated	147/307 (47.9)
Complicated (lymphobrochial disease)	
Compression	25/307 (8.1)
Consolidation	62/307 (20.6)
Pleurisy	**24/307 (7.8)**
Pericarditis	**1/307 (0.3)**
Disseminated (miliary) disease	**15/307 (4.9)**
Adult-type disease	**14/307 (4.6)**
Extra-thoracic tuberculosis	**72 (16.4)**
Peripheral lymphadenitis	
Cervical	35/72 (48.6)
Other	1/72 (1.4)
Central nervous system involvement	
Meningitis	14/72 (19.4)
Tuberculoma	2/72 (2.8
Abdominal TB	**1/72 (1.4)**
Osteo-articular disease	
Vertebral spondylitis	4/72 (5.6)
Other	7/72 (9.7)
Skin	**8/72 (11.1)**
[Intra- + Extra-thoracic disease]	**[25 (5.7)]**

Not tuberculosis – Chest radiograph not truly suggestive, no bacteriologic or histological proof and no extra-thoracic disease
Children with both intra and extra-thoracic disease manifestations were included in both groups

receive preventive chemotherapy (prophylaxis). A more appropriate term is 'incubation phase' TB, emphasizing that timely intervention will halt progression to disease.

Intra-thoracic lymphadenopathy
These children usually have documented recent exposure to a tuberculosis source case, a positive TST and hilar or paratracheal lymphadenopathy on chest radiograph. In the complete absence of symptoms or other signs indicative of disease, intra-thoracic adenopathy essentially indicates recent primary infection. However, due to the increased risk if left untreated, children should receive treatment rather than single-drug prophylaxis. In the presence of respiratory and/or constitutional symptoms, intra-thoracic adenopathy is almost pathognomonic of tuberculosis, although other conditions such as lymphoma should also be considered, especially with paratracheal adenopathy in the absence of documented tuberculosis exposure and/or infection.

Progressive primary focus
It is unusual for the primary focus to be visible on chest radiograph since it is transient; however, it often becomes visible later after calcification. In very young and/or immune compromised children who are unable to contain the organism at the point of entry, the primary focus may progress to fill a whole lobe or segment and even undergo cavitation.

Lymphobronchial tuberculosis
Intra-thoracic lymph nodes are in close apposition to the airways. Therefore diseased lymph nodes may have a wide spectrum of consequences. Narrowing of an airway may lead to distal collapse or, if a ball-valve mechanism develops, to hyperinflation and lobar emphysema. Ulceration of a node and discharge of its contents into a bronchus may trigger a hypersensitivity response in the affected segment or lobe. This may be seen radiologically as 'collapse-consolidation' or if viable bacilli are aspirated, as an expansile caseating pneumonia with/without visible cavitation. Although the complications of lymphobronchial tuberculosis may develop at any age, they are more common in younger children, possibly due to the smaller diameter of the airways and a greater tendency for regional

lymph node enlargement and inflammation. With appropriate treatment these lesions resolve clinically over two to three months, but enlarged nodes may remain radiologically visible for a prolonged period of time. Rarely, permanently collapsed or fibrosed segments or lobes may contain areas of bronchiectasis or bronchostenosis; usually as a result of extensive caseating pneumonia. It is important not to try and prognosticate given the initial severity of disease, since most children show a remarkable degree of recovery.

Adult-type tuberculosis

Adult-type tuberculosis, with involvement of the lung apices and cavitation, is more frequently seen at puberty, posing as great an infection risk as that in adult patients. This type of tuberculosis may develop shortly after primary infection, but also from reactivation of Simon's foci in the lungs or following re-infection. Re-infection is particularly likely in communities with a very high incidence of tuberculosis.

The bronchial spread of bacilli from a cavity may cause localized or widespread dissemination of bacilli throughout the lungs with a typical 'tree in bud' bronchopneumonic picture on chest radiograph. At times this complication may be indistinguishable from advanced miliary infection of the lungs.

Pleural effusion

A small effusion or thickening of the pleura is frequently seen in conjunction with the primary focus. It is, however, unusual to see a large pleural effusion in young children (<5 years of age), without significant underlying lung pathology. In older children, large exudative, straw-coloured, lymphocytic effusions occur more frequently and represent a pleural hyperreactivity response following recent primary infection. Rarely bacilli multiply in the pleural cavity causing caseating empyema.

Extra-thoracic tuberculosis

Disseminated (miliary) tuberculosis

Occult haematogenous dissemination occurs with most primary infection events, but is usually controlled by the development of specific cellular immunity. In disseminated (miliary) tuberculosis, this process escapes control. It occurs most often within the first few months after primary infection, and is most common in very young,

malnourished or immune compromised children. Haematogenous dissemination may also follow advanced lung disease. Physical signs include wasting, hepatosplenomegaly and generalized lymphadenopathy. Respiratory symptoms are often minimal, mainly tachypnoea, and auscultation is usually normal, although fine crepitations may be heard. As the clinical appearance may be very subtle, a high index of suspicion is required, especially in young vulnerable children exposed to a source case. Fever, poor feeding and lethargy without obvious cause may be the only symptoms. Splenomegaly under these circumstances is suggestive and retinal involvement may be visible. A chest radiograph is mandatory. The radiological 'snow-storm' appearance of a diffuse reticulonodular (miliary) pattern throughout both lung fields is highly suggestive, but may be mimicked by conditions such as lymphocytic interstitial pneumonitis (LIP), histoplasmosis, and sarcoidosis (typical non-caseating granulamas – very rare in children). Patients with miliary lung disease rarely have clubbing, the presence of which should raise the suspicion of LIP instead. Mental changes such as apathy and irritability may herald the onset of tuberculous meningitis (TBM), which is frequently associated with disseminated (miliary) tuberculosis. Disseminated (miliary) tuberculosis may also occur with a normal-appearing chest radiograph, to be confirmed by bone marrow or liver biopsy.

Tuberculous meningitis (TBM)

During occult dissemination, bacilli may lodge near the surface of the cortex or in the meninges and give rise to the so-called 'Rich focus' facilitating entry across the blood brain barrier into the cerebrospinal fluid (CSF). There is also a close association between miliary tuberculosis and TBM. Less commonly, TBM may develop from a tuberculous process in the middle ear, mastoid bone or spinal column. These subcortical or meningeal foci undergo caseation and discharge their contents into the CSF. This process may take at least two to three months.

> TBM is the most dangerous complication of TB. It causes considerable mortality and morbidity (severe cerebral palsy and mental retardation) in developing countries.

Therefore TBM is very unusual during the first three months of life (although congenital infection with early TBM may rarely occur). In most cases TBM develops within three to six months of primary infection; but sometimes the Rich focus is first contained and only later breaks down to give rise to TBM. The breakdown of such an established focus may be unexplained or due to immunosuppression. The discharge of bacilli and tuberculous antigens into the CSF elicits an inflammatory response leading to a thick proteinaceous exudate covering the base of the brain, enveloping the cranial nerves and blood vessels, and obstructing the flow of CSF. Obstructive hydrocephalus, which may be communicating or non-communicating, is present in approximately 80 per cent of children at diagnosis. The resultant raised intracranial pressure compromises cerebral blood flow and may cause cranial nerve palsies. The inflammatory process also causes vasculitis of the cerebral blood vessels leading to brain infarction (strokes).

The onset of TBM is gradual with non-specific signs such as irritability, lassitude, headache and vomiting. As the disease progresses, increasing apathy may culminate in focal neurological signs or convulsions. Clinically disease progression may be classified into three stages:

- Stage I: Signs of meningeal irritation; but fully conscious with no focal neurological signs or hydrocephalus
- Stage II: Confusion and/or focal neurological signs (squints, hemiparesis)
- Stage III: Stupor or delirium with/without focal neurological signs.

Early diagnosis and the prompt institution of appropriate treatment are essential for an optimal outcome. There is no place for a 'wait and see' approach. Tragically, very few cases are diagnosed at Stage I, when the prognosis is at its best. Progression from Stage I to III can occur over one to two days.

Diagnostic features. Most children with TBM are below three years of age and have a history of close contact with an adult with pulmonary tuberculosis, but have either received no prophylaxis or had non-adherent care-givers. Most children have clear evidence of failure to thrive preceding the onset of TBM, usually missed by healthcare personnel. A positive TST is obtained in 70–80 per cent of children with TBM, less so if they are HIV-infected or severely malnourished. (One should not wait for a TST result before beginning treatment.) Two thirds of children with TBM have a chest radiograph showing features of primary tuberculosis. Head computerized tomography (CT), if available, usually provides valuable supporting evidence. Various combinations of infarctions, particularly of the middle cerebral artery, hydrocephalus and tuberculoma may be found. Periventricular oedema may indicate non-communicating obstructed CSF that requires urgent shunting. On a contrasted CT scan, basal enhancement may be seen as a result of the tuberculous vasculitis, although this is less prominent in HIV-infected children and in early cases the CT may be normal. Magnetic resonance imaging, particularly for the evaluation of spinal involvement and in the extent of ischaemic damage, is helpful for prognosis.

Cerebrospinal fluid (CSF) changes. Typically the CSF will be clear and a clot may form if the tube is left standing on the bench. The cell count will be low ($<500 \times 10^6/l$) with a predominance of lymphocytes. Sometimes polymorphonuclear leukocyte predominance may cause considerable confusion. The glucose is typically low (<2.2 mmol/L), but is normal in about 25 per cent of cases. The protein concentration will usually be >1.2 g/L, but in approximately 20 per cent of cases may be lower, or even normal and compatible with viral meningitis.

Acid-fast bacilli are rarely seen on microscopy, but the success of this test depends on the amount of CSF obtained, the number of samples collected, and the care spent on searching for organisms. CSF culture yields are low and results are not available for weeks or more. For children, limited quantities of CSF are best submitted for culture rather than staining.

A variety of CSF tests have been evaluated, including biochemical tests (adenosine deaminase activity, lactate dehydrogenase, lactate, tryptophan colour test, and AFB-specific compounds detected by gas chromatography), radioisotope studies (bromide partition test), and immunological tests (for detection of antigen, antibody, or acute phase reactants). None provide high clinical utility and clinical judgment remains essential. Polymerase chain reaction (PCR)-based tests are specific and reasonably sensitive in adult studies, but have not yet fulfilled their promise in clinical practice. A useful distinguishing feature is that CSF values take weeks to months to return to normal, while rapid normalization is the rule with viral meningitis and effectively treated bacterial meningitis. In high burden settings, in any case of meningitis with slow onset over days or where the Gram stain and culture of the cerebrospinal fluid and blood are negative for pyogenic bacteria, a diagnosis of TBM should be considered.

If in any doubt, rather start TBM treatment and reconsider the diagnosis when additional results become available, since any delay in therapy may be catastrophic. In uncertain cases it may be useful to repeat the CSF analysis after 10–14 days. In most other forms of bacterial meningitis CSF values should have normalized by then. The continued presence of abnormalities, despite appropriate antibiotic treatment for other forms of bacterial meningitis, justifies a decision to complete TBM treatment.

Superficial lymphadenitis
Superficial lymphadenitis usually involves the cervical nodes, but occasionally axillary or inguinal nodes. Cervical lymphadenitis is the most common extra-thoracic manifestation of tuberculosis in children and may result from a primary focus in the upper or lower respiratory tract; the site of the affected nodes provides some indication of its location. Right sided axillary nodes are frequently associated with BCG vaccination, especially in infants. Diseased lymph nodes are painless, firm and adherent ('matted'), due to significant periadenitis and fibrosis. Caseation may lead to 'cold abscess' formation with softening, changes in the overlying skin and a draining sinus. Warm, tender nodes, except for BCG IRIS, are unlikely to be tuberculous, although secondary bacterial infection may occur. In endemic areas, a visible neck mass with the features described and without visible scalp or skin lesions is likely to tuberculous. (*see* Table 17.3) summarizes the clinical characteristics of children diagnosed with tuberculous lymphadenitis.

Histological and/or bacteriological confirmation can be achieved by performing a simple fine needle aspiration biopsy as an outpatient procedure. Important diseases to consider in the differential diagnosis include:

Table 17.3 Clinical characteristics of children with TB lymphadenitis (n=35)

Lymph node characteristics	Number (%)
Persistence (present for >4 weeks, no response to antibiotics)	35 (100)
Size	
<2×2 cm	4 (11.4)
(2–4) × (2–4) cm	25 (71.5)
>4×4 cm	6 (17.1)
Character	
Single	5 (14.3)
Multiple – discreet	14 (40.0)
– matted	16 (45.7)
Solid	28 (80.0)
Fluctuant – without secondary bacterial infection	5 (14.3)
– with secondary bacterial infection (red and warm)	2 (5.7)
Associated findings	
Tuberculin skin test (TST)	
0 mm	2 (5.7)
1–9 mm	0
≥10 mm	33 (94.3)
≥15 mm	32 (91.4)
Mean response 19.1 mm (standard deviation 2.9 mm)	
Constitutional symptoms	
Any symptom	21 (60.0)
Fever	7 (20.0)
Cough	9 (25.7)
Night sweats	8 (22.8)
Fatigue	19 (54.3)
Failure to thrive	10 (28.6)
Chest radiograph	
Suggestive of tuberculosis	13 (37.1)
Lymph node disease – uncomplicated	8 (22.8)
– with airway compression	1 (2.9)
– with parenchymal consolidation	4 (11.4)

Size – transverse diameter of the largest cervical mass.
Fatigue – less playful and active since the mass was first noted.
Failure to thrive – crossing at least one centile line in the preceding three months or having lost more than 10 per cent of bodyweight (minimum 1 kg) over any time interval

+ Malignancies, especially lymphoma
+ Acute pyogenic infections
+ Chronic fungal infection.

Abdominal tuberculosis

Abdominal tuberculosis may arise by haematogenous or lymphogenic dissemination, secondary spread due to swallowed bacilli from pulmonary disease, primary infection from cow's milk due to *M. bovis* (rare in South Africa), and rarely by extension from pelvic disease (post-menarche).

Following ingestion, bacilli spread along the following pathway: intestinal mucosa, mesenteric glands, peri-adenitis and leakage of caseous material from lymph nodes, low-grade peritonitis, and infection of serosa and bowel wall. Intestinal tuberculosis is less common in children, while lymph node involvement and peritonitis is more common than in adults.

There are usually four clinical forms of abdominal tuberculosis:

- Intestinal tuberculosis (mostly terminal ileum and caecum but any part of gastrointestinal tract may be involved)
- Abdominal lymphadenopathy
- Peritoneal disease (wet type with ascites, an encysted type, and a fibrotic type)
- Solid organ tuberculosis (liver, spleen– *see below*).

The most common symptoms are abdominal distension, fever, loss of weight, diarrhoea, and abdominal pain. Deep palpation often reveals masses due to enlarged lymph nodes or matted mesenteric and omental clumping in the right iliac fossa, centrally, or along both sides of the spine. Thickened adherent bowel, low-grade peritonitis, swollen omentum and nodal masses may produce a doughy feel. Acute or subacute intestinal obstruction may be caused by strictures (single or multiple), peritoneal or omental adhesions or compression by lymph node masses. Some children may present with acute abdomen due to perforation. Occasionally interluminal fistulae are found, causing chronic diarrhoea. Umbilical fistula and chronic fistula-in-ano may occur. Massive ascites is another potential complication. Obstruction of intestinal lymphatics can cause protein-losing enteropathy, steatorrhoea, and chylous ascites. Compression of the inferior vena cava may cause oedema of the lower limbs. Tuberculomas of the caecum may present as a tumour and ulcerative lesions can cause blood in the stools.

The differential diagnosis must include lymphoma for abdominal masses and other causes of intestinal obstruction, ascites, malabsorption, protein-losing enteropathy (PLE), and blood in the stools.

An abdominal ultrasound and/or CT scan may help to confirm enlarged intra-abdominal nodes with caseating centres. Laparoscopic biopsy for histology and culture may be required for precise diagnosis.

Liver and spleen

Hepatosplenomegaly is frequent and may be a non-specific reticulo-endothelial response to infection. Alternatively it is due to tuberculous granuloma formation in these organs. Mycobacteria reach the liver by miliary spread, through occult dissemination or from intra-abdominal lesions. Occasionally the spleen enlarges in the absence of hepatomegaly. Symptoms include abdominal pain, fever, and weight loss. Rarely there is obstructive jaundice or acute hepatitis. An isolated tuberculoma may present as a hepatic nodule.

Tuberculous pericarditis

The pericardium is infected from adjacent lymph nodes and by haematogenous spread. This results in pericarditis with effusion and long term constriction of the heart due to fibrinous organization or calcification of the pericardium. The early signs are a pericardial friction rub, increased cardiac dullness, an impalpable apex beat, and muffled heart sounds. With cardiac tamponade or constriction, the jugular venous pressure becomes raised, the liver enlarges markedly, and there is peripheral oedema. Important investigations are chest radiograph and echo cardiography. Pericardiocentesis may be required therapeutically and may assist with establishing a definitive diagnosis.

Upper respiratory tract disease

Primary lesions of the mouth and tonsils can occur, especially via a contaminated 'comforter/dummy' or following ingestion of contaminated milk. Tonsils are asymmetrically enlarged and red, with small yellow nodules and shallow grey ulcers. Submandibular adenitis is typically seen. Spread to the middle ear may occur via local extension along the Eustachian tube. Painless dental ulcers may occur as well as involvement of the adenoids, or larynx.

Eyes

Tuberculosis rarely causes conjunctival infection, presenting as conjunctivitis, lachrymation, swelling and reddening of eyelids and sclera. The everted eyelid reveals thick granulation with yellow areas. Pre-auricular or tonsillar nodes enlarge. Phlyctens, small grey nodules at the limbus into which drain a leash of conjunctival vessels, are rare manifestations of an excessive hypersensitivity response following recent primary infection. Other sites that may be involved include the cornea, lachrymal gland, iris, uvea, and retina (haemorrhages); choroidal tubercles may be seen with disseminated (miliary) disease.

Ears and mastoids

Tubercles may appear on the ear-drum, causing multiple perforations (especially in the lower half of the drum), but the most common sign is a chronic painless discharge (otorrhoea). Enlargement of the lymph node between the mastoid and angle of the mandible may result in the insidious development of conductive deafness and/or facial nerve palsy (especially in those below two years of age). The most serious complication is spread to the central nervous system.

Skin involvement

Tuberculous skin lesions are best grouped according to the site of infection. The skin may be the primary focus, in which case the infection has been passed on through direct contact. This results in a tuberculous chancre or wart. Haematogenous spread may produce multiple nodular lesions, papulonecrotic tuberculids, a single large plaque or ulcer, multiple abscesses or a chronic indurated destructive lesion of the cheek, nose, or ear (lupus vulgaris). Sinuses or fistulae may develop over underlying adenitis. Erythema nodosum is a skin manifestation of hypersensitivity most common in adolescent girls (also associated with other infections).

Osteo-articular (bone and joint) disease

Vertebral involvement (Pott's disease) is most common (50 per cent of all osteo-articular tuberculosis), followed by disease of the weight-bearing joints, especially the hip and knee. Tuberculous dactylitis manifests as indurated, reddened fingers with thickened phalanges. The radiological features are of decreased density of bones, cysts, and periostitis. Syphilis, salmonella, and sickle-cell anaemia must be considered in the differential diagnosis. Multi-joint reactive arthritis (Poncet's arthritis) is a rare hypersensitivity type reaction.

Adrenals

Infection of the adrenals is rare and is usually not associated with dysfunction. Addison's disease may present many years after bilateral infection and is therefore mostly seen in adults.

Blood changes

In general, there are no consistent patterns and haematological features are those common to any chronic infection. When it disseminates to bone marrow, tuberculosis can result in a wide range of haematological abnormalities including normocytic, normochromic anaemia, aplastic anaemia, pancytopaenia, neutrophil leucocytosis, a leucoerythroblastic reaction, and blood pictures resembling leukaemia and myelosclerosis. Haemophagocytosis may also occur.

Urogenital tuberculosis

With haematogenous dissemination, tubercle bacilli may be found in the urine without affecting the kidney. Renal lesions are rare in children; these include tubercles on the surface and/or within the kidney, abscesses, calcified lesions, and widespread destruction of parenchyma. Incidental discovery of sterile pyuria should lead to an active search for tuberculosis.

Genital lesions are equally rare before the onset of puberty. Epididymitis may be associated with renal tuberculosis; involvement is usually bilateral with hard and irregular cords. Orchitis may cause enlargement of a testicle. Penile tuberculosis has been recorded as a rare complication of circumcision that was not performed under aseptic conditions. Vulval and vaginal involvement may give rise to inguinal adenitis. Salpingitis may cause abdominal pain, irregular menses, and a lower abdominal mass.

Congenital and neonatal tuberculosis

Tuberculosis is common in pregnant women from endemic areas, facilitated by the mildly immunosuppressive effect of pregnancy. HIV-infected women and their infants are especially at risk. The risk is highest with undiagnosed maternal tuberculosis or where the mother has been treated for less than two months at the time of delivery.

True congenital infection occurs via haematogenous spread across the placenta and is usually seen in mothers with disseminated (miliary) disease or following recent primary infection with occult bacillary dissemination. Examination of the placenta or endometrial fluid/biopsy for culture and histology may confirm the diagnosis. Intrauterine growth retardation and prematurity may occur, with the infant developing additional symptoms during the first month of life. Both abdominal and/or respiratory disease may be present. With intra-uterine infection the primary focus is in the liver and non-specific abdominal symptoms tend to predominate. Abdominal distension, ascites, hepatosplenomegaly and obstructive jaundice occur commonly, as does disseminated (miliary) disease with or without central nervous system involvement.

Neonatal infection (which is frequently included with congenital disease) occurs during delivery, with swallowing or aspiration of infected amniotic fluid, or after delivery, with inhalation of infectious droplets from the mother or another close contact. Premature babies cared for in kangaroo units are particularly vulnerable and every effort should be made to ensure that mothers with symptoms suggestive of tuberculosis are not admitted to kangaroo care wards without first excluding active disease. Disease presentation is similar to congenital infection with high risk of disseminated (miliary) disease, or presentation may be delayed (three to six months) when respiratory disease predominates.

Diagnosis

It is *essential* to always document a history of contact with a potential source case in the past year. Ask about all people known to have tuberculosis, but also about adults with symptoms suspicious of active disease. In high burden areas tuberculosis exposure may occur outside the household or immediate family. Ask about the health of all household members, including neighbours and frequent visitors. If a potential source case is identified always enquire about known drug resistance or their treatment history, since retreatment and/or poor adherence to therapy are strongly associated with drug resistance.

In regions with a high prevalence of tuberculosis the following three symptoms and signs are highly predictive of TB, especially in immune competent children.

- Documented failure to thrive or weight loss (crossing of percentile lines or 'flattening off of the growth trajectory')
- Persistent, non-remitting cough and/or wheeze (>2 weeks duration and not responding to a course of antibiotics)
- Unusual fatigue (reduced playfulness).

In very small children fatigue is difficult to discern: therefore the first two symptoms are most informative. With airway involvement children may also experience large airway wheezing unresponsive to bronchodilators. In case of uncertainty, clinical follow-up remains highly informative, since natural symptom resolution does not occur with active tuberculosis and rapid disease progression is rare, unless children are very young or immune compromised.

Other clinical pointers include:

- Prolonged unexplained fever
- Organomegaly and/or lymphadenopathy
- Lethargy or altered level of consciousness, with or without vomiting, headache or convulsions
- Poorly defined symptoms and signs of any organ system, as discussed above.

Tuberculin skin test (TST)
A positive TST indicates delayed type hypersensitivity to tuberculoprotein. A positive test indicates likely infection with *M.tb* and provides essentially the same information as close exposure to an infectious index case; it is not necessarily indicative of active disease. If the child is very young (<3–5 years), it can be assumed that not only is the child infected, but that infection took place recently and that the child is probably still in the period of greatest danger for the development of disease (the first year) following primary infection. These children should receive preventive chemotherapy (prophylaxis). If the child is ill this increases the probability that the

A source case is the likely source of infection, while an index case is the first case of tuberculosis identified

Table 17.4 Interpretation of skin test results*

Interpretation	Mantoux induration (mm)	Mono test induration (mm)	Tine test description
Negative	0–4	<2	Papules <2 mm
Atypical Mycobacteria or BCG	0–9	2–3	Papules >2mm
BCG or M. tuberculosis	10–14	4–7	Coalescence of two or more papules
M. tuberculosis	≥15	≥8	Ring of confluence

*In the presence of HIV infection any induration ≥5 mm or its equivalent is regarded as indicative of M. tuberculosis infection

illness may be due to tuberculosis and active disease should be excluded.

It must be emphasized that a negative TST does not exclude the possibility of active tuberculosis, since it may be falsely negative.

TST is carried out with purified protein derivative (PPD), using the Mantoux method. Intradermal injection of two tuberculin units (2TU; 0.1 ml) of PPD RT23 or 5TU of Japanese PPD is usually done on the flexor surface of the left forearm. If done correctly, a temporary wheal of 7–8 mm should be raised. The test response is measured after 48–72 hours, documenting the transverse diameter of induration (swelling), not redness. The 'ball-point method' is helpful and

Reasons for a false negative Tuberculin Skin Test include:

- Poor technique: if, for example, Mantoux solution is injected subcutaneously instead of intradermally
- Performed within three months of exposure. Since it is not known when exposure occurred, all children in close contact with an adult index case must receive prophylaxis, regardless of the TST reaction, if active disease has been ruled out
- Immune compromise of any origin
  - HIV/AIDS
  - Protein-energy malnutrition (PEM)
  - Measles, other viral infections or recent immunization with live vaccines
  - Overwhelming disease (e.g. disseminated (miliary) tuberculosis)
  - Immunosuppressive medicines such as steroids.

all results should be documented as millimeter induration on the Road to Health card.

Exposure to other mycobacteria may complicate TST interpretation because of cross-reactivity. Neonatal BCG immunization may elicit a TST response, but this usually wanes within the first one to two years of life. Exposure to other non-tuberculous mycobacteria (NTM) may also cause a positive reaction. In general though, induration ≥10 mm is highly suggestive of infection with *M.tb*. In fact, the majority of children with *M.tb* infection, irrespective of BCG vaccination or HIV status, have an induration of ≥15 mm. In HIV-infected individuals it is recommended that all indurations ≥5 mm should be regarded as positive. Disposable TSTs such as the Tine® and the Mono® tests are not as accurate as the Mantoux method, but have the advantages of convenience and ease of administration.

Chest radiography

A segmental opacity, cavitation, bronchopneumonia and/or a pleural effusion may all suggest the possibility of tuberculosis, but it is only lymphadenopathy and a miliary pattern that can be considered diagnostic and even these findings may occasionally be caused by other conditions. In clinical practice, a diagnosis of probable tuberculosis frequently rests upon documented exposure (a history of close contact with an adult with infectious pulmonary tuberculosis) or infection (a positive TST), a constellation of clinical symptoms and a chest radiograph (in the case of intrathoracic disease) suggestive of tuberculosis.

Bacteriological confirmation

Bacteriological confirmation is complicated by the difficulty of specimen collection and the fact

Table 17.5 Summary of various bacteriologic specimen collection methods

Specimen collection method	Problems/ Benefits	Potential clinical application
Sputum	Not feasible in very young children who cannot expectorate; assistance and supervision improves the quality of the specimen	Routine sample to be collected in children >7 yrs of age (all children who can produce a good quality specimen)
Induced sputum	Increased yield compared to gastric aspirate; no age restriction; specialized technique, requiring well trained personnel, nebulization and suction facilities; potential transmission risk	To be considered in the hospital setting on an in- or out-patient basis
Gastric aspirate	Difficult and invasive procedure; not easily performed on an outpatient basis; requires prolonged fasting; Sample collection advised on 3 consecutive days	Routine sample to be collected in hospitalized children who cannot produce a good quality sputum specimen
Nasopharyngeal aspiration	Less invasive than gastric aspirate; no fasting required; comparable yield to gastric aspirate	To be considered in primary health care clinics or on an outpatient basis
String test	Less invasive than gastric aspirate; Tolerated well in children >4 years; bacteriologic yield and feasibility require further investigation	May become the sample of choice in children who can swallow the capsule, but cannot produce a good quality sputum specimen
Broncho-alveolar lavage	Extremely invasive, no proven advantage over gastric aspirate	Only for use in patients who are intubated or who require diagnostic bronchoscopy
Urine /stool	Not invasive; excretion of *M. tuberculosis* well documented	Being evaluated for use with novel sensitive bacteriologic or antigen-based tests
Blood / bone marrow	Good sample sources to consider in the case of probable disseminated TB	To be considered for the confirmation of probable disseminated TB in hospitalized patients
Cerebrospinal fluid (CSF)	Fairly invasive; bacteriologic yield low	To be considered if signs of tuberculous meningitis
Fine needle aspiration biopsy (FNAB)	Minimally invasive using a fine 23G needle; excellent bacteriologic yield, minimal side-effects	Procedure of choice in children with superficial lymphadenopathy

that children usually have paucibacillary (smear-negative) disease. Culture is more sensitive than smear microscopy, but clinically less helpful since it may take four to eight weeks and requires some laboratory support, frequently unavailable in tuberculosis endemic areas. Children tend to swallow rather than spit out their sputum. Therefore, examination of early-morning gastric aspirates and/or induced sputum specimens are most helpful. *M.tb* may be recovered from other

Table 17.6 Summary of traditional and novel diagnostic approaches

Traditional approaches	Application	Problems/ Benefits	Validation
TB culture using solid or liquid media	Bacteriologic confirmation of active TB	Slow 'turn around' time for solid media; liquid media too expensive for most poor countries	Accepted gold standard; liquid media more sensitive and quicker for results
Chest radiography	Diagnosis of probable active TB	Rarely available in endemic areas with limited resources; accurate disease classification important	Reliable in expert hands and in presence of suspicious symptoms
Symptom-based approaches	Diagnosis of probable active TB	Poor symptom definition	Not validated
Tuberculin skin test (TST)	Diagnosis of *M. tuberculosis* infection	Rarely available in endemic areas; does not differentiate latent TB infection (LTBI) from active disease; insensitive in immune compromised children; simple to use and less expensive than blood-based tests	Various cut-offs advised in different settings Mantoux is 'Gold Standard' Tine test easier but less sensitive
Novel approaches Symptom-based	**Application**	**Problems/Benefits**	**Validation**
Symptom-based screening	Screening child contacts of adult TB cases	Limited resources required; should improve access to preventive chemotherapy for asymptomatic high-risk contacts in endemic areas	Currently advised in resource-limited settings; requires further validation
Refined symptom-based diagnosis	Diagnosis of probable active TB	Limited resources required; should improve access to chemotherapy in resource-limited settings; poor performance in HIV-infected children	Additional validation required
Immune-based	**Application**	**Problems/Benefits**	**Validation**
Antibody-based assays	Diagnosis of probable active TB	Simple, point of care testing, variable accuracy and difficulty in distinguishing LTBI from active TB	Further development required

continued

Table 17.6 *continued*

Organism-based	Application	Problems/Benefits	Validation
T-cell assays	Diagnosis of LTBI	Limited data in children, inability to differentiate LTBI from active TB; blood volume required (3–5 ml); expensive; may have particular relevance in high-risk children, where LTBI treatment is warranted	Not well validated in children
Bacteriophage-based tests	Diagnosis of probable active TB, and detection of rifampicin resistance	Requires laboratory infrastructure; performs relatively poorly when used on clinical specimens	Not well validated in children Less accurate than PCR-based tests
Microscopic observation drug susceptibility (MODS) assay	Diagnosis of probable active TB, and detection of drug resistance	Simple and feasible, limited resources required	Well validated in adults, but not in children
PCR-based tests	Diagnosis of probable active TB, and detection of drug resistance	Requires good laboratory infrastructure and excellent quality control measures Sensitivity tends to be poor in paucibacillary TB Requires systems	Well validated in adults, but not in children
Antigen-based assays	Diagnosis of probable active TB	Simple, point of care testing; limited clinical data on accuracy	Further development required

infected tissues (e.g. pus, cerebrospinal fluid, bone marrow, pleural and ascitic fluids). Fine needle aspiration biopsy (FNAB) is a minimally invasive procedure with excellent bacteriological yield in cases with superficial lymphadenitis.

HIV-testing

Diagnosis of tuberculosis is usually quite straightforward in an HIV-uninfected child if the above mentioned diagnostic principles and tests are used, but HIV infection and its related conditions can mimic many of the symptoms, signs and investigations for TB. All children with suspected tuberculosis should, therefore, be tested for HIV after appropriate counselling.

Due to the difficulty of establishing an accurate diagnosis, especially in HIV-infected children, every effort should be made to achieve bacteriological confirmation. With the rising prevalence of drug-resistant tuberculosis, obtaining material for culture has additional value to evaluate drug susceptibility. Table 17.5 provides an overview of various bacteriologic specimen collection methods and Table 17.6 provides a concise summary of traditional and novel diagnostic approaches.

Diagnostic dilemmas

The varying degree of certainty with which TB is diagnosed in childhood, coupled with the wide spectrum of manifestations, creates a dilemma for the clinician. In a sick young infant it may be appropriate to start treatment for tuberculosis without delay, with relatively little diagnostic information, whereas in an older child who is not acutely ill one might choose to delay treatment until greater diagnostic certainty is obtained. HIV infection has added a further complication, as many of the clinical features that lead the clinician to suspect tuberculosis, such as malnutrition, persistent respiratory signs and symptoms, lymphadenopathy and hepatosplenomegaly occur in HIV-infected children. Inevitably many HIV-infected children who may not have confirmed tuberculosis will receive antituberculosis treatment. Such cases require careful consideration of all the available diagnostic evidence and the clinical course may eventually permit a decision to stop antituberculosis treatment, although a 'trial of treatment' is never advised.

Management

This requires an integrated view of the factors involved in the spread of TB and must therefore involve consideration of the specific community, as well as the individual case and his or her contact with source cases.

Protecting any community against TB should include:

* Improvement of socio-economic living conditions
* Community participation in health care and health education
* Pasteurization of milk
* BCG vaccination.

BCG vaccination has produced variable efficacy, but there is general consensus that neonatal vaccination provides some protection (60–70 per cent) against disseminated forms of TB early in childhood. However, a protective effect has not been demonstrated in HIV-infected children. BCG is a live vaccine that poses a risk to immune compromised individuals and should not be administered to children known to be HIV-infected. However, as infants are routinely immunized at birth, when the HIV status of HIV-exposed infants is not yet known, they should still be immunized, as >95 per cent of these infants will be HIV-uninfected.

Detection and treatment of high-risk contacts

This is very important, since most children are infected following documented contact with an adult or adolescent source case. Since TB exposure is ubiquitous in endemic settings, public health efforts focus on preventive therapy for those at highest risk of progressing

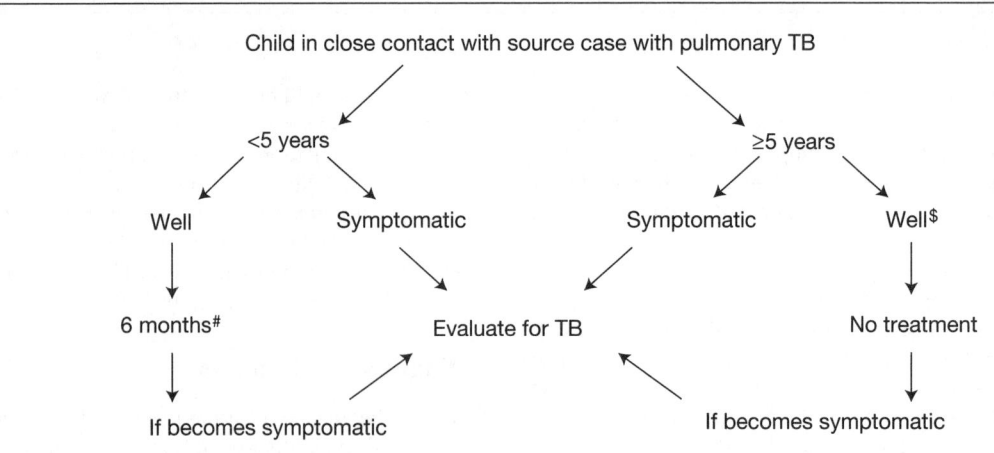

Figure 17.2 Suggested approach (WHO 2006) to contact management when chest radiograph and tuberculin skin testing are not readily available

Child in close contact with source case with pulmonary TB

<5 years

≥5 years

Well

Symptomatic

Symptomatic

Well$

6 months#

Evaluate for TB

No treatment

If becomes symptomatic

If becomes symptomatic

#Isoniazid 10 mg/kg daily for 6 months
$If the child is HIV-infected, give isoniazid (10 mg/kg daily) for 6 months

to active disease. The most vulnerable are very young (<3–5 years of age) and/or immune compromised children. The majority of children in close contact with an infectious case will have live tubercle bacilli within them, even without being obviously ill. All children less than five years of age or immune compromised (HIV-infected) should receive preventive therapy after *each* documented exposure, once active disease has been ruled out. In resource-limited settings, a simple symptom-based screening tool should be used. (*See* Figure 17.2)

In addition, any child under five years of age with a significant Mantoux reaction (>10 mm, or >5 mm if HIV-infected) should also receive preventive therapy if not clinically diseased and not previously treated for infection or tuberculosis. Contact detection and investigation may seem tedious and time-consuming, but is vital to reduce the burden of paediatric TB.

Figure 17.3 Flow diagram to guide the diagnosis and appropriate management of children with suspected tuberculosis

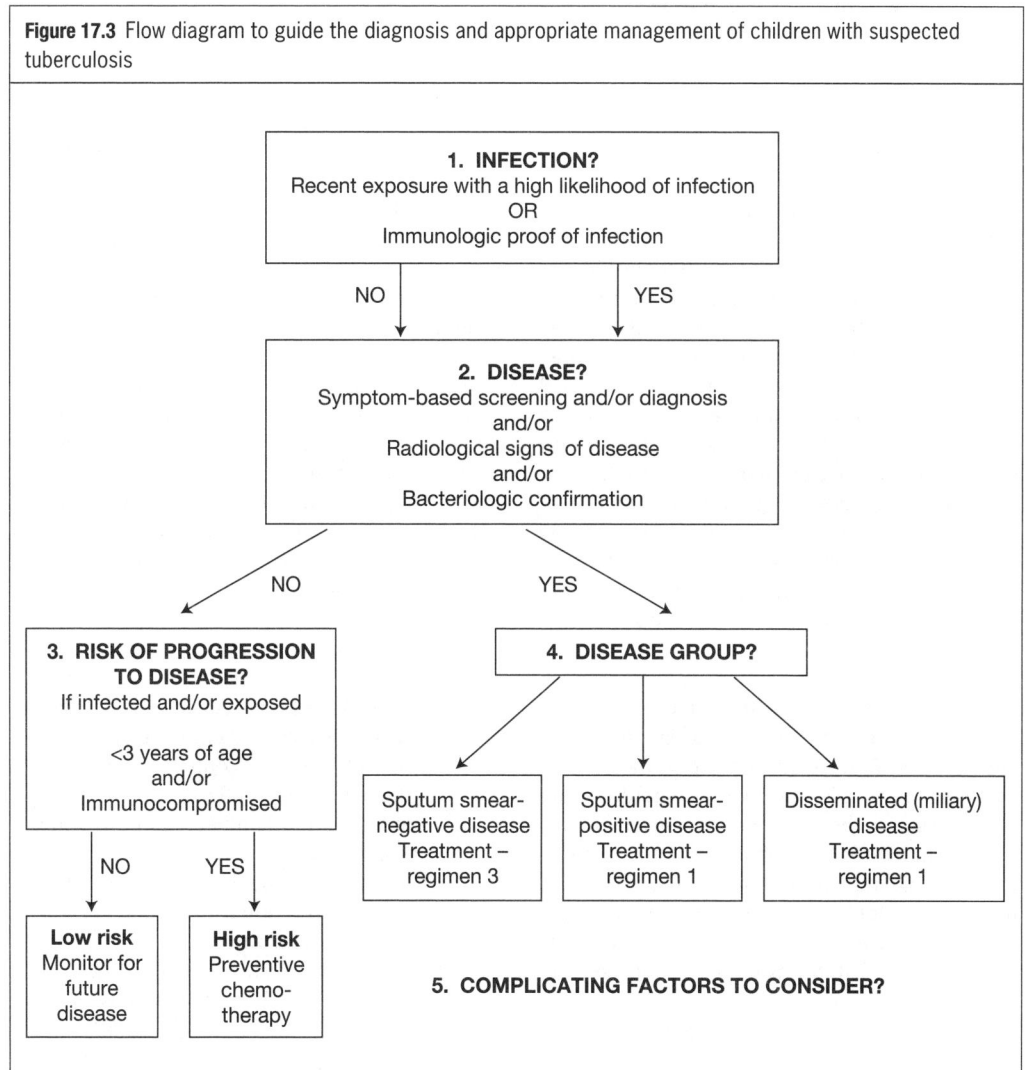

Case management

Case-finding

There are two ways in which children suffering from tuberculosis can be identified:

- Detection when presenting for healthcare (passive case finding))
- Tracing contacts of adults with pulmonary TB (*see above*) with screening of at-risk groups (active case finding).

More extensive active case finding is not cost-effective.

Passive case-finding can be improved by increasing awareness of the common symptoms and signs of TB through health education and by improving health care access.

Case management

Figure 17.3 contains a flow diagram to guide the management of children with suspected TB.

Isoniazid (INH) remains the most potent bactericidal agent. In adults, INH reduces the number of organisms expectorated by 90 per cent within two days. Rifampicin (RMP) and ethambutol (EMB) are less active against actively metabolizing organisms, while pyrazinamide (PZA) has almost no role in their killing. RMP and PZA are, however, key agents for sterilizing lesions, essential for successful short-course chemotherapy. Without them six-month therapy is not possible, necessitating prolonged treatment for 9–12 months. EMB, an important supporting agent for high bacterial loads (extensive or cavitary lesions), has only moderate bactericidal or sterilizing properties, but assists the prevention of drug-resistant TB.

Treatment commences with a bactericidal, intensive phase consisting of INH, RMP and PZA (EMB included with high bacterial loads) for two months. EMB is often omitted in children as most forms of childhood tuberculosis are paucibacillary. The continuation phase consists of INH and RMP for four months and aims to eliminate all remaining viable organisms. The number of medicines available for the treatment of TB is limited and they should be used with due care. Table 17.7 lists the available first and second line agents.

There is general agreement on the optimal first line regimens for the management of TB (*see* Table 17.8).

The aims of antituberculosis treatment are as follows:

- Rapid elimination of actively metabolizing organisms to reduce infectivity and limit morbidity and mortality.
- Prevention of future relapse disease by killing the remaining population of dormant or intermittently metabolizing organisms (sterilization).
- Prevention of acquired drug resistance; achieved with multi-drug regimens and fixed dose combination tablets.
- Accomplishing the above aims with minimal toxicity.

Treatment guidelines

Adherence refers not only to the manner in which the patient follows treatment instructions, but equally to the degree to which health workers observe national guidelines for the management and reporting of tuberculosis cases.

Treatment must be supervised. Adherence is the most important factor influencing response to treatment. Where children are managed on an ambulatory basis, strict adherence to the treatment schedule can be assured only through an extensive network of primary health care centres and trained community health workers to assist the family with directly observed therapy. Health professionals and local authorities must comply with national guidelines for diagnosis, treatment and follow-up.

Points to remember:

- Drug toxicity is less common in children than in adults. Hepatotoxicity, especially, is rare; however, should jaundice occur, stop treatment with all potentially hepatotoxic medicines immediately. A combination of amikacin, EMB and a fluoroquinolone, (e.g. ofloxacin) may be substituted while expert advice is sought. Always consider alternative common causes such as hepatitis A infection.
- Use child-friendly formulations, such as dispersible fixed dose combination tablets. If unavailable and the child cannot swallow tablets or capsules, crush the former or empty the latter into a spoon, flavour with an acceptable vehicle, and administer. Do

Table 17.7 First and second line antituberculosis medicines and recommended dosages in children

1st line Medicines	Mode of action	Dosage [mg/kg/dose] (maximum)
		Daily
Isoniazid	bactericidal	10 range 10–20 (300 mg)
Rifampicin	bactericidal and sterilizing	10–20 (600 mg)
Pyrazinamide	sterilizing	30 range 20–40 (2 000 mg)
Ethambutol&	bacteriostatic	20 range 15–25 (1 200 mg)
Streptomycin	bacteriostatic	15 range 12–18 (1 000 mg)
2nd line Medicines		
Aminoglycosides Kanamycin Amikacin Polypeptide Capreomycin	bacteriostatic	15–30 (1 000 mg) 15–30 (1 000 mg) 15–30 (1 000 mg)
Ethionamide or prothionamide	bactericidal	15–20 (750 mg)
Fluoroquinolones# Ofloxacin Levofloxacin Moxifloxacin	bactericidal	10–20 (800 mg) 7.5–10 (750 mg) 7.5 (400 mg) 30–40 (1 500 mg)
Cycloserine or terizidone	bacteriostatic	10–20 (1 000 mg)
Para-aminosalisylic acid (PAS)	bacteriostatic	150–200 (8–12 g)

& Ethambutol should be used with caution in children <7 years of age where visual acuity cannot be evaluated. It seems safe at recommended doses of 15–25 mg/kg.
# Ciprofloxacin is the least active against tuberculosis, and should not be used. Ofloxacin is currently the fluoroquinolone of choice; reports on the use of levofloxacin and moxafloxacin in children are eagerly awaited.

Table 17.8 Recommended treatment regimens for different disease categories

Category	Treatment regimen	
	Intensive phase	Continuation phase
I New sputum smear-positive or smear-negative TB with extensive lung involvement	2 months INH, RMP, PZA, EMB	4 months INH, RMP
II Previously treated pulmonary TB#	2 months INH, RMP, PZA, EMB SM followed by 1 month INH, RMP, PZA, EMB	5 months INH, RMP, PZA, EMB
III Sputum smear-negative TB or less severe forms of extra-pulmonary TB*	2 months INH, RPMP, PZA	4 months INH, RMP

INH = isoniazid, RMP = rifampicin, PZA = pyrazinamide, EMB = ethambutol, ETH = ethionamide, SM = streptomycin.
#Regimen 2 is not used in children, retreatment cases receive the same regimen as indicated for first time treatment
*Most children will fall into category III. Where cavities or extensive lung lesions are present (even if 'smear-negative'), children should be treated with regimen I.

Directly observed treatment (DOT) consists of the following:

- No medicines are given to the patient to take home.
- No self-administration of medicines is allowed.
- An observer (reliable lay or professional person with a strong sense of responsibility) must see the patients swallowing the medicines.
- Medicines should be pre-packed in individual dosages.
- Use the correct combination of antituberculosis medicines.
- Patient/parental education and support (including socio-economic support where indicated).
- Take treatment seven days a week.

not allow the medicines to stand in vitamin preparations for more than a few minutes, as this inactivates RMP.

- Children with smear-positive tuberculosis or cavitary disease should, however, be isolated until smear-negative sputum is obtained to avoid nosocomial spread.

Monitoring progress

Follow clinical response to treatment. The following are signs of progress:

- Appetite returning with good weight gain. Children should be weighed monthly while on treatment and drug dosages adjusted accordingly.
- Resolution of symptoms.
- Radiographic signs may take many months to improve and a repeat chest radiograph is only indicated when a child fails to improve clinically.
- Follow-up with smear and/or cultures are essential in drug-resistant tuberculosis cases and recommended in all smear-positve cases, especially HIV-infected children.

Possible causes of failure to respond to treatment include:

- Poor treatment adherence
  - Check administration of medicine.
  - Check that medicine is not being vomited.
- Poor drug absorption
  - A useful aid is the orange colour of the urine with RMP treatment. In unusual

cases it may be necessary to perform drug levels and parenteral administration of certain medicines may be necessary. HIV-infected children are more likely to experience inadequate drug absorption.

- Anorexia due to ethionamide (ETH) or other drug related adverse events.
- Wrong diagnosis (consider alternative diagnoses as relevant) or intercurrent infection.
- Drug-resistant tuberculosis. Enquire about history of contact with drug-resistant or treatment failure/retreatment in a source case.
- Paradoxical worsening (IRIS)
  - To be considered following nutritional rehabilitation or recent institution of antiretroviral therapy.

Special circumstances for treatment of TB

Osteo-articular tuberculosis

General principles of treatment apply, including keeping the affected joint initially at rest (by splinting) with later mobilization. Incision and evacuation may be necessary and is frequently done to confirm the diagnosis. Despite lack of rigorous evidence, most clinicians prefer to give a longer duration of treatment of 9–12 months, especially in spinal tuberculosis cases.

Abdominal tuberculosis

This frequently presents with complications such as protein losing enteropathy, peritonitis, and intestinal obstruction, all of which may cause impaired absorption. Parenteral administration of medicines may be required initially.

Tuberculous meningitis (TBM)

Brain and cerebrospinal fluid penetration of medicines is crucial in the treatment of TBM. This explains why increased drug dosages are used and ETH is added as the fourth drug of choice. In South Africa the preferred regimen is INH (15–20 mg/kg body weight/day to a maximum of 300 mg), RMP (20 mg/kg body weight/day to a maximum of 600 mg), PZA (30–40 mg/kg body weight to a maximum of 2 g) and ETH (20 mg/kg body weight/day to a maximum of 750 mg), given daily for total of six months.

Obstructive hydrocephalus, communicating in approximately 80 per cent of cases is an important complication of TBM. If available, a computed tomography (CT) scan of the head should be performed to help confirm TBM and exclude space-occupying lesions. An air encephalogram remains the most reliable way to differentiate communicating from non-communicating hydrocephalus. Air injected while performing a lumbar puncture should be visible in the ventricles on a skull radiograph taken straight afterwards. For communicating hydrocephalus the raised intra-cranial pressure will usually respond to furosemide (1 mg/kg body weight/day) and acetazolamide (100 mg/kg/body weight/day) given at six- to eight-hourly intervals. Should the hydrocephalus be non-communicating, an urgent ventricular shunt operation is indicated.

Adjuvant steroid therapy
Controlled clinical trials have confirmed the benefit of adjuvant steroid therapy in TBM and tuberculous pericarditis where it reduces the long-term sequelae of constrictive pericarditis. Prednisone at 2 mg/kg/body weight, or its equivalent, is routinely used for a month where after the dose is tapered over two to four weeks.

Other conditions where steroids may be beneficial or lead to more rapid symptomatic response include large pleural effusions, massive lymph node enlargement with severe narrowing of the airways, tuberculous laryngitis with life-threatening obstruction and IRIS. Steroids are also rarely used with tuberculosis of the adrenal glands that affect endogenous steroid production and in renal tract tuberculosis to prevent ureteric scarring.

HIV and TB co-infection

> TB is the most common opportunistic infection of HIV-infected South African children. TB and HIV exacerbate each other. The CD4 depletion from HIV increases the vulnerability to TB. TB infection accelerates viral replication, leading to further suppression of CD4 cells. The diagnosis and management of TB is complicated in co-infected children.

HIV-infected children have an increased mortality rate, probably related to HIV and not to failure of antituberculosis treatment.

In HIV infected children the following problems are observed (*see* also Chapter 18, HIV infection):

- Increased rates of TB infection and repeated episodes of disease due to primary infection, re-infection and reactivation. Increased vulnerability due to CD4 depletion and young age leads to high rates of primary disease and reactivation. There is a high risk for re-infection due to increased exposure to TB in households with adult HIV-infected contacts. There may be a delay in diagnosis of TB in HIV infected adults, and there may be an increased risk of drug resistant forms of TB due to the higher rates of resistance in HIV infected adults.
- Diagnosis of TB is complicated by overlapping symptoms of TB and HIV. Chronic cough, failure to gain weight and fatigue are all symptoms of HIV as well as TB. Tuberculosis may present as acute bacterial pneumonia. There is a high prevalence of chronic lung disease and of severe pulmonary disease, especially of cavitations. There is a reduced reliability of PPD skin testing in the presence of HIV.
- Treatment of tuberculosis is more complicated in the presence of HIV. Malabsorption of TB drugs, especially RMP, is well documented in HIV-infected individuals. Failure of resolution of clinical and/radiological features and persistent positive cultures are well documented after six months of therapy. Therefore, many experts agree that children with severe tuberculosis should be managed for nine rather than six months. Where possible, clinical and radiological review and follow-up cultures should be performed prior to stopping TB therapy. Resolution should be documented. Due to the severity of TB disease in HIV, children may require management with more drugs than usual.
- TB carries higher mortality rates in HIV infected children.

Co-treatment of HIV and TB is complicated by:
- High pill burden, which increases the risk for poor adherence.

Table 17.9 Adverse events shared by antituberculosis drugs and antiretroviral drugs

Adverse effect	Antituberculous Drugs	Antiretroviral	Intervention
Rash	PZA, RMP, INH	NVP, EFV, ABC	Clinical monitoring and pre treatment guidance
Nausea and vomiting	ETH, EMB, PZA, RMP, INH	AZT, RTV, Kaletra	
Hepatitis	PZA, RMP, INH, ETH	NVP, all PIs, EFV	Regular monitoring of ALT
Bone marrow	INH, RMP	AZT	Symptomatic therapy
Peripheral neuropathy	INH	D4T / DDI	Add Vitamin B6 to management in all children

- Overlapping toxicity. Adult data suggests that HIV infected persons experience a higher rate of adverse events when treated for TB. Limited paediatric data suggests that the risk of adverse events relates to the number of drugs used. In addition, TB drugs and antiretroviral therapy share many side effects, especially hepatic, haematological and cutaneous (*see* Table 17.9).
- Rifampicin is a potent inducer of the cytochrome p450 enzyme and p-glycoprotein. This could lead to subtherapeutic levels of protease inhibitors and nevirapine, which increases the risk of resistance and failure of antiretroviral therapy. Reduced plasma levels of non-nucleoside reverse transcriptase inhibitors (NNRTI) are well documented and more frequent with nevirapine than efavirenz. For children on lopinavir/ritonavir, added ritonavir reduces this problem. Co-administration of nevirapine and RMP is not recommended. Drug adjustments are therefore required.

The following is therefore recommended:

1 **Child presents with TB before starting anti-retroviral therapy**:

   For many children with HIV, TB is their presenting illness and therefore they will have not yet started antiretroviral therapy:
   - Children >3 years and >10 kg: 2 NRTIs plus efavirenz. There is no need to adjust the dose of efavirenz.
   - Children <10 kg and 3 years: 2NRTI and

Table 17.10 Recommendation on the timing of antiretroviral therapy in patients on TB treatment for children >1 year

Stage	When to initiate antiretroviral therapy if on TB therapy
4	Start antiretroviral therapy 2–8 weeks later
3	Severe advanced suppression Start antiretroviral therapy 2–8 weeks later Mild or moderate suppression Evaluate the possibility of delaying antiretroviral therapy till after completion of TB treatment. If poor response to TB treatment antiretroviral therapy should be started

LPV/r with added RTV at the same dose of LPV. For each ml of LPV/r, add 0.75 ml RTV. RTV has a short shelf life and a vile taste. It may also increase gastrointestinal discomfort and vomiting. Parents of children on four antiretrovirals require additional supportive counselling. Discontinue extra RTV two weeks after stopping TB treatment. This allows for a washout period where there may still be rapid metabolism of LPV.

- For children <1 year of age, in those with advanced immunosuppression or Stage 3 or 4 HIV disease, antiretroviral therapy should be initiated shortly (as soon as two weeks) after beginning antituberculosis treatment.

2 The child develops TB while on antiretroviral therapy:

Although the risk of TB is decreased for children on antiretroviral therapy, children are still at higher risk than the general population. The options depend on the current regimen, as class changes should be avoided. The options are as follows:

- If on LPV/r, add RTV
- If on nevirapine and,
- >3 years of age and weight >10 kg, switch to efavirenz.
- If <3 years of age or weight <10 kg, switch to LPV/r and RTV if fully suppressed. Alternatively, where LPV/r is unavailable, use NVP at the maximum dosage for body surface area. In children not fully virally suppressed, consult an expert.

3 The immune reconstitution inflammatory syndrome (IRIS) is a paradoxical worsening of inflammation usually due to TB infection after antiretroviral-induced improvement in the patient's immune status. Although seldom fatal, morbidity includes prolonged hospitalization and significant diagnostic confusion. The risk is highest in children with disseminated TB, severe immune suppression and a short interval between TB treatment and antiretroviral initiation. Despite risk of IRIS, delaying antiretroviral therapy may lead to death and a poor response to antituberculosis therapy.

Drug-resistant tuberculosis

Any population of *M.tb* will contain a small number of resistant organisms arising at a relatively low but constant rate by spontaneous mutation. Monotherapy, either intentional or unintentional (for example, one active agent in child with unsuspected multidrug resistance), kills off susceptible bacteria, thereby allowing the resistant organisms to proliferate, replacing the former. Large tuberculous lesions penetrated by low concentrations of a single drug will rapidly lead to excessive multiplication of drug-resistant organisms, whereas even low concentra-

tions of two medicines can inhibit such growth. Development of resistance through inadequate medication, is termed 'previously treated' (or acquired) resistance. Inadequate chemotherapy is most often due to either poor prescribing practices or to failure to comply by the patient/caregiver.

Patients without prior antituberculosis therapy may be infected by bacilli from a drug-resistant source case and have 'new' (or primary) drug resistance, i.e. transmitted resistance. Most drug resistance in childhood will be transmitted resistance, because children usually have paucibacillary (low bacillary load) tuberculosis, making the development of drug resistance unlikely.

Resistance to one first-line drug is referred to as monoresistance; poly-drug resistance is resistance to two or more first-line medicines, but not to both INH and RMP; multidrug resistance (MDR) is resistance to both INH and RMP with or without other medicines, and extensive drug resistance (XDR) is MDR tuberculosis plus resistance to the fluoroquinolones and one or more of the second-line injectables agents (kanamycin, amikacin and/or capreomycin).

Drug resistance is a microbiological diagnosis-culture and drug susceptibility test (DST) result from either the child or the adult source case is necessary to confirm the diagnosis. Clinical and radiological features do not distinguish between susceptible and resistant TB.

Drug-resistant (and especially MDR) TB is diagnosed as follows:

- Confirmed drug resistance: Drug Susceptibility Test from the child's *M.tb* isolate confirms drug resistance
- Probable drug resistance: Infectious (adult) source case has confirmed drug-resistant tuberculosis
- Suspected drug resistance: Child with TB not responding to treatment while adherence to antituberculosis treatment is good or; contact with an infectious pulmonary TB case who fails treatment, is a retreatment case or has chronic tuberculosis.

When drug resistance is suspected, every effort should be made to obtain a culture of *M.tb* for DST. If known in either the child or adult source case, a treatment regimen should be constructed considering the DST result as well as previous antituberculosis medicines used, When drug resistance is a possibility (not confirmed in child or source case) the initiation of treatment should await the results of DST in the child or source case. When this is not advisable due to the seriousness of disease a regimen should be constructed using three or preferably four agents to which neither the child nor the source case have been exposed.

The following important points should be considered when treating MDR- or XDR-TB cases:

- To prevent further worsening of drug resistance, single agents should *never* be added to a failing regimen.
- Only daily treatment with directly observed therapy should be used.
- Three, or preferably four, medicines to which the isolate is susceptible or naïve (not previously used in patient or source case) should be used. The regimen should further take into account different drug groups and possible cross-resistance between medicines.
- Counselling and patient motivation is important, as parents find it difficult to understand why children need to be treated for 12–18 months or more.

- Treatment of MDR and XDR tuberculosis should preferably be managed in a centre with expertise, as the treatment and adverse events are complicated.

Management of child contacts of drug-resistant source cases

Child contacts of drug-resistant TB cases should be screened the same way as those in contact with susceptible TB. Contacts of INH-monoresistant source cases (<5 years or HIV-infected) should receive RMP 10 mg/kg/day for six months. Current national guidelines recommend that child contacts of MDR and XDR tuberculosis cases should receive INH prophylaxis only (as they may have also had contact with a drug susceptible case) and careful follow-up (at least two-monthly) should continue for a minimum of 12 months. If disease develops, they should be started on a MDR-/XDR tuberculosis treatment regimen. Some experts advise an alternative preventive treatment regimen of high-dose INH (15–20 mg/kg/day) with (in MDR TB contacts) or without (in XDR TB contacts) two medicines to which the source case is susceptible, usually a fluoroquinolone (ofloxacin) plus EMB or ETH (if source case resistant to EMB).

18

Human Immuno-deficiency Virus Infection

The human immunodeficiency viruses (HIV) belong to a large family of related retroviruses. Members of the retrovirus group have been known to cause immunodeficiency, malignancy, and central nervous system degeneration in other animals. The core of the human immunodeficiency virus (*see* Figure 18.1) contains RNA and the enzyme reverse transcriptase. The outer coat contains lipid and glycoprotein 120 (gp 120).

Epidemiology

The first cases of AIDS in Africa were described in 1983, and by 1987 comprised only 9.6 per cent of the known AIDS cases worldwide. The virus has since spread rapidly to produce a pandemic affecting every country in the world. HIV/AIDS is most serious in Africa and spreading rapidly; about 70 per cent of the world's AIDS burden is borne by Africa.

Some of the factors that have contributed to the severity of this epidemic in Africa are:
- Migrant labour, especially from one country to another, and from rural to urban areas
- Social and economic devastation
- Poor access to health and educational services
- Erosion of traditional values and breakdown of family life
- Cultural practices.

Almost 90 per cent of all HIV-infected children live in sub-Saharan Africa. Every day in sub-Saharan Africa, about 1 000 children acquire HIV-1 infection from their mothers. It was

Figure 18.1 Human immunodeficiency virus (HIV)

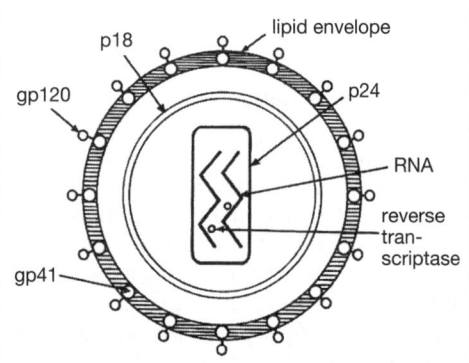

The glycoproteins (gp) and proteins (p) are important, as they are the antigens which stimulate the immune systems to generate specific antibodies.
(Adapted from 'Explaining the nature of the virus that causes AIDS'; AIDS Action, issue 3.) © Dr Don Jeffries, Virology Dept., St. Bartholomews Hospital.

estimated that in 2007, 370 000 children became HIV-infected, and 270 000 children under 15 years of age died from HIV/AIDS (UNAIDS).

In children, transmission of HIV infection occurs in the following ways:
- Mother-to-Child Transmission (MTCT or *vertical transmission*): accounts for the large majority (>95 per cent) of HIV infection in children. Infection may occur through intra-uterine transmission, intrapartum transmission, or postnatally through breastfeeding

- Sexual abuse: the child is sexually abused by an HIV infected adult or adolescent
- Blood transfusion: all blood/blood products in SA are screened
- Scarification/body piercings with unsterile instruments
- Horizontal transmission: in sexually active adolescents.

World-wide, vertically acquired HIV infection of children now presents in two distinct epidemiological patterns.

In the more developed world mother-to-child transmission is now uncommon because of effective antenatal care and diagnosis, antiretroviral prophylaxis, elective Caesarean section and formula feeding.

In resource-poor and developing countries, on the other hand, many barriers exist to effective implementation of programmes to reduce mother-to-child transmission of HIV, leading to a persistently high infection rate of infants. The biggest challenge exists at the community level where family and community systems are breaking down around children infected or affected by HIV/AIDS. Furthermore, the acknowledged risk of breast milk transmission is a major social and nutritional dilemma in countries where most of the advances in infant mortality rates have been due to campaigns in support of breast feeding. If availability, safety and nutritional adequacy of replacement feeding cannot be guaranteed, a lowered HIV transmission rate due to formula feeding could well be cancelled out by increased morbidity and mortality from enteral infection and malnutrition (see Table 18.1).

Transmission

The risk of vertical transmission is influenced by a number of identified factors:
- A high maternal viral load
- A high viral load in vaginal and cervical secretions
- Chorioamnionitis
- Maternal vitamin A deficiency
- Vaginal delivery
- Duration of ruptured membranes longer than four hours
- Instrumentation during delivery
- Prematurity
- A high viral load in breast milk

- Local breast pathology such as mastitis or cracked nipples
- Local mouth factors of baby such as oral thrush or sores
- Mixed (non-exclusive) breastfeeding
- Longer duration of breastfeeding.

These enable targeted interventions to reduce the risk (See Table 18.2).

Prevention of transmission

HIV has direct and indirect impacts on both maternal and child survival. HIV-positive mothers suffer an increased risk of dying within two years after giving birth, compared with HIV-negative mothers. This places their infants at risk of increased mortality independent of the child's own HIV-infection status.

Most of childhood HIV/AIDS is acquired through mother-to-child-transmission. Prevention of heterosexual transmission in young adults and adolescents will therefore reduce childhood HIV. Programmes to combat sexually transmitted infections have a positive influence on the

Table 18.1 Epidemiological patterns of paediatric HIV

Developed countries	Developing countries
Effective prevention of mother-to-child transmission, therefore a low infection rate <2%. The emphasis in HIV management shifts to ▪ *Missed opportunities of prevention* ▪ *Effects of intra-uterine antiretroviral therapy exposure* ▪ *Optimized individual therapy*	Persisting high level epidemic in underserved populations with an overwhelming impact on community-wide patterns of morbidity and mortality. ▪ *Emphasize strategies of prevention of mother-to-child-transmission and of access to resources and care* ▪ *The risk of MTCT from breastfeeding is a major social, nutritional and medical dilemma*

Table 18.2 Interventions to reduce the risk of mother-to-child-transmission

Risk category	Interventions
Maternal status during antenatal care	■ Initiate antiretroviral therapy or antiretroviral prophylaxis for PMTCT according to the most appropriate protocol for local circumstances ■ Personal hygiene and health care with special emphasis on adequate and early treatment of sexually transmitted and inflammatory conditions of the genital tract ■ Counselling and support on nutrition including improving vitamin A status and providing food and nutrient supplementation in circumstances of potential deficiency
Fetal status *in utero*	■ Prevent premature delivery ■ Manage clinical and subclinical chorioamnionitis with appropriate antibiotics
Labour and delivery	■ Consider Caesarian section delivery before labour and before rupture of membranes ■ Delay rupture of membranes ■ Antiseptic and virucidal cleansing of vaginal canal ■ Limit instrumentation during delivery and episiotomy as far as possible ■ Reduce fetal exposure to maternal blood
Infant exposure to infection	■ Pre- and post-exposure antiretroviral prophylaxis during labour and after delivery ■ Exclusive breastfeeding for up to six months with rapid weaning or alternatively exclusive formula feeding ■ Pasteurise or flash heat expressed breast milk ■ Early treatment of oral thrush or sores
Post-partum mother	■ Counselling and support on infant feeding

reduction of HIV prevalence and are therefore important strategies for prevention.

In the absence of a cure or vaccine, prevention is the only method available at present to help reduce the spread of HIV/AIDS. Prevention programmes should take into account local cultural beliefs and attitudes, but it has been shown that antiretroviral prophylaxis administered to a woman during pregnancy and delivery, and to her infant shortly following birth sharply reduces the likelihood of the mother passing HIV infection to her baby.

Prerequisites to the prevention of MTCT are an efficient system of identification of infected women during the antenatal period by informed counselling and voluntary testing, and all the issues surrounding access, counselling on availability of therapy options, compliance and support. The most serious impediment to the introduction of cost-effective strategies is a lack of capacity and infrastructure. Large numbers of women deliver prematurely or outside the healthcare setting in remote rural areas or urban slums. Poor geographical service reach, aggravated by weak health systems, and the fear, stigma and denial that discourage many women from being tested for HIV are significant barriers to wider PMTCT coverage.

Accordingly, the appropriate place for a programme for the prevention of mother-to-child-transmission (PMTCT) is in the antenatal services, where it should be integrated with the maternal, newborn and child health (MNCH) programmes and should have direct linkages to the local HIV services for the ongoing management of both mother and child.

Table 18.3 Essential components of an integrated PMTCT programme

Services for antenatal care	Services for HIV-positive women in the postpartum period
<ul><li>Essential antenatal care including routine offer of HIV testing and counselling</li><li>Clinical and immunological assessment of HIV-positive women</li><li>Initiation of antiretroviral treatment and prophylaxis for PMTCT</li><li>Screening, prevention and treatment of TB</li></ul>	<ul><li>Provide counselling and support on infant feeding</li><li>Provide follow-up care for mother and infant:</li></ul> *HIV-related care and antiretroviral therapy when indicated* *Cotrimoxazole prophylaxis for women and their infants*
<ul><li>Screening, prevention and management of STIs</li><li>Screening for and management of liver disease</li><li>Screening for and management of injecting drug use</li><li>Cotrimoxazole and isoniazid prophylaxis</li><li>Counselling and support on nutrition</li><li>Counselling and support on infant feeding</li><li>Management of malaria in stable malaria areas</li></ul>	*Sexual and reproductive health services* *Counselling and support on feeding and nutrition* *Diagnosis of HIV infection in infants* <ul><li>Adherence support for women receiving antiretroviral therapy</li></ul>

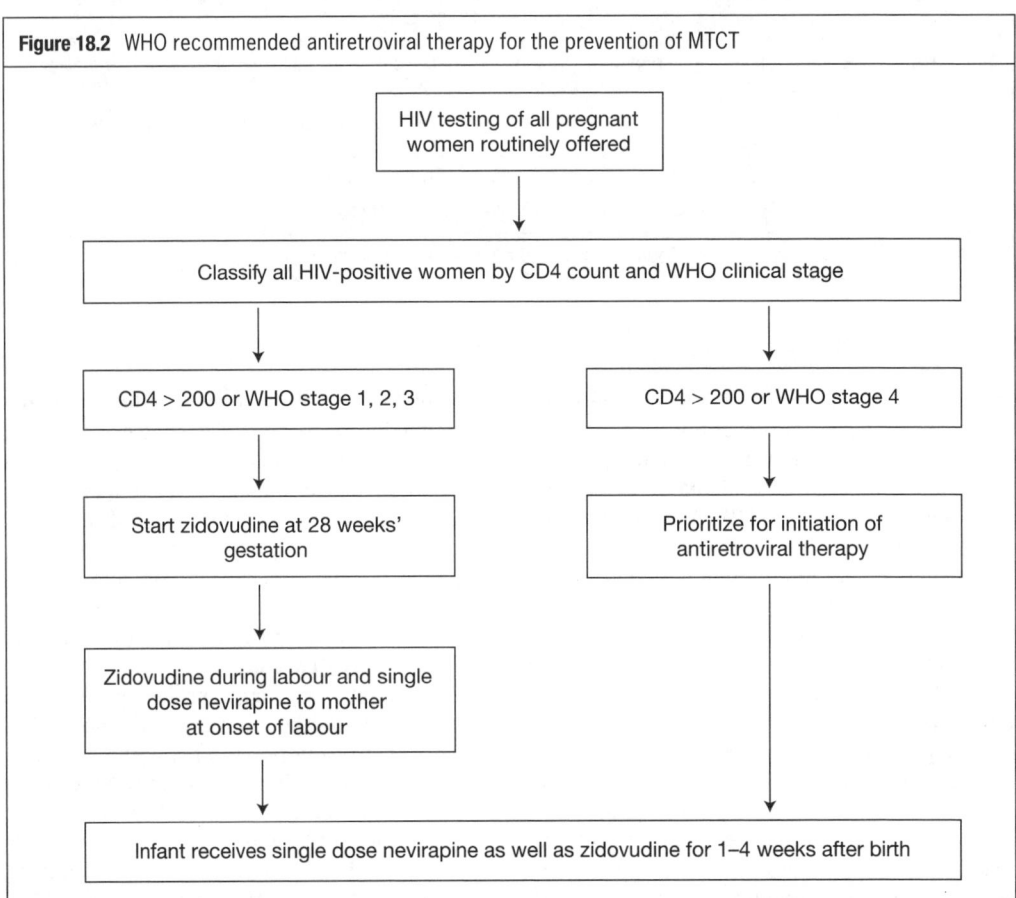

Figure 18.2 WHO recommended antiretroviral therapy for the prevention of MTCT

HIV testing of all pregnant women routinely offered

Classify all HIV-positive women by CD4 count and WHO clinical stage

CD4 > 200 or WHO stage 1, 2, 3 | CD4 > 200 or WHO stage 4

Start zidovudine at 28 weeks' gestation | Prioritize for initiation of antiretroviral therapy

Zidovudine during labour and single dose nevirapine to mother at onset of labour

Infant receives single dose nevirapine as well as zidovudine for 1–4 weeks after birth

Community mobilization and family support, especially from men, for women who are HIV-positive remain urgent priorities.

Pathogenesis and diagnosis

The human immunodeficiency virus infects the helper-inducer T_4 or CD_4+ subset of T-lymphocytes, macrophages, and other cells. The external envelope glycoprotein gp120 of HIV has great affinity for the CD_4 molecule, which is present on the surface of these cells.

The gut is the commonest portal of entry for vertically acquired postnatal HIV infection. As gut epithelial cells do not express the CD4 receptor, the HI virus gains entry to the lamina propria by means of additional receptors and co-receptors. These co-receptors include CCR5 (used by virus that penetrates macrophages, e.g. in the gut) and CXCR4 (used by viruses that penetrate T-cells). Ongoing viral replication in lymphoid tissue and the release of inflammatory mediators results in physiological alterations and features of immune dysregulation and immune-mediated disorders, even before immune deficiency is clinically obvious.

HIV irreversibly infects cells; these die (apoptosis) or are destroyed. When a large proportion of these lymphocytes have been destroyed this results in immunodeficiency or immune collapse, which leads to the clinical manifestations of AIDS.

Immunological abnormalities in paediatric AIDS:

T-cells:
- Total lymphopaenia
- CD4 lymphopaenia
- Reversal of CD4:CD8 ratio.

B-cells:
- Hypergamma-globulinaemia (early abnormality)
- Abnormal antibody response to variety of antigens.

Polymorphonuclear neutrophils:
- Neutropaenia
- Impaired chemotaxis and phagocytosis.

Clinical suspicion

HIV infection is commonly associated with the following circumstances:

At birth:
- HIV-infected mother
- Low birth weight and prematurity

Infancy and early childhood:
- Recurrent infections
- Infections with unusual organisms
- Unusual presentation or course of a common infection
- Unexplained failure to thrive, or wasting
- Resistant oral thrush
- Unexplained hepatosplenomegaly and generalized lymphadenopathy
- Unexplained tone disturbances

Childhood:
- Cardiomyopathy
- Nephropathy
- Lymphocytic interstitial pneumonitis
- Encephalopathy
- Unexplained multisystemic symptoms or signs
- Unusual haematological disturbances and malignancies.

Suspect HIV infection if three or more of the following clinical conditions are found together:

- Pneumonia
- Ear discharge at any stage,
- Low weight-for-age or unsatisfactory weight gain
- Persistent diarrhoea now or in the past three months
- Enlarged lymph glands in two or more sites
- Oral thrush
- Parotid enlargement.

Laboratory diagnosis of HIV infection

It is important to identify HIV infection in pregnant women as an HIV-infected mother can transmit the infection to her offspring. Therefore every pregnant mother must be offered counselling and testing. It is important to make an early diagnosis in an HIV-exposed baby before symptoms develop. This could help the family deal with the diagnosis, or be reassured if the child is uninfected. An infant who is confirmed HIV positive should be followed up regularly (see Comprehensive clinical care), while the care giver of an infant who is confirmed HIV negative should be counselled and supported so that she adheres to feeding options that reduce the risk of HIV transmission.

All infants born to HIV infected women are 'exposed' to HIV infection. Even though they may or may not become infected, they will all test positive by serological (antibody) tests as they acquire maternal HIV antibodies transplacentally. These infants are termed 'HIV-exposed' and the transferred antibodies (IgG) may persist for up to 18 months. Therefore antibody tests alone are not diagnostic of infection in this age group. The preferred method of testing in these young infants is therefore detection of viral particles by Polymerase Chain Reaction (PCR) for the HIV-1 DNA or RNA, performed after four to six weeks of age. Other methods of testing in infants include HIV-1 viral culture and HIV-1 P24 antigen detection.

HIV-1 infection in children >18 months of age can be confirmed by serological tests alone, which detect antibodies to groups of viral proteins, as in adults. The Enzyme-Linked Immunosorbent Assay (ELISA) is the preferred method of testing. Using the Rapid test (must have two positive tests) provides a quick and reliable method of confirming the diagnosis.

DIAGNOSIS OF HIV-1 INFECTION:

Children <18 months:
 Positive HIV-1 DNA or RNA PCR or
 Positive HIV-1 P24 antigen (infant
 >1month or
 Positve HIV-1 culture
Children >18 months:
Positive HIV-1 antibody detection (positive ELISA
or repeatedly positive Rapid Test or confirmatory
Western Blot or immunofluorescence assay)

A breastfeeding infant continues to be at risk of acquiring infection, therefore a negative HIV-1 DNA/RNA PCR (if <18 months) or antibody test (if >18 months) should be repeated at least six weeks after breastfeeding has stopped. All HIV-exposed infants should have a confirmatory serological test at 18 months of age.

Before performing laboratory tests it is important that informed parental consent be obtained and confidentiality maintained at all times. It is essential for the mother to understand that an HIV test on her baby is an indirect test of her own status. As this might have far-reaching implications for the mother, pre-test and post-test counselling is an essential part of diagnostic testing. In particular, the doctor should be certain that the caregiver (e.g. grandmother) is indeed appropriate and competent to be approached for consent. This can raise serious ethical issues.

Staging

Once an infant or child has been diagnosed as HIV infected, he/she should be allocated a clinical and immunological disease stage according to the criteria listed in Tables 18.4 and 18.5. Staging is important because:

- It helps to determine the prognosis.
- It guides the management and consideration for antiretroviral therapy.

Clinical staging of HIV Infection: Two classification systems are available: the World Health Organization (WHO) classification and the Centres for Disease Control and Prevention (CDC) classification. The recently revised WHO clinical staging system (*see* Table 18.4) is based on the presence of a number of indicator or AIDS-defining clinical and laboratory conditions in four clinical categories, ranging from asymptomatic to severe. It is widely used in resource-limited settings. The CDC paediatric HIV staging system is based on a composite of four clinical and three immunological categories.

Immunological staging of HIV Infection: The CDC in the USA has established strict criteria for the definition of paediatric AIDS. Decreasing numbers of CD4 lymphocytes, and inverted CD4:CD8 ratios are the immunological hallmarks of an advancing HIV infection. Total CD4 counts vary according to age, and in infants and younger children the CD4 percentage, rather than the absolute count, is the best indicator of the state of the immune system. (*see* Table 18.5)

Natural history and clinical manifestations

Untreated, HIV infection progresses from asymptomatic infection to symptomatic disease to full-blown AIDS. This progression occurs more rapidly in children than in adults. The course

Table 18.4. WHO clinical staging of HIV/AIDS
(For persons under 15 years of age with confirmed laboratory evidence of HIV infection)

Stage I	▪ Asymptomatic ▪ Persistent generalized lymphadenopathy
Stage II	▪ Hepatosplenomegaly ▪ Papular pruritic eruptions ▪ Seborrhoeic dermatitis ▪ Extensive human papilloma virus infection ▪ Extensive molluscum contagiosum ▪ Fungal nail infections ▪ Recurrent oral ulcerations ▪ Lineal gingival erythema (LGE) ▪ Angular cheilitis ▪ Parotid enlargement ▪ Herpes zoster ▪ Recurrent or chronic RTIs (otitis media, otorrhoea, sinusitis)
Stage III	▪ Moderate unexplained malnutrition not adequately responding to standard therapy ▪ Unexplained persistent diarrhoea (14 days or more) ▪ Unexplained persistent fever (intermittent or constant, for longer than one month) ▪ Oral candidiasis (outside neonatal period) ▪ Oral hairy leukoplakia ▪ Acute necrotizing ulcerative gingivitis/periodontitis ▪ Pulmonary TB ▪ Tuberculous lymphadenopathy (axillary, cervical or inguinal) ▪ Severe recurrent presumed bacterial pneumonia ▪ Unexplained anaemia (<8 gm/dl), and/or neutropaenia (<500/mm³) and/or thrombocytopaenia (<50 000/mm³) for more than one month ▪ Chronic HIV-associated lung disease including bronchiectasis ▪ Symptomatic lymphoid interstitial pneumonitis (LIP)
Stage IV	▪ Unexplained severe wasting or severe malnutrition not adequately responding to standard therapy ▪ Pneumocystis pneumonia ▪ Recurrent severe presumed bacterial infection (e.g. empyema, pyomyositis, bone or joint infection, meningitis, but excluding pneumonia) ▪ Chronic herpes simplex infection (orolabial or cutaneous of more than one month's duration) ▪ Extrapulmonary TB ▪ Kaposi's sarcoma ▪ Oesophageal candidiasis ▪ CNS toxoplasmosis (outside the neonatal period) ▪ HIV encephalopathy ▪ CMV infection (CMV retinitis or CMV infection of organs other than liver, spleen or lymph nodes; onset at the age of 1 month or more) ▪ Extrapulmonary cryptococcosis including meningitis ▪ Any disseminated endemic mycosis (e.g. extrapulmonary histoplasmosis, coccidiomycosis, penicilliosis) ▪ Cryptosporidiosis ▪ Isosporiasis

Table 18.4. *continued*	
Stage IV	▪ Disseminated non-tuberculous mycobacterial infection
	▪ Candida of trachea, bronchi or lungs
	▪ Visceral herpes simplex infection
	▪ Acquired HIV-associated rectal fistula
	▪ Cerebral or B cell non-Hodgkin's lymphoma
	▪ Progressive multifocal leukoencephalopathy (PML)
	▪ HIV-associated cardiomyopathy or HIV-associated nephropathy

Table 18.5 Immunological categories of paediatric HIV

	Age of child					
Immunologic category	<12 months		1–5 years		6–12 years	
	CD4/ml	(%)	CD4/ml	(%)	CD4/ml	(%)
1: No immunosuppression	≥1500	(≥25)	≥1000	(≥25)	≥500	(≥25)
2: Moderate immunosuppression	750–1 499	(15–24)	500–999	(15–24)	200–499	(15–24)
3: Severe immunosuppression	<750	(<15)	<500	(<15)	<200	(<15)

From: Centres for Disease Control and Prevention: MMWR 43(RR–12): 1–19, 1994

of the disease is quite variable; some patients deteriorate rapidly within the first few months of life (*fast progressors*), most progress more slowly (*intermediate progressors*), and a few perinatally infected babies have survived to adolescence (*slow progressors*).

The timing of infection, as well as a number of other factors, appear to determine the duration of the incubation period and the rate of disease progression:

- Children with perinatal infection are assumed to be infected *in utero* or at birth. Those infected *in utero* may have more severe disease and rapid disease progression. The incubation period is usually between four and six months; however, in some instances it has been found to be much shorter, or as long as seven years. Approximately 50 per cent of paediatric cases are diagnosed during the first year of life and up to 80 per cent by two years of age.
- Many babies are born with a low birth weight for gestational age; this may reflect

a poor maternal status with obstetric complications or early infection. Many such infants present with AIDS-defining conditions within the first few months of life.

- The low level of transplacentally acquired maternal antibodies associated with prematurity is associated with a higher risk of disease and more rapid progression of disease.
- The immunosuppressive effect of poor nutrition or repeated intercurrent infections may contribute to a rapid evolution of the disease.
- Some predictors of poor early outcome can be identified at birth, such as a lower mean birth weight, asphyxia, neonatal jaundice and infections.

Clinical manifestations

The clinical manifestations of HIV infection are wide-ranging. By three months of age, 60 per cent of HIV-infected infants manifest some signs and symptoms of disease.

Earliest manifestations

The earliest manifestations of infection include:

- Thrush
- Lymphadenopathy
- Growth failure
- Tone disturbances.
- More severe early manifestations include *Pneumocystis jirovecii* pneumonia, cytomegalovirus virus infection, and tuberculosis.

Generalized lymphadenopathy/hepatosplenomegaly

Generalized lymphadenopathy, often with large but discrete nodes, with or without hepatosplenomegaly, is one of the commonest presentations in children with symptomatic HIV. This is most frequently due to the immune reaction to HIV, but tuberculosis, cytomegalovirus and other herpes groups must be considered. Generalized lymphadenopathy and parotid and other salivary gland enlargement are also associated with lymphocytic interstitial pneumonitis.

Failure to thrive

Growth failure is usual and early, but typical kwashiorkor is seen less frequently than severe wasting. Even where diarrhoea is not a major feature, patients may remain anorexic and lose weight or fail to thrive. In many patients admitted with apparent protein-energy malnutrition, there are unusual features such as the degree of subcutaneous wasting, or the persistence of relatively normal-looking hair in spite of apparently severe protein deficiency, which point to malnutrition acquired secondarily to an underlying disease process.

Recurrent infections

Common problems such as septicaemia, pneumonia, meningitis, and abscesses may occur before any other features of HIV infection are evident. These infections are recurrent and severe, but usually respond well to antibiotic therapy. Infecting organisms include *Streptococcus pneumoniae*, *Haemophilus influenzae*, *Staphylococcus aureus*, and Gram-negative organisms, including salmonella. Chronic suppurative otitis media is a very common complication.

Opportunistic and viral infections cause complications in children with more established HIV disease. Candida, *Pneumocystis jirovecii*, Epstein

Barr virus (EBV), cytomegalovirus (CMV), Herpes simplex, adenovirus, and cryptosporidium have been isolated from these patients. Tuberculosis has a particularly strong association with HIV.

Respiratory system

Pulmonary disease is a frequent, and often the first, presentation in childhood HIV. It is associated with high morbidity and mortality. Multiple opportunistic pathogens may be present in infants presenting with severe pneumonia. Bacterial pneumonia is frequent in children and may be associated with bacteraemia. (*See* Chapter 25, Respiratory tract disorders.)

Pneumocystis jirovecii, a fungus, causes opportunistic infection in immunosuppressed patients. A common presentation is acute onset of tachypnoea, fever, and non-productive cough. Hypoxaemia is frequently present.

A presumptive diagnosis of *P. jirovecii* pneumonia should be made in infants in the following cases:

- There is no improvement after three days of locally recommended antimicrobial therapy.
- A high concentration of oxygen is needed to correct the cyanosis.
- The serum LDH is elevated above 500 IU/l.

Tuberculosis

In developing countries, tuberculosis is frequently found in adults and children with HIV infection. There is extensive overlap between the clinical features of the two diseases, tuberculin skin testing is often unsuccessful due to the suppression of delayed hypersensitivity in HIV, and therefore the diagnosis is difficult. Strenuous efforts should be made to diagnose or exclude TB in all HIV infected children, as antiretroviral therapy is also more complex in the face of co-existing TB. (*see* Chapter 17, Tuberculosis).

Lymphocytic interstitial pneumonitis (LIP) is a chronic, progressive pulmonary disorder, usually presenting after the first year of life. Cough is present with normal auscultatory findings. Hypoxaemia is frequently present. Digital clubbing occurs as the disease progresses. Generalized lymphadenopathy and parotid and other salivary gland enlargement are usually present. The pathogenesis is unclear. A diffuse nodular pattern, with or without hilar or paratracheal lymph node enlargement, may be present on the chest X-ray (*see* Chapter 25, Respiratory tract disorders).

Gastrointestinal tract

Gastrointestinal symptoms including anorexia, vomiting and diarrhoea are extremely common. Associated oral thrush, generalized lymphade-nopathy, hepatosplenomegaly and respiratory symptoms are very suggestive of HIV-related diarrhoea. In the developing world, these occur against the background of a very high incidence of acute infective diarrhoea. There may be acute watery diarrhoea, which can lead to dehydration, or persistent diarrhoea with failure to thrive. The stools may contain frank blood or red cells may be found together with faecal leucocytes on stool dipstick examination. Combinations of malabsorptive features may be found including lactose or monosaccharide malabsorption and increased stool fat (*see* Chapter 24, Gastrointestinal disorders).

Neurological system

A large number of children with HIV infection will develop neurological involvement. Features include HIV encephalopathy (triad of micro-cephaly, developmental delay or regression of milestones and tone disturbances), seizures, secondary CNS infections (e.g. bacterial menin-gitis), and cryptococcal meningitis (*see* Chapter 26, Neurological and muscular disorders).

Haematological abnormalities/malignancies

Several abnormalities have been reported, of which immune thrombocytopaenia is the most serious. Others are anaemia, lymphopaenia, and neutropaenia.

Kaposi's sarcoma, T-cell lymphomas, and leu-kaemia appear to be affecting younger children. (*See* Chapter 22, Neoplastic disorders.)

Cardiovascular system

HIV-associated cardiomyopathy, pericardial effusion, and conduction abnormalities have been reported in children. These generally manifest later in childhood.

Renal disease

Abnormal urinalyses are a frequent finding. Urinary tract infection occurs commonly. HIV-associated nephropathy (mainly glomerulosclerosis)

is uncommon, but, when it occurs, the prognosis appears to be poor.

Management of the HIV infected child

Comprehensive clinical care consists of:

- Counselling and support of mothers and care-givers
- Counselling and support on infant feeding choices
- Nutritional advice and routine micronutrient supplementation
- Growth monitoring
- Immunization
- *Pneumocystis jirovecii* prophylaxis
- Routine treatment for intestinal worms
- Prompt and adequate treatment of intercurrent infections
- Antiretroviral therapy
- Monitoring and follow-up

Counselling the mother

The mother needs to be counselled about the implications of the diagnosis for herself and her child. Often, she is not aware of her own status when the diagnosis is made in her child. She may therefore experience the double shock of being told of HIV infection in her child and herself, so the health worker must be aware of the normal emotional reactions that mothers may experience in response to bad news, and be prepared to repeat the information at several subsequent sessions. Any queries that the mother or care giver has, should be addressed.

The treatment outcomes are strongly dependent on the mother's compliance in giving treatment and bringing the child for follow-up appointments. A strong effort should therefore be made to ensure mother's understanding, trust and commitment.

A clear follow-up schedule should be devised. Ideally all HIV-exposed infants should be followed up monthly for the first year of life. At six weeks, PJP prophylaxis is initiated and the infant's status determined by PCR. The care giver should be educated about possible signs and symptoms of HIV disease and in the event, the need to seek earlier medical attention.

Many families still experience stigmatization and ostracism in their communities. Health workers must be sensitive to these issues in their dealings with patients and families, but at the same time maintain a non-judgmental frankness and openness. Mothers must understand that denying or hiding their child's diagnosis is to the child's disadvantage; healthworkers must maintain patient confidentiality at all times.

Infant feeding choices

(*See* Chapter 9, Feeding of infants and young children)

HIV may be transmitted by breast milk and can confer an additional 5–16 per cent risk of infection after birth, depending on the pattern and duration of breastfeeding. The risk is increased when there is mixed feeding, i.e. giving breast milk and something else such as formula, porridge, water.

HIV-infected women should be counselled during pregnancy about their infant feeding choices.

> The most appropriate infant feeding option for a mother with HIV depends on her individual circumstances, including her health and her local family circumstances.

Health professionals should ensure that the mother is able to make a fully informed choice, but should guard against assuming that they can impose their advice on mothers, and should be prepared to support the mother in her own choice.

- Exclusive breastfeeding is recommended for HIV-infected mothers for the first six months of the child's life unless replacement feeding is acceptable, affordable, sustainable and safe for them and their infants before that time.
- When replacement feeding is acceptable, feasible, affordable, sustainable and safe, avoidance of all breastfeeding by HIV-infected mothers is recommended.
- All HIV-exposed infants should receive regular follow-up care and periodic re-assessment of infant feeding choices,

particularly at the time of infant diagnosis and at six months.

Exclusive formula feeding may be difficult where water, fuel or cleaning utensils and materials are scarce or where the family expects the mother to breastfeed. Formula feeding under such circumstances subjects the infants to the risk of developing potentially fatal gastroenteritis and other infections.

The HIV-positive mother who has chosen not to breastfeed must be shown how to prepare feeds, must know what volume and strength of feed to prepare, how often to feed the infant and how to use a cup rather than a bottle. Cup feeding should be promoted as cups are easy to clean.

Flash heating of expressed breast milk is a safe method of replacement feeding for HIV-positive mothers. Heat treating breast milk inactivates the HIV virus and will eliminate titres of most other viruses, thus ensuring a safe supply of breast milk from HIV-positive mothers to their own infants. Studies have shown that mothers who have been breastfeeding in the first six months can then switch to expressing and heat treatment of their breast milk to prevent any risk of HIV transmission while maintaining the nutritional and immunological benefits of breast milk.

Method of heat treating expressed breast milk

1 Express between 50–120 ml milk into a clean 450 ml glass jar.
2 Place jar of milk (without lid) in a 1 l aluminium pot with sufficient water to cover the level of breastmilk (about two fingers above).
3 Place the pot on a heat source and allow the water to boil. When the water is boiling rapidly take the jar of milk out of the water, place the lid on and allow to cool before feeding to the baby.

Growth monitoring and nutritional advice

HIV infection can impair the nutritional status of infected children from early in life. Length and height are reduced in almost all infected children and growth faltering often occurs even before opportunistic infections or other symptoms. In children, growth is a good reflection of a child's 'lean body tissue' – the total amount of muscle and non-fat tissue in the body. Another good indicator of a child's general nutritional status is the mid-upper-arm circumference (MUAC). When children with HIV infection become malnourished they lose more muscle compared to malnourished children without HIV infection. Both groups of children can also lose fat reserves.

Monitoring of growth parameters should be done at every visit including monitoring of weight, height and occipital-frontal circumference. Weight should be recorded and plotted on appropriate growth charts. Static weight, weight crossing a percentile or weight below the third percentile are danger signs and require assessment and intervention. Children with severe growth failure and loss of muscle (lean body tissue) are at an increased risk of death. If there is growth failure, an assessment for HIV related features and treatable causes such as acute or chronic infections (e.g. respiratory, gastrointestinal, urinary tract infections or TB) should be performed.

Antiretroviral treatment, when clinically indicated, improves weight, growth and development of infected children and improves their life expectancy.

Routine micronutrient supplementation

All HIV-exposed children should receive routine multivitamin supplements daily and vitamin A supplementation according to the following schedule:

Table 18.6 Target group dosage schedule for vitamin A		
Target	**Age**	**Dose**
Non-breastfed infants	0 to 5 months	50 000 IU single dose at age 6 weeks
All infants	6 to 11 months	100 000 IU single dose at age between 6 to 11 months (preferably at 9 months when child comes for immunisation)
All children	1 to 5 years	200 000 IU single dose at 12 months and then every 6 months until the age of 5 years

---

Management of growth failure in HIV:

- Treat underlying infections
- Provide food supplementation
- Consider initiation of antiretroviral therapy.

Immunization

HIV-infected and HIV-exposed children should be immunized according to the routine national immunisation schedule. There is concern regarding the safety of BCG in HIV-infected infants, based on several cases of local and disseminated BCG disease reported in HIV-infected infants. The Global Advisory Committee of the WHO states that BCG is contraindicated in HIV-infected infants. However, the benefits of BCG vaccine in uninfected, but HIV-exposed infants are considerable. Current South African policy still recommends routine BCG vaccination at birth in HIV-exposed infants. Otherwise, HIV-positive children should receive all routine vaccinations, including live vaccines.

Routine treatment for worms

Routine treatment of intestinal parasites has been shown to be associated with an improved outcome. Accordingly, all HIV infected children older than one year receive regular deworming treatment. Up to age two years, children are given mebendazole, 100 mg twice daily for three days every six months, and over two years, a single 500 mg dose of mebendazole is given if there has not been a dose in the preceding six months.

Pneumocystis jirovecii pneumonia (PJP) prophylaxis

All HIV-exposed infants should be started on PJP prophylaxis at six weeks of age. Trimethoprim–sulfamethoxazole (cotrimoxazole), 5 mg/kg/day is the drug of choice. PJP prophylaxis should be stopped only if:

- The infant is confirmed HIV-negative (*see* HIV diagnosis).
- An HIV-positive child on antiretroviral therapy has two consecutive normal CD4 counts.

Antiretroviral therapy

Antiretroviral medications function at different points in the lifecycle of the virus as it infects the CD4 cell (*see* Figure 18.3)

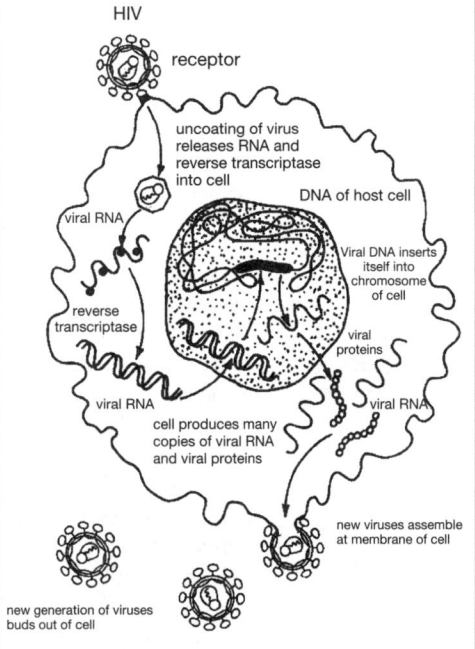

Figure 18.3 Host cell invaded by HIV: viral RNA forms viral DNA by means of reverse transcriptase. Viral DNA inserts itself into ribosome where viral proteins are generated

HIV
receptor
uncoating of virus releases RNA and reverse transcriptase into cell
viral RNA
DNA of host cell
Viral DNA inserts itself into chromosome of cell
reverse transcriptase
viral proteins
viral RNA
viral RNA
cell produces many copies of viral RNA and viral proteins
new viruses assemble at membrane of cell
new generation of viruses buds out of cell

The antiretroviral medications registered in South Africa are shown in Table 18.7. Antiretroviral therapy, however, is not a cure but a treatment and aims to suppresses viral replication and thereby prevent CD4 cell destruction. If the antiretroviral drugs are stopped or doses missed, the HI virus in reservoir sites will started replicating again allowing for the selection of viruses that are resistant to the drugs. Over 96 per cent adherence to therapy is required in order to maintain viral suppression and prevent the emergence of viral resistance. This means that the patient can, at maximum, miss only one dose every two weeks. Maintaining this degree of treatment adherence requires intense counselling and support before the initiation of therapy and throughout the duration of the therapy.

> Once antiretroviral therapy is started the child will remain on therapy for the rest of his or her life.

The aims of antiretroviral therapy are:
- Suppression of viral load below detectable levels.
- Promotion of growth.
- Decrease in the number of opportunistic infections.
- Improvement in cognitive function.
- Achievement of developmental milestones.

When to start antiretroviral therapy in children

The timing of the initiation of antiretroviral therapy is based on weighing the benefits of early initiation (preservation of the immune system and decreased mortality and morbidity) versus delayed initiation (shorter total duration on therapy and therefore decreased side-effect profile, lowered risk of development of resistance and decreased financial and resource costs). Guidelines regarding timing of initiation of antiretroviral therapy vary from country to country and change over time, therefore it is important to keep up-to-date with the local guidelines. The South African National Department of Health guidelines are available at www.doh.gov.za.

Recent evidence suggests that infants younger than 12 months with proven HIV infection should urgently commence antiretroviral therapy on diagnosis, and that the CD4 criteria should be applied to those older than one year, along with three-monthly monitoring and WHO staging criteria. It may happen that symptomatic patients who are WHO stages 3 or 4 do not yet qualify for antiretroviral therapy on CD4 criteria. Under such circumstances, it is advised to apply the clinical criteria in the treatment decision (*see* Table 18.8).

Baseline investigations prior to initiating antiretroviral therapy

Prior to starting antiretroviral therapy in an HIV-infected child, certain baseline data must be available to confirm a child's suitability for and likely success with treatment.

A complete evaluation includes growth charting and surface area calculation as well as

Table 18.7 Antiretroviral therapy registered (or soon to be registered) in South Africa

Generic name/ Trade name ® Strength	Dosage	Major toxicities	Other comments
Nucleoside reverse transcriptase inhibitors (NRTIs)			
Zidovudine (AZT) Retrovir® Syrup: 10 mg/ml Capsules: 100 mg	$180-240$ mg/m^2 Capsules: 100 mg 12 hourly (all ages) from 4 wk. Neonates: 2 mg/kg 6 hourly Premature: 1.5 mg/kg 12 hourly for 2 wk., then 2 mg/kg 8 hourly IV: 120 mg/m^2 6 hourly or 20 mg/m^2/hr	Neutropaenia Anaemia Headaches Myopathy (rare)	Double dose for HIV encephalopathy (180 mg/m^2 6 hourly)
Lamivudine (3TC) 3TC® Syrup: 10 mg/ml Tablets: 150 mg (can be broken)	4 mg/kg 12 hourly Neonates <30 d.: 2 mg/kg 12 hourly >50 kg: 150 mg 12 hourly (can use Combivir®) AZT 300 mg and 3TC 150 mg)	Headache Abdominal pain Pancreatitis Peripheral neuropathy and neutropenia (all rare)	Well tolerated. Store at room temperature (use within 1 mo. of opening)
Didanosine (ddI) Solution: 10 mg/ml Tablets: 25, 50, 100, 150, and 200 mg	2 weeks to 8 m 100 mg/m^2 12 hourly After 8 months 120 mg/m^2 12 hourly Adolescents daily <60 kg: 250 mg >60 kg: 400 mg daily	Pancreatitis and Peripheral neuropathy rare (dose related) Diarrhoea and abdominal pain	Dosage can be combined for single daily dose on empty stomach, 1h before or 2h after food Tablets can be dissolved in water Suspension must be refrigerated (stable for 30 d). To obtain sufficient antacid buffer use 2 tablets; if cost is a consideration give 1 tablet with 10 ml antacid as ddI is inactivated by acid in the stomach
Stavudine (d4T) Zerit® Solution: 1 mg/ml Capsules: 20, 30, and 40 mg	1 mg/kg 12 hourly 30-60 kg: 30 mg 12 hourly >60 kg: 40 mg 12 hourly	Headache GI upset Peripheral, neuropathy and pancreatitis (both rare)	Large volume of suspension: must be refrigerated, stable for 30 d. Capsules can be well tolerated opened up
Abacavir (ABC) Ziagen® Solution: 20 mg/ml Tablet: 300 mg	8 mg/kg/ 12 hourly	1–3% develop hypersensitivity – fever, malaise, mucositis ± rashes, usually in first 6 wk. Stop drug – do not rechallenge	Can crush tablets

Table 18.7 *continued*

Generic name/Trade name®/Strength	Dosage	Major toxicities	Other comments
Non nucleoside reverse transcriptase inhibitors			
Nevirapine Viramune® Solution: 10 mg/ml Tablet: 200 mg	Start at 200 mg/m² daily ×14 days; then if no rash, increase in first 2 wk. to 200 mg/m² 12 hourly (maximum daily dosage 400 mg) <2 mo. of age: 120 mg/m² for daily and 12 hourly dosages)	Rash most common Do not increase dosage until rash resolves Intense monitoring of liver functions necessary in first 3 mo., then less frequently	Store at room temperature. Can give with food. Rifampicin reduces levels
Efavirenz Stocrin® 50 mg and 200 mg capsules	15 mg/kg daily or 10–15 kg: 200 mg 15–20kg: 250 mg 20–25 kg: 300 mg 25–33 kg: 350 mg 33–40 kg: 400 mg >40 kg: 600 mg daily	Sleepiness Abnormal dreams Skin rash	Take at night to decrease CNS side effects. Avoid taking with high-fat meal. Can open capsule and give with stewed apple and other foods or drinks. Limited pharmaco-kinetic data <3 yr. Avoid in children under 3 yr
Protease Inhibitors			
Nelfinavir Viracept® Tablet: 250 mg	<10 kg: 75 mg/kg twice daily 10–19.9 kg: 60 mg/kg twice daily Adolescent: 1 250 mg twice daily	Diarrhoea Vomiting Rash Abnormal lipids	Take with food to increase absorption. Crush tablets. Powder formulation not recommended
Indinavir Crixivan® Capsules (hard gel capsules): 200 mg	33 mg/kg 8 hourly	Nausea Hyper-bilirubinaemia Abnormal lipids	Fasting or with low-fat snack. Drink lots of water daily. Avoid Coke. Avoid in neonates
Ritonavir Norvir® Suspension: 80 mg/ml Capsules: 100 mg	>3 mo. of age/ start at 250 mg/m² 12 hourly; increase over 5 d. to 400 mg/m² 12 hourly	Nausea Vomiting Abdominal pain (severe) Increase in liver enzymes Abnormal lipids	Food improves tolerability. Can try to coat mouth with peanut butter prior to medication
*Lopinavir/Ritonavir Kaletra® Solution: 80/20 mg/ml Capsules: 133/33 mg	230/57.5 mg/m² 12 hourly 300/75 mg/m² 12 hourly, if used with nevirapine or efavirenz, or if PI experienced	Diarrhoea Nausea Abnormal lipids	Take with a meal to increase absorption. Solution has a bitter taste

For 'boosted' Kaletra®, add 0.75 ml Ritonavir for each ml of Kaletra®

Table 18.8 Immunological marker criteria for starting antiretroviral therapy in children (WHO)

Age	Infants <12 months	Children 12–36 months	Children 36–56 months	Children over 6 years
CD4 %		<20	<15	<15
CD4 count (cells/mm³)	ALL	<750	<350	As in adults (<200)
WHO Stage		3 and 4	3 and 4	3 and 4

Criteria to be met before starting antiretroviral therapy in children:

- Diagnosis is confirmed.
- Clinical and immunological criteria are met.
- Social criteria: adherence to treatment is probable.
- Baseline investigations have been performed.

the following baseline investigations: full blood count and differential white count, serum liver enzymes, CD4 count and HI viral load, exclusion of tuberculosis.

Adherence

Maintaining adherence to the treatment regimen over long periods of time is extremely challenging, especially if there is poor social support. Adherence counselling should start before the initiation of therapy, ensuring that care givers understand and accept the importance of maintaining 100 per cent compliance. In general, a responsible adult must have been identified to administer the medicine, who is contactable and who will attend the clinic.

Disclosure of the diagnosis to the father and other family-members should be encouraged, so ensuring that medications can be given openly to the child at home and that additional treatment supporters are available when the primary care giver is not available.

Additional adherence tools include treatment diary cards, calendars, alarm clocks, cellular phone alarms, pill-boxes and linking treatment with daily tasks such as breakfast and supper or brushing teeth in the morning and evening.

Adherence should be reinforced at every patient visit and compliance reviewed by assessing diary cards and pill counts. Social circumstances can change eg the caregiver may become ill or family income may decrease, therefore caregivers should be encouraged to seek assistance to ensure compliance.

The child should be encouraged to take partial responsibility for taking medications when this is age appropriate, but should always be supervised by caregivers to ensure compliance.

What medication to start

Antiretroviral therapy consists of at least three drugs from different antiretroviral drug classes used in combination in order to limit the development of resistance. Acceptable combinations include:

Table 18.9 Antiretroviral combinations

Two NRTIs	+	One NNRTI:
abacavir + 3TC		
d4T + 3TC		nevirapine or efavirenz
abacavir + AZT		
Two NRTIs	**+**	**One PI**
abacavir + 3TC		
d4T + 3TC		Kaletra® (lopinavir/ritonovir)
AZT + ddI		

Abacavir and AZT are available for substitution if toxicity occurs.

South African guidelines currently recommend:

- d4T + 3TC + Kaletra® for infants <3 years
- d4T + 3TC + efavirenz for children >3 years.

In public health programmes with universal access to antiretroviral therapy, standard regimens are used to ensure sustainable usage of available drugs, a continuous supply of drugs and to limit the cost of the medications. Table 18.10 shows NRTI drug combinations to be avoided.

The current recommended WHO first-line paediatric regimens are shown in Table 18.11. Common side effects are shown in Table 18.20.

Monitoring

The aim of monitoring is to ensure clinical and laboratory response to treatment and to monitor for side effects or adverse events.

Response to treatment is judged as follows:
- Clinical response: Weight gain, growth, developmental progress, opportunistic infections and adjusted modified WHO staging
- Laboratory response: CD4 count, viral load

Side-effects are documented according to:
- Clinical signs and symptoms (*see* Table 18.12)
- Haematological and biochemical derangements of blood count, liver function tests, blood glucose and serum cholesterol and triglycerides (especially in patients on protease inhibitors).

Tuberculosis and HIV
(*see* also Chapter 17, Tuberculosis)

If a child presents with tuberculosis before starting antiretroviral therapy, the TB therapy should be completed before commencing antiretroviral therapy, if possible. However, if the child is severely immunocompromised or symptomatic, antiretroviral therapy should be delayed for between two weeks to two months. Due to the induction of the cytochrome P450 system by rifamycin, the serum levels of Kaletra® and efavirenz are decreased and the dose should therefore be adjusted accordingly. The patients' alanine transaminase (ALT) should be monitored monthly during the course of the therapy.

Due to potential combined hepatotoxicity, patients on nevirapine should be switched to efavirenz and the ALT monitored monthly. If the child is unable to tolerate the large number of drugs, the antiretroviral therapy may have to be interrupted until TB therapy has been completed.

Patients co-infected with *Mycobacterium tuberculosis* and HIV pose a unique challenge due to:

- Shared toxicity of antiretroviral drugs and antituberculosis therapy.
- Drug interactions between antiretroviral drugs and antituberculosis therapy.
- Development of IRIS.
- High pill burden with associated poor adherence.

Immune reconstitution inflammatory syndrome (IRIS)

IRIS refers to the paradoxical clinical deterioration following immunological and virologi-

Table 18.10 NRTI drug combinations to be avoided

Combinations	Reason
d4T + AZT	Both drugs work through common metabolic pathways
d4T + ddl	These drugs have overlapping toxicities

Table 18.11 First-line antiretroviral combinations for children

Population	<12 months / No PMTCT or NVP exposure	<12 months PMTCT or NVP exposure	1–4 years	>5 years
Regimen	2 NRTI + NVP	2 NRTI + Protease Inhibitor	2 NRTI + NVP or EFV	2 NRTI + NVP or EFV
Example	D4T + 3TC + NVP	D4T + 3TC + Kaletra®	D4T + 3TC + NVP or EFV	D4T + 3TC + NVP or EFV

Table 18.12 Common side effects of antiretroviral drugs

Clinical symptoms and signs	Drugs responsible	Time of onset	Pathophysiological basis	Severity and risk	Management
Skin					
Maculopapular itchy rashes	NNRTIs (eg *nevirapine*, *efavirenz*) PI (eg lopinavir/ ritonavir – rare) *NRTI (e.g. stavudine)*	First few weeks	Hypersensitivity	Not serious	Local management of itch Local steroid
Stevens Johnson syndrome	NNRTIs (eg *Nevirapine* NRTI (eg abacavir)	Any time	Hypersensitivity	Serious	Stop drug
Abdominal and Metabolic					
Abdominal pain	NRTI (eg *stavudine lamivudine*, didanosine, zidovudine) PI (eg *lopinavir/ ritonavir*	Any time	Pancreatitis Hepatitis Hyperlactataemia Lactic acidosis	Serious	Investigate and stop drugs if Grade IV toxicity
GIT upset nausea, diarrhoea	NRTI (eg *lamivudine stavudine didanosine*) PI (eg *ritonavir*, lopinavir/ritonavir)	Any time	Drug reaction	Affects compliance	Antiemetic
Liver enlargement	NRTI (eg *stavudine*, *didanosine*, zidovudine) NNRTI (eg *nevirapine*)	Any time	Mitochondrial toxicity with steatosis, hepatitis, lactic acidosis	Serious	Investigate alternative drugs if persistent or progressive
Abnormal lipids	PI (eg *ritonavir*, *lopinavir/ritonavir*)	Any time	Drug reaction	Unknown	Monitor, use cholesterol lowering methods eg fibrates
CNS and Neuromuscular					
Neuromuscular symptoms, eg myopathy or peripheral neuropathy	NRTI (eg *zidovudine*, stavudine, didanosine, lamivudine)	Any time	Drug reaction (often dose dependent)	Serious	Reduce dose

Table 18.12 continued					
Clinical symptoms and signs	Drugs responsible	Time of onset	Pathophysiological basis	Severity and risk	Management
Headache	NRTI (eg *stavudine, lamivudine,* zidovudine) PI (eg ritonavir)	Any time	Drug reaction	Moderate	Analgesics
Sleep disturbance, confusion	NNRTI (eg *efavirenz*)	Any time	Drug reaction	Moderate	Monitor, reduce dose or stop
Haematological					
Neutropaenia	NRTI (eg *zidovudine,* lamivudine)	Any time	Drug reaction with bone marrow suppression	Serious	Reduce dose or stop
Anaemia	NRTI (eg *zidovudine*) PI (eg **lopinavir/ ritonavir**) Indinavir	Any time	Drug reaction with bone marrow suppression or Haemolysis	Serious	Reduce dose
Drugs commonly associated are indicated in bold italic					

cal response after the initiation of antiretroviral therapy. This deterioration has been ascribed to the recovery of an appropriate host immune response and consequent ability to recognize latent infective and non-infective antigens. The diagnosis is based on the presence of three primary characteristics:

- Identification of an antigen that has elicited the response.
- Change in the host immunity (either increasing CD4 count or decreasing viral load).
- Exclusion of other possible explanations for the clinical syndrome, e.g. treatment failure, adverse drug reactions and acute opportunistic infections.

Risk factors for the development of IRIS include a very low CD4 count or high viral load at initiation of antiretroviral therapy, the presence of an active or latent infection and a genetic susceptibility for the development of IRIS. The clinical presentation may vary depending on the offending antigen. *Mycobacterium tuberculosis* IRIS is commonly encountered in tuberculosis-endemic areas. Common clinical presentations of TB IRIS include high fever, cervical and intra-thoracic lymphadenopathy and new or deteriorating pulmonary infiltrates.

Management of IRIS includes the treatment of the underlying opportunistic infection, continuation of antiretroviral therapy and the use of non-steroidal anti-inflammatory drugs (NSAID) or corticosteroids either locally (e.g. intra-ocular for CMV IRIS) or systemically in selected cases. If the IRIS is life-threatening the antiretroviral therapy may rarely have to be temporarily stopped.

Treatment failure

Failure of clinical or laboratory response to antiretroviral therapy usually indicates the presence of viral resistance. Viral resistance may emerge as a primary event (i.e. the child is infected with a drug-resistant HIV strain) or as a secondary event (i.e. the child develops resistance while on antiretrovirals). Primary resistance is uncom-

Clinical presentations of IRIS:

- Infectious IRIS:
  Mycobacterium TB IRIS
  Mycobacterium bovis (BCG) IRIS
  Mycobacterium avium complex (MAC) IRIS
  Cryptococcal IRIS
  PJP IRIS
  Cytomegalovirus IRIS
  Varicella zoster/ Herpes simplex IRIS
- Non-infectious IRIS:
  Kaposi's sarcoma IRIS
  Autoimmune IRIS
  Sarcoid IRIS

mon in resource-limited countries due to the limited access to antiretrovirals, but will emerge as a problem with increased antiretroviral use for PMTCT and adult treatment. Secondary resistance can develop due to:

- Non-adherence to therapy
- Sub-optimal dosage
- Drug-interactions resulting in decreased serum concentrations of antiretroviral drugs.

Treatment failure can manifest as clinical failure, immunological failure or virological failure (*see* Table 18.13).

Management of treatment failure

- Assessment of adherence, antiretroviral drug dosages and concomitant medications or opportunistic infections.
- Intensive adherence counselling
- Repeat viral load, and if persistently >1 000 copies/ml, consider change in treatment regimen
- The treatment regimen can be changed based on an HIV-viral resistance test (genotypic or phenotypic resistance test) result, or empirically by changing from a first line regimen to a second line regimen.

Prognosis

Infant mortality and morbidity due to common childhood illnesses such as pneumonia and gastroenteritis are much higher in children infected with HIV than in those not infected. The HIV epidemic has resulted in an increase of child mortality rates in most sub-Saharan African countries, causing up to a third of young child deaths in these areas (*see* Chapter 4, Community paediatrics, child health and survival).

In the absence of antiretroviral therapy, a third of the HIV-infected babies may have died by one year of age and most by five years. Studies documenting the rapid clinical and immunological deterioration of HIV-infected infants have resulted in recent changes in the treatment guidelines, allowing for the treatment of all HIV infected infants <1 year of age, irrespective of clinical or immunological stage.

Table 18.13 Treatment failure on antiretroviral therapy

Clinical failure	Treatment failure	Virological failure
Growth failure	Confirmed return of CD4 % to baseline prior to initiation of therapy	Failure to achieve viral suppression
Loss of neuro-developmental milestones	More than 50% decline in CD4 % from peak	Reappearance of any detectable viral load
Disease progression: • To additional disease in the current stage; or • To the next stage		Rebound of viral load to baseline prior to antiretroviral therapy
Recurrence of prior opportunistic infections		

Once a child is commenced on antiretroviral therapy, this has to be seen as lifelong treatment. Even though the treatment of HIV-infected children with antiretroviral therapy is associated with a significant reduction in short term morbidity and mortality, HIV at present is not a curable condition.

For HIV-infected children, the use of antiretroviral therapy is associated with improved growth and neurodevelopment, and a substantial reduction in the frequency of opportunistic infections and hospitalizations associated with HIV. Paediatric HIV should therefore be optimally treated as any other chronic medical condition.

Management of HIV-affected children in the community

The impact of the AIDS epidemic extends far beyond that of the HIV infection on the children directly involved. As a general rule, each infected child has an infected mother, who may herself begin to develop the symptoms of AIDS. This may severely affect her own ability to care for both her ill child and for any other members of the family in several different ways, including income-generating potential, working in food production, and the strength to feed or take her children for preventive or curative healthcare.

Infants born to HIV-infected mothers are at a higher-than-average risk of morbidity and mortality irrespective of whether they are HIV-infected or not. In a study from Central Africa the mortality of HIV-exposed but uninfected infants was already double that of those who were not HIV-exposed by six months of age. The possible explanations for the increased mortality in HIV-exposed uninfected infants include increased exposure to pathogens from an HIV-infected mother, lowered caring capacity by HIV-infected mothers, suboptimal nutrition and greater socioeconomic deprivation due to the family impact of HIV. Furthermore, if the HIV-infected mother should die, the HIV-uninfected children suffer a three to four times increased risk of mortality.

HIV infection of the mother therefore carries an enormous health risk for her children, irrespective of their HIV infection status. It is encumbent on health professionals to pay particular attention to all HIV-exposed infants. Every assessment of the infant should include an enquiry into the health status of the parents, their recent CD4 counts and their access to treatment and support. Ensuring appropriate referral for social support such as support grants, food relief programmes and placement/fostering if necessary is important for the health of the child.

The uninfected family members also face a number of important psychosocial issues, such as:

- Coping with a potentially fatal illness
- Emotional and financial demands of chronic ill health
- Disruption of normal family life
- Guilt, anxiety, and depression
- Stigmatisation and ostracism by the community and other family members
- Early death of the infected parent/parents.

Easy access to counselling services and ready support from other groups, such as social workers, psychologists, churches and religious communities, may help the family to cope better. AIDS epidemics have begun to overburden traditional hospital-based health care services. There is an urgent need to reorientate the present health services towards primary healthcare. Health workers should be trained to provide the following services to the community:

- Education and information regarding HIV infection and its prevention
- Early detection
- Counselling
- Care of the infected child at home and at clinic level
- Care of the dying child.

Talking to children infected and affected by HIV

The experience of chronic and progressive illness associated with HIV raises many questions that children must be able to talk about. Parents and healthcare workers often find it very difficult to anticipate and respond to children's questions about their disease. This may be aggravated by the adult's own unresolved fears and emotions. As a consequence, children may become emotionally very isolated.

The most important support for the child is its relationship of trust with its care giver. Health professionals must advise and help the care giver to maintain a caring reassurance and presence towards the child right through to possible terminal illness. Continued counselling and support of the care giver is required throughout this process.

Children react to the emotional cues from the reactions of their care givers to their disease. So it is important that caregivers should not lie to them. On the other hand, children are more concerned with the present discomfort or fear than with the more abstract thoughts of death that the parent is concerned with. Questions raised by the child should be answered as honestly as possible with terminology and content that is appropriate to the child's emotional and intellectual development. It is best to proceed in a step-wise manner that begins with informing the child that he/she has an infection that needs treatment, before moving to more detailed information concerning HIV in an age-appropriate manner.

AIDS orphans

(*See* also Chapter 5, Social paediatrics.)

A huge number of children are orphaned by the premature deaths of parents and care givers. It has been estimated that the number of orphaned children under 14 years of age has far exceeded two million, of whom 95 per cent are from Africa. These children are not only faced with the loss of family support and nurturing during their own growth and development, but also with physical, social, and economic deprivation. While the extended families of these children are generally willing to assume parental responsibility, the additional mouths to feed are an economic burden on people living in generally impoverished circumstances. In many instances there are no family members to turn to, leaving some children to fend for themselves (child-headed households). Some children who have lost both parents are being looked after by their elderly grandparents, who themselves have a limited or no income, while others have become 'street children' and therefore constantly at risk of sexually transmitted infections and HIV.

It is important, therefore, that health workers and national policy-makers formulate plans to care for the growing number of AIDS orphans.

PART 6

Disorders of regulation and immune control

19

Endocrine disorders

The endocrine system is one of the regulatory systems of the body, which, together with the nervous system and the immune system, serves to promote and regulate the maintenance of the body's internal environment, as well as its energy balance, growth, development at puberty, and reproduction.

Endocrine disorders may be suspected in the presence of classic constellations of signs and symptoms (e.g. Graves disease). On the other hand, many features of an endocrinopathy may be quite non-specific, e.g. disorders of growth or development. Persistent unexplained biochemical abnormalities (e.g. abnormal serum urea and electrolytes) lead to the suspicion of an endocrinopathy. Although screening is not widely available, some disorders (e.g. congenital hypothyroidism) may be detected before clinical disease occurs.

Development of the endocrine system in childhood

The time from conception through intra-uterine growth and postnatal development, childhood and adolescence, is a period of progressive biological change. The genetically controlled differentiation of cells into tissues, organs and endocrine glands is followed by progressive growth and maturation. With differentiation, the hormone-producing cell gains the ability to secrete before the controlling loops and reactions (feed-back control, periodicity, sleep-wake cyc-

ling, seasonality) are established. In all of these, the state of nutrition has an important additional function through its influence on substrate availability.

The patterns of hormone secretion are established with growth and maturation. Just before birth, there is a rapid increase in adrenocorticotrophin (ACTH) secretion, which results in an increased output of cortisol. This is thought to be associated with rapid maturation of enzyme systems, including those of the lungs, in preparation for birth and extra-uterine existence.

The baby's birth is followed by an increase in antidiuretic hormone (ADH), renin and angiotensin levels. Postnatally, there is elevated catecholamine secretion, particularly noradrenaline, which helps to maintain the blood glucose level by its effect on the metabolism of brown fat before feeding is initiated.

The stress of birth is followed by a surge in thyrotropin activity, which results in high levels of circulating thyroid hormone levels. These drop to normal levels only by the end of the first week. Premature or small-for-dates babies have thyroid hormone levels that are lower than, but parallel to, those of full-term infants.

Even the sex hormones are higher in the newborn baby than at any other time until puberty. This period of increased gonadotrophin and sex hormone output lasts for a few months. It may be associated with symptoms: in some girls there is a vaginal discharge and occasionally even a withdrawal bleed. Many babies develop gynaecomastia (enlargement of the breasts) and many newborn boys have quite pigmented rugous scrotal skin.

Childhood is quite a stable period endocrinologically. Between early childhood and the age of about eight to nine years, the hypothalamo-pituitary-gonadal axis is dormant, with strong negative feedbacks inhibiting the release of both gonadotrophin and sex hormones. At the start of puberty, a gradual increase in sleep-associated pulsatile luteinizing hormone (LH) release occurs, followed by extension to day time by mid-puberty. Cyclic secretion and a change to a positive feed forward loop heralds the onset of menarche. The girl's body mass has an influence on the pulsatile release of LH releasing hormone (LHRH). In general, menarche occurs only after a mass of 46.5 kg has been achieved, with a specific ratio of fat to lean body mass.

During puberty, the secretion of growth hormone again increases and, together with the release of sex hormones, is responsible for the puberty growth spurt. After puberty, growth hormone secretion persists at low levels.

The cellular responses to hormone actions are modulated through their binding to specific receptors and intracellular second-messenger mechanisms. Normal homeostasis is thus maintained by integrated autonomic, endocrine, immune, and metabolic responses. For example, the effect of growth hormone is mediated through IGF-1; this is acutely decreased by fasting, indicating the interaction between endocrine and nutritional events.

Linkages between regulatory systems

The different systems receive input from each other to fine-tune homeostatic control. Some neurons release chemical substances into the bloodstream to act as hormones (e.g. hypothalamic releasing factors). The innervation of endocrine glands influences their secretion rate. In addition, hormones have an influence on immune reactions, while cytokines have an influence on neuroendocrine function.

One example of the above is the interaction between inflammation and hormone response: the pro-inflammatory mediator interleukin 1 (IL-1) is released from lymphocytes in response to infection. This has an influence in the hypothalamus, where it increases the secretion of ACTH. This in turn results in increased cortisol secretion. The effect of cortisol is to increase the numbers of polymorph neutrophils and to decrease the numbers of lymphocytes, thus decreasing the production of IL-1 and antibodies and so limiting the degree of inflammatory damage. In some patients IL-1 secretion does not result in increased cortisol and some have been seen to develop progressive inflammation and arthritis, which responds to treatment with cortisol.

Measurement and evaluation

Endocrine organs are commonly assessed by sonographic measurement. This depends on observer experience and the appropriate use of age-related standards.

The measurement of hormone blood levels demands a good laboratory and an understanding of the dynamic nature of the levels obtained, some of which can change acutely even in response to the anxiety of having blood taken. The blood level of any hormone reflects its balance at that particular moment in relation to pulsatility, circadian rhythm, and stress-mediated surges, as well as the influence of substrate and any opposing hormone. Random blood samples are of very little use (e.g. to measure growth hormone). A properly planned dynamic test of hormone response to a releasing stress is much more likely to yield diagnostically useful information, and should be performed with proper consultation. When the treatment of a suspected endocrine disorder cannot wait for laboratory confirmation (e.g. adrenal collapse), a frozen sample of separated serum is all that is necessary before a therapeutic trial is started. After telephonic consultation, the frozen samples could be transported to a distant main laboratory for confirmation of the diagnosis, which usually involves a radio-immuno-assay procedure.

In infancy and childhood the blood levels of many hormones are much higher than the usual normal adult range. It follows that the interpretation of hormone levels is dependent on the child's age. The normal ranges of hormone levels are therefore difficult to interpret in childhood. Ideally the relationship of the members of feedback loops should be measured together, such as T_4 and thyroid stimulating hormone (TSH), insulin and blood glucose, vasopressin and plasma osmolality, and testosterone and LH.

In developing countries, under-recognition of endocrine disorders may be attributed to the higher incidence of infective and nutritional disorders in these communities. However, there may also be genetic factors that explain differences in the incidence of endocrine disorders in different communities.

Hypoglycaemia

(*see* chapter 10, Metabolic disorders)

Both metabolic abnormalities and endocrine disorders can result in hypoglycaemia. Infants and children at high risk for hypoglycaemia include those who are premature, who have intrauterine growth retardation, who are born to diabetic mothers, or who present with septicaemia or severe illness. Hypoglycaemia may be due to defects involving hepatic glycogen release or storage, gluconeogenesis, carnitine metabolism or fatty acid oxidation, as well as mixed or unknown conditions such as ketotic hypoglycaemia. Endocrine abnormalities that can result in hypoglycaemia include hyperinsulinism, and cortisol or growth hormone deficiency.

Symptoms of hypoglycaemia may be non-specific and include poor feeding, lethargy, apnoea, cyanotic spells, hypothermia, seizures and coma.

In order to identify the cause of hypoglycaemia, a careful history and physical examination, coupled with laboratory investigations, are necessary.

Laboratory evaluation of hypoglycaemia

Although hypoglycaemia can be screened for by using the fingerstick reagent strips, hypoglycaemia should be documented by measuring the true serum glucose level. A sample of blood collected at the time of hypoglycaemia constitutes a part of the 'critical sample'. Such an archival sample of blood may be saved and stored for future laboratory tests. In addition, the urinalysis helps to distinguish disorders of increased glucose utilization from disorders of glucose production by the absence or presence of ketones, respectively (*see* Table 19.1).

Growth disorders

Normal growth

Growth is a dynamic process, involving a change in length or height as a function of time. It is a sensitive barometer of health. Not only is growth monitoring important in order to assess the general health of a child, but the recognition of poor growth should alert the clinician to look for a treatable condition. Growth follows a predictable pattern throughout childhood and adolescence. In the first year of life, the child grows at a rate of up to 25 cm per year; in the second year the growth rate is 12 cm per year; thereafter the rate reduces to 5 cm per year until puberty.

Phases of growth

Infantile growth

From conception and into the first year of life, the growth process is almost entirely dependent on nutrition. Intra-uterine growth retardation (IUGR) and malnutrition have profound effects on stature.

Childhood growth

The childhood growth phase includes a component of basic growth that is influenced by genetic factors, along with a component that is growth-hormone dependent.

Around the age of six to eight years children have an increase in the rate of growth, called the mid-childhood growth spurt, which is thought to be mediated by adrenal androgens.

Pubertal growth

The pubertal portion of growth is regulated by both growth hormone and the sex steroids

Table 19.1 Laboratory evaluation of hypoglycaemia	
Critical sample	**Archival sample**
True blood glucose Liver function tests Electrolytes Serum bicarbonate Urinalysis, including presence or absence of ketones	Serum for insulin, ketones, growth hormone, cortisol C peptide Carnitine profile Amino acids Toxins (e.g. ethanol) Urine amino and organic acids

(testosterone and oestrogens). The pubertal growth spurt occurs earlier in girls than in boys. The two year delay before the onset of the male growth spurt and a 3 cm greater total growth during puberty, accounts for the average 13 cm difference in the final height between adult males and females.

Growth assessment

The study of the growth of an individual child requires both accuracy and insight in interpreting the data collected.

Height should be accurately measured with a stadiometer in children over two years of age; the length of those less than two years of age should be measured with an infant stadiometer (measuring board). Comparison of body segments (upper segment or sitting height with lower segment) are important in assessing if the growth disorder is secondary to a skeletal abnormality.

Maturational changes in the skeleton with advancing chronological age can be quantified and represented as bone age (assessed by X-rays of the left hand and wrist, see Figure 19.1).

A widely-used system for estimating skeletal maturity is the Greulich and Pyle atlas. Bone age is used to estimate the amount of growth that is left until adult height is achieved (when the epiphyses have fused).

In addition to standard distance centile charts, growth velocity centile charts are invaluable in the assessment of growth disorders (see Chapter 2, Growth and development). The growth velocity is the difference between two measurements of growth made over a period of time (not less than

six months apart), expressed as centimetres per year. The longer the growth velocity remains below the 50th percentile, the more likely it is that investigation will reveal a growth abnormality.

The Standard Deviation Score (z score) is often used to compare mathematically the growth of individual children to the population mean, but does not contribute as much to the appreciation of the growth of an individual child as do growth velocity and midparental height (see below).

The short child

In a population of children two standard deviations below the mean for height (-2SD) about 20 per cent may be expected to have pathological short stature, with the remaining 80 per cent about equally divided between familial short stature and constitutional delay. In contrast, most children at –3SD below the population mean for height have pathological short stature.

In **familial short stature**, the height age (the chronological age corresponding to the 50th percentile for the child's height) may be delayed several years, but the skeletal age is similar to the chronological age. Many family members may be short, and the child will grow at his or her genetic potential.

In **constitutional delay** of growth and maturation, the height age and skeletal age are equally retarded with respect to the chronological age. The members of the family are generally normal in height, but often have a history of delayed growth and delayed sexual maturation.

One may more accurately identify children with growth disorders by the evaluation of the growth velocity. Height velocity standard curves should be used to assess growth rate. Children

Table 19.2 Basic data required for the diagnostic evaluation of short stature		
History	**Examination**	**Investigations**
Birth weight	Accurate height, weight, span	Urine dipstix and stool microscopy
Gestational age	measurements	Haemoglobin
Detailed family history and both	Careful plotting of present and	Serum albumin and blood urea
parents' heights	previous measurements on growth	T_4 and TSH
Detailed feeding history	chart	Radiological bone age
Detailed history of growth and	Clinical examination of nutritional	
development	state, development and organ	
	systems	

Figure 19.1 Ossification centres of the hand and age appearance

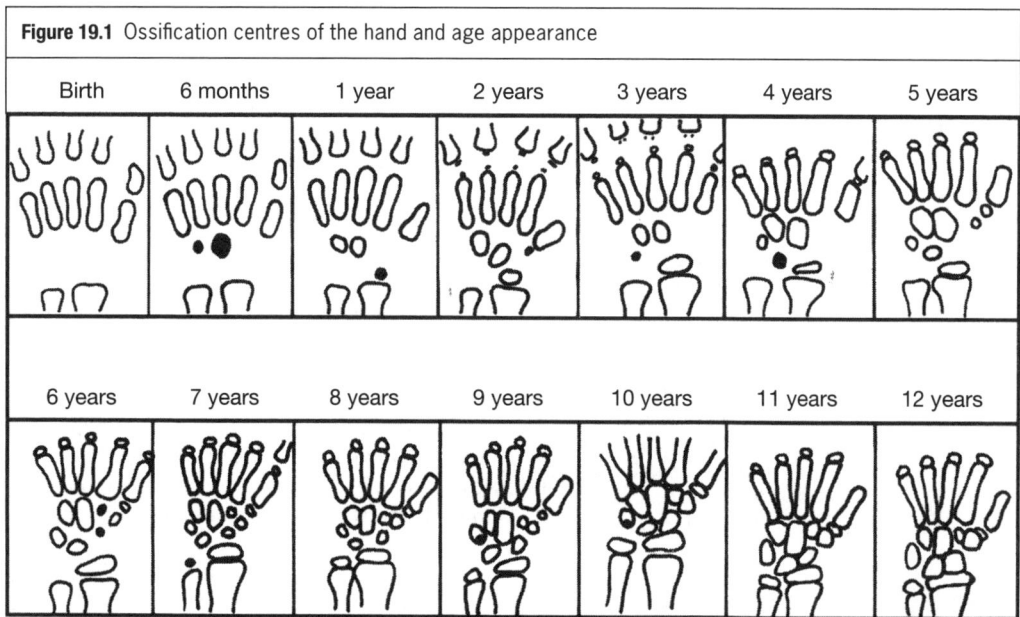

| Birth | 6 months | 1 year | 2 years | 3 years | 4 years | 5 years |

| 6 years | 7 years | 8 years | 9 years | 10 years | 11 years | 12 years |

---

should maintain their growth channels from two years of age until puberty.

The midparental or target height is calculated by averaging the heights of the parents and adding or subtracting 6.5 cm for boys and girls respectively. If the child's final predicted height according to its percentile is more than 5 cm outside the target height, this may warrant further investigation.

Systemic illness as a cause of growth failure

Normal growth is an indicator of good health. Malnutrition and illness are associated with a decreased growth rate. When evaluating growth failure, nutritional deficiencies and systemic illness must be excluded.

> Children with a height less than −3SD below the mean, a subnormal growth velocity crossing growth channels, or a height percentile substantially different from that of the midparental height plotted on the gender-specific percentile chart should be evaluated for a growth disturbance.

A careful clinical examination is necessary to rule out systemic disease. Gastrointestinal disorders (e.g. coeliac disease), genetic disorders (e.g. Turner's syndrome), rickets, metabolic disease (e.g. renal tubular acidosis); cardiac, pulmonary, hepatic, renal, haematological and collagen vascular disease can all compromise growth. Abnormal growth may also be a reflection of suboptimal therapy of a chronic condition (e.g. asthma). Growth failure is a common feature of infectious disease, including HIV infection.

All diseases impair growth, so a child who is not growing needs a diagnosis and treatment. A short child growing at a rate appropriate for his age may need a diagnosis to explain why he is short, but an active disease process is unlikely in such a child.

A systematic approach is needed to a child presenting with short stature in order to arrive at a diagnosis. After excluding systemic disease, genetic conditions (e.g. Turner's syndrome), malnutrition and having considered the possibility of 'normal' variants (specifically constitutional

> The single most important cause of growth retardation worldwide is malnutrition.

Table 19.3 Differential dignosis of short stature	
NORMAL VARIANTS	**PATHOLOGICAL**
I Familial short stature	I Proportionate short stature a Prenatal onset e.g. IUGR, dysmorphic syndromes (e.g. Silver-Russel syndrome), chromosomosal disorder (e.g. Turner's syndrome) b Postnatal onset e.g. Psycho-social dwarfism, malnutrition, gastrointestinal disorders (e.g. coeliac disease), renal disorders, cardiopulmonary disease, chronic anaemia, endocrine diseases
II Constitutional delay of growth	II Disproportionate short stature Rickets Skeletal dysplasias

delay of puberty and familial short stature), an endocrine cause for the short stature may be considered. Clinical clues to the presence of an endocrine cause include a 'cherubic' appearance of the face (in growth hormone deficiency) and an increased weight to height ratio, with the child appearing to be obese. Neonatal clues to growth hormone deficiency include hypoglycaemia and micropenis.

Endocrine causes of short stature

Hypopituitarism and growth hormone deficiency

This disorder is characterized by a deficiency of one, some, or all, of the peptide hormones secreted by the pituitary gland. The following circumstances may be associated with malfunction of the pituitary gland:

- Cranial malformations, such as holoprosencephaly, septo-optic dysplasia, midline craniocerebral or midfacial abnormalities.
- Embryonic defects, such as pituitary hypoplasia, pituitary aplasia, and congenital absence of the pituitary gland.

Many of these defects have a genetic basis.

- Long term survivors of childhood cancers may be at risk for hypopituitarism if the pituitary has not been shielded during cranial irradiation.
- Infectious damage from meningitis or encephalitis.
- Infiltrative disorders such as histiocytosis.
- Trauma can lead to hypopituitarism.

It is important to distinguish the patient with multiple anterior pituitary hormone deficiencies (i.e deficiencies of TSH, ACTH and GH) from a patient with an isolated deficiency (e.g. GH deficiency only). Patients with suspected hypopituitarism should be investigated using stimulation tests at a referral centre. Appropriate laboratory investigations would include thyroid function tests, serum cortisol, and insulin-like growth factor (IGF). The evaluation of the growth hormone secretory status is complex, but it is possible to accurately assess GH secretion in the majority of children. As GH is relatively expensive, the decision to treat with GH must be made after careful evaluation of the possible benefits.

Hypothyroidism

Untreated congenital hypothyroidism and acquired hypothyroidism result in poor growth.

Precocious puberty

Initially patients with precocious puberty may be taller than their peers but end up with a diminished adult height because of earlier closure of epiphyses.

Congenital adrenal hyperplasia (CAH)

Excessive doses of steroids or inadequate treatment with consequent androgen-induced advancement of bone age can result in short stature.

Cushing syndrome

Glucocortoid excess in Cushing's syndrome can retard bone maturation and most affected children will be short.

Pseudohypoparathyroidism

End-organ resistance to parathyroid hormone may present with a distinct phenotype, that is short stature, truncal obesity, short metacarpals, round face and mental retardation.

Poorly controlled diabetes mellitus

Children with poorly controlled diabetes exhibit poor growth. The combination of severe growth failure and hepatosplenomegaly due to excess hepatic deposition of glycogen in poorly-controlled diabetics is known as Mauriac syndrome.

Psychosocial aspects of short stature

Parents, children and their doctors may be concerned about the prospect of short stature. The impact of short stature on the child or his family depends on a number of social concerns. Severe short stature can be a social handicap and early evaluation is important.

An important condition that may be overlooked is psycho-social deprivation, which not only can lead to poor growth, but also can affect the growth hormone secretory status.

Tall stature

The differential diagnosis of tall stature includes familial tall stature, obesity, thyrotoxicosis, precocious puberty, genetic syndromes (e.g. Marfan's syndrome), chromosomal disorders (e.g. Klinefelter's syndrome), and, very rarely, conditions of growth hormone excess.

Obesity

(*see* also chapter 13, Nutritional disorders)

Obesity is emerging as a serious public health concern in the 21st century. The most commonly used measure of obesity is the body mass index (BMI) defined as kilogram of body weight per height in meters squared (kg/m^2). In the paediatric age group the BMI percentiles vary by age and sex. Children are defined as overweight if the BMI is greater than the 95th percentile and at risk for overweight if the BMI percentile is between the 85th to 95th percentile. Children with a BMI greater than the 85th percentile should receive a medical evaluation (to recognize individuals with obesity secondary to hormonal disorders or genetic syndromes). Approximately 5 per cent of cases of obesity referred for evaluation are due to endocrine disorders, genetic syndromes, hypothalamic lesions and single gene mutations.

The clinical features and associated growth failure (short stature) of hypothyroidism, hypopituitarism and hypercortisolism enable these conditions to be ruled out on clinical grounds in the vast majority of cases. Likewise, most dysmorphic syndromes associated with obesity (e.g. Prader Willi Syndrome) are also associated with short stature and distinct phenotypic characteristics. A normal or increased growth velocity suggests 'idiopathic/simple' obesity.

Overweight children (i.e BMI greater than the 95th percentile) should be routinely evaluated for the presence of co-morbid conditions (e.g. Type 2 diabetes mellitus and obstructive sleep apnoea).

> Endocrine or genetic tests only need to be performed in obese children who are also short and/or not growing.

Disorders of sex development

A new classification of intersexual conditions has recently been proposed. The term 'Disorders of Sex Development" (DSD) is now being used to describe abnormalities of genital development that arise with atypical chromosomal, gonadal and anatomic sex (*see* Table 19.4).

Investigation and management of DSD

Any ambiguity of a newborn infant's external genitalia requires assessment, consultation with experts, and a plan of action *prior to discharge*.

In order to get optimal clinical care, individuals with DSD should not be assigned a gender until expert evaluation is carried out at a centre with an experienced multidisciplinary team. The family should participate in the decision-making process. Family concerns should be respected. It should be explained to the parents that the best course of action may not initially be clear, but that the health care team will work with the family to reach the best possible set of decisions in the circumstance (*see* Table 19.5).

Disorders of puberty

Puberty is the developmental process that gives rise to secondary sexual characteristics and the capacity to reproduce. The age of onset of puberty

Table 19.4 Disorders of sexual development classification

Sex chromosome DSD	45, X/XY (mixed gonadal dysgenesis) 47, XXY (Klinefelter's syndrome) 45, X (Turner's syndrome)
46, XY DSD	Disorders of gonadal (testicular) development Disorder of androgen synthesis or action Other (cloacal extrophy, severe hypospadias)
46, XX DSD	Disorder of gonadal (ovarian) development (e.g. ovotesticular DSD or 'true hermaphrodite') Androgen excess (e.g. congenital adrenal hyperplasia) Other (cloacal extrophy, vaginal atresia)

varies and is more closely correlated with bone age than with chronological age. In girls, puberty begins with breast development between eight and 13 years of age. In boys, puberty begins with testicular enlargement, between nine and 14 years of age. The age at which children enter puberty is decreasing, perhaps related to increased weight and adiposity.

Table 19.5 An approach to ambiguous genitalia

What is the phenotypic sex and functional anatomy?	What is the aetiological diagnosis?
Clinical examination (presence of gonads?) Ultrasound Exploratory laparotomy	Chromosome analysis Sodium and potassium balance Plasma 17-OH progesterone Gonadal biopsy

Variations of pubertal development

Premature thelarche
Unilateral or bilateral breast enlargement without other signs of sexual maturation (especially without signs of oestrogenization) occurs commonly in girls up to two years of age and rarely after four years. Most regress between six months and six years after diagnosis. Significant nipple development is absent and there is no evidence of oestrogen-induced thickening and dulling of the vaginal mucosa or enlargement of the uterus on ultrasonography. Stature is normal. Premature thelarche is usually a benign self-limited disorder.

Premature adrenarche
This term applies to the appearance of sexual hair before the age of eight years in girls and nine years in boys, without other evidence of maturation. Premature adrenarche is an early maturational event of adrenal androgen production. It is usually a benign condition that requires no therapy.

Adolescent gynaecomastia
Transient breast enlargement occurs in approximately one third of normal males during early to midpuberty. Management is reassurance and psychological support, provided physical examination shows him to be normal and progressing in puberty.

Precocious puberty

Precocious puberty is the appearance of any signs of secondary sexual maturation before the age of eight years in girls and the age of nine years in boys.

True or central precocious puberty
This results from premature activation of the hypothalamic–pituitary–gonadal axis. Gonadotrophin-dependent precocious puberty occurs at least ten times more frequently in girls than in boys. In more than 90 per cent of girls, sexual precocity is idiopathic. In males with central precocious puberty, there is a high incidence of intracranial pathology and one should therefore have a low threshold for neurological investigations.

Peripheral, 'pseudoprecocious' puberty
Secondary sex characteristics develop as a result of increased sex steroid activity, independent of the hypothalamic gonadotrophin releasing hormone pulse generator. This may be iso- or

heterosexual. A number of tumours, including gonadal and adrenal tumours, may secrete sex hormones. These cases require referral for specialist opinion.

Delayed puberty

The absence of signs of puberty at 14 years in a boy and at 13 years in a girl constitutes delayed puberty. The cause of delayed puberty can be classified into two groups:

- Temporary disorders: constitutional delay in puberty, chronic disease and nutritional disorders.
- Permanent disorders: permanent hypogonadotrophic hypogonadism or hypergonadotrophic hypogonadism.

Disorders of water balance

Syndrome of inappropriate antidiuretic hormone secretion (SIADH)

This is associated with a variety of intracranial and extracranial conditions, but is most commonly seen in severe meningitis (mainly tuberculous), head injury, pulmonary disorders, and with vincristine therapy. Increased renal tubular water reabsorption results in diminished output of highly concentrated urine in the face of plasma hypo-osmolality, leading to dilutional hyponatraemia without dehydration. The clinical features are those of water intoxication: nausea, vomiting, muscle weakness, neurological irritability, convulsions, and coma. A number of patients develop oedema.

In conditions known to predispose to SIADH, excessive oral and intravenous fluids should be avoided. The mainstay of treatment consists of restriction of water intake and provision of enough sodium until a steady rise in serum sodium and a loss of body weight occur. In emergency situations, the slow intravenous administration of 3% saline (5 ml/kg) combined with furosemide therapy (0.5 to 1 mg/kg) may help for a while.

Diabetes insipidus

The symptoms of this disorder include polyuria, thirst, chronic dehydration, and growth failure.

The passage of large amounts of dilute, glucose-free, pale-coloured urine may be due to a deficiency of ADH or to a lack of its effect on the kidneys. The diagnosis is confirmed when inappropriately dilute urine is excreted in the presence of serum hypertonicity. Overnight water deprivation tests may be dangerous in children suspected of having diabetes insipidus (DI). The test is best done in the morning when fluids can be totally withheld under supervision, preferably in a secondary or tertiary institution. In DI, the test leads to rapid dehydration with a rise in plasma osmolality and sodium, but with little change in urine output, urine osmolality, or specific gravity. If the defect can be corrected with vasopressin administration, a central nervous system cause is implicated.

Central diabetes insipidus

The lack of ADH secretion by the posterior pituitary may be partial or complete. Rarely, this is inherited or idiopathic but it is more commonly acquired as a result of organic lesions of the hypothalamo-pituitary area, such as trauma, craniopharyngioma and other tumours, histiocytosis, and following neurosurgery. On occasions, the ADH deficiency may precede the symptoms of the underlying pathology; hence a computerized tomography (CT) scan is essential if no obvious cause is found. Older children are not dehydrated unless the thirst centre is also involved. When plasma osmolality or sodium is normal, the condition must be distinguished from compulsive water drinking.

The treatment consists of hormone replacement, either with lysine vasopressin or desamino-D-arginine vasopressin (DDAVP), given as intranasal spray. DDAVP needs to be refrigerated to ensure stability, has a long (12- to 24-hour) duration of action, and excessive administration carries a risk of water intoxication.

Nephrogenic diabetes insipidus

ADH insensitivity at the renal tubular level is a familial condition and occurs mainly in boys as an X-linked dominant trait. Heterozygous girls may also rarely be affected clinically. Soon after birth, the infants present with vomiting, constipation, hypotonia, failure to thrive, and recurrent hypertonic dehydration. Occasionally, the condition may be mimicked by chronic hypokalaemia due to kwashiorkor or long-standing diarrhoea.

There is no response to vasopressin administration. Treatment is difficult and must always include a high water intake with frequent feeding, even during the night. A low-salt diet, hydrochlorothiazide (3 mg/kg/d) with indomethacin (1.5 to 3 mg/kg/d), reduces the urine losses only partially but helps to prevent recurrent admissions for dehydration and also promotes weight gain.

Diabetes mellitus

It is estimated that there are about half a million children with diabetes in the world. Diagnostic criteria for diabetes are based on blood glucose measurements and the presence or absence of symptoms. Type 1 diabetes, the commonest form of diabetes in childhood, is caused by the destruction of beta cells leading to absolute deficiency of insulin. Most cases are primarily due to T-cell mediated pancreatic b-cell destruction. Patients become symptomatic when approximately 90% of the pancreatic beta cells are destroyed.

Type 2 diabetes, due to insulin resistance, is being recognized in children who are overweight, particularly around the time of puberty.

Diagnosis

The diagnosis is straightforward in children with classical symptoms. Such patients present with polyuria, polydipsia, blurring of vision, and weight loss, in association with glycosuria and ketonuria. If management is not instituted early, ketoacidosis may develop and lead to stupor and coma. The diagnosis is confirmed by an elevated blood glucose concentration.

If the diagnosis of diabetes is suspected in a child with minimal symptoms, confirmatory tests include a fasting glucose greater than 7 mmol/L or a two hour post prandial glucose greater than 11.1 mmol/L. In the absence of symptoms, hyperglycaemia detected incidentally or during acute stress situations, should not be regarded as diagnostic of diabetes.

In order to confirm the diagnosis of Type 1 diabetes, one needs to measure specific antibod-

ies, (e.g. islet cell and GAD antibodies) although these tests are not widely available.

With the increased prevalence of obesity, type 2 diabetes mellitus has recently been recognized as an important entity in children and adolescents. The risks for developing type 2 diabetes are high if the BMI is above the 85th percentile for age, especially if there is a positive family history of diabetes. Type 2 diabetes occurs typically in adolescents during puberty. Insulin secretion becomes inadequate to meet the increased demand posed by insulin resistance. Other features of insulin resistance include hyperlipidaemia, hypertension, acanthosis nigricans, non–alcoholic fatty liver disease and polycystic ovarian hyperandrogenism. Occasionally patients with type 2 diabetes may be misdiagnosed as type 1, particularly if the initial presentation is with ketoacidosis. Although these patients can be managed with insulin initially, the insulin requirements decrease as the diabetes is controlled and the patients should then be referred to a specialist for further evaluation and therapy.

Diabetic ketoacidosis

Diabetic ketoacidosis (DKA) results from absolute or relative deficiency of insulin and increased levels of counterregulatory hormones (catecholamines, glucagon, cortisol, and growth hormone). Absolute insulin deficiency occurs in a previously undiagnosed diabetic, or when an injection of insulin (particularly the basal insulin) is omitted in a known diabetic. Relative insulin deficiency occurs in stress situations (e.g. sepsis, trauma) when the counterregulatory hormones increase in response to the stress. The combination of low serum insulin and high counterregulatory hormone concentrations results in a catabolic state with increased glucose production by the liver and kidney (via glycogenolysis and gluconeogenesis), impaired peripheral glucose utilization resulting in hyperglycaemia and hyperosmolality, and increased lipolysis and ketogenesis.

The clinical features of diabetic ketoacidosis (DKA) include acidotic breathing (rapid, deep, sighing respiration) nausea, vomiting, abdominal pain, depressed level of consciousness and coma. If one does not have a high index of suspicion, the presentation may be confused with an acute abdominal emergency. Diabetes must be considered in any dehydrated and acidotic patient, as failure to institute urgent therapy can be fatal. The biochemical criteria for the diagnosis of DKA include hyperglycaemia (blood glucose >11 mmol/L), a venous pH <7.3, a serum bicarbonate level <15 mmol/L, and ketonuria.

Management of DKA

Intravenous fluids (0.9% saline) should be administered as soon as possible to restore adequate perfusion. Typically, an intravenous bolus of 10–20 ml/kg is required. The degree of fluid deficit is usually estimated to be 7.5 per cent to 10 per cent of body weight. This estimated deficit, along with maintenance fluid requirements, should be replaced evenly over 36 to 48 hours using 0.45% or 0.9% saline, depending on the 'corrected sodium', calculated according to the formula:

$$\text{Corrected Na} = \text{measured Na} + \frac{(2\,(\text{Glucose}-5.5)}{5.5}$$

Patients with a corrected sodium above 150 mmol/L should receive 0.45% saline.

Insulin should be administered at a rate of 0.1 unit/kg/hour. When the glucose concentration drops to 11 mmol/L dextrose should be added to the intravenous fluids to avoid hypoglycaemia, while the insulin infusion is continued to promote resolution of ketosis and acidosis. With insulin treatment, there is substantial movement of potassium from the extracellular space into the intracellular space. Potassium should therefore be added to the intravenous fluids, provided that the renal function is adequate. Treatment with bicarbonate should not be given routinely to children with DKA because acidosis can usually be corrected with insulin and fluids alone. Children with DKA should ideally be managed in a high care area with frequent monitoring of vital signs and hourly estimations of glucose and electrolytes. The IV infusion is discontinued when the patient is clinically stable and a substantial improvement in acidosis and ketonaemia has occurred. The first maintenance insulin dose should be given two hours before discontinuing the intravenous insulin infusion, in order to allow for absorption of the insulin, which is administered subcutaneously in divided doses. A combination of rapid and intermediate acting insulin is required at a usual dose of 0.5 to 0.7 units/kg/24hr. The regimen chosen should be individualized.

A potentially serious, though rare, complication of DKA is cerebral oedema. Symptoms and signs of cerebral oedema include headache, altered mental status, vomiting, hypertension and inappropriate slowing of the heart rate. Cerebral oedema should be recognized immediately and managed with IV mannitol 1 to 2 g/kg.

Long term care

The evaluation and management of a child with diabetes is challenging, particularly in settings where healthcare systems do not have specialized diabetes centres. Ideally the care of a child with diabetes should be provided by a multidisciplinary team consisting of a paediatrician, a diabetic educator, a dietician, a paediatric social worker and a psychologist with knowledge about paediatric diabetes. As a multidisciplinary team is very unlikely to be available in remote areas, contact by telephone or the internet may be necessary. Skills for self-management have to be learnt by the child and family in order to optimize control. The parents have to assume responsibility for all aspects of care and without active parental involvement the care is likely to be suboptimal. The child can only grasp concepts appropriate to his or her level of maturity. Parents should anticipate power struggles that may occur at each childhood developmental stage. The increased concentrations of counterregulatory hormones during puberty may be associated with metabolic decompensation unless the total daily dose of insulin dose is increased. Consistent, repeated educational advice regarding injection technique, home glucose monitoring, dietary adjustments, coping with intercurrent infections, making adjustments for anticipated exercise and recognizing the symptoms of hypoglycaemia and hyperglycaemia improve self management skills. Health professionals must be aware of psychosocial factors, including food security, or else control of the diabetes will be compromised.

The risk for long term microvascular complications in diabetic children can be reduced by good glycaemic control. Treatment regimens that reduce HbA1c levels protect against the development and progression of retinopathy, nephropathy, and neuropathy. In order to achieve optimal glycaemic targets, sufficient time and education needs to be devoted by the diabetes team, adapted to the individual child and family. Regular supervision is essential to maintain glucose control, and monitoring of risk factors of acute and chronic complications including the HbA1c, should be undertaken in consultation with a centre specializing in diabetes. Improving glycaemic targets should go hand in hand with the skills to recognize and manage hypoglycaemia. Children, particularly under six years of age, generally are not capable of self management and are reliant on supervision from an adult.

Children may fail to recognise that they are hypoglycaemic when neuroglycopaenia (impaired thinking, mood changes, irritability, dizziness, tiredness) occurs before autonomic activation.

Newer insulin analogues (both rapid acting and longer acting 'basal' insulins) have been shown to be of benefit in the paediatric population. Technological advances, such as the use of insulin pumps requires intensive education. The well motivated child and family with a good grasp of the insulin action profiles can achieve good glycaemic control despite not being able to afford insulin pumps.

Disorders of the thyroid

Congenital hypothyroidism

Without a screening programme, congenital hypothyroidism is usually missed, as many of the clinical features do not become apparent until two or three months of age. Instituting therapy at that time does not prevent neurological sequelae.

Only 10 to 15 per cent of hypothyroid newborns present with a suspicious clinical picture. The most reliable signs are an open posterior fontanelle (greater than 1 cm), an umbilical hernia, coarse facial features, and poor sucking. In the absence of systematic screening programmes, a high index of awareness may be maintained by the use of a congenital hypothyroidism score (see Table 19.6). Although jaundice is not highly weighted in the scoring system, being a common occurrence in the first week of life, prolonged unconjugated hyperbilirubinaemia lasting a few weeks should raise suspicion of congenital hypothyroidism. Patients should preferably be referred to a specialist.

Screening programmes use dried blood spots on filter paper to measure TSH. As there is normally a surge in TSH in the first 24 hours after

Table 19.6 Congenital hypothyroidism score

Symptom	Score
Hernia, umbilical	2
Hypothermia	1
Coarse facial features	2
Enlarged tongue	1
Hypotonia	1
Jaundice (>3 days)	1
Dry skin	1
Wide posterior fontanelle	1
Constipation	2
Duration of gestation >40 wk	1
Birth weight >3.5 kg	1
Female sex	1
Total	15

Score >5 suggests hypothyroidism

birth, screening should only be performed after the first 24 hours of life. Neonates with elevated TSH after the first 24 hours should be evaluated for congenital hypothyroidism. The laboratory diagnosis is not difficult. Serum T_4 is low to low normal and the thyroid-stimulating hormone (TSH) value is always significantly elevated except in the rare instance of secondary pituitary hypothyroidism.

The causes of hypothyroidism are shown in Table 19.7.

Patients with dysgenesis and secondary hypothyroidism have no goitre. Delayed skeletal maturation, as assessed by the size of the distal femoral epiphysis on an X-ray of the knee, can provide an added argument in favour of a therapeutic trial if no reliable laboratory is available.

Treatment can always be stopped in the second year of life, when brain development is no longer vulnerable, to allow for retesting. When hypothyroidism occurs after infancy, there is much less severe brain damage, but these children are sluggish in their movements, have a puffy appearance, and grow slowly. The treatment of congenital hypothyroism is thyroxine 10–15 µg/kg/day in the first year. Growth, bone age, and measurement of T_4 and TSH may be used to monitor the adequacy of dosage.

Hyperthyroidism

Thyroid hyperfunction is rare in children but

Table 19.7 Causes of hypothyroidism
Dysgenesis
Aplasia
Maldescent
Iodine deficiency
Familial enzyme defect
Ingestion of goitrogens
• Antenatal
iodide-containing cough mixtures
antithyroid drugs
para-amino-salicylic acid
• Postnatal
iodide-containing cough mixtures
Auto-immune thyroiditis
Secondary hypothyroidism
Hypothalamic or pituitary disease

Table 19.8 Adrenocortical insufficiency
Aplasia/hypoplasia
Enzyme defect
Congenital adrenal hyperplasia
Destruction
Haemorrhage
Infection (TB)
Waterhouse-Friderichsen syndrome
Auto-immune disease
X-linked adrenoleukodystrophy
Suppression of pituitary-adrenal axis
Iatrogenic: steroid therapy
ACTH deficiency
Hypothalamic/pituitary damage
Congenital unresponsiveness to ACTH

may occur at all ages, including the neonatal period, when it is caused by the transplacental passage of thyroid-stimulating immunoglobulins from a mother with Graves disease. The main presenting features in children are emotional lability, nervousness, behavioural disturbances, sweating and nocturnal enuresis, but a large goitre and severe ophthalmopathy are rare. The diagnosis is confirmed by an elevated serum T_4 and a suppressed TSH. The various methods available for treatment are antithyroid drugs, subtotal thyroidectomy, and radioactive iodine.

Disorders of the adrenal cortex

Acute adrenal insufficiency

An adrenal crisis may be the presenting feature of any of the conditions listed in Table 19.8, or it may occur in treated patients as a result of acute stress. Inadequate secretion of glucocorticoids and mineralocorticoids results in **salt loss**, **hypoglycaemia**, and **circulatory collapse**. The serum potassium is high, the sodium low to low normal, and there is a poorly compensated metabolic acidosis.

Acute management

- Take blood samples for electrolytes, acid base, urea, and glucose, and freeze extra serum for plasma cortisol assay.
- Fluid and electrolyte replacement to re-expand the blood volume and elevate the blood pressure: Ringer's lactate, plasma or Haemaccel® must be infused intravenously for severe shock, otherwise 0.9% sodium chloride in 5% dextrose is given at the rate of 10 to 20 ml/kg over the first hour; thereafter at a maintenance rate to deliver 60 ml/kg over the following 24 hours.
- Hydrocortisone sodium succinate (Solu-Cortef®) is given as an IV bolus (50 mg for small children and 100 mg for larger children) followed by 50–100 mg/24 hr added to the IV maintenance solution.
- 9a-fluorohydrocortisone (Florinef®) 0.05–0.1 mg/d orally.
- Monitor circulation, electrolytes, and glucose levels.

Congenital adrenal hyperplasia

This is an autosomal recessive condition due to a partial or severe deficiency of an enzyme in the biosynthetic pathway of cortisol and in 50 per cent of cases also of aldosterone. It is being recognized more frequently in black African

> Acute adrenal insufficiency is an acute medical emergency requiring immediate treatment before any transfer.

babies. Cortisol deficiency is present early in fetal life, resulting in stimulation of excessive ACTH release, which causes hyperplasia of the adrenal cortex and virilization of the external genitalia by androgenic precursors. The most common type is due to 21-hydroxylase deficiency. The diagnosis should be suspected in any newborn with intersexuality in whom gonads are not palpable, or in any male infant who presents with a salt-wasting syndrome soon after birth. The electrolytes will be abnormal (high potassium, low sodium, low bicarbonate and low glucose) only if salt loss is present. Pre-treatment serum has to be stored in a deep-freeze for later confirmation of the diagnosis, which will rest on finding increased levels of 17-OH progesterone and adrenal androgens. About two-thirds of cases do not have symptoms and signs of adrenal insufficiency because the adrenal hyperplasia compensates for the enzyme deficiency.

After acute management as for adrenal crisis, life-long maintenance is started with oral hydrocortisone or cortisone acetate (20–25 mg/m^2/d in divided doses) in all infants, and 9a-fluorohydrocortisone (0.05–0.1 mg once daily) with added dietary salt if necessary for the salt-losers.

The child is issued with an identity disc with the diagnosis engraved on it. When stable, the infant should be referred to a tertiary centre for a review of the diagnosis, assessment of the need for surgical repair of the intersexed genitalia in female patients, and for genetic counselling. With good follow-up care and constant availability of medication, long-term survival may be ensured.

Antenatal diagnosis is possible in tertiary centres, where careful genetic counselling and first trimester steroid treatment may be offered to reduce the chance of virilization of an affected female fetus.

Addison's disease

The adrenal cortex may atrophy as part of an auto-immune or metabolic disorder or be destroyed by tuberculous infection. The patients are weak, anorectic, and may present with vomiting, diarrhoea, dehydration, and hypotension. There is an increase in pigmentation of the skin, buccal mucosa, and nails. The biochemical features of hypo-adrenalism are present and, although

basal cortisol may be low normal, there is a poor response to an ACTH stimulation test.

Life-long maintenance treatment is similar to that of congenital adrenal hyperplasia. With intercurrent illness or stress, the hydrocortisone dose should be doubled or tripled until the illness has resolved.

Hyperadrenocorticism

Hyperfunction of the adrenal cortex may present clinically with Cushing's syndrome or with marked virilization, depending on the specific steroid secretion.

Cushing's syndrome is caused by:
- Excess steroid therapy (the most common cause)
- Adrenal tumour: onset of symptoms occurs before eight years of age, usually in early childhood and is associated with virilization; often malignant
- ACTH-secreting micro-adenoma: more frequent in adolescence
- Ectopic ACTH-secreting tumours: very rare.

The moon face, truncal obesity, and 'buffalo hump' are characteristic. Growth failure with retarded bone age is an important point in differentiation from nutritional obesity, unless androgens are also excessively secreted. Muscle wasting and weakness, thinning of the skin with purple striae, personality changes, hypertension, and virilization may be present.

Florid cases should be referred to a tertiary care centre without delay. In a doubtful case, there may be a place for attempting to confirm or exclude the presence of an elevated cortisol secretion. Useful screening laboratory tests are the estimation of a 24-hour urinary free cortisol excretion and the overnight dexamethasone adrenal suppression test (dexamethasone 0.3 mg/m^2 is given orally at 11 pm and plasma cortisol is measured the next morning at 08:00). Adrenal tumour localization may be made by ultrasonography, IVP, or CT scan.

The predominantly virilizing adrenal tumours have to be differentiated from adrenal hyperplasia by the lack of suppressibility of the elevated androgens by dexamethasone, and by radiological localization.

Surgical resection, either by unilateral adrenalectomy or transsphenoidal micro-adenodectomy, should only be attempted in a very specialized centre with experienced surgeons and endocrinologists.

Disorders of the parathyroid glands

Parathyroid hormone (PTH) is intimately linked to the maintenance of normal serum calcium and is therefore an important factor in the development of metabolic bone disease (*see* Chapter 12, Rickets and metabolic bone diseases).

Primary hyperparathyroidism

Hypercalcaemia caused by hyperfunctioning parathyroid glands is uncommon in children. Familial parathyroid hyperplasia may occur on its own or as part of dominantly inherited multiple endocrine adenomatosis. Solitary adenomas are even more rare, and present in later childhood or adolescence, usually with long-standing symptoms representing a poor awareness of the disorder and the lack of routine biochemical screening in children. Malaise, gastrointestinal symptoms, abdominal pains, nephrolithiasis, bone pain, and fractures are the most common presenting symptoms. An elevated serum calcium and a lowered serum phosphorus level in the presence of a normal urea strongly suggest the diagnosis, which can be confirmed by finding raised PTH levels. Surgical removal is curative but only an experienced surgeon should attempt the neck exploration.

Hypercalcaemia may also be due to vitamin D intoxication, malignant bony secondary deposits, and leukaemia.

Secondary hyperparathyroidism

This is much more common than primary hyperparathyroidism in children and is due to a chronically decreased serum calcium, such as occurs in vitamin D deficiency or chronic renal failure. This results in stimulation of parathyroid hyperplasia. Excessive bony resorption with deformities and fractures may ensue. The serum calcium is at low normal levels, the serum phosphorus is decreased in patients with normal renal function, and the alkaline phosphatase is elevated. Treatment consists of vitamin D or its active metabolites in order to maintain serum calcium levels as close to normal as possible.

Hypoparathyroidism

Transient neonatal hypoparathyroidism may occur in association with maternal hyperparathyroidism or diabetes. It presents with hypocalcaemic convulsions and apnoeic spells. The treatment is intravenous calcium for convulsions.

Congenital hypoparathyroidism

- Sex-linked recessive type: onset with hypocalcaemia occurs at a few days to a few months of age.
- Hypoplasia: associated with heart and thymus defect, e.g. Di George syndrome.

Idiopathic acquired hypoparathyroidism

This presents after one year of age and may be associated with other auto-immune conditions (Addison's disease, thyroiditis) presenting later in life. Patients present with tetany, convulsions, intellectual impairment, dental enamel hypoplasia, and cataracts, and may have mucocutaneous candidiasis. Another form is secondary to hypomagnesaemia.

The diagnosis is suspected on the findings of a low serum calcium, a high serum phosphorus, and a normal alkaline phosphatase and urea, together with X-ray evidence of metaphyseal density and intracranial basal ganglia calcification.

Vitamin D or its active metabolites, extra calcium, and phosphate binders such as calcium carbonate are the prescribed treatment, with regular monitoring of serum calcium levels to avoid hypercalcaemia.

Parathyroid resistance syndrome

This comprises a group of disorders with the clinical and biochemical picture of hypoparathyroidism, but with normal or raised PTH levels. Not all patients have the typical features of Albright's hereditary osteodystrophy, which comprise short stature, mental retardation, and skeletal changes. Treatment is as for hypoparathyroidism.

20

Allergic disorders

An allergic reaction is a hypersensitivity response mediated by immunological mechanisms. The precipitating factors are antigens or allergens, most of which are proteins in nature. The Gell and Coombs classification of allergy reminds us that there are many immunological mechanisms in allergy. IgE mediated allergy is the commonest form but non-IgE mediated allergy is often responsible for food allergy, drug allergy and chronic urticaria.

Atopy is defined as the inherited tendency to produce IgE in response to allergen exposure and then to produce a clinical disease such as asthma, allergic rhinitis or eczema. This definition employs the concepts of IgE-mediated allergy in the context of an inflammatory disease state.

The following conditions often have an allergic basis:

- Acute collapse: anaphylaxis
- Hives (urticaria) and swelling (angio-oedema)
- Eczema
- Chronic rhinitis (blocked or runny nose)
- Hay fever and sneezing
- Conjunctivitis (red, itchy eyes)
- Asthma and wheezing

The immunological mechanisms of allergy include:

- Immediate hypersensitivity (IgE mediated)
- Complement mediated hypersensitivity
- Antigen-antibody reactions (IgG mediated)
- Cell-mediated (delayed hypersensitivity).

- Vomiting, abdominal pains, diarrhoea (food allergy).

Pathology (IgE mediated allergy)

Once an allergic individual has been sensitized to a specific allergen, e.g. grass pollen or house-dust mites (*Dermatophagoides pteronyssinus*), specific antibodies of the IgE subclass develop. The combination of allergen and IgE antibody located on specialized cells, called mast cells situated in the respiratory, gastrointestinal tract and in the skin results in the release of potent chemical mediators from granules contained in these cells. Among these mediators are histamine, tryptase and a wide range of cytokines. This part of the reaction occurs rapidly and is known as the *early phase of the allergic reaction*. Some hours later products of arachidonic acid metabolism occurring in the mast cell membrane release potent, smooth muscle constrictors and inflammatory agents. Depending on the pathway of arachidonic acid metabolism, i.e. cycloxygenase or lipoxygenase, leukotrienes or prostaglandins are released into the surrounding tissues. The recruitment of inflammatory cells such as eosinophils and neutrophils to the site of the reaction results in local tissue damage and inflammation, through the release of substances such as major basic protein. This phase of the reaction is the *late phase allergic reaction* and occurs six to eight hours after the initiation of the allergic reaction. Prolonged inflammation of the affected tissues occurs, which accounts for the characteristic pathological changes associated with the common allergic disorders, which include asthma, allergic rhinitis, atopic eczema, urticaria, angioedema, and food allergies.

Epidemiology and factors influencing allergy

There has been an increase in the prevalence of allergic disorders. Possibly as many as three in every ten children suffer from one or another allergic disorder. The reason for this increase is unknown, but many environmental factors contribute to the sensitization of an allergy-prone individual in early life. An important factor may be lack of exposure to environmental microbial organisms with a change from infection-fighting immunity to allergy-producing immunity in young children. Familial inheritance of allergy suggests a genetic cause, but the specific genes are not known, suggesting a polygenic mode of inheritance. Most allergic children have a strong family history.

The allergic march

Allergic manifestations tend to vary with the age of the child, a phenomenon that is called the 'allergic march'. Gastrointestinal and skin allergies are usually the first of the disorders to present in infancy and often manifest in the first few weeks of life. Food allergy appears to be the primary problem accounting for these early conditions. Both of these disorders tend to become less severe by the second or third year of life. At this stage asthma and allergic rhinitis usually present for the first time. Fully 80 per cent of asthmatic children have had their first attack by the age of five years. There is a strong tendency for many children to develop atopic eczema in infancy and later for allergic rhinitis and asthma to become a problem in the same child.

Climate, weather, and location

Climatic conditions have a great effect on allergic diseases. The climate will determine which pollens and fungal spore exposure occurs. Weather conditions, e.g. cold air, may strongly affect susceptible children. A damp climate favours the growth of highly allergenic fungal spores. Many children who are sensitive to fungal spores will be at their worst during humid weather. Sudden weather changes also cause worsening of symptoms in many allergic children. These weather conditions are also conducive to the child being susceptible to infection with respiratory viruses, such as respiratory syncitial virus (RSV) or rhinoviruses. These viruses have been implicated in initiating allergic respiratory illnesses in atopic children.

Intensity and frequency of exposure to allergens

The intensity and frequency of exposure to allergens plays a large part in the development of allergic disorders. It is not enough to be an allergic individual exposed to potentially sensitizing allergens. The two must be in close contact for a long enough period for sensitization to occur. The most important allergens are those encountered most often either in homes, out of doors, or at school or day-care centres, and which occur in abundance in the environment. Some foods and other allergens may cause reactions by contact, e.g. clothing, leather goods, dyes, or metals.

Approach to the potentially allergic child

A careful allergy history should ideally be obtained from the child's mother to help identify the child's allergic disorder, as well as to identify possible allergens in his or her environment. Four areas need to be carefully considered:

- The circumstances, place, and timing of the onset of symptoms
- The home, especially the child's bedroom
- The classroom or day-care centre
- The diet.

Table 20.1 lists the most common allergens affecting allergic children and their usual place of occurrence. There are a number of pointers to allergy which may be identified on clinical examination.

Physical examination of the allergic child

Many allergic children are unhappy or irritable and many have the characteristic allergic facies. They are often extremely pale and have dark blue rings under their eyes known as 'allergic shiners'. A nasal crease is often noted

Table 20.1 Allergens of importance in allergic children and their source

Home	School	Diet	Outdoor and seasonal
Housedust	Dust	Milk	Trees
Mites	Small pets, e.g.	Wheat	Grasses
Cats	guinea pigs, mice,	Eggs	Weeds, e.g. plantain
Dogs	hamsters	Soya	Fungal spores
Birds	Fungal spores	Peanuts	Flowers
Fungal spores		Fish	Shrubs
		Nuts	
		Pork	

where the bony and cartilaginous portions of the nose meet – the 'allergic crease'. This is due to the child continuously rubbing the tip of the nose in an upward direction to relieve nasal itching and obstruction. This manoeuvre is one of the common allergic mannerisms and is known as the 'allergic salute'. Face pulling and nose twitching is also common. Allergic children are often mouth-breathers and they may have a gaping appearance. Their lips are often dry and cracked as a result of chronic mouth-breathing.

The ear, nose, throat and respiratory systems require careful examination. Assessment of the appearance of the nasal mucous membrane requires experience. Nasal mucosal swelling, changes in colour of the mucosa, and the nature of the mucus discharge should be noted. Postnasal mucus drip is common, as is a rather granular appearance of the posterior pharyngeal wall due to lymphoid hyperplasia. Serous otitis media, also known as 'glue ear', is commonly associated with nasal allergy. Air bubbles may be noted behind the eardrum in the early stages of this condition.

Chest deformities are fairly common. Barrel chest, pigeon chest, and pectus excavatum are the most common deformities in asthmatic children. Hyperinflation of the chest is often present, even between obvious attacks of asthma. Unless the chest is carefully auscultated with the child breathing out forcibly, the expiratory wheeze may be missed.

The skin and exposed mucosal surfaces are often affected in allergic children. The conjunctivae should be checked for 'pavement slabbing' of the mucosa, which is typical of allergic conjunctivitis. Special note should be taken of the flex-ures of the arms and legs, the neck, feet, and back for possible atopic eczema.

Investigations in allergy diagnosis

There are many conditions that may mimic allergic disorders in children. This is especially the case with asthma, allergic rhinitis, and suspected food allergies. Skin tests or CAP-RAST, provocation tests, and elimination diets will help to identify those allergens most likely to be causing clinical symptoms.

Skin tests

Skin tests are simple to perform, and are cheap and accurate. They are preferably performed on the child's forearms. Antihistamine and bronchodilator therapy should be discontinued for 24 to 48 hours prior to these tests. Test sites are marked out 1–2 cm apart using a felt-tip pen. A drop of each of the allergic testing solutions is placed at each mark and a special lancet, which prevents deeper entry of the point than 1 mm, is inserted through each drop in turn. A new lancet should be used for each drop or the point can simply be wiped clean each time prior to proceeding to the next test drop. It is important not to prick too deeply and not to draw blood. Many false positive reactions occur because

The common allergy tests are:

- Skin tests
- CAP-RAST
- Provocation tests
- Elimination diets.

of poor technique. After 15 minutes, observe the test sites for erythema and weal formation. The average (greatest and smallest) or largest diameter of the weal in millimetres should be noted and compared with controls. If a large weal (>15 mm) appears in less than 10 minutes, wipe the allergen from that test site.

A negative control using the saline diluent solution alone should always be included to assess excessive local skin reaction to mechanical trauma. This occurs especially in children who have a tendency to develop dermatographism. A 0.1 per cent histamine solution serves as a positive control. This histamine positive control aids in interpreting skin tests (a standard 3+ reaction) and demonstrates diminished or absent skin reactivity to histamine found in some infants and in children who have inadvertently taken antihistaminics.

Skin tests for foods are less accurate than for the inhalant allergens and a larger weal size, careful history, limited CAP-RAST tests, or elimination diets may be required for diagnosis. Provocation tests require specialized facilities and are not advised unless adequate facilities and expertise are available.

Further special investigations are directed towards establishing that the child is definitely an allergic individual and also towards excluding some of the more common conditions encountered in southern Africa, which should always be included in the differential diagnosis of allergic disorders (*see* Table 20.2).

Allergy emergencies

Anaphylaxis

Anaphylaxis is an acute allergic reaction caused by the administration of an allergen or antigen to which the patient is sensitive. These include many drugs, e.g. aspirin, antibiotics, especially penicillin, vaccines, sera, and insect bites and stings. The onset is usually unexpected and may occur within seconds to minutes after exposure to the allergen. The child may collapse and rapidly enter a state of shock and possible respiratory arrest. In general, allergic reactions which occur abruptly are the most severe and may well be fatal.

> A successful outcome depends on immediate therapy of anaphylaxis.

Treatment

In the following order, give immediately:

- Adrenaline 1:1 000, 0.3–0.5 ml IM. The dose may be repeated at intervals of 20 minutes if necessary.
- Antihistamine, e.g. promethazine (Phenergan®), 0.25–0.5 mg/kg IM.
- IV fluids – shock is due to hypovolaemia secondary to massive exudation of intravascular fluid. Maintenance of normal intravascular volume by IV fluids is essential, e.g. normal saline or Ringer's solution.
- Oxygen is given by face mask or nasal catheter to prevent hypoxaemia.
- Aminophylline is administered if bronchospasm develops. It must be given slowly IV in a dose of 4 mg/kg.
- Intubation if there is airway obstruction due to angioedema. This is fortunately seldom necessary.

Next:

- Steroids are only administered following the immediate and urgent steps outlined above. Steroids have a slow onset of action. Administer hydrocortisone 100–200 mg IV four- to six-hourly for 24 hours or longer if required.

Asthma

Asthma is a chronic inflammatory condition of the airways in which there are episodes of reversible narrowing of the airways in response to various stimuli. It is characterized by cough, wheezing, and dyspnoea. A more practical definition has been proposed:

> Any child, regardless of age, with recurrent (three or more) episodes of wheezing and/or dyspnoea that respond to a bronchodilator should be considered as having asthma until proven otherwise.

Table 20.2 Special investigations in the diagnosis of allergic disorders

Diagnostic tests	Positive results	Interpretation
Phadiotop	Positive or negative	A new screening test to detect the allergic child. Eliminates problems of interpretation found with total IgE estimation. Rather expensive
Blood eosinophils	>6% on peripheral count or 400 cells/mm³ on total count	Suggests allergy. Not specific. Parasitic infestation will also cause elevated counts. Examine stools
Nasal mucus stained with Hansel's stain	Clumps of eosinophils seen on slide	Allergic rhinitis, but normal in young infants
Sweat test	Raised sweat chloride, above 70 mEq/l	Suggests cystic fibrosis – important in differential diagnosis
Immunoglobulins	**Positive results**	**Interpretation**
IgA IgG IgE	Range for age	If low, may account for recurrent respiratory infections If raised, indicates allergy or worm infestation. Examine stools
Radiographs	**Positive results**	**Interpretation**
Chest	Hyperinflation in quiescent periods	Chronic asthma (always hyperinflated in acute attacks)
Postnasal space	Enlarged adenoids	Common cause of nasal obstruction
Paranasal sinuses	Mucosal thickening or opacification	Infection, or associated with allergic rhinitis
RAST		Detects IgE directed against common allergens. May be useful in young children, those with extensive eczema, or where anti-histamines have not been discontinued. Expensive. Use appropriately

An essential feature of asthma is the extreme sensitivity of the airways to environmental and other factors. This increased sensitivity is known as bronchial hyperreactivity.

The onset of asthma may be as early as the first few weeks of life, but is most common between the ages of two and five years. It is often initially confused with bronchiolitis in infants. A health professional faced by a wheezing child should establish whether there is a family history of asthma and other allergic disorders. Most helpful in diagnosis is the recurrent nature of the wheezing episodes. The old saying that 'all that wheezes is not asthma' is certainly true in developing countries, but to this should still be added 'but usually is asthma in children over three years'. As asthma episodes become more frequent and severe, and where schooling, sport, exercise, and sleep are interfered with, these children must be referred for regular treatment of their asthma.

Prevalence

Studies indicate a prevalence rate of between 13 and 20 per cent in South African children. Asthma may be slightly less common in children from rural areas compared with those living in large urban areas. Admissions to hospital of children with acute asthma attacks appear to be on the increase, a trend which has also been reported in many developed countries.

Pathology

Asthma is considered to be an inflammatory disease of the airways. Airway narrowing and obstruction are caused by a combination of the following abnormalities:

- Airway smooth muscle spasm
- Inflammation, which may involve the following:
  - Eosinophil and lymphocyte infiltration
  - Mast cell activation
  - Subepithelial collagen deposition
  - Damage to the airway epithelium
- Mucus plugging of smaller airways.

Following exposure to allergens and other irritants, mast cells in the airway mucosa appear to initiate both an immediate bronchospastic response and a later inflammatory response, which results in a two-phase alteration in the airway reactivity. Mast cell-derived mediators, such as histamine and leukotrienes produce immediate bronchoconstriction. This appears to be the major feature of the immediate response. Interleukins, especially IL-5, attract eosinophils and neutrophils to the airway mucosa. Eosino-phils release major basic protein which damages airway epithelium, and induce mast cell mediator release.

Precipitating factors

There are many factors that may precipitate asthma attacks (*see* Figure 20.1).

Diagnosis

The first approach to asthma diagnosis should always be an adequate history followed by the physical examination. The history includes the family history and the patient's symptoms. This helps to exclude conditions which mimic asthma (*see* Table 20.3). Investigations should include simple pulmonary function tests using a peak flow meter. The Mini Wright Peak Flow Meter is reasonably priced and gives accurate readings. If airflow obstruction is present, the diagnosis can be confirmed by demonstrating significant improvement (>15 per cent) in the peak flow reading, following an inhaled beta$_2$ agonist bronchodilator. Most children from about five years are able to perform these studies well, but younger children are often unable to blow adequately on the peak flow meter.

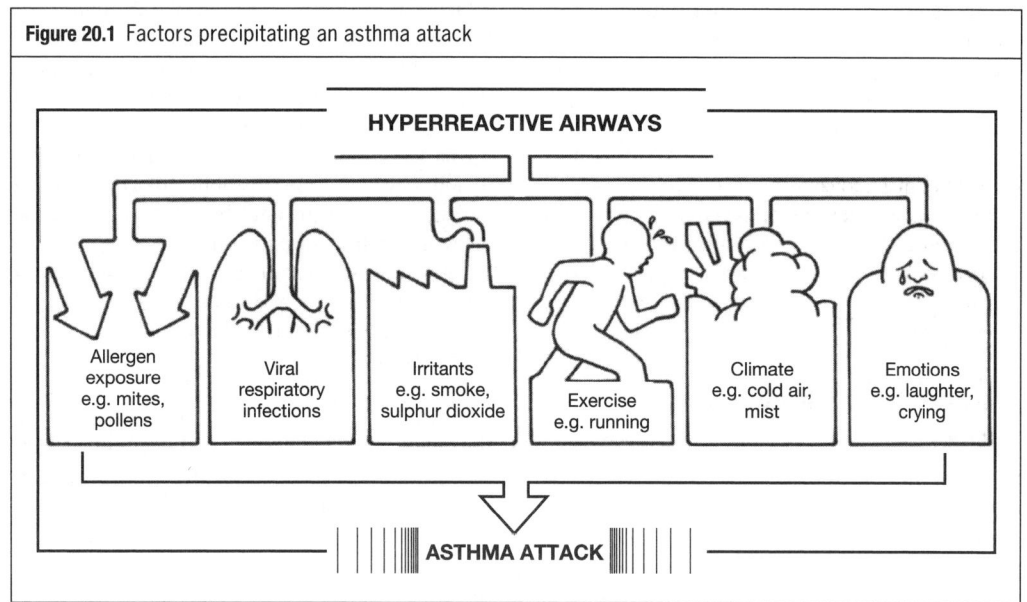

Figure 20.1 Factors precipitating an asthma attack

HYPERREACTIVE AIRWAYS

Allergen exposure e.g. mites, pollens

Viral respiratory infections

Irritants e.g. smoke, sulphur dioxide

Exercise e.g. running

Climate e.g. cold air, mist

Emotions e.g. laughter, crying

ASTHMA ATTACK

Table 20.3 Differential diagnosis of asthma in infants and children

- **Foreign bodies in the airway** – unilateral wheezing may be noted, but not in all cases

- **Supraglottic causes**
  Retropharyngeal abscess
  Tonsillar abscess
  Epiglottitis

- **Laryngeal causes**
  Croup
  Stenosis
  Tetany
  Vocal cord paralysis
  Angioedema of larynx

- **Tracheal causes**
  Tracheomalacia
  Tracheitis
  Vascular rings
  Lymph node compression

- **Bronchial causes**
  Bronchiolitis
  Bronchitis
  Bronchiectasis
  Lymph node compression, e.g. tuberculosis

- **Pulmonary causes**
  Pneumonia
  Cystic fibrosis
  Tuberculosis
  Pertussis
  Atelectasis
  Congenital lobar emphysema
  Hypersensitivity pneumonitis
  Loeffler's syndrome

- **Other causes**
  Congestive cardiac failure
  Gastro-oesophageal reflux
  Hyperventilation

Another diagnostic technique is a therapeutic trial with a bronchodilator. A record of changes in peak flow rates measured at home and entered in a carefully kept asthma diary (*see* Figure 20.2) will show response to medication. This approach yields as much definitive information as an exercise or histamine challenge.

Limited skin testing is useful to determine possible sensitization to environmental allergens. Once the offending allergen is identified, parents can be advised on ways to limit exposure. Recommended skin tests for this region include housedust mites (*D. pteronyssinus*), cats, dogs, South African grasses, Bermuda grass and cockroach. CAP-RAST tests are a useful alternative where skin tests cannot be performed, but are expensive.

Treatment of asthma: the acute attack

Do not underestimate the severity of an asthma attack. Signs of a severe attack include anxiety, restlessness, tachycardia, and intense wheezing on auscultation. Whispering speech and pulsus paradoxus indicate severe airway obstruction. The peak flow is the most useful objective measurement of the degree of airway obstruction.

Beta$_2$ agonist bronchodilators in inhaled form are the most useful drugs for treating acute attacks of asthma. Salbutamol (Ventolin®) or fenoterol (Berotec®) puffs given by metered dose inhaler (MDI) with a spacer may be administered frequently. Each puff is given separately, one at a time, to a maximum of 6–10 puffs. The powder forms of these inhalers require active inhalation, which may be beyond the ability of a child with a bad attack of asthma and should therefore not be used under these circumstances.

If there is no response to the inhaler either initially or after several doses over a period of one hour the child should be treated as for acute severe asthma.

Nebulization. Nebulization remains useful in the management of acute asthma, but oxygen should be used to nebulize the bronchodilator. Several electronically driven home nebulizers are available. They are simple air compressors, which can nebulize salbutamol or fenoterol respirator solution via a face mask nebulizer.

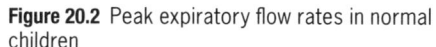

Figure 20.2 Peak expiratory flow rates in normal children

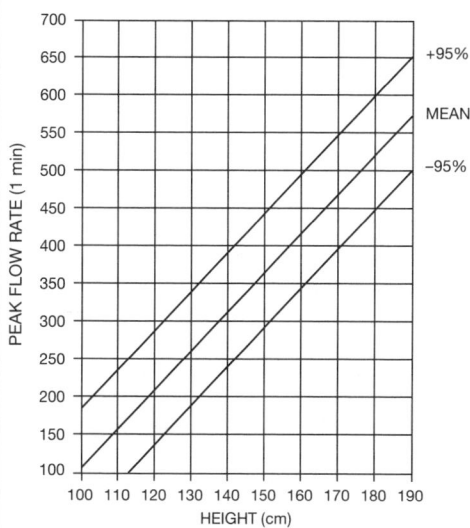

Source: Godfrey et al., British Journal of Diseases of the Chest, vol. 64, no. 15 (1970). By permission of Elsevier.

Home nebulisers are not useful because they don't employ oxygen.

If there is no response to two nebulizations given one hour apart, the child must be managed as for acute severe asthma.

Acute severe asthma

Acute severe asthma may occur in any asthmatic child, usually quite suddenly. There is no response to the usual methods of treatment, probably due to severe inflammation of the airway mucosa and plugging by tenacious mucus. Precipitating factors include allergen exposure, viral infections, weather changes, or emotional upsets. Not uncommonly, no cause may be found.

Physical findings include:

♦ An anxious patient with laboured breathing, audible wheeze, and tachypnoea, which interferes with speech
♦ Marked hyperinflation of the chest with use of accessory muscles of respiration
♦ Markedly diminished breath sounds with intense wheezing on auscultation
♦ Pulsus paradoxus >10 mmHg during inspiration.

Treatment of acute severe asthma

♦ Hospitalize, preferably in an intensive care unit
♦ Treat hypoxaemia: give oxygen by face mask or nasal prongs at low flow
♦ Nebulize with beta$_2$ agonist preparations. Give: 1 ml salbutamol or fenoterol respirator solution diluted with 1 ml of normal saline in the nebulizer. Repeat continuously
♦ Administer steroids: Oral steroids (prednisone 1–2mg/kg) or hydrocortisone 2 mg/kg IV; this is irrespective of whether or not the child has previously had steroid therapy. The dose is repeated daily if oral, or every six hours if iv. The majority of children improve by this time. Convert to an oral prednisone course for 10 days after an episode of acute severe asthma. Improvement should be monitored using a peak flow meter
♦ Aminophylline must only be used with great caution as severe side-effects may occur in children. It should only be used where facilities for measuring the serum levels are available.

Note:

1 If the patient responds poorly to therapy, arterial blood gases should be monitored as necessary.
2 ECG monitoring is essential if IV aminophylline is being given.
3 Do not overhydrate the patient.
4 Monitor peak flow levels at least every six hours.

Acute severe asthma must be regarded as a medical emergency. It is diagnosed when:

▪ There is no response to two puffs of beta$_2$ agonist bronchodilator given 30 minutes apart.
▪ There is no response to two nebulizations with a beta$_2$ agonist bronchodilator.

Asthma maintenance treatment programme

(*See* Figure 20.3: Asthma action plan.)

Modes of delivery. Delivery of the drug by inhalation is always preferable. Dry powder or metered dose inhalers (MDI) are usually used. Direct delivery of medication to the airways allows lower doses to be used, which reduces the likelihood of side-effects. However, leukotriene receptor antagonists are given as oral therapy.

MDIs with spacers. These are simple devices ideal for use in children from any age. Younger children accept these spacer devices very readily. The spacer device is attached to the MDI, e.g. Aerochamber® with a soft face mask. A very effective spacer device may be constructed out of a plastic cola bottle. A hole large enough to take the mouthpiece of the MDI is cut in the end of the bottle. Three to six puffs of the MDI are then introduced into the bottle. The child simply has to pant or breathe in and out of the spout of the bottle to inhale an adequate dose of medication.

Treatment schedules

Asthma therapy aims to achieve as normal a quality of life for the child as possible. Children must be free of symptoms, hardly need relief

> **Maintenance treatment of asthma falls into two main categories:**
>
> - anti-inflammatory or 'controller' agents, such as inhaled corticosteroids, or leukotriene receptor antagonists and
> - bronchodilators or 'relievers' such as beta$_2$ agonists

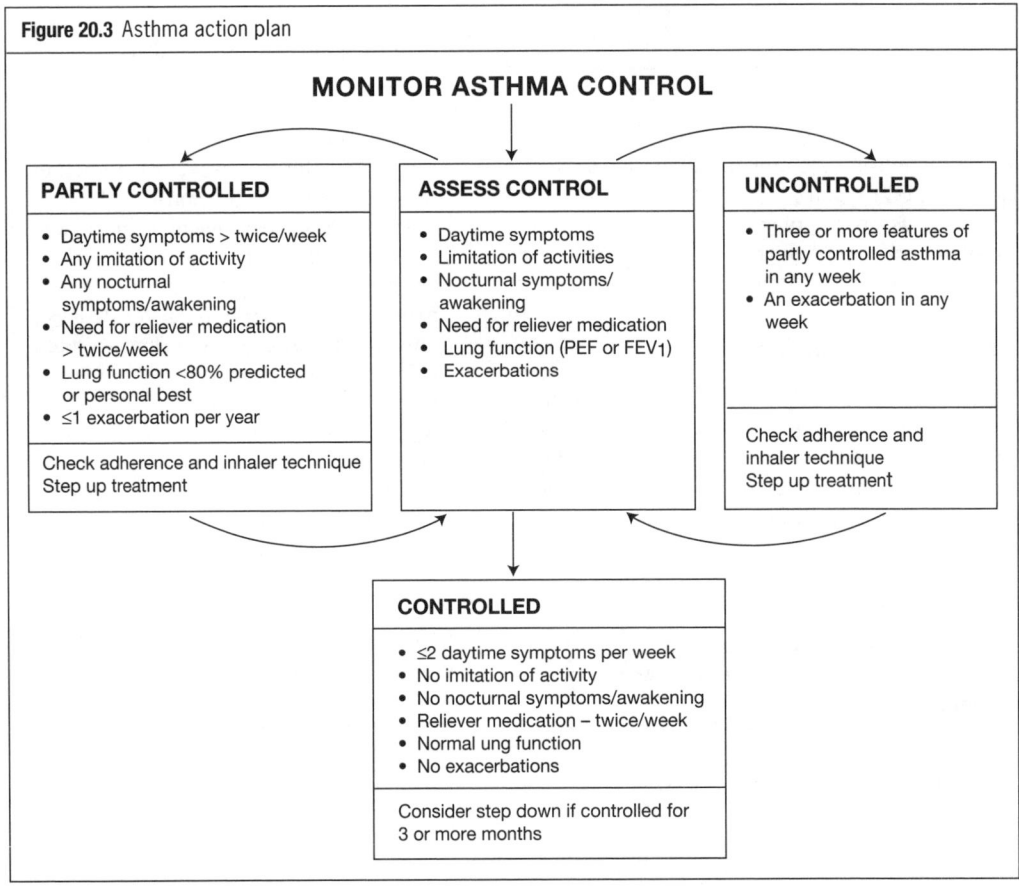

Figure 20.3 Asthma action plan

MONITOR ASTHMA CONTROL

PARTLY CONTROLLED
- Daytime symptoms > twice/week
- Any imitation of activity
- Any nocturnal symptoms/awakening
- Need for reliever medication > twice/week
- Lung function <80% predicted or personal best
- ≤1 exacerbation per year

Check adherence and inhaler technique
Step up treatment

ASSESS CONTROL
- Daytime symptoms
- Limitation of activities
- Nocturnal symptoms/awakening
- Need for reliever medication
- Lung function (PEF or FEV$_1$)
- Exacerbations

UNCONTROLLED
- Three or more features of partly controlled asthma in any week
- An exacerbation in any week

Check adherence and inhaler technique
Step up treatment

CONTROLLED
- ≤2 daytime symptoms per week
- No imitation of activity
- No nocturnal symptoms/awakening
- Reliever medication – twice/week
- Normal ung function
- No exacerbations

Consider step down if controlled for 3 or more months

medication and not have attacks of asthma. The child should be able to participate in sport, attend school regularly, and sleep well at night. Treatment programmes vary according to the frequency and severity of the child's symptoms. Careful monitoring of the child's growth and attention to possible side-effects of treatment is essential. The most important determinant of asthma treatment is control of the disease. In addition objective tests for asthma control should be applied and include patient centred questionnaires, peak flow and spirometry and measures of airway inflammation such as exhaled nitric oxide.

Mild persistent asthma is common in children. Symptoms of asthma such as cough and wheeze occur once or twice a week. Low-dose inhaled corticosteroid is recommended, preferably in MDI form with a spacer. The dose for inhaled beclomethasone, budesonide or fluticasone should not exceed 800 mcg daily. An alternative treatment for mildly asthmatic children is oral leukotriene receptor antagonists.

Moderate persistent asthma requires combinations of asthma drugs, either an inhaled corticosteroid plus a long-acting beta agonist or an inhaled corticosteroid plus a leukotriene receptor antagonist.

Children with difficult-to-manage asthma should always been seen by a paediatrician.

Common problems in asthma management

Infants and small children

Treatment may be difficult for various reasons. A spacer with face mask, e.g. Aerochamber® to which an MDI device is attached, is probably the most effective way of delivering drugs. Inhaled steroid preparations should be used in difficult cases. It should be remembered that asthma is only one cause of a wheezy infant and a trial of asthma therapy may work for asthmatics, but should be stopped if not solving the problem.

Exercise-induced bronchospasm (EIB)

Most asthmatic children have symptoms with exercise if not well controlled. The most important response to EIB is to improve overall asthma control. EIB may be controlled with an inhaled beta$_2$ agonist used five to ten minutes before exercise. If there is a poor response to the use of a beta$_2$ agonist, suspect poor asthma control in that child.

Nocturnal asthma

Regular episodes of coughing and wheezing at night (usually in the early hours of the morning) indicate poor asthma control and the need for more effective therapy. Once appropriate daytime therapy has been prescribed, attention should be paid to any possible nocturnal symptoms. Attention to environmental control in children with sensitivity to household allergens must be recommended. Long-acting theophyllines or the long-acting beta$_2$ agonists, e.g. salmeterol (Serevent®) or fomoterol (Oxis®), may be effective in eliminating this problem.

Poor asthma control impairs quality of life and increases cost through the need to manage regular exacerbations.

Allergic rhinitis

There are two forms of allergic rhinitis; the intermittent or seasonal form (also known as hay fever), and the persistent form with year-round symptoms. Intense sneezing, watery rhinitis, nasal congestion, and conjunctivitis are the main symptoms. Itching is especially found in the seasonal form. Symptoms may often mimic a cold but the persistence of symptoms or their seasonal nature helps in making a diagnosis.

Intermittent or seasonal allergic rhinitis

Symptoms are usually precipitated by exposure to seasonal windborne pollens, e.g. tree pollens or fungal spores. These usually occur in spring, early summer, and at the change of seasons. There is intense sneezing, watery nasal discharge, and itching. There is also itching of the palate and the auditory canals. The diagnosis is usually made easily. The allergen is identified by means of a history, skin testing, or CAP-RAST. Clumping of eosinophils will be seen on smears of nasal mucus stained with Hansel's stain.

Treatment

It is usually impossible to avoid the allergens causing seasonal allergic rhinitis.

- Short-acting non-sedating antihistamines such as cetirizine (Zyrtec®) and loratidine (Clarityne®) may give successful results. The older antihistamines with their sedative side-effects are not recommended.
- Beclomethasone, budesonide, or fluticasone nasal sprays are very effective. These are intranasal steroids. Children prefer the aqueous form of these preparations.
- Desensitization is very effective, especially for grass pollen allergy where virtually all children will benefit from desensitization. This form of treatment should be reserved for centres with adequate expertise. Sublingual desensitization (SLIT) to pollens is very useful in children.

Persistent allergic rhinitis

Perennial allergic rhinitis is usually due to sensitivity to allergens present in the environment throughout the year, e.g. grass pollen, housedust mite, pet allergens, or fungal spores. Nasal itching is not common but obstruction and watery nasal discharge are troublesome. Children usually have a typical pale allergic facies with blue discoloration of the lower eyelids ('allergic shiners'). A nasal crease is often noted. Repeated upward rubbing of the nose ('the allergic salute') produces the crease. Allergic mannerisms, such as pulling the face and the 'salute', are common. The nasal mucous membrane is swollen and paler than normal. The turbinates appear wet and a watery nasal discharge may be present. Secondary complications result from the mucosal swelling including maxillary sinusitis and serous otitis media ('glue ear').

> Nasal decongestant drops of any type should not be used for prolonged periods. Even though the danger of rebound chemical rhinitis is unlikely with some preparations, prolonged use is not recommended

Treatment

- Environmental control is an essential component of treatment. Simple schemes to reduce indoor mite, mould, and pet allergen exposure are often very effective.

- Beclomethasone, budesonide, or fluticasone nasal sprays are highly effective in this form of rhinitis. Oral steroids are not recommended unless symptoms are very severe and response to therapy is poor. This is unlikely with the range of treatments now available.
- Desensitization is often successful, especially if the child is sensitive to a single unavoidable allergen, e.g. housedust mite. The procedure is ineffective when more than two allergens are combined in the vaccine. It is not intended as a substitute for removal of avoidable allergens, e.g. dogs and cats.

Food allergy

Food allergy is thought to affect only 1–4 per cent of the paediatric population, especially infants and young children. It becomes less common after the age of two to three years.

There is often a family history of food allergy or other atopic disorders which helps in the diagnosis. Gastrointestinal symptoms such as vomiting and diarrhoea are the most common manifestations of food allergy, but skin reactions, such as urticaria and atopic eczema, and angioedema and respiratory symptoms, including nasal obstruction or wheezing, may occur.

Few foods have been implicated in food allergy in infants. These include egg white, cow's milk, soya, peanuts, wheat, and fish. Sensitivity to shellfish and nuts occurs later and may persist throughout life.

A careful history, skin test, or CAP-RAST may be helpful in establishing the diagnosis and identifying the offending food. Where there is any difficulty, elimination diets, oligoallergenic diets, or rarely double-blind placebo-controlled food challenge tests may be indicated. These measures should be performed in special units only.

> True food allergy always involves an immune mechanism and should not be confused with the many cases of intolerance to foods, such as tyramine in cheeses or toxins contained in contaminated foods.

Treatment is usually effective if the offending food is eliminated from the diet, e.g. a milk- or egg-free diet. However for truly allergic children strict avoidance of all hidden food ingredients of that allergen is required.

Some children have a non-IgE mediated food allergy (especially to milk and soya), where tests based on detecting IgE are not useful. In infants with persistent gastro-intestinal symptoms and/or failure to thrive as well as skin symptoms, food allergy should be considered. In these infants an avoidance diet is useful. Young children may require an extensively hydrolysed milk and some require an initial period of an amino acid formula. However, one should ensure a correct diagnosis in an experienced unit before embarking on highly expensive or nutritionally risky diets.

Natural history of allergic conditions

The vast majority of children with atopic eczema will outgrow their illness before they have reached their teens. This applies especially to boys and to those children in whom the illness first manifests in the early years of childhood. Most asthmatics, including those who have required prolonged steroid therapy, are less likely to outgrow their condition. Children with intermittent and persistent allergic rhinitis are often troubled in adult life by these illnesses unless they are adequately treated in their early years.

Table 20.4 Allergy clinic advice to parents on environmental control

- Do not keep dried flowers, books, or stuffed toys in the child's bedroom.
- Your child must not make up the bed or help with dusting.
- Avoid bedspreads and heavy curtains.
- If there is a double bunk, let the allergic child sleep on top.
- Do not allow animals or birds in the bedroom and preferably not in the house.
- When visiting or on trips take the child's pillow along.
- Do not use enzyme-containing washing powders.
- Avoid using insecticide or deodorant sprays in the child's presence.
- Avoid ice-cold drinks and drinks preserved with sulphur dioxide.
- Do not let your child eat in bed.

21

Immune and connective tissue disorders

Immune deficiencies

An increased susceptibility to infection, re-sulting in severe, persistent, recurrent or unusual infections with poor or incomplete response to antimicrobial therapy is the hall-mark of immune deficiency (*see* Table 21.1). Most immune deficiencies are attributable to exogenous factors and are referred to as *secondary immunodeficiency diseases*. Exo-genous factors that may impair immune function include protein-energy malnutrition, protein-losing states such as protein-losing enteropathy and nephrotic syndrome, HIV infection, measles, influenza, CMV infection and other infections, and immunosuppresive agents

Secondary immune deficiencies are much more common than primary immunodeficiency diseases.

such as glucocorticosteroids, methotrexate and cyclophosphamide.

The *primary immunodeficiency diseases* (PIDs) are a rare group of genetic conditions that result in a spectrum of intrinsic immunological defects. The incidence of PIDs, excluding IgA deficiency (frequency of 1 in 500) is about 1 in 10 000. More than 200 PIDs have been identified and the genetic mechanisms of more than 120 have been characterized. These conditions may affect vari-

Table 21.1 Clinical manifestations of immunodeficiency

Common warning signs	Other features
Eight or more ear infections per annum	Infection caused by unusual organisms
Two or more serious sinus infections per annum	Bronchiectasis
Two or more months of antibiotics with little effect	Diarrhoea and malabsorption
Two or more episodes of pneumonia within 1 year	Evidence of autoimmunity
Failure to thrive	Recurrent fever
Recurrent deep-seated or organ abscesses	Hepatosplenomegaly
Persistent thrush of mouth, nails or skin	Severe viral infection
Two or more deep-seated infections, e.g.	Chronic liver disease
osteomyelitis, meningitis, septicaemia	Arthralgia and arthritis
Family history of primary immunodeficiency disease	Chronic encephalitis
	Adverse reactions to vaccines
	Delayed umbilical cord separation
	Syndromes associated with immunodeficiency

ous components of immune function, including humoral immunity (antibody deficiencies and combined disorders), cell-mediated immunity (T-cell deficiencies and combined disorders), complement function (complement deficiencies), and phagocytic function (neutrophil and macrophage disorders). Antibody deficiencies are the most common group, accounting for more than 50 per cent of all PIDs (*see* Tables 21.2 and 21.3).

Recurrent infection

Recurrent infection is a common manifestation

of primary and secondary immunodeficiency diseases. However, there are several other groups of conditions in which recurrent infection is a feature:

- Healthy pre-school children experience an average of six infections per annum, but as many as 12 per annum are within two standard deviations of the mean. These infections are usually upper respiratory and self-limiting in nature.
- Children who attend nursery school or day-care centres may experience more infections.
- Socioeconomic factors, such as limited

Table 21.2 The frequency and pattern of infections in PIDs

Immune category	Frequency (%)	Common Infections
Antibody deficiencies	50–65	Encapsulated bacterial infections, e.g. *Pneumococcus, H. influenzae* *Mycoplasma* infections Chronic enterovirus infections
Predominantly T-cell disorders	10–15	Wide spectrum of viral, bacterial, fungal, and coccidial infections
Combined T- and B-cell deficiencies	10–15	
Complement deficiencies	1–5	Early component deficiencies: encapsulated bacterial Infections Terminal component deficiencies (C6 – C9): recurrent neisserial infections
Phagocytic disorders	7–15	Catalase positive bacterial infections, e.g. *S. aureus, S. marcescens, E. coli, Pseudomonas* spp. Fungal infections, e.g. *Aspergillus* spp.

Table 21.3: Common PIDs

Antibody deficiencies	T-cell / Combined T- and B-cell deficiencies	Complement deficiencies	Neutrophil disorders	Syndromes with immunodeficiency
Common variable immunodeficiency	TB plus severe combined	C6 deficiency C1-esterase	Severe congenital neutropaenia	DiGeorge syndrome
X-linked agammaglobulinaemia	immunodeficiency	inhibitor deficiency	Cyclical neutropaenia	Ataxia telangiectasia
Isolated IgG subclass deficiency IgA deficiency Transient hypogammaglobulinaemia of infancy	TB without SCID		Chronic granulomatous disease	Wiskott-Aldrich syndrome

access to clean running water, inadequate human waste disposal, overcrowding, exposure to cigarette smoke and other aero-pollutants increase the risk for recurrent infection.

- Anatomic or functional defects involving a single organ system may cause recurrent infection at a single site, e.g. a saccroccoxygeal sinus results in recurrent meningitis, and gastro-oesophageal reflux or a tracheo-oesophageal fistula causes recurrent aspiration pneumonia.
- Diseases affecting the primary immune barriers (skin and mucosal surfaces) may predispose to recurrent infection, e.g. extensive eczema is associated with skin and soft tissue infections and bacteraemias, and vitamin A deficiency disrupts mucosal integrity, increasing the risk for respiratory infection and gastroenteritis.
- Delayed development of the immune system or immunological immaturity may be responsible for a transient increased susceptibility to infection during the first few years of life. Transient hypogammaglobulinaemia of infancy is an example of delayed immunological maturity in which there is a delay in the development of humoral immunity,

resulting in transiently low immunoglobulin concentrations.

Investigations for PIDs

Before specialized investigations for the PIDs are requested the other causes of recurrent infection should be considered, and the child should be screened for HIV infection. Classically, the different categories of PIDs are associated with different groups of infections (*see* Table 21.2). To screen for PIDs a general screen is completed (*see* Table 21.4, steps 1–3). The interpretation of the results may require assistance from a trained clinician or immunologist. A clinical immunologist should direct more sophisticated testing (*see* Table 21. 4, step 4).

Treatment of PIDs

Treatment depends on the type of PID. Many antibody deficiencies and combined deficiencies require immunoglobulin replacement therapy (IVIG). The intravenous route is the preferred route of administration. Generally 300-600 mg per kg every three to four weeks is recommended. Life-long replacement is recommended for severe, genetically confirmed deficiencies. In conditions without a molecular genetic diagnosis, IVIG should initially be administered for one to five years, followed by re-evaluation of

Table 21.4 Immunological testing, adapted from the approach of the Jeffery Modell Foundation			
Step 1	**Step 2**	**Step 3**	**Step 4**
History, physical examination, mass and height	Specific antibody responses (tetanus, diphtheria)	Lymphocyte subsets (CD3, CD4, CD8, CD19, CD16/56)	Complement screen (CH50)
			Enzyme measurements (adenosine deaminase, purine nucleoside phosphorylase)
Exclude HIV infection Full blood count and differential count	Response to pneumococcal vaccine (pre- and post- titres)	Lymphocyte proliferative responses (using mitogen and antigen stimulation)	
			Phagocytic studies (surface glycoproteins, mobility, phago-cytosis)
Immunoglobulin levels (IgA, IgM, IgG, IgE)	IgG subclass analysis	Neutrophil oxidation burst	NK cytotoxicity studies
			Further complement studies, AH50
			Neo antigen to test antibody production
			Other surface/cytoplasmic molecules
			Cytokine receptor studies Family/genetic studies

serum immunoglobulin concentrations since hypogammaglobulinaemia may be transient and resolve spontaneously. IVIG is not indicated for IgA deficiency. In milder conditions, e.g. IgA deficiency and transient hypogammaglobulinaemia of infancy, recurrent infections may be controlled with prophylactic antibiotics. Bone marrow transplantation (BMT) is the treatment of choice for severe immunodeficiencies, such as severe combined immunodeficiency (SCID) or T-cell deficiencies. During the pre-BMT phase children with SCID may benefit from broad spectrum antimicrobial prophylaxis plus IVIG. Other therapies include cytokines, such as interferon-γ for chronic granulomatous disease, myeloid haematopoietic growth factors for congenital and cyclical neutropaenia, and enzyme replacement for adenosine deaminase deficiency.

Connective tissue disorders

Rheumatic diseases manifest with acute and chronic inflammation of the connective tissues of the musculoskeletal system, skin and blood vessels. Therefore, many different organs may be affected. Paediatric rheumatology includes the study of inflammatory as well as non-inflammatory disorders of connective tissues; the commonest condition is **juvenile idiopathic arthritis** (JIA). The frequency of connective tissue disorders in South Africa is not known, but ranges from 20 to 400/100 000 in other regions of the world. The incidence rate for JIA ranges from 4 to 23/100 000. The incidence is higher in African-Americans than in Caucasians. The frequency of rheumatic disease in developing countries is probably higher than commonly reported.

Disease mechanisms

The aetiology of connective tissue disorders is largely unknown, but is thought to be due to genetic predisposition and disordered immunity resulting in an autoimmune process. An aberrant genetically regulated immune response to environmental antigens probably initiates the autoimmune process. Various hypotheses, such as superantigen activation, bystander activation and molecular mimicry attempt to explain how infections can trigger autoimmunity. In healthy persons, recognition of self antigens in the context of self MHC (major histocompatibility complex) molecules, forms part of the normal adaptive immune response by B- and T-cells. Defective recognition of 'self' from 'non-self' or failure to downregulate this response results in autoimmunity (*see* Figure 21.1).

The generation of auto-reactive antibodies and T-cells fuels a chronic inflammatory response affecting joints, connective tissues and blood vessels. Several mechanisms are involved in the loss of self-tolerance, including impaired clearance of dead cell debris and impaired elimination of autoreactive cells by apoptosis. This is believed to be strongly influenced by genetic factors with complex interactions between multiple genes, and microbial or non-microbial environmental factors. Human leukocyte antigen (HLA) genes have been shown to associate with most autoimmune diseases. Around 40 genes have been linked to human and animal autoimmune disease. A recognized association is that of HLA B27 positivity and ankylosing spondylitis. Whereas only few autoimmune diseases are caused by single gene defects the mutations of several genes are involved in conditions such as the autoinflammatory diseases e.g. familial Mediterranean fever (MEFV) or with the susceptibility to Crohn's disease. New genetic tools such as genome-wide scans continue to identify additional genetic risk factors.

Advances in understanding the immune mediated mechanisms of inflammation have led to the development of specific 'biologic' agents. This has ushered in a challenging era of new treatment options in which powerful, targeted immune suppression is balanced against best clinical outcome.

Some rheumatic diseases have different clinical expressions in children and adults, e.g. inflammatory myosis. A narrow age at onset of some of these conditions, e.g. Kawasaki Syndrome (usually during the first five years of life), may reflect specific childhood modifying factors, possibly linked to initial pathogen exposure in the absence of protective immunity. Other clinical differences may be associated with skeletal immaturity, epiphyses which are not fused causing growth abnormalities in an arthritic limb and stunting in widespread arthritis.

The broad clinical spectrum of juvenile arthritis is probably the result of different immunological mechanisms causing different clinical subtypes.

Figure 21.1 Development of autoimmune disease

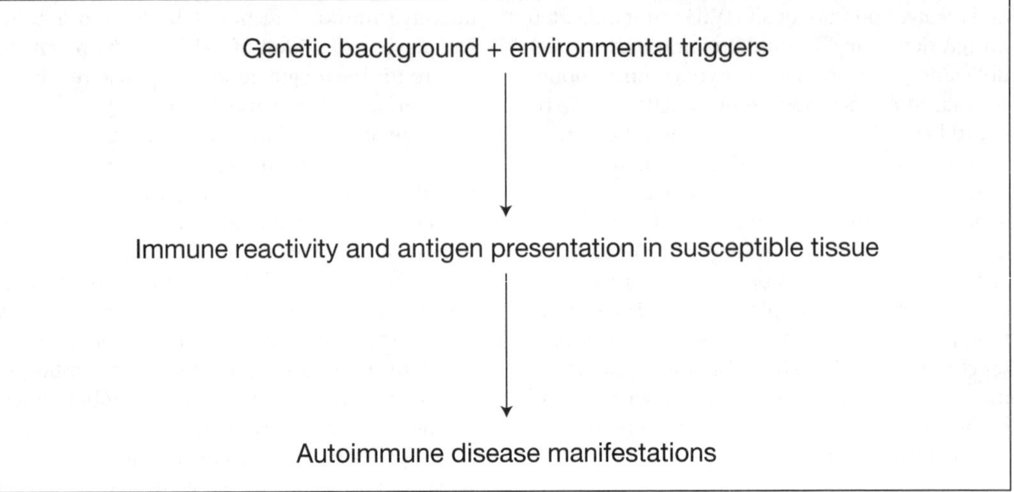

Genetic background + environmental triggers

↓

Immune reactivity and antigen presentation in susceptible tissue

↓

Autoimmune disease manifestations

For example, Systemic onset JIA or Still's disease is distinct from arthritic forms of JIA, and is considered a variant of the auto-inflammatory diseases.

Systemic vasculitis is characterized by inflammation and fibrinoid necrosis of blood vessel walls. The pathogenesis may involve cell-mediated inflammation, immune complex-mediated inflammation or anti-neutrophil cytoplasmic antibody-mediated inflammation. For example, immune complex formation appears to be the major pathogenesis event in Henoch-Schönlein purpura, whereas Takayasu's arteritis is essentially a T-cell driven process, probably triggered by an infectious agent. Vasculitis may occur in autoimmune diseases such as JIA and systemic lupus erythematosus (SLE). Vasculitis in patients with SLE is associated with the presence of co-existent anti-Ro-SSA, HLA and DR3 antibodies and more rarely anti-DNA, anti-Sm and anti-RNP antibodies. In both JIA and SLE autoantibodies are induced against endothelial antigens, including anti-endothelial cell antibodies and antibodies against endothelial expressed adhesion molecules.

Clinical manifestations

The different connective tissue diseases can present with similar, often nonspecific, clinical features especially during the early stages. This frequently makes specific diagnosis difficult. These diseases tend to be chronic or recurrent; exceptions are Kawasaki disease and Henoch-Schönlein purpura, which are mostly self-limited acute disorders.

Common *symptoms* in children include:
- Fever, which may manifest as pyrexia of unknown origin (PUO)
- Weight loss
- Irritability and disturbed sleep pattern
- Fatigue
- Rashes
- Musculoskeletal aches and pains.

The following *system involvements* may be seen:
- Eyes: conjunctivitis, uveitis
- Skin: palmar erythema and desquamation, maculopapular or linear rashes, pain, thickening, immobility, tightening, nodules
- Joints: mono- or polyarthritis
- Reticulo-endothelial system activation: lymph nodes, not matted together, hepatosplenomegaly
- Organ dysfunction of any organ system.

Differential diagnosis of presenting problems

PUO, i.e. persistent fever of more than three weeks duration and uncertain diagnosis despite intensive investigation:

- Infections. Sepsis often causes high swinging fever and toxicity: search for hidden abscesses, chronic infection (e.g. tuberculosis, HIV, brucellosis) must be actively excluded and may show much overlap with chronic inflammatory conditions
- Non-infective inflammation cannot be proven by specific laboratory parameters, but markers of inflammation (acute phase responses) are frequently elevated
- Malignancy
- Drug fever
- Hereditary periodic fever syndromes.

Musculoskeletal complaints
- Injury
- Malignancy

Table 21.5 Differential diagnosis of arthritis

Monoarthritis: acute onset

Condition	Supportive evidence
Septic arthritis	Joint aspiration yields pus for bacterial culture
Malignancy	Pain is adjacent to joint
Trauma	History
Non-accidental injury	Story and findings do not match
Haemophilia	Boy with other evidence of bleeding disorder
Slipped upper femoral epiphysis	Adolescent, often obese, acute onset usually without trauma
Reactive arthritis	Prior infection
Pauci-articular onset juvenile idiopathic arthritis (JIA)	Rarely present with acute onset, diagnosed in retrospect
Enthesitis related arthritis	Enthesitis related arthritis
Osteochondritis	Enthesitis and inflammatory spinal pain
Osteonecrosis (including Perthes' disease)	
Idiopathic osteolysis of the hip	

Monoarthritis: gradual onset

Condition	Supportive evidence
Pauci-articular onset JIA	Pre-school girl, develops further joint involvement later
Enthesitis related arthritis	Back pain or buttock pain
Tuberculosis	Other evidence of tuberculosis, biopsy and culture
Other conditions	Usually need biopsy and culture to diagnose

Polyarthritis

Condition	Supportive evidence
Acute rheumatic fever	According to modified Jones' criteria
Reactive arthritis	Recent infection
JIA	Often symmetrical, large and small joints, non-erosive arthritis
Enthesitis-related arthritis	Back pain and enthesitis usually associated
Systemic lupus erythematosus	Associated skin changes
Osteochondritis/osteonecrosis (including Perthes')	Better after rest, becomes worse with exercise
Slipped upper femoral epiphyses	Adolescent, often obese, acute onset usually without trauma
Other conditions	Need biopsy to diagnose

◆ Chronic infections, eg. tuberculosis of the vertebra (Pott's disease)
◆ Juvenile arthritis or other connective tissue disorder–when children complain of backache there may be a serious underlying problem and tumour or infiltration of the spinal cord or spinal column, or other space-occupying lesion must be excluded as indicated.

A careful clinical and neurological examination is indicated. After a plain X-ray, ultrasonography, computerized tomography (CT) or magnetic resonance imaging (MRI) scans may be considered.

The differential diagnosis of arthritis is considered in relation to the number of joints affected, and to manner of onset (*see* Table 21.5).

Skin rashes

The skin rashes of connective tissue disorders have to be differentiated from eczema and infective rashes.

The distribution may be typical for a specific connective tissue entity, such as on the upper eyelids and over the knuckles in dermatomyositis or on the 'butterfly' area of the face in systemic lupus erythematosis. An evanescent erythematous salmon coloured rash over the trunk may suggest systemic onset juvenile idiopathic arthritis (sJIA).

Multisystem disease

Dysfunction or abnormality of more than one organ system may occur in connective tissue diseases, but should be differentiated from other diseases, such as infections (e.g. tuberculosis, HIV), or malignancy (e.g. leukaemia).

Classification of childhood rheumatological conditions

The spectrum of the rheumatological disorders of childhood is given in Table 21.6. Because the aetiology and pathogenesis of many of these conditions are uncertain, there are ongoing revisions in the classification. Some categories are not mutually exclusive, i.e. some conditions fall into more than one category of the classification.

Chronic arthritis of childhood

This is one of the common chronic disorders of childhood. The diagnosis in Africa is often delayed because the disease is not recognized and because it is not commonly fatal. Early diagnosis is important because treatment can improve symptoms, restore function and quality of life and minimize muscle wasting, joint deformities and growth disturbances and other complications.

The following sections briefly describe the most important conditions and their different clinical patterns and complications. Since the chronic arthritides of childhood share a common approach to treatment, this is dealt with below the category section. Finally, the differential diagnoses of common presentations are discussed.

Juvenile idiopathic arthritis (JIA)

The Juvenile Idiopathic Arthritis (JIA) classification by the International League against Rheumatism (ILAR) (Durban 1997) and subsequent revision has unified the older juvenile rheumatoid arthritis (JRA) and juvenile chronic arthritis (JCA) (*see* Table 21.6). This has enabled multicentre collaborative research aimed at increasing the understanding of clinical, therapeutic and prognostic outcomes.

JIA ranges from a mild condition to a serious, disabling and disfiguring, but rarely fatal disease. Early diagnosis and appropriate treatment are most important for good outcome. The hallmark symptoms of inflammatory as opposed to mechanical arthritis are stiffness and pain that are *worse after resting*, typically resulting in early morning stiffness. Relief of symptoms *with rest* is more common in mechanical or degenerative arthritis.

The general definition of JIA:
◆ Exclusion of other known conditions
◆ Aetiology of the arthritis unknown
◆ Age of onset <16 years
◆ Arthritis in one or more joints
◆ Duration of disease >six weeks
◆ Different onset patterns are classified in categories according to clinical presentation.

Table 21.6 Spectrum of rheumatic disorders of childhood

Juvenile idiopathic arthritis (JIA) – International League against Rheumatism (ILAR) classification – 2001 Edmonton modification
Systemic onset JIA
Oligoarticular JIA
– Persistent
– Extended
Polyarthritis – rheumatoid factor (RF) negative
Polyarthritis – RF positive
Psoriatic arthritis
Enthesitis-related arthritis
Other arthritis
– Fits no other category
– Fits more than one category

Infectious and post-infectious arthritis
Viral: transient synovitis, hepatitis B, HIV, parvovirus B19, rubella, mumps
Reiter's syndrome: arthritis, uveitis, urethritis
Streptococcal: streptococcal arthritis, acute rheumatic fever

Mechanical disorders
Hypermobility syndrome: generalized and localized
Other structural disorders, overuse syndromes

Pain amplification syndromes
'Growing pains'
Fibromyalgia, fibrositis
Other

Connective tissue diseases
Systemic lupus erythematosus (SLE)
Juvenile dermatomyositis
Scleroderma
Other

Vasculitides
see Table 21.8

Skeletal dysplasias
Osteochondroses: Perthes' disease of the hips, other osteochondritis/osteonecrosis
Other

Other arthritides and miscellaneous conditions

Definition of selected terms

- **Arthritis**: Objective joint swelling, or effusion, or at least two of the following signs: limited range of movement, pain on movement, or warmth.
- **Arthralgia**; Subjective feeling of painful joint without clinical signs.
- **Enthesitis**: Tenderness at entheses, which are sites of insertion of ligament, tendon, fascia or joint capsule into bone. Occurs especially in heel pad, ball of foot, tibial tuberosity, back of heel – Achilles tendon insertion.
- **Spondyloarthritis**: Inflammation of the joints of the axial skeleton and the entheses, commonly associated with uveitis. Rheumatoid and antinuclear factor negative, high frequency of HLA-B27 positivity.
- **Apophyses**: Sites of growth cartilage where tendons insert.
- **Osteochondroses**: A group of diseases, including variants of normal ossification, relating to stress injuries or avascular necrosis, which affect the primary or secondary ossification centres.
- **Anterior uveitis**: Commonly iridocyclitis: inflammation of the iris and ciliary body.
- **Chronic uveitis**: Synechiae: adhesions of the iris to the lens, keratic deposits, cataracts, glaucoma.
- **Antinuclear antibody** (ANA): Associated with oligoarthritis, female gender, uveitis and younger age.
- **Rheumatoid factor** (RF): associated with adult pattern of rheumatoid arthritis.
- **Anti-citrullinated peptide antibody** (Anti-CCP): An early laboratory marker associated with higher predictive value for emergence of rheumatoid arthritis than RF.
- **DMARDs**: Disease modifying anti-rheumatic drugs, e.g. methotrexate.
- **NSAIDs**: Non steroidal anti-inflammatory drugs.
- **Biologicals**: More specifically targeted anti-inflmmatory and disease modifying drugs, e.g. tumour necrosis factor antagonists, CD20 blockers, interleukin antagonists.
- **Cytokines**: Signalling molecules involved in host immune defence with pro- as well as anti-inflammatory activity.

Categories of JIA (Second revision, Edmonton, 2001):

- **Systemic**: Arthritis may coexist with, or be preceded by persistent high spiking fever of at least two weeks duration, with temperature spikes for at least three consecutive days (quotidian). These features are accompanied by one or more of:
  - Hepatomegaly and/or splenomegaly
  - Generalized lymphadenopathy
  - Evanescent (nonfixed) rash with erythematous macules 2–5 mm in size
  - Serositis (pericarditis, pleuritis).

This group makes up about 10–20 per cent of JIA. Most patients present in early childhood and the most striking features are extra-articular (outside the joints) which makes the diagnosis difficult at onset. Male to female distribution is equal, unlike the female predominance in most other rheumatological disorders. Uveitis is uncommon. About 50 per cent of children with systemic onset JIA will develop destructive polyarthritis that responds poorly to conventional treatment. Treatment with specific cytokine blockade (anti-IL1, anti-IL6) may improve outcome.

- **Oligoarthritis persistent**: arthritis in up to four, usually larger, joints throughout the disease course. This is the common subtype in the Caucasian population. High risk for uveitis, which can be asymptomatic and destructive with synechiae and cataract formation, particularly in young girls. Iridocyclitis is diagnosed by special slit-lamp examination. Prognosis is good with early diagnosis and good management.
- **Oligoarthritis extended**: Affects a cumulative total of five or more joints (polyarthritis) after the first six months of disease. The arthritis tends to become chronic and destructive, requiring more aggressive treatment options and consequently the prognosis is poorer than for the persistent form.
- **Polyarthritis**: arthritis in five or more joints within the first six months, subdivided into rheumatoid factor (+) or (–). Multiple large and small joints may be affected including those of fingers and toes. Involvement of the temporomandibular and spinal joints may be overlooked.
- **RF (–)**: About 30 per cent of Caucasian patients fall into this category but this is the commonest subtype in the Asian and African populations. Young girls are commonly affected and better outcome depends on more aggressive treatments, which may include biologic agents such as tumour necrosis factor alpha (TNF-α) blockade in well resourced settings.
- **RF (+)**: This group constitutes about 5 per cent of JIA. It is the childhood onset form of adult rheumatoid arthritis (RA), usually in adolescent girls with symmetric large and small joint involvement. Two or more tests for RF at least three months apart during the first six months of disease must be positive. The arthritis tends to be aggressive but the prognosis is improving with very early use of DMARDs, and the possibility of using biologic agents in the future.
- **Enthesitis related arthritis**: Arthritis and/or enthesitis with at least two of the following :
  - The presence of a history of sacroiliac joint tenderness and/or inflammatory lumbosacral pain
  - The presence of HLA-B27 positivity
  - Onset in a boy after the age of six years of age
  - Acute (symptomatic) anterior uveitis
  - A relevant medical history in a first-degree relative, e.g. ankylosing spondylitis or enthesitis

The sub-group with the HLA-B27 positivity and anterior uveitis probably represents the childhood equivalent of adult ankylosing spondyloarthritis and reactive arthritis. But peripheral, usually asymmetric arthritis and not sacroiliitis, is the main clinical feature.

- **Psoriatic arthritis**: Arthritis and psoriasis, or arthritis and at least two of:
  - Psoriasis in a first-degree relative
  - Dactylitis ('Sausage' shaped arthritis of digits)
  - Nail abnormalities, e.g. pitting

This form of arthritis tends to be chronic and relapsing. The absence of psoriatic skin lesions in the child can delay the diagnosis significantly. Early and aggressive therapy can prolong reasonably good quality life. The adult type may respond to TNF-α antagonist therapy.

- **Other 'undifferentiated' arthritis**: arthritis of unknown cause that persists for at least six weeks and that does not fulfill the criteria for one or more of the above categories.

Complications of persistent arthritis in children

Complications include:
- Generalized growth failure and anaemia of chronic disease
- Localized over- or undergrowth of limbs
- Joint destruction and deformities with contractures, resulting in impaired mobility
- Complications of chronic uveitis including blindness
- Complications of treatment, particularly infections due to immunosuppression
- Macrophage activation syndrome (MAS) which may be fatal in systemic juvenile arthritis
- Osteoporosis due to steroid treatment or the underlying the disease.

Special investigations

Diagnosis of connective tissue diseases rely predominantly on the clinical findings. Investigations may support the diagnosis. Blood tests are more commonly used to monitor side effects of medication. Screening and monitoring tests are the white cell count, platelet count, erythrocyte sedimentation rate (ESR) and C-reactive protein (CRP). These are unlikely to be normal in the presence of infection or malignancy, but may be moderately raised or normal in chronic inflammatory conditions. Rheumatoid factor (RF) and antinuclear antibodies (ANA) have rather low sensitivities and specificities but can be helpful in the differential diagnosis and prognosis. Anti-CCP measurements appear to have greater specificity than RF for the diagnosis of rheumatoid arthritis. Arthroscopy and synovial biopsy are specifically indicated where infective causes are suspected, particularly in monoarthritis and especially in the very young child or infant. Imaging can assist in resolving the differential diagnosis, and in assessing control or disease progression. Plain X-rays are commonly used, but are not very informative during the first months of disease, unless trauma or malignancy is suspected. Ultrasound performed by an experienced radiologist has become a useful tool in evaluating inflamed joints. Rheumatologists may request tomography, arthrograms, radio-active imaging, CT scanning, and MRI imaging in selective circumstances.

Management of persistent arthritis in children

The goals of treatment should be set in conjunction with the patient and parents. They should include:
- Relief of symptoms
- Maintenance of joint range of motion
- Maintenance of muscle strength
- Rehabilitation to best quality of life.

Monitoring progress

The control of disease activity and the impact of the disease on the family should be monitored regularly and it is helpful to involve all members of the therapeutic team in this process. Specialist rheumatology referral should be requested for a treatment plan for the newly diagnosed child where possible. Children with active inflammation should be seen monthly or more frequently. Those in whom the disease is well controlled or in remission need only be seen three- to six-monthly. Small children sometimes do not express pain in the way that adults do, as they may have grown up with pain. In these children, arthritis may present with refusal to move or use a limb, rather than by verbalizing pain. Face cartoons (smiling or sad face) and parent questionnaires can be useful in monitoring response to therapy in the small child. Formal childhood health assessment questionnaires (CHAQ) with a core set of outcome criteria, physician scores, joint scores and inflammatory markers are critical for evaluating and adjusting treatment in the older child.

The range of motion of affected joints, the muscle bulk of affected limbs, and the ability to function at home, in the school, and socially should be recorded at least annually. All children with persistent arthritis should have a slit-lamp examination by an ophthalmologist on diagnosis and then as indicated per category However, ANA-positive girls with oligoarthritis onset JIA should have slit-lamp examinations three-monthly or more frequently. A child-friendly physiotherapist or occupational therapist can be invaluable in monitoring disease and preventing disability.

Drug therapy

Treatment strategies for the specific categories of JIA have replaced the pyramid approach to treatment. Identification of poor prognostic factors and improved knowledge of the inflammatory process has promoted targeted drug interventions.

Non-steroidal anti-inflammatory drugs (NSAIDs)

The mainstay of initial analgesic and mildly anti-inflammatory therapy for children with JIA are the NSAIDs. The commonly used NSAIDs are listed in Table 21.7. On the basis of effectiveness, cost, and convenience, ibuprofen and indomethacin are the prefered NSAIDs. Diclofenac is one of the most widely used agents. Children tolerate NSAIDs better than adults. The most common adverse effect of NSAIDs is abdominal pain. Therefore, NSAIDs should be taken with meals. If the abdominal pain occurs, an antacid is usually effective. Other problems may include headache, changes in mood, rashes and, rarely, interstitial nephritis. Care should be taken when giving NSAIDs to a patient with renal disease, and the combination of methotrexate and NSAIDs should be avoided if renal function is impaired.

Glucocorticosteroids

Long-term oral glucocorticoids are avoided where possible because of their adverse effects. Growth failure and suppression of the hypothalamic-pituitary-adrenal axis are the main concerns. 'Low-dose' prednisone (0.3–0.5 mg/kg/d) may be added to an NSAID and methotrexate when the disease is not adequately con-trolled or for the systemic phase of systemic onset JIA. Some disease-modifying activity has been ascribed to low dose maintenance treatment with prednisone. Higher doses (2 mg/kg/d) may be used for a week or two to gain control of an acute flare-up. So-called pulse therapy with very high doses given orally (prednisone) or intravenously (methylprednisolone) over one to three days is occasionally used for a severe exacerbation of JIA. Pulse therapy is potentially dangerous and should only be given where the patient can be closely monitored for hypertension, and changes in serum glucose and electrolytes. Prolonged steroid therapy requires additional intake of calcium and Vitamin D to prevent osteoporosis.

Disease modifying anti-rheumatic drugs (DMARDs)

Cytotoxic agents

Methotrexate is added rapidly if the arthritis is not adequately controlled by NSAIDs: 0.3 mg/kg/week taken as a single dose on an empty stomach is the usual starting dose. This is increased until there is a satisfactory response or the maximum dose of 1 mg/kg/week or 25 mg/week is reached. Intramuscular or subcutaneous injections may improve absorption and the clinical response. Adverse effects may be minimized by splitting the dose into two per week within 24 hours and by adding folic acid 5 mg twice weekly. Adverse effects include nausea, mood changes, mouth ulcers, raised liver enzymes, bone marrow toxicity, and blood or protein in the urine. Patients should be monitored three to four monthly with history, clinical examination, and laboratory tests for liver enzymes (ALT screen),

Table 21.7 Commonly used NSAIDs			
NSAID	**Dose mg/kg/d**	**Number of doses/day**	**Comment**
Naproxen	10	2	For school aged children BD dosage useful
Ibuprofen	40	3	Mild anti-inflammatory
Indomethacin	1–2.5	3	Potent; oral, slow-release, and suppository
Diclofenac	1–3	3	Potent; injection for acute flare, also suppository and drop form

full blood count, and urine blood and protein.

Other cytotoxic drugs such as cyclophosph-amide and cyclosporin may be considered if methotrexate fails.

The DMARDs, chloroquine, sulfasalazine and azathioprine play a lesser role in drug therapy of JIA and should be reserved for specialist rheumatologists to prescribe.

Biological DMARDS

These genetically engineered drugs work by selectively blocking the effects of cytokines. They are an important treatment option for DMARD-refractory JIA patients. Antagonists to TNF-α, Interleukin 1, Interleukin 6, CD20 and others are commercially available but at significant cost, which places them currently out of reach for most children in developing countries. Drugs such as etanercept (TNF-α blocker), the first registered agent for use in children, produce substantial health gains in treatment-resistant polyarticular JIA. Biologic treatment options have to be carefully considered because of rare potential adverse effects, especially serious infections and malignancy. Treatment must be supervised by a rheumatologist. Emerging evidence on the use of other biologic agents will guide future treat-ment options.

Intra-articular injection

Intra-articular injections of long-acting steroids such as triamcinolone hexacetonide are indicated to alleviate pain and suppress inflammation in a joint, tendon or bursa that is inflamed out of proportion to other tissues, or is not responsive to non-invasive anti-inflammatory therapy. This may prove the treatment of choice for oligoarticular arthritis and may also be used to limit systemic glucorticosteroid administra-tion, to decrease swelling of inflamed soft tissue, or relieve nerve entrapment, e.g. carpal tunnel syndrome.

Physiotherapy and occupational therapy

Occupational therapy and physiotherapy are vital to the management of rheumatic diseases in childhood for maintaining function and preventing contractures. These services can provide:

- Exercises to increase range of movement of joints and to increase muscle bulk
- Splinting (e.g. nocturnal resting splints, working splints, and dynamic splints) for pain relief and the prevention of contractures
- Shoe inserts for pain relief from tender heels or sensitive metatarsal heads
- Shoe raise for a short leg to prevent contracture in the longer leg
- Advice on aids for activities of daily living
- Specialized assessments to monitor the course of the disease, measure its impact, and evaluate potential for employment in adolescents.

Orthopaedic surgery

An orthopaedic surgeon may be needed to:
- Perform diagnostic arthroscopy and synovial biopsy
- Restore function or relieve pain in severely damaged joints with:
  - Replacement (arthroplasty)
  - Fusion (arthrodesis)
  - Re-alignment (osteotomy).
  - Removing synovium (synovectomy)
- Inject or aspirate joints
- Institute traction to relieve pain and restore alignment, particularly for the hip joint
- Tendon releases may be required.

Ophthalmology

Regular monitoring for uveitis is essential, as about 20 per cent of JIA patients will have ocular inflammation. ANA positive oligoarticular arthri-tis carries the highest risk of uveitis, which may have an asymptomatic onset and require fre-quent follow up assessments, unlike the low risk systemic arthritis.

Infectious and post-infectious arthritis

Children with *septic arthritis* are usually very ill with high fever and a swollen joint that is hot and has markedly restricted range of movement. *S. aureus* is the usual cause. Less frequently, *S. pneumoniae* and *H. influenzae* cause pyogenic arthritis. More recently, *Kingella kingae* has been recognised to be an important cause of septic arthritis.

Tuberculosis infection of a joint is not uncommon and must be ruled out by biopsy in any persistent monoarthritis. Tuberculosis may also cause a symmetrical polyarthritis that is sterile. This was described by Poncet (Poncet's disease).

Reactive (or post-infectious) arthritis may follow invasive bacterial infection in children. It is defined as a non-suppurative arthritis that occurs in close temporal association with a non-articular infection. Bacteria associated with reactive arthritis include *S. pyogenes*, *N. meningitidis*, *Salmonella* spp., *Shigella* spp., and *Campylobacter* spp. Reactive arthritis most frequently occurs in HLA-B27-positive individuals.

Acute rheumatic fever follows infection with a group A beta-haemolytic streptococcus. Clinical features and management are described in Chapter 28, Cardiovascular disorders, since joint symptoms are seldom the dominating problem for long. If acute rheumatic fever has been ruled out, the other reactive and post-infectious arthritides can be treated symptomatically with non-steroidal anti-inflammatory drugs. The patient should be followed up to ensure that the arthritis resolves within three months. Proven post-streptococcal arthritis without carditis should be treated with prophylactic penicillin.

Summary of diagnosis and management of JIA

Diagnosis
Arthritis for more than six weeks in a child under 16 years of age
No cause found
One or more joints may be involved, typically with inflammatory pain which is worse after rest.

Management
Support patient, family, and teacher
Relieve symptoms; control inflammation
- NSAIDs, methotrexate, prednisone and intra-articular steroids are the mainstay of treatment
Maintain joint and muscle function
Monitor for complications
- Anterior uveitis
- Treatment complications.

HIV arthritis may present as monoarthritis, oligoarthritis or polyarthritis affecting both small and large joints. The large joints of the lower limbs are the most frequently affected. Arthritis occurs at any stage of HIV disease and ranges from a transient synovitis to a severely destructive form of disease. Spondyloarthropathy, enthesitis and dactylitis are common features of HIV-related arthritis. Non-steroidal anti-inflammatory drugs, sulphasalazine, hydroxychloroquine and antiretrovirals are used in the treatment of HIV arthritis.

Mechanical disorders

Symptoms in mechanical disorders, such as *avascular necrosis* (i.e. osteonecrosis) and *osteochondritis*, overuse, and the *hypermobility syndrome*, are usually related to physical activity and are more common in adolescents. In contrast to inflammatory joint disease, the symptoms tend to worsen during the day. The knee, ankle, hip, and back are most commonly involved.

The benign hypermobility syndrome is a term applied to musculoskeletal pain without any associated congenital syndrome or abnormality of connective tissue. This may be an extreme variation of normal. It may be associated with mild recurrent arthritis and it may predispose to injury but the prognosis is good.

A diagnosis of hypermobility syndrome can be made if at least six or more points are obtained on the Beighton Scale:
- Apposition of thumbs to flexor aspect of forearm   (2)
- Hyperextension of 5th metacarpo-phalangeal joints to 90°   (2)
- Hyperextension of elbows greater than 10°   (2)
- Hyperextension of knees greater than 10°   (2)
- Touch palms to floor with knees straight   (1)

Non-accidental injury

Joint swelling from non-accidental injury may result from traumatic periostitis, haemorrhage, or fracture of the epiphysis. If the history does not fit with the examination, the possibility of non-accidental injury should be investigated with a more detailed history and possibly a radiographic skeletal survey and bone scan.

Pain amplification syndromes

Growing pains

A common problem in the primary health clinic is a young child (from four to twelve years old) who complains of recurrent evening or night pain. These pains are intermittent and are classically in the lower limbs, behind the knee, in the calves and thigh areas, shins, and occasionally in the upper extremities. The pain may interfere with sleep but resolves by the morning and daytime activity is normal. Growth, development, physical examination and laboratory investigations are completely normal. The parents and child can be reassured that he or she will grow out of the problem, that symptomatic treatment with mild analgesics and comfort measures like local heat and rubbing the limb is all that is required. Laboratory tests are usually not indicated, but an ESR and full blood count (FBC) might be useful to screen for inflammatory or malignant conditions.

Fibromyalgia and fibrositis

Fibromyalgia is characterized by diffuse, often ill-defined musculoskeletal aching and stiffness, and multiple tender points in characteristic locations. Sleep is disturbed and the patient is often anxious and depressed. The syndrome is well recognized in adults. It sometimes occurs in adolescent girls, but is very rare in boys. Treatment is difficult. The parents and patient should be reassured that, although the pain is real, there is no underlying serious disorder. Physiotherapy, NSAIDs, and low-dose tricyclic antidepressants, (e.g. amitryptyline 10 mg nocte) may be offered. A normal ESR would tend to rule out inflammatory conditions.

Other connective tissue diseases in childhood

Systemic lupus erythematosus (SLE)

The diagnosis of SLE is made when at least four of the following modified ACR criteria are present, either simultaneously or serially:

- Malar rash
- Discoid lupus rash
- Photosensitivity
- Oral or nasopharyngeal ulcers
- Arthritis
- Pleuritis or pericarditis
- Nephritis - proteinuria or cellular casts
- Anaemia, leucopaenia ($<4\,000/mm^3$), lymphopaenia ($<1\,500/mm^3$), or thrombocytopaenia ($<15\,0000/mm^3$)
- Positive immunoserology : Antibodies to dsDNA or to Sm nuclear antigen, positive finding of antiphospholipid antibodies such as false positive syphilis serology, lupus anticoagulant or anticardiolipin antibodies
- Antinuclear antibody
- Neurologic manifestations: psychosis, convulsions.

SLE is an auto-immune disease that may involve nearly every organ system. It is rare in childhood, most commonly affects adolescent girls, and the clinical picture closely resembles SLE in adults. In children under five years it is exceedingly rare, affects both sexes, and has a very poor prognosis. The prevalence of SLE is higher among black adults and children than in whites in the USA, UK, and the Caribbean. In Africa, however, the disorder has been infrequently reported among black adults and is rare in black children; the exception being the Western Cape, where the disease occurs more often in mixed races and black women than in white women. SLE usually presents as chronic polyarthritis or arthralgia, fever, and a characteristic rash. The rash is typically chronic, maculo-papular, erythematous, and distributed over the malar area of the face and bridge of the nose in a butterfly distribution, but it may mimic many other rashes.

SLE is a multisystem disease in which the underlying pathology is a widespread vasculitis affecting small blood vessels associated with circulating soluble immune complexes. Areas of infarction and thrombosis due to the underlying vasculitis may be evident in the fingers, palms, soles, and mucous membranes. The renal system is commonly affected by the vasculitis and this can progress to chronic nephritis and renal failure. Hepatomegaly, lymphadenopathy, pericarditis, polyserositis, and neurological and haematological dysfunction are frequent complications.

The diagnosis is usually suspected when chronic arthritis is associated with the typical rash, or in adolescent girls with multisystem disease including purpura, nephritis, and migraine in the presence of a positive antinuclear antibody test. Laboratory tests may provide confirmatory evidence and antinuclear and anti-DNA antibodies are often present. The Coombs' test may be positive. In the acute phase, complement levels may be low, the ESR is raised and there is often anaemia, leucopaenia, and thrombocytopaenia. These patients should be managed at a specialized referral centre.

Neonatal SLE is seen in infants whose mothers have SLE, which may be unrecognized. It is due to the placental transfer of maternal auto-antibodies. The infant may develop a fever and skin rashes in the first few weeks of life but the most important consequence is congenital heart block, which can be permanent. Congenital heart block can be detected *in utero* and the mothers of all newborns with congenital heart block should be investigated for SLE.

Drug induced SLE is a reversible form of SLE that may be induced by certain drugs, e.g. hydrallazine, carbamazepine; 95 per cent of patients have antihistone antibodies. SLE resolves when the drug is withdrawn.

Treatment

SLE is difficult to treat and the prognosis is not good. Non-steroidal anti-inflammatory drugs can control arthritic symptoms but high-dose corticosteroids are usually required for renal, haematological, and neurological involvement. The disease usually progresses and renal failure frequently develops. Immunosuppressive drugs may be used but, as with steroids, side effects are serious and children with SLE should be referred to a specialist centre for assessment and advice.

Juvenile dermatomyositis

Dermatomyositis should be suspected in children with progressive symmetrical muscle weakness and characteristic skin lesions. The typical skin changes are a violaceous or purplish discoloration of the upper eyelids associated with periorbital oedema, and chronic, atrophic, scaly, mauve lesions over the dorsal surfaces of the metacarpo-phalangeal and inter-phalangeal joints, elbows, and knees. The myositis may be painful and affects mainly proximal muscles. The onset may be acute, subacute, or chronic but it is insidiously progressive and may affect swallowing and breathing. There is often a low-grade fever, and these children are irritable and miserable. The underlying pathology is a vasculitis of small blood vessels.

The diagnosis is largely clinical and all laboratory tests may be negative. However, a raised creatine phosphokinase (CPK) and other liver enzymes, increased urinary creatine-to-creatinine ratio, an abnormal EMG, and muscle biopsy may help to confirm the diagnosis. Subcutaneous and muscular dystrophic calcinosis may develop later in the disease. The differential diagnosis includes other forms of myositis (viral infections, trichinosis, toxoplasmosis), and infectious polyneuritis.

Prognosis without treatment is poor and it is most important to make the diagnosis early, and promptly start high-dose corticosteroids (2 mg/kg/d). This usually prevents progression, controls symptoms, and leads to long-lasting remission. Failure of steroid treatment or steroid dependency forces the use of other immunosuppressive drugs. Careful monitoring of muscle weakness, respiratory failure, and swallowing problems is essential, and early physiotherapy and occupational therapy prevent contractures. All patients should be referred to a unit specializing in the management of the disease.

Scleroderma

Scleroderma may be localized, with areas of fibrosis, atrophy, and synovitis. The rarer systemic form or systemic sclerosis has signs of generalized fibrosis of the subcutaneous tissues, skin, oesophagus, and internal organs, and Raynaud's phenomenon is common. Therapy of scleroderma is difficult but corticosteroids may control symptoms.

Mixed connective tissue disease

Mixed connective tissue disease is an overlap syndrome, which combines some of the features of SLE, dermatomyositis, scleroderma, and JIA. Antibodies to ribonucleoprotein (RNP) give a speckled antinuclear pattern in tissue sections and are frequently but not invariably present. Therapy of mixed connective tissue disease is difficult but corticosteroids may control symptoms.

Vasculitides

The vasculitides are rare in children, except for Henoch-Schönlein purpura, Kawasaki disease and to a lesser extent Takayasu's arteritis (*see* Table 21.8). Revised consensus criteria for classifying common childhood vasculitides were recently published (*see* Table 21.9).

Henoch-Schönlein purpura (HSP)

HSP is the most common vasculitis in childhood, occurring characteristically between the ages of three and 10 years. Over 50 per cent of all cases occur before the age of five years. The typical patient presents with abdominal pain, palpable purpura over the buttocks and pressure-bearing areas, and large-joint arthritis (*see* Table 21.9). In atypical cases the rash is maculopapular or urticarial, and may be mistaken for SLE, meningococcaemia or dermatitis herpetiformis. The symptoms may develop in any order and renal involvement may only become apparent several weeks after presentation. Clinically significant nephritis develops in about 30 per cent of cases of HSP. The abdominal pain, rash, and arthritis are self-limited but renal disease may persist. Microscopic haematuria without proteinuria and with normal blood pressure will resolve, but this may take up to two years. About 25 per cent of children who have macroscopic haematuria and/or proteinuria and/or hypertension will go on to chronic renal failure. Progress to end-stage renal failure is less common.

There are no diagnostic laboratory tests for HSP. The platelet count is normal or increased. Treatment is supportive with control of pain, maintenance of hydration and nutrition and, if nephritis develops, control of blood pressure. Severe gastrointestinal tract or joint involvement may respond to prednisone 2 mg/ kg/d. Acute nephritic syndrome or nephrotic syndrome should be referred to a specialist centre for treat-

Table 21.8 International Consensus Classification of Childhood Vasculitides, 2008		
I	Predominantly large vessel vasculitis	Takayasu arteritis
II	Predominantly medium-sized vessel vasculitis	Childhood polyarteritis nodosa Cutaneous polyarteritis Kawasaki disease
III	Predominantly small vessel vasculitis	A. Granulomatous Wegener's granulomatosis Churg-Strauss syndrome B. Non-granulomatous Microscopic polyangiitis Henoch-Schönlein purpura Isolated cutaneous leukocytoclastic vasculitis Hypocomplementaemic urticarial vasculitis
IV	Other vasculitides	Bechet's disease Vasculitis secondary to infection (Including hepatitis B-associated polyarteritis nodosa), malignancies, and drugs, including hypersentitivity vasculitis Vasculitis associated with connective tissue diseases Isolated vasculitis of the CNS Cogan's syndrome Unclassified

ment with steroids and/or azathioprine and/ or intravenous immunoglobulin.

In two-thirds of cases the disease is transient. In about 50 per cent of cases it recurs one or more times with diminishing severity on each occasion. Relapses are often associated with upper respiratory tract infections and may be prevented with prophylactic penicillin.

Takayasu's arteritis

This form of arteritis is confined to the aorta and large vessels, and occurs mainly in older girls. The condition is found worldwide but the highest prevalence is in Japan and the Far East, and it is not uncommon in southern Africa. Many affected children are undernourished and are from impoverished communities. Immune deposits have been detected in affected vessels but the relative roles of infection, immunity, nutrition and genetics are not known. An association has been noted with a strongly reactive tuberculin test but no other signs of tuberculosis are usually present.

In the acute phase the condition is often missed because the symptoms are non-specific: fever, arthralgia, myalgia, and fatigue. Laboratory studies show a raised ESR and IgG. Hypertension is the most common presenting feature, followed by cardiac failure, bruits, and absent pulses (*see* Table 21.9). Many children present late in the disease when the underlying vasculitis has led to stenosis, thrombosis, or aneurysmal dilation of the aorta and its branch vessels, and symptoms secondary to arterial occlusion develop. When the abdominal aorta and renal arteries are affected, severe hypertension and its complications, and symptoms of visceral ischaemia develop.

Table 21.9 Consensus criteria for diagnosing common childhood vasculitides		
I	Henoch-Schönlein purpura	Palpable purpura (mandatory) in the presence of at least one of the following four features: • Diffuse abdominal pain • Any biopsy showing IgA deposition • Arthritis or arthralgia • Renal Involvement (any haematuria and/or proteinuria)
II	Takayasu arteritis	Angiographic abnormalities (conventional, CT, or MRI) of the aorta or its main branches (mandatory), plus at least one of the following four features: • Decreased peripheral artery pulses and/or claudication of extremities • Blood pressure difference >10 mmHg • Bruits over aorta and/or main branches • Hypertension (related to childhood normative data)
III	Kawasaki disease	Fever persisting for at least five days (mandatory) plus four of the following five features: • Changes in peripheral extremities (erythema and/or oedema of palms and soles; during the later stages periungual desquamation) or perineal area • Polymorphous exanthema • Bilateral conjunctival injection • Changes in lips and oral cavity (red fissured lips, strawberry tongue, injection of oral and pharyngeal mucosa) • Cervical lymphadenopathy In the presence of coronary artery involvement and fever, fewer than four of the remaining five criteria are sufficient

Involvement of the carotid arteries leads to cerebral anoxic symptoms and focal neurological signs. Absent or reduced pulses are frequently detected (pulseless disease) in one or more of the limbs and bruits may be heard.

The disease has been classified according to the anatomical distribution:

- Type I: disease is confined to the aortic arch
- Type II: disease of descending thoracic and abdominal aorta
- Type III: is a combination of types I and II
- Type IV: Any of the previous types with pulmonary artery involvement
- Type V: Isolated peripheral arterial disease.

Angiography (conventional, CT or MRI) is the most important investigation for assessing the extent of the arterial disease. Treatment is aimed at controlling symptoms, e.g. hypertension and seizures. If there are signs of active inflammation, corticosteroids, cyclophosphamide, methotrexate or mycophenolate mofetil are used to control the inflammatory response. Antituberculosis therapy has been advocated but there is no evidence that it alters the course of the disease, which is slowly progressive but may arrest at any stage. Surgical correction of vascular stenosis or the removal of an ischaemic kidney may be indicated, particularly when renovascular hypertension is present.

Kawasaki disease

Kawasaki disease is an acute multisystem disease predominantly affecting young children. Approximately 85 per cent of patients are under five years of age. The disease is uncommon in patients aged less than three months or more than five years. The disease has a worldwide distribution with the highest incidence recorded among Japanese children. Although the aetiology is unknown an infectious agent is strongly suspected on epidemiological grounds: particularly pronounced seasonality, clustering of cases, and occurrence of epidemics. The pathology is due to a vasculitis affecting predominately medium-sized arteries of which coronary artery involvement is most important. Symptoms usually last for two to four weeks and resolve spontaneously. The children are characteristically toxic looking, irritable, and may experience pain in their hands and feet. Typical clinical manifestations are described in Table 21.9. Approximately 20 per cent of untreated children develop coronary artery aneurysms. Some of these resolve spontaneously but acute and residual coronary artery insufficiency may result in death or severe cardiac disability. Other features include uveitis, sterile pyuria, arthritis or arthralgia, aseptic meningitis, pericardial effusion, and gallbladder inflammation.

There are no specific diagnostic tests for Kawasaki disease. The diagnosis is based on the presence of at least five clinical criteria (*see* Table 21.9). The differential diagnosis includes group A streptococcal infections, staphylococcal toxin syndromes, measles, drug reactions, rickettsial infections, infectious mononucleosis, and other rheumatic diseases. Laboratory investigations are non-specific but a high level of acute phase markers (ESR, CRP), elevated WCC with neutrophil leukocytosis, white blood cells seen on urinalysis, elevated transaminases or bilirubin and a negative ASOT may be documented. An elevated platelet count starting 10–14 days after the onset of the illness may be seen.

Treatment

Both intravenous immunoglobulin (IVIG) and aspirin are recommended. Corticosteroids have not been shown to be effective. Intravenous immunoglobulin (IVIG) administered during the first 10 days of the illness reduces the incidence of coronary artery aneurysms to about 5 per cent. A single infusion of 2 g/kg over 10–12 hours should be given as soon as the clinical diagnosis has been established. Care must be taken to prevent fluid overload. High-dose aspirin (30-50 mg/kg/d) is given for the first two weeks and followed by low-dose aspirin (3 to 5 mg/kg/d) for a further six to eight weeks to inhibit platelet aggregation. Aspirin reduces the duration and severity of symptoms but has no effect on the development of coronary artery vasculitis. Peeling fingers and sore lips should be treated with emollients and lip balm respectively.

Following the administration of IVIG there usually rapid defervescence. Persistent or recurrent fever may benefit from a second dose of IVIG. There are no clear guidelines for the treatment of refractory disease, but immunosuppressive agents have been used.

Coronary artery involvement is detected by

echocardiography and follow-up studies should be performed at six to eight weeks. Children with coronary artery aneuryms require long-term aspirin and cardiology follow-up. Most lesions ultimately resolve. There is a small risk for persistent coronary artery lesions and myocardial infarction.

Polyarteritis nodosa

This is a rare multisystem disease characterized by fever, Raynaud's phenomenon, arthralgia, myalgia, and erythematous skin rashes. The underlying pathology is a generalized inflammatory vasculitis of medium-sized vessels, which may affect any organ, but renal and neurologic involvement is the most serious. The aetiology is believed to be immune complex mediated and evidence of preceding streptococcal and hepatitis B infection may be obtained in a proportion of cases. Diagnosis requires a biopsy showing small and mid-sized artery necrotizing vasculitis or angiographic abnormalities (aneurysms or occlusions) in addition to systemic features. The prognosis is not good, but steroid treatment helps to control symptoms and cytotoxic drugs such as cyclophosphamide are sometimes indicated.

Clinical problems posed by chronic conditions

In caring for a patient with a chronic disorder, the problems faced by the practitioner fall into three categories: the 'new' patient, the 'known' patient who needs routine care, and the 'known' patient who has a severe flare of disease. The different demands imposed on the health care team by these three situations are discussed below.

New patient

The challenges facing the doctor in the management of a new patient revolve around the following aspects:
- Making the diagnosis
- Breaking the news
- Adherence to medication
- Controlling the disease.

'Known' patients: routine visit

The regular follow-up visits of a patient with an established diagnosis require the following to be done:
- **Assess disease activity**. The history, examination and, where appropriate, special tests should assess the current activity of the disease and answer the question 'Is the disease adequately controlled?'
- **Assess disease impact**. A chronic disease has an impact on the patient and family, which should be assessed; on activities of the patient's daily life, such as school attendance, participation in social events, writing, dressing, feeding, and washing. The social and financial impact on the family (parents and siblings) should also be assessed. The impact of the treatment should be assessed in terms of side-effects of medication, and in terms of compliance with appointments and therapy.
- **Manage disease and monitor progression and drug side-effects**. Treatment will be adjusted or maintained according to the control of disease activity and the impact of the disease.
- **Support the patient, family, and school teacher**. The patient and family will need constant support and the school teacher needs to be brought into the health care team.
- **Be aware of 'alternative' medicine**. The more chronic and severe the disease, the more certain it is that the patient or parents will want to try 'alternative' or 'complementary' medicine. This should be discussed with them at the earliest opportunity and regularly at follow-up visits. Acupuncture is finding a place in orthodox medicine in the treatment of chronic pain and patients may be referred for this. Other modalities such as diets, copper bracelets, and homeopathy have not been tested in clinical trials nor found to have any useful effect.

'Known' patient with a chronic disorder who has 'new' signs and symptoms

The 'known' patient who has an acute exacerbation of the disease, or new signs and symptoms, poses a different set of challenges. It has to be decided if this is a flare-up in the disease, if it is a complication of the treatment, or if it is a new and unrelated disease. This demands continued vigilance and care in taking the history and in clinical examination.

Many chronic diseases are life-long. Care needs of older children and adolescents should be considered. The clinic environment should be supportive. Adolescents have specific health issues relating to their growth, development and sexual maturation, and experience social challenges including drug and alcohol-related problems. Furthermore, ensuring seamless transition from paediatric to adult services is essential to maintain optimal treatment and ensure quality of life.

22 Neoplastic disorders

One in 600 children will develop cancer before the age of 15 years. Cancer is the most important cause of death in childhood in Western countries after trauma.

Successful clinical trials in paediatric oncology in the last 40 years have changed the outcome from definite death to survival in nearly 80 per cent of children. More than two-thirds of children can potentially be cured, but many children in the developing world remain undiagnosed or die because of the unavailability of modern oncotherapy or delay in referral to a paediatric oncology unit while the child still has limited disease. Doctors, primary healthcare workers, parents and guardians must be educated about the warning signs and symptoms of childhood cancer, and be encouraged to seek expert advice without delay in the presence of these signs or symptoms (*see* box below).

Future developments will include the use of biological agents, with the aim of improving the survival of children who have cancers that are not currently curable. Furthermore, it is important to improve access to care for the majority of children in developing countries, who currently are not receiving cancer treatment or receive inadequate treatment.

Knowledge of the molecular basis of cancer is rapidly increasing. The genetic information of the cancer cell is different from the normal cell counterpart, leading to genomic instability with the formation of novel proteins or dysregulation of existing genes. Genomic instability can be increased or decreased by genetic and environmental factors. These chromosomal changes can be characterized by DNA analysis. There is a large variety of known altered transcriptional genes, which contribute to the development of leukaemias and solid tumours.

This molecular knowledge is applied to make a diagnosis, determine prognosis, measure the presence of clinically occult disease, and/or provide genetic counselling. Current novel therapies include drugs targeting the genetic changes that cause cancer. One example is acute myeloid leukaemia FAB type 3, where primary treatment with all-trans retinoic acid often induces remission. This compound binds to the abnormal gene, and allows the cancerous myelocytes to develop into microscopically normal cells. Potential 'targeted' molecular treatment of cancer will change treat-

---

Exclude cancer when the following signs or symptoms are present:

- A visible or palpable swelling that is not obviously due to a localized infection
- Enlarged lymph nodes (>1 cm) persisting for more than three weeks
- Acute-onset neurological symptoms not due to infection (e.g. early morning headache with nausea and vomiting, convulsions, deterioration in school work)
- Unexplained skin bruises
- Anaemia that does not respond to treatment as expected
- Unexplained fever lasting more than two weeks
- Unexplained persistent pain (especially pain waking the child up in the night)
- A white pupil reflex (absent normal red pupil reflex).

ment protocols in the future and hopefully further improve the cure rate.

Childhood cancer affects different organs to those affected by cancer in adults. Nephroblastoma, neuroblastoma, and retinoblastoma occur only in children, while the bronchus, gastrointestinal tract, and breast are the main sites of cancers in adults. The relative incidence of childhood cancers differs also between continents and between countries. Burkitt's lymphoma and retinoblastoma are notably more, and brain tumours notably less, common in some countries in Africa than they are in developed countries such as the USA and England. A population-based tumour registry of a defined geographic area is the only scientific way to obtain accurate epidemiological data about cancer in children. A hospital tumour registry reflects all cases treated at that hospital (*see* Table 22.1).

All children with cancer should be managed in a regional or national paediatric cancer unit. This is the only way to provide the necessary expertise regarding the investigations, modern drugs, paediatric surgery, radiotherapy, comprehensive supportive care, and a good chance of cure to children in the public health arena. However, in the majority of developing countries, the cost of non-generic drugs, modern diagnostic facilities, and optimal supportive care makes it impossible to provide the gold standard of treatment of industrialized countries. It is therefore important to use simple, relatively inexpensive diagnostic techniques such as ultrasound and fine needle aspirates, and to develop treatment strategies that are affordable and sustainable, while still providing a good chance of cure. The services of a social worker, physiotherapist, occupational therapist, psychologist, hospital teacher, and the support of the community all add to the chances of successful treatment. If therapeutic resources

Aetiological factors in childhood tumours

- Infections: Burkitt's lymphoma (Epstein-Barr virus and malaria), hepatocellular carcinoma (Hep B virus)
- Kaposi's sarcoma (human herpes virus 8 or HHP8)
- Genetic: Bilateral retinoblastoma, familial cancer syndromes
- Chromosomal: Down's syndrome, Fanconi's anaemia confer an increased risk of cancer
- Environmental: Skin cancer (sun exposure), lung cancer (smoking)
- Immune deficiency states (inherited, post transplantation, HIV infection).

Table 22.1 Relative frequency (%) of tumours

Diagnostic group	England and Wales	Uganda	Tygerberg Hospital (South Africa)
	1981–1990	1992–1995	1983–2001
Leukaemias	32.6	5.6	24.8
Lymphomas	10.0	28.2	15.9
Brain and spinal cord	22.5	1.2	20.1
Sympathetic nervous system	7.0	0.6	7.6
Retinoblastoma	2.7	6.5	4.7
Renal tumours	5.8	4.7	9.8
Hepatic tumours	0.9	1.5	1.2
Malignant bone tumours	4.8	2.9	3.7
Soft tissue sarcoma	6.8	40.6*	5.2
Germ cell and gonadal tumours	3.5	0.9	2.7
Carcinoma and epithelial tumours	3.0	3.8	2.0
Other and unspecified	0.4	3.5	1.0
*Mainly Kaposi's sarcoma			

are limited, children with an almost hopeless prognosis at the time of diagnosis, e.g. stage IV neuroblastoma, and children with recurrent disease, should probably receive only palliative care. Although modern oncotherapy can cure the majority of children, the treatment itself may have major long-term side-effects, which necessitates meticulous long-term follow-up of these children.

The challenge is to cure the child of cancer with the least harmful combination of treatment and to maintain normal growth and development. Of equal importance is the provision of good palliative care in children with incurable disease.

Long-term side-effects of oncotherapy

- Alkylating agents: Infertility, second malignancies
- Radiotherapy: Second malignancies, damage to growing bone, muscle, and subcutaneous tissue
- Cranial irradiation: Intellectual and endocrine damage
- Anthracyclines (doxorubicin): Cardiomyopathy
- Bleomycin: Lung fibrosis
- Platinum compounds: Deafness, renal failure
- Aggressive surgery: Mutilation.

Leukaemia

The acute leukaemias are characterized by uncontrolled proliferation or defective maturation of white blood cells. They account for >20 per cent of neoplastic disorders in children in South Africa. The majority of leukaemias in children are the acute variety of which acute lymphoblastic leukaemia (ALL) is the most common leukaemia in white children (>80 per cent), followed by acute non-lymphocytic leukaemia (ANLL). Black children have a relatively lower and Hispanic children a relatively higher ALL incidence rate than white children. In black children in Africa and other countries ANLL may account for up to half the cases of acute childhood leukaemia. Although the ultimate cause is unknown, we know that children with structural chromosomal defects, such as Down's syndrome and Fanconi's anaemia, have a higher incidence

of acute leukaemia, and that there is a relationship between chromosomal aberrations and the activation of proto-oncogenes.

Chronic myelocytic leukaemia is rare in children and can occur as either the chronic, adult Philadelphia chromosome positive variety, or as a more fulminant juvenile form. Chronic lymphocytic leukaemia does not occur in children.

Clinical features

ALL has a peak incidence between one and five years of age but may occur at any age. ANLL has no comparable age peak. Males have a slightly higher incidence of both ALL and ANLL than females.

Following a short history of days to weeks, children present with the following symptoms and signs:

Symptoms and signs of leukaemia

Fatigue and pallor	88%
Hepatosplenomegaly	80%
Fever	61%
Bleeding or bruising	48%
Lymphadenopathy	40%
Bone pain	23%

There may be thymic enlargement on X-ray, radiological bone lesions, and central nervous system involvement with blast cells in the cerebrospinal fluid present at diagnosis. The symptoms and signs are the result of leukaemia cells that occupy and replace the normal bone marrow and tissue of other organs, disturbing normal body functions.

The early symptoms may be indistinguishable from common viral infections. Bone and joint pains are often a feature of ALL, which may be mistaken for rheumatic fever. Pain in the bones may be mistaken for 'growing pains'. Gingival hypertrophy and ulcerative oropharyngeal lesions occur more commonly in ANLL. Orbital chloromata may be a feature of ANLL in black children, but are rarely seen in white children. Infection at presentation is more common in ANLL than ALL. In advanced disease, the clinical picture of fever, lymphadenopathy, hepatosplenomegaly, and wasting, in conjunction with pulmonary or abdominal symptoms, may mimic disseminated tuberculosis, chronic bacterial or parasitic infections, and AIDS. Patients with lytic bone lesions and periosteal reactions, which occur mainly in ALL, may be misdiagnosed as osteomyelitis or neuroblastoma.

Diagnosis

The laboratory diagnosis is suspected on the basis of abnormalities in the blood count. A Coulter count may show a normal, raised, or low white cell count with usually a normochromic, normocytic anaemia (80 per cent) (Hb <10 g/dl),and thrombocytopaenia (platelets <100 × 10^9/l). These findings should prompt the laboratory to examine a blood smear and recognize and report the presence of abnormal white cells (blasts). It is absolutely essential to perform a bone marrow aspirate. This is mainly to confirm the diagnosis of leukaemia, and secondly, to obtain tissue to characterize the exact biological nature of the disease. Identification of the morphologic, cytochemical, immunological (surface marker), and cytogenetic characteristics of the blast cells is necessary for the correct classification into subtypes of ALL and ANLL. Treatment and prognosis is dependent on the subtype of leukaemia and it is therefore preferable that these special investigations are done in a centre with all the necessary laboratory services.

In ALL, the treatment and outcome differs for T cell, B cell, and pre-B cell plus pre-pre-B cell (the so-called common ALL) leukaemia. Specific chromosomal translocations correlate with specific ALL immunophenotypes. The t(9;21) translocation is associated with a poor prognosis. In South Africa, we use the French-American-British (FAB) morphological and cytochemical classification for ANLL subtypes. (*See* Table 22.2)

Other investigations

Before commencing therapy it is important to establish that the patient has normal coagulation, normal renal function, and normal liver function. A chest radiograph is used to assess mediastinal involvement, and the cerebrospinal fluid is examined for the presence of blasts. A tuberculin test and base-line culture of nose and throat swabs, stool, and urine form part of an initial infectious screening. It is useful to know if the child has antibodies against varicella, measles, hepatitis B, cytomegalovirus and HIV. Histo-compatibility leucocyte antigen (HLA) typing is needed if a bone marrow transplant is considered.

Early morbidity

The most dangerous complications in the first week after diagnosis are haemorrhage (including cerebral bleeding), severe infections, and metabolic disturbances secondary to the tumour lysis syndrome.

Management

Management of childhood leukaemia includes medical treatment of the disease, as well as provision of constant support, guidance and encouragement to the child and family.

Specific therapy

Chemotherapy is designed to provide a combination of drugs that kill leukaemic cells by inter-

Table 22.2 Classification systems for acute leukaemia		
FAB classification of ANLL		**Classification of ALL based on immunophenotype**
M0	no maturation	B cell lineage
M1	minimal maturation	Pro-B/Early B cell ALL
M2	with maturation	Common ALL (cALL)
M3	promyelocytic	Pre-B ALL
M4	myelomonocytic	B ALL
M5A	monoblastic (undifferentiated)	T cell lineage
M5B	monocytic (differentiated)	Pro-T ALL
M6	erythroleukaemic	Pre-T ALL
M7	megakaryoblastic	Common T ALL
MDS	myelodysplastic syndrome	

fering with different phases of DNA synthesis or cell metabolism, and which have their greatest effect on immature or dividing cells. The dosage of the drugs used is limited by their immediate and long-term side-effects on normal tissues.

The first intensive phase of chemotherapy, which is called the induction, will eliminate all measurable disease in 90 per cent of patients. This is followed by a second phase of intensive chemotherapy, called consolidation, which is meant to obliterate occult disease. Intrathecal cytostatics are given to eradicate occult disease in the central nervous system (CNS). Only children with very high-risk disease are nowadays given limited cranial radiotherapy as additional CNS prophylaxis. Patients are subsequently given continuous low-dose maintenance chemotherapy for two to three years after which all treatment is stopped. A bone marrow transplant improves the chance of cure in some children with subtypes of ALL or ANLL that are known to respond poorly to chemotherapy or in children who have relapsed.

Supportive treatment

Families of children with cancer are at high risk of developing marital stress and psychological problems among family members, and carry an enormous additional financial burden. A supportive team consisting of medical and nursing personnel, a social worker, and religious and psychological advisers is therefore essential. The child him or herself may additionally need a physiotherapist, occupational therapist, nutritionist, and school teacher.

Tumour lysis syndrome during induction therapy is prevented by using allopurinol and by meticulous attention to renal function, fluid, electrolyte and mineral balance. Fatal haemorrhage associated with severe thrombocytopaenia (platelets $<20 \times 10^9/l$) can be prevented with platelet transfusions, and haemorrhagic shock prevented by the timeous transfusion of red cells. The patient's suppressed immune status and therapy-induced neutropaenia make life-threatening bacterial, fungal, and viral infections a constant hazard. In principle, all children with $<0.5 \times 10^9/l$ neutrophils and a single documented fever of 38.5 °C, or two episodes of 38 °C in a 24-hour period, should be empirically started on treatment with broad-spectrum antibiotics (e.g. ceftriaxone and amikacin) while awaiting the outcome of blood and other cultures. Antibiotics that are effective against staphylococci and fungi are added if there is no satisfactory response. Growth factors (G-CSF and erythropoietin) are used only in very special circumstances.

Acyclovir is effective treatment for chickenpox, herpes zoster, and herpes simplex. A high index of suspicion for tuberculosis should be maintained. All children are given oral cotrimoxazole as prophylaxis against *Pneumocystis jirovecii* for the full duration of treatment. Separate isolation units are unnecessary for these children if all members of staff enforce simple rules to prevent sepsis, such as hand washing. The majority of children suffering from cancer do not maintain an adequate intake of calories despite the concerted efforts of medical staff and family. It is therefore mandatory to check the daily food intake, and not to hesitate to supplement this with nasogastric feeds (and sometimes parenteral nutrition) if the dietary intake is inadequate. An indwelling venous line (Broviac® or Port-o-cath® type) facilitates treatment, but carries the risk of infection and needs good supervision.

Prognosis

More than 70 per cent of children with ALL are cured permanently with modern chemotherapy and supportive care. A reduction in the blast count in the peripheral blood to $<1.0 \times 10^9/l$ after a week of prednisone therapy, indicates a good prognosis. For reasons thus far unexplained, black children have a poorer outcome despite receiving the same therapy. Poor prognostic factors include age, e.g. less than <1 year and >10 years at diagnosis; initial white cell count exceeding $20 \times 10^9/l$; and sex, where boys do worse than girls. Certain chromosomal aberrations also fare worse. B-cell ALL and involvement of the CNS at diagnosis adversely influence outcome. In ANLL the chance of disease-free survival is approaching 50 per cent with optimal treatment. The outcome differs in various subtypes.

Complications

These complications include disease recurrence in the marrow, CNS, or testes relapse, and the morbidity during the actual treatment, as well as known treatment-related long-term effects. For example high dose methotrexate and radiotherapy may damage cognitive functions, causing learning disabilities. The hypothalamic-pituitary axis may also be adversely affected by cranial irradiation with resultant growth retardation.

Lymphomas

The malignant lymphomas have a wide range of cell types and histological patterns involving lymphoreticular tissue. A biopsy specimen or fine needle aspirate enables the pathologist to perform a proper histological and immunological assessment and diagnosis. Non-Hodgkin's lymphoma and Hodgkin's disease are unrelated disorders.

Non-Hodgkin's lymphomas (NHL)

The Non-Hodgkin's lymphomas (NHL) can be divided into lymphomas that originate from either precursor lymphoblastic cells or from mature cells, further subdivided into either B-cell or T-cell/NK-cell lineage (WHO classification). These lymphomas account for approximately 10 per cent of childhood tumours in South Africa. Children suffer mainly from one of the following four types of NHL (WHO classification):

* Mature B-cell lymphomas (including several subtypes, especially Burkitt's lymphoma)
* Mature T-cell and Natural Killer-cell lymphomas
* Precursor pre-B lymphoblastic lymphoma and
* Precursor T-cell lymphoblastic lymphoma.

The diagnosis is confirmed on biopsy, fine needle aspirate or other cytology. Lymphomas are staged using the Murphy (St Jude) classification and for this purpose a thorough clinical examination, a chest X-ray, ultrasonography, computerized tomography (CT) scan (if available), a bone marrow examination, and a cerebrospinal fluid (CSF) examination should be done to determine the stage of the disease.

Burkitt's lymphomas

Burkitt's lymphoma (BL) is the most common type of cancer in central African countries within 15° latitude of the equator. In Malawi, endemic Burkitt's lymphoma accounts for 50 per cent of all childhood malignancies. Clinically, BL

Murphy staging system of lymphoma

* *Stage I*: Single nodal or extranodal site (not in the mediastinum or abdomen)
* *Stage II*: One or more extranodal sites plus regional nodes, or two extranodal sites on the same side of the diaphragm
* *Stage III*: Two or more sites on both sides of the diaphragm, including all primary intrathoracic and extensive abdominal tumours
* *Stage IV*: I to III plus bone marrow involvement (<25 per cent infiltration) and/or CNS disease.

---

presents as two types, which have differences at the molecular level: endemic Burkitt's lymphoma (BL), which occurs mainly in Africa, and sporadic BL, which occurs in Europe, North America, and in other continents. Both types occur in children of all ethnic groups in South Africa, although the sporadic type is more common. The histology and the initial response to treatment is the same for both endemic and sporadic BL. It is thought that infection with Epstein-Barr virus (EBV) in Africa at a young age may immortalize and stimulate the proliferation of B-cells. This in turn may lead to translocations of chromosome 8 with deregulation of the c-Myc oncogene, which is involved in the control of cellular proliferation. This disease has a very aggressive growth pattern and can double in size within a day.

Endemic Burkitt's lymphoma

The peak age is seven years with a marked male predominance. The most common presentation is a fast-growing swelling of the maxilla or mandible with extension into the nasopharynx, nose and orbit. A loose tooth is often the first presenting symptom. Abdominal disease with ascites and infiltration of retroperitoneal organs (kidney, ovaries) is also a common presentation. The bone marrow is involved in 10 per cent and the CNS in 25 per cent of children at diagnosis. CNS involvement can manifest clinically as paraplegia or cranial nerve palsies with tumour cells present in the cerebrospinal fluid (CSF).

Sporadic B-cell lymphoma

The median age and male predominance are the same as in African Burkitt's. Two-thirds of children present with an abdominal mass. The primary site is usually in the ileocaecal region. Primary tumours of the head and neck region and of superficial lymph nodes constitute the other third.

Treatment. This is the same for all B-cell lymphomas. Major surgery to debulk the tumour (surgical excision), is not indicated due to the sensitivity of the tumour to chemotherapy. The intensity of treatment varies with the stage of disease and more than 80 per cent of children can be cured with five months of intensive chemotherapy (e.g. the French LMB type protocols). This intensive chemotherapy must be accompanied by appropriate supportive care, such as critical laboratory investigations, blood products, antibiotics, antifungal agents, antiviral agents, and parenteral nutritional support to prevent death due to treatment complications. Chemotherapy is started at a low dose for the first week of treatment to prevent rapid tumour break-down and renal metabolic complications. The prevention of tumour lysis syndrome and complications of therapy are managed as in leukaemia. The therapy is intensive and expensive. Many countries in Africa simply cannot provide optimal drugs and supportive care to indigent patients, and have to tailor therapy according to what is locally available. Cure rates of 25–60 per cent have been recorded with less intensive treatment protocols. Disease-free survival for 12 months after completed therapy carries a >95 per cent probability of permanent cure.

Diffuse Large B-cell lymphoma (DLBCLs)

This lymphoma has a diverse clinical presentation, varying from tumours in the gastrointestinal tract, other sites in the abdomen and the head and neck region (especially Waldeyer's ring). These lymphomas are also associated with immunodeficiency and may occur in unusual sites such as bone or CNS. The treatment is the same as for Burkitt's lymphoma.

Precursor B and precursor T Lymphoblastic Lymphomas (B-LL and T-LL)

A third of lymphomas in childhood fall into this category and these lymphomas are indistinguishable from their related ALLs. Children with T-LL (T-cell origin) present at an older age than children with BL and also show a male prepon-

derance. The most common clinical finding is a mediastinal mass. The tumour can rapidly cause obstruction of the big vessels, particularly superior vena cava obstruction with life-threatening airway obstruction, necessitating emergency treatment. The clinical features of this oncology emergency are dyspnoea, dysphagia and pain with swelling of the neck, face and upper limbs. The empirical emergency treatment includes either low dose radiotherapy or steroids. Pleural and pericardial effusions are not uncommon. Rapidly enlarging painless cervical, supraclavicular, and axillary lymph nodes are a common presenting complaint.

LL of precursor B-cell origin usually presents as limited disease with frequent involvement of bone. If the bone marrow is involved and contains >25 per cent blasts, the diagnosis is technically changed to lymphoblastic leukaemia, although it is in essence the same disease entity.

Treatment. More than 70 per cent of children are cured with either a German (BFM-based) T-cell leukaemia protocol or an American lymphoma protocol (LSA2-L2). The duration of therapy is longer than the treatment of BL. The same precautions to prevent metabolic derangements and to manage morbidity apply as in acute leukaemia.

Anaplastic large-cell lymphoma (ALCL)

This is the most uncommon NHL of childhood, which originates from mature T-cell and NK-cells. The disease presents in two clinical forms, either as primary systemic ALCL (usually the clinical picture in children) and primary cutaneous ALCL. It occurs in older children, has a male preponderance, and is associated with inherited and acquired immune-deficiency states. The children usually present with advanced stage disease with fever and weight loss. The disease has various primary nodal sites, which include the mediastinum, gastrointestinal tract and bone. The disease has a relatively favourable prognosis with modern chemotherapy.

Hodgkin's lymphoma (HL)

HL constitutes between 5 and 11 per cent of childhood cancers in different countries in Africa. It results from the transformation of lymphocytes into the typical Reed-Sternberg multinucleated giant cells, which is the histological hallmark of HL. Epstein-Barr virus infection is probably involved in this malignant transformation. The World Health Organization (WHO) classification divides HL into nodular lymphocyte predominant (<5 per cent of all cases) and classical HL (95 per cent of cases) which has four histological subtypes: lymphocyte-rich, nodular sclerosis (the most common subtype), mixed cellularity, and lymphocyte-depleted. Usually HL has a bimodal age distribution with an early peak in young adults (20s) and another peak after 50 years of age in developed countries. The incidence of HL is, however, influenced by socio-economic factors. Children from a poor socio-economic environment develop HL at a younger age (early peak is before adolescence), and have a high incidence of mixed cellularity histology compared with children from an advantaged background who have a high incidence of nodular sclerosis histology. HL is rare before the age of three years. There is a slight male predominance. The progress of the disease is slow. The diagnosis is established on an excision lymph node biopsy or a fine needle aspirate.

Clinically, 75 per cent of children present with painless cervical lymphadenopathy, 25 per cent with axillary or inguinal lymphadenopathy, and 25 per cent with an enlarged liver and/or spleen, or an abdominal mass at diagnosis. Systemic signs such as weight loss, night sweats, pruritus, or pyrexia are present in 50 per cent of cases. There is also evidence of mediastinal lymphadenopathy on chest X-ray in 67 per cent of children at diagnosis. Patients in South Africa are often wrongly treated for tuberculosis and early biopsy or fine needle aspirate should be done for painless enlarged lymph glands, which persist for more than three weeks.

Treatment is given according to the stage of disease and it is important to accurately define and classify HL according to the Ann Arbor clinical staging system. This requires a good clinical examination, complete blood count, serum chemistry, chest X-ray, abdominal ultrasound, bone marrow examination and lymph node biopsy. A Gallium scan shows radionuclide uptake in tumour in two-thirds of patients. A CT or magnetic resonance imaging (MRI) scan may help to define the extent of disease. Lymphangiography and splenectomy are definitely not indicated in children.

The treatment consists of chemotherapy and

Ann Arbor staging system of Hodgkins lymphoma with Cotswald modifications

Stage

- 1 Involvement of one lymph-node region or lymphoid structure (e.g. spleen, thymus, Waldeyer ring)
- 2 Two or more lymph-node regions on the same side of the diaphragm
- 3 Lymph-node regions on both sides of the diaphragm
- 3_1: with splenic hilar, coeliac or portal nodes
- 3_2: with para-aortic, iliac, or mesenteric nodes
- 4 Involvement of extranodal site(s) beyond that designated E.

Modifying features

- A No symptoms
- B Fever, drenching night sweats, weight loss greater than 10 per cent in six months
- C Bulky disease: greater than a third widening of mediastinum
- D greater than 10 cm maximum diameter of nodal mass
- E Involvement of single, contiguous, or proximal extranodal site

---

the addition of limited dose radiotherapy to the involved field. Stage I HL can, however, be cured by radiotherapy alone and a large proportion of all stages of HL, by chemotherapy alone. A complete remission must be obtained at the onset, and full treatment compliance is necessary to achieve a cure. Well-tried chemotherapy protocols known as MOPP and ABVD give comparable long-term survival rates, but differ in their long-term adverse side-effects on the heart and gonads. Patients are at increased risk to develop herpes zoster. The recorded survival in South African children was 95 per cent in stages I and II, and 70 per cent in stages III and IV of the disease.

Malignant solid tumours

Nephroblastoma (Wilm's tumour)

Wilm's tumour (WT) is the most common and curable solid tumour and accounts for >10 per cent of all childhood cancer in South Africa, Namibia and Zimbabwe. Boys and girls are equally affected and the peak age is between one and five years. Associated congenital abnormalities are present in 20 per cent, of which the most common abnormalties are aniridia, hemihypertrophy, and urogenital abnormalities. The genetic basis of WT is complex and partly located in genes on chromosome 11. Histological subtypes are important because they relate to outcome (cure rate). The tumour may grow into the renal vein, spread locally into adjacent organs and along the ureter, and through the lymphatics to the para-aortic nodes. Haematogenous spread may be to the lungs, liver, bones, and brain.

Clinically the most common presentation is that of an abdominal mass, which is noticed by the parents or a health worker. It is large, firm, irregular, usually painless and often a fixed tumour. Fever, abdominal pain, haematuria, and hypertension may be present. In South Africa patients are often malnourished and large tumours are common at diagnosis. About 5 per cent of children present with bilateral tumours. Investigations include a full blood count, urea and electrolyte estimation, liver function tests, and urinalysis for the presence of blood, protein, white blood cells, and level of catecholamine excretion (to exclude neuroblastoma). Ultrasound examination is mandatory for the examination of all abdominal tumours in children and is a fast, inexpensive, safe and non-invasive investigation. It will distinguish cystic and solid tumours and can demonstrate tumours in the opposite kidney, tumour thrombi in the inferior vena cava, and metastases to the liver and abdomen. An intravenous pyelogram (optional) will demonstrate an intra-renal mass and distortion of the kidney, while computerized axial tomography or MRI (if available and affordable) are useful to define the tumour margins and anatomical changes. An antero-posterior and lateral chest X-ray are essential to detect pulmonary metastasis. A fine needle aspirate or percutaneous core needle biopsy will confirm the diagnosis, but needs a skilled pathologist to evaluate.

The differential diagnosis includes neuroblastoma, which can compress and displace the kidney, hydronephrosis, and polycystic kidneys, which are discernible on ultrasound, and other rare renal tumours. Mesoblastic nephroma is a benign tumour, which normally occurs in children aged under six months.

It is essential to assess and record the stage of the WT at the time of surgery according to the USA National Wilm's Tumour Study System (NWTS) or the International Society of Paediatric Oncology (SIOP) classification. Tumours are further classified histologically into favourable and unfavourable groups.

Treatment intensity is determined by stage and histology. The tumour is shrunk with four to six weeks of chemotherapy before attempting complete surgical resection (SIOP approach). Smaller tumours are easier to resect, and less likely to be ruptured intra-operatively. This approach gives the same survival probability as a primary resection, but at a lower cost and morbidity. All children need postoperative chemotherapy, which varies according to the stage and histology. Radiotherapy to the tumour bed is added in some stage II, and all stage III and IV patients. Patients who have recurrence of disease after completion of therapy can sometimes be cured with a different combination of chemotherapy.

Survival at five years exceeds 90 per cent for stage I and 50 per cent for stage IV disease if either SIOP or NWTS protocols are followed meticulously. The morbidity of treatment is higher in children with concomitant malnutrition or infectious diseases.

Neuroblastoma

This tumour can develop anywhere in the sympathetic nervous system in primitive sympathetic cells, which migrate from the neural crest of the embryo to form the sympathetic nervous system in the fetus. The adrenal gland is the

---

NWTS staging system (simplified)

- *Stage I:* Tumour limited to the kidney and completely resected
- *Stage II:* Tumour extends beyond the kidney in the abdomen, but is completely resected
- *Stage III:* Residual tumour confined to the abdomen
- *Stage IV:* Haematogenous metastases
- *Stage V:* Bilateral renal involvement.

most common primary site, followed by other abdominal sites, the thorax, the cervical region, and the pelvis. The spinal cord may be compressed by so-called 'dumb-bell' tumours, which extend through the neural foramina of the vertebrae. Neuroblastoma may differentiate spontaneously or after treatment into ganglioneuroblastoma or ganglioneuroma (a benign tumour). Eighty per cent of neuroblastomas produce catecholamines. This is detected by measuring the metabolites homovanillic acid (HVA) and vanillyl mandelic acid (VMA) in the urine. Although it is the most common solid tumour of children in Europe, the incidence in Africa varies from extremely rare in some countries to being the second most common solid tumour in South Africa. Half of the tumours present before the age of two years and 75 per cent before the age of four years. Clinical outcome can be predicted according to histological and molecular examination of tumour tissue. Loss of chromosome 1p, the presence of n-Myc amplification and high TRKB expression indicate a rapidly progressive disease with poor prognosis. Age above one year and advanced stage at diagnosis are also related to a poorer outcome. The majority of children present with advanced disease. The International Neuroblastoma Study Group (INNS) staging system is in general use.

The **clinical findings** depend on the site of the tumour. Abdominal disease presents as a large irregular mass, which often crosses the midline and may be associated with digestive symptoms and pain. Thoracic tumours cause respiratory symptoms. In the head and neck area visible tumour may be associated with a Horner syndrome. Pelvic tumours may disturb micturition and defaecation. Neuroblastoma of the paraspinal area may extend through the neural foramina and these so-called dumb-bell tumours can compress the spinal cord. This may cause pain, paralysis, and disturbances in bladder and bowel function, depending on the level of compression. Many children unfortunately present with disseminated disease without an identifiable primary tumour. Such patients may have prominent swellings on the skull, proptosis with peri-orbital blue discoloration, disseminated skin metastases, painful skeletal lesions, or gross and irregular hepatomegaly. Fever, anaemia, and bone pain are common. Very occasionally children present with chronic diarrhoea or ataxia and opsimyoclonus.

The **diagnostic criteria** are a histological diagnosis or the combination of marrow infiltration plus raised catecholamines in the urine. An abdominal X-ray may show calcification in the tumour. Skeletal X-rays will demonstrate metastatic lesions. Abdominal ultrasound is essential and computerized axial tomography (CAT) or MRI (if available) useful to determine the extent of disease. A bone marrow aspirate and trephine are necessary for accurate staging. Marrow infiltration can also be demonstrated by nuclear magnetic imaging. I^{131} MIBG is an isotope that binds to catecholamine-secreting tissue, and is useful to demonstrate primary and metastatic neuroblastoma. Electron microscopy may confirm the diagnosis if routine histology is unable to do so. A raised serum ferritin at diagnosis is an unfavourable finding.

In view of the extremely poor prognosis of advanced disease, and the recent ability to identify patients who will respond favourably to therapy by examining tumour tissue for 1p deletion and n-Myc amplification, these investigations should ideally be performed routinely. This will make it possible to allocate limited resources to children who can be cured.

Treatment consists of surgery only for stages I and IIA disease. Children with stages IIB and III disease are given chemotherapy followed by resection if possible. Children with stage IV disease should receive palliative therapy only if

INNS staging system (simplified)

- *Stage I:* Localized tumour, completely macroscopically excised
- *Stage IIA:* Unilateral tumour, incomplete gross excision, but no involvement of ipsilateral regional lymph nodes
- *Stage IIB:* Like IIA, with positive ipsilateral regional lymph nodes
- *Stage III:* Unresectable tumour; crosses midline or is unilateral with regional lymph node involvement on the other or both sides
- *Stage IV:* Spread of tumour to distant lymph nodes, bone marrow, bone, liver, and/or other organs
- *Stage IVS:* Localized primary tumour with spread limited to liver, skin, and/or bone marrow and infants <1 year of age (no bone metastasis).

a bone marrow transplant is not possible. Stage IVS is treated with no or little chemotherapy. Therapeutic doses of I¹³¹ MIBG can provide fast pain relief and transient resolution of tumour. Low-dose radiotherapy is useful for the control of local disease and pain. Chemotherapy followed by a bone marrow transplant will save the life of a minority of children with unfavourable disease.

The **prognosis** depends on the age and stage, and the risk factors previously mentioned. More than 90 per cent of local South African children with stages I and II, 50 per cent of children with stages III and IVS, and no children with stage IV disease are disease-free survivors five years after diagnosis.

Rhabdomyosarcoma

Rhabdomyosarcoma is the most common soft-tissue sarcoma of childhood. It can arise from embryonic precursor cells in any part of the body where striated muscle is found. The median age at diagnosis is five years. The families of some children carry an autosomal dominant inherited risk to develop a variety of malignant tumours (Li Fraumeni syndrome). Embryonal and alveolar histological subtypes have different clinical presentations and prognoses. Almost half of the tumours occur in the head and neck region (orbit, nasopharynx, middle ear, face), a quarter in the genito-urinary system (bladder, prostate, vagina, uterus, paratesticular), and the remainder in the extremities, trunk, or retroperitoneum. Metastases occur early to regional lymph nodes and haematogenously to the lung, bones, and marrow.

Tumours in the ear, nose, bladder, uterus, or vagina may present as polypoid lesions, which cause obstruction or a blood-stained or offensive discharge. On the trunk and extremities the tumour presents as a soft-tissue mass, which may be tender and is easily confused with an acute abscess. Orbital swelling may be mistaken for a retinoblastoma, neuroblastoma, or Burkitt's lymphoma. The brain and cerebrospinal fluid may be infiltrated with parameningeal tumours.

The **diagnosis** is established by fine needle aspirate or surgical biopsy of the lesion. The local extent of disease and all potential sites for metastatic spread must be fully investigated.

Treatment includes surgery, chemotherapy, and radiotherapy. Primary total surgical resection followed by chemotherapy, or chemotherapy followed by complete resection of residual tumour, offers the best chance of cure. Mutilating surgery must be minimized by first shrinking unresectable tumours with chemotherapy. Radiotherapy is necessary to tumour sites where surgical removal has not been microscopically complete. Approximately 50 per cent of all children are cured with modern treatment.

Liver tumours

The two main primary malignant liver tumours, hepatoblastoma and hepatocellular carcinoma, usually present with abdominal swelling and an enlarged irregular, firm liver, which may be tender. Both conditions are rare. The serum alpha-fetoprotein is elevated in 80 per cent of children with hepatoblastoma, and in some children with hepatocellular carcinomas. Routine vaccination of infants against hepatitis B will reduce the incidence of hepatocellular carcinoma in the future.

Hepatoblastoma predominates in males and generally occurs before the age of three years. The right lobe of the liver is usually involved. Other anomalies, e.g. hemihypertrophy and virilization, may be present. Hepatocellular carcinoma rarely occurs before the age of six years. Both tumours can spread locally and give rise to lung metastases.

The presence of tumour on abdominal sonar, together with a raised serum alpha-fetoprotein (AFP) in a child aged three years or less, fulfils the criteria for the diagnosis of hepatoblastoma and makes a biopsy unnecessary. Lung metastases must be excluded. Two-thirds of hepatoblastomas can be cured by completely resecting the tumour after shrinking it to an operable size with chemotherapy (platinum compounds), followed by more chemotherapy. The same approach will cure a much smaller percentage of children with hepatocellular carcinoma. A liver transplant may save the life of some children with unresectable disease.

Germ cell tumours

These are relatively rare tumours, which develop from the primordial germ cells of the embryo which are normally destined to produce sperm or ova. The signs and symptoms depend on the tumour location. They may present as an ovarian or testicular tumour or in an extra-gonadal site. The sacrococcygeal region is the commonest extra-gonadal site. Other sites are the retroperitoneum, vagina, mediastinum, and the pineal region.

Most of these tumours secrete the tumour marker, alpha-fetoprotein (the highest level is seen in yolk-sac tumours). Human chorionic gonadotrophin (HCG) is another tumour marker, which may be secreted by choriocarcinoma. These markers are useful for diagnosis, to assess the response to treatment, and to monitor the patient for tumour recurrence.

These tumours are usually very sensitive to modern chemotherapy combinations. The combination of chemotherapy and primary or delayed total surgical resection can cure the majority of children. Radiotherapy can cure intra-cranial tumours.

Retinoblastoma

Retinoblastoma (RB) is an aggressive tumour of the retina, which accounts for 3 per cent of cancers in children under the age of 15 years. The tumour usually occurs in children under the age of two years and causes vision loss, and even death in advanced disease. RB seems to be more common in Africa, India and Latin America. The majority of RB occurs sporadically, while in a minority the disease is familial or inherited. Retinoblastoma is caused by the loss of both of a pair of tumour suppressor genes (anti-oncogenes), one of which is situated on the long arm of each chromosome 13, in the developing retinal cell.

Two-thirds of children with retinoblastoma have developed two random mutations, which result in the loss of both tumour suppressor genes in one retinal cell after birth. They usually develop unilateral disease at a median age of 24 months.

The remaining one-third of children have, at birth, already lost the pair of tumour suppressor genes in every body cell by autosomal dominant inheritance, or by a mutation at the time of conception. They develop multiple and bilateral retinoblastoma, which presents at a median age of 12 months.

The survival of these patients has improved with treatment that involves a multimodality approach. The earliest stage is intraocular and is one of the most curable childhood cancers

> ## The WHO classification of germ cell tumours
>
> - Mature teratoma
> - Embryonal carcinoma
> - Immature teratoma
> - Yolk-sac tumours (endodermal sinus tumour, orchioblastoma, infantile adenocarcinoma)
> - Germinoma (seminoma of testis, dysgerminoma of ovary).

with an overall survival of more than 90 per cent. Advanced extraocular disease presents with either local extension into the CNS or distant metastasis, and has a very poor prognosis. The mother normally complains of a white spot in the pupil (leukocoria or 'cat's eye reflex'), a squint, or proptosis. Gross proptosis or a large orbital mass is a common presentation. The differential diagnosis is rhabdomyosarcoma, neuroblastoma, Burkitt's lymphoma, and visceral larva migrans of the eye.

Investigation should include an ophthalmo-logical examination under anaesthesia, a local X-ray and skeletal survey, CT or MRI scan of the brain. Examination of the bone marrow and microscopy of cerebrospinal fluid for malignant cells are essential tests for advanced disease.

Treatment depends on the extent of disease. Small lesions can be cured with photocoagulation or localized radiotherapy (brachytherapy) with preservation of vision. Enucleation is adequate therapy in more advanced disease, which is limited to the eyeball. Chemotherapy with or without radiotherapy are added in advanced disease. The outcome in advanced and metastatic disease is usually unfavourable, and may justify the use of a palliative treatment approach. Frequent ophthalmological screening until the age of five years is essential to ensure early diagnosis of a second tumour or recurrence. The risk for children of survivors of retinoblastoma to develop retinoblastoma is one in two in bilateral (inherited) and one in 20 in sporadic (unilateral) disease.

Brain tumours

(*See* Chapter 26, Neurological and muscular disorders.)

Bone tumours

Osteogenic sarcoma is the most common primary bone tumour in children, coinciding with the growth spurt with a median onset at 12 years of age. Aetiology is unknown, but irradiation is the only known environmental agent to cause bone sarcomas. Localized swelling and pain are the commonest presentation. The femur (50 per cent), tibia (30 per cent), and humerus (10 per cent) are most commonly affected. Lung metastases can occur. The differential diagnosis includes osteomyelitis, traumatic fracture, lymphoma, and eosinophilic granuloma. A biopsy is essential. Chest X-rays and a technetium bone scan are needed to detect metastases. A CT scan and MRI are useful to define the extent of tissue involvement. Significant reduction in tumour size is possible with chemotherapy. A resection/amputation in combination with chemotherapy is necessary to obtain a cure and can be combined with a variety of limb-sparing techniques. Approximately half the patients can be cured.

Ewing's sarcoma of bone and soft tissue primitive neuro-ectodermal tumours (PNET) share a characteristic t(11;22) translocation and should be grouped together. Ewing's sarcoma most commonly involves the pelvis, femur, humerus, and rib and presents with local pain or swelling. A biopsy is necessary and the same investigations as for osteosarcoma are indicated. The outcome is influenced by the initial volume of the disease, the site, and the ability to completely resect the tumour after chemotherapy. Radiotherapy is used for unresectable sites. The survival in children with limited disease is 60 per cent.

The histiocytic disorders

The term histiocytosis refers to disorders of the mononuclear phagocytic system. They are classified as follows:

- *Class I:* Langerhans cell histiocytosis
- *Class II:* Sinus histiocytosis with massive lymphadenopathy
  - Virus-associated haemophagocytic syndrome
  - Familial haemophagocytic lymphohistiocytosis
- *Class III*: Acute monocytic leukaemia
  - Malignant histiocytosis
  - True histiocytic lymphomas.

The class I and II histiocytic disorders are reactive conditions and not primary malignant disorders. They can nevertheless result in death, and cytostatic agents are often used in their treatment. A biopsy is essential for the diagnosis.

Langerhans cell histiocytosis

This term includes a spectrum of diseases. Histologically they all demonstrate abnormal proliferation of histiocytes associated with specific immunohistochemical characteristics, and the presence of cytoplasmic Birbeck granules in the histiocytes on electron microscopy. The management and outcome in children with localized and those with generalized disease is different.

Half of the patients present with localized disease. Single or multiple lesions of the membranous bones may present in older children as painful swellings or a pathological fracture, and on X-ray show a well-demarcated lytic lesion. Secondary diabetes insipidus is possible due to hypothalamic involvement from adjacent bony lesions. Local therapy consists of curettage, intralesional steroid injection, or low-dose radiotherapy. Isolated skin involvement in infants is often mistaken for and treated as seborrhoeic eczema. Spontaneous regression may occur or topical steroids can cure. Young children can develop lymphadenopathy, which tends to recur and resolve spontaneously. The prognosis of localized disease is excellent.

Generalized disease is common in younger children under two years of age. It can consist of a combination of bone and/or skin and/or lymph gland involvement, together with any combination of hepatomegaly, splenomegaly, pulmonary infiltrate, marrow involvement, and cytopaenia, diarrhoea and failure to thrive, and diabetes insipidus and growth retardation. These children are treated with a combination of methylprednisolone and cytostatics for at least six months. The drugs are slowly tapered once the child is in remission. Repeated recurrences over time are not unusual and one-third of children may eventually die of the disease.

Kaposi's sarcoma (KS)

In 1872, Moriz Kaposi described the disease as 'idiopathic multiple pigmented sarcomas of the skin'. Histopathological features include interweaving bands of spindle cells and vascular structures embedded in a network of reticular and collagen fibres. It used to be a rare disease except in certain endemic regions and populations, such as the black inhabitants of the highland areas in DR Congo, Kenya, and Tanzania. Children with classical KS presented mainly with lymphadenopathy. The relative incidence of KS (as a percentage of childhood malignancy) has increased from 2.63 per cent in 1982, to 19 per cent in 1992 in Zambia. This change from endemic to epidemic proportions has been caused by AIDS. In Uganda, KS has become the most common malignancy and the most important cause of generalized lymphadenopathy in children. Herpes hominis virus 8 is present in all tumour cells. These children have associated wasting and anaemia, and are almost all serologically HIV positive. The clinical course is progressive and they die within weeks. The clinical diagnosis must be confirmed on biopsy, tuberculosis excluded, and chest X-ray and the HIV status assessed after counselling. The disease does improve temporarily when full antiretroviral therapy is instituted. Surgical excision of a single lesion offers the only current hope of complete cure. The general approach is to provide the best available palliative care.

PART 7

System-based disorders

23

Disorders of the blood

Blood disorders present in two main ways: as pallor (pale mucous membranes or hand palms) or as a bleeding disorder. Because pallor is the clinical sign of anaemia, an ability to recognise it and measure the haemoglobin (Hb) is the most important primary care skill in the management of haematological disorders. Indications to measure Hb include the following:

Six points from the history	Six clinical findings
Pica	Pale mucosa/pallor
Intestinal parasites	Clinical malnutrition
Infants who had a low birth weight	Bleeding in skin or mucosa
Blood loss	Jaundice
Family history of anaemia	Lymphadenopathy
Ingestion of drugs or poisons	Enlarged liver and/ or spleen

Normal values

The diagnosis of anaemia in infancy and childhood is based upon knowledge of the changes in Hb, haematocrit (HCT), and red cell characteristics which occur during growth and development (*see* Table 23.1 and Figure 23.1). The high Hb level ('physiological polycythaemia') at birth reflects recent exposure to the relatively hypoxic intra-uterine environment.

Delay in clamping the cord can increase the blood volume by more than 20 ml/kg. The Hb level of capillary blood may be 2 g/dl more than that of venous blood. A further increase in Hb on the first day is due to postnatal reduction in plasma volume. The progressive postnatal decrease in Hb, which reaches a nadir between six and twelve weeks ('physiological anaemia') is a physiological adjustment, more marked in preterm infants. It is not due to iron deficiency nor is it corrected by iron therapy.

Reference values for haematological parameters should be available to all primary care practitioners, to facilitate management and referral.

Anaemia

Anaemia is defined as a decrease in haemoglobin (Hb) or haematocrit (HCT) below the normal value for age and sex.

Indications for referral for investigation

- Presumed iron deficiency anaemia which does not respond to treatment
- Unexplained anaemia and/or a macrocytic anaemia after the neonatal period
- Haemolytic anaemia
- Thrombocytopaenia
- Pancytopaenia
- Lymphadenopathy or hepatosplenomegaly which is not due to common infections
- Unexplained bleeding disorders.

The main pathogenetic mechanisms are:

- ◆ Impaired or ineffective blood production
- ◆ Haemorrhage
- ◆ Haemolysis – increased red cell destruction.

Table 23.1 Normal blood values in infancy and childhood

	Hb (g/dl)	HCT (%)	MCV (fl)	MCH (pg)	Retics (%)
Cord	16.5	52.0	108	36	5
1 day	19.6	61.0	107	37	5
1 week	18.2	58.0	198	33	1
1 month	14.5	44.0	196	32	1
2 months	11.5	35.0	194	30	1
6 months	11.6	35.0	190	30	1
1 year	11.5	35.0	178	27	1.5
2–5 years	12.5	37.0	180	27	1.5
6–12 years	13.5	40.0	185	29	1.5
Adolescent					
Male	15–17	46–52	78–98	26–32	0.5–2
Female	13–15	40–46	78–98	26–32	0.5–2

Hb = haemoglobin   HCT = haematocrit   MCV = mean cell volume   MCH = mean cell haemoglobin   Retics = reticulocytes

Figure 23.1 Changes in haemoglobin levels in early infancy

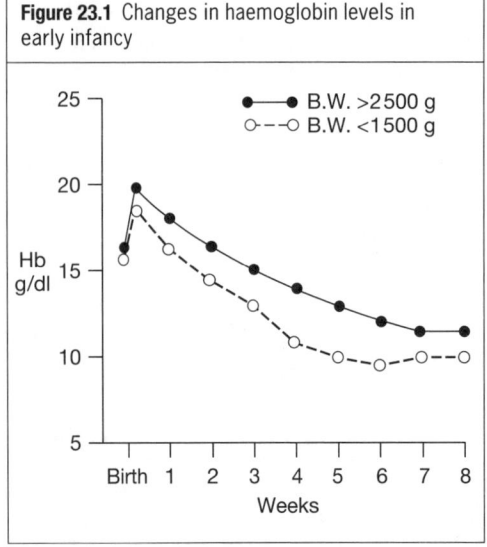

Anaemia is not a disease in itself but a manifestation of an underlying disorder. In developing populations more than one cause is often present in the same patient, e.g. nutritional deficiency, infection, or parasites causing blood loss. A high prevalence of low birth weight results in a large number of infants at risk of developing nutritional (iron deficiency) anaemia. The cause of anaemia must always be established before treatment is given.

Anaemia in the newborn

(*See also* Chapter 7, Care of the newborn.)

In South Africa this is defined as a Hb less than 13.5 g/dl in the full-term infant and is most commonly due to haemolysis, blood loss, or infection (*see* Table 23.2).

The mean cell volume (MCV) at birth is higher ('physiological macrocytosis') and may fall to lower than adult levels by about three months. The red cells tend to be microcytic from three months to approximately six years and could be mistaken for those of iron-deficiency anaemia or thalassaemia minor. (As a rough guide the normal MCV is equal to 70 + 1 for each year of age up to six years.) The reticulocyte count is approximately 5 per cent at birth and declines to below 1 per cent at one week. Hypoplastic anaemia is rare. Evaluation of the aetiology includes a detailed history of pregnancy and delivery with particular reference to infections, blood loss, and drug ingestion. The family's ethnic background and a history of previously anaemic or jaundiced infants, miscarriages, blood transfusions, or splenectomies are particularly important in relationship to hereditary haemolytic anaemias, Rhesus (Rh), and ABO incompatibility. Jaundice and hepatosplenomegaly suggest haemolysis or infection, whereas pallor, shock, or overt bleeding indicate blood loss anaemia (*see* Table 23.2). Cephalhaematoma and bleeding into organs (e.g. spleen, liver) should be excluded.

Table 23.2 Important causes of anaemia in infancy and childhood

	Newborn	Infancy and pre-school	Later childhood
Impaired production	—	Iron deficiency PEM Folate deficiency	Iron deficiency Folate deficiency Vitamin B$_{12}$ deficiency

	Infections
	  TORCH
	  HIV
	Red cell aplasia
		Infection
		
		Acquired (infection, idiopathic, drugs)
			Infection
			Systemic disease
			
			Acquired (infection, idiopathic, drugs)

		Fanconi's	Fanconi's
	Congenital leukaemia	Acute leukaemia Solid tumours	Acute leukaemia Lymphoma Solid tumours

Blood loss	Feto-maternal
	Twin-twin
	Cord
	Cephalhaematoma
	Haemorrhagic disease
	Blood sampling
		Gastrointestinal
		  (malformations,
		  polyps, parasites)
		Platelet/coagulation
		  abnormalities
			Gastrointestinal
			  (malformations, ulcer,
			  parasites)
			Urogenital (bilharzia)
			Platelet/coagulation
			  abnormalities

Haemolysis	Rh/ABO
	Infection
	Hereditary
	  – Spherocytosis
	  – G6PD deficiency
		Infection
		  – Malaria
		Auto-immune
		Hereditary
		  – Spherocytosis
		  – G6PD deficiency
			Infection
			  – Malaria
			Auto-immune
			Hereditary
			  – Spherocytosis
			  – Hb-pathies
			  – Thalassaemia
			  – G6PD deficiency

The placenta should always be examined as a possible site of the haemorrhage. In twin births, twin-to-twin haemorrhage may occur, resulting in anaemia in one and polycythaemia in the other. Feto-maternal transfusions may cause chronic anaemia in the neonate.

As the profoundly anaemic, jaundiced, or sick neonate requires immediate intervention, it is important to have a logical approach to the differential diagnosis. *See* Figure 23.2.

If possible, the results of appropriate investigations should be available before any form of treatment is started. Sometimes, however, it may be more prudent to treat and to do investigations when the child is bigger and older.

The reticulocyte count is the most useful test to differentiate hypoplastic anaemia from anaemia due to haemolysis or blood loss. A direct Coombs' test will differentiate the immune (Rh/ABO) from non-immune haemolytic anaemias (hereditary or infective). (For more information *see* Chapter 7, Care of the newborn.)

Infection must be considered in the first instance when a jaundiced and anaemic infant with hepatosplenomegaly shows no evidence of blood group incompatibility. Hereditary haemolytic anaemia should be suspected if there are specific red cell morphological abnormalities: spherocytes (hereditary spherocytosis), elliptocytes (hereditary elliptocytosis), or pykno-

Figure 23.2 Approach to anaemia in the newborn

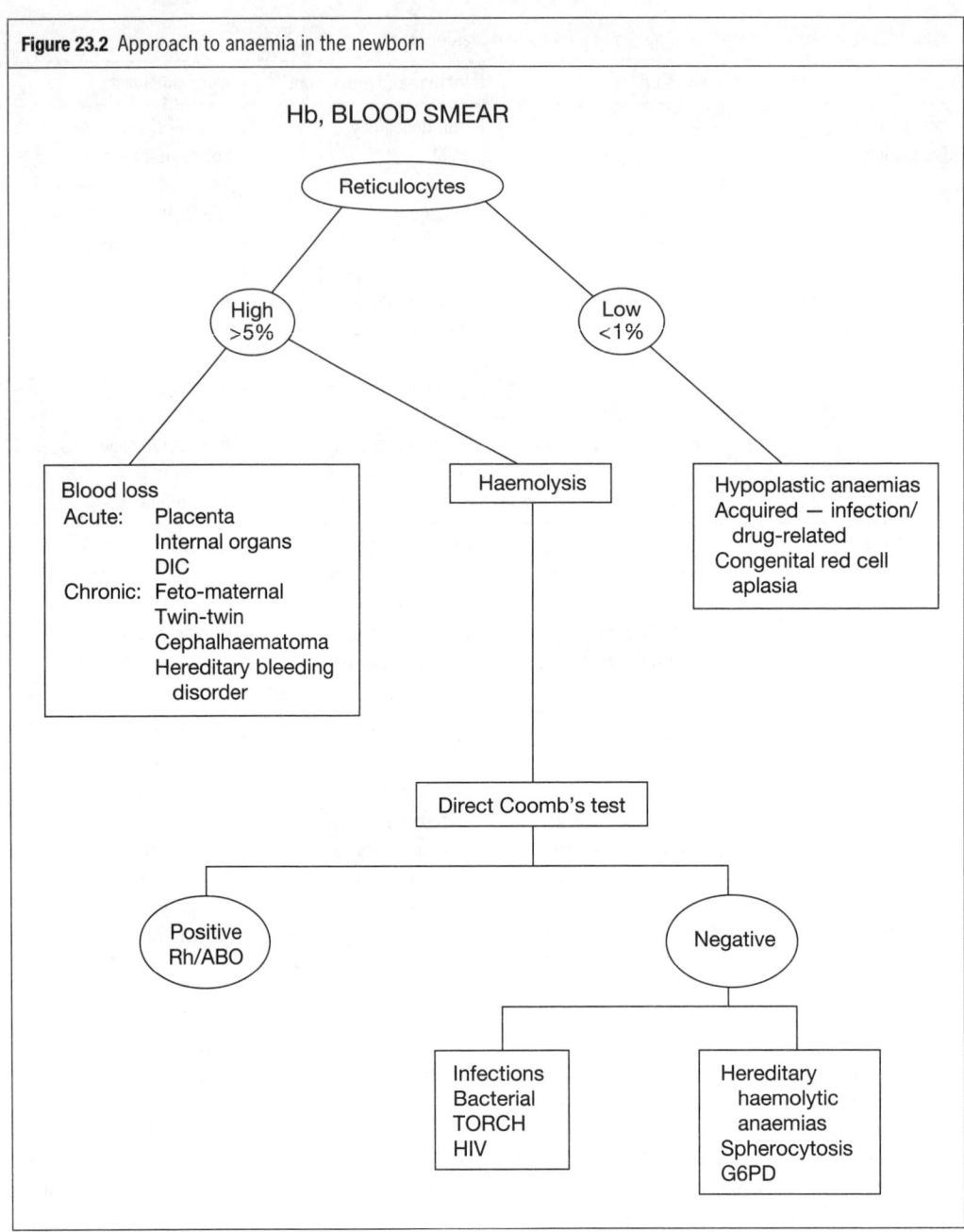

cytes (glucose-6-phosphate dehydrogenase deficiency). The more common haemoglobin-opathies (HbS, HbC) and beta-thalassaemia are asymptomatic at birth. Anaemia develops only at three to six months, as fetal Hb F is replaced by adult Hb A, which contains the defective globin chains. Alpha-thalassaemia may be present at birth as alpha chains are present. (*See* Haemo-globinopathies, *below*.)

If an **emergency blood transfusion** has to be given before a definitive diagnosis has been made, certain rules should be followed:

- The transfused blood must be compatible with both mother and baby in case maternal antibodies are present in the infant's circulation.
- Diagnostic blood samples must be taken before transfusion and should include:
  (i) 1 ml clotted blood for a Coomb's test,
  (ii) 1 ml EDTA blood for a full blood count, blood smear, and reticulocyte count,
  (iii) 2.5 ml EDTA blood for red cell studies (osmotic fragility and G6PD),
  (iv) 2.5 ml citrated blood for coagulation studies, where appropriate.

Serological tests for congenital infections (TORCH) can be performed after the transfusion if indicated. In unexplained anaemia, the Kleihauer test should be done on the mother's blood to detect feto-maternal bleeding.

Haemolytic disease of the newborn (erythroblastosis fetalis)

(*See* Chapter 7, Care of the newborn.)

Anaemia in infancy and later childhood

The most common causes of childhood anaemia are outlined in Table 23.2. In developing countries nutritional deficiencies and anaemias secondary to infection, systemic disease, and parasites predominate. The most common cause of anaemia is iron deficiency, caused by inadequate nutrition, low birth weight or parasites. The diet should be improved, parasites eliminated, and empirical treatment commenced with ferro drops or ferrous sulphate suspension for three weeks, when the Hb should be measured again. If the Hb has not improved referral to a competent centre is required.

At all ages blood loss must be excluded. However, the cause of the anaemia is often multifactorial. Hereditary haemolytic anaemias are less common but cause significant morbidity and mortality in certain well-defined population groups. A schematic approach to the differential diagnosis is given in Figure 23.3, based on the morphological characteristics of the red blood cells and the reticulocyte count. From the age of six months anaemia may be classified according to cause or to the size and shape of the red cells.

Two values easily remembered are below 70 fl and above 90 fl for microcytic and macrocytic anaemia respectively.

Iron-deficiency anaemia

Iron deficiency is the most common cause of anaemia in early childhood. Prenatal predisposing factors include maternal multiparity, twin births, low birth weight, and blood loss, which result in depleted iron stores at birth. Full-term babies usually have adequate iron reserves for three months of life after which they are dependent on the iron in their food.

As the total body iron stores at birth are directly related to birth weight, all low-birth-weight (LBW) infants start life with deficient stores. The single most important postnatal cause of iron deficiency is inadequate dietary intake relative to rapid growth. LBW infants, even if breastfed, will become iron deficient unless they are given supplementary iron from the age of two months. Additional contributory factors include bacterial, viral, and parasitic infections, which impair iron uptake and utilization, or cause chronic blood loss. The age groups at greatest risk are six months to three years and then in adolescence.

The incidence of iron deficiency varies inversely with socio-economic status ranging from less than 5 per cent in affluent Western societies to more than 50 per cent in developing countries.

Clinical manifestations

Initial symptoms and signs are vague and non-specific, e.g. tiredness and lethargy. Irritability, anorexia, and pica are common. Frequently the child presents with an intercurrent infection with anaemia as an incidental finding. As the development of anaemia is a gradual process, children may adapt to haemoglobin levels even below 5 g/dl with minimal systemic upset. Varying degrees of pallor, koilonychia, moderate splenomegaly, and a soft ejection systolic murmur may be the only abnormal physical findings. Parietal bossing of the skull may be present in patients with iron deficiency due to chronic blood loss. Other signs of suboptimal nutrition may be present.

Haematological findings

The characteristic blood findings in iron deficiency are microcytosis (MCV <70 fl),

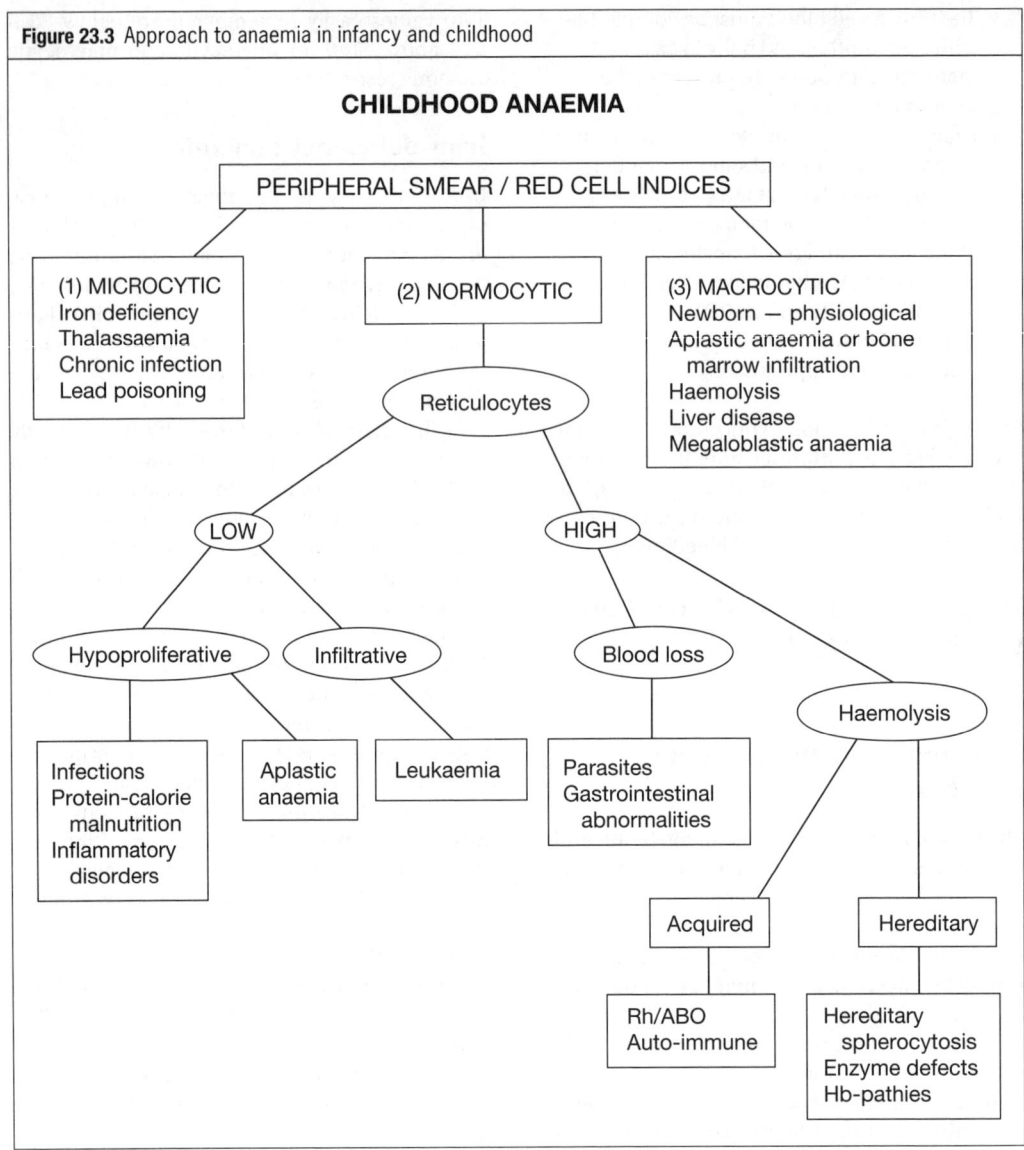

Figure 23.3 Approach to anaemia in infancy and childhood

hypochromia (MCH <26 pg), reduced serum iron (<40 µg/dl), increased iron-binding capacity (>450 µg/dl), decreased transferrin saturation (<16 per cent) and decreased serum ferritin (<10 ng/ml). The free erythrocyte protoporphyrin level (FEP) and red cell distribution width (RDW) is increased. These changes precede the development of anaemia. The reticulocyte count is increased where blood loss is the cause but is low when nutritional factors are to blame. A response to iron treatment usually confirms the diagnosis.

Differential diagnosis

A hypochromic, microcytic blood picture occurring in a child aged six months to three years with a poor dietary history or low birth weight is usually accepted as sufficient evidence for a diagnosis of nutritional iron deficiency. Biochemical tests need not be done routinely. The diagnosis can be confirmed with a therapeutic trial of oral ferrous sulphate provided follow-up is possible. In areas where intestinal parasites are common, stools should be examined for occult blood and ova. A source of blood loss should always be sought in children with recurrent episodes of hypochromic anaemia and in older children with a good dietary history who present with an iron-deficient blood picture. Raw cow's milk may cause chronic subclinical intestinal blood loss: heating or boiling the milk denatures the protein and hence obviates this problem. Pulmonary haemosiderosis should be suspected in infants who relapse despite adequate iron therapy, or in older children with repeated respiratory problems and associated iron deficiency. Lead poisoning was a common accompaniment of iron deficiency in certain urban populations, and can be confirmed by blood lead level estimation.

Other disorders giving a hypochromic, microcytic anaemia are the thalassaemia syndromes and long-standing chronic infections or inflammatory disorders (*see below*).

Treatment

Oral ferrous sulphate (citrate, gluconate, or fumarate), in a dose of 6 mg of elemental Fe^{++}/ kg/day, will correct nutritional iron deficiency anaemia within four weeks in over 90 per cent of cases. Symptoms of lethargy and irritability improve within days of commencing treatment – a feature which is confirmatory of the diagnosis. The minimal acceptable response is a rise in haemoglobin of 2 g/dl in three weeks. Lack of response is usually due to poor drug compliance or incorrect diagnosis. Slow or incomplete response may be due to intercurrent infection, impaired absorption, or continuing blood loss, occult folate deficiency or inadequate dosage.

Parenteral iron therapy is rarely indicated for medical reasons, but may be necessary in cases of poor compliance with oral therapy or in malabsorptive states. It should not be given to patients with active infections or underlying systemic disease.

Blood transfusion is not recommended for chronic iron deficiency anaemia unless it is very severe (Hb <4 g/dl), and there are cardiopulmonary symptoms, or continuing blood loss or severe infection is present. Packed red cells 5–10 ml/kg should be transfused slowly with a diuretic given simultaneously.

Dietary factors. Milk is a poor source of iron, but the iron in breastmilk is more readily absorbed than that in cow's milk, and fully breastfed infants rarely develop iron deficiency. The haem iron present in meat is better absorbed than the inorganic iron in cereals and vegetables. The availability of iron from iron-fortified foods varies widely. Rice is a poor source. Egg iron is very poorly absorbed and the addition of eggs to a mixed meal will retard the absorption of iron from other foods. Citrus fruits or medicinal vitamin C significantly enhance the availability of dietary iron.

Iron requirements and prevention of iron deficiency. A minimal daily intake of 1 mg Fe^{++}/ kg/d (maximum 15 mg/d) is recommended for full-term infants and 2 mg/kg/d for prematures. Promotion of breastfeeding, the introduction of mixed feeding by six months of age, and appropriate advice regarding iron-rich foods are the most important factors in prevention of iron deficiency. LBW infants, however, require additional iron supplementation by six to eight weeks of age. This can be given as medicinal iron, or as iron-fortified formula in non-breastfed infants. Supplementation from birth is not indicated and may be harmful. Term infants who are fed on cow's milk formula from birth and who receive mainly cereals and vegetables as weaning foods require iron supplements from the age of three months to prevent iron deficiency.

Megaloblastic anaemias

These are uncommon in children, but more prevalent in some areas of developing countries. The main cause is dietary folate deficiency.

This is most often due to decreased intake or absorption associated with general malnutrition, chronic diarrhoeal disorders, and intercurrent infection. Other aetiological factors are chronic haemolytic anaemias, where there is an increased requirement due to rapid red cell turnover, and anti-convulsant therapy which impairs folate absorption. LBW infants who grow rapidly have an increased demand for folate and are at risk. Goat's milk is a poor source of folate.

Vitamin B_{12} deficiency occurs rarely in children. The most common causes are extreme vegetarian diets, chronic ileal disease, resection of the lower ileum, and deficient or abnormal gastric intrinsic factor. Megaloblastic anaemia due to Vitamin B_{12} deficiency may suggest malabsorption due to giardia infestation. Juvenile pernicious anaemia and inherited disorders of B_{12} metabolism are extremely rare.

Confirmatory diagnostic tests include determination of serum vitamin B_{12}, Schilling test of B_{12} absorption, and investigation for gastrointestinal pathology.

Clinical features

The age group at greatest risk is six months to three years and, in particular, malnourished (kwashiorkor) or LBW infants. Presenting signs include pallor, occasionally mild icterus, and, in severe cases, a petechial rash. Children with megaloblastic anaemia are usually more ill than those with iron deficiency and a comparable degree of anaemia.

Haematological findings

Anaemia is often severe with Hb levels below 7 g/dl. The MCV is usually more than 100 fl, but may be misleadingly low due to marked variation in cell size and shape or concomitant iron deficiency. The peripheral smear frequently shows a combination of oval macrocytes, normochromic, normocytic cells, and microcytes. Leucopaenia and thrombocytopaenia may occur and hypersegmentation of neutrophils is characteristic. Serum folate is below 3 ng/ml, red cell folate below 160 µg/ml, and serum iron is elevated. Bone marrow examination confirms the presence of megaloblastic changes in both red and white cell precursors.

Prevention and treatment

The minimum daily requirement of folic acid is 50 µg. Good dietary sources are liver, eggs, fresh green vegetables, yeast, and nuts. Breastmilk and cow's milk have small but adequate amounts of folate for young infants. Goat's milk is markedly deficient. Folate is heat labile and thus destroyed by cooking.

Treatment with folic acid, 1 mg daily for 10 to 14 days, will correct the anaemia. Further supplementation for approximately one month is recommended to replenish stores. The diet should be adequate for protein and iron. Before commencing folate treatment, vitamin B_{12} levels should be checked.

In patients with vitamin B_{12} deficiency, long-term replacement therapy with parenteral vitamin B_{12} 50 to 1000 µg monthly is usually required.

Anaemia of protein-energy malnutrition (PEM)

(*See also* Chapter 13, Nutritional disorders.)

Anaemia is a regular feature of PEM. Numerous factors contribute to the aetiology, varying in different geographical areas. Protein deficiency *per se* causes anaemia. Iron deficiency is uncommon at presentation but develops in most cases during recovery as growth requirements increase. Folate deficiency is less common than iron deficiency, but frank megaloblastic anaemia can occur. Other contributing factors are bacterial and parasitic infections, dilutional effects due to blood volume changes, and variable vitamin and trace element deficiencies.

Haematological features

The anaemia of protein deficiency is moderate, Hb 8–10 g/dl, normocytic and normochromic. Reticulocytosis develops within seven to ten days of dietary rehabilitation. A transient decrease in Hb coincides with loss of oedema and plasma volume expansion. Bone marrow iron stores are frequently increased on admission, but decrease rapidly during dietary rehabilitation. Overt iron deficiency with hypochromia and microcytosis commonly develops within four weeks. The (WBC) varies with the presence or absence of infection. Thrombocytopaenia may occur in severely ill, infected patients.

The presence of severe anaemia suggests coincidental folate or iron deficiency or infection.

Treatment

Treatment is directed towards nutritional rehabilitation and control of intercurrent infection.

Folic acid supplementation, 1–5 mg daily for 10 days, is advisable early in the therapeutic regimen. Iron supplementation should be deferred until infections are controlled and initiation of transferrin regeneration within two to three weeks. Transfusion of packed red cells may be required in severely anaemic patients or if infection is present.

Anaemia of infection

Anaemia associated with acute infection is usually haemolytic in type and/or due to impaired iron utilization. Transient red cell aplasia can also occur. Chronic infections are a common cause of low-grade anaemia in children, particularly chronic respiratory, urinary, and parasitic infections.

> An underlying infection should always be excluded in an anaemic child.

Anaemia of chronic systemic diseases

Rheumatoid arthritis, renal, hepatic, endocrine disorders, malignancy and chronic infections are also associated with chronic anaemia, which varies with the activity of the underlying disease. The anaemia is usually present from early on in the disease and then remains constant.

The characteristic features are a moderate normocytic, normochromic anaemia (Hb 8–10 g/dl) with evidence of subclinical haemolysis,

impaired marrow response to anaemia, and impaired iron utilization. In long-standing cases, microcytosis and hypochromia may develop. Serum iron and transferrin are both decreased. The RDW may be normal. Serum ferritin and bone marrow iron are increased. These features distinguish this type of anaemia from iron eficiency with which it is often confused (*see* Figure 23.4).

As absorption and utilization of iron are impaired, iron therapy is ineffective and contra-indicated. The treatment is that of the underlying disease. Once this is controlled the anaemia will also resolve.

Aplastic anaemia

Acquired aplastic anaemia

The most common causes of acquired aplastic anaemia are listed in Table 23.3. In the majority of cases no precipitating factor can be identified.

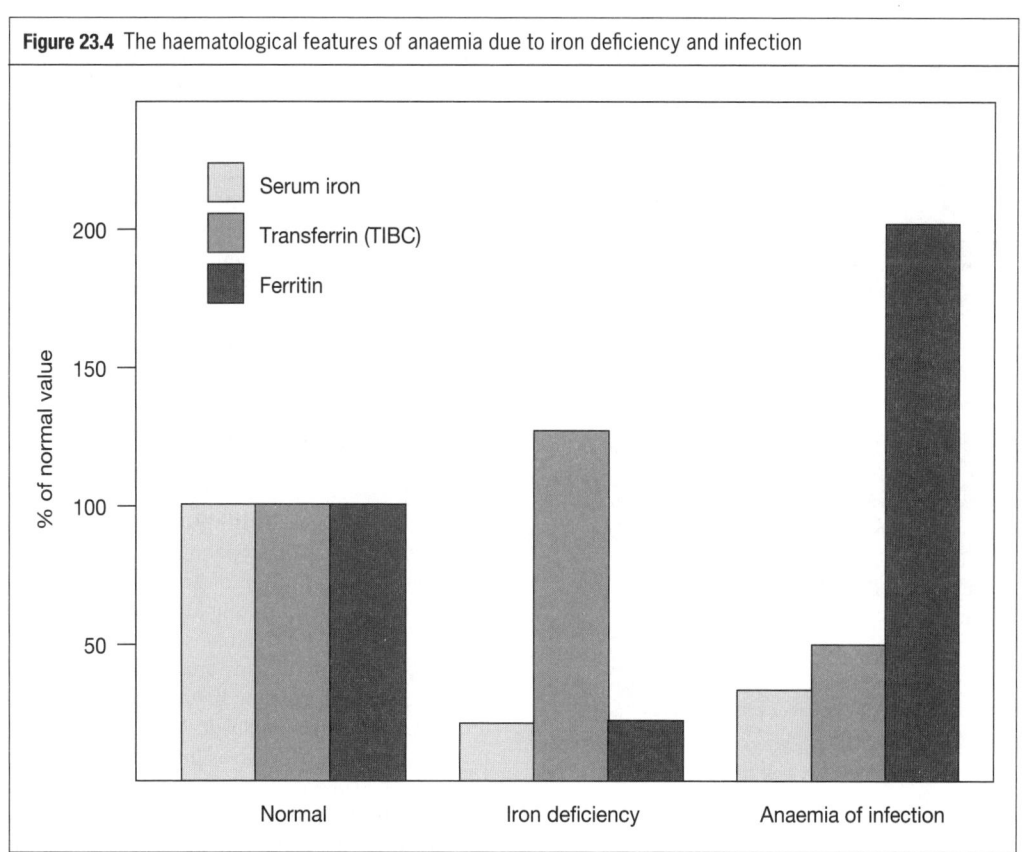

Figure 23.4 The haematological features of anaemia due to iron deficiency and infection

There is increasing evidence that immunological factors play an important aetiological role

Clinical and haematological features. The onset is usually insidious with pallor, lethargy, easy bruising, and petechiae progressing to overt haemorrhage and serious intercurrent infection.

Hepatosplenomegaly is rarely seen in acquired aplastic anaemia and hence is a useful differentiating feature from acute leukaemia, which may otherwise have a similar clinical presentation.

The blood picture is one of peripheral pancytopaenia. Diagnosis is confirmed by bone marrow aspirate and trephine biopsy.

Treatment. The treatment of choice in severe aplasia is bone marrow transplantation from a histocompatible sibling. Where this is not feasible, immunosuppressive therapy (anti-thymocyte globulin, cyclosporin-A, corticosteroids) and/or androgens are indicated. Supportive use of granulocyte colony stimulating factor (G-CSF) as well as transfusions of red blood cells and platelets should be reserved for life-threatening situations, as bone marrow transplantation is most successful in those who have had the least transfusions. Early referral to a competent centre is therefore also important.

The prognosis depends on which treatment option is possible. Approximately 15 per cent of patients make a complete spontaneous haematological recovery. With bone marrow transplantation, approximately 70–90 per cent survive in full haematological remission for longer than two years. The major complication is the development of graft versus host reaction. Survival after immune therapy ranges from 50–70 per cent.

> Aplastic anaemia occurs due to bone marrow failure, which may be either hereditary or acquired, and usually affects all haemopoietic elements to give rise to pancytopaenia.

Table 23.3 Causes of acquired aplastic anaemia

Idiopathic
Antibiotics
   chloramphenicol, sulfonamides
Anticonvulsants
   phenobarbitone, phenytoin
Antimalarials
   quinine, amodiaquine
Cancer chemotherapeutic agents
Chemicals
   benzene, carbon tetrachloride, glue
Insecticides
   DDT, chlordane, parathion, lindane
Infections
   Hepatitis A, HIV, EBV, rubella, measles, mumps, influenza
Protein-energy malnutrition (PEM)
Irradiation
Pre-leukaemic conditions

Fanconi's anaemia

This familial hypoplastic anaemia is inherited as an autosomal recessive trait. A high prevalence has been recorded in some geographical areas in South Africa (Bloemfontein) among certain white and black population groups. Associated physical abnormalities in order of frequency are pigmentary skin changes (76 per cent), low birth weight, short stature, thumb anomalies, microcephaly, hypogenitalism, renal anomalies, other skeletal anomalies, strabismus, hyperreflexia, microphthalmia, mental retardation, deafness, and congenital heart disease. The bone marrow is hypocellular, and chromosomal analysis typically reveals chromosomal breakages and structural abnormalities.

Pancytopaenia rarely develops before four years of age and may temporarily respond to androgens and steroids. Bone marrow transplants have been performed with some success and are the best treatment option. Patients have a high risk to develop myeloid leukaemia and cancer. Repeated transfusions are associated with iron overload. The life expectancy is markedly shortened.

Acquired red cell aplasia

Transient erythroblastopaenia of childhood (TEC) is a rare condition of unknown aetiology. The anaemia is self limiting and red cell aplasia usually lasts no more than seven to ten days but may cause significant anaemia. In patients with pre-existing chronic haemolytic anaemias, a similar transient aplastic episode may be precipitated by a parvovirus infection and result in sudden severe anaemia requiring blood transfusion. A decrease in reticulocyte count is usually the first sign of impending crisis in these patients. Both conditions may be treated with blood transfusions and supportive care.

Congenital pure red cell aplasia (Blackfan-Diamond syndrome)

This is a rare disorder in which a selective aplasia of erythroid precursors is present at birth but the condition may only be diagnosed at a later date. Treatment with corticosteroids is effective and long-term maintenance therapy is required but may influence growth.

Haemolytic anaemias

Haemolytic anaemias are characterized by evidence of increased red cell destruction (anaemia, jaundice, urobilinogenuria, or hae-moglobinuria), and a compensatory increase in bone marrow erythropoeisis (reticulocytosis). In long-standing haemolytic anaemia, extramedullary haemopoeisis in liver and spleen may contribute to hepatosplenomegaly, and expanded bone marrow cavities from erythroid hyperplasia will cause skull bossing and thinning of the cortices of long bones.

When red cell destruction occurs mainly extravascularly in the spleen and reticulo-endothelial system, the predominant clinical feature is jaundice. When destruction is mainly intravascular, the main features are pallor and haemoglobinuria.

The most common causes are listed in Table 23.4.

Hereditary spherocytosis (HS)

This is the most common inherited haemolytic anaemia in South Africa. The inheritance pattern is autosomal dominant. In 25 per cent of cases it is due to a new mutation with no family history. The red cells are spherocytic in shape. The basic defect is in the red cell membrane, which is deficient in spectrin and is associated with increased permeability to sodium. The degree of spectrin deficiency correlates closely with the severity of disease and the degree of spherocytosis. The spherocytes are trapped and destroyed in the venous sinuses of the spleen, hence splenectomy will cure the anaemia.

Clinical features
These are very variable, ranging from an asymptomatic, compensated haemolytic process to

Haemolytic anaemias may be due either to hereditary intrinsic defects of the red cell membrane, enzymes, or haemoglobin, or to acquired extrinsic factors such as infections, antibodies, and mechanical trauma.

Table 23.4 Classification of haemolytic anaemia

Hereditary
Membrane defect
  Hereditary spherocytosis
Enzyme deficiencies
  Glucose-6-phosphate dehydrogenase (G6PD)
  Haemoglobin abnormalities
  Sickle-cell anaemia
  Thalassaemia

Acquired
Iso-immune
  Haemolytic disease of newborn
Auto-immune
  Viral infection
  Bacterial septicaemia
  Penicillin, sulphonamide, cephalosporin,
    rifampicin
Non-immune
  Malaria
  Burns
  Hypersplenism

severe recurrent anaemia requiring transfusion. Most cases exhibit jaundice in the newborn period. Differentiation from ABO haemolytic disease may be difficult but the Coomb's test will be of help. In HS the persistence of spherocytes beyond the neonatal period, together with evidence of increased osmotic fragility in the infant and one parent, confirms the diagnosis.

In later childhood, episodic jaundice precipitated by infection is a common presentation, frequently associated with splenomegaly. Complications include transient aplastic crises, which are usually precipitated by infection (e.g. parvovirus) and resolve spontaneously with a brisk reticulocytosis. Gallstones and leg ulcers are uncommon complications in young children, but become increasingly prevalent from adolescence onwards.

Haematological features

Anaemia can be moderate (Hb 8–10 g/dl), but may become severe (Hb 3–5 g/dl), during aplastic or hyperhaemolytic crises usually due to parvovirus. Reticulocytes range from 5–15 per cent. Diagnosis is based on the finding of spherocytes, increased red cell osmotic fragility, and increased autohaemolysis corrected (*in vitro*) by glucose. In most instances one parent will show similar abnormalities. Auto-immune haemolytic anaemia, which also has spherocytes, can be excluded by a negative Coombs' test.

Treatment

Splenectomy effectively controls haemolysis by removing the main site of red cell destruction. The intrinsic abnormality of the red cell is unchanged. The most severe post-splenectomy complication is overwhelming pneumococcal septicaemia. Risk of this complication is minimized, firstly by deferring the operation until the child is five years of age, and secondly by giving preoperative pneumococcal vaccine and prophylactic penicillin postoperatively.

Hereditary elliptocytosis

This is characterized by oval-shaped red cells (elliptocytes), and is due to abnormality of the red cell skeletal membrane. In the majority of patients (85–90 per cent), inheritance is autosomal dominant and the disease is asymptomatic. A mild compensated haemolytic anaemia may be present. In the remainder it appears to be autosomal recessive and characterized by moderate to severe haemolysis. Splenectomy is effective in ameliorating haemolysis in severe cases.

Enzyme deficiencies

The most common red cell enzyme deficiencies causing clinical haemolysis are, in order of frequency, glucose-6-phosphate dehydrogenase (G6PD), pyruvate kinase (PK), glucose-phosphate-isomerase (GPI), and hexokinase (HX) deficiency.

G-6PD deficiency occurs worldwide, with particular prevalence in people originating from areas endemic for falciparum malaria. The deficiency provides a limited protective effect against the development of falciparum malaria. There are numerous genetic mutants of the G-6PD enzyme throughout the world. The enzyme deficiency is associated with a reduction in the red cell life-span. The magnitude of this effect depends on the particular gene mutation and the enzyme levels. In Caucasians the incidence ranges from approximately 3 per cent in Greeks to more than 50 per cent in Sephardic Jews. In American blacks the incidence is 10 per cent and in South African blacks 3–5 per cent, depending on the tribal group. The gene for G-6PD is carried on the X-chromosome and transmitted as a sex-linked recessive. Female heterozygotes are asymptomatic carriers and may have both normal and abnormal G-6PD In their red-cells. Affected males and homozygous females show full expression of the disease.

Clinical and haematological features

Expression varies and neonatal jaundice is often the presenting feature. In Caucasians, enzyme levels are usually lower than in blacks and they exhibit a low-grade, compensated haemolytic anaemia with increased reticulocytes and occasional splenomegaly. Blacks usually show no clinical or haematological abnormalities until exposed to oxidant stress. The typical acute haemolytic episode develops three to four days after ingestion of oxidant drugs or the development of infection (*see* Table 23.5).

Jaundice and haemoglobinuria are followed by a sharp drop in Hb. Brisk reticulocytosis develops within three to seven days and Hb returns to normal over one to two weeks. Neonates may develop haemolysis from substances excreted in the breast milk. Diagnosis is confirmed by G-6PD screening tests or quantitative assay in red cells.

Treatment

This involves avoidance of oxidant drugs and the use of blood transfusion during acute haemolytic episodes. Splenectomy is not helpful.

Pyruvate kinase (PK) deficiency is a rare autosomal recessive disorder occurring mainly in people of northern European stock. Diagnosis is confirmed by an enzyme screening test or red cell assay. Hemolysis may also be precipitated by infections.

Glucose-6-phosphate isomerase (GPI) and hexokinase (HX) deficiency are rare disorders, transmitted in an autosomal recessive manner, and not restricted to any specific ethnic group. Diagnosis is confirmed by red cell enzyme assay. Both conditions respond to splenectomy.

Table 23.5 Causes of haemolysis in G6PD deficiency

Drugs:	Antimalarials
	Sulphonamides
	Chloramphenicol
	Nitrofurantoin
	Nalidixic acid
	Aspirin/phenacetin compounds
	Vitamin K (large doses)
Chemicals:	Naphthalene moth balls
	Benzene
Food:	Fava beans
Infections:	Bacterial
	Viral
Metabolic:	Diabetic acidosis

Acquired haemolytic anaemias

Infections

It is important to remember that infections or drug therapy may also precipitate or exaggerate haemolysis in children with hereditary haemolytic anaemia, such as G-6PD deficiency. Therapy consists of treatment of the child for the underlying disease with effective therapy and supportive transfusion of packed red cells as necessary.

Auto-immune haemolytic anaemia

This is uncommon in children, but may occur as a very acute, mostly self-limiting episode in association with viral or mycoplasma infections. Steroid therapy is the treatment of choice. Chronic auto-immune haemolytic anaemia is usually a manifestation of underlying lymphoma, generalized auto-immune disease, or immune-deficiency disorder and may necessitate splenectomy.

Haemoglobinopathies and thalassaemia syndromes

(*See* Table 23.6.)

Normal adult haemoglobin has three components, Hb A, Hb A2, and Hb F, with Hb A comprising more than 95 per cent of the total. Hb F (with four alpha and two gamma and two delta chains) is the major component at birth and decreases by 3–4 per cent per week to reach adult levels by approximately six months of age.

The alpha globin chains are common to all the normal haemoglobins. Defects of alpha chains will therefore be manifest from birth, whereas defects of beta chains will not manifest clinically until three to six months of age when beta chain synthesis predominates.

The most common haemoglobinopathy, sickle-cell disease (Hb SS), is the result of the inherited substitution of valine for glutamic acid in the 6th position of the beta chain. This renders the Hb less soluble on deoxygenation. Tactoids form within the red cell, distorting its shape, impeding passage through small capillaries, and causing vaso-occlusive crises and haemolytic anaemia. Other beta chain defects causing less severe haemolysis are Hb C, D, and E.

Sickle-cell disease

This condition represents the homozygous state for the sickle-cell gene (Hb SS). Heterozygote

---

Acquired haemolytic anaemia may complicate septicaemia due to *Escherichia coli, H. influenzae,* staphylococci or streptococci, particularly in infants and young children. Haemolysis is a regular feature of malarial infection and may be the presenting feature.

Abnormalities of haemoglobin that cause clinical disease are due either to substitutions or deletions of amino acids in the globin chains, or to impaired rates of globin chain synthesis.

Table 23.6 Haemoglobin composition and concentration related to age

Haemoglobin	Globin chains	Birth %	6 months %	Adult %
Hb A	α2β2	10–35	92	>95
Hb A2	α2β2	0–1.8	1–3	2–3
Hb F	α2γ2	65–90	<5	<1

carriers have sickle-cell trait (approximately 40 per cent of Hb S) (Hb AS). The disease is inherited as an autosomal co-dominant.

It is the most common severe inherited disease in Africa generally, except in South Africa. Approximately 10 per cent of American blacks have sickle-cell trait. In Africa the incidence is highest in West Africa (30–40 per cent) and lowest in South Africa (1 per cent). The gene is also prevalent in certain peoples of Mediterranean, Saudi Arabian, and Asiatic origin. The geographical distribution tends to parallel that of falciparum malaria.

Clinical and haematological features

The characteristic features of sickle-cell disease are those of a chronic haemolytic anaemia, punctuated by painful crises due to vaso-occlusive episodes. The clinical picture varies with age and environmental factors. In infancy, painful swelling of hands and feet (so-called hand and foot syndrome) may be the presenting feature while the acute chest syndrome, which may cause considerable morbidity, is more common in the older child. Varying degrees of pallor, jaundice, and hepatosplenomegaly will also be noted.

Intravascular sickling, with or without infarctive episodes involving mesenteric, renal, cerebral, skeletal, or pulmonary capillaries, give rise to a wide variety of clinical signs, ranging from acute abdominal pain, haematuria, and hemiplegia, to bone pains and haemoptysis. Repeated infarcts in the spleen result in progressive splenic hypofunction and atrophy by about five years of age. Intravascular sickling crises may be precipitated by acute infections, hypoxia, shock, dehydration, acidosis, or exposure to cold. In addition, patients may develop aplastic crises or hyperhaemolytic crises associated with worsening of the anaemia. Acute exacerbation of anaemia with a rapid increase in the size of the spleen occurs in sequestration crises and requires an urgent blood transfusion. Patients with sickle-cell disease are also particularly prone to pneumococcal and *Haemophilus influenzae* infections and to salmonella osteomyelitis, which simulate infarction of the bone.

In the steady state, the anaemia may be moderate or severe (Hb 5–9 g/dl), but tends to be relatively constant for each individual. Reticulocytes are increased. Sickle cells are usually demonstrable on the blood smear. The diagnosis is confirmed by Hb electrophoresis. Hb S constitutes over 80 per cent of the total haemoglobin and the remainder is Hb F. Both parents will show sickle-cell trait (Hb AS), and are usually asymptomatic, but sickling crises can be provoked by anaesthesia or anoxic stress.

Treatment

There is no curative treatment for sickle-cell disease. Management is difficult and best done in cooperation with and the supervision of a competent centre. Treatment of sickling crises is supportive and aimed at correcting dehydration and acidosis, relieving pain, and controlling underlying infection. Blood transfusion may be required in aplastic or hyperhaemolytic crises, but is not indicated on a regular basis for anaemia. Folic acid in a dose of 5 mg/d has been shown to improve growth and the Hb level.

Thalassaemia syndromes

The thalassaemia syndromes are a heterogenous group of hereditary disorders, caused by deficiencies in the production of one or more of the types of globin chains that serve as sub-units of normal Hb. They are characterized by abnormalities of haem synthesis, resulting in ineffective microcytic, hypochromic erythropoeisis and, in severe cases, chronic haemolytic anaemia and progressive haemosiderosis. Defective production or translation of the mRNA controlling globin chains, results in decreased synthesis of either α, β, δ, or β chains. The most common form is β-thalassaemia. In the most severe type, no β-chains are sythesized at all. Hb A is absent and the predominant haemoglobin is Hb F.

The β-thalassaemias are characterized by decreased β chain synthesis. Homozygous β-thalassaemia is incompatible with life. In these cases, the predominant haemoglobin at birth is Hb Barts (β 4). Heterozygotes may exhibit transient Hb Barts at birth or Hb H (β 4) in later life.

β-thalassaemia is most prevalent in people of Mediterranean, Middle Eastern, and Asiatic origin. Clusters of patients with β-thalassaemia are seen in the Indian community in KwaZulu-Natal and Gauteng in South Africa, but it is rare in blacks. Thalassaemia major (Cooley's anaemia) is the term used for individuals homozygous for the β-thalassaemia gene, with severe clinical disease. Thalassaemia minor indicates the heterozygous state and is usually asymptomatic. The red cells may be microcytic and hypochromic.

Individuals doubly heterozygous for two different thalassaemia genes have clinical manifestations of variable severity and are classified as thalassaemia intermedia.

Clinical and haematological features

Signs of β-thalassaemia major are usually evident within the first year of life, most patients presenting between the ages of four to six months. The disease is characterized by pallor, mild jaundice, fever, failure to thrive, abdominal distension, and hepatosplenomegaly, which progresses to a severe transfusion-dependent haemolytic anaemia. Skull bossing and maxillary hypertrophy develop within the first two years, resulting in a typical facies. Progressive haemosiderosis results in hepatic, cardiac, and endocrine dysfunction. Growth is stunted and intercurrent infections are common. Few patients survive beyond the first decade without treatment.

Anaemia is severe (Hb 4–7 g/dl). The red cells are microcytic and hypochromic with bizarre poikilocytes, target cells, stippled cells, normoblasts, and increased reticulocytes. Serum iron, transferrin saturation, serum ferritin, and bone marrow iron are all increased.

Hb F is markedly increased (60–90 per cent), Hb A is decreased or absent, and Hb A2 variable.

Treatment

All new patients with Hb greater than 7 g/dl should be investigated to make sure that they do not have thalassaemia intermedia. If the child is asymptomatic and growing well, regular blood transfusions should not be given. Severe forms of thalassaemia require regular transfusions designed to maintain the Hb at 10–14 g/dl. On this regimen, skull bossing, skeletal deformities, and growth retardation are minimized. Patients feel and look well and can participate in normal activities. Iron-chelating agents such as desferrioxamine, given by continuous overnight subcutaneous infusion, promote urinary iron excretion and delay the progression of haemosiderosis. An oral iron-chelator is now available. Splenectomy may be required in patients with gross splenomegaly and increasing transfusion requirements.

Prevention

Screening for thalassaemia trait should be

Table 23.7 Features of thalassaemia trait and iron-deficiency anaemia

	β-thalassaemia minor	Iron deficiency
Anaemia	Mild or absent	Mild to severe
Hb g/dl	Rarely <10 g	Frequently <10 g
MCV fl	Often >65	<72
MCV/RBC ratio	<11.5	>13.5
RDW	Normal	Increased
Serum iron	Normal	Decreased
Serum ferritin	Normal	Decreased
FEP*	Normal	Increased
HB A2	Increased	Normal
Hb F	Usually increased	Normal

FEP–Free erythrocyte protoporhyrin

encouraged in high-risk population groups. Appropriate pre-marital counselling of affected couples is recommended, and consanguinous marriages should be discouraged. Prenatal diagnosis can be made either from direct fetal blood sampling or from skin fibroblasts obtained by amniocentesis.

β-thalassaemia minor (trait) is associated with mild anaemia and rarely causes clinical symptoms. It is frequently misdiagnosed as iron deficiency. In communities where both conditions are common, it is important to be able to distinguish between the two (*see* Table 23.7).

Iron therapy is ineffective in thalassaemia minor and is contra-indicated.

If both parents have thalassaemia minor there is a 25 per cent chance of transmitting thalassaemia major and a 50 per cent chance of thalassaemia minor. (*See* Chapter 3, Medical genetics and birth defects)

Leucocyte disorders

Quantitative or qualitative changes in the white blood cells accompany a wide variety of childhood illnesses. The significance must be interpreted in relationship to the normal

Table 23.8 Normal white blood cell counts in infancy and childhood

	WBC x 10^9/l		Neutrophils %	Lymphocytes %
	BWt >2.5 kg	BWt <2.5 kg		
Cord blood	16.0*	9.3	70	30
1 day (capillary)	20.5	14.9	75	25
1 week	15.6		60	40
1 month	10.6		40	60
1 year	10.0		40	60
2–5 years	5.0–15.0**		50	50
6–14 years	5.0–10.0**		65	35

*Mean value   **Range*

variations in white cells which occur during growth and development (*see* Table 23.8).

Neutrophil leucocytosis is a physiological finding at birth and persists for 24–72 hours. Thereafter there is a progressive decrease in total white cell count and neutrophils. Lymphocytes are the predominant cells from one month to three years of age. By four years of age, equal proportions of granulocytes and lymphocytes are present. Thereafter granulocytes predominate.

The total granulocyte mass is distributed between:

* The bone marrow reserve pool
* The marginating granulocyte pool lining blood vessel walls
* The circulating granulocytes and
* Tissue granulocytes.

Changes in the peripheral white cell count may result from an absolute increase or decrease in bone marrow production, or from a re-distribution of cells between the four sites mentioned above.

Leucocytosis

Infection is the most common cause of an increased WBC in children. The predominant cell type frequently indicates the type of infection. Neutrophils predominate in bacterial infections, lymphocytes in viral infections and whooping-cough, and eosinophils in parasitic and allergic disorders.

Other causes of leucocytosis are summarized in Table 23.9 (the important causes are in **bold** type).

Leukaemoid and leuco-erythroblastic reactions are relatively common in developing countries where severe and recurrent infections are prevalent in children.

Myeloid leukaemoid reactions (WBC >50,0 × 10^9/l and/or >5 per cent immature cells in the peripheral blood) are most often associated with overwhelming bacterial infections (*E. coli*, staphylococcus, shigella) and congenital syphilis; less commonly with tuberculosis, haemolytic anaemias, and neoplastic disorders.

Lymphocytic leukaemoid reactions are usually due to whooping cough. Leukaemia and neoplastic disorders are discussed in Chapter 22, Neoplastic disorders.

Leucopaenia

A reduction in total WBC to below 15 000 per ml results in that person being very susceptible to bacterial infections and may be caused by typhoid fever, brucellosis, and severe or prolonged bacterial infections, which deplete both peripheral granulocytes and the marrow storage pool. These patients are usually febrile, sick, and toxic. Leucopaenia in the newborn is often a manifestation of septicaemia. Immune neutropaenia, due to antibodies derived from the mother, is a cause of transient neutropaenia in the newborn period, causing minimal systemic upset. Acquired bone marrow aplasia due to drug therapy alone or in conjunction with infection may cause severe neutropaenia. Hereditary aplasia and neutropaenia are rare conditions characterized by severe, recurrent bacterial infections.

Table 23.9 Causes of leucocytosis (important causes are in bold)

	Neutrophils	Monocytes	Lymphocytes	Eosinophils
Physiological	**Newborns** Stress, anxiety Exercise	**Recovery phase acute infections**	**Early childhood (1 month–4 yrs)**	Recovery from shock/infection
Infections	**Bacterial** **Fungal** Syphilis Endotoxin	Tuberculosis SBE Congenital syphilis	**Viral:** Infectious mononucleosis Cytomegalovirus Whooping cough Acute infectious lymphocytosis	**Parasitic:** Ascariasis Strongyloidiasis Ankylostomiasis Toxocariasis Trichinosis
Drugs	**Steroids** Epinephrine	–	–	Penicillin and others **(hypersensitivity reaction)**
Haematological/ neoplastic	Haemorrhage Haemolytic anaemias Transfusion reactions Metastatic tumours Myeloblastic leukaemias (immature cells)	Hodgkin's lymphoma Histiocytosis Monoblastic leukaemia **Neutropaenic states**	Lymphoblastic leukaemia Lymphomas Aplastic anaemia Neutropaenias	Histiocytosis Hodgkin's lymphoma Metastatic tumours
Miscellaneous	Connective tissue disease Diabetic acidosis Chronic inflammatory disorders Post-splenectomy	Connective tissue disorder Sprue Regional ileitis	Thyrotoxicosis	**Allergic disorders** Pulmonary eosinophilia Idiopathic hyper- eosinophilic syndrome

Copper deficiency is often an unrecognized but correctable cause of neutropaenia in malnourished, infected infants and those receiving hyperalimentation. Approximately 20 per cent of blacks exhibit leucopaenia (WBC <4.0 10^9/l) due to neutropaenia which appears to be genetic in origin and is not associated with an increased susceptibility to infection.

Hereditary or acquired defects of chemotaxis, opsonization, phagocytosis, and bacterial killing result in increased susceptibility to bacterial and/ or fungal infections.

Functional disorders of neutrophils

The ability of neutrophils to eradicate infection by destruction of bacteria involves four major functions.

Treatment

The management of the child with leucocytosis is essentially that of addressing the underlying disease. Neutropaenia and functional neutrophil disorders call for eradication of bacterial infections by appropriate antibiotic therapy. Children with hereditary neutropaenic disorders or those on long-term cancer chemotherapy should be protected from exposure to infections.

Oral hygiene and the use of oral antiseptic and antifungal agents are important. Biological substances such as erythropoietins, granulocyte and granulocyte monocytic colony stimulating factors (G-CSF and GM-CSF), and interleukin III which influence growth and function of haematopoeitic cells are being used in clinical practice for cytopaenias. However, the cost is exorbitant. Prophylactic antibiotics are also used.

Bleeding disorders

The basic mechanism of haemostasis depends on three major components:

- Integrity of the vessel wall resulting in vasoconstriction
- Platelets forming the primary haemostatic plug
- Coagulation factors which form the fibrin clot, plus pro-coagulants and fibrinolysis.

These disorders often present as emergencies. Prompt diagnosis and treatment can modify a life-threatening haemorrhage to a moderate one.

The abnormality may be quantitative or qualitative, and the cause can be inherited or acquired. The diagnosis is based on the history, clinical findings, and four basic laboratory tests.

History

A recent history of trauma and the severity of the injury should be elicited. One needs to enquire about previous operations, symptoms of infections, about drug ingestion such as aspirin, and possible inadequate vitamin C and K intake. The site of the bleeding must be established, namely joints, muscles, mucous membrane, and/or skin.

In the past history, age of onset and prolonged bleeding following minor trauma or surgery are important. Conversely, a negative response excludes an abnormality unless the missing

> Bleeding disorders are characterized by persistent or excessive bleeding following minor trauma, dental extractions or surgical operations, or by spontaneous bleeding into the skin or joints, recurrent epistaxis, or by a family history of a bleeding tendency.

factor(s) had been inadvertently replaced. Recurrent bleeding from a single orifice such as the nose or rectum may be due to a bleeding disorder, but a local cause should always be excluded.

A recent past history of a viral infection is important for the diagnosis of idiopathic thrombocytopaenic purpura (ITP). A family history of abnormal bleeding suggests an inherited cause. If only male siblings and maternal uncles are involved, haemophilia A or B should be suspected. A negative history, however, does not rule out haemophilia, as 30 per cent of cases are due to spontaneous mutation.

Clinical signs

On examination, every attempt should be made to make a clinical diagnosis (*see* Table 23.10).

Anaemia or signs of shock may be present, with severe bleeding. An acquired cause is more likely if the child looks ill; on the other hand, a child with an inherited cause usually looks well. Other signs suggestive of an acquired disorder are fever, jaundice, bone tenderness, lymphadenopathy, hepatosplenomegaly, and arthritis.

The type and site of bleeding and the sex of the patient may throw further light on the possible cause. Purpura means bleeding into the skin ('dry purpura') or mucous membranes ('wet purpura'). Bleeding may be superficial as in platelet or small vessel defects, or deep as in coagulation defects. Petechiae or pinhead-sized purpuric lesions, which tend to occur over pressure sites, are highly suggestive of the former and are rare in coagulation disorders. Ecchymotic lesions alone suggest a coagulation disorder. Coexisting petechiae and ecchymoses occur in severe platelet deficiency. Vascular purpura is often due to inherited diseases of the connective tissue, but acquired disorders, like Henoch Schönlein Purpura with a characteristic rash, may also occur.

Multiple bleeding sites are common in acquired causes as in disseminated intravascular coagulation (DIC). Bleeding into joints and/or muscles is the hallmark of haemophilia. Gastrointestinal bleeding occurs frequently in vitamin K deficiency, severe liver disease, and platelet abnormalities.

If the patient is a male, haemophilia is likely.

The four basic screening tests outlined in Table 23.11 are needed to localize the defect in the haemostatic mechanism. As a guide, if a single coagulation test is abnormal, an inherited cause is

Table 23.10 The clinical diagnostic approach to bleeding disorders

Physical findings	Level of disorder	Disease
Petechiae, superficial ecchymoses, mucous membrane bleeding	Platelets	Platelets: – quantitative defect, e.g. ITP – qualitative defect, e.g. drugs
	Blood vessels	Scurvy, vasculitis, etc.
Palpable purpura	Blood vessels	Hypersensitivity, vasculitis, e.g. Henoch-Schönlein purpura

Haemarthrosis
  deep ecchymosis
  ± mucous membrane
	Coagulation factors (VIII, IX)	Haemophilia A & B,
		  Von Willebrand's disease

Other signs, e.g. fever, jaundice, hepatosplenomegaly, etc.	Combinations of above	Leukaemia, liver disease,
		  portal hypertension,
		  DIC, SLE, etc.

most likely, e.g. prolonged partial thromboplastin time (PTT) in haemophilia. Conversely, multiple abnormal tests suggest an acquired cause.

The full blood count and smear will detect the severity of the anaemia, thrombocytopaenia, red cell and leucocyte abnormalities, e.g. leukaemia. Megathrombocytes in the peripheral smear are indicative of increased platelet production due to destruction, consumption, or sequestration as in ITP, DIC, or hypersplenism. Bone marrow aspiration is necessary if thrombocytopaenia, pancytopaenia, macrocytosis, or blasts are present in order to elucidate the cause or confirm diagnosis.

Determination of the bleeding time is unnecessary and contra-indicated in the presence of severe thrombocytopaenia. The bleeding time is performed when there are clinical signs indicating a platelet problem, e.g. petechiae, but the platelet count is normal.

In the absence of suitable laboratory facilities, a provisional diagnosis can be based on the bleeding time, the Hess test, and clotting time. The PTT and the INR (PT) help to identify and diagnose a particular coagulation factor problem.

Haemophilia must always be considered as a possible cause in a boy with a bleeding disorder.

Table 23.11 Four basic screening tests

Test	Evaluates
Platelet count (part of FBC)	Platelet numbers and size
Bleeding time	Quantitative and qualitative platelet defects Vessel wall
Prothrombin time (PT)	Coagulation factors – extrinsic pathway: factors VII, X, V, II, I
Partial thrombo-plastin time (PTT)	Intrinsic pathway: factors XII, XI, IX, VIII, X, V, II, I

Blood vessel disorders

The following are discussed in detail in other chapters: Henoch-Schönlein purpura, systemic lupus erythematosus (SLE) (Chapter 21, Immune and connective tissue disorders); infections (Chapters 14, Principles of infection in children and 15, Systemic infections), scurvy (Chapter 13, Nutritional disorders).

Purpuric and petechial rashes occur in many diseases. Pseudomonas, rickettsiae, arbovirus and EBV infections and SLE may result in low platelet counts with identifiable bleeds. Purpura fulminans is seen occasionally with severe extensive vasculitis usually involving the buttocks and skin of the lower extremities. It may follow on measles, viral and bacterial infections but the precise cause is unknown. It is often fatal and probably represents a severe immunological reaction involving vessel walls.

Quantitative platelet disorders

Thrombocytopaenia is defined as a platelet count below $100 \times 10^9/l$ but is usually only symptomatic when the count is $< 20 \times 10^9/l$.

Bleeding may occur if the platelet count falls below $20 \times 10^9/l$. Bone marrow aspiration may be indicated to establish if the megakaryocytes are decreased, normal, or increased, and to exclude abnormalities of the red and white cell series.

Fanconi's anaemia and congenital mega-karyocytic aplasia are rare congenital causes of defective production of megakaryocytes. More commonly this is acquired due to marrow damage by infections, drugs, chemicals, or irradiation. It may also be due to marrow infiltration as in leukaemia or neuroblastoma.

The most common cause for thrombocyto-paenia is probably infection resulting in marrow damage, immunological destruction, or consumption (DIC). It is postulated, however, that bacteria and their endotoxic products may cause direct injury to the platelets or alter the vascular endothelium, resulting in adhesion of platelets.

Drugs may also induce immune thrombocyto-paenia, with recovery on withdrawal of the offending drug. Falciparum malaria is associated with IgG and IgM platelet antibodies and thrombocytopaenia in the acute phase. The platelet count recovers following appropriate therapy.

A rare immunological process is involved when maternal iso-immune antibodies are formed in response to fetal platelet antigens, as in Rh blood group incompatibilities. On the other hand, auto-immune antibodies may be transferred across the placenta from a mother with idiopathic thrombocytopaenic purpura or SLE. Intra-uterine infections are a common cause of neonatal thrombocytopaenia. Hence the mother's full blood count (FBC) and platelet count and a screen for congenital infection are called for.

Idiopathic thrombocytopaenic purpura (ITP)

ITP is the commonest cause of thrombocyto-paenia in children between two and six years in Western countries, but appears to be less common in the South African black population. This may be genetic or due to under-diagnosis. A history of a viral infection in the preceding three weeks is often present.

ITP can be acute or chronic: in both instances it has an immunological basis. In childhood the acute self-limiting disease usually occurs following viral infections. In this condition platelets are destroyed as innocent bystanders in an interaction of antigen-antibody complexes related to the infective agent. There is an inverse relation between the decline in level of platelet associated IgG antibodies and the recovery in the platelet count. In chronic ITP, however, platelet antibodies are formed, resulting in an insiduous onset of purpura and a protracted course. An underlying cause, such as SLE, should always be excluded.

Clinical picture
There is an acute onset of spontaneous bruising, petechial mucous membrane bleeding from the gums and nose, and sometimes bleeding in the urinary or gastrointestinal tract. Pressure areas and the palate should be inspected for petechiae. Cerebral haemorrhage occurs in less than 1 per cent of patients. Blood loss is seldom severe enough to warrant a blood transfusion. The child is apyrexial and otherwise well. Petechiae and ecchymoses are easily missed in dark-skinned patients. Black patients may also present with anaemia or shock due to delay in diagnosis.

Laboratory investigations
The platelet count is normally below 50 X $10^9/l$ with megathrombocytes and normal red and white cells in the peripheral blood. The bone mar-

> Thrombocytopaenia may be the result of diminished bone marrow production, excessive destruction or consumption, excessive pooling as in an enlarged spleen, or ineffective thrombopoiesis (as in folate and vitamin B_{12} deficiency).

row aspirate, if indicated, demonstrates normal or increased numbers of active megakaryocytes and normal white cell and red cell precursors. Platelet antibody determinations are of no use in patient management. Children over 10 years, especially girls, should be investigated for auto-immune disorders such as SLE. HIV infection may be associated with immune thrombocyto-paenia and should be excluded.

Course and treatment
Eighty per cent of children recover within one month without specific therapy. Patients should be observed until spontaneous or treatment-induced recovery occurs. Treatment is indicated only if significant mucous membrane haemor-rhage is present. Epistaxis can often be con-trolled effectively with a nasal plug. Prednisone 4 mg/kg/d is given for four to seven days. Intra-venous high-dose immunoglobulin will effect a transient rise in platelet count in the majority of patients in a shorter time, but general use is lim-ited due to the high cost. A splenectomy is indi-cated in patients who bleed excessively despite medical treatment and those who remain both symptomatic and thrombocytopaenic after one year. Cytostatics and immune-regulating drugs are not routinely indicated. Platelet transfusions are not helpful because of the extremely short platelet survival due to platelet antibodies.

Neonates of mothers with ITP have a 33 per cent chance of transient thrombocytopaenia at birth, because maternal platelet antibodies may cross the placenta.

Hypersplenism

This is the term used for a lowered platelet, red cell, and white cell count, single or in any combination, which results from pooling or increased destruction of blood cells in an enlarged spleen. Production of the various elements by the bone marrow is normal or increased and the peripheral cell count reverts to normal after splenectomy.

Qualitative platelet disorders

These disorders may be congenital or acquired. The former variety is very rare (e.g. Glanzmann's thrombasthenia, storage pool disease).

Acquired platelet function defects occur

> **The diagnosis of ITP is made on the following diagnostic criteria :**
>
> - Presence of spontaneous purpura
> - A platelet count of less than $100 \times 10^9/l$
> - Normal white and red cells
> - Absence of pathological cells in peripheral blood or marrow
> - Normal clotting and prothrombin times,
> - No history of drug ingestion or disease which may produce thrombocytopaenia and
> - No enlargement of lymph nodes.

following drug ingestion such as aspirin and in patients with uraemia. Characteristically the bleeding time is prolonged but the platelet count, INR (PT), and PTT are normal. Platelet function tests are abnormal.

Coagulation disorders

Defective coagulation occurs as a result of inherited clotting defects, such as haemophilia, or there may be an acquired problem as in DIC or vitamin K deficiency.

Haemophilia

Haemophilia A is caused by a deficiency of fac-tor VIII with reduced clotting activity. Haemo-philia B (Christmas disease) is due to deficiency of factor IX. The former is four to five times more frequent and both have X-linked recessive inher-itance. Haemophilia C (factor XI deficiency) is an autosomal-recessive disease with a high frequency in the Jewish population. Character-istically, in haemophilia the PTT is prolonged. About 30 per cent of cases of haemophilia A occur sporadically, because the disease was pre-viously unrecognized in the family or because of a mutation. Carrier females may be detected as they may possess an excess of immuno-reactive factor VIII in comparison with the amount of clotting-activity factor VIII.

Severity is inversely proportional to factor levels in haemophilia A and B: mild bleeding after trauma occurs when levels are between 30 and 5 per cent; moderate bleeding usually after trauma occurs with levels of 5–2 per cent; and severe symptoms or spontaneous bleeds occur when the level is less than 2 per cent.

Haemorrhage may develop during the neonatal period, but nearly always during the first few years of life, when the child begins to crawl and walk. While bleeding can occur from any site, the hallmarks of haemophilia are haemarthrosis and intramuscular haematoma. During the first year of life bleeding occurs mainly into muscles and subcutaneous tissues. The most serious bleeding is intracranial, which may be spontaneous and lethal. Bleeding into the forearm may cause neurovascular occlusion and result in Volkmann's ischaemic contracture. Paralytic ileus may result from retroperitoneal bleeding; compression of the femoral nerve may occur if blood tracks down behind the inguinal ligament. Respiratory obstruction and dysphagia are the result of bleeding into the posterior pharyngeal wall. Haematuria can be a problem.

Haemophilia B has similar clinical problems; severity corresponds to factor IX levels. Haemophilia C is a milder disease.

Management

The parents and the child must be fully informed about the disease. Genetic counselling is clearly very important after investigation of family members. The child should wear an identity disc which displays the diagnosis of the disease.

Local pressure must be applied whenever feasible. Replacement therapy aims at raising the factor VIII level in haemophilia A to between 30 and 60 per cent of normal depending on the severity and site of the bleed. As the half-life of factor VIII is eight to twelve hours, treatment should initially be repeated at 12-hourly intervals. Fresh frozen plasma, 15–20 ml/kg given every 12 hours raises the level to about 30 per cent but can lead to volume overload. Factor VIII concentrates 15–40 units/kg raise the level to 30–80 per cent respectively. Treatment usually has to be continued for three days or more but can be discontinued if there is no further evidence of haemorrhage or continuing pain.

Acute knee arthrosis requires additional attention. The patient should be admitted and weight-bearing avoided. A plaster of Paris or similar back-slab must be applied to immobilize the joint in slight flexion. Aspiration may be indicated if the joint is tense and very painful. The procedure must be performed in a competent

The following must be strictly avoided before factor replacement in haemophilia:

- Jugular or femoral vein puncture
- Lumbar puncture
- Intramuscular injections
- Any form of surgery
- Aspirin should never be given.

(preferably tertiary) centre with strict aseptic precautions and factor VIII concentrate must be administered immediately prior to the aspiration. A short course of steroids (prednisone 2 mg/kg/d for three days) accelerates the reduction of pain and swelling. Fresh frozen plasma, 15–20 ml/kg is used for haemophilia C

Surgical procedures and dental extractions should be preceded by administration of 20–40 factor units/kg. Antifibrinolytic agents (e.g. epsilon-amino-caproic acid) should be given before and after dental extraction. The presence of inhibitors must always be excluded preoperatively. Replacement therapy must continue for five to ten to thirty days postoperatively depending on the particular procedure. A multidisciplinary approach – involving a paediatrician, haematologist, physiotherapist, orthopaedic surgeon, and psychologist – is desirable.

As a therapeutic or prophylactic measure factor VIII can be given by the family at home or in a clinic on a regular basis. Factor IX concentrate or prothrombin complex concentrates 20–40 units/kg can be used for Haemophilia B.

Mild cases of haemophilia and Von Willebrand's disease can be treated with desamino-D-arginine vasopressin (DDAVP) which raises the level of factor VIII.

Von Willebrand's disease

This is an autosomal dominant disorder in which there is a qualitative or quantitative Von Willebrand's factor deficiency, which results in decreased platelet adhesiveness. The bleeding time is therefore often increased and the PTT may be prolonged. The most frequent presentation is mucosal bleeding and epistaxis. Treatment is similar to that for haemophilia A except that highly purified factor VIII concentrates are not used.

Vitamin K deficiency

This vitamin is required by the liver for the activation of factors II, VII, IX, and X. The natural K vitamins are synthesized by intestinal flora. Being fat-soluble they require bile for absorption and are not stored in the body. In vitamin K deficiency the liver synthesizes abnormal proteins known as PIVKAs which are inactive and may cause inhibition of coagulation. The INR (PT) and PTT are characteristically prolonged.

Bleeding occurs on the second or third day of life, or later in breastfed babies due to a deficiency of factors II, VII, IX, and X. Melaena, haematemesis, and umbilical cord bleeding may occur. In overt bleeding 1–5 mg of vitamin K stops bleeding within two to four hours. Should bleeding continue, 10–15 ml/kg of fresh plasma should be given and DIC must be excluded. This can be prevented by giving 1 mg of vitamin K IM or IV at birth to the baby or before delivery to the mother.

Other causes of Vitamin K deficiency are obstructive jaundice, malabsorption syndromes, prolonged use of broad-spectrum antibiotics, oral anticoagulants, and a diet deficient in vitamin K.

> Haemorrhagic disease of the newborn is due to functional immaturity of the liver and poor stores of vitamin K, because the infant's gut flora has not been established and breastmilk contains very little vitamin K.

Liver disease

All coagulation factors, except factor VIII, are synthesized in the liver; blood levels of the latter are therefore normal or even raised in liver failure. Coagulation factor deficiencies may occur in both acute and chronic liver disease. The liver also degrades activated clotting factors and fibrinolytic enzymes. Failure of this procedure may trigger off DIC and cause excessive fibrinolysis. The levels of vitamin K-dependent factors are the first to fall, followed by factor V and fibrinogen. The INR (PT), PTT, and possibly thrombin time are prolonged. Thrombocytopaenia may also occur secondary to portal hypertension and hypersplenism. Bleeding may also be due to a local cause, e.g. varices in portal hypertension.

The treatment is fresh frozen plasma. Prothrombin complex should be avoided.

Disseminated intravascular coagulation (DIC)

It complicates a number of conditions such as septicaemia, viraemia, shock, hypoxia, burns, malignancy (e.g. promyelocytic leukaemia), and postoperative states. The newborn is particularly susceptible (*see* Chapter 7, Care of the newborn).

Episodes of DIC result from intravascular activation of the coagulation system with consequent widespread deposition of platelets and altered fibrinogen in the micro-circulation. If it is severe this results in generalized haemorrhage and/or end-organ failure due to blockage of the microvessels by thrombi. The kidneys are most susceptible to this ischaemic damage as are the brain, heart, and adrenals, resulting in renal failure and micro-angiopathic haemolytic anaemia.

All four basic screening tests may be abnormal due to consumption of clotting factors and platelets, which are the first to fall. In addition, the thrombin time is prolonged, the fibrinogen is low, and there are increased fibrin degradation products (FDPs). As this is a dynamic process of consumption and regeneration, these parameters may not always be abnormal. Factor assays are not always necessary, but factor VIII is low in contrast to liver disease.

In severe DIC the FDPs are not elevated, due to inhibition of the fibrinolytic response; this indicates a poor outcome with irreversible organ failure.

The management is controversial but the first step is to treat for the underlying cause. If the bleeding is severe, platelet concentrates, fresh frozen plasma, and cryoprecipitate should be given. Heparin may be used after replacement therapy for purpura fulminans, and in acute promyelocytic leukaemia to prevent DIC.

> DIC is the most common acquired cause of severe life-threatening bleeding.

24

Gastrointestinal disorders

Vomiting and regurgitation

Vomiting is a common, often distressing symptom in infancy and childhood. Some of the numerous causes are relatively benign and only require supportive management while others are serious and require urgent attention.

Afferent signals from the gastrointestinal tract, vestibular apparatus, visual cortex, higher cortical centres, and a variety of chemical stimuli are able to initiate vomiting.

An episode of vomiting is preceded by retrograde contraction of the proximal small bowel with regurgitation of duodenal contents into the stomach. This is followed by contraction of abdominal muscles and the diaphragm, relaxation of the lower oesophageal sphincter and forceful expulsion of gastric contents. Usually this is accompanied by autonomic symptoms such as an increase in heart and respiratory rate and hypersalivation.

Infants who are thriving and who retain their appetite are unlikely to have a serious underlying disease. Conversely, dehydration, weight loss, and associated electrolyte and acid base abnormalities indicate significant vomiting.

The causes of vomiting can be classified according to the patient's age, the system involved (e.g. urinary tract), or the associated symptoms and signs.

The management is both supportive and focused on the underlying cause, rather than on providing anti-emetic medication.

A detailed *history and examination* will usually establish the cause of vomiting or guide the clinician to appropriate investigations.

Contents of vomitus

Undigested food in the vomitus suggests abnormalities such as oesophageal strictures and achalasia. Fresh blood or 'coffee ground' vomitus is usually due to swallowed blood, gastritis, oesophagitis, oesophageal or gastric varices. Bilious vomiting requires assessment for intestinal obstruction distal to the second part of the duodenum.

Relationship to meals and time of day

Association with specific foods such as cow's milk or infant formula suggest food allergy. Vomiting, often accompanied by pain, also occurs in children with peptic ulcers. Rarely, inherited metabolic diseases may present with vomiting after meals (e.g. hereditary fructose intolerance). Early morning vomiting is a feature of raised intracranial pressure.

Associated symptoms and signs

Dysphagia or odynophagia occur in children

Vomiting is a complex centrally controlled reflex. Conditions outside the gastrointestinal tract may also cause vomiting. Vomiting must be distinguished from regurgitation which is an effortless process not accompanied by muscle contraction or autonomic symptoms.

Table 24.1 Causes of vomiting in infancy and childhood

A Vomiting in the first week of life
Common causes
- Gastric irritation
  - Ingestion of blood/mucus
- Feeding faults
  - Overfeeding/underfeeding

Less common causes
- Infections
  - Gastroenteritis, oral thrush, urinary tract infection (UTI), meningitis, septicaemia, necrotizing enterocolitis
- Raised intracranial pressure
  - Hydrocephalus, intracranial bleed, kernicterus
- Intestinal malformation and obstruction
  - Hiatus hernia, intestinal atresia, malrotation, meconium ileus, volvulus, intestinal duplication, annular pancreas, Hirschsprung's disease
- Toxic and metabolic disorders
  - Cardiac failure, drugs, inborn errors of metabolism

B Vomiting in early infancy
Common causes
- Gastro-oesophageal reflux
- Feeding faults
  - Overfeeding/underfeeding, emotional deprivation
- Common infections
  - Upper respiratory tract infection, gastroenteritis, oral candidiasis

Less common causes
- Infections
  - UTI, meningitis, encephalitis, hepatitis, pertussis
- Intestinal malformation and obstructions
  - Hypertrophic pyloric stenosis, lactobezoar, malrotation, volvulus, intestinal duplications, Hirschsprung's disease
- Intracranial pathology
  - hydrocephalus, kernicterus

- Toxic and metabolic disorders
  - Cardiac failure, drugs, uraemia, hypercalcaemia, inborn errors of metabolism

C Vomiting in late infancy
Common causes
- Infections
  - Gastroenteritis, respiratory tract infection, UTI

Less common causes
- Infections
  - Meningitis, hepatitis, encephalitis, pertussis
- Intestinal malformation and obstruction
  - Intussusception, malrotation, gastro-oesophageal reflux
- Food intolerance
  - Cow's milk protein sensitivity, coeliac disease
- Toxic and metabolic disorders
  - Poisoning, drugs, uraemia, Reye's syndrome

D Vomiting in childhood
Common causes
- Acute causes
  - Gastroenteritis, upper respiratory tract infection, food poisoning
- Acute dietary indiscretion

Less common causes
- Infection
  - UTI, meningitis, hepatitis, encephalitis
- Digestive tract disorders
  - Peptic ulcers, appendicitis, intussusception, malrotation, childhood Menetrier's disease, achalasia
- Toxic and metabolic disorders
  - Drugs, poisons, Reye's syndrome, uraemia, diabetes mellitus, hypercalcaemia
- Raised intracranial pressure
  - Hypertensive encephalopathy, tumors, hydrocephalus
- Psychogenic/other
  - Migraine, cyclic vomiting, bulimia

with oesophagitis and oesophageal strictures. Associated diarrhoea may indicate infectious diarrhoea, food allergy, or partial intestinal obstruction. Abdominal distension may indicate intestinal obstruction. Visible peristaltic waves and a pyloric tumour are characteristic of pyloric stenosis. Abdominal tenderness is a feature of peritonitis and specific organ disease such as hepatitis. An abdominal mass is a frequent sign in tuberculosis of the abdomen and tumours. Sites of hernias should be examined for an incarcerated hernia.

Symptoms and signs of other organ disease

Jaundice and tender hepatomegaly suggest hepatitis. Headache or signs of raised intracranial pressure point to meningitis, migraine, inherited metabolic disease, space occupying lesions, toxins and drugs. Diseases of urinary tract, respiratory, or heart may be associated with vomiting. Bouts of coughing (such as occur in pertussis) may be followed by vomiting.

Medication

Toxic effects of drugs such as theophylline and digitalis may manifest initially with vomiting.

Gastro-oesophageal reflux

Gastro-oesophageal reflux (GOR) is the passage of gastric contents into the oesophagus. This is usually due to transient relaxation of the lower oesophageal sphincter (LES). Less often GOR may be the result of low LES tone (chalasia). Regurgitation occurs when the reflux material passes into the mouth.

Natural history

Regurgitation is common in infancy. Approximately 60 per cent of infants regurgitate their milk feeds at the age of three months. By the age of one year this has resolved in more than 90 per cent of infants. In the vast majority of infants this regurgitation is not pathological and does not require specific treatment. In a small proportion of infants however, complications may arise.

Complications

When complications occur, regurgitation is termed *gastro-oesophageal reflux disease* (GORD). These include oesophagitis, respiratory disease, and at times failure to thrive. Peptic oesophagitis causes pain, refusal of feeds, posturing, and less frequently haematemesis and iron deficiency anaemia. Severe long standing GORD may cause peptic strictures of the oesophagus. Intestinal metaplasia (Barret's oesophagus), a rare complication in childhood, is a precursor to oesophageal adenocarcinoma in adults. The natural history of Barret's oesophagus in childhood is unknown.

Stridor, hoarseness, chronic cough, aspiration pneumonia, recurrent wheezing and

Table 24.2 Danger signs in the vomiting child
Bile-stained or faeculent vomiting
Blood in the vomit
Projectile vomiting
Dehydration
Acid base and electrolyte abnormalities (e.g. alkalosis and hypochloraemia)
Weight loss
Signs of intestinal obstruction
Fever and other signs of systemic infection
Central nervous system symptoms (e.g. drowsiness, headache, signs of raised intracranial pressure)

Regurgitation is common in infancy; more than 90 per cent resolve by one year.

Important complications are:
- Reflux oesophagitis (present with dysphagia, rarely haematemesis)
- Respiratory complications
- Failure to thrive

Most infants are effectively managed conservatively:
- Parental reassurance
- Feeding technique and thickening of feeds
- Positioning of the infant.

Proton pump inhibitors are the most effective antacid treatment.

Surgery is reserved for GORD that does not respond to optimal medical management.

bronchiectasis are the respiratory complications associated with GORD. Asthma may be aggravated by GORD and controlling acid reflux may improve asthma control. Steroid dependant asthmatics should be evaluated for GORD, particularly those with complaints of heartburn. Other conditions with which the association with GORD is less well established are otitis media and sinusitis.

Historically, failure to thrive has been associated with severe GORD. Children with poor weight gain or wasting should be thoroughly investigated for other causes of malnutrition before ascribing the malnutrition to GOR.

Athetoid movements and posturing associated with GORD (Sandifer syndrome) may be confused with seizures and occur most commonly in children with brain injury. Children with cerebral palsy often have severe GORD that is resistant to medical and surgical treatment. These children are more likely to have erosive oesophagitis and to develop oesophageal strictures.

Diagnosis

A thorough history and physical examination for complications are usually all that are required for the evaluation of infants with functional GOR. Signs of raised intracranial pressure, intestinal obstruction (e.g. projectile vomiting, abdominal distention) and urinary tract infection (urine examination) should be excluded. A barium swallow allows evaluation of the oesophageal anatomy, gastric outlet obstruction, and proximal small bowel obstruction. Twenty-four hour oesophageal pH-metry is indicated where the diagnosis of GOR is uncertain (e.g. 'silent GOR' in respiratory disease) or where the effect of therapy needs to be assessed. Oesophagoscopy with oesophageal biopsies allows assessment of the distal oesophagus for signs of peptic oesophagitis and other mucosal abnormalities. Biopsies of the oesophageal mucosa may demonstrate the features of peptic oesophagitis or other diseases of the oesophagus such as eosinophilic oesophagitis. The application of newer investigations such as oesophageal impedance in the evaluation of children with GORD still needs to be defined.

Other causes of chronic respiratory disease should be excluded before ascribing these to GOR. In particular oropharyngeal incoordination and anatomic abnormalities such as tracheo-oesophageal fistula should be excluded in children with chronic aspiration syndromes.

Treatment

A stepwise approach to the treatment of GOR is followed according to the severity of the symptoms.

Functional regurgitation

Parental reassurance and advice regarding feeding technique are adequate for the management of most of these infants. Parents should take care not to overfeed their infants. Regular, equally sized feeds are recommended and the correct teat size and burping technique also should be ensured. Thickening feeds reduce the frequency of regurgitation. Thickeners may be added to formula feeds or specialised anti-reflux infant formula may be used in non-breastfed infants.

Infants regurgitate less in the prone position. This is however in conflict with current guidelines to prevent sudden infant death syndrome (SIDS) so the prone position is only recommended in infants who are no longer at risk of SIDS (over the age of one year). Placing the baby on the left or right side may provide some relief.

Gastro-oesophageal reflux disease

Young infants with severe malnutrition or respiratory complications of GOR initially receive transpyloric feeds. This reduces the risk of GOR and allows nutritional rehabilitation and recovery of the respiratory complaints.

Acid related complications are treated with proton pump inhibitors. These provide the most effective inhibition of acid secretion. Histamine receptor antagonists may also be used. Surgery is reserved for infants and children who do not respond to optimal medical therapy.

Diarrhoea

Diarrhoea is characterized by an increased frequency and volume of stool and a decreased consistency. Children usually experience numerous episodes of diarrhoea during the first five years of life. Most are due to infections and although most episodes are self-limiting, they can be associated with significant complications and mortality, with diarrhoea being responsible for up to 2.5 million deaths in young children worldwide each year. Other causes include inherited and acquired disorders of digestion and absorption, motility disturbances, drugs and food intolerance.

Pathophysiology

Diarrhoea results when there is decreased water and electrolyte absorption in the intestine. Normal infants and young children lose only about 5–10 g/kg of water daily in their stool. This relatively small loss of water is the result of extremely effective absorption of electrolytes and water in the small intestine and colon. Under normal conditions the small intestine reabsorbs 80–90 per cent of the water that is ingested or secreted into it. Most of the remaining water and electrolytes are absorbed by the colon. It is important to remember that the intestine is constantly absorbing and secreting water.

When this normal process is disturbed, the stool content of water and electrolytes increases. This may be the result of decreased absorption of water and/or increased secretion. When the net absorption of water by the small bowel is decreased the colon is still able to compensate by increasing absorption. Only when the absorptive capacity of the colon is exceeded or colonic absorption is decreased (e.g. in the presence of colonic disease) does diarrhoea ensue.

Osmotic diarrhoea occurs when there is increased intraluminal osmolality due to sugar malabsorption or the ingestion of non-absorbable sugars such as sorbitol, which decrease the net absorption of water.

Secretory diarrhoea is the result of increased secretion of water and electrolytes induced by a variety of stimuli such as bacterial toxins (e.g. enterotoxins of *Vibrio cholera* and enterotoxogenic *E. coli*), viral proteins (e.g. NSP4 of rotavirus), or hormones (e.g. VIP).

Inflammation (often secondary to direct mucosal invasion by bacteria, e.g. shigella) causes mucosal injury that reduces the absorptive capacity of the intestine, and increases fluid secretion and loss of endogenous proteins. Increased intestinal permeability may also decrease water and electrolyte absorption.

In addition to the loss of water and electrolytes, the absorption of nutrients is decreased. This can lead to significant malnutrition, particularly when the diarrhoea is prolonged.

Carbohydrate malabsorption

Congenital disaccharidase deficiencies are extremely rare. The acquired forms are most commonly secondary to mucosal injury following an acute infectious insult. Carbohydrate malabsorption may be suspected from the description of the stools, which characteristically are watery and expelled forcefully together with a lot of gas. The older child may describe abdominal cramps, which are relieved by the passage of a stool, while the young infant may be irritable and cry a lot just prior to stooling. The stools are acidic and may cause severe excoriation of the patient's buttocks. The diagnosis is confirmed by demonstrating a stool pH <4, positive reducing substances in the faecal water and abnormal breath hydrogen test following ingestion of the specific dietary sugar. Where testing facilities are not available, a therapeutic trial of removing the carbohydrate from the diet should be instituted. If carbohydrate malabsorption is causing the symptoms, there will be an abrupt resolution following removal of the offending sugar from the diet.

Lactase is the most vulnerable brush border enzyme and secondary lactose intolerance occurs after insults such as acute diarrhoea, malnutrition and untreated coeliac disease. It can cause significant osmotic diarrhoea. Removal of lactose from the diet results in rapid resolution of the diarrhoea.

Fat malabsorption

Fat malabsorption may be due either to intraluminal factors affecting digestion, or to factors affecting uptake across the mucosa and subsequent transport in the lymphatics. Intraluminal digestion is largely dependent on delivery of adequate exocrine pancreatic enzymes and bile salts. In Caucasian populations, cystic fibrosis is by far the most common cause of exocrine pancreatic insufficiency in childhood. Deficiency of bile salts is most commonly associated with chronic liver disease. Worldwide, coeliac disease is the most common cause of a mucosal abnormality causing fat malabsorption in children. In disadvantaged communities other conditions which have to be considered are heavy infestation with *Giardia lamblia*, and abdominal tuberculosis which can cause obstruction to lymphatic flow from the gut. Investigations to detect fat malabsorption include stool microscopy stained to detect fat droplets, steatocrit or three-day stool faecal fat quantitation. If present, additional tests will be required to identify the cause of the malabsorption.

Investigations

Patients with uncomplicated acute diarrhoeal disease do not require special investigations to determine the aetiology. Infants and children with complicated and chronic diarrhoea require further investigation and often in-hospital management.

Stool microbiology

Routine culture, microscopy and viral studies of stools are not indicated in the management of children with acute diarrhoea. These investigations are, however, useful in the management of persistent and chronic diarrhoea and if an opportunistic infection is suspected in an immune deficient child. Stool cultures and viral studies are also performed during diarrhoea epidemics and as part of surveillance programmes.

When stools are sent for culture, care should be taken to ensure that the sample is adequate and reaches the laboratory promptly. The laboratory should be alerted if specific organisms such as cryptosporidium parvum or cholera are suspected.

The diagnosis of *Clostridium difficile* infection is confirmed by demonstrating the presence of the toxin in the stool.

Stool microscopy may show leucocytes (often in patients with colitis), red cells (colitis, other causes of intestinal bleeding), and protozoa (*Giardia lamblia*, amoeba, *Cryptosporidium parvum*) and helminth eggs

Cryptosporidium infection is diagnosed by a number of techniques: using stains such as the modified Ziehl-Neelsen or safranine methylene blue stains, or by antigen detection such as ELISA or PCR.

Faecal osmolar gap

Calculation of the faecal osmolar gap (FOG) can aid in the distinction between osmotic and secretory diarrhoea. The faecal osmolar gap (FOG) is calculated by the following formula: $280 - \{2 \times ([Na] + [k])\}$.

The FOG is less than 50 mosmol/l in pure secretory diarrhoea. In the case of severe osmotic diarrhoea the FOG usually exceeds 100-125 mosmol/l. In the case of a mixed osmotic and secretory diarrhoea or moderate carbohydrate malabsorption an intermediate FOG is found. Osmotic diarrhoea resolves rapidly when oral feeds are interrupted while diarrhoea persists in patients with a secretory diarrhoea.

Reducing sugars

Reducing sugars can be detected in the stool with the Clinitest® reagent. For this test five drops of stool are mixed with 10 drops of water. A clinitest tablet is added and an effervescent reaction follows. The colour change that occurs allows the presence of reducing substances to be quantified on a scale ranging from a trace to 4+ according to a colour strip. It should be remembered that sucrose is not a reducing sugar. A stool pH of less than 5.5 also suggests sugar malabsorption. The stool pH of young breast infants may however normally be 5.0. A more precise evaluation of sugar in the stool (e.g. lactose) can be done by chromatography.

Breath hydrogen test
The breath hydrogen test is also used to test for sugar malabsorption. This may be technically challenging in infants and requires specialized equipment that is often not available in developing countries.

Pancreatic elastase-1
Pancreatic elastase-1 is a pancreas-specific protease that resists degradation and is found in very high concentrations in the stool. It is a sensitive and specific test for moderate to severe pancreatic insufficiency. It can be used as a screening test for cystic fibrosis. Low levels (<160 μg/g) make pancreatic insufficiency likely. It is not influenced by oral enzyme replacement, but is often falsely low in watery stools.

Determination of stool fat
In the presence of fat malabsorption fat droplets may be observed with stool microscopy. Visualisation of the droplets is improved with the use of dyes (e.g. Sudan stain). This test is not very specific and requires confirmation with other investigations.

The acid steatocrit is a simple investigation that allows measurement of stool fat content.

It shows good correlation with formal stool fat measurement and is a useful screening test.

A 72 hour stool fat measurement has been the gold standard to assess stool fat content. This test requires complete collection of stool from children on a diet with a controlled fat content. The accurate collection of stool in children is difficult so the simpler alternative tests are usually used.

Stool alpha-1-antitrypsin

Alpha-1-antitrypsin is an endogenous protein that normally occurs in small quantities in the stool. Increased loss of alpha-1-antitrypsin in the stool indicates an increased intestinal loss of endogenous protein (e.g. in protein losing enteropathy).

- Diarrhoea is an important cause of death in young children.
- Early replacement of water and electrolyte losses prevents most deaths and serious complications.
- Feeds, in particular breastfeeding, should not be interrupted unnecessarily.
- Comorbid disease contributes to mortality and morbidity (malnutrition, pneumonia, HIV, bacteraemia) and should be treated promptly.
- Breastfeeding and vitamin A and zinc supplementation reduce the mortality and morbidity of diarrhoea.
- Antibiotics are only used for specific indications.
- Antidiarrhoeal drugs are not used.

Acute infectious diarrhoea

Acute diarrhoeal disease is a leading cause of infant death and morbidity in developing countries. Poor sanitation and hygiene, and contaminated water and food lead to faecal-oral spread of infection. Early weaning and the use of incorrect weaning feeds predispose to diarrhoea and malnutrition. In poor communities children experience on average up to five episodes of diarrhoea per year.

Dehydration, shock and electrolyte abnormalities (such as hypokalaemia and hypernatraemia) are the most important causes of death. The mortality is also increased in children with comorbid conditions, in particular pneumonia, bacteraemia, and malnutrition.

A variety of infectious agents cause diarrhoea. In developed countries most acute diarrhoeal disease is caused by viral infections. World-wide, rotavirus is the most important virus that causes diarrhoea. Bacterial diarrhoea is more common in developing countries. *E coli*, *Salmonella* spp., shigella, and campylobacter are some of the common organisms. In endemic areas cholera is an important pathogen. Cryptosporidium and *Giardia lamblia* are the two most important protozoa causing diarrhoea.

Clinical evaluation

Children with diarrhoea are evaluated for signs of hypovolaemic shock and dehydration (*see* Table 24.4). The clinical evaluation of dehydration is imprecise and does not rely on the evaluation of a single sign. Rather, the degree of dehydration is estimated using a combination of signs. Weight loss provides the most accurate estimate if the child's weight shortly before the onset of diarrhoea is known. Initially there are no signs of dehydration present.

As the child becomes more dehydrated, signs and symptoms become apparent. Initially the children are thirsty and irritable. Subsequently, other signs of dehydration can be elicited, such as decreased skin turgor and sunken eyes and fontanelle (in infants). It is important to

Table 24.3 Common pathogens causing acute diarrhoea in childhood	
Viruses	Human rotavirus, Norovirus, enteric adenovirus, calicivirus, astrovirus
Bacteria	*Escherichia coli*, vibrios (cholera), salmonella, shigella, campylobacter, *Clostridium difficile*, yersinia, pseudomonas, klebsiella, staphylococcus
Parasitic	Protozoa (giardia, cryptosporidium, microsporidium, isospora, *Entamoeba histolytica*, *Balantidium coli*). Helminths (schistosoma, trichuris, strongyloides, trichinella, trematodes)

remember that skin turgor overestimates the degree of dehydration in wasted children and conversely underestimates dehydration in obese children and those with hypernatraemic dehydration.

As the dehydration becomes more severe, signs of hypovolaemic shock develop. These include a decreased level of conciousness, cool extremities, decreased or absent urine output, and low volume peripheral pulses. Hypotension is a late sign. If the fluid loss is very rapid a child may be shocked without features of severe dehydration.

Important comorbid conditions that should be excluded are bacteraemia, pneumonia, and malnutrition. Infants and young children with these conditions are more likely to develop serious complications and die and should be treated aggressively. Immune compromised children (as a result of HIV infection and rare primary immune deficiencies) also require special attention as they are more likely to require hospitalisation and often have a prolonged course and an increased mortality.

Dysentery refers to the passage of blood and

Table 24.4 Assessment and management of dehydration due to diarrhoea

Degree of Dehydration	Signs	Comments	Treatment
Hypovolaemic shock **OR** **severe dehydration** (the management of hypovolaemic shock and severe dehydration are similar)	Cold extremities Delayed capillary refill Low volume (thready) pulse Lethargic or unconscious Hypotension Two of the following signs: Lethargic or unconscious Sunken eyes Not able to drink or drinking poorly Skin pinch goes back very slowly	Urgent attention required (may indicate associated disease) Signs of shock may be present in the absence of signs of dehydration Consider other causes of shock, e.g. septic shock Ask the caregiver what the child's eyes normally look like Regular assessments (including weight measurement) essential	Intravenous resuscitation: Fluid: Ringer's Lactate Normal saline Volume 20 ml/kg rapidly – Remember to continue with rehydration after initial resuscitation and replace ongoing losses
Moderate (some dehydration)	Restless, irritable	Consider other causes, e.g. meningitis. See above See comments in 'Important points to remember'	**Oral rehydration** 20 ml/kg/hour until rehydrated. If not rehydrated after 6 hours: Consider IV rehydration Reconsider diagnosis **Maintenance** Up to 2 years: 50–100 ml ORS after each loose stool. 2 years and more: 100–200 ml after each loose stool

Modified from WHO, IMCI and CDC Recommendations

mucus in the stool. Although the vast majority of cases of dysentery are infective in origin (shigella, salmonella, campylobacter), non-infectious causes of dysentery occasionally occur in childhood. Conditions such as allergic proctocolitis and colonic lymphoid nodular hyperplasia should be considered. When blood and mucus are passed without any faecal matter, intussusception must be considered, which may occur *de novo* or as a complication of acute infective diarrhoea or dysentery of any cause. Other causes of rectal bleeding that should be considered include: Henoch-Schönlein purpura, Meckel's diverticulum, inflammatory bowel disease and polyps. Blood on the surface of the stool is likely to be caused by ano-rectal pathology, e.g. fissure *in ano*. In the newborn, necrotizing enterocolitis presents with bleeding per rectum.

Complications

Biochemical abnormalities
(*see* Chapter 10, Metabolic disorders)

Potassium
Hypokalaemia is a serious complication. Infants with hypokalaemia may be hypotonic, develop a paralytic ileus, bradycardia and respiratory failure. It occurs more commonly in children with prolonged or recurrent episodes of diarrhoea and malnutrition. Potassium is supplemented intravenously or orally.

Hyperkalaemia occurs in patients with renal failure and is aggravated by the presence of a metabolic acidosis. This is a serious complication that leads to cardiac arrythmia and death and should be treated promptly.

Table 24.5 Complications of acute diarrhoeal disease

Dehydration	Hypoglycaemia
Shock	Renal failure
Electrolyte	Haemolytic uraemic
abnormalities	syndrome
Hypernatraemia	Rhabdomyolysis
Hyponatraemia	CNS
Hypokalaemia	Convulsions
Hypocalcaemia	Venous sinus
Hypomagnesaemia	thrombosis

Sodium
Hypernatraemia and hyponatraemia are also electrolyte abnormalities that may have severe complications. Neurological manifestations such as irritability and seizures occur. Complications include cerebral vein thrombosis, cerebral oedema, central pontine myelinolysis, sub-arachnoid haemorrhage, rhabdomyolysis, and renal failure. The diagnosis relies on biochemical evaluation.

Hypernatraemia occurs when free water loss exceeds sodium loss or when excess sodium is given to infants with diarrhoea. This occurs with the incorrect mixing of oral rehydration fluid. Correction of dehydration in these patients should be more gradual as a too rapid decrease in serum sodium concentration may lead to cerebral oedema.

Hyponatraemia is frequently encountered in patients with a secretory diarrhoea (e.g. shigella and cholera infections) and malnourished patients. A sodium level below 120 mmol/l should be corrected with a fluid containing a higher sodium content than that of half-strength Darrow's solution, especially if the patient has neurological symptoms.

Other electrolyte abnormalities
Hypocalcaemia and hypomagnesaemia occur particularly in children with secretory diarrhoea.

Metabolic acidosis
Metabolic acidosis frequently occurs in patients with diarrhoea and dehydration. This is due to a combination of loss of base in the stools, poor tissue perfusion, and decreased renal hydrogen clearance. Correction of shock and dehydration with fluid replacement are the mainstays of the treatment of acidosis in this situation. Bicarbonate is only administered in the presence of severe metabolic acidosis that does not respond to rehydration.

Hypoglycaemia and hyperglycaemia
Blood sugar disturbances are frequently observed. Hypoglycaemia is seen in malnourished, septicaemic, and hypothermic infants, as well as in those who have been starved for some time.

Hyperglycaemia is usually due to stress-related catecholamine release. It is often associated with hypernatraemia. The differentiation from diabetes mellitus is made by the presence of severe ketoacidosis and polyuria in the latter condition. With correction of dehydration and electrolyte disturbance, the blood sugar returns to normal and insulin is usually not required.

Renal failure

Prerenal failure is a common complication of severe dehydration. Correction of the dehydration reverses this complication. Shock and prolonged severe dehydration may cause renal injury leading to acute tubular necrosis or cortical necrosis in severe cases. The haemolytic uraemic syndrome (manifesting with anuria or oliguria, severe anaemia, and thrombocytopaenia) may follow infection with verotoxin-producing *E. coli (E. coli O157)* or shigatoxin-producing *S. dysenteriae* 1. (*see* Chapter 27, Renal and urinary tract disorders)

Convulsions

These are relatively common in patients with diarrhoea. Numerous causes should be considered: febrile seizures, hypoglycaemia, electrolyte abnormalities (hypo- or hypernatraemia), cerebral venous thrombosis, meningitis, encephalitis, and cerebral oedema secondary to too rapid correction of hypernatraemia. Hypocalcaemia and hypomagnesaemia cause tetany that must be distinguished from true seizures.

Management of infectious diarrhoea

Fluid management is guided by the presence of shock and the degree of dehydration. The response to treatment must be re-evaluated regularly and children are monitored for recurrence of dehydration every 4–6 hours. (*see* Table 24.4)

Shock
Children with hypovolaemic shock and severe dehydration should be promptly identified on presentation to health care facilities. Intravenous fluids (e.g. Ringers lactate or normal saline) are rapidly administered to shocked children. Where intravenous access is not possible, an intra-osseus line should be used.

Rehydration

The vast majority of infants and children with diarrhoea can effectively be rehydrated with oral rehydration solutions. Caregivers are instructed to start oral rehydration as soon as their child develops diarrhoea. Early introduction of rehydration fluids can prevent the development of dehydration in most children. It is consequently important that all mothers with young children should be familiar with the principles of oral rehydration and have written instructions available on the preparation of oral rehydration solutions.

Children who refuse oral rehydration or who vomit repeatedly can usually be effectively rehydrated through a nasogastric tube. Intravenous rehydration is initiated in those patients who

Table 24.6 Composition of the SAPA* and WHO recommended ORS formulae compared with half-strength Darrow's/dextrose solution

	SAPA-ORS	WHO-ORS Standard	WHO-ORS Reduced osmolarity	$\frac{1}{2}$ Darrow's Dextrose
Sodium (mmol/l)	64	90	75	61
Potassium (mmol/l)	20	20	20	17
Chloride (mmol/l)	54	80	65	51
Base (mmol/l)**	30	30	10	27
Glucose	2%	2%	1.35% (anhydrous)	5%

*   *South African Paediatric Association*
** *Lactate is being used in place of bicarbonate in half-strength Darrows solution. Citrate is replacing bicarbonate in ORS powder mixtures as it increases the shelf-life and is equally effective as a base.*

have failed to improve with optimal oral rehydration therapy, who have severe dehydration or shock, or where there is a contraindication to the administration of oral fluids (e.g. paralytic ileus).

Once children are rehydrated, administration of ORS to replace ongoing losses should continue until the diarrhoea has resolved.

Feeding during diarrhoea

During an episode of diarrhoea children often lose their appetite and may develop secondary malabsorption of nutrients. This leads to weight loss and may precipitate severe malnutrition, particularly when the diarrhoea is prolonged or when there are recurrent episodes of diarrhoea.

Normal feeds should be continued as far as the child's appetite will allow. Offering regular small feeds is often successful in achieving adequate intake. In particular breastfeeding should not be interrupted as continued breastfeeding may shorten the duration of diarrhoea and minimise the nutritional effects of the disease. Diluted formula should not be given. Once the diarrhoea has resolved, the child is offered additional feeds to allow recovery of the nutritional deficit that has developed.

Antibiotics

Antibiotics are not routinely given to children with diarrhoea. Children with dysentery and those with cholera complicated with severe dehydration should receive antibiotics. Co-existent conditions, such as pneumonia and bacteraemia will also require systemic antibiotic therapy.

The degree of dehydration can be underestimated in:

- Overweight infants
- Hypernatraemia
- Poor technique when assessing skin turgor.

The degree of dehydration can be overestimated in:

- Wasted infants.

Gradual rehydration is safer for infants with:

- Hypernatraemia
- Severe malnutrition
- Significant cardiac or respiratory disease
- Age less than 3 months.

Children at high risk of bacteraemia are also initially treated with antibiotics. This includes children with severe immune deficiency (e.g. AIDS), severe malnutrition, and children under the age of three months of age. Specific infections such as amoebiasis and giardiasis are also treated with the appropriate antimicrobial agent.

Probiotics

Supplementation with certain probiotics reduces the risk of developing nosocomial diarrhoea, antibiotic associated diarrhoea and diarrhoea in day-care centres. Probiotics can also provide a moderate reduction in the duration of diarrhoea from causes such as rotavirus infection. For probiotics to be effective an adequate dose (greater than 100 million CFU) of viable organisms must be given daily. Not all probiotics are equally effective and the choice of probiotic is guided by available clinical trials.

Antidiarrhoeal drugs

Antidiarrhoeal drugs are not recommended in the treatment of acute diarrhoea in children. They may prolong the duration of symptoms in patients with dysentery and have been associated with serious complications, such as toxic megacolon. Some of these drugs may also have serious systemic side effects.

Occasionally antidiarrhoeal drugs may be used to provide symptomatic relief for children with chronic diarrhoea not responding to treatment. Care should be taken to use an agent that has an acceptable side-effect profile.

Newer drugs such as the encephalinase inhibitors may have some value in reducing stool losses. These drugs are however not yet available in South Africa. Octreotide, a somatostatin analogue, has anti-secretory properties. A trial of treatment is indicated in children with resistent severe secretory diarrhoea.

Antiemetics

Antiemetics are not indicated, as the vomiting is due to local factors in the gut or starvation ketosis and responds well to simple measures of fluid therapy. The usual antiemetic drugs also have significant side-effects.

Vitamin A supplementation

Regular vitamin A supplementation to children in countries with a high prevalence of vitamin

A deficiency has been shown to reduce the 'all cause' mortality of children under the age of five years and specifically to reduce the morbidity and mortality of diarrhoeal disease. Children at risk of vitamin A deficiency should consequently receive regular vitamin A supplementation.

Zinc

Zinc supplementation reduces the duration of both acute and persistent diarrhoeal disease in developing countries. Zinc should be given to children on admission and continued for two weeks after discharge.

Prevention of diarrhoeal disease

Rotavirus vaccine

Oral rotavirus vaccines have been developed recently and are included in the routine vaccination schedule. They are administered to infants during the first six months and have been shown to dramatically reduce the incidence of rotavirus diarrhoea, in particular severe episodes that require hospital admission.

Water/sanitation/breastfeeding

Public health measures such as improved housing, safe water supply, sanitation, and waste disposal decrease the risk of developing diarrhoea. Preventative measures, including those suggested by WHO, are:
  ◆ Exclusive breastfeeding for at least four to six months
  ◆ Introduction of appropriate complementary foods at six months. These should be nutritious and hygienically prepared.
  ◆ Use of safe water.
  ◆ Hand washing. All family members should wash hands before preparing food, before eating, after defaecation and after cleaning and disposing of a baby's faeces.
  ◆ Food safety. Steps are taken to prevent contamination of food, e.g. hand washing, thorough cooking of food, and cleaning of cooking utensils.
  ◆ Use of latrines and safe disposal of stools.
  ◆ Early identification of and nutritional intervention for malnutrition.
  ◆ Immunization, especially against rotavirus and measles, which is frequently complicated by diarrhoea.

  ◆ Maternal education to promote an understanding of hygiene and optimal use of available resources.

Specific enteric infections

Salmonella infections

Clinical manifestations
(*See also* Chapter 15, Systemic infections). An incubation period of 12–24 hours is followed by abrupt onset of diarrhoea, vomiting, abdominal pain, and fever. Stools are usually watery, but may contain blood and mucus.

The severity of the illness varies from a mild self-limited attack of diarrhoea and vomiting, which lasts a few days, to that in which the child is acutely ill with high fever and severe dehydration. Irritability, meningism, encephalopathy, and convulsions may occur. Extra-intestinal complications (septicaemia, meningitis, osteitis, arthritis and pneumonia) occur commonly in patients with sickle cell anaemia,

Treatment
Antibiotics are not indicated in infections localized to the bowel in immune-competent children. Young infants, severely immune-compromised children and those with extra-intestinal complications should receive antibiotic treatment. Salmonellae are increasingly resistant to the commonly used chemotherapeutic agents. The drug of choice will depend on the sensitivity of the organisms.

Escherichia coli infections

E. coli is one of the most common bacterial causes of diarrhoea. A variety of strains that cause diarrhoea have been identified. Entero-invasive *E. coli* serogroups (EIEC) behave like shigella and produce dysentery following adherence and invasion of the gut epithelium. The entero-haemorrhagic *E. coli* 0157:H7 (EHEC) produce a shiga-like toxin, which causes dysentery and, in a small proportion of cases, haemolytic uraemic syndrome (HUS) may result. EHEC outbreaks have usually occurred following ingestion of contaminated meat. Other pathogenic strains are enteropathogenic (EPEC), enterotoxigenic (ETEC), enteroaggregative and enteroadherent *E. coli*.

Campylobacter infections

Campylobacter jejuni is the main species causing intestinal disease. It is a common cause of diarrhoea in travellers. Infection usually follows ingestion of contaminated food, water, or milk. After an incubation period of three to five days, fever, nausea, vomiting, and abdominal pain precede the onset of diarrhoea with watery stools, which may contain blood and mucus. Colitis may be indistinguishable from other causes of inflammatory bowel disease and occasionally it may mimic an acute abdomen. Reactive arthritis and Guillain-Barrè syndrome have been associated with *C. jejuni* infections. In AIDS, severe protracted diarrhoea with extra-intestinal manifestations may occur.

As it is usually a self-limiting disease, antibiotics are not indicated, but erythromycin may be beneficial in certain severe forms.

Yersinia enterocolitica

This organism is a recognized cause of diarrhoea in children, and commonly invades the terminal ileum, but may cause dysentery. Animals are the reservoir for the infection. Complications include erythema nodosum, reactive arthritis, and thrombocytopaenia. Antibiotics are not indicated.

Cholera

Cholera is an acute watery diarrhoeal illness caused by *Vibrio cholerae*. It must be suspected in the presence of profuse watery diarrhoea plus vomiting without nausea.

Epidemiology

Vibrios are spread by the faecal-oral route through contaminated food and water and therefore cause disease in impoverished communities with poor sanitation. Human carriers and mild cases spread the disease (there are no animal hosts).

Pathogenesis

Vibrio cholera infection is confined to the intestinal lumen. An enterotoxin, which consists of two subunits: A, the active component, and B, the cell-binding component, is released. The toxin inhibits sodium absorption and stimulates chloride and water secretion leading to severe secretory diarrhoea.

Clinical features

An incubation period of one to five days is followed by a profuse secretory diarrhoea. The stools quickly become colourless with mucus ('rice water'). There is often associated vomiting without nausea. Severe dehydration, shock and electrolyte abnormalities ensue. The diarrhoea usually resolves within three days but in exceptional circumstances lasts for up to 10 days. With rapid replacement of fluid and electrolytes, hospital mortality rate is 1–2 per cent. Mortality can exceed 50 per cent when fluid replacement is inadequate.

Diagnosis

The clinical picture is almost pathognomonic during outbreaks and treatment should not be delayed pending confirmation of the diagnosis. *Vibrio cholera* is best cultured on specialized media but stool specimens must reach the laboratory promptly. Additional diagnostic techniques include dark-field and phase contrast microscopy. Agglutinating or toxin-neutralizing antibodies can be detected in the serum.

Management

The management of cholera can be summarised as follows:

- Observe enteric precautions.
- Rapid fluid replacement and rehydration. Intravenous rehydration is required in children with circulatory collapse, continued vomiting or severe dehydration.
- The routine use of antibiotics in the treatment of cholera is not recommended. They are however given to patients with severe dehydration as they shorten the duration of diarrhoea. The choice of antibiotics is guided by local resistance patterns. In South Africa a three day course of ciprofloxacin is given to children under the age of eight years and tetracycline to children over the age of eight years. These guidelines are regularly reviewed according to local resistance patterns and clinicians need to familiarise themselves with local recommendations.
- Strict input/output charting, frequent blood pressure readings, and serum urea and electrolyte measurements are necessary.

Prevention

Measures that prevent the contamination of food and water control the spread of cholera. These include clean water supply, sanitation and personal hygiene. Water can be sterilized by boiling or the addition of household bleach.

Oral vaccines are available for cholera. Immunity however wanes after 6–12 months. They are indicated for travelers to a cholera endemic area or persons living in areas with a high risk of cholera, e.g. refugee camps where there is a high possibility of a cholera outbreak. Currently the Department of Health in South Africa does not recommend the use of cholera vaccines.

Rotavirus

The wheel-like double stranded RNA virus is predominantly spread by the faecal–oral route although there is evidence that transmission by respiratory droplets also occurs. It is the most important viral cause of diarrhoea in children. The virus infects mature enterocytes on the villus tips in the small intestine. Enterocyte injury, compensatory crypt cell proliferation, and toxic effects of viral proteins lead to decreased carbohydrate absorption (in particular lactose) and increased net intestinal water secretion.

After an incubation period of one to two days there is a sudden onset of symptoms. Fever and vomiting are followed by non-bloody watery diarrhoea. Febrile seizures, severe dehydration and electrolyte abnormalities are important complications.

Treatment is supportive with attention to fluid therapy and early reintroduction of feeds. Effective vaccines are available. Probiotic supplementation may result in a modest reduction in the duration of diarrhoea.

> Rotavirus causes a combination of secretory and osmotic diarrhoea.

Diagnosis

Enzyme immunoassays offer high sensitivity and specificity, and stool electron microscopy will show the typical appearance.

Shigella dysentery

Four serogroups are responsible for bacillary dysentery: *Shigella dysenteriae* (sd1), *Shigella flexneri, Shigella boydii, Shigella sonnei.*

Epidemiology

S. flexneri is the most common cause of shigella dysentery in South Africa. Outbreaks of Sd1 occur that cause severe disease. The infecting dose is small and spread from person to person is particularly likely to occur in overcrowded home conditions or in institutions. Children with diarrhoea are more likely to spread infection than asymptomatic carriers. In the tropics, infection may be spread by flies or by contaminated food and water.

Pathogenesis

Shigellae are invasive organisms that cause ulceration of the colonic mucosa. They also produce an enterotoxin that causes a watery diarrhoea. Sd1 also elaborates an exotoxin (shigatoxin) which is responsible for the severe manifestations such as haemolytic-uraemic syndrome.

Clinical picture

After a short incubation period of one to four days, there is an abrupt onset of fever, abdominal pain, and watery stools which often, but not invariably, contain blood and mucus. The severity of the illness varies from a mild self-limiting disease to severe diarrhoea with dehydration, shock and extra-intestinal complications. Hyponatraemia is a common electrolyte abnormality. Extra-intestinal manifestations such as encephalopathy, meningism, convulsions and reactive arthritis may occur. Disseminated intravascular coagulation and haemolytic-uraemic syndrome are common complications of Sd1 infection. Immune compromised patients, young infants, and malnourished children may develop a shigella septicaemia with a high mortality.

Management

Mild cases require no specific therapy. Replacement of fluid and electrolytes is necessary. High-risk patients are admitted to hospital. Antibiotics are given according to the sensitivity of the local strains. Presently the WHO recommends treatment with ciprofloxacin or ceftriaxone. In some regions (e.g. South Africa) shigella remains sensitive to nalidixic acid.

Cryptosporidium

Cryptosporidium infection accounts for up to 10 per cent of diarrhoea in children in developing countries. The organism is water-borne with most infections occurring in warm wet months of the year.

Epidemiology
Transmission is by the faecal-oral route. Person-to-person spread occurs in daycare centres and households. Nosocomial infection has been documented but is easily prevented by maintaining basic hygiene measures. Contamination of drinking water and recreational water (e.g. swimming pools) has led to large outbreaks. Spread from farm animals (e.g. cattle) and household pets also occurs. Filtration or boiling of water is required to prevent infection as the organism is not killed by standard chlorination.

In developing countries symptomatic infection predominantly occurs in children under the age of five years. In developed countries adults become symptomatic after travel related exposure. Immune compromised patients are at particular risk of infection and serious disease.

Clinical picture
After an incubation period of approximately one week (1–30 days) patients develop diarrhoea. This is often severe watery diarrhoea that leads to profound loss of water and electrolytes. Other symptoms include abdominal cramps, fever and occasionally vomiting. Weight loss may be severe and young children in developing countries are at risk of developing severe malnutrition. Most immune-competent children recover by 7–10 days although some children may develop persistent diarrhoea lasting longer than 14 days.

Immune compromised children often have an adverse course. There is significant mortality in these children and they are more likely to develop chronic diarrhoea and extra-intestinal complications. Of these, biliary tract complications such as sclerosing cholangitis are the most important. Treatment with antiretroviral therapy greatly reduces the risk of these complications in HIV-infected children. Children with severe malnutrition are also at increased risk and have a high mortality.

Diagnosis usually relies on stool microscopy. Occasionally the organism is identified in histological specimens.

Management
Treatment is predominantly supportive, providing adequate fluid and nutritional support.

No reliable antimicrobial treatment is available. A number of agents that have been used with limited success include azithromycin, clarithromycin, nitazoxanide, and paromomycin. Opiate agonists have been used in adults to control symptoms. These drugs should be used with caution in infants and children as they often have severe side-effects. Octreotide, a somatostatin analogue, is an anti-secretory agent that may alleviate symptoms in some patients.

Chronic diarrhoea

Chronic diarrhoea is defined as the passage of abnormal, unformed stools for a period of 14 days or longer.

The most important type of chronic diarrhoea in developing countries is that following an episode of acute diarrhoea. Other causes include inherited diseases of the intestinal mucosa, protein sensitisation, anatomic abnormalities of the intestine, motility disturbances, immune deficiencies, and chronic inflammatory diseases.

The management of children with this complaint is one of the most difficult challenges in paediatrics. This group of conditions has a high morbidity and mortality and requires early diagnosis and management.

The causes of chronic diarrhoea vary according to the age of onset, but there is considerable overlap depending on the specific society and environment.

Some of these conditions may present with typical dehydrating diarrhoea and varying degrees of malabsorption. Alternatively, other conditions present predominantly with malabsorption and no or little dehydration. However, conditions such as coeliac disease and cystic fibrosis that usually present as a malabsorption syndrome may occasionally present with severe electrolyte abnormalities and dehydration.

Malabsorption refers to the inefficient transfer of one or more nutrients from the intestinal lumen into the body resulting in excessive faecal losses of these substances. It may be due to a specific defect in absorption such as protein (e.g. enterokinase deficiency), carbohydrate (e.g. lactose intolerance), fat (e.g. abetalipoproteinaemia) or vitamins (B_{12}). Generalised malabsorption is however more common.

Table 24.7 Disorders associated with chronic diarrhoea in childhood

Congenital diarrhoea Congenital chloride diarrhoea Microvillus inclusion disease Epithelial dysplasia or Tufting enteropathy Autoimmune enteropathy	**Pancreatic insufficiency** Cystic fibrosis Schwachman-Diamond syndrome Congenital lipase deficiency
Mucosal damage and abnormalities Infections (viral, bacterial, protozoal) Post-enteritis enteropathy Coeliac disease Protein-sensitive enteropathy Eosinophilic gastro-enteropathy Intestinal lymphangiectasia (congenital and acquired)	**Anatomic abnormalities** Short bowel syndrome Stagnant loop syndrome Malrotation **Enzyme deficiencies** Secondary disaccharidase deficiencies Adult-type lactase deficiency Congenital disaccharidase deficiency Enterokinase deficiency
Immune deficiency HIV Primary immune deficiency	**Metabolic and endocrine abnormalities** Acrodermatitis enteropathica Abetalipoproteinaemia
Endocrine disorders VIP secreting tumours e.g. VIPoma (usually in pancreas), ganglioneuroblastomas, ganglioneuromas Zollinger-Ellison syndrome Carcinoid tumours Thyrotoxicosis	Wolman's disease Hypoparathyroidism Hyperparathyroidism **Other** Small bowel bacterial overgrowth

Evaluation

The evaluation of a child with chronic diarrhoea requires a systematic approach. Firstly it is important to determine if the diarrhoea is functionally important (affects on nutrition, hydration and metabolic state). Clues to the diagnosis are sought in the history and physical examination. Basic special investigations may further assist in confirming the diagnosis. In some patients invasive investigations such as intestinal biopsies are required. A therapeutic trial of a hypoallergenic formula may be of value in children with food allergy .

Intestinal infections, cystic fibrosis, severe malnutrition and coeliac disease account for more than 90 per cent of causes of malabsorption. This leads to failure to thrive and chronic diarrhoea.

History
Some of the important points to elicit in the history are:

♦ Maternal history: HIV status, infections during pregnancy, polyhydramnios (associated with congenital enteropathy)
♦ Neonatal history: surgical conditions (e.g. meconium peritonitis, necrotizing enterocolitis, intestinal resection), neonatal diarrhoea
♦ Previous medical history: recurrent infections, previous episodes of diarrhoea
♦ Family history: previous deaths in infancy or childhood (suggestive of inherited diseases), allergy, lactose intolerance
♦ Diet: association of diarrhoea with specific feeds (e.g. dairy products for children with lactose intolerance), fruit juice (may cause an osmotic diarrhoea), breast or formula fed
♦ Systemic symptoms: fever, arthritis

(reactive arthritis, inflammatory bowel disease), rash (IBD)

- Characteristics of the stool: watery (secretory or osmotic), pale, foul smelling, greasy stools (steatorrhoea), blood and mucus (colitis), undigested vegetable matter (non-specific chronic diarrhoea). When children have severe fat malabsorption oil droplets may be seen surrounding the faeces.

Physical examination

The examination includes assessment of nutrition and hydration, and the presence of pathological lymph nodes, arthritis and rash. Children with significant malabsorption, in particular fat malabsorption, have decreased subcutaneous fat and muscle wasting.

The abdomen must be examined for abdominal masses (e.g. TB abdomen, faeces), distention (fat malabsorption, motility disturbances, subtotal intestinal obstruction), organomegaly and other signs of intestinal obstruction. Hepatomegaly may be due to fatty infiltration. Perianal fistula, fissures, and peri-anal cellulits are sought. A nappy rash may be due to contact dermatitis, candida infections, or nutritional deficiencies such as zinc.

Special investigations

The investigations performed for the evaluation of acute diarrhoea are also appropriate in the evaluation of chronic diarrhoea. Stool microscopy and culture should be performed, as certain bacteria and protozoa may cause chronic diarrhoea. Stool analysis may also be useful to demonstrate carbohydrate malabsorption (reducing substances in the stool, stool chromatography, FOG, breath hydrogen test), fat malabsorption (stool microscopy for fat droplets, steatocrit, 72-hour stool fat determination), exocrine pancreatic function (faecal elastase), and loss of endogenous protein (alpha-one-antitrypsin). Additional investigations include: full blood count, biochemistry (serum albumin, calcium, phosphate, and magnesium), immunological evaluation (HIV and primary immune deficiency) and radiology of the abdomen (ultrasound, contrast imaging). Some patients will require endoscopy and biopsy of the small and large intestine. Depending on clinical suspicion and initial test results further testing may include a sweat test and coeliac screen.

Persistent diarrhoea

Persistent diarrhoea (PD) refers to episodes of acute onset diarrhoea that last longer than 14 days. In developed countries very few children with acute diarrhoea will progress to persistent diarrhoea. In developing countries however, the proportion of children with acute diarrhoea who develop persistent diarrhoea may exceed 10 per cent. The mortality and morbidity associated with persistent diarrhoea is far higher than that of acute diarrhoea and accounts for up to 50 per cent of diarrhoeal disease deaths in children.

Risk factors

A number of organisms have been associated with progression to PD. These include non-typhoid salmonella, shigella, entero-adherent and entero-aggregative *E. coli*, and *Cryptosporidium parvum*. Young children, those with recurrent episodes of diarrhoea and who are malnourished are more likely to develop PD. In addition immune compromised children, particularly those with HIV infection, are more likely to develop PD. Early weaning from breastmilk, inappropriate weaning feeds, and incorrect management of acute diarrhoea also predispose to PD.

Pathophysiology

It is generally accepted that mucosal injury is central to the pathogenesis. Factors that contribute to the injury include re-infection, small bowel bacterial overgrowth, the deconjugation and dehydroxylation of bile salts (which causes secretory diarrhoea), micronutrient deficiency, and protein sensitisation. Lactose malabsorption is a common feature of PD. Rarely children may become sucrose intolerant and even develop acquired monosaccharide intolerance.

- Chronic diarrhoea has a higher mortality and morbidity than acute diarrhoea.
- Persistent diarrhoea is the most important cause of chronic diarrhoea in developing countries.
- In addition to replacement of water and electrolyte losses, nutritional support of these children is very important.
- History and physical examination often provide valuable clues to the diagnosis.
- Always consider HIV infection in children with chronic diarrhoea.

Treatment

Maintaining hydration and correction of electrolyte abnormalities can usually be achieved with oral rehydration therapy. Children with severe secretory diarrhoea or acquired monosaccharide intolerance may require intravenous rehydration.

Nutritional support

Nutritional support is essential in the management of PD. Breastmilk should not be interrupted if possible. Formula-fed infants will often tolerate a normal lactose-containing formula. Those who are lactose intolerant are given a low lactose feed. Commercially available formula can be used but these are more expensive than standard feeds. If they are not available feeds prepared with fermented milk are often well tolerated. Regardless of the feed that is used, it is important to ensure that energy and protein intake is adequate.

Micronutrient supplementation, in particular zinc, may enhance recovery. Other supplements that may be of value are vitamin A and folate.

Children who have protein sensitisation will benefit from the use of hydrolysed formula. These

are expensive and their use should be reserved for selected patients in a resource constrained environment.

The rare patient who does not respond to treatment and continues to lose weight and dehydrate will require parenteral nutrition. This should only be performed in centres with adequate expertise and facilities.

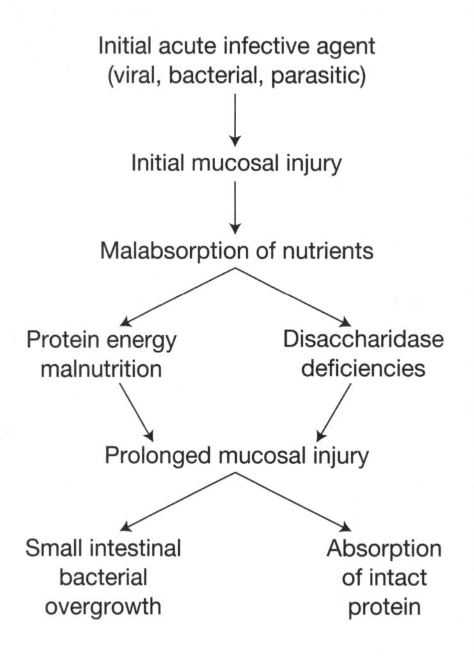

Drug support

Oral antibiotics (e.g. aminoglycosides and metronidazole) may be used in children with suspected small bowel bacterial over growth. This is often combined with cholestyramine, a bile salt binding resin.

Urinary tract infections and bacteraemia often occur in the setting of PD and may delay recovery. They require appropriate investigation and systemic antibiotic treatment.

Diarrhoea in HIV infected children

More than 50 per cent of the total body lymphocytes are found in the intestinal mucosa. These are infected early in the course of HIV infection, with rapid depletion of mucosal lymphocytes. After acute HIV infection the intestinal mucosa serves as a reservoir for chronic HIV replication. Histological changes in the intestine include villous blunting, crypt hyperplasia, and an inflammatory infiltrate of the lamina propria. After initiation of antiretroviral treatment these changes improve but may not fully recover. There are also a number of functional changes such as increased intestinal permeability and protein loss, and iron and carbohydrate malabsorption (in particular lactose).

Diarrhoea is consequently one of the common complications of HIV infection. It is more severe than in HIV-uninfected children, frequently follows a prolonged course, is often recurrent and has a high mortality. Factors that influence the prognosis in these children are their immune status, whether they are receiving antiretroviral therapy, malnutrition, and the presence of co-morbid conditions.

The pathogenesis is multifold. Common stool pathogens are initially responsible for most episodes of diarrhoea while opportunistic infections (OI) are important in children with advanced disease. Malabsorption of sugars and fat, and bacterial overgrowth contribute to diarrhoeal disease.

Figure 24.1 Pathogenesis of chronic diarrhoea

Initial acute infective agent
(viral, bacterial, parasitic)

↓

Initial mucosal injury

↓

Malabsorption of nutrients

Protein energy malnutrition

Disaccharidase deficiencies

Prolonged mucosal injury

Small intestinal bacterial overgrowth

Absorption of intact protein

A number of drugs, in particular protease inhibitor drugs (e.g. nelfinavir, amprenavir, ritonavir, saquinavir), may also cause diarrhoea.

The management of children with HIV infection who present with diarrhoea largely follows the same principles as the management of non-HIV infected children. These children are however at increased risk of bacteraemia, so antibiotics are given sooner than in other children. The diarrhoea is also more likely to follow a prolonged course. They should consequently be followed closely and many will require admission. OIs should be sought in children who are severely immune compromised and who have persistent diarrhoea. This includes organisms such as cryptosporidium (remember to alert the laboratory so they will do the appropriate stains) and cytomegalovirus (CMV). The diagnosis of CMV relies on histology and tissue culture. This requires endoscopy with mucosal biopsies.

HIV infected children with recurrent episodes of diarrhoea or chronic diarrhoea should be considered for antiretroviral treatment. Vitamin A supplementation may reduce the risk of developing severe diarrhoea. The child's caregivers should be instructed in the hygienic preparation of feeds and water should be boiled before use.

Protein allergy

The most common food allergy in childhood is cow's milk protein allergy with an estimated prevalence of 2–7.5 per cent. Allergy to other food proteins in childhood includes soya bean (including soya infant formula), egg, nuts, peanuts and seafood. The allergic reaction may be IgE or non-IgE mediated. The most important types of intestinal presentation are briefly discussed here. The extra-intestinal manifestations and diagnosis of allergy are discussed in Chapter 20, Allergic disorders.

Food protein induced (FPI) enteropathy presents in the first year of life with vomiting one to two hours after a meal, diarrhoea, abdominal distention and failure to thrive. With severe intestinal involvement associated malabsorption may lead to severe malnutrition and anaemia.

FPI colitis and proctitis typically present with rectal bleeding, often in the first weeks of life. Most of these infants are otherwise asymptomatic although some may develop iron deficiency anaemia. With combined colitis and enteropathy (FPI enterocolitis) failure to thrive is more prominent.

In rare cases allergens secreted in the breastmilk may cause FPI enterocolitis or colitis. In most patients breastmilk feeding can be continued. However, if the infant becomes anaemic or fails to gain weight, the mother may be placed on a dairy exclusion diet. If symptoms persist an extensively hydrolysed infant formula is indicated.

Cow's milk protein allergy tends to resolve with age. By the age of three years 90 per cent will have complete resolution of their symptoms. IgE-mediated allergy (particularly in the presence of high IgE levels) is more likely to persist and these children are also more likely to develop allergies to other antigens.

Other intestinal manifestations of food protein allergy are eosinophilic oesophagitis, gastritis, and gastroenteritis. Infants with these conditions present with dysphagia, bolus obstruction of the oesophagus, vomiting, diarrhoea and malabsorption. The diagnosis requires biopsy of the oesophageal, gastric and small bowel mucosa to demonstrate eosinophilic infiltration.

Chronic diarrhoea due to inherited diseases of the intestinal mucosa

Inherited diseases of the intestine usually present within the first months of life. These conditions may be divided into those that are associated with villous blunting and those that have normal mucosal histology. These diseases are due to transport defects (e.g. sodium-glucose cotransporter defect), enzyme deficiencies (enterokinase deficiency), or enterocyte abnormalities (e.g. microvillous inclusion disease).

Onset of symptoms is often within the first few days after birth. Some mothers will give a history of polyhydramnios. There may be a family history of previous infant deaths or similar symptoms. The diarrhoea may be osmotic (e.g. sodium glucose cotransporter defect) or secretory (e.g. congenital microvillous inclusion disease). Attention to providing early adequate nutritional support and correcting dehydration and elec-trolyte abnormalities improves the prognosis. Many of these infants will require specialized investigations and parenteral nutrition. They should be referred to centres experienced in their management as soon as possible.

Non-specific chronic diarrhoea

This entity, sometimes called 'toddler's diarrhoea', occurs in children between the ages of one and three years. It is often preceded by an episode of acute infectious diarrhoea. The children pass large unformed stools during the day but not at night. The stools often contain undigested vegetable material (e.g. carrots and peas) but no blood. Despite the diarrhoea, the children gain weight normally and appear healthy. Symptoms tend to be intermittent and usually resolve by the age of four years.

It is important to elicit a dietary history. Ingestion of nonabsorbable carbohydrates such as sorbitol cause a similar presentation. These are used as artificial sweeteners and are present in some fruit juices. An unbalanced diet, rich in carbohydrates, may also cause frequent unformed stools. Correction of the diet and elimination of nonabsorbable carbohydrates often resolves the symptoms. Lactose intolerance should also be considered. Chronic *Giardia lamblia* infection should also be excluded as this may be confused with non-specific chronic diarrhoea.

Treatment of these children includes reassurance of the caregivers and dietary manipulation. Reducing the carbohydrate and increasing the fat content in the diet often provide symptomatic improvement.

Protein–losing enteropathy

An increased loss of plasma proteins through the gut mucosa can occur in many gastrointestinal and non-gastrointestinal diseases because of increased mucosal permeability to protein or due to abnormalities of lymph flow.

Increased mucosal permeability is most frequently due to intestinal infections (acute infections and chronic infections like tuberculosis). Other causes include food protein induced enteropathy, inflammatory bowel disease and eosinophilic enteropathy. Protein loss from lymphatics may be due to primary or secondary intestinal lymphangiectasia. The latter results from lymphatic obstruction secondary to conditions such as tuberculosis and lymphoma or due to cardiac conditions such as constrictive pericarditis and after certain types of cardiac surgery (e.g. Fontan procedure).

Clinical features are those relating to the underlying cause but in addition include hypoproteinaemic oedema, ascites and pleural effusion. Such patients may be misdiagnosed as suffering from kwashiorkor, but do not have other features of malnutrition and are often under six months of age. The hallmark of the condition is a panhypoproteinaemia with both albumin and globulin being reduced. It is important to exclude cirrhosis and renal protein loss. Stool alpha-1-antitrypsin clearance is a simple measure of stool protein. If the protein loss is from the lymphatics lymphopaenia is common. The site of the protein loss may be defined by endoscopy and biopsy. The treatment is that of the underlying condition. An albumin (20 per cent) infusion may be required to correct the hypoalbuminaemia and oedema.

Coeliac disease (CD)

Coeliac disease is an immune mediated enteropathy triggered by the ingestion of gluten (contained in wheat, rye, barley, and oats) in genetically susceptible people. An inappropriate T-cell response leads to proximal small intestinal mucosal injury causing villous atrophy. The major predisposing HLA genes are DQ2 and DQ8 occurring in 98 per cent of patients with CD.

Clinical manifestations may be gastrointestinal (typical), non-gastrointestinal (atypical) or asymptomatic. Children typically present with failure to thrive, chronic diarrhoea, abdominal distension, muscle wasting, hypotonia and poor appetite up to 6-24 months after the introduction of gluten containing cereals, but can present later with atypical findings such as iron deficiency anaemia, growth failure, osteopaenia, pubertal delay or abnormalities in liver function. There is an increased association of CD with Type 1 diabetes, IgA deficiency, autoimmune disorders, Trisomy 21, and dermatitis herpetiformis.

The diagnosis is suggested with positive tissue transglutaminase (tTG) screening test, but confirmed on demonstrating villous atrophy on jejunal biopsy which subsequently improves with dietary elimination of gluten.

Treatment is a gluten-free diet for life. This is difficult to achieve and requires the assistance of a dietitian to ensure that the all sources of gluten are avoided and that the diet is nutritionally complete. Multivitamin, folate, vitamin D, calcium and iron supplements are indicated initially.

Cystic fibrosis

Cystic fibrosis is an autosomal recessive condition arising from mutations in the gene for cystic fibrosis transmembrane conductance regulator (CFTR) on chromosome 7. It is common in Caucasian populations (commonest mutation △F508), and is increasingly recognised in the other population groups in South Africa (commonest mutation 3120+1G→A). Abnormally viscous mucus leads to obstruction of tubular structures in multiple organ systems. The pancreas, intestine, liver and gallbladder may be involved. Neonates may present with intestinal obstruction at birth (meconium ileus) or obstructive jaundice. Affected children typically present with a combination of failure to thrive with chronic foul-smelling diarrhoea (steatorrhoea due to pancreatic insufficiency), together with recurrent respiratory infections usually leading to bronchiectasis (*see* Chapter 25, Respiratory tract disorders). They can have electrolyte derangements, typically hyponatraemia with hypochloraemic metabolic alkalosis. There may be a positive family history. A high index of suspicion must be maintained in any child presenting with one or a combination of these features at any age. Affected children may go on to develop cirrhosis with portal hypertension and insulin dependent diabetes mellitus.

Cystic fibrosis is suspected in any child presenting with one or more of:

- Neonatal intestinal obstruction or neonatal obstructive jaundice
- Poor growth despite adequate intake
- steatorrhoea
- Recurrent chest infections especially with *S. aureus* or pseudomonas, bronchiectasis
- Hypochloraemic metabolic alkalosis
- Rectal prolapse
- Nasal polyps with or without a positive family history.

Diagnosis

The diagnosis is confirmed on the basis of an abnormally elevated sweat chloride, or if the child tests homozygous for two CFTR mutations. Screening for cystic fibrosis can be performed either with sweat conductivity or by detecting low faecal elastase levels.

Management

The prognosis has improved significantly over the past 20 years with aggressive management. Management includes pancreatic enzyme replacement therapy (Creon®) with all feeds, together with aggressive nutritional support and fat soluble vitamin supplementation. Referral to a specialised centre for workup and multidisciplinary management by a paediatric pulmonologist, a paediatric gastroenterologist, physiotherapist, dietician and social worker is essential to optimise care and improve survival.

Constipation and faecal impaction

Functional constipation is very common in children. In addition to hard, infrequent stools, children may complain of recurrent abdominal pain, have a poor appetite and have faecal incontinence. The cause of constipation and subsequently faecal impaction is often multifactorial. It may have been initiated by a period of voluntary stool withholding early in the child's life, when the urge to defaecate had been resisted either due to fear of pain on defaecation (from a fissure-in-ano or an episode of acute constipation); rebellion against rigorous toilet training; refusal to use public toilet facilities; or disinclination to interrupt enjoyable activities. This may be aggravated by a sedentary way of life, and poor eating habits with diets containing little natural fibre and poor fluid intake. There is progressive accumulation of stool until the rectum habituates to the stimulus of the enlarging faecal mass and the urge to defecate subsides. In severe cases there is faecal incontinence due to overflow from faecal impaction. Although most cases are functional, organic causes of constipation should be excluded by a thorough history and examination.

Important *organic causes* include Hirschsprung's disease (*see* Chapter 8, Surgical conditions of the newborn), metabolic conditions such as hypothyroidism and hypocalcaemia, anatomic malformations, neuronal intestinal dysplasia, drug ingestion and neuropathic conditions such as a tethered cord.

Physical examination

Physical examination should include an assessment of growth, an abdominal examination looking for distension and fecal masses, inspection of the rectum and perianal area and a rectal examination, as well as a thorough neurological examination. Children with functional constipation are usually well grown and appear healthy, with a soft flat abdomen but faeces may be palpable in the left iliac fossa or caecum.

Table 24.8 Constipation: Important aspects of the history and examination	
History	**Examination**
Delayed passage of meconium after birth	Growth (weight and height)
Age of onset of constipation	Thyroid, skin, hair
Diet	Spine
Painful defaecation	Tendon reflexes (ankle)
Blood on stool	Abdominal examination
Withholding behaviour	Anus (fissures, tone, skin tags, erythema)
Toilet training, toilet habit	Rectal examination (faeces in rectum, masses)
History of allergy	

Suspect an organic cause of constipation with the following:

- Delayed passage of meconium and abnormal bowel movements after birth (Hirschprung's disease)
- Explosive stool release after rectal examination
- Occult blood in stool
- Failure to thrive, abdominal distension and obstructive symptoms
- Thyromegaly
- Abnormalities of lumbosacral area and perineum and
- Abnormal neurological findings.

Investigations

No investigations are usually needed in simple functional constipation, although a straight X-ray of the abdomen in the supine position may demonstrate a large amount of faecal matter throughout the colon.

Management

Management begins with counselling and education of the child and parents about the underlying aetiology and the need for continued therapy and regular follow-up for many months.

An associated anal fissure should be treated with applications of anaesthetic creams to the anal verge.

If faecal impaction is present, initial clearance is best achieved with oral administration of large volumes of a balanced electrolyte/polyethylene glycol solution (Golytely®) or Pegicol/Movicol®), or repeated Fleet® or Microlax® enemas daily for three days. Clearance can be checked clinically and if necessary confirmed with repeat abdominal X-rays.

Preventing the re-accumulation of stool involves three steps:

- Dietary modification to increase the intake of foods rich in natural fibre (bran, fruits and vegetable), or supplementary fibre, together with increased fluid intake.
- A regular toilet regimen must be established as these children frequently do not sense the need to defecate and it takes time for normal rectal sensation to return. Reward systems like star charts can be useful adjuncts to management.
- Maintenance medication is essential, to help establish regular bowel habits. Commonly used agents include osmotic laxatives like sorbitol/lactulose , stool lubricants (mineral oil), or PEG containing products(Movicol/Pegicol®). Stimulant laxatives (Senokot® and Dulcolax®) are not usually required or recommended in children.

The aim is to first clear faecal impaction , commence maintenance therapy to soften stools and prevent re-accumulation, and to modify behaviour and diet.

Regular follow-up to ensure compliance and monitor progress is essential. Cases associated with faecal incontinence can be particularly challenging to manage and may need referral to a specialised unit

Peptic ulcer disease

The incidence of peptic ulcer disease (PUD) in children is not known but with greater use of endoscopy it is being increasingly diagnosed. Peptic ulcers can occur at any age. In infants and young children gastric ulcers predominate, while duodenal ulcers are five times more common than gastric ulcers in children over six years. The clinical features vary with the age of the patient. Younger children with PUD may feed poorly, have crying spells, or present with haematemesis, melaena or signs of gastric perforation. Children over eight years of age are more likely to complain of abdominal pain with PUD. The pain is typically epigastric, occurring two to three hours after meals and relieved by food in about 50 per cent of cases. Pain that wakes the patient at night, or is present on rising in the morning, is highly suggestive of PUD. Many patients have atypical symptoms such as poorly localized pain, anorexia or vomiting. A positive family history of PUD, particularly if in a first-degree relative, is an important diagnostic clue. Examination of the abdomen often reveals marked tenderness to deep palpation in the epigastrium. Anaemia and occult blood-positive stools are supportive findings. If the history and physical examination suggest PUD, the patient should be referred for gastroscopy. There are a number of causes for PUD in children. H. pylori infection is the most common cause. Other causes that need to be considered are: hypergastrinaemia, stress ulceration, Crohn's disease, medication (e.g. NSAIDS), and infections such as CMV (particularly in immune compromised children). Medical treatment is to inhibit gastric acid secretion (proton pump inhibitors, H_2 Receptor antagonists), to coat the ulcer base using sucralfate and to treat the underlying cause. Surgical therapy is indicated if there is perforation or uncontrolled bleeding.

Helicobacter pylori

H. pylori is a major cause of gastritis in children and is particularly prevalent in developing countries. The majority of infected individuals do not experience any symptoms and in most children, the presence of the bacterium does not lead to disease. In children symptoms of nausea, vomiting or epigastric pain are indicative of gastritis or peptic ulcer disease. Diagnostic tests for H. pylori include histology, culture, stool antigen tests, serology or the urea breath test. Treatment is triple therapy consisting of a proton pump inhibitor plus two antibiotics (clarithromycin or amoxicillin or metronidazole) for 14 days. Chronic H. pylori is associated with the development of gastric lymphoma and adenocarcinoma.

Chronic abdominal pain

Abdominal pain is a common complaint in childhood and adolescence. The differential diagnosis is wide; therefore a thorough history and physical examination should be done, taking into account the patient's age.

On history it is important to ask about the site and nature of the pain and whether it is associated with specific triggers (e.g. meals). Pain from the liver, pancreas, biliary tree, stomach and upper bowel is felt in the epigastrium; from the distal small bowel, caecum, appendix or proximal colon at the umbilicus, and pain from the distal large bowel, urinary tract or pelvic organs is usually suprapubic.

Abdominal pain may be visceral or somatic in origin. Visceral pain is caused by distension of a hollow muscular organ and somatic pain originates from the skin, muscles or parietal peritoneum. Occasionally abdominal pain can be referred from structures inside the chest.

Abdominal pain can be divided into acute onset abdominal pain or chronic abdominal pain. Chronic abdominal pain is either due to pathological or functional disorders. One of the challenges in managing these children is distinguishing between those children with a functional disorder and those with an identifiable organic disease.

Aetiology

There are many causes of chronic or recurrent episodes of abdominal pain in childhood (*see* Table 24.9). Constipation is one of the most common conditions presenting with abdominal pain, but in the remainder, an organic cause for chronic abdominal pain is seldom found. These children suffer from a functional disorder.

Functional disorders

Functional gastrointestinal disorders are gastrointestinal symptoms that can not be explained by structural or biochemical abnormalities. The diagnosis relies on an assessment of symptoms and exclusion of other disorders.

Typically children between 5 and 14 years of age are affected. To fulfill the criteria, symptoms must be present at least once per week for at least two months in the absence of evidence of an inflammatory, anatomic, metabolic, or neoplastic process that explains the symptoms.

Table 24.9 Causes of recurrent episodes of abdominal pain

Disorder	Symptoms	Evaluation
Nonorganic		
Functional abdominal pain	Periumbilical	History and examination
GI Tract		
Faecal loading/constipation	Stool retention, evidence of constipation	History and examination, Abdominal XRay
Parasitic infection (ascaris,giardia)	Bloating, gas, cramps, diarrhoea	Stool microscopy, immunoassay
Infection (abdominal TB, yersinia)	Distension, vague abdominal pain	Ultrasound abdomen
Lactose intolerance	Bloating, gas, cramps, diarrhoea on exposure to lactose	Trial of lactose free diet, lactose breath hydrogen test
Peptic ulcer	Burning or gnawing epigastric pain, worse on awakening or before meals, relieved with antacids	Gastroscopy or upper GI contrast studies
Oesophagitis	Epigastric pain, substernal burning	Gastroscopy
Excess fructose or sorbitol ingestion	Bloating, gas, diarrhoea	History of large intake of apples, fruit juice or chewing gum
Crohn's disease	Cramps, bloody stools	Colonoscopy
Meckel's diverticulum	Periumbilical or lower abdominal pain, may have blood in the stool	Meckel scan
Recurrent intussusception	Paroxysmal severe cramping, abdominal pain, blood may be present in stool	Contrast studies, ultrasound
Internal, inguinal, abdominal wall hernia	Dull abdomen, abdominal wall pain	Physical examination, CT of abdominal wall
Chronic appendicitis, appendiceal mucocele	Recurrent right lower quadrant pain	Barium enema, CT
Gallbladder and pancreas		
Cholelithiasis	RUQ pain, may worsen with meals	Ultrasound of gallbladder
		continued

In addition to pain, other symptoms may be present: headache, pallor, nausea, dizziness, fatigue and low grade fever.

The family history is strongly positive for functional disorder, including spastic colon, irritable bowel syndrome, anxiety attacks, mental disorders and migraine. These children are usually well grown and appear healthy. The abdomen is not distended and soft to palpation. Examination of the other systems is normal.

Diagnosis

A full blood count, ESR, urine analysis and stool analysis for parasites and occult blood are done,

Table 24.9 Causes of recurrent episodes of abdominal pain *continued*		
Disorder	**Symptoms**	**Evaluation**
Choledochal cyst	RUQ pain, mass + or − increased bilirubin	Ultrasound or CT
Recurrent pancreatitis	Persistent boring pain may radiate to back, vomiting	Serum amylase and lipase, trypsinogen, ultrasound
Genitourinary tract		
UTI	Suprapubic or flank pain	Urinalysis, culture, renal ultrasound
Hydronephrosis	Unilateral abdominal pain, flank pain	Renal ultrasound
Urolithiasis	Severe pain, flank to inguinal region	Urinalysis, ultrasound, IVP, CT
Miscellaneous causes		
Abdominal migraine	Nausea, family history of migraine	History
Abdominal epilepsy	May have seizure prodrome	EEG
Gilbert Syndrome	Mild abdominal pain, slightly elevated unconjugated bilirubin	Serum bilirubin
Sickle cell crisis	Anaemia	Haematologic evaluation
Familial Mediterranean Fever	Paroxysmal episodes of fever, severe abdominal pain and tenderness with other evidence of polyserositis	History and examination DNA diagnosis
Lead poisoning	Vague abdominal pain, constipation	Blood lead level
Henoch-Schönlein purpura	Recurrent severe crampy abdominal pain, occult blood positive, purpura and arthritis	History and examination, urinalysis
Angioneurotic oedema	Swelling of face or airway, crampy pain	History and examination Upper GI contrast studies Serum C1 esterase inhibitor
Acute intermittent porphyria	Precipitated by drugs, fasting or infections	Urine spot test for porphyrins

Functional disorders associated with abdominal pain are

- Functional dyspepsia
- Irritable bowel syndrome
- Childhood functional abdominal pain
- Abdominal migraine.

but unnecessary investigations increase parental and patient fears and therefore should be kept to a minimum.

Negative investigations and a suggestive history and examination should lead to a firm diagnosis. Features that should alert the physician to the possibility of an organic disorder for the pain are listed in Table 24.10.

Management

It is essential to reassure the patient and the parents that no serious organic pathology exists. Medications have very little place in the management. Some patients benefit from dietary modification which includes increasing the dietary fibre.

Table 24.10 Features suggesting an organic cause abdominal pain

Age of onset: <5 years or >14 years of age
Pain localization: away from umbilicus
Nocturnal pain
Food intake aggravates or relieves pain
Associated features: fever, arthralgia, rash, jaundice
Loss of appetite, weight loss
Alteration in bowel habit
Positive family history of peptic ulcer or inflammatory bowel disease
Abdominal distension, mass or visceromegaly
Faecal soiling
Anal skin tags
Occult blood positive stool

With firm reassurance by the physician symptoms resolve in 30–50 per cent of children within six weeks of presentation.

Parasitic infestations

Ascaris infestation may cause abdominal pain either by bowel obstruction or by migration of a worm up the biliary tract.

Giardiasis is usually described as a diffuse discomfort. It may be accompanied by anorexia, nausea, abdominal distension and diarrhoea. Symptoms may fluctuate in severity and even disappear for variable periods of time.

Inflammmatory bowel disease (IBD)

Inflammatory bowel disease is a heterogeneous group of diseases of which ulcerative colitis and Crohn's disease are the major forms. Although the aetiology is poorly understood, genetic and environmental factors seem to be involved in the pathogenesis. Although both these conditions occur more frequently in adolescents and young adults, they may also occur in young children.

The presenting symptoms include abdominal pain, anorexia, weight loss, diarrhoea and blood in the stool. Often this is initially mistakenly diagnosed as an infectious colitis. Extra-intestinal symptoms are often present, particularly in children with Crohn's Disease. These include arthritis, arthralgia, rash, fever, and lethargy. Anaemia and a raised ESR are also associated. The clinical course is characterised by exacerbations and remissions.

Crohn's disease involves any part of the gastrointestinal tract, with involvement of the terminal ileum and colon being the most common. Involvement is segmental with disease-free areas between the involved mucosa. Important complications include fistula formation (including peri-anal fistula) and intestinal strictures.

Ulcerative colitis involves the colon. Involvement of the colon is continuous, extending from the rectum proximally for a varying length.

In a small proportion of patients the colitis cannot be categorised as ulcerative colitis or Crohn's disease, these patients are said to have indeterminate colitis.

The diagnosis is often delayed, particularly in children with Crohn's disease, due to the subtlety of the initial presentation. Clinicians should consider the diagnosis in children presenting with chronic abdominal pain, abnormal stools, or unexplained failure to thrive.

The diagnosis does not rely on a single investigation, rather it depends on

- The presence of a compatible clinical presentation
- Suggestive radiological examination
- Endoscopic appearance
- Mucosal histology.

in the absence of other causes of chronic intestinal inflammation. In particular, intestinal tuberculosis and HIV infection should be considered in developing countries. Serological investigations (pANCA and ASCA) may have some value as screening tests. They can however not replace more invasive investigations.

Inflammatory bowel disease is a chronic disease that requires multidisciplinary management involving the primary care physician, gastroenterologist, dietician, psychiatrist or psychologist, social worker and surgeon. The aims of treatment are to control symptoms, to optimise growth and development, encourage normal social development, to prevent complications of the disease and to avoid side-effects of treatment.

Nutritional support is an important aspect of the treatment as most of these children have some degree of malnutrition at presentation. Exclusive enteral nutrition has been used to induce remission in children with Crohn's disease. Occasionally children will require parenteral nutrition for a few weeks.

Drug therapy is with aminosalicylates, immunosuppressive agents (e.g. steroids, azathioprine and methotrexate), immune modulating drugs (e.g. infliximab) and antibiotics. Surgery is indicated for complications such as intestinal obstruction in Crohn's disease and uncontrolled ulcerative colitis.

Table 24.11 Comparison of Crohn's disease and ulcerative colitis

Feature	Crohn's disease	Ulcerative colitis
Rectal disease	Occasional	Common
Abdominal mass	Common	Not present
Ileal involvement	Common	None (backwash ileitis)
Perianal disease	Common	Unusual
Strictures	Common	Unusual
Fistula	Common	Unusual
Transmural involvement	Common	Unusual
Crypt abscesses	Less common	Common
Granulomas	Common	Unusual
Risk of colonic cancer	Slightly increased	Greatly increased

25

Respiratory tract disorders

> The most important clinical sign of significant respiratory disease is tachypnoea. Respiratory distress is the name given to the subjective sensation of inadequate oxygenation.

A careful history often leads to the correct diagnosis. In children, special attention must be given to a history of contact with an adult with active tuberculosis (TB), parental smoking, recurrent infections suggesting immune deficiency, overcrowded and polluted surroundings, nutritional status, feeding difficulties (aspiration pneumonia), parental asthma or atopy, and the infant's birth weight.

Apart from acute respiratory infection, which can happen at any age, the age of onset is a useful indicator of the cause of respiratory disease. Acute airway obstruction present from birth indicates a congenital airway problem, while in the three- to four-month-old age group acute viral bronchiolitis is more likely and in the two- to three-year age group asthma is the most likely diagnosis.

The most common respiratory symptoms and signs among children are described in the following sections.

Cough

The characteristic of the cough is often a clue as to where the pathology is located. A barking cough is indicative of subglottic pathology, while a brassy cough indicates tracheal compression. The timing of the cough may also help in the diagnosis. If a child coughs soon after being put to bed, this indicates upper airway pathology with a postnasal drip. A child with asthma wakes coughing early in the morning or coughs after exercise. Children with asthma often have a wheezy cough. A productive cough with a copious amount of purulent sputum is indicative of bronchiectasis. A paroxysmal cough with an inspiratory whoop is suggestive of whooping cough (pertussis).

Cough may also be a referred symptom of pathology elsewhere (via the vagus nerve) and a psychogenic symptom (often called a 'honking cough').

Chronic cough

A cough that lasts for longer than 14 days is regarded as a chronic cough. The cough is a symptom of an underlying disease and therefore should not be suppressed if the cause has not been determined. (*See* Table 25.11.)

Tachypnoea

The respiratory rate of small children is faster than that of older children and adults. When respiratory disease occurs the respiratory rate increases because small children are not able to increase their tidal volume. It is more efficient for them to increase their minute volume by increasing their respiratory rate. For this reason tachypnoea is a very sensitive sign of respiratory disease. Tachypnoea is defined as a respiratory rate of greater than 60 breaths per minute in a child under three months of age, greater than 50 between three months and one year of age, and greater than 40 for children between one and five years of age. The respiratory rate must be counted for a full minute when the child is at rest and not feeding, as children are inclined to breathe periodically, especially when they are upset. It is important to note that a slower than normal rate may reflect deterioration, pre-apnoea, or some central nervous system disease or metabolic disorder.

Wheeze

A wheezy chest is a common complaint and sign. Wheezing can be the result of either small or large airway disease. Small airways obstruction is distinguished from large airway obstruction by the fact that the wheeze is not as prominent (best heard with a stethoscope), and the presence of associated crackles and airtrapping giving rise to a hyperinflated barrel-shaped chest. The most common small airway disease is acute viral bronchiolitis. In large airway obstruction, the wheeze is normally so loud that it can easily be heard without a stethoscope and is often audible in both inspiration and expiration.

Stridor

Stridor is most easily heard as a high pitched sound during inspiration, but as the obstruction becomes more severe it is audible in both inspiration and expiration. The high-pitched inspiratory sound is mostly the result of extrathoracic airway obstruction. Croup is the most common cause of stridor.

Crackles

These are interrupted sounds associated with the movement of air through inflammatory secretions within the airways or air spaces. They are usually associated with airway conditions such as bronchiolitis, bronchopneumonia or other causes of interstitial and alveolar disease, e.g. lobar pneumonia, cardiac failure.

Chest wall and sternal retraction

When there is severe respiratory disease, rib and sternal retraction occur. This is due to the decreased compliance of the chest wall in small children. Rib and sternal retraction occur with extensive alveolar disease and airway obstruction. Another feature of the compliant chest wall is that severe chest trauma can occur without any rib fractures being present. Subcostal and lower costal retractions are a result of a

Table 25.1 Normal respiratory rates (RR) for children

Age	RR
Neonates	40–50
Infants	25–40
1–5 years	20–30
5–10 years	15–25
10–16 years	15–20

flattened diaphragm, which, when present for a prolonged period, results in a groove called Harrison's sulcus.

Clubbing of the fingers

Clubbing of the fingers indicates, among other conditions, the presence of suppurative lung disease, lymphocytic interstitial pneumonia which is associated with HIV disease, cyanotic congenital heart disease, or infective endocarditis. Bronchiectasis, the most common suppurative lung disease in children, is a common cause of chronic pulmonary symptoms in under-privileged children.

Chest wall deformity

A barrel- or funnel-shaped chest, marked Harrison's sulcus, and rounded high shoulders all indicate chronic airway obstruction, the most common cause being untreated or poorly treated asthma.

Respiratory distress and failure

This refers to a constellation of clinical symptoms and signs that include tachypnoea, chest recession, grunting, use of accessory neck muscles, alae nasi flaring, and cyanosis. It is graded into mild, moderate, or severe based on the magnitude of these signs. Restlessness, agitation, drowsiness, pallor, or central cyanosis give an indication of the severity of deranged gas exchange. These signs indicate severe hypoxia and that requires immediate supplemental oxygen. Hypercapnoea results in bounding pulses and peripheral vaso-dilatation. Pulsus paradoxus, the exaggerated fall in systemic arterial pressure on inspiration, occurs during severe airway obstruction and is a useful sign in determining the severity of asthma and croup.

Acute respiratory infection (ARI)

Acute respiratory infections (ARIs) are the leading cause of death in children living in the developing world. In South Africa, ARIs are responsible for 20 per cent of the deaths under the age of five years. Of these, acute pneumonia is responsible for about 90 per cent of the fatalities. The death rate from ARI in black children is as much as 270 times higher than that of white children in certain areas, but that of white and Asian children in South Africa is still seven times higher than that of children in the developed world.

ARI is responsible for between 20-60 per cent of all out-patient visits and 12-45 per cent of hospital admissions of children.

The upper respiratory tract (*See* Chapter 34, Disorders of the ear, nose, and throat) is separated from the lower respiratory tract by the base of the epiglottis. Common respiratory infections and their aetiology are shown in Table 25.2.

It is normal for a child to develop six to eight respiratory tract infections per annum for the first two to three years of life. The majority of these infections involve only the upper respiratory tract with rhinitis being the most common infection. The lower respiratory tract is also involved in about 20-30 per cent of the upper respiratory infections, the most common being bronchitis, pneumonia and bronchiolitis.

Factors that influence the incidence of respiratory tract infections include:

♦ **Breastfeeding and early weaning**. There is a decreased incidence of ARI and case fatality rate from pneumonia in breastfed children, while early weaning is associated with increased incidence and mortality from ARI. Prolonged breastfeeding decreases the incidence of atopy.

♦ **Poor nutritional status**. Pneumonia is 12 times more common in malnourished than well-nourished children. Vitamin A deficiency and low birth weight also increase the incidence and the mortality.

♦ **Poor socio-economic status**. Poverty, overcrowding, and the indoor use of wood or coal fires for heating and cooking.

♦ **HIV incidence**. HIV-infected infants have an increased incidence of both usual and unusual respiratory tract infections.

♦ **Immunization**. Up to 25 per cent of the deaths from respiratory disease can be prevented by immunizing against measles, diphtheria, pertussis, *Haemophilus influenzae*, *Streptococcus pneumoniae*, and administering BCG vaccination.

> ARI mortality is highest in children under two years of age who are severely malnourished, HIV infected, weaned early, and whose parents do not have easy access to health care.

Table 25.2 Acute respiratory tract infections

	Diagnosis	Common aetiology
Upper respiratory tract	Rhinitis	Viral
	Otitis media	Bacterial (*S. pneumoniae*; *H. influenzae*)
	Tonsillitis	Bacterial (β-Haemolytic streptococcus)
	Pharyngitis	Bacterial (Streptococcus)
	Sinusitis	Viral
		Bacterial (*S. pneumoniae*; *H. influenzae*)
Lower respiratory tract	Laryngotracheo-bronchitis	Viral (para-influenza, measles)
	Tracheobronchitis	Viral
	Bronchiolitis	Viral (RSV)
	Pneumonia	Bacterial and viral (*H. influenzae*; *S. pneumoniae*)

- **Parental smoking**. The number and seriousness of pneumonia, bronchiolitis, and asthma attacks are increased in children who passively inhale tobacco smoke.
- **Parasitic infection**. The inflammatory changes in the lung associated with the pulmonary migration of ascaris larvae predispose to bacterial superinfection.
- **Structural abnormalities** such as congenital cysts or sequestration make children more susceptible to respiratory tract infections.
- **Rainy and cold weather** is associated with an increased incidence of acute respiratory infections.

Airway obstruction

Obstruction of the airway can occur at many levels in the airways. It is clinically classified into extrathoracic and intrathoracic airway

Respiratory illnesses are serious and require immediate attention in the following situations:

- Under two months of age
- Depressed level of consciousness
- Stridor when calm
- Severe malnutrition
- Associated symptomatic HIV/AIDS.

obstruction. Extrathoracic airway obstruction is characterized by the clinical finding of inspiratory stridor and intrathoracic obstruction by the presence of an expiratory wheeze. When critical or fixed airway obstruction is present then the stridor or wheeze is heard in both inspiration and expiration. (*see* Figure 25.1).

Extrathoracic airway obstruction can be caused by either acute disease or chronic anatomical abnormalities. (*See* Table 25.3)

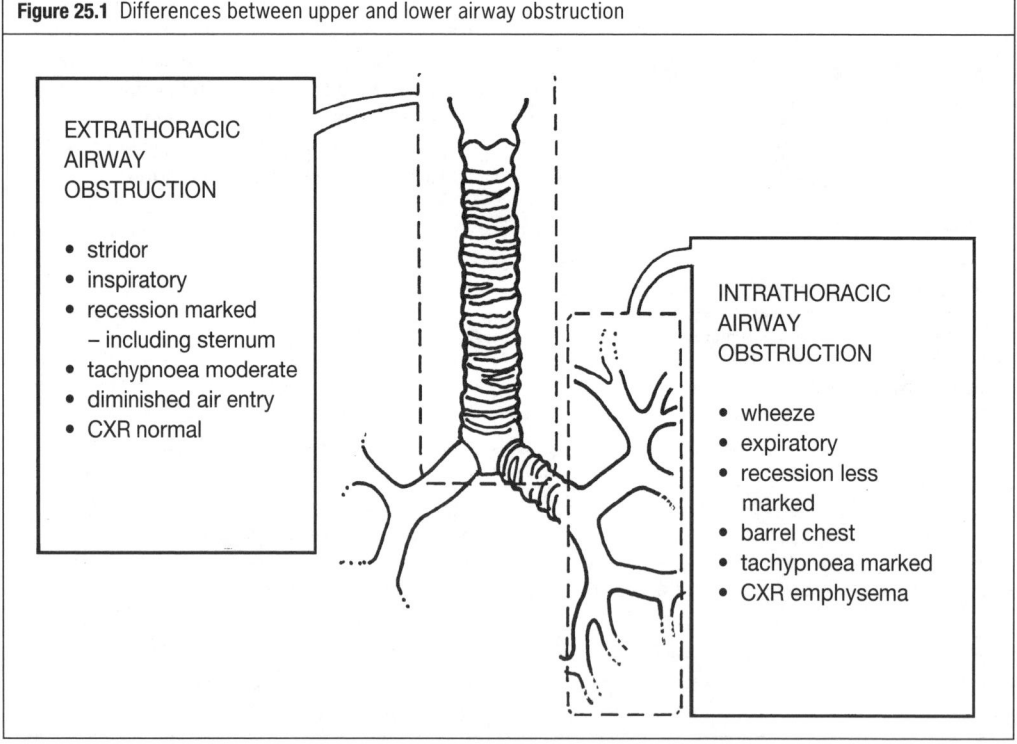

Figure 25.1 Differences between upper and lower airway obstruction

EXTRATHORACIC AIRWAY OBSTRUCTION

- stridor
- inspiratory
- recession marked
  – including sternum
- tachypnoea moderate
- diminished air entry
- CXR normal

INTRATHORACIC AIRWAY OBSTRUCTION

- wheeze
- expiratory
- recession less marked
- barrel chest
- tachypnoea marked
- CXR emphysema

Table 25.3 Common causes of upper airway obstruction

	Condition
Acute	*Infectious* Laryngo-tracheo-bronchitis Epiglottitis Bacterial tracheitis Retropharyngeal abscess Paratracheal gland enlargement *Mechanical* Foreign body *Allergic* Angioneurotic oedema *Trauma* Intubation injury Thermal injury
Chronic	*Congenital* Laryngomalacia Laryngeal cysts *Infectious* Laryngeal papillomatosis Hypertrophy of tonsils and adenoids *Trauma* Subglottic stenosis

Causes of acute upper airway obstruction

Acute laryngo-tracheo-bronchitis (croup)

Acute laryngo-tracheo-bronchitis (LTB) is the most common cause of stridor in children between six months and two years. It is almost always caused by viral infections, most commonly parainfluenza viruses. In developing countries, measles and Herpes simplex infection of the larynx are still common causes of severe croup. Herpes simplex virus infection of the larynx is difficult to diagnose as only about 50 per cent of these children have herpetiform lesions in their mouths. HIV infected children often have additional causes of acute upper airway obstruction which includes oropharyngeal candidiasis and tuberculosis.

Clinical picture. Two to three days after an acute upper respiratory tract infection the child develops stridor with a characteristic bark-like cough and a hoarse voice. The child is not febrile and does not appear toxically ill. As the upper airway obstruction (UAO) worsens, the stridor is heard in expiration, the patient develops a pulsus paradoxus and uses its abdominal muscles during expiration to overcome the airway obstruction. With severe airway obstruction the child becomes hypoxic which results in tachycardia, restlessness, and confusion. Severe exhaustion from the work of breathing can result in the stridor being less prominent with no decrease in the airway obstruction. This is an ominous sign and requires immediate attention.

Treatment is instituted according to the grading system of Klein (*see* Table 25.4). It should be stressed that this grading is only applicable to acute LTB. A child with grade 2 or worse airway obstruction should be transferred to a hospital where nebulized adrenaline can be administered.

- Nebulized adrenaline (1:1 000 solution 1 ml in 1 ml saline) should be repeated every 20 to 30 minutes.
- Parenteral steroids (dexamethasone 0.6 mg/kg as a single dose or prednisone 1–2 mg/kg as a single dose) are of benefit to children with grade 2 or worse stridor but are contraindicated in children with measles and herpes LTB.

Table 25.4 Acute laryngo-tracheo-bronchitis: grading and treatment

Grade	Criteria	Treatment
Grade 1	Inspiratory stridor	Observe
Grade 2	Inspiratory and expiratory stridor	Nebulized adrenaline
Grade 3	Inspiratory and expiratory stridor and pulsus paradoxus	Continuous nebulized adrenaline; if no improvement, intubate
Grade 4	Impending apnoea	Intubate

♦ Nebulized steroids are of equal benefit but are expensive.

Children with grade 3 stridor should be referred to a hospital where nasotracheal intubation or tracheotomy can be performed. Children with grade 3 and 4 obstruction should be intubated immediately before transfer to a hospital where high care is available. Nasotracheal intubation is the treatment of choice.

No child with uncomplicated LTB should be denied intubation due to lack of ICU facilities as the overall prognosis is excellent with a short duration of illness (five days). Herpes LTB requires a longer duration of intubation and needs to be treated with acyclovir for 14 days.

LTB is a more severe condition with a higher mortality rate in the developing world compared with that in developed communities because:

♦ The obstruction is severe enough to warrant relief by intubation in a larger percentage of cases.
♦ A significantly greater number of cases have coexisting lower respiratory tract infections that are probably related to immunodepression from malnutrition, HIV disease, measles and iron deficiency anaemia.

Acute bacterial epiglottitis

This is an uncommon cause of airway obstruction but the mortality is extremely high if the disease is not immediately recognized. It occurs mainly in two- to five-year-old children and is mostly caused by *H. influenzae B*.

Clinical picture. This is an acute *H. influenzae* infection of the supraglottic region leading to severe dysphagia, drooling, and airway obstruction. The patients have a high fever and are toxic due to the accompanying septicaemia. The airway patency is protected by sitting in a characteristic tripod position with the head forward, the cervical spine held straight, and the upper bodies supported with the arms. Any disturbance of this position during examination of the throat or positioning the child for neck radiographs can lead to immediate complete airway obstruction.

Acute epiglottitis is a medical emergency.

The characteristic 'cherry red' swollen epiglottis confirms the diagnosis but is not always readily visible. Further examination must then be avoided as complete airway obstruction may be precipitated. A lateral neck radiograph shows a swollen epiglottis and aryepiglottal folds giving the appearance of a 'hitch-hiker's thumb'. The hypopharynx is overdistended with air and the cervical vertebrae held in a straight position.

As soon as the diagnosis is suspected, the child must be moved to an area where intubation and resuscitation can be performed under conditions optional for that facility. The causative organism can be isolated from a blood culture or throat swab which should only be taken after the child has been intubated.

Management. Nasotracheal intubation is carried out under general anaesthesia. If facilities are inadequate to ensure that the tube will remain in position, a tracheotomy is a safer procedure. If the child's airway obstructs before intubation, adequate ventilation can be achieved by positive pressure ventilation with a resuscitation bag.

Amoxycillin (200 mg/kg/d IV) or ceftriaxone (100 mg/kg/d) should be started immediately. The oedema normally subsides quickly and most of the children can be safely extubated after 36 to 48 hours.

Foreign body aspiration

Foreign body aspiration is suspected when a healthy child suddenly develops stridor and severe airway obstruction requiring immediate therapy. If life-threatening airway obstruction is present and the foreign body can not be removed by a Heimlich manoeuvre, or by placing the child over the knee and giving a few hard thumps on the back, the child must be intubated immediately and the foreign body forced into one of the bronchi. This relieves the laryngeal obstruction and the child can be transported safely to a hospital where bronchoscopy can be performed to remove the obstruction.

Oesophageal foreign bodies also cause stridor by displacing the tracheo-oesophageal membrane anteriorly into the lumen of the trachea.

Retropharyngeal abscess

Lymph nodes in the prevertebral space drain the nasopharynx and posterior nasal passages. Abscess formation in these glands can lead to obstruction of the upper airways. The child is toxic, has dysphagia, hyperextension of the head, noisy breathing, and enlarged submandibular and cervical glands. On examination of the throat, the large retropharyngeal mass is visible. This can be confirmed on a lateral neck radiograph with the distance between the anterior vertebral body wall and the air column increased. Treatment is by broad-spectrum antibiotics and surgical drainage of the abscess under general anaesthesia.

Bacterial tracheitis

Severe infection of the trachea by *S. aureus,* or *H. influenzae* can lead to variable airway obstruction with stridor. The child has a high fever and coughs up large amounts of tenacious, yellow sputum. The treatment of choice is intravenous amoxycillin (200 mg/kg/d) and cloxacillin (100 mg/kg/d). Intubation might be required. In a child who has not been immunized, diphtheria should be suspected.

Subglottic oedema after intubation

The cricoid, the only complete cartilage ring in the airway, is the narrowest part in a child's airway. The cricoid is often injured during intubation if an inappropriately large endotracheal tube is used. This can be prevented if an endotracheal tube of the correct size is used; always ensure that a small air leak is present immediately after intubation. If an air leak is not present, a smaller tube is required.

Causes of persistent upper airway obstruction

Laryngomalacia

The most common cause of upper airway obstruction that occurs in the first month of life is laryngomalacia. The stridor has a typical sound, often referred to as cogwheel stridor, which is often less prominent if the child is nursed prone. Laryngomalacia is due to prominent aryepiglottal tissue which is sucked into the laryngeal opening during inspiration, causing the obstruction. The stridor is more prominent during fever or activity. The stridor becomes less audible as the first year of life progresses and in the majority of cases is no longer audible after one year. The diagnosis is confirmed by laryngoscopy. In the vast majority of cases no further intervention is required.

Vocal cord palsy

Unilateral vocal cord palsy is common in children with hydrocephalus and raised intracranial pressure. The diagnosis is confirmed by direct laryngoscopy.

Subglottic stenosis

In children intubated with a too large an endotracheal tube or ventilated for a prolonged period of time, necrosis of the mucosa occurs in the subglottic region, which heals by fibrosis, leading to narrowing of the subglottic region. The obstruction can become progressively more severe, requiring a tracheostomy. The diagnosis is confirmed by bronchoscopy and needs complicated surgical correction.

Laryngeal papillomatosis

Warty tumours may grow in any portion of the larynx and usually involve the vocal cords. Airway obstruction may occur, especially if viral upper respiratory infection is superimposed. These symptoms are usually preceded by a period of hoarseness or aphonia. These lesions occur more commonly in HIV Infected children. They require laser treatment to remove them, but may re-occur after treatment.

Obstructive sleep apnoea

Snoring in children is abnormal and is mostly the result of upper airway obstruction. In some children this obstruction is so severe that they have apnoeic spells. The mother often reports this as snoring followed by a period of silence after which the child wakes up. As a result of the obstruction the child hypoventilates, this results in the arterial pCO_2 rising and the pO_2 to fall. The resulting hypoxia causes pulmonary arterial vasoconstriction leading to pulmonary hypertension and in some cases congestive cardiac failure. The diagnosis is made by observing the sleeping child. The snoring can be seen to be followed by a period in which the child attempts to breath but there is no air movement. The most common causes of sleep apnoea are enlarged tonsils and adenoids.

Treatment. If there is substantial obstruction, low flow (0.5 to 2.0 l/min) oxygen delivered by means of a thin nasopharyngeal tube can often relieve the obstruction (Constant Inflation of the Pharanyx (CIP)). Tonsillectomy and adenoidectomy often correct the problem.

Intrathoracic airway obstruction

Lower airway obstruction is characterized by expiratory wheezing and caused by obstruction of either the small (bronchioles) or larger airways (*see* Table 25.5). Small airway obstruction is characterized by airtrapping which presents with a barrel chest, decreased cardiac dullness, downward displacement of the liver and an expiratory wheeze audible with a stethoscope. In large airway obstruction, by contrast, the wheeze is so prominent that it is heard without the aid of a stethoscope and air trapping is less prominent. The most common cause of lower airway obstruction in children less than one year is acute viral bronchiolitis, while asthma is the most common cause in older children.

Wheezing in children

About 50 per cent of children wheeze during the first three years of life. In 30 per cent of children the wheezing only occurs in the first three years of life and then disappears. These children are more likely to be low-birth-weight infants born to mothers who smoke. It has been shown that they have decreased lung function and wheeze during viral infections. Those that continue to wheeze after three years of age, or begin wheezing then, are more likely to have asthma.

Causes of lower airway obstruction

Acute viral bronchiolitis

Respiratory syncytial virus (RSV), a paramyxovirus, is the most important cause of respiratory tract infection in infants up to two years of age. It has a peak incidence in children between three and four months of age in developed countries

and a few months later in developing countries. Children particularly at risk include preterm infants and children with congenital heart or chronic lung disease. Transmission is via droplet spread. The incubation period is about three to seven days and children remain infectious for about a week after the symptoms subside. Annual epidemics occur in winter. About 50 per cent of susceptible infants contract their primary infection in each epidemic. Reinfection can occur and RSV is also a common cause of nosocomial infections in hospital.

RSV infection causes mucosal oedema and epithelial desquamation of the bronchioli which lead to small airway obstruction, increased airway resistance and air trapping. Adenovirus bronchiolitis is also common in poor communities.

Clinical picture. The disease starts with an upper respiratory tract infection (URTI), especially if other family members have a cold. The child develops a cough, tachypnoea, a low-grade fever, and in severe cases feeding difficulties.

On examination the child has a barrel chest as a result of air trapping, widespread expiratory wheeze, and bilateral crackles. Only children with severe tachypnoea (>50/minute), chest wall indrawing or feeding difficulties require admission to hospital. Severe airway obstruction resolves within three to five days.

The **diagnosis** is clinical, with the identification of the virus of little practical importance. Definitive diagnosis can be made by culture of RSV from nasopharyngeal aspirates or detection of antigen by ELISA or immunofluorescent tests (IFAT). A chest radiograph is useful in excluding other causes of airway obstruction but is not routinely indicated. The radiological picture of acute bronchiolitis is that of air trapping as illustrated by flat diaphragms and air visible in the retrosternal space on a lateral chest radiograph. Mucous plugging can cause segmental and lobar collapse which is often confused with the radiological picture of broncho- or lobar pneumonia. The severity can be determined by establishing the transcutaneous oxygen saturation.

The **treatment** is supportive:
- Supplemental oxygen is given to prevent hypoxia.
- Fluids are given per mouth or nasogastric tube except in the tachypnoeic children.

Table 25.5 Intrathoracic airway obstruction	
Large airways	**Small airways**
Foreign body inhalation	Acute viral bronchiolitis
TB gland obstruction	Asthma
Congenital	Pneumonia with
abnormalities	eosinophilia
Anomalous artery	Aspiration pneumonia
Bronchogenic cyst	Cardiac failure
Tracheomalacia	Cystic fibrosis
	Bronchiectasis

Intravenous fluid is restricted to 60 ml/kg/d due to inappropriate ADH secretion.

- A trial with nebulized adrenaline or β_2-agonists is warranted as 30 per cent of children treated with these drugs improve. Nebulization is discontinued in those who do not respond.
- Steroids are controversial and generally not helpful.
- Antibiotics are not indicated unless:
  - white cell count is >15.0 × 10^9/l
  - temperature is >38.5 °C
  - there is patchy opacification on a chest radiograph.
- Ventilation for respiratory failure (this rarely occurs).

Prevention. RSV immunoglobulin prophylaxis on a monthly basis has been shown to be effective in reducing the risk of disease in at-risk children. Mostly restricted to high risk premature babies less than 34 weeks gestational age. However, such therapy is expensive. No vaccine is available.

Long-term sequelae. About 50 per cent of the children will have further attacks of lower airway obstruction which in most cases respond to bronchodilators.

Bronchiolitis obliterans develops in a proportion following adenovirus infection. These children remain symptomatic for months after the acute attack with constant expiratory wheezing and bilateral crackles. The chest radiograph shows air trapping with perihilar streaking. Some children present with repeated attacks of pneumonia. The diagnosis can be confirmed by means of a chest computer tomogram which demonstrates areas of air trapping. These children sometimes respond to oral prednisone (1 mg/kg/d), inhaled steroids, and bronchodilators. In certain cases bronchiolitis obliterans leads to bronchiectasis.

Asthma

Asthma is very common in children and often underdiagnosed. Asthma should be considered in all children with recurrent airway obstruction especially if the obstruction is relieved by a bronchodilator or the parents have asthma or are atopic. (*See* Chapter 20, Allergic disorders.)

Cardiac failure

(*See also* Chapter 28, Cardiovascular disorders.)

Children, especially those younger than two years, with left-sided cardiac failure may present with expiratory wheezing which results from bronchial mucosal oedema causing increased airway resistance. Narrowing of the left main bronchus by an enlarged left atrium may contribute to the expiratory wheeze. Alveolar opacification as a result of lung oedema is difficult to differentiate from pneumonia.

Cystic fibrosis

Cystic fibrosis (CF) is one of the most common genetic defects in Caucasian children, occurring in 1:2 000 live births. The most common gene deletion occurs at position 508 on chromosome 7, but is uncommon in the developing world. A variety of other mutations occurs in black African children and may be responsible for a somewhat different phenotype. The chronic respiratory symptoms usually start in the first year of life but this can be considerably delayed. There is persistent cough, recurring pneumonia, chronic upper respiratory tract infections, chronic sinusitis and chronic airway obstruction. Eventually, bronchiectasis develops as a result of recurrent *P. aeruginosa* and *S. aureus* infections. Accompanying or preceding the respiratory symptoms, these children develop malabsorption due to pancreatic insufficiency. They have bulky, foul-smelling stools containing large amounts of fat. Neonates may present with prolonged neonatal jaundice due to obstruction of the biliary tree by viscid secretions, or with meconium ileus and neonatal constipation or intestinal obstruction.

The **diagnosis** is confirmed by a positive sweat test (>60 mmol/l chloride) or demonstration of one of the genetic deletions.

The **treatment** of CF is specialized and it is therefore advisable to refer the child to a specialized unit. The cornerstones of treatment are: regular home chest physiotherapy with postural drainage, aggressive treatment of respiratory tract infections, pancreatic enzyme replacement, high calorie and high protein diets, vitamin supplementation, immunization against infections, and education of the parents and children. New developments in prophylactic treatment (nebu-

Consider cystic fibrosis in any child who fails to thrive or has recurrent respiratory symptoms.

lized tobramicin) are receiving more attention in an attempt to decrease lung damage.

The pulmonary disease is progressive, leading to chronic respiratory failure and cor pulmonale. The mean survival of patients in cystic fibrosis clinics has increased to over 30 years. This increase in survival means that physicians looking after adult patients also need to be knowledgeable about CF care.

Foreign body inhalation

Although children of all ages inhale foreign bodies it is most common in boys under the age of three years. The typical history is that of a healthy child who choked while playing, started coughing, turned blue, and was short of breath for a period of time. The classical clinical triad of unilateral wheeze, decreased unilateral ventilation, and lung collapse is found in the minority only. The most common clinical sign is an area of decreased ventilation over a lung or lobe of the lung. A normal physical examination does not exclude the diagnosis.

Radiology. Only 10–30 per cent of foreign bodies are radio-opaque. Indirect evidence of foreign body aspiration is lobar collapse, lobar hyperinflation, and decreased vasculature in a lung as a result of hypoxic vasoconstriction. Further evidence of foreign body aspiration is obtained if there is no difference in the volume of a lung on radiographs taken in inspiration and expiration due to a ball valve effect causing the air trapping. A normal chest radiograph does not exclude foreign body inhalation.

Treatment. Rigid bronchoscopy is essential for diagnostic and therapeutic reasons. All children

---

Foreign body inhalation should be considered in the differential diagnosis of the following clinical pictures:

- Stridor not responding to therapy
- Asthma not responding to bronchodilators
- Pneumonia not responding to treatment
- Repeated episodes of pneumonia occurring in the same lobe
- Unexplained respiratory failure of sudden onset
- Chronic cough
- Unexplained lobar collapse
- Localized bronchiectasis.

---

suspected of inhaling a foreign body should undergo bronchoscopy.

Pneumonia

Pneumonia is a common serious respiratory infection. In the developing world it is the most common cause of death in children under five years of age. In developed countries childhood pneumonia is mostly caused by viral infections and has a low morbidity and mortality. On the other hand, in developing communities bacteria and now *Pneumocystis jirovecii* are responsible for about 65 per cent of pneumonia cases.

Many children who develop pneumonia will be diagnosed and treated in a clinic. Therefore a system of classification and management of acute respiratory infections (ARI) has been developed by the World Health Organization (WHO) to optimize treatment of children who have limited access to health care. These ARI case management programmes have resulted in up to 84 per cent reduction in mortality from pneumonia. They utilize the *respiratory rate at rest, intercostal and sternal recession, and ability to drink* (see Table 25.6) to classify children with ARI.

Based on severity, treatment algorithms have been devised. Amoxicillin is the recommended antibiotic because it is cheap, can be given orally, and is effective against the bacteria commonly responsible for community acquired pneumonia, namely *Streptococcus pneumoniae* and *Haemophilus influenzae*.

All mothers of children with ARI treated at home require education regarding the symptoms and signs of deterioration, and the value of regular follow-up. If there is deterioration of the child's symptoms the child should immediately be brought back to the clinic. If the cough persists after 14 days, the child should be referred to exclude chronic respiratory problems such as pulmonary tuberculosis, foreign body inhalation, complications of pneumonia (empyema, lung abscess, or bronchiectasis) or increasingly, an unusual pneumonia in an HIV-infected child.

Organisms responsible for pneumonia

The following pathogens are specifically responsible for respiratory symptoms:

- *Bordetella pertussis* and parapertussis

Table 25.6 Acute respiratory tract infections: classification and management		
Severity	**Criteria**	**Management**
1 No pneumonia	Cough No tachypnoea	Supportive measures Antipyretic No antibiotics
2 Pneumonia	Cough Tachypnoea No rib or sternal retraction	Supportive measures Antipyretic (paracetamol) Antibiotics
3 Severe pneumonia	Cough Tachypnoea Rib and sternal retraction	Supportive measures Antibiotics Refer to hospital
4 Very severe pneumonia	Cough Tachypnoea Chest wall retraction Unable to drink Cyanosis	Supportive measures Oxygen Antibiotic Immediate referral to secondary or tertiary hospital

If a child has severe or very severe pneumonia, the following measures should be carried out before and during transfer to hospital:

- Give antipyretics where necessary.
- Remove nasal secretions with a syringe or suction apparatus after softening with drops of sodium bicarbonate or saline.
- Give oxygen (40 per cent) by nasal prongs after clearing the nasal passages.
- Use a stomach tube to decompress the stomach from swallowed air and to give fluids (50–80 ml/kg/d) if needed.
- If the child is severely distressed, give fluids intravenously (60 ml/kg/24 hours if not dehydrated).
- Before transferring the child it is recommended to administer intravenous penicillin or preferably ceftriaxone (100 mg/kg).

- Bacteria: *Streptococcus pneumoniae, Haemophilus influenzae, Staphylococcus aureus, Mycobacterium tuberculosis*
- *Chlamydia pneumoniae, Mycoplasma pneumoniae*
- Respiratory viruses, including respiratory syncitial virus (RSV), influenza virus and adenovirus

- *Pneumocystis jirovecii* and cytomegalovirus (CMV) in immunosuppressed children
- Other unusual organisms can also be responsible in immunosuppressed children: *Cryptococcus* and *Aspergillus*.

The organisms responsible for pneumonia vary according to the age and immune status of the child and where the pneumonia was contracted. Community-acquired pneumonia (CAP) is the most common and is caused by the organisms described below. Hospital-acquired pneumonia (nosocomial pneumonia) is mostly caused by highly resistant Gram-negative organisms and methicillin resistant *Staphylococcus aureus*.

In developing countries *S. pneumoniae, H. influenzae*, and *S. aureus* are the organisms most commonly involved. Viral infections are responsible for approximately 40 per cent of pneumonia in children. The same respiratory viruses (RSV and adenovirus) occur as in the developed world although measles pneumonia is still alarmingly common. Other organisms such as *Mycoplasma pneumoniae, Moraxella catarrhalis*, and *Chlamydia pneumoniae* occur, but their precise role is uncertain.

In developed communities respiratory syncytial virus, adenovirus, para-influenza, and influenza viruses are the most common causative agents. *M. pneumoniae* and *C. pneumoniae* are common in school-going children, causing the so-called atypical pneumonia. Bacteria cause only between 5 and 10 per cent of pneumonia, with *S. pneumoniae* and *H. influenzae* remaining the commonest. As outlined in Table 25.7, other pathogens are involved under special circumstances in certain groups of children, or in association with HIV disease (*see below*).

Clinical picture

The clinical picture is determined by the age of the child and the causative organism. Neonates may present only with non-specific signs: lethargy, failure to feed, fever or temperature instability, tachypnoea, and sometimes with apnoea and cyanosis (*see* Chapter 7, Care of the newborn).

Older children often begin with the runny nose and sore throat of an upper respiratory infection followed by a cough, fever, and tachypnoea. In most children, altered breath sounds and crackles are present on auscultation. The classical signs of lobar consolidation, namely dullness to percussion and bronchial breathing, are found in a minority of cases. Bronchopneumonia is far more common.

Mild pneumonia is characterized by the child only having tachypnoea. As the pneumonia progresses there is in addition to tachypnoea, rib and sternal retraction leading to feeding difficulties. Occasionally respiratory failure supervenes.

The best non-invasive way of judging the severity of hypoxia is by measuring the transcutaneous oxygen saturation. A pulse oximeter reading of <90 per cent indicates respiratory failure and the use of supplemental oxygen. Arterial blood gases are seldom required to asses the severity of pneumonia. A sudden deterioration during the course of pneumonia is suggestive of a complication such as pneumothorax or pyopneumothorax which requires immediate drainage.

Special investigations

Radiological picture. Routine chest radiographs are not necessary in uncomplicated pneumonia as findings do not impact on treatment. Chest X-ray should be ordered when complications are suspected, tuberculosis is considered (order lateral X-ray as well), or where there is poor response to standard antibiotic treatment. Bacterial pneumonia in children is normally characterized by widespread, poorly demarcated, alveolar opacities with air bronchograms. The classical lobar or segmental opacification with air bronchograms is less common. Viral pneumonia, on the other hand, causes perihilar streaking, interstitial changes, and air trapping. Mucous plugging in viral pneumonia results in lobar or segmental collapse which is easily confused with a lobar or segmental bacterial pneumonia. Although these features are useful they are not specific enough to differentiate between viral and bacterial pneumonia on radiological features alone.

Radiological clues of causative organisms:

- Staphylococcal pneumonia often shows progression of areas of break-down to pneumatocele formation, lung abscesses, empyema, or pyopneumothorax.
- Klebsiella, anaerobes, *H. influenzae*, and *Mycobacterium tuberculosis* can cause cavitating or expansile pneumonia.
- *Mycobacterium tuberculosis, S. aureus, H. influenzae,* and anaerobic pneumonia may present with pleural effusion and empyema.

Pneumatoceles are thin-walled air-filled spaces mostly without an air-fluid level. They can rupture, causing a pneumothorax or become so large that they compress the rest of the lung causing respiratory embarrassment. The majority of cases clear spontaneously within three months. Other causes of pneumatoceles are *H. influenzae* pneumonia, hydrocarbon inhalation pneumonia, and lung contusion.

Other diagnostic aids:

- A high **white cell count** with a leucocytosis and shift to the left on the differential white cell count and positive C-reactive protein are often indirect evidence of bacterial pneumonia. However, viral pneumonia can also cause a high white cell count and children that are very ill from a bacterial pneumonia often fail to show these features.
- **Blood cultures** prior to treatment are extremely valuable in isolating the organism in severe pneumonia, although they isolate the causative organism in only 25 per cent of cases of bacterial pneumonia. A negative blood culture does not exclude a bacterial infection. Organisms cultured from pleural fluid are always pathological.
- **Throat swabs or pharyngeal aspirates** are not specific as the specimen is usually contaminated by upper respiratory tract organisms and are not useful. A *sputum*

specimen in older children, if correctly collected and analysed according to Light's criteria, can be useful. Sputum can be induced by inhalation of hypertonic saline. This is useful for the diagnosis of TB and *P. jirovecii*.

- **Transtracheal and lung aspirates, as well as non-bronchoscopic broncho-alveolar lavage** are specific tests but should only be performed in institutions with the necessary expertise.
- A **tuberculin skin test** should always be done especially if the child has been in contact with an adult with newly diagnosed TB, the patient does not respond to treatment or has unusual radiological features.
- **Viruses** can either be cultured from nasopharyngeal aspirates or demonstrated using immunofluorescent techniques.

Treatment

The mainstays of treatment are antibiotics and oxygen.

Correct antibiotic choice. Amoxycillin is the antibiotic of choice at the primary care level. Referral is essential if the child has rib retraction, is unable to drink, or shows evidence of respiratory distress.

District and regional hospitals. Amoxycillin (200 mg/kg/d) is given in four divided doses unless staphylococcal pneumonia is suspected, when cloxacillin (100 mg/kg/d in four divided doses) is added. In children over five years parenteral penicillin can be used as *S. pneumoniae* is the most likely cause. *For severe pneumonia, parenteral penicillin for two days followed by oral amoxycillin is recommended if the child has responded well to treatment. Penicillin together with an aminoglycoside (gentamicin) is indicated in very severe pneumonia.* If the child is supected of having an atypical course, erythromycin (40 mg/kg/d) should be given for 10–14 days.

Once the child is fever-free for three days the antibiotics can be discontinued. Although the exact duration of antibiotics to be given for pneumonia is not known, most patients respond within 3–5 days. Patients with a lung abscess or empyema should be treated for 21 days. Parenteral antibiotics are only indicated in severely ill patients and those with gastro-intestinal upsets.

Children under the age of three months, severely malnourished children, children with hospital-acquired pneumonia, or with severe immune suppression will require different antibiotic regimes. (*see* Table 25.7).

Oxygen administration. All children with severe pneumonia who present with cyanosis, grunting, restlessness, inability to drink, severe chest and sternal retraction and tacchypnoea of >70 breaths per minute should be given oxygen unless the transcutaneous saturation can be

Table 25.7 Aetiology and treatment of pneumonia in special groups of children

Group	Organisms	Antibiotic
Immune-compromised	Gram-negative	Ampicillin
	Staphylococcus aureus	+
	Opportunistic organisms	Co-trimoxazole
	Pneumocystis jirovecii,	+
	M. tuberculosis	Aminoglycoside
Less than 3 months	Gram-negative organism	Ampicillin
	Group B streptococcus	+
	Staphylococcus aureus	Aminoglycoside
Hospital-acquired pneumonia	Gram-negative organism	Aminoglycoside
	Methicillin-resistant	+
	Staphylococcus aureus	Piperacillin + tazobactam
		+
		Vancomycin (if staphyloccocal infection suspected)

measured. In most children, adequate oxygenation is achieved by means of a low flow (0.5–2 l/min) of oxygen through nasal prongs. If a child fails to improve after this oxygen administration, the child should be transferred to a hospital where ventilatory support can be offered. Other methods of delivering oxygen include nasopharyngeal tubes. Face masks are ineffective in delivering oxygen to young children.

Blood transfusion. The amount of oxygen delivered to the tissues can be improved by maintaining the haematocrit above 30 per cent in patients with very severe pneumonia.

Hydration. If the child is unable to drink, a nasogastric tube can be passed but in severely distressed children intravenous maintenance fluid (50–80 ml/kg/d) is required.

Temperature control. Children with a temperature greater than 38 °C should receive paracetamol (30 mg/kg/d) in four to six divided doses.

Airway obstruction. Many children with bronchopneumonia have lower airway obstruction, in which case a β_2 agonist is given via a spacer.

Nutritional support. The extra energy requirement for children with pneumonia is an additional 50 to 60 kcal/kg/day. Zinc supplementation decreases the duration of hospitalization.

Antipyretics and analgesia. Pain should be treated aggressively. Antipyretics should only be used in patients with a temperature greater than 38 °C to reduce the risk of febrile convulsions.

Other supportive measures. Children with measles pneumonia and HIV disease require vitamin A. The nasal passages are kept clear with saline nasal drops and suctioning.

Treatments of **no proven benefit** in uncomplicated acute pneumonia include:

- Mucolytics
- Chest physiotherapy
- Postural drainage
- Nebulized therapy.

Failure to respond to therapy may be due to the following factors:

- Incorrect choice of antibiotic or the dose is inadequate.
- The pneumonia is not caused by the suspected organism or the organism is resistant to the antibiotics used. Knowledge of the local antibiotic sensitivity patterns of organisms is helpful.
- Development of an empyema or other complication.
- The pneumonia is caused by *Mycobacterium tuberculosis.*
- Suppressed immunity (often due to malnutrition or HIV infection) may lead to infection by an opportunistic organism.
- Underlying cause for the pneumonia, e.g. foreign body aspiration or bronchiectasis.
- Left-sided cardiac failure commonly masquerades as pneumonia.

Prognosis

Most children recover from pneumonia without any residual damage. Incorrectly treated pneumonia can lead to lung tissue destruction and bronchiectasis. About half of the children who develop pneumonia secondary to measles or adenovirus have persistent airway obstruction and reduced lung function as a result of small airway disease.

Other causes of pneumonia

Chlamydia pneumoniae

(*See* Table 25.8.)

This obligate intracellular bacterium has been recognized as a relatively frequent cause of atypical pneumonia in children older than three years. After an insidious onset with fever, malaise, headache, cough becomes worse and the patient develops signs of a pneumonia. Treatment consists of erythromycin, newer macrolides or quinolones, but treatment may have to be prolonged because of slow response.

Mycoplasma pneumoniae

Not strictly a bacterium, this smallest self-replicating organism is dependent on attachment to host cells for survival. It has worldwide endemicity and is one of the commonest causes of pneumonia in school-aged children, but rare in those younger than three to four years. Onset is with headache, fever, rhinitis, and sore throat.

The child should be referred to the next level hospital if the temperature has not settled after three to five days and the cause has not been identified, or if the child maintains a cough or wheeze for longer than 14 days.

Table 25.8 Other causes of pneumonia*

Pulmonary tuberculosis
Hydrocarbon inhalation
Atypical pneumonia
   Mycoplasma pneumoniae
   Chlamydia trachomatis
Eosinophilic pneumonia (Loeffler's)
Aspiration
   Premature infants
   Neurological defects
   Palatopharyngeal incoordination
   Gastro-oesophageal reflux
   Anatomical defects
   Tracheo-oesphageal fistula
   Cleft palate
Infectious diseases
   HIV disease
   Pneumocystis jirovecii,
   Lymphocytic interstitial pneumonitis
   Measles with secondary bacterial and viral
   infection
   Pertussis
   Legionnaires disease

*See text for the common causes of pneumonia.

Cough develops into lower respiratory symptoms over a period of about two weeks. This is one of the prototypes of 'atypical pneumonia' because clinical severity is much worse than suggested by the findings on examination. Patients produce frothy white sputum. The disease responds well to erythromycin and the newer macrolide antibiotics.

Pulmonary tuberculosis

(*See* Chapter 17, Tuberculosis.)

In any child with an unusual or non-responding pneumonia, TB must be considered, especially if the child has been in contact with an adult with newly diagnosed TB or is from a community with a high incidence of TB. Children of any age can develop TB but it is especially common in children younger than four years. Other risk factors for the development of TB are HIV disease, malignancies, children receiving immunosuppressive treatment, and children with congenital and acquired heart disease. Tuberculin skin testing should be done in every child who fails to respond to treatment. Radiological changes include hilar or mediastinal lymphadenopathy, lobar collapse or hyperinflation, cavitation and pleural effusion. It is also most useful to do a chest radiograph of the parents as one of them often has active TB.

Hydrocarbon inhalation pneumonia

Paraffin, petrol, and other volatile hydrocarbons used for cooking and heating are often stored in unmarked bottles. Children accidentally drink from these bottles and inhale the vapours. Twenty to 40 per cent of these children will develop chemical pneumonitis. Normally the child develops signs of respiratory distress within 30 minutes which can become progressively worse over the next 24–48 hours, but there can be a delay of up to six hours before the signs of pneumonia appear. Secondary bacterial pneumonia may follow the chemical pneumonitis. This is not prevented by prophylactic antibiotics. Ingestion of large amounts of hydrocarbons may cause neurological signs (confusion, loss of consciousness, convulsions). Other complications are pneumothorax and pneumatocele formation. The chest radiograph shows widespread alveolar opacification which often appears worse than the clinical picture of the child. (*See also* Chapter 11, Poisoning.)

Treatment. Adequate oxygenation and close observation for deterioration are essential as extensive involvement may require mechanical ventilation. Induced vomiting is contra-indicated as this can lead to increased hydrocarbon inhalation. Antibiotics are only indicated if a secondary bacterial infection is suspected. Steroids do not change the course of the disease.

Pulmonary eosinophilia (PIE)

Pulmonary infiltrates with eosinophilia on peripheral blood occur fairly frequently in children subjected to poor living conditions as they have a high prevalence of parasitic infestation.

Common causes of pulmonary eosinophilia are:

- *Simple PIE (Loeffler's):* symptoms lasting no longer than a month.
- *Prolonged PIE:* definite, recurrent pulmonary symptoms of two to six months' duration; but with eventual recovery.
- *Tropical eosinophilia:* applied to those where eosinophilic lung granulomas contain degenerating microfilaria.

- *Other rare causes* include polyarteritis
  nodosa, Hodgkin's lymphoma, asthma, and
  drugs such as nitrofurantoin, penicillin, or
  imipramine.

In many cases an aetiological agent cannot be
demonstrated. Simple PIE (Loeffler's) occurs
more often in children with a personal or family
history of allergy. If a specific cause is found, it
is usually a nematode (ascaris or toxocara) but
amoebiasis, trichinosis, hookworm infestation,
and strongyloidosis may cause PIE.

Diagnosis. The child has a cough or wheeze
with occasional crackles, the chest radiograph
shows migratory and transient pulmonary infiltrates, and occasionally atelectasis. The blood
eosinophil count is 10–50 per cent of white cells.
It is difficult to establish a definitive diagnosis as
symptoms may occur before ova or adult ascaris
appear in stool and larval toxocara become
encysted in tissue (including lung) and never
reach the gut to produce ova.

Treatment is symptomatic as the disease is
self-limiting, but giving a broad-spectrum ver-
micide (mebendazole or albendazole) may help.
If symptoms are troublesome, a short course of
prednisone will accelerate resolution of pulmonary infiltrates.

Aspiration pneumonia

Aspiration pneumonia is a reasonably common
cause of recurrent pneumonia or a wheezy chest
in toddlers. The causes include the following:

- *Palatopharyngeal incoordination.* The
  incoordination of swallowing is especially
  common in children with severe neurological
  disease and in patients with a cleft palate.
  These children choke and cough while they
  swallow.
- *Tracheo-oesophageal fistula.* This is a rare
  congenital lesion which presents with
  recurrent pneumonia and coughing during
  feeding.
- *Gastro-oesophageal reflux.* The reflux
  can occur as the result of a functional
  abnormality of the cardiac sphincter
  which is particularly common among
  premature babies or in conjunction
  with anatomical anomalies such as a
  diaphragmatic hernia.

Diagnosis. The diagnosis is often made from the
history or from watching the child feed. Chest
radiograph changes are usually in upper lobes
in the infant under six months. The diagnosis
is confirmed by a combination of a barium
swallow, radio-isotope milk scan, and oesophageal pH studies.

Treatment. Gastro-oesophageal reflux is
treated medically initially (*see* Chapter 24, Gastrointestinal disorders, and Chapter 30, Paediatric surgical disorders), but if the respiratory
symptoms persist for longer than six to eight
weeks in spite of intensive therapy, then fundoplication is indicated.

Smoke inhalation (thermal trauma)

Acute upper airway obstruction (UAO) from
laryngeal and/or tracheal oedema, or pneumonia
can occur following inhalation of hot air, smoke,
or chemical fumes, especially if the patient is
confined in a closed space. Various noxious
gases may be generated from the material burnt.
Combustion of wood generates carbon monoxide,
which combines with haemoglobin, resulting
in low arterial oxygen content with possible
hypoxaemic cerebral damage in the absence
of cyanosis. Other gases (e.g. aldehydes) cause
local pulmonary tissue damage. Bronchiolitis
and alveolitis may also occur, with wheezing
and crackles. There may be an interval of some
hours between smoke inhalation and onset of
respiratory manifestations.

Treatment. Breathing pure oxygen will reverse
carbon monoxide intoxication. If burns of the
face and mouth are present, UAO is very likely to
develop and early intubation is recommended. If
respiratory insufficiency supervenes from thermal trauma to the lung, mechanical ventilation
is also needed. Bronchodilators by nebulization
may be helpful, but the use of steroids for an
anti-inflammatory action has not been shown to
be useful.

Lung involvement in HIV disease

The lungs of HIV-infected children are often
affected by opportunistic infections; over two-
thirds of patients will have at least one respiratory
episode during the course of their disease, and
many succumb from these diseases. The lungs
of about 90 per cent of HIV-infected patients

are affected by infectious and non-infectious complications (AIDS-related) at necropsy (*see* Table 25.9).

Infectious diseases

Bacterial pneumonia occurs more frequently in HIV-infected children than in the general population and accounts for 38–57 per cent of HIV-related lung disease. The spectrum of pathogens is similar to that of the non-HIV-infected population (*S. pneumoniae, H. influenzae, S. aureus*, and Gram-negatives). The clinical presentation is often more aggressive and chest radiographs may be atypical. There is a high rate of complications, including cavity formation, empyema, and abscess formation. Antimicrobial therapy may be required for longer periods and relapse of infection has been noted despite appropriate antibiotic therapy. The outcome of infection is often poor. Some cases develop chronic lung damage.

Pneumocystis jirovecii pneumonia accounts for about a third to half of severe acute pulmonary HIV-related disease. The clinical presentation includes young, well-nourished infants with an insidious onset of progressive tachypnoea, fever, and non-productive cough. On examination they show varying degrees of respiratory distress with hypoxia out of proportion to the chest findings. There may be very few auscultatory findings, but occasionally fine crackles are heard. Chest radiographs show bilateral perihilar interstitial infiltrates which may progress to diffuse confluent alveolar shadowing over a period of several days. The serum lactate dehydrogenase (LDH) is commonly raised. The diagnosis is confirmed by ELISA, PCR or methenamine silver stains on induced sputum or broncho-alveolar lavage specimens. Treatment with high-dose co-trimoxazole (twice the normal dose) is indicated. Side-effects have been noted with co-trimoxazole but are uncommon. Primary and secondary prophylaxis with co-trimoxazole for *P. jirovecii* pneumonia is beneficial (*see* Chapter 18, HIV infection).

Cytomegalovirus (CMV) infection of the lung is common in HIV infected children. It occurs in isolation or may be present in association with *P. jirovecii*. The clinical presentation is similar to *P. jirovecii* and it is impossible to distinguish between these diseases; both seem to coexist. Diagnosis of CMV of the lung is supported by a positive IgM serological test, CMV DNA polymerase chain reaction, culture of the organism from the urine and histology of lung biopsies. Prolonged treatment with ganciclovir has been advocated.

Mycobacterium tuberculosis infection occurs in 11–52 per cent of HIV-infected children. Both HIV disease and TB share common complaints and the tuberculin test is often negative in HIV-positive children, making the diagnosis extremely difficult. Owing to the immune suppression, a Mantoux skin test of greater than 5 mm induration is accepted as positive. The clinical presentation in HIV-positive children depends on the state of the immune suppression. Early in HIV disease a typical primary picture is found but as the immunity is suppressed the picture becomes more atypical. The chest radiograph is often not diagnostic as the picture is atypical. The yield of AFB from gastric aspirate or sputum for TB from HIV-infected children is low; a negative AFB stain should not exclude the diagnosis of TB. All specimens must be sent for mycobacterial culture. TB acts as a potent further suppressor of immunity and accelerates the natural progression of HIV disease. Treatment is by conventional anti-tuberculosis drug regimes. Children with HIV and TB have a poorer outcome than children with TB alone. Directly observed therapy is essential to ensure drug adherence and prevent the development of multidrug resistant TB. (*See* Chapter 17, Tuberculosis.)

Other opportunistic infections such as *Candida albicans* and *Cryptococcus neoformans* pulmonary infections are uncommon with non-specific clinical and radiological appearances. *Mycobacterium avium intracellulare* rarely presents in children.

Table 25.9 HIV-related lung disease	
Cause	**Pneumonia**
Infectious	Bacterial
	Pneumocystis jirovecii
	Tuberculosis
	Cytomegalovirus
Non-infectious	Lymphocytic interstitial
	pneumonitis
	Lymphoma
	Kaposi's sarcoma

Non-infectious lung disease

Lymphocytic interstitial pneumonitis (LIP) is common in children between one and five years of age. The condition arises from the infiltration of lymphocytes into different organs. The clinical presentation is usually one of slowly progressive dyspnoea, cough, and signs of chronic lung disease, namely clubbing and chest deformity. Other associated signs include generalised lymphadenopathy, parotid enlargement and hepatomegaly. Chest radiographs show reticulonodular shadowing; a pattern very similar to miliary tuberculosis. LIP is a clinical diagnosis but can be confirmed by transbronchial or open lung biopsy. Treatment with prednisolone and antiretroviral therapy is effective resulting in resolution of the symptoms and chest radiographic changes. **Lymphomas**, both B- and T-cell, have been associated with HIV infection. The outcome is poor; median survival is less than one year without antiretroviral therapy.

Kaposi's sarcoma rarely presents in HIV-infected children. The disease often involves the trachea, bronchi, lung parenchyma, pleura, skin, and lymph nodes. Diagnosis is suspected if oral haemorrhagic lesions are present and proven by biopsy. The lesions are very haemorrhagic and care should be exercised during biopsy. Treatment is with chemotherapy and antiretroviral therapy. The outcome is poor.

Approach to a child with recurrent or persistent pneumonia

(*See* Table 25.10)

Recurrent pneumonia is diagnosed when a child develops more than two episodes of pneumonia within 18 months, while persistent pneumonia refers to lung parenchymal infection for 30 days despite the use of antimicrobials. In most children the clinical symptoms of acute pneumonia disappear within 5–14 days and the chest radiograph reverts to normal within four weeks.

In infants aspiration pneumonia is relatively more common while cystic fibrosis is more frequent in children with associated failure to thrive.

Diagnostic pointers when assessing a child with recurrent or persistent pneumonia:

♦ *Widespread disease.* The pneumonia is not limited to one anatomical part of the

Table 25.10 Causes of recurrent and persistent pneumonia

Widespread involvement
Allergy
Undiagnosed asthma
Pulmonary infiltrates with eosinophilia
Inflammation
Airway damage by viral or bacterial infections
Recurrent aspiration
Sucking or swallowing abnormalities
Tracheo-oesophageal fistula
Gastro-oesophageal reflux
Muco-ciliary clearance defects
Cystic fibrosis
Immotile cilia syndrome
Immunodeficiencies
Acquired
   Severe malnutrition
   HIV disease
Congenital
   T-lymphocyte deficiencies
   Agamma-globulinaemia
   Complement deficiencies
   Neutrophil abnormalities
Passive smoking

Anatomically localized
Foreign body
Extrinsic compression, e.g. TB lymph nodes
Bronchiectasis
Congenital lung lesions, e.g. lobar sequestration

lung or recur in various lobes of the lung. These patients are most likely to have an abnormality of their cough mechanism (neurologically impaired patients), aspiration pneumonia, abnormal mucus or mucous clearance (cystic fibrosis or cilia abnormalities), acquired (HIV disease or malnutrition) or congenital

The most common causes of recurrent pneumonia or persistent pneumonia are pulmonary TB, foreign body aspiration, misdiagnosed or inappropriately treated asthma, HIV associated lung disease, and bronchiectasis.

immune abnormalities. After severe adenovirus or measles pneumonia there is damage to the small airways which gives rise to recurrent pneumonia.

◆ *Localized disease.* If the pneumonia occurs in the same radiological lobe, then the most likely cause is an anatomical abnormality of the bronchus or lung parenchyma. Common causes are TB, foreign body aspiration, or localized bronchiectasis. In rare cases, congenital anomalies of the respiratory system present in this way. The history is that of pneumonia followed by recurrent chest symptoms. Chest radiograph shadows usually persist in the same anatomical position. These patients benefit by determining the cause of the anatomical abnormality by bronchoscopy and/or chest computerized tomography (CT).

Approach. After a careful history, clinical and radiological examination, the cause is normally apparent. If not, then TB, foreign body aspiration, asthma, and HIV disease should be excluded. Antibiotics are of no use unless there is pyrexia due to super-added infection. Chest physiotherapy is helpful if there is collapse or structural damage that prevents clearance of secretions. Bronchial hyperreactivity, which responds to a bronchodilator, is present in some cases. If the diagnosis is still uncertain the child should be referred to a specialist centre as further investigations are needed.

Undiagnosed or undertreated asthma is often confused with recurrent pneumonia. The chest radiographic changes are the result of mucus plugging of the airways, leading to segmental or lobar collapse being diagnosed as pneumonia. A trial of asthma therapy is often beneficial if the child has features suggestive of asthma. (*see* Chapter 20, Allergic disorders).

Suppurative lung disease

The two main causes of chronic suppurative lung disease are bronchiectasis and lung abscess, neither of which are common in children.

Bronchiectasis

Bronchiectasis occurs when there is permanent destruction of the bronchial walls and lung tissue due to chronic infection. There are three mechanisms:

◆ Bronchial lumen obstruction, e.g. tuberculous glands and a foreign body. In the developing world, pertussis is an important additional cause.

◆ Parenchymal destruction from necrotizing pneumonia usually caused by bacteria (staphylococci, klebsiella, anaerobes, tuberculosis) and respiratory viruses, especially measles and adenovirus.

◆ Repeated respiratory tract infections are an important cause in malnourished children, those with cystic fibrosis, generalized immune deficiencies including HIV infection, and those with aspiration pneumonia.

Dyskinesia of the cilia is a rare cause of bronchiectasis. These children have associated dextrocardia and chronic sinusitis.

Clinical picture. These children are seen repeatedly or admitted to hospital with lower respiratory tract infections. Characteristically they have a cough productive of copious amounts of infected sputum. The history of sputum production is difficult to assess as children swallow sputum immediately after coughing it up. Haemoptysis is rare in children. On examination only those with severe long-standing involvement have clubbing, halitosis, and are growth-retarded. On auscultation of the chest, widespread crackles and wheezes are heard although in some cases the signs can be localized to the affected lobe. The expiratory wheeze does not always respond to bronchodilators due to airway destruction. A sign of advanced disease is pulmonary hypertension which eventually leads to cor pulmonale. The diagnosis is suspected on the basis of the clinical picture and chest radiograph (honeycomb appearance) and confirmed by computer tomography.

The chest radiograph can be non-specific or show an area of opacification which fails to resolve. A honey-comb appearance (small cysts) may be seen in the affected area, which is the result of destroyed bronchi and parenchyma. Alternately, there may be widespread destruction of the lung with fibrosis and loss of volume. In rare cases the chest radiograph can be normal. Computer tomography is indicated if there is uncertainty about the diagnosis or if surgery is planned.

Treatment. Bronchiectasis can be prevented by immunization of children, the correct treatment of pneumonia and foreign body inhalation, early detection and treatment of tuberculosis and antiretroviral therapy. The cornerstone of medical treatment is physiotherapy with postural drainage. This technique must be taught to the parents and continued daily at home.

Appropriate antibiotics must be prescribed for acute lung infections and the child immunized against influenza each winter. The conjugate pneumococcal vaccine should also be administered. A certain proportion of children benefit from bronchodilation.

Surgical treatment is indicated if the disease is unilateral, lung function maintained and pulmonary hypertension not present. Clinical indications of compromised lung function are

Table 25.11 Chronic cough: causes and associated features

	Aetiology	Other signs, symptoms	Radiograph
Upper airway	Allergic rhinitis	Enlarged tonsils, adenoids	Normal or thickened bronchi at bases
	Pharyngitis	Postnasal drip	Normal
	Sinusitis	Postnasal drip	Opaque sinus
Lower airway	Asthma	Wheezy, night cough, expiratory wheeze, chest deformity	Hyperinflation
	Bronchitis (viral)	Wheeze	Normal or increased basal bronchial markings
	Aspiration	Wheeze	Increased bronchial marking commonly
	Cigarette smoke	Nil	Normal
	Pulmonary TB	Loss of weight	Peripheral and hilar opacity, mediastinal glands
	Pertussis	Apnoea in infants, paroxysmal cough	'Shaggy heart'
	Mycoplasma pneumoniae	Paroxysmal cough, often clinical clear chest	Diffuse subsegmental or patchy consolidation
	Chronic lung disease: Bronchiectasis	Crackles, wheezes, clubbing	Hyperinflation, ring shadows
	Obliterative bronchiolitis	Wheezes	Hyperinflation, segmental atelectasis
	Cystic fibrosis	Failure to thrive, chronic diarrhoea, clubbing	Hyperinflation, disseminated densities, lobar atelectasis
	Focal lesions: Foreign body	Onset with choking Localized wheeze	Radio-opaque foreign body Atelectasis + localized emphysema
	Mediastinal mass	Localized wheeze	Mediastinal mass Atelectasis
Psychogenic		Honking cough Ceases with sleep	Normal

tachypnoea, chest wall deformity and hypoxia in room air.

Lung abscess

Lung abscesses mostly follow *S. aureus, H. influenzae, Klebsiella pneumoniae, M. tuberculosis,* anaerobic and sometimes *S. pneumoniae* infections. The children are toxic, have a high swinging fever, produce foul-smelling sputum, and respond poorly to antibiotics. Amphoric breathing is often heard over the abscess. The chest radiograph shows a cavity with a fluid level which must be differentiated from a loculated pyopneumothorax, diaphragmatic hernia, and echinococcus (hydatid) cyst. Treatment consists of postural drainage and intravenous antibiotics (penicillin, and aminoglycoside). If the lung abscess does not drain, the child must be referred to a tertiary hospital to exclude an obstruction of the bronchus and consider transthoracic drainage of the abscess.

Chronic cough

(*See* Table 25.11)

The most common cause of a chronic cough is undiagnosed or undertreated asthma. Pulmonary tuberculosis, HIV associated lung diseases, and pertussis are frequent causes in developing countries.

Children with HIV disease often have a chronic cough caused by repeated infections, TB, and lymphocytic interstitial pneumonia (LIP). Children exposed to parental tobacco smoke have a higher incidence of pneumonia, asthma, and other respiratory infections. Indoor pollution from wood fires used for heating and cooking may cause chronic bronchitis and repeated attacks of pneumonia. Undiagnosed foreign body aspiration or bronchiectasis can present with a chronic cough. A chest radiograph is mandatory in all children with a chronic cough. If the child is old enough, asthma can be objectively diagnosed by demonstrating airway reversibility.

Lobar and segmental collapse

Lobar collapse is clinically suspected where dullness to percussion and decreased air entry is present and the trachea is displaced to the same side. Segmental collapse is seldom diagnosed clinically. On chest radiography there is lung volume loss, displacement of the fissures, and a dense opacification without air bronchograms. The most common causes of lobar and segmental collapse are seen in Table 25.12.

Treatment. A suspected foreign body calls for urgent bronchoscopy. Other causes of collapse are treated by physiotherapy with specific treatment for the primary cause. Most cases of collapse resolve with physiotherapy. Bronchoscopy is indicated where this does not occur within four weeks, if the patient deteriorates clinically, or the cause is uncertain.

Diseases of the pleural cavity

Pleural fluid

Fluid in the pleural cavity can be either a transudate or an exudate, which require differentiation as their causes differ and an exudate might need to be drained. An exudate has one or more of the following characteristics:

- The ratio of protein in the pleural fluid to the protein in serum is greater than 0.5.
- The ratio of lactic dehydrogenase (LDH) in the pleural fluid to that in serum is greater than 0.6.
- The LDH in pleural fluid is greater than 250 IU/l.

A diagnostic tap is necessary to determine the nature of the fluid and aspiration is done over the point of maximal dullness after confirmation of effusion by a chest radiograph. The aspirated fluid must be sent for chemical analysis, microbiological culture, and cytology. Before

Table 25.12 Lobar and segmental collapse: common causes

TB gland obstruction
Mucous plugging in pneumonia
Foreign body inhalation
Aspiration pneumonia
Bronchial stenosis (acquired and congenital)
Bronchiectasis

needle aspiration other causes of an opaque chest, such as total lung collapse, pneumonectomy, diaphragmatic paralysis, and diaphragmatic hernia should be considered and excluded clinically and radiologically.

Common causes of an **exudate** are pulmonary tuberculosis and bacterial pleurisy complicating pneumococcal, staphylococcal, haemophilus, or anaerobic pneumonia. Subdiaphragmatic pathology (amoebic liver abscess or a subphrenic abscess) less commonly causes empyema. Most of the cells in the exudate caused by a bacterial infection are polymorphonuclear leucocytes whilst in tuberculosis lymphocytes predominate. A very low sugar on the pleural fluid performed on a glucometer suggests a bacterial cause of effusion or empyema.

Most children with empyema are successfully **treated** with antibiotics and intercostal drainage. If in spite of this treatment the fever does not resolve or the empyema is loculated, an open drainage under general anaesthesia is needed.

Tuberculous effusions do not usually need intercostal drainage. If the child is very short of breath, drainage by needle aspiration is usually sufficient (*see* Chapter 17, Tuberculosis).

A transudate is usually associated with conditions of fluid overload or severe hypoproteinaemia. The most common causes are left-sided cardiac failure, nephrosis, renal, and liver failure. Transudates have very few cells in them and do not need drainage except if the patient is very short of breath.

Pneumothorax

Spontaneous pneumothoraces occur during staphylococcal pneumonia, an acute asthma attack, pneumatocele rupture, or following hydrocarbon inhalation pneumonia. Chest wall trauma or mechanical ventilation injury to the lung may cause a pneumothorax. Clinical signs are sudden dyspnoea, tympanic note on chest percussion with decreased air entry, and shifting of the trachea to the opposite side.

A **tension pneumothorax** is present when shock results from a decrease in venous return to the right side of the heart. The diagnosis is confirmed on chest radiograph. Tension pneumothorax requires immediate needle aspiration of pleural air. The needle is inserted into the 2nd or 3rd intercostal space, between mid-clavicular and anterior axillary lines. This is followed by chest tube insertion and underwater seal.

Miscellaneous conditions

Congenital abnormalities of the respiratory system

Congenital abnormalities should be considered in children who present with:
+ Unexplained stridor
+ Unexplained shortness of breath
+ Repeated respiratory tract infections, especially if cavities are seen on the chest radiograph
+ Expiratory wheeze not responding to bronchodilators
+ Unexplained opacification on chest radiograph especially if it has been present since birth.

The most common congenital abnormalities are choanal atresia, subglottic stenosis, congenital lobar emphysema, bronchogenic cyst, lobar sequestration, diaphragmatic hernia, and eventration of the diaphragm.

Smoking and the child's lungs

Young children exposed to environmental tobacco smoke in their households are more likely to develop bronchiolitis, asthma and pneumonia. Not only are the diseases more common but the disease is more severe in children exposed to tobacco smoke. They require more medical attention, clinic visits, and hospitalization.

Infant and neonatal mortality rates are increased. Infants born to mothers who smoke weigh on average 200 g less than those born to mothers who do not smoke. These infants have smaller lungs and wheeze more frequently with viral infections.

Most active smoking starts in adolescence and is more likely to occur if the parents smoke. All efforts should be made at this age to prevent smoking by teaching children skills to withstand peer pressure, preventing advertising aimed at adolescents, and preventing the sale of cigarettes to teenagers.

Near drowning

Hypoxaemia begins within seconds of submersion; ineffective circulation within two to four minutes, and irreversible brain damage about five minutes later. The above depends on the water temperature, as hypothermia prolongs the time during which survival is possible. Laryngospasm initially prevents water aspiration but when this relaxes water enters the lungs.

Emergency treatment. Remove foreign material from the airway, determine if the child is breathing and initiate mouth-to-mouth ventilation if needed. If no palpable pulse is present, start external cardiac massage while continuing mouth-to-mouth ventilation. Call for help and give supplemental oxygen at the earliest possible opportunity.

Hospital management. These children need to be treated for respiratory failure, cerebral oedema, and electrolyte imbalance. All children, irrespective of their clinical condition, should be kept in hospital overnight as lung oedema can occur in the first 24 hours. A good prognosis can be predicted for children breathing spontaneously when admitted to hospital.

Lung therapeutics

Supplemental oxygen

The outcome of children with moderate and severe lung disease is improved by supplemental oxygen. The method of oxygen delivery is important. Commonly utilized methods of oxygen delivery include face mask, head box, nasal prongs and nasopharyngeal tube. The preferred method of oxygen delivery is via nasal prongs because the flow required to deliver a particular concentration of oxygen is much lower (0.5–2 l/min) and therefore cheaper. The patients find nasal prongs more comfortable, the oxygen is delivered during feeding, the risk of oxygen toxicity is minimal and no humidification is needed. The maximum concentration delivered by this method is about 35 per cent.

In newborn infants receiving supplemental oxygen the oxygen saturation must be kept at about 92 per cent as higher concentrations in especially prematures can lead to retinopathy of prematurity and permanent blindness.

Fluids and feeds

Fluids and feeds are an important part of management of most respiratory conditions. Calculation of the amount of fluid required is complicated by the increased insensible fluid loss as a result of a raised temperature and hyperventilation which is counteracted by the increased secretion of antidiuretic hormone (ADH). It is recommended that the intravenous fluid volume be restricted to 60 per cent of the daily requirements in patients with severe respiratory distress from pneumonia, bronchiolitis, or asthma. Nasogastric or oral feeds at normal daily requirement volumes should be commenced as soon as the child is stable.

Physiotherapy

This is indicated in children with mucous plugging leading to collapse, bronchiectasis, those with a poor cough reflex secondary to neuromuscular disease, and in children being ventilated. In uncomplicated pneumonia or bronchiolitis, physiotherapy does not change the course of the disease. During an acute asthma attack physiotherapy is contra-indicated.

Mucolytics and cough suppressants

Mucolytics are of no benefit. Most cough suppressants have sedatives as a constituent and should not be used in children with lung disease as they are not beneficial and can be harmful.

Aerosol and powder devices

The use of aerosol and powder devices to deliver medication to the site of inflammation or infection in the airways is beneficial. Commonly utilized means are metered-dose inhalers (MDI) which can be used with spacer devices, dry powder devices, and nebulization. The correct device must be used and measures taken to ensure that the patient can use them. Bronchodilators, inhaled corticosteroids and antibiotics could be given via nebulizers.

Long-term effects of respiratory disease

A high proportion of adults suffering from chronic bronchitis have symptoms dating back to childhood. New evidence suggests that a larger portion of these patients were low-birth-weight infants who had repeated respiratory tract infections.

Long-term effects can be prevented by immunization of children, parental education about acute respiratory infections, limiting the use of biofuels for heating and cooking by electrification of homes, limiting environmental pollution, making parents aware of the hazards of tobacco smoking, and having health care available and accessible so that children with acute respiratory infections can receive immediate attention.

26

Neurological and muscular disorders

Neurology is a clinical discipline. A detailed history of the course of the illness, its prodrome and associated features, along with a meticulous neurological examination will, in most instances, enable the clinician to narrow down the possible differential diagnoses. The proper management of children presenting with a neurological problem requires an intimate knowledge of the developing neuro-anatomy and neurophysiology of the child's central nervous system (CNS).

Disorders of the CNS present with the following symptom complexes.

Headache

This common symptom is often overlooked *(see below)*.

Meningeal irritation

Neck stiffness is caused by meningitis, subarachnoid haemorrhage, posterior fossa lesions, spinal lesions, and paraspinal inflammatory reactions including apical pneumonia, paravertebral or paraspinal and perinephric abscesses. The clinical signs are:
- A positive Kernig sign
- A positive Brudzinski sign: passive neck flexion ('chin on the chest') causes reflex flexion of legs and arms as well as pain.

Raised intracranial pressure

This is due to intracranial space-occupying lesions (abscess or tumour), cerebral oedema (inflammatory, vasogenic, cytotoxic), progressive hydrocephalus, and haemorrhage. The symptoms include:

- Headache and vomiting (especially early in the morning)
- Visual disturbances (papilloedema may not always be present)
- Relative bradycardia and hypertension (Cushing's reflex)
- Change in level of consciousness.

Coma and encephalopathy

Altered levels of consciousness are usually symptomatic of a serious underlying neurological or metabolic disorder. The causes of coma may be classified into three broad groups:
- Diseases that cause no focal neurological signs or cerebrospinal fluid (CSF) abnormality
- Diseases that cause meningeal irritation with blood or white cells in the CSF
- Diseases that cause focal neurological signs without CSF changes.

Seizures

Seizures are caused by a wide variety of cerebral insults including structural and developmental abnormalities, metabolic disorders, genetic and infections. Neonatal seizures are sometimes very subtle but important to diagnose.

Strokes

Cerebrovascular accidents arise as a result of embolism, thrombosis or haemorrhage and present commonly with convulsions, hemiplegia or both. Similar acute focal neurological deficits can be caused by Todd's paresis (after epileptic seizure), arteriovascular malformations, hydrocephalus or space-occupying lesions.

Disturbances of tone and power

Generalized hypotonia ('floppy infant') may occur with disorders of lower motor neuron, upper motor neuron (cerebellar lesions), syndromic and metabolic disorders.

Ataxia and incoordination

Ataxic disorders of children occur due to acute, chronic progressive, and chronic non-progressive conditions affecting the cerebellum.

Movement disorders

Abnormalities of structure or biochemical function of basal ganglia lead to involuntary movement disorders.

Disorders of motor function

Cerebral palsy is a motor disability due to a non-progressive insult or damage of the developing motor brain.

Specific developmental delays

May be due to specific defects, e.g. mental retardation, deafness, and language delay.

Developmental regression

Loss of developmental abilities, which had previously been present, indicates a progressive disorder involving the brain, such as subacute sclerosing panencephalitis (SSPE), HIV encephalopathy, and inherited metabolic disease involving the brain, infections, and tumours. Regression also occurs with severe wasting disease and with severe emotional disturbance or deprivation.

Headache

Headache is common in children, becoming more frequent with increasing age. The vast majority of headaches in children are not associated with organic structural disease, but there are certain warning features of a potential organic brain lesion. Both the physical as well as the psychological factors in the aetiology of headaches need to be considered.

Headaches may be classified according to the temporal pattern, as shown in Table 26.1

Conditions such as sinusitis, otitis media, orbital problems (optic and retrobulbar neuritis) and dental disorders are rare causes of headaches

Features associated with an organic brain lesion:

- Severe headache of recent onset
- Chronic and progressive
- Localized pain
- Wakes the child at night
- Exacerbated by straining, valsalva manoevre, or a change in position
- Associated with neurological symptoms and signs
- A change in headache pattern or severity.

in children but need to be excluded. These can usually be diagnosed by a careful history and examination. It is essential to rule out a more serious cause of an acute headache and not miss meningitis, intracranial haemorrhage or a space-occupying lesion. Neurological symptoms or signs need to be thoroughly investigated.

Acute recurrent headaches

Migraine is the most common form of headache in childhood. It is a specific disorder characterized by episodic, periodic paroxysmal attacks of vasoconstriction and vasodilatation of cerebral blood vessels. In 50 per cent of all migraine sufferers, the attacks start before the age of 20 years and 20 per cent of the patients have had an attack before the age of five years. In many children, the onset of headaches has been preceded by colic, recurrent abdominal pain, vomiting or motion sickness starting as early as two years of age. In childhood, boys are affected more frequently than girls, but from puberty, girls are affected more frequently. After symptom-free intervals, attacks are often precipitated by certain trigger phenomena (*see* Table 26.2).

The headaches have several of the following features: they are throbbing in nature; have a unilateral location (but can be bilateral and alternating in sides); relief after sleep is classical; presence of an aura; associated abdominal pain (may be the only symptom in the younger child); associated nausea and vomiting; and a family history (usually the mother or aunt) of a similar condition. The incidence of migraine increases with age. Migraine is divided into three different types.

Table 26.1 Temporal classification of headaches

Temporal pattern	Cause of headache	Headache type
Acute	Infections and fever Toxins Post convulsions Anaemia, hypoxia Electrolyte imbalance, hypoglycaemia Hypertension, hunger, trauma, emboli, thrombosis, haemorrhage Post lumbar puncture	If associated with neurological signs and symptoms, prompt diagnosis is essential
Acute and recurrent	Migraine	

Chronic progressive	Raised intracranial pressure
	Traction headaches
	Brain tumours
	Space-occupying lesions – brain
	    abscess, hydrocephalus, subdural
	    haemorrhages
	Benign raised intracranial pressure
		Recur periodically
		Increase in frequency and severity over
		    time
		Neurological symptoms and signs appear
		    over 6–8 weeks

Chronic non-progressive	Tension headaches
	Psychogenic headaches
		Occur several times weekly, daily, or
		    constantly, without significant changes
		    in severity
		Usually not associated with neurological
		    symptoms or signs

Classic migraine (migraine with aura) is less common in children than in adults. The aura may be preceded by prodromes, which may be visual, consisting of flashing lights, blurred vision, scotomata, transient blindness or hemianopsia,

Table 26.2 Trigger/precipitating factors in migraine

Anxiety	
Fatigue	Lack of sleep
Stress	Headache occurs after the stress during relaxation
Head trauma	Common precipitator in males
Exercise	Either during or after
Menstruation	At menarche or associated with pre-menstrual tension

Diet	Tyramine-containing foods
	    (release of serotonin)
	    ice cream, red wine, cheeses

Medication	Contraceptive pill (high oestrogen and then withdrawal)

or include sensations of parasthesias of both hands or the perioral area and rarely, auditory or olfactory symptoms. In some children the aura may occur alone without the headache. The description of an aura may be difficult to obtain, particularly in a young child. Classic migraine tends to be biphasic in that the attack begins with an aura due to the vasoconstriction, which is then followed by the headache due to vasodilatation.

Common migraine (without aura) is a frequent form in children. There is usually no well-defined aura but autonomic features are common, comprising anorexia, nausea, vomiting and abdominal pain, facial pallor and 'dark rings' under the eyes. Sometimes the autonomic features are more prominent than the headache. Sleep is effective in relieving migraine headaches and is often of diagnostic value although many children may resist sleep during the attack. The headache may be unilateral or bilateral, lasting an average of two to six hours. The attacks are seldom more frequent than once or twice a week.

Complicated migraine is usually more common in children than in adults. The overall frequency of complicated migraine varies between 5 and 10 per cent. This type can be associated with neurological deficits, which are presumably due to prolonged vasoconstriction and ischaemia of that particular area of the brain with a spreading depression through the surrounding neurons. Classically, the deficit precedes the headache, but may follow it and can last for several days. The term applies to hemiplegic and aphasic migraine, ophthalmoplegic migraine, confusional states, and basilar migraine.

The **periodic syndromes** include benign paroxysmal vertigo and cyclic vomiting. Both these conditions have a strong association with migraine. Benign paroxysmal vertigo occurs in children between the ages of two and seven years. The attacks are sudden and brief (lasting 1–2 minutes), when the child becomes unsteady and cannot maintain his posture, but sits down and holds on tightly during the attack, acting in a tearful and fearful manner.

Cyclic vomiting consists of episodes of unexplained paroxysmal abdominal pain and vomiting. Classic or common migraine may develop later.

Cluster headaches are very uncommon before 10 years of age. They are more common in males and consist of intense, non-throbbing periorbital pain with lacrimation, unilateral conjunctival injection, nasal stuffiness and facial flushing. The pain is brief, usually very severe and can spread to the hemicranium. The headaches may recur for a few days to weeks in clusters and then not appear for a year or more. The attacks tend to occur more commonly at night.

Chronic progressive headache

This includes conditions in which the pathology is within the cranial vault and where there is raised intracranial pressure, which causes traction on the intracranial pain-sensitive structures. If physical examination reveals localizing neurological signs, then a computerized tomography (CT) or magnetic resonance imaging (MRI) scan of the brain is indicated. The location of the headache in brain tumours rarely has any localizing value. Benign raised intracranial pressure presents with signs of raised pressure with papilloedema. Testing of the visual fields may reveal an enlarged blind spot. Lumbar puncture will reveal high pressure with a normal chemistry.

Chronic non-progressive headache

This includes conditions such as tension headaches and psychogenic headaches. Tension headache is thought to result from sustained contraction of muscles of the neck and scalp, and is one of the most common headaches in adolescence and adulthood. These headaches are characterized by a sensation of a tightness, pressure or constriction like a band about the head.

Psychogenic or functional headaches are due to depression, conversion reactions, and hypochondriacal states. These headaches may be accompanied by mood changes, withdrawal, poor school performance, sleep disturbance, lack of energy, and weight loss.

Management of headache
- Get a reliable and complete history
- Do a thorough systemic and neurological examination
- Look for sites of related pain (ears, eyes, sinuses, teeth)
- X-ray sinuses
- If signs and symptoms are suggestive of an organic lesion, do a CT scan of the brain
- Reassure the parents and child when appropriate
- Give adequate analgesics (usually only necessary for a short time)
- Avoid narcotic analgesics
- Prescribe prophylactic medication if migraine attacks are debilitating and frequent.

Treatment should always include reassurance of the child and parent in the cases of non-organic headaches. The most widely used and successful analgesic in childhood headaches is paracetamol which is very efficacious when given in the correct doses (15–20 mg/kg/dose). The narcotic analgesics should only be used when warranted by the severity of the headache and only for short periods. Rest and sleep is important for most migraine suffers and some children may require anti-emetics if vomiting is a problem. In the vast majority of paediatric migraine patients, prophylaxis is unnecessary and should only be considered if the attacks become severe and debilitating. Trigger factors should be looked for and removed; often these are dietary items or some form of stress and anxiety. There are numerous drugs that may be used in the more severe cases and these include propranolol, pizotifen, cyproheptadine, amitriptyline, and anti-convulsants (e.g. sodium valproate).

Coma and acute encephalopathies

Encephalopathy refers to an involvement of the central nervous system such that it is unable to function at optimal levels. The usual presentation of severe acute encephalopathy in children is either convulsions, coma, or both. Consciousness is the awareness of self and the environment. This is regulated in two areas of the brain – the cerebral hemispheres, which control the content of consciousness, and the ascending reticular activating system (ARAS) in the brainstem, which maintains the person in a suitably aroused state. Altered or reduced states of consciousness reflect either diffuse and bilateral impairment of cerebral hemispheres or failure of the brainstem ARAS, or both.

It is important to avoid an early assumed diagnosis before carefully and diligently excluding other conditions in which the management might be quite different. Coma is often a life-threatening situation and a good approach to the problem is essential because time may be of the essence. A good history is needed of the onset, course of events and any precipitating factors.

Aetiology and assessment

Coma may be classified into three broad groups depending on the presence or absence of focal neurological signs and the state of the CSF (*see* Table 26.3).

- Treat the treatable as soon as possible. The ABC of resuscitation should apply, with a full and adequate history and a detailed neurological examination undertaken. Check the serum glucose, remove toxins (either those ingested or on the skin), control status epilepticus, ensure normal blood pressure and perfusion, look for signs and sites of infection and institute appropriate treatment.
- If the child is in a coma, refer to secondary or tertiary level of care as a matter of urgency.

Table 26.3 Causes of coma

Diseases that cause no focal neurological signs or CSF abnormality	Intoxications Metabolic Infections Shock Epilepsy Hypertensive encephalopathy Hyper/hypothermia Concussion
Diseases that cause meningeal irritation with blood or white cells in the CSF	Subarachnoid haemorrhage Bacterial meningitis Viral encephalitis
Diseases that cause focal neurological signs without CSF changes	Brain haemorrhage Cerebral infarction Brain abscess or empyema Subdural or epidural haemorrhage Brain tumour Miscellaneous

In one series the following causes of acute encephalopathy/coma were found: infections (34 per cent); anoxia/ischaemia (21 per cent); toxic/metabolic (12 per cent); intracranial hae-morrhage (16 per cent); miscellaneous (burns, cardio-respiratory, leukaemia, nephritis, hepatic, diabetic ketoacidosis) (17 per cent).

It is important to treat what is treatable as soon as possible, perhaps even before the cause of the coma has been established, in order to avoid potentially treatable fatal or permanent brain damage.

There are a number of important questions that one should ask. Is there a lesion and where is it? Is it focal or diffuse? There are certain clinical guidelines that will help one decide. Focal hemisphere lesions may produce focal neuro-logical signs, but one needs a bilateral hemi-sphere lesion to produce coma. Small focal lesions must be in the brainstem to produce coma directly. The pattern of changes in the following five physiological variables give valu-able information about what level of the brain is involved, the nature of the involvement, and the direction that the disease process is going:

- State of consciousness
- Pattern of respiration
- Pupillary reactions
- Eye movements and oculovestibular responses
- Motor function.

State of consciousness

The best and most informative way to document the level of consciousness is to describe it as fully as possible in regard to the child's responses to external stimuli. The Glasgow coma scale is extensively used in older children and this has been modified to be more applicable to infants and small children (see Table 26.4).

Table 26.4 Adult and paediatric coma scales				
Adult scale–Glasgow coma scale (Teasdale & Jennet, 1974)		**Paediatric scale **** (Simpson & Reilly, 1982)		
Eyes open				
Spontaneously	4			
To speech	3	As in adult scale		
To pain	2			
None	1			
Best verbal response		Orientated		5
Orientated	5	Words		4
Confused	4	Vocal sounds		3
Inappropriate words	3	Cries		2
Incomprehensible sounds	2	None		1
None	1			
Best motor response				
Obeys commands	6			
Localizes pain	5			
Withdraws	4	As in adult scale		
Flexion to pain	3			
Extension to pain	2			
None	1			
Normal aggregate score	15	**Normal aggregate scores:		
		0–6 months		9
		6–12 months		11
		1–2 years		12
		2–5 years		13

Both scales are used more commonly in patients with head injuries. In very young infants the diagnosis of coma may be confirmed by the absence of sleep/wake cycles on continuous electroencephalograph (EEG) tracings.

Some conditions appear coma-like but differ in a number of ways.

The **persistent vegetative** state occurs when the cerebral cortex is so extensively damaged that it cannot be aroused and sustain normal cognitive function. The eyes open in response to verbal stimuli and sleep/wake cycles exist, but these patients show no discrete localizing motor responses and cannot obey any verbal commands.

Akinetic mutism is a condition of silent, alert-appearing immobility in which sleep/wake cycles have returned, but where there is no external evidence of mental activity and very little, if any, motor activity present. The child is fully conscious and may only be able to communicate by moving the eyes and opening and closing them. This condition usually occurs following a discrete lesion at the top of the brainstem. This is similar to the locked-in syndrome.

Pattern of respiration

It is important to realise that the control of respiration is integrated at many levels and this control is regulated through both metabolic and neurogenic factors. The pattern and type of respiration observed in a comatose child can give valuable clues as to the neurological localization of the lesion. These patterns usually follow a cephalo-caudal progression:

- **Post hyperventilation apnoea (PHVA)**. Normally, if carbon dioxide (pCO_2) is lowered by a brief period of hyperventilation, awake subjects will resume regular breathing without a delay. Patients with metabolic or bilateral structural forebrain disease will demonstrate a period of apnoea.
- **Cheyne-Stokes respiration (CSR)** is a neurogenic alteration in respiratory control that usually results from an intracranial cause located bilaterally deep in the cerebral hemispheres, basal ganglia or internal capsule. Diffuse metabolic brain dysfunction can also result in CSR. The pattern of CSR that is clinically observed is hyperpnoea that increases in rate over

a few seconds, then slowly decreases to a short period of apnoea and then the cycle is repeated (also seen in hypoxaemia and congested lungs).
- **Central neurogenic hyperventilation (CNH)** is extremely rare and consists of sustained, rapid and fairly deep hyperpnoea due to a lesion in the mid-pons.
- **Apneustic breathing** is a prolonged inspiratory cramp, which may also occur in expiration. The site of the lesion is in the mid- to caudal pontine area and involves damage to the respiratory centres, associated with pontine infarction, hypoglycaemia, anoxia, and severe meningitis.
- **Ataxic breathing** has a completely irregular pattern in which both deep and shallow breaths occur randomly. It represents damage to the medullary neurons that generate the respiratory rhythm, including the reticular formation of the dorsomedial part of the medulla.

Pupillary reactions

Because the brainstem areas controlling consciousness are anatomically adjacent to those controlling the pupils, pupillary reactions are a valuable guide to the location of brainstem lesions causing coma. The pupillary pathways are relatively resistant to metabolic insults, thus the presence or absence of the 'light reflex' is the single most important physical sign distinguishing structural from metabolic causes of coma. One should always consider a metabolic cause of coma, in the first instance, if there is a light reflex present in a patient showing other signs of severe midbrain depression. At a hypothalamic level, a Horner's syndrome may be present (miosis, anhydrosis, ptosis) on the ipsilateral side. Midbrain damage at a dorsal tectal level will interrupt the light reflex, the pupils will be mid position, fixed to light, but regular in shape. At a nuclear midbrain level, pupils are mid position, fixed, slightly irregular and unequal. Pontine lesions interrupt the sympathetic pathways, leaving the parasympathetic pathways intact. The pupils will be very small, but the light reflex will be present. During resuscitation, drugs are infused which may have an effect on the size and reactivity of the pupils. Atropine, in large amounts, produces fully dilated and fixed pupils, whereas morphine will result in small pupils, but which react normally to light (use a magnifying glass). Anoxia or ischaemic damage results in wide, fixed pupils. Hypothermia and barbiturates will give rise to fixed pupils.

Eye movements and oculovestibular responses

The two most important reflexes are the oculo-cephalic (Doll's eye movement) and oculovestib-ular reflexes. **The Doll's eye reflex is only valid in comatose states**. It is evoked by turning the child's head from side to side (once it is established that the child does not have an injured neck), or vertically, and observing the movement of the eyes.

The oculovestibular reflex (caloric stimulation) is the response of the eyes to cold or warm water instilled into the ears. (Make sure that the eardrums are intact before performing this test). In an intact oculovestibular system, the eyes will move slowly towards the cold stimulus. In severe brainstem injury or deep metabolic coma, there is loss of response to caloric stimulation.

Eyes that are directed straight ahead have no localizing value in coma. Conjugate deviation (horizontally) may either mean an ipsilateral hemisphere lesion or a contralateral pontine lesion. If the eyes can then be brought beyond the midline by head turning or the caloric response, this points towards a hemispherical lesion. If the eyes cannot be brought beyond the midline, then this suggests a pontine lesion. Eyes that are conjugately deviated down imply that the lesion is either a compressive or metabolic one, causing depression on the diencephalon. If the eyes can be raised above the horizontal by the caloric response or by head tilting, this then suggests a metabolic cause and if not, a compressive lesion. Except for mild strabismus, dysconjugate ocular deviation in coma means a structural brainstem lesion.

If the Doll's eye reflex is intact, the eyes will move in the opposite direction to the direction in which the head is turned. If the eyes remain still, looking straight ahead as the head is turned, then the Doll's eye reflex is absent, implying the loss of that brainstem connection and function.

Motor function

The motor dysfunction usually gives an idea of the site of the lesion. Perhaps the most important motor responses to look for in coma are the postural responses to pain.

Decorticate posturing, which involves flexion of the arms and extension of the legs, is found in lesions of the internal capsule or the rostral cerebral peduncles. Decerebrate posturing, which involves extension of both the arms and legs, involves the area extending from the brainstem to the midpons. This posturing can occur either from direct damage, pressure from above or severe metabolic disorders. Decerebrate posturing of the upper limbs and flexion of the lower limbs imply a lesion of the lower pons. A flaccid posture implies depression of the central motor mechanisms in the medullopontine reticular formation.

Management

- Treatment must take place, to some extent, independent of a diagnosis. The maxim 'treat what is treatable' is very important in the management of children with an acute encephalopathy or those in coma. This involves five main areas:
  - Infection – diagnose (LP may be deferred until space occupying lesion excluded on CT/MRI scan) and treat meningitis promptly with the appropriate antibiotics. If herpes encephalitis is suspected, acyclovir (or equivalent) should be started as soon as possible.
  - Control seizures – *see* the section on Status epilepticus, *below*.
  - Detect and treat raised intracranial pressure (ICP). Raised intracranial pressure is basically due to an increase in the volume of one or more of the intracranial compartments, which means either too much CSF (hydrocephalus), too much brain (oedema, mass), or too much blood (congestion, hyperviscosity, vasodilatation, haemorrhage). The raised pressure can also interfere with cerebral circulation and this will lead to both ischaemia and hypoxia of cerebral tissue. If the cerebral blood flow drops below

20 ml/100g/min, ischaemic damage will occur. Cerebral perfusion pressure (CPP) is defined in terms of the mean blood pressure (MBP) minus intracranial pressure (ICP) and is dependent on both the systemic blood pressure and the intracranial pressure. If the systemic pressure falls out of the range of 60–150 mmHg, then autoregulation of the cerebral blood vessels fails and the CBF will be severely affected.

- Maintain microcirculation – control blood pressure, reduce ICP, reduce haematocrit, prevent platelet aggregation, prevent excessive hyperventilation.
- Maintain homeostasis–electrolyte, glucose, acid base, respiratory, cardiovascular balance.

Methods to reduce intracranial pressure include:
- Avoid constrictions around the neck, keep the head up at a 30-degree angle, maintain the pH and pCO_2 in normal range and make sure that the airways are clear.
- Remove CSF.
- Steroids stabilise lysosomal membranes; inhibit prostaglandin formation; reduce endothelial permeability, leucocyte diapedesis, and CSF formation. Steroids are more effective in vasogenic oedema, but should be avoided in herpes encephalitis. It is important to withdraw steroids slowly.
- The use of hyperosmolar agents, such as mannitol, to induce an osmotic diuresis and thereby reduce cerebral oedema. Mannitol should be used in combination with dexamethasone to prevent the mannitol from entering the neurons and adding to the oedematous state. Mannitol should not be used in the face of dehydration and it is important to restrict fluid requirements to 60–70 per cent of daily requirements.
- Hyperventilation is a very effective short-term means of controlling ICP and should be used when mannitol and dexamethasone have failed. The ideal is to maintain the pCO_2 as near normal as possible, 35–38 mmHg, which prevents excessive vasoconstriction or vasodilatation.

The gold standard in the management of raised intracranial pressure is the ability to assess the pressure accurately at all times. There are only a few centres that can measure intracranial pressure directly. Unless this is available, one can only guess at what is happening to the ICP. It is the perfusion of cerebral tissues that is of ultimate importance and intracranial pressure monitoring gives one an indirect means of assessing perfusion pressure. (*See* Table 26.5.)

Hydrocephalus

Hydrocephalus means an excessive amount of CSF in all or part of the intracranial fluid spaces which is or has been under increased pressure, at least in the initial stages of the disorder. Excessive CSF due to brain atrophy or dysgenesis (*ex vacuo* dilatation) is not referred to as hydrocephalus.

CSF is produced by the choroid plexus in the lateral ventricles. From there it flows through the foramina of Monro into the 3rd ventricle, down the Sylvian aqueduct into the 4th ventricle and then out through the foramina of Luschka and Magendie into the cisterna magnum and then it bathes the brain via a number of

Table 26.5 Ideal parameters to aim for in the management of coma	
PaO_2	90–120 mmHg
$PaCO_2$	35–38 mmHg
Haemoglobin	12 g/dl
Haematocrit	35
Mean arterial pressure (MAP)	>60 mmHg <90 mmHg
CVP	4–6 mmHg
CPP = MAP–ICP	50 mmHg or >
CBF	Must remain >18–20 ml/100 g/min (Normal = 50–100 ml/100 g/min)

cisterns. Approximately 10–15 per cent of the CSF travels down the spinal pathways. It is eventually reabsorbed through the subarachnoid granulations and into the sagittal sinus. The rate of CSF formation ranges from 0.3–0.4 ml/minute and continues even when the intraventricular pressure is increased. Total CSF volume in the newborn is approximately 50 ml, increasing with age to an adult volume of approximately 150 ml. Normal lumbar CSF pressure is 50–120 mm H$_2$O in the recumbent child.

The clinical signs and symptoms of hydrocephalus in children are as follows:

- A large head or a progressively enlarging head circumference is common. This should be monitored by regular head circumference measurements and plotted on a head circumference growth chart. Any circumference that crosses centiles is highly suspicious.
- Raised intracranial pressure may present with symptoms of irritability, drowsiness, vomiting or jitteriness. A tense anterior fontanelle, splayed sutures, distension of scalp veins, sun-setting eyes or loss of upward gaze, neck retraction or neck stiffness, and pyramidal tract signs are the more common clinical signs of hydrocephalus.

Symptoms vary according to the age of the child (sutures remain open in the young child allowing relative enlargement of the head before compression of intracranial contents occur), the severity and rate of progression. Look for a possible cause: posterior fossa tumour, post meningitis (TBM, pneumoccocal), myelomeningocele (NTD), and congenital aqueduct stenosis.

Management of hydrocephalus entails making a definitive diagnosis. Trans-illumination of the skull by a bright light shone through the anterior fontanelle in a darkened room may be very suggestive of a large hydrocephalus. If the anterior fontanelle is still patent an ultrasound examination is helpful and most suited for follow-up examinations. However, most neurosurgeons will require a CT or MRI scan of the brain in acquired hydrocephalus to better elucidate the possible cause. Measurement of CSF pressure may be required in acute cases and the neurosurgeon will require the CSF/intraventricular pressure to assist in choosing a particular shunt. A lumbar puncture may be indicated in certain instances to rule out meningitis.

The treatment depends on the rate of progression and enlargement of the ventricles and skull circumference and the resultant intracranial pressure effects on neural tissue. Ideally, one would wish to reduce intracranial pressure by

Table 26.6 Classification of hydrocephalus

Mechanism	Cause

Obstruction of CSF pathways:
Intraventricular block:
    Foramen of Monro
    3rd ventricle
    Sylvian aqueduct
 	
    4th ventricle
	
	Tumour, cyst
	Tumour, cyst
	Tumour, inflammation, haemorrhage, congenital aqueduct stenosis
	Posterior fossa tumour/cyst (Dandy-Walker), neural tube defect

Extraventricular block: Basal block	Inflammation (meningitis), tumours

Deficient reabsorption:
    Arachnoid villi abnormalities
    Venous hypertension
	Chemical arachnoiditis (blood, infection)

Over-secretion of CSF	Choroid plexus papilloma (rare)

Adapted from: Aicardi J. 1992. Diseases of the Nervous System in Childhood, by permission of MacKeith Press.

either diverting CSF flow (surgical) or reducing CSF production (medical, primarily diuretics). The decision to intervene surgically, either by a temporary external CSF shunt or a more permanent internal shunt is never an easy one. In the neonatal period, repeated lumbar puncture may be of some help to relieve the pressure but generally has not been of much long-term benefit. Most shunting procedures use the ventriculoperitoneal route rather than the lumbo-peritoneal route. Shunting is a relatively simple surgical procedure but is often associated with a number of complications.

When there is doubt as what to do, it is essential to refer the child to a tertiary care institution as soon as possible for specialized management.

Seizures in childhood

Classification

The childhood epilepsies have been recently classified according to 'syndromes' based primarily on clinical and EEG features. Childhood epilepsies often appear in the form of age-related electroclinical syndromes, in which seizures present as the leading symptom. The type of epileptic syndrome usually determines the initial management plan. These syndromes consist of age-related clinical seizures, specific EEG characteristics and associated neurological signs. The new classification of childhood epilepsies is confusing, but the epilepsies are divided into four main groups:

- Localization-related (focal, partial) epilepsies and syndromes
- Generalized epilepsies and syndromes
- Undetermined epilepsies and syndromes
- Specific syndromes (febrile convulsions).

These groups are further subdivided into an idiopathic, symptomatic, and cryptogenic group.

The influence of age on epilepsy

The epilepsies of childhood are very much age-related and influenced by the rate and stage of maturation of the developing brain. Thus, the same type of insult occurring at different ages may present with very different epileptic syndromes.

Clinical epileptic syndromes are classified according to four main age-related periods:
- Neonatal (birth to three months)
- Infancy and early childhood (three months to three years)
- Childhood to early adolescence
- Nine years to adulthood.

Neonatal seizures

Seizures in the newborn may take many subtle forms due to the relatively undeveloped cortex, e.g. facial grimacing; nystagmus; intermittent apnoeic episodes; myoclonus; sudden loss of muscle tone; eye blinking and chewing. 'Febrile seizures' are not observed. One needs to consider a structural CNS abnormality in many cases.

It is important to differentiate seizures from jitteriness in the newborn. The frequency of a jitter is faster than a clonic fit, and one can usually abort jitteriness by moving or flexing the limb.

Causes of neonatal seizures:
- Perinatal–anoxia, trauma, intracranial haemorrhage
- Metabolic:
  - Hypoglycaemia, hypocalcaemia, hypomagnesaemia
  - Hyper/hyponatraemia, kernicterus
  - Pyridoxine deficiency, disorders of amino acids or organic acids
- Infections, e.g. bacterial meningitis
- Developmental/structural abnormalities
- Drug withdrawal (substance-abusing mother).

It is important to identify the metabolic causes, as many of them can be readily corrected.

Some other neonatal epileptic syndromes are:
- Benign idiopathic neonatal convulsions
- Early myoclonic encephalopathy
- Early-infantile epileptic encephalopathy with suppression-bursts ('Ohtahara syndrome').

Infancy and early childhood

The CNS is more susceptible to extrinsic changes, such as fever. Specific types of seizures are observed in this period, e.g. infantile spasms and the Lennox-Gastaut syndrome. Myoclonic seizures and status epilepticus are frequently seen.

Febrile convulsions

These are generalized seizures that occur in association with a significant fever. There are specific criteria that should be present to make the diagnosis.

Criteria for 'benign' febrile fits:
- Age: six months to five years
- Extracranial cause of fever
- Family history of febrile convulsions
- Significant temperature (greater than 38.5 °C)
- Generalized convulsion, duration not longer than 15 minutes
- No neurological deficit pre- or post-convulsion
- Normal EEG after one week (usually unnecessary to perform).

Prognosis: About 40 per cent will have a second febrile seizure (that means 60 per cent will not). Certain risk factors are associated with a greater chance of the child having a subsequent non-febrile convulsion. The chance increases with the number of risk factors that may be present. Perhaps the most important of these is the association of complicated seizures, particularly when the seizure becomes prolonged.

Risk factors of having a non-febrile seizure subsequent to a febrile convulsion:
- Family history of non-febrile seizures
- Associated neurological deficit
- Complicated seizure (prolonged; focal; recurrent).

If non-febrile seizures occur, most will do so in the first year following a febrile seizure and 75 per cent begin within three years.

Long-term prophylactic treatment of febrile seizures is controversial and only indicated if there are one or more risk factors present. The drug of choice is sodium valproate or phenobarbitone. Intermittent diazepam (Valium®), either orally or per rectum, given at the time of the fever, is now being widely used, but only when properly explained to the parent or caregiver.

Note: Prophylaxis will decrease the occurrence of febrile seizures but not that of non-febrile seizures.

Infantile spasms (West's syndrome)

Infantile spasms are a unique form of seizure limited almost entirely to infants in their first year of life (age range: three months to one year). West's syndrome comprises a triad:
- Flexor or extensor spasms (Salaam attacks)
- Hypsarrhythmia on EEG
- Mental retardation.

The seizures consist mainly of large spasms (flexor predominating over extensor) and are characteristically repetitive, bilateral and symmetrical. They may occur in clusters of 'minor movements' (head nodding, eye deviation, crying, and facial flushing) especially seen on awakening and falling asleep. Concurrent seizures take the form of atonic, tonic, atypical absences, and partial motor fits.

Mental retardation may in fact precede the spasms and appear as behavioural regression. The onset of the myoclonic spasms may worsen the mental retardation.

Infantile spasms have a variety of causes, are strongly age-dependent, and are very resistant to conventional anti-convulsant therapy. The syndrome has broadly been divided into two categories, namely symptomatic and cryptogenic. The symptomatic group comprises those causes of infantile spasms that have been identified (*see* Table 26.7).

The cryptogenic group consists of causes that have not yet been identified and where the child has usually developed normally before the onset of the spasms. The cryptogenic group carries a

---

Table 26.7 Main causes of infantile spasms

- **Dysgenetic**
  Migrational disorders
  Tuberous sclerosis; neurofibromatosis; Sturge-Weber syndrome; incontinentia pigmenti; heterotopias; Aicardi's syndrome
- **Hypoxic/ischaemic**
  Prenatal; perinatal; postnatal
- **Infections**
  CMV; rubella; toxoplasmosis; meningitis; encephalitis; brain abscess
- **Haemorrhage and trauma**
- **Metabolic and toxic**
  Inborn errors of metabolism; degenerative diseases; hypoglycaemia; lead toxicity

slightly better prognosis than the symptomatic group. Treatment comprises various anticonvulsants – benzodiazepines, valproate, vigabatrin and steroids. The use of steroids is usually confined to the cryptogenic group only. Relapses occur commonly and may be preceded by EEG abnormalities. Prognosis is usually grave, with a 20 per cent mortality and a high morbidity. Cerebral palsy occurs in 33–50 per cent, mental retardation in 70–85 per cent, and psychiatric disturbances in 28 per cent of cases.

Lennox-Gastaut syndrome (LGS)
This is a group of early childhood epileptic encephalopathies consisting of a triad of characteristic seizure types, interictal slow spike-wave discharges on the EEG, and mental retardation. The seizures in LGS are known as 'stare, jerk and fall' epilepsy and are always of several types:
- Brief tonic (activated by non-rem sleep)
- Atonic drop attack (one to four seconds and may be precipitated by a myoclonic jerk)
- Myoclonic attacks
- Atypical absences
- Status–absence, myoclonic, clonic, tonic.

The 'stare' is attributable to the absence, the 'jerk' to the myoclonus, and the 'fall' to the atonic drop attack. Attacks are usually precipitated by inactivity and drowsiness and one needs to guard against over-sedation with too many anticonvulsants. Valproate and the benzodiazepines are the most commonly used drugs. More recently, lamotrigine and topiramate have been used as an add-on therapy. Steroids in the form of ACTH or prednisone may be used for short periods, but have not shown much success. A protective helmet is essential to protect the head from the sudden myoclonic and atonic drop attacks.

LGS, which forms 70 per cent of all the childhood intractable epilepsies, is one of the worst form of all the childhood epilepsies, only surpassed by Dravet's syndrome. The prognosis is poor. Eighty per cent will continue to have seizures, which are extremely resistant to normal anti-convulsant therapy. The aetiology of LGS is very similar to that of infantile spasms. In 25 per cent of cases, infantile spasms will progress to the LGS. There has also been an association with frontal lobe lesions and certain HLA haplotypes.

Other types of epileptic syndromes at this age:
- Benign myoclonic epilepsy in infants
- Severe myoclonic epilepsy in infants (Dravet's syndrome)
- Myoclonic epilepsy in non-progressive encephalopathy
- Epilepsy and inborn error of metabolism.

Childhood
There is a predominance of cryptogenic epilepsies and genetic factors play a part. Some well-defined syndromes are seen, viz. typical absences (petit mal), benign rolandic epilepsy, and the emergence of partial complex (temporal lobe) epilepsy.

Typical absences (petit mal)
Petit mal epilepsy occurs specifically in the age group of 5–15 years. These spells consist of brief lapses of consciousness that may be associated with staring, eye fluttering and fine movements of the perioral muscles. The patient does not lose body tone, but may drop objects held in the hand. The episodes last less than 10 seconds and the child is usually able to resume pre-seizure activity. Episodes may occur frequently throughout the day, and patients usually have no recall of the episode.

EEG. Classical generalized, three per second spike and wave. Hyperventilation for one to three minutes will invariably cause both the clinical and EEG phenomena. The nature and course of these seizures is usually benign. There is, however, an association with later onset of tonic clonic seizures. It is thought that the later the onset of petit mal, the greater the likelihood of developing tonic clonic seizures later in life. Treatment consists of valproate, ethosuximide or lamotrigine.

Temporal lobe epilepsy (TLE)
Complex partial seizures can occur at an early age, but are usually first observed in young children. This syndrome comprises seizures arising from the temporal lobes and their connections. Thus, these seizures manifest in the form of olfactory, gustatory, psychosensory (visual and auditory hallucinations), and autonomic symptoms. Memory distortions and emotions may also be involved. Sensations of extreme pleasure or displeasure, fears, intense depression, anger, temper tantrums, or inane laughter may occur, as

may visceral manifestations, a hollow feeling in the stomach, rising sensation with nausea, choking, palpitations, salivation, pallor or flushing, pilo-erection, and pupil dilation. These seizures may manifest with impaired consciousness as well as tonic/clonic seizures.

Benign partial epilepsy with rolandic/centro-temporal spikes (BECRS/BECTS)

The syndrome is characterized by the onset of seizures between two and fourteen years of age (peak five to eight years), simple focal motor fits as an exclusive or dominant type in the vast majority of cases, an EEG showing spikes in the lower rolandic (sylvian fissure) area on an otherwise normal background, and the absence of neurological or intellectual impairment.

The clinical features include partial fits, which are brief and involve preferentially, **one side of the face** (tonic contraction of one side of the face, and clonic jerks of the cheek and eyelids), **oropharyngeal muscles** (guttural sounds, movement of the mouth, contraction of the jaw, feelings of suffocation, profuse salivation, paraesthesias in and around the mouth), and **the upper limbs**. Consciousness is maintained in most instances. An inability to speak is common. Although the children know what they want to say they can only utter inarticulate sounds. Seizures are nocturnal, occurring commonly in the early hours of the morning and the association with sleep is striking. Most seizures are brief, but the longer ones may result in a Todd's paresis. The frequency of seizures in BECRS is low. When seizures are frequent, they tend to occur in clusters with long intervals between the clusters. In younger children, the seizures tend to be less localized and are more nocturnal.

The interictal form of the EEG forms an essential part of the syndrome. The waveform consists of a negative, sharp wave with a relatively blunted peak, followed by a positive wave whose amplitude might be 50 per cent of the preceding sharp wave. The sharp waves are often grouped in short bursts. These waveforms occur on a normal background. These findings are enhanced by sleep. These EEG changes are usually not affected by anti-epileptic drugs (AEDs). Fluctuations in the location, activity, severity and number of EEG paroxysms are not related to frequency of seizures.

BECRS usually remits by the age of 15 years.

Normalization of the EEG usually occurs after the clinical remission. The prognosis for BECRS is very good. Genetic factors play a major role in the aetiology. Treatment consists of the use of carbamazepine (Tegretol®) or valproate (Epilim®). However, because of the benign nature of the condition and the low frequency of seizures, many workers would choose not to treat with AEDs.

Other childhood epileptic syndromes at this age are:

- Epilepsy with myoclonic absences
- Epilepsies with generalized tonic–clonic seizures
- Syndromes of acquired aphasia with seizure disorders
- Epilepsy with continuous spikes and waves during slow sleep.

Childhood and adolescence

The epileptic syndromes occurring during the childhood and adolescence phase begin to take the form of the adult type of epilepsies. Focal epilepsy is more commonly associated with brain injury. There is also the emergence of certain specific epileptic syndromes:

- Reading epilepsy
- Photosensitive epilepsies
- Juvenile absence epilepsy
- Epilepsy with grand mal on awakening
- Benign partial epilepsy of adolescence
- Epilepsia partialis continua in children
- Progressive myoclonic epilepsies in childhood and adolescence.

Anti-convulsant therapy

Principles of anticonvulsant therapy

- Prevent seizures without over-sedating the child. The most appropriate anti-convulsant for a particular child is the drug which has the most favourable effect with minimal side-effects. The more established, 'older' anti-convulsants should be chosen first as they are successful in 80 per cent of the common childhood epileptic syndromes and are less expensive than the 'newer' ones. These should be reserved for those syndromes which are resistant or intractable to conventional therapy and for those children who suffer unacceptable side-effects.

- Avoid precipitating factors such as sleep deprivation, antihistamines, over-hydration, over-sedation; emotional upsets, or alcohol.
- One drug to be added or changed at a time. Use one drug to maximum dose before adding a second drug or changing a drug. Allow time for the drug to reach a steady state (5 x half-life). Try to avoid using two drugs from the same chemical group. Polypharmacy is reserved for the few really resistant childhood epilepsies as it leads to interactions resulting in agonistic or antagonistic effects of the drugs and this will have a direct effect on the drug levels and control of the epileptic syndrome. Space drugs properly according to their half-lives. This means that a drug with a half-life of 8 –12 hours should be administered twice to three times per 24 hours.
- Therapy to be continued for at least two years after last attack. Once deciding to stop, wean slowly. If seizures recur, place the child back on the original dose of the medication just prior to the break-through fit.

Status epilepticus

Status epilepticus is defined as an epileptic seizure that is sufficiently prolonged or repeated at sufficiently brief intervals so as to produce a varying and enduring epileptic condition, either in terms of convulsions or mental state (i.e they do not recover to their original state of awareness - consciousness). Status epilepticus is diagnosed if the episodes of continuous cerebral dysrhythmia last 30 minutes or longer with no recovery of consciousness between seizures. The seizures may be generalized or partial, convulsive or non-convulsive. In fact, status epilepticus may occur with any type of seizure. The most severe form of status epilepticus that is often associated with severe brain damage is generalized tonic–clonic status. It most commonly occurs in the first two years of life and represents the first seizure in many children. The causes of status epilepticus are categorized as either idiopathic, cryptogenic, or symptomatic.

Treatment

Convulsive status epilepticus is regarded as a medical emergency. Prompt and appropriate therapy is mandatory in order to prevent neurological damage. The brain responds to prolonged seizures by going into a compensatory phase, where there is an attempt to increase the

Table 26.8 Anti-epileptic drugs in children

	Dose mg/kg/day	Half-life (hrs)
Generalised and focal seizures		
Phenobarbitone	5–10	98
Phenytoin	4–8	24
Carbamazepine	15–30 (20)	8–12
Sodium valproate	20–40	8
Specialist intiated drugs		
Lamotrigine	1–8 (titrate slowly with valproate)	24+
Topiramate	1–8 (titrate slowly)	12
Vigabatrin	40–100	3–5 days
Gabapentin	10–25	6
Typical absences		
Sodium valproate	20–40	8
Ethosuximide	20–35	40
Specialist intiated drug		
Lamotrigine	1–8 (titrate slowly with valproate)	24+
Complex partial seizures (focal)		
Carbamazepine	15–30 (20)	8–12
Phenytoin	4–8	24
Febrile seizures		
Diazepam (intermittent rectal/oral)	0.5	
Phenobarbitone (seldom used)	5–10	
Sodium valproate (seldom used)	20–40	
Myoclonic seizures		
Sodium valproate	20–40	8
Clonazepam	0.03–0.05	30
Clobazam	0.5–2.0	
Nitrazepam	0.2–0.5	
ACTH	10–60 units/day	

Classification of status epilepticus

	Convulsive	Non-convulsive
Generalized	Tonic–clonic	Typical absences
	Clonic	Atypical absences
	Myoclonic	Tonic (Lennox-Gastaut (LGS))
Partial	Simple (epilepsia partialis continua)	Complex partial

blood flow to the brain by increasing cardiac output (tachycardia; hypertension; rise in central venous pressure). A build-up of lactic acid also occurs. This compensatory phase is eventually replaced by a decompensated phase, where there is a fall in cardiac output, cerebral congestion and oedema, raised intracranial pressure, metabolic acidosis, SIADH, and eventually cell death.

The objectives of management are to maintain vital functions (blood pressure, perfusion, airways, and oxygenation) and to identify and treat causal or precipitating factors. The next step is to terminate seizure activity.

Suggested drug regime for status epilepticus:

♦ Diazepam (Valium®). 0.25–0.5 mg/kg (IVI); 0.5–0.75 mg/kg (rectally). Diazepam is a very lipid soluble and is rapidly taken up by the body fat, with a resulting fall in blood levels. It may cause respiratory depression, especially when administered with phenobarbitone. This initial dose of diazepam may be repeated. Many neurologists prefer lorazepam (0.1 mg/kg) to diazepam, given as an IVI infusion at a rate of 1–2 mg per minute, to a maximum dose of 8 mg

♦ Phenytoin (Epanutin®). The loading dose can be either one of the following: 15–20 mg/kg slow infusion (max rate of infusion = 1 mg/kg/min, OR 10 mg/kg slow IVI infusion, then 5 mg/kg in six hours, then 5 mg/kg in a further six hours
NB: Never give phenytoin intramuscularly
It may be used in conjunction with diazepam.
   Use with saline solution as it precipitates out in glucose-containing solutions.

♦ A further loading dose of phenytoin (an additional 5 mg/kg by slow infusion) may be given if convulsions have not stopped. Obtaining serum phenytoin levels at the time will help to optimally load the child and prevent toxic levels of the drug being reached. However, if the seizure has not been brought under control by 15 minutes, then arrangements for an ICU bed should be made and a thiopentone infusion instituted as soon as possible.

♦ Midazolam (Dormicum®) – bolus 0.15 mg/kg followed by continuous infusion of 0.02–0.4 mg/kg/hr increasing to 1.8 mg/kg/hr. (may be given intranasally if battling to get ivi line).

♦ Phenobarbitone. Loading dose of 5–10 mg/kg IVI; neonates 10–20 mg/kg IVI. The drawback of using phenobarbitone as a drug in status epilepticus, is that it penetrates the CNS very slowly and may cause severe respiratory depression, especially when combined with benzodiazepines. Most workers will only use phenobarb for status epilepticus in the neonatal and early infancy period.

♦ Paraldehyde. 0.1–0.15 ml/kg rectally (max 0.4 mg/kg). Paraldehyde is very corrosive and needs to be diluted, either with Aracus oil 2:1 or normal saline. This drug has a wide safety margin and the dose can be repeated safely. The rectal preparation has proved to be a useful adjuvant when diazepam and phenytoin have failed to control the status and when one is waiting for an ICU bed.

♦ Lidocaine. Initial dose 2–3 mg/kg, then infusion 3–10 mg/kg/hr. The anti-epileptic action is transient. One needs to beware of high doses.

♦ General anaesthesia. Once the above medications have failed to stop the fit, general anaesthesia needs to be considered. This will require ventilatory support. Thiopentone is the most common form used. The dose is usually assessed on titration. The starting infusion dose is 1–3 mg/kg/hr and one may need to go as high as 5–7 mg/kg/hr. However, phenobarb has a much better anti-convulsant property than the shorter acting barbiturates.

Note – in children under three years, consider pyridoxine 50–100 mg IVI/oral in intractable seizures.

Most cases of status epilepticus can be controlled on the regimen of initial diazepam followed by a correct loading of phenytoin and maintaining the serum level of the medication for long enough for the acute aggravating factors to subside. Ongoing treatment will depend on the pre-existing condition of the child. If the child is a known epileptic then he/she needs to continue with prophylactic medication. If the cause of the status epilepticus is relatively benign (biochemical or infective) then slow weaning of the anti-convulsant should occur over the next few weeks.

Paroxysmal non-epileptic disorders

These are a group of disorders that may be confused with epilepsy. It is important to recognize these episodes as being non-epileptic to avoid unnecessary long-term anti-convulsant therapy. Sometimes the parent, caregiver or witness to a child having a fit is unable to describe the episode properly. If one asks the witness to *mimic* what they observed, the clinical picture often becomes more representative and accurate. One should ask about pre-seizure sensations and post-ictal phenomena, such as confusion, drowsiness, or sleep.

Classification of paroxysmal non-epileptic disorders

Anoxic-ischaemic
 ◆ Apnoeic spells (newborn)
 ◆ Breath-holding spells (six months to two years) there are two types:
   – **Cyanotic:** crying and cyanosis precedes unconsciousness and there is no change in cardiac rhythm. The young child often experiences a minor irritation and may have a temper tantrum, cry and hold its breath, fall down, may go stiff and have a few clonic jerks.
   – **Pallid:** there is only a brief or silent cry followed by pallor, associated with a bradycardia and at times asystole. This is a presumed vasovagal episode. Prognosis is good in both types and no treatment, apart from reassuring the parents, is indicated.

 ◆ Syncope: cardiac, tussive, micturition
 ◆ Orthostatic hypotension
 ◆ Hypertensive encephalopathy
 ◆ Transient encephalopathy
 ◆ Migraine.

Psychological
 ◆ Conversion reaction
 ◆ Malingering
 ◆ Masturbation
 ◆ Hyperventilation.

Sleep disorders
 ◆ Narcolepsy
 ◆ Pickwickian syndrome
 ◆ Enuresis
 ◆ Somnambulism
 ◆ Night terrors.

Movement disorder
 ◆ Familial paroxysmal choreoathetosis
 ◆ Sandifer syndrome
 ◆ Shuddering attacks.

Toxic
 ◆ Paroxysmal dystonia.

Other
 ◆ Recurrent vertigo.

The 'floppy infant' and disorders of the lower motor neuron

The 'floppy child' displays signs of hypotonia, which may be manifest as an unusual frog-like posture in infancy. When pulled from supine to the sitting position, the head flops back or flexes forward with the chin on the chest. In the child of six months and older, the back will be rounded instead of straight when attempting to sit. When the child is suspended in the ventral position, the arms, head and legs hang down like a 'raggedy Ann doll'. Muscle tone is low and there is an excessive range of movement around the joints, causing the knees and elbows to hyperextend, and the wrist and ankles to be placed in strange postures. The infants remain relatively immobile and the older child may have delayed motor milestones.

The first decision to make when assessing a floppy child is whether there is weakness or

Table 26.9 Paralytic and non-paralytic conditions associated with hypotonia

- **Anterior horn cells**
  Infantile spinal muscular atrophy (SMA)
  Types 1, 2 and 3
  Poliomyelitis
- **Nerve roots**
  Guillain-Barré syndrome
- **Neuropathies**
  Hereditary motor & sensory neuropathies (CMT)
- **Myasthenia gravis**
  Neonatal/juvenile/congenital)
- **Myopathies**
  Congenital myopathies:
  Myotubular myopathy
  Nemaline myopathy
  Central core disease
  Congenital fibre type disproportion
- **Dystrophies**
  Muscular dystrophy
  Myotonic dystrophy
  Metabolic myopathies:
  Glycogenoses (types 2, 3, 4, 5, 7)
  Mitochondrial myopathy
  Lipid storage myopathy
  Periodic paralysis

- **Disorders of the CNS**
  Mental retardation
  Birth asphyxia/trauma
  Hypotonic cerebral palsy
  Chromosomal disorders (Down's syndrome)
  Metabolic disorders:
  Lipidoses
  Leukodystrophies
  Mucopolysaccharidoses
  Aminoacidurias
  Leigh's syndrome
- **Connective tissue disorders**
  Congenital ligament laxity
  Ehlers-Danlos syndrome
  Marfan's syndrome
  Osteogenesis imperfecta
- **Prader-Willi syndrome**
- **Metabolic disorders**
  Organic acidaemias
  Hypercalcaemia
  Rickets
  Hypothyroidism
  Renal tubular acidosis
  Coeliac disease

not, that is, is the condition paralytic or non-paralytic? This can be assessed by observing whether the infant can move its limbs against gravity or withdraw them from noxious stimuli or not. Thereafter, the diagnostic problems of the floppy child are approached according to the anatomical site of the lesion (*see* Table 26.9).

One needs to assess whether the problem is due to an upper or lower motor neuron lesion. The combination of motor as well as intellectual delay usually points towards a central lesion. The presence of brisk deep tendon reflexes, with truncal hypotonia might suggest a diagnosis of hypotonic cerebral palsy. Most of the causes of a floppy child will be due to a lower motor neuron problem. Upper motor neuron causes of hypotonia will be due to diseases of the cerebellum. The dysmorphic features of Down's, Prader-Willi, Marfan's and Ehlers-Danlos syndromes should not be over-looked. There is a wide range of apparently normal states of

ligament laxity in the general population and congenital laxity of the ligaments is common. Additional clinical signs such as rickets or acidosis may lead one to suspect a generalized metabolic or endocrine disorder.

Lesions of the lower motor neuron system are associated with hypotonia, reduced or absent reflexes, wasting (usually an early sign), and a degree of weakness, either in a proximal or distal distribution. Associated features can be helpful in pointing to some of the disorders.

- Facial muscle involvement – seen in some of the congenital myopathies (myotubular myopathy; central core myopathy; nemaline myopathy); SMA; mitochondrial myopathy; myasthenia gravis and myotonic dystrophy.
- Ocular muscle involvement – involvement of the external ocular muscles is seen in myotubular myopathy; mitochondrial myopathy; myasthenia gravis, and dystrophica myotonia.
- Arthrogryposis – is more likely in congenital

muscular dystrophy and congenital myotonic dystrophy.

- Contractures – commonly found in congenital muscular dystrophy; congenital myotonic dystrophy and in cases of SMA as a result of immobility of a limb due to extreme weakness.
- Sucking and swallowing difficulties – common in SMA (types 1 and 2); congenital myotonic dystrophy; myotubular myopathy; nemaline myopathy; neonatal myasthenia; Prader-Willi syndrome, and birth asphyxia.

Anterior horn cell

Infantile spinal muscular atrophy (SMA)

Infantile SMA is the most common neuromuscular disorder of childhood. It is a group of hereditary disorders affecting proximal symmetrical muscular atrophy associated with progressive degeneration of the anterior horn cells of the spinal cord and brainstem motor neurons. The clinical features include a proximal muscle weakness and wasting of varying intensity, the legs affected more than the arms. Facial weakness is seen in 50 per cent of cases if carefully looked for. Fasciculations of the tongue and small muscles of the hand (minimyoclonus) are often seen. Tendon reflexes are reduced to absent, and in the severe types marked hypotonia is observed. For practical purposes, the clinical spectrum can be divided into three main groups (mild, intermediate, and severe; *see also* Table 26.10) based on the ability of the child to sit or stand and walk unaided.

Type 1 SMA usually presents within the first few weeks of life. The mother may have noticed decreased fetal movements in a minority of cases. The infant shows generalized hypotonia with marked weakness and wasting of the limbs and trunk with poor head control, the legs more involved than the arms. Bulbar weakness is often present with difficulties in sucking and swallowing. The intercostal muscles are severely affected, making breathing difficult. The chest takes on a bell-shaped appearance. There is often intercostal recession with rib crowding on a plain chest X-ray. The cry and cough are weak. The infants are prone to recurrent pneumonias accounting for repeated admissions to hospital. Cardiac muscle is not involved. Tendon reflexes are invariably absent and contractures may be seen as a result of the immobility of the limbs. The arms may be characteristically internally rotated due to the internal rotation of the shoulders giving the 'jug-handle' position of the arms with the hands facing outwards. Sweating of the soles and palms is frequently seen in all three types of SMA.

Type 2 SMA presents within the first few months of life. The course of the disease is slower and less progressive and the clinical features not as marked as they are in type 1 SMA. The tendon reflexes are reduced rather than absent and fasciculations are seen more readily, particularly in the tongue. The course is more benign with a slow progression of weakness. The single most important prognostic sign is the involvement of the respiratory system.

Type 3 SMA patients usually have normal milestones in the first year of life, but tend to walk at a somewhat later stage. They present with features of a proximal muscle weakness similar to a patient with Duchenne's muscular dystrophy. They walk flat-footed with the foot everted. Tremor of the hands (minimyoclonus) is commonly seen and tendon reflexes may initially be normal. The prognosis is good with most children reaching adulthood as the decline is very gradual. In some cases, there may in fact be improvement in function as there may be compensatory re-innervation of the muscles.

Table 26.10 Clinical classification of SMA			
Type	**Onset**	**Course**	**Age of death**
1 Severe (Werdnig-Hoffmann)	Birth to 6 months	Never sit	<2 years
2 Intermediate (Werdnig-Hoffmann)	<18 months	Never stand	>2 years
3 Mild (Kugelberg-Welander)	>18 months	Stand alone	Adult

Source: Dubowitz V. 1995. Muscle disorders of childhood (2nd edition). By permission of Elsevier.

Special investigations. The muscle enzymes (CPK) are usually normal. Ultrasonography of the muscles will show an increased echo in the muscle with a loss of muscle bulk. ECG may show signs of fasciculations on the tracing from the underlying intercostal muscles. Electromyography (EMG) may reveal evidence of a neurogenic atrophy and fibrillation potentials as well as large polyphasic potentials at rest. Muscle biopsy shows atrophic type 1 and 2 muscle fibres which tend to be rounded in outline and clustered in groups, interspersed with fascicles of markedly hypertrophied fibres (mainly type 1 fibres reinnervated) and fascicles of normal muscle fibres. It is often difficult to assess the severity of the condition from the muscle biopsy and some of the milder forms show less characteristic histopathological features.

Genetics. Infantile spinal muscular atrophy is autosomal recessively inherited with a recurrence risk of 1:4. The gene (SMN) for SMA has been located on chromosome 5. These findings make antenatal diagnosis possible, confirming clinical impressions.

Treatment. This remains supportive in the severe forms with the active and appropriate treatment of respiratory infections. Physiotherapy is useful, particularly in the intermediate and mild forms.

Poliomyelitis

This viral disease affects the anterior horn cells. The illness is usually preceded by mild GIT symptoms, followed by fever, headache, nausea, and pain in the neck, back and limbs. This is followed within a week or two with an ascending, often asymmetrical motor paralysis, usually associated with muscle spasm. The weakness may be so extensive as to involve a total flaccid quadriplegia and there may also be bulbar and respiratory involvement, which can be life-threatening. EMG shows evidence of denervation; the CSF reveals an elevated protein and a mild lymphocytosis. Culture of the virus from the CSF confirms the diagnosis. Failing this, a rise of the virus antibody titres is helpful. The other enteroviruses, coxsackie and echovirus can give rise to similar features. Treatment is supportive. Hopefully, poliomyelitis will soon be eradicated worldwide through immunization.

Nerve roots

Guillain-Barré syndrome (acute polyradiculoneuritis)

This is a demyelinating neuropathy of the anterior and posterior nerve roots, induced by an immune process. The motor signs, which tend to dominate the clinical features, are preceded by an upper respiratory tract infection a week or two earlier, usually viral (coxsackie, echo, and herpes virus). In more than 60 per cent of cases, there is an initial paraesthesia of the fingers and toes, which often goes undetected unless one specifically enquires about it. The onset in children is usually acute and rapid, often over a few hours, but may be insidious, with the emergence of an ascending, usually symmetrical motor paralysis of the legs extending variably to involve the trunk, upper limbs, respiratory, bulbar and facial muscles. This weakness is often accompanied by muscle pain. Reflexes are reduced to absent. Because the anterior and posterior roots carry motor, sensory and autonomic fibres (in cervical and sacral segments), sensory loss may be present,

Table 26.11 Peripheral neuropathies in children

Drugs
- Isoniazid
- Vincristine

Toxins
- Lead; mercury; gold; thallium; arsenic; glue; benzine

Hereditary motor and sensory neuropathy (HSN)

Chronic inflammatory demyelinating polyradiculopathy

Congenital hypomyelination neuropathy

Giant axonal neuropathy

Friedreich's ataxia

Krabbe disease

Metabolic neuropathies
- Diabetes
- Uraemic neuropathy
- Acute intermittent porphyria
- Vitamin deficiency (B_1, B_{12})
- Abeta-lipoproteinaemia
- Alpha-lipoprotein deficiency
- Metachromatic leukodystrophy
- Refsum disease

Diphtheria

usually in a glove and stocking distribution. There may also be instability of autonomic function with wide swings in blood pressure, heart rate and urinary incontinence or retention. The important life-threatening feature is the onset of respiratory failure leading to a need for ventilatory assistance.

The finding of an elevated protein in the CSF which is otherwise normal, assists the diagnosis. Nerve conduction studies show delayed conductance in keeping with a demyelinating condition. Management is supportive; the respiratory status needs to be monitored at all times. Physiotherapy plays an important role, especially in the children who are immobile and recover slowly. The use of intravenous gammaglobulin, either in a dose of 400 mg/kg/d for four to five days or more preferably 1 g/kg/d for two days, is often followed by a dramatic response. The prognosis is generally good with more than 80 per cent showing complete recovery. However, in a few cases, recovery may take many months to a year. In 5 per cent of cases there will be a residual weakness.

Peripheral nerves

Peripheral neuropathies are relatively uncommon in children. Possible conditions are listed in Table 26.11.

Neuromuscular junction

Acquired juvenile myasthenia gravis

This is the most common myasthenic disorder, and is due to antibodies that attach to acetylcholine receptors and compete with acetylcholine for binding sites on these post-synaptic receptors. The characteristic clinical feature is weakness and an abnormal fatigue after repeated or sustained activity and by improvement after rest. The weakness affects the extra-ocular muscles most commonly (clinically presenting with ptosis and extra-ocular muscle weakness), but may also involve facial muscles, neck, trunk, and extremities. There is a predominance of female patients. The diagnosis can be made clinically by fatiguing certain muscle groups, measuring the power in these muscles before and after fatigue. This can be confirmed by giving intramuscular neostigmine and observing an improvement in the power within 5–15 minutes. The fatigability of the muscles can also be demonstrated by a decrement in the muscle action potentials after repetitive stimulation of the nerve, recorded by surface electrodes. Serum anti-AChR antibodies can usually be detected in 65–75 per cent of patients with generalized myasthenia gravis and in about 50 per cent of those with pure ocular myasthenia. There is an incidence of associated disorders, such as thyroid disease, diabetes and arthritis. Treatment consists of longer acting anticholinesterase drugs such as pyridostigmine (Mestinon®) 15–60 mg four-hourly except at night. This form of therapy is only symptomatic and improves the neuromuscular transmission. Thymectomy and immunosuppressive therapy is more definitive, but controversy exists as to which children require thymectomy. In general, the earlier that thymectomy is performed, the better the results. Children whose weakness is confined to the eye muscles usually do not require thymectomies, but rather those who have a more extensive disease and those children in whom the disease is still progressing. Plasma exchange or intravenous gammaglobulin therapy can be used in myasthenic crises. Steroid therapy has also been used, but long-term steroid therapy in children is not without complications. Certain drugs may produce an exacerbation of symptoms in children with myasthenia gravis. These include muscle relaxants (curare, Flaxedil®, decamethonium, and succinylcholine); quinine, quinidine and aminoglycoside antibiotics (aminoglycosides) (increase neuromuscular block).

There are several types of myasthenia gravis. A **transient neonatal** form occurs as a result of maternal antibodies (IgG) crossing the placenta in a mother who has the adult type of myasthenia gravis. The baby may present with marked hypotonia, apnoeic attacks, bulbar weakness, and pooling of saliva. Symptoms are transient with a full recovery in three to five weeks. A rare group of **congenital myasthenic syndromes** are genetically determined and some patients may present in the neonatal period or sometime later. This rare group will demonstrate defects in the synthesis, storage, release and degradation of acetylcholine as well as defects in the postsynaptic membrane. Most of them will respond to acetylcholinesterase inhibitors.

Botulism

Botulism presents as acute hypotonia and weakness in infants between the ages of three to eighteen months. The botulinum toxin is ingested from contaminated food, especially honey, giving rise to generalized weakness, opthalmoplegia and bulbar weakness. The toxin affects neuromuscular transmission.

Organophosphate poisoning

Organophosphate poisoning occurs either from ingestion or absorption through the skin of the insecticide. The toxin is an acetylcholinesterase inhibitor, which may result in serious cholinergic signs in the form of salivation, lacrimation, and bronchospasm (muscarinic manifestations). The nicotinic signs include muscle weakness, muscle fasciculation and decreased respiratory effort. The CNS signs are anxiety, restlessness, confusion, headache, slurred speech, ataxia, and generalized seizures. Treatment consists of decontamination, atropine to reverse the cho-linergic signs, and pralidoxime (2-PAM or proto-pam), a cholinesterase reactivator that reverses the neuromuscular effects and restores muscle strength and respiratory effort (*See* Chapter 11, Poisoning).

Muscle disorders

Muscle disorders may be classified as:
- Congenital myopathies
- Muscular dystrophies
- Myotonic disorders
- Metabolic/inflammatory myopathies.

Congenital myopathies

The pathology is present at birth, but the clinical features are relatively non-progressive, or very slowly progressive. They are characterized by structural abnormalities in the muscle and are usually of genetic origin, most following an auto-somal-dominant pattern of inheritance. There are six morphologically distinct types which usu-ally cannot readily be distinguished from one another on clinical grounds and need a muscle biopsy for further differentiation.
- **Central core disease** presents in early infancy or later in childhood with a non-progressive proximal muscle weakness and muscle cramps after exercise. In a few cases, the weakness has been more generalized. There may also be a mild degree of facial weakness. Histologically, the cores seem to have a predilection for type 1 fibres. There

is a stronger association with malignant hyperpyrexia than in the other myopathies. Inheritance is autosomal-dominant with sporadic break-throughs occurring.
- **Minicore disease** usually presents with mild, non-progressive weakness. Associated diaphragmatic weakness may cause nocturnal hypoventilation leading to disturbed sleep and early-morning headaches. The nocturnal hypoventilation can be severe enough to be life-threatening. It can usually be treated with the use of nasal oxygen or home ventilation at night. Mild facial weakness may be present. Inheritance is autosomal-recessive.
- **Nemaline myopathy** ('rod-body' myopathy). There is a wide variation in the degree of weakness observed in this condition. There are also associated dysmorphic features that characterize this myopathy, including skeletal dysmorphism with kyphoscoliosis, pes cavus, high arched palate, and a long face. There is a high incidence of respiratory problems due to diaphragmatic involvement and they may suffer from nocturnal hypoventilation as in central core disease. Swallowing difficulties are often encountered in the neonate and infant. Cardiomyopathy has been reported in late-onset nemaline myopathy and is extremely rare in the infantile cases. Prognosis depends to a large extent on the respiratory deficiency. Inheritance is both autosomal-recessive (more common), and dominant with sporadic mutations occurring and a variable clinical expression.
- **Myotubular myopathy** (centronuclear myopathy). These patients present with a varying degree of weakness, often including ptosis and weakness of the extraocular muscles, facial as well as the axial musculature. Inheritance is either autosomal-dominant or X-linked recessive.
- **Congenital fibre type disproportion.** These children present with floppiness shortly after birth with contractures of the muscles of the feet and hands and some having dislocation of the hips. There is a wide range in the degree of weakness observed affecting mainly the muscle of the trunk and extremities. After an initial progression, the disease seems to become static from the age

of two years, and many show improvement. It is important to confirm the diagnosis as it generally has a good prognosis and needs to be differentiated from conditions like SMA and congenital myotonic dystrophy.

* **Congenital myopathies** with abnormalities of subcellular organelles. There are groups of myopathies in which organelles within the cells have been observed and include finger-print myopathy; sarcotubular myopathy; zebra-body myopathy; reducing body myopathy; cytoplasmic body myopathy; and hyaline body myopathy.

Muscular dystrophies

These are defined as 'a group of genetically determined disorders with progressive degeneration of skeletal muscle and no structural abnormality in the central or peripheral nervous system, and have been subdivided into various types on the basis of the clinical distribution and severity of muscle weakness and pattern of inheritance' (Dubowitz, *Muscle disorders of childhood*, 2nd edition, 1995).

Duchenne's muscular dystrophy is by far the most common dystrophy affecting children and can be defined as an X-linked disorder characterized by progressive weakness of predominantly proximal muscles due to a deficiency of the membrane protein dystrophin. The onset is usually insidious, occurring at the time when the child first starts walking, but signs may only become apparent after five years of age. There is an abnormality of gait, frequent falls, difficulty in climbing stairs, and usually some delay in motor milestones. The distribution of weakness affects the proximal muscles initially, causing the child to adopt a waddling gait, a lordotic posture, and a tendency to 'toe walk'. There is progressive difficulty in getting up out of a chair and in rising from lying or sitting on the floor. Gower's sign consists of the manoeuvre by which the child goes from a supine to a prone position, then into a knee-elbow position, followed by extending the knees and elbows and then drawing the hands and feet closer together and then slowly climbing up his legs by supporting himself with hands on his knees and thighs. Gower's manoeuvre is not pathognomonic of Duchenne's muscular dystrophy but will occur in any condition where there is significant proximal weakness of the lower limbs. Pain in the muscles, especially

in the calves and particularly following exercise, is common. Pseudohypertrophy of the muscles occurs commonly and is seen more obviously in the earlier stages of the disease. It involves the calves as well as the triceps, deltoids, and masseter muscles. Progressive weakness leads to failure to walk during the early teens. The weakness causes deformities of the spine with scoliosis and contractures of the ankles, knee and hip flexors, as well as the elbows. The tendon reflexes become reduced and absent from early on in the disease with the ankle jerks preserved for some time. Weak intercostal muscles and the worsening scoliosis cause respiratory problems. The vital capacity begins to decline in the early teens and death usually results from a respiratory tract infection, which can progress extremely rapidly. Cardiomyopathy may be an associated manifestation of the disorder presenting with right ventricular strain on ECG. The mean IQ in most series of Duchenne's muscular dystrophy is in the region of 85, suggesting a slight intellectual impairment.

Special investigations include serum muscle enzymes. There is a gross elevation of the CPK, particularly in the earlier stages of the disease with the levels reaching 50–100 times normal. EMG shows a characteristic myopathic pattern of low amplitude, to short-duration polyphasic motor unit action potentials. Muscle biopsy remains the definitive means of confirming the tissue diagnosis. Dystrophin, the gene product, can be measured both qualitatively and quantitatively from the biopsy as well as from serum in certain laboratories. Absence of dystrophin confirms the diagnosis, whereas the presence of altered size or abundance of dystrophin suggests a Becker-type of dystrophy. DNA testing has recently become much more specific in confirming the diagnosis.

Management involves attempts to keep the child as mobile and ambulant for as long as possible. Once the child has lost ambulation, he becomes more prone to the various complications such as muscle contractures and deformities. Rehabilitation includes physiotherapy (night splints, passive exercises, and proper positioning). The correct timing and the benefits of surgical intervention for the various contractures and scoliosis remain controversial. A number of clinical trials have shown an improvement in muscle power, muscle mass, and a fall in the rate of muscle breakdown with steroid treatment.

Female carriers of the X-linked Duchenne gene may be detected by a slight to moderate elevation of CPK (in 70 per cent of cases) and by recombinant DNA technology.

Becker's muscular dystrophy is very similar to Duchenne's dystrophy in clinical appearance and distribution of weakness but milder in severity. It has the same location on the Xp21 chromosome as Duchenne's dystrophy and is thus allelic. Duchenne's and Becker's dystrophy are due to deletions or other mutations at the same gene locus and are now referred to as the 'dystrophinopathies'. The onset of symptoms occurs later, with a more benign course, ambulation continuing well into adolescence and even adult life.

Congenital muscular dystrophy (CMD) consists of a group of dystrophies affecting infants with muscle weakness at birth or within a few months of life. They often present with hypotonia and on occasions may present with arthrogryposis. The condition usually remains static but cases have been known to show considerable functional improvement. Respiratory and swallowing problems may accompany the weakness. The CPK may be moderately elevated and muscle biopsy shows dystrophy and a marked replacement of muscle by adipose and connective tissue. Most of the CMDs can now be diagnosed genetically.

Myotonic syndromes

Myotonia is a state of delayed relaxation, or sustained contraction of skeletal muscle due to instability of the muscle cell membrane. This is manifested clinically after a sustained contraction of the muscles, such as when asking the child to hold her hand in a tight fist and then to rapidly open the hand, observing delayed relaxation with an inability to open the hand quickly. Clinical myotonia can be confirmed on EMG by the insertion of a concentric needle which produces insertional irritability and myotonic bursts which can be precipitated by percussing the muscle. There are a number of myotonic disorders:

Myotonic dystrophy (Steinert's disease). The classic form occurs in adolescents and adults, with myotonia, dystrophy of the facial muscles, shoulder girdle, brachioradialis and the anterior compartment of the leg muscle. Associated features include baldness, testicular atrophy, hyperinsulinism,

peripheral neuropathy, growth hormone disturbances, posterior cataracts, and intellectual impairment. It is autosomal-dominant in inheritance, the gene located on chromosome 19.

There is a neonatal form, onset is prenatal, and the fetus may present with hydramnios. Babies are commonly born small for gestational age, and arthrogryposis, weakness (especially facial), hypotonia, and pes cavus are the usual clinical features. Myotonia is uncommon before three to four years of age. Because of the dominant inheritance, it is important to look for myotonia in the mother or father.

Myotonia congenita. There are two forms of this condition. The first is an autosomal-dominant form, Thomsen's disease, and the second, the autosomal-recessive variety, Becker's disease. They differ slightly in their respective clinical features, both demonstrating myotonia and muscle hypertrophy. In Thomsen's disease, the course is more benign, especially the extent of the muscle hypertrophy. The myotonia usually first manifests when the child has difficulty in moving their limbs after a period of prolonged rest and is often worse on wakening in the morning, tending to improve during the day. Cold, fatigue, and mood (fright or tension) may aggravate the myotonia. In the recessive form, the myotonia is usually later in onset, progresses more slowly, but is more marked and more generalized, affecting the legs before the arms and face. The muscle hypertrophy and weakness is more striking than in the dominant form. Muscle biopsy is not very helpful in either form.

Paramyotonia congenita (Eulenburg's disease) is characterized by myotonia that is brought on or aggravated by cold. The myotonia is mild and affects the eyelids, face, and hands and responds rapidly to warming.

Chondrodystrophic myotonia (Schwartz-Jampel syndrome) consists of myotonia, chondrodysplasia, and short stature. Children with this kind of myotonia display a striking facial appearance of blepharospasm, narrow palpebral fissures, micrognathia, and flattened facies. The muscles are hypertrophied and stiff with limitations of joint movements.

Metabolic/inflammatory muscle disorders

This is a large group of disorders, as listed in Table 26.12.

Table 26.12 Metabolic, endocrine, and inflammatory myopathies

Metabolic myopathies	Endocrine myopathies
• Glycogenoses (Types 2, 3, 4, 5, 7, 8, 9, 10, 11)	• Thyroid disorders
• Lipid disorders	Thyrotoxicosis (thyrotoxic myopathy, myasthenia,
• Carnitine disorders	periodic paralysis, exophthalmic ophthalmoplegia)
Acyl-CoA dehydrogenase deficiency	Hypothyroidism (Kocher-Debre-Semelaigne
• Glutaric aciduria type 2	syndrome, Hoffmann's syndrome)
• Mitochondrial disorders	• Pituitary and adrenal
• Periodic paralysis	Hypo/hyperpituitarism, Cushing's syndrome, steroid
Hypokalaemic periodic paralysis	myopathy, Addison's disease, hyperaldosteronism
Hyperkalaemic periodic paralysis	
	Inflammatory myopathies
Nutritional myopathies	Dermatomyositis/polymyositis
Protein-energy malnutrition	Focal myositis
Rickets	Inclusion body myositis
	Reducing body myositis
	Viral myositis

Ataxic disorders

The term ataxia indicates an incoordination of postural control and gait as well as an incoordination of the skilled movements involved in fine hand movements and speech. The cerebellum is vital for the control of movement patterns and is also involved in motor learning. It allows one to judge the speed, force and direction that is required in a particular movement. The extra pyramidal system and the cerebellum together give the ability to rapidly stop and start a movement and to execute a movement with ease and fluidity. The cerebellum is a postnatally maturing organ and thus many of the signs which in an adult would be regarded as indicating disease of the cerebellum, can be taken as being normal in children at certain stages of their development. The developing child is in fact displaying 'physiological cerebellar signs' and these should not be interpreted as being signs and symptoms of cerebellar disease.

The cerebellum is a vast coordinator of information and receives approximately 40 times more afferent than efferent fibres. It is able to analyse the current situation of the muscles of the body (information from muscle spindles, joint receptors, pressure receptors; together with the position of the head and its relationship to the body and the motion of the body via the labyrinths; together with information from the

eyes and body image from the parietal cortex). This allows the cerebellum a total picture of the body's position in space, motion, head position, and limb position, as well as the state of the contraction of different muscles, all to be available if needed to allow a cortical movement to occur and that movement to be adjusted in speed, force or direction, as well as stabilizing other parts of the body against imbalance produced by that movement.

Clinical features

Truncal ataxia is a disorder of posture, tone, locomotion, and equilibrium and is seen in midline disorders of the cerebellum such as congenital absence of the vermis, vermis tumours (medulloblastomas), some causes of hydrocephalus, and perinatal asphyxia. The child is floppy with exaggerated joint angles and the development of posture is retarded with head lag and truncal hypotonia. Congenital ataxia results in a developmental delay in motor skills. The cerebellum is part of the motor circuit necessary for skilled learned motor movements and disease of the cerebellum can interfere with motor learning. This is seen especially in speech where instead of observing a dysarthria, one finds a developmental delay in articulation. The learned motor skills are delayed as seen in hand function in fastening buttons, laces, and assembling objects. This is not only clumsiness but also a dyspraxia. Righting reactions may be affected with the child having difficulty in rolling, getting up from lying to sitting and eventually standing.

Volitional ataxia. If the cerebellum is diseased, movement is clumsy with poor adjustment of speed, force, and direction and this is shown clinically as an intention tremor. Dysmetria is present due to the difficulty in judging distance. Difficulty in starting and stopping a movement rapidly is often manifested as dysdiadochokinesia or by pendular tendon reflexes. In particular, the child's speech will be slurred, dysarthric or explosive, staccato. Nystagmus is often seen in acquired ataxia but is absent in congenital ataxia. There is a degree of hypotonia but not to the same extent as that seen in truncal ataxia.

Hypotonia is the most important of the cerebellar signs and one should seriously reconsider the diagnosis of a cerebellar disorder if hypotonia is not among the signs.

Ataxia may be divided into three broad categories: acute, chronic static, and chronic progressive. The presentation of **acute ataxia** can be dramatic and frightening to the child. The child may be unable to walk or will stagger and reel about. If the limbs are involved then the child may be unable to feed and be severely clumsy with a marked tremor. Nystagmus is unusual in acute-onset ataxia and speech is usually dysarthric. The approach to a child presenting with an acute onset of cerebellar signs and symptoms is to assess, as soon as possible, whether one is dealing with a relatively benign self-limiting condition or a more severe life-threatening disorder. If the cerebellar signs are symmetrical on either side of the body with no other localizing neurological signs or signs of raised intracranial pressure, then the likelihood of a more benign condition is higher. One needs to look for signs of recent infection (post-chickenpox staining of the skin) and obtain a comprehensive history of any past trauma or possible intoxication. Signs and symptoms of other CNS involvement would strongly suggest the need for a CT or MRI scan of the brain as soon as possible.

Chronic non-progressive ataxias are better known as the ataxic/hypotonic cerebral palsies. These conditions are static and do not progress. There are a number of conditions that cause this group of disorders (*see* Table 26.14), most of them being congenital malformations of the cerebellum.

Chronic progressive ataxia may be due to lesions in the cerebellum with loss of Purkinje cells, cerebellar nuclei, or in one of the abundant afferent or efferent pathways entering or leaving the cerebellum such as olivary atrophy, spinocerebellar degeneration, posterior column demyelination, or a peripheral nerve lesion with a sensory neuropathy. It is therefore necessary to consider the vestibular, cerebellar, proprioceptive, and peripheral nerve functions in all cases of chronic ataxia.

Friedreich's ataxia is one of the more common spinocerebellar ataxias with onset before 20 years, an autosomal recessive inheritance, and the combined involvement of large sensory fibres in peripheral nerves, cerebellar tracts, pyramidal tracts and posterior columns. Clinical features are varied and consist of progressive ataxia, often presenting initially as progressive gait difficulties, the ataxia affecting both the limbs and gait. Nystagmus is not a common accompanying sign but speech will be affected in almost 100 per cent of cases. The involvement of the corticospinal tracts will present with weakness, a positive Babinski response but with absent knee and ankle jerks (may be present initially). The limbs show a distal wasting affecting the calf muscles in the leg and the small muscles of the hand. Posterior column involvement shows as a loss of position and vibration sense and a positive Romberg test, but may not be obvious in the early stages of the disease. Bladder dysfunction in the form of a spastic bladder is not an uncommon symptom. Involvement of cranial nerves often occurs. Scoliosis is present in over 75 per cent of cases and can be severe enough to cause marked respiratory embarrassment. A characteristic feature of Friedreich's ataxia is the presence of talipes equinovarus and pes cavus. There may also be a claw hand deformity. Cardiomyopathies are the most common accompanying cardiac abnormalities and often progressive in nature. There are ECG abnormalities (deep Q waves, low wave QRS complexes, T-wave inversion, and S-T segment changes) and symmetric ventricular hypertrophy is frequent. Associated findings may include diabetes mellitus with an abnormal glucose tolerance curve and insulin resistance appears to be the explanation.

Diagnosis may be confirmed on DNA studies for the Frataxin gene, chromosome 9q13.

Table 26.13 Selected causes of acute ataxia in childhood

Infections
Viral cerebellitis (chicken-pox; polio; coxsackie; Epstein Barr; echo; influenza; mumps; measles)
Bacterial (diphtheria; pertussis; scarlet fever; typhoid)
Cerebellar abscess
Toxic/metabolic
Alcohol
Drugs – phenytoin; carbamazapine; phenobarbitone; Hartnup disease; argininosuccinic aminoaciduria; Maple syrup urine disease; hyperammonaemia Hypoglycaemia; organic acidurias; Leigh's encephalopathy; lead; glue; mercury; tic paralysis poisoning; methotrexate; vitamin A
Posterior fossa tumours
Trauma (Cerebellar haemorrhage)
Vascular–rare (Embolism; thrombosis; AVM's)
Basilar migraine
Pseudo-ataxia (motor weakness; non-convulsive status epilepticus)

Table 26.14 Chronic non-progressive cerebellar ataxias

Perinatal insults
- Birth asphyxia
- Metabolic (hypoglycaemia; hyperbilirubinaemia)
- Intraventricular haemorrhage; meningitis
Congenital malformations
- Primary cerebellar hypoplasia
- Hydrocephalus: (Dandy Walker syndrome; Arnold Chiari malformation; platybasia; chromosomal disorders 8, 18)
Fetal alcohol syndrome
Joubert syndrome
Cerebellar/kidney associations
- Cerebellar/renal cystic disease syndrome
- Meckel-Gruber syndrome
- Cerebro-hepatorenal syndrome of Zellweger
- Von Hippel-Lindau syndrome (cerebellar haemangioblastoma and hypernephroid tumours)
Postnatally acquired
- Hypoxic insults
- Hypoglycaemia; chronic phenytoin; thiamine deficiency; thyroid deficiency
- Trauma

Ataxia telangiectasia (Louis-Bar disease). Clinically, the two most striking and cardinal features are a progressive ataxia with onset between one and four years of age and abnormal eye movements. There is often an associated choreoathetosis with dystonic posturing, particularly of the hands, and facial grimacing with a slow spreading smile. Speech may be dysarthric and cerebellar in nature. Abnormal eye movements take the form of an oculomotor apraxia. Saccades are slowly initiated and hypometric, so that fixation of a target is obtained by head rather than eye deviation, often associated with a head thrust or forced eye blinking. Eye deviation lags behind head turning and is saccadic, often halting midway through a movement.

The telangiectasia usually appears a little later in the disease with a wide range in time of onset from about three years of age and sometimes not until adolescence. They occur in the outer part of the bulbar conjunctivae, back of ears, exposed parts of the neck, cheeks, bridge of nose, popliteal and antecubital fossae. Other cutaneous manifestations consist of cafe-au-lait spots, vitiligo, and sclerodermoid changes. There is a higher risk of these patients developing malignancies, particularly lymphomas and gliomas. There is an abnormality in both cellular and humoral immunity due to a decreased synthesis of immunoglobulins and a thymic hypoplasia. The most consistent marker is an elevated alpha fetoprotein level. The immunoglobulins IgA, IgE, and IgG are usually low. There is no specific therapy for these patients, although prompt treatment of infections is important. Treatment of the neurological manifestations is disappointing.

Involuntary movement disorders in children

These movements occur at rest and in the absence of volitional movement, although physical, emotional, and mental stress may aggravate the involuntary movements. The movements are without apparent purpose, but often the child may attempt to turn the purposeless involuntary

Movement disorders are attributable to abnormalities in the structural and biochemical function of the nuclear masses of the basal ganglia. They are not under voluntary control and the patient usually cannot stop them at will.

movement into a voluntary one as seen in certain forms of chorea.

There is no easy way of classifying diseases which cause movement disorders. However, it is useful to classify them into three broad clinical groups (see Table 26.15).

In disease states, the biochemical balance of the neurotransmitters (dopamine, acetylcholine, serotonin, histamine, GABA, glutamate, and substance P) is interfered with and may result in a synergistic or antagonistic response at the different receptor sites. This inhibition or exci-

tation of the receptors may lead to involuntary movements.

In the hypokinetic (akinetic-rigid syndromes) there is a dopaminergic under-activity in the brain. In the hyperkinetic disorders, one finds an excess of movement and these movements are attributable to either an over-activity of cerebral dopaminergic mechanisms or a cholinergic under-activity.

Generally speaking, hyperkinetic disorders are treated with dopamine antagonists and cholinergics, while the hypokinetic disorders are treated with dopamine replacement therapy and anticholinergics.

The hyperkinetic disorders (tics, chorea, tremors, and myoclonus) are more commonly seen in children than the hypokinetic disorders. The movements tend to involve the upper limbs and face more commonly than the lower limbs. Often there is an overlap of the different types of movements in the same patient (e.g. chorea and tics), one usually predominating over the other.

Hyperkinetic disorders (dyskinesias)

Chorea is a flow of brief, rapid, and irregular jerks that are random in place and time, flitting unpredictably from one part of the body to another. The movements are characterized by their irregularity and failure to be repetitive at a single site. The areas of the basal ganglia that are thought to be involved are the caudate nucleus and sub-thalamic nuclei. Hypotonia often accompanies chorea and may be extreme at times. Hyperpronation of the outstretched hands is seen with the palms pointing outwards and the waxing and waning of the intensity of a hand grip is common.

Table 26.15 Classification of involuntary movement disorders in children

Hyperkinetic	Chorea
	Myoclonus
	Tics
	Tremors
Hypokinetic	Akinetic rigid syndrome
	Juvenile parkinsonism
	Progressive pallidal degenerations
Dystonia	Post-encephalitic parkinsonism
	Extensor dystonia
	Athetosis

Table 26.16 Some causes of chorea

Sydenham's chorea	Symptomatic chorea	Drug-induced
Cerebral palsy	Thyrotoxicosis	Phenytoin
Huntington's chorea–juvenile form	SLE	Phenothiazine
Benign hereditary chorea	Henoch-Schönlein purpura	Alcohol
Choreo-acanthocytosis	Polycythaemia rubra vera	Lithium
Ataxia telangiectasia	Hypernatraemia	Phenobarbitone
Encephalitis lethargica	Hypoparathyroidism	
	Subdural haematoma	
	Wilson's disease	
	Post-asphyxial states	

The most common cause of chorea in children in South Africa is **Sydenham's chorea**. There are numerous other causes, which are listed in Table 26.16.

Sydenham's chorea is one of the five major signs of rheumatic fever (Jones's criteria) and classically presents some time after the initial infection has occurred. As a result, these patients are usually afebrile, the ESR is usually normal and the anti-streptococcal antibody titres are not raised. Approximately a third of the patients will have evidence of cardiac involvement. The three cardinal features of Sydenham's chorea are chorea, emotional lability and hypotonia, and the combination of chorea and hypotonia may be so severe to render the child helpless. The chorea develops insidiously, is generalized in 80 per cent but may remain as hemi-chorea in some. After the first few weeks, the chorea usually begins to subside with recovery occurring over the next three to six months. Approximately 25 per cent of cases will experience one or more recurrences over the next two to three years. Treatment of Sydenham's chorea involves the usual prophylactic treatment required for rheumatic fever (penicillin until the age of 20 years). During the acute illness, the chorea may be severe enough to warrant the use of one of the dopamine antagonists.

Hemiballism is a form of chorea in which the movements are much more coarse and ballistic in nature, where the limbs on one side of the body will be 'flung' like a ballistic missile. Hemiballism is seen on rare occasions as an accompaniment of Sydenham's chorea, stroke, cerebral tumours, and trauma.

Myoclonus consists of rapid shock like muscle jerks, often repetitive and sometimes rhythmic. Myoclonus may be spontaneous or triggered by tactile, proprioceptive, visual or auditory stimuli, or by movement. Clinically, myoclonic jerks may be divided into generalized or focal, rhythmic or arrhythmic, spontaneous or stimulus sensitive. They may be physiological, as in sleep or with hiccoughs, or pathological (e.g. epileptic; symptomatic of an underlying CNS disorder).

Tics are rapid, repetitive, and stereotyped movements which can be suppressed in the child by an effort of will. The various tics range from simple developmental tics to more severe types like the Gilles de la Tourette syndrome. Approximately 25–30 per cent of children

between the ages of eight and twelve years will manifest insignificant developmental tics that are transient. Manneristic tics are commonly seen in patients with mental retardation and in autism. Multiple tics may result from certain drugs, including L-dopa and methylphenidate (Ritalin®). It is not unusual to see tics associated with Sydenham's chorea.

Gilles de la Tourette syndrome is a syndrome affecting males more frequently than females with onset between the ages of 5–15 years. Criteria for diagnosis need to be met in every case, in order to prevent misdiagnosis and unnecessary treatment (*see* Table 26.17).

The illness is usually life-long and the course of the disease fluctuates with time, often becoming less severe with age. The patient develops a wide variety of motor tics, affecting mainly the face, neck, and shoulders. These tics can be suppressed for a period of time, are aggravated by stress, and wax and wane. Vocal tics are essential to the diagnosis and may take the form of grunts, barks, sucking in of air, coughs, clearing of the throat, and sniffing. Some of the patients may display a wide variety of complex neuro-behavioural disorders. Coprolalia (bad language) is a relatively common feature and one that most medical students remember the syndrome by!

Tremor is the sinusoidal movement of a body part due to rhythmic muscle contraction and may occur at rest or on action. A **physiological tremor** (8–12 Hz) usually goes unnoticed, but may be exaggerated by stress, anxiety, hypoglycaemia, betamimetic drugs, and thyrotoxicosis. **Benign essential tremor** (4–8 Hz) characteristically affects the hands and is made worse by attempting to maintain a posture. A family history is present in over 50 per cent of cases. A **flapping tremor** may be found in such conditions as liver failure, renal failure, hyperammonaemia,

---

Table 26.17 Criteria for diagnosis of Tourette syndrome

- Multiple motor tics and one or more vocal tics present at some time, not necessarily concurrently
- Frequent tics for more than a year
- Location, number, frequency, complexity, and severity of tics change over time
- Onset before 21 years of age

Wilson's disease, or CO_2 narcosis. **Cerebellar tremor** (4–5 Hz) is an intention tremor, which is characteristically heightened as the patient attempts to reach the target (as in the finger-to-nose test). A **parkinsonian tremor** (5 Hz) is one of the few tremors that is present at rest, improving on movement.

Dystonia

Dystonia is due to sustained contraction of various muscle groups that is repetitive in nature and distorts parts of the body into dystonic positions. It is characterized by simultaneous contraction of agonist and antagonist muscles. Dystonic movements are slow and laboured.

Clinically, dystonia may present either as a flexion dystonia or an extensor dystonia which is the type most commonly seen in cerebral palsy.

Athetosis is a form of alternating dystonia with the tone alternating between flexion and extension. Athetosis involves the distal musculature more than the proximal and the movements are slow, writhing, and sinuous. Dystonia may present as a manifestation of a number of diseases due to hereditary or idiopathic causes, or be symptomatic of a wide variety of pathological traumatic, infectious, vascular, metabolic, and degenerative conditions.

The pharmacological management of the chronic movement disorders is difficult and requires referral to a centre where there is suitable expertise in the handling of such cases.

Cerebrovascular disorders

Stroke is more common in children than originally suspected. Recognition of the cause of the cerebrovascular insult is important, because the likelihood of a recurrence depends to a large extent on the underlying abnormality and the available treatment. A thorough investigation will yield a result in 60–70 per cent of cases.

The term **'infantile hemiplegia'** refers to a sudden onset of childhood stroke, especially where no specific cause can be found. Infants most frequently present with epileptic fits and motor signs may be minimal. The older infant may present with a history of abnormal hand preference due to the emerging hemiplegia.

Cerebrovascular disorders can be classified

> Strokes in children have a number of different clinical presentations that vary with the child's age. The most common cause of stroke in children is heart disease with a right to left shunt that can cause polycythaemia and emboli.

on pathophysiological grounds into four main groups of vascular dysfunction. There are clinical features of each type.

Embolism usually presents with a sudden loss of neurological function; this loss may be fragmentary as the embolic fragments break up and occlude vessels further down the line. Reperfusion often occurs, resulting in a higher incidence of secondary haemorrhage into the infarcted area. Small emboli will give rise to a lacunar infarct of one of the penetrating blood vessels in the basal ganglia, thalamus, pons, and white matter of the cerebrum and cerebellum.

Arterial thrombosis usually takes longer to develop than an embolism and a stuttering course may be evident in some cases. Transient ischaemic episodes may precede the occlusion, but these are uncommon in children. Arterial thrombosis in children is usually due to a vasculopathy of the cerebral vessels, infection, dehydration, haemoglobinopathies, and certain malignancies.

Venous thrombosis tends to be more common in children than in adults. Seizures, altered mental state, signs of raised intracranial pressure, and focal neurological deficits accompany the insult.

Cerebral haemorrhage has a dramatic onset of headache, vomiting, and a progressive deterioration of neurological function. Trauma, vascular malformations, inflammatory diseases, and haematological disorders are the usual causes.

There are many **non-vascular lesions** that may cause an acute neurological deficit similar to that seen in a stroke.

- Todd's paresis and other focal deficits may follow a prolonged epileptic fit. These deficits seldom last beyond 24 hours.
- Complicated migraine or hemiplegic migraine is sometimes seen in children.
- A vascular lesion, such as an AVM, can give rise to a focal seizure and this may prove to be confusing.
- A neoplasm can mimic a vascular lesion

either due to a haemorrhage into a tumour, or herniation of brain tissue from the mass.

♦ Hydrocephalus either primary or secondary to a cerebral tumour can give rise to acute neurological signs. Other masses that may do likewise, are intracerebral abscess or a tuberculoma.

Most of the disorders listed in Table 26.18 are unusual.

Moyamoya syndrome is a rare cause of stroke. It results from progressive intracranial arterial occlusions usually involving the vessels around the circle of Willis with secondary collaterals distal to the occlusions. The syndrome is a radiological diagnosis and the defect is only seen on angiography when the collaterals appear as a 'puff of smoke'. Recurrent transient neurological deficits are common, especially alternating hemiplegias. Neurofibromatosis, tuberculosis (TB), sickle-cell disease, and cranial irradiation are commonly linked to Moyamoya disease.

Mitochondrial cytopathy, especially the MELAS syndrome (**m**itochondrial myopathy, **e**ncephalopathy, **l**actic **a**cidosis, and **s**troke-like episodes), has been incriminated in the cause of strokes usually beginning in the second decade of life.

Assessment and management

A systematic approach is needed in the diagnosis of cerebrovascular disease in children due to the many possible causes. This should be done in a stepwise manner progressing from the less to the more invasive. As far as possible it is important to find a cause because of the potential recurrence of the stroke and the possibility of treatment and cure. The evaluation should be organized in stages, with each step influenced by the information from the history, physical examination and previous tests.

A CT scan or MRI of the brain is the most informative investigation. However, simpler laboratory investigations should be obtained as soon as possible and these should include a full blood count and platelet count, prothrombin time and partial thromboplastin time, haemoglobin electrophoresis, and sedimentation rate. If the CT scan or MRI reveals an infarct, then one should proceed to an ECG, echocardiogram, and chest X-ray. A lumbar puncture should be done to exclude infective processes such as bacterial or tuberculous meningitis, provided the child does not have raised intracranial pressure or suspicion of a space-occupying lesion. A vasculitis screen, collagen vascular screen, serum

---

Table 26.18 Causes of stroke in children

Congenital heart disease	**Vasospastic disorders**
Acquired heart disease	Migraine; subarachnoid haemorrhage
Rheumatic heart disease; endocarditis;	**Haematological disorders**
Kawasaki's disease; cardiomyopathy; myocarditis;	Haemoglobinopathies; ITP; TTP; polycythaemia;
prosthetic heart valves; atrial myxoma	DIC; leukaemia; antithrombin 3 deficiency; protein
Systemic vascular disease	C & protein S deficiency; lupus anticoagulant;
Hypertension; atherosclerosis; diabetes;	anticardiolipin antibodies; vitamin K deficiency;
fibromuscular dysplasia; volume depletion	pregnancy; the Pill; congenital coagulation defects;
Vasculitis	liver dysfunction; thrombosis
Meningitis; collagen vascular disorders; (SLE, poly-	**Vascular malformations**
arteritis nodosa); Takayasu's arteritis; haemolytic	Arterio-venous malformations; aneurysms; vein of
uraemic syndrome; rheumatoid arthritis; drug	Galen abnormalities; Sturge-Weber syndrome
abuse; Marfan's syndrome; Ehlers-Danlos syndrome	**Trauma**
(type 4)	Air/fat embolism; carotid dissection; vertebral
Vasculopathies	occlusion; penetrating trauma; post- catheterization
Moyamoya syndrome; homocystinuria; Fabry's	emboli
disease; pseudoxanthoma elasticum; mitochondrial	
encephalomyopathies (MELAS)	

and urine amino acids, antithrombin 3, protein C and S, anticardiolipin antibody, cholesterol and triglycerides, lactate and pyruvate should also be performed. If the scan reveals a haemorrhage, then a coagulation screen should be undertaken. A cerebral angiogram should be considered if the cause for the stroke remains unclear, especially if there is a bleed. This becomes important when an AVM or vasculitis is suspected.

Cerebral palsy

Cerebral palsy (CP) is one of the more common of the neurological disorders of childhood. Cerebral palsy has been defined as a disability of motor function due to a non-progressive insult or damage to a developing motor brain. The insult affects the motor brain and its pathways while they are developing. It is generally accepted that this includes the period soon after conception up to approximately five years of age. The areas of the brain that control motor function include motor cortex, cerebellum, basal ganglia, brainstem and their various pathways. The motor manifestations of brain damage include spasticity from involvement of the cerebral cortex; involvement of the cerebellum results in hypotonia with or without ataxia, and involvement of the basal ganglia results in dyskinesias (athetosis/chorea) and dystonia. Although the damage to the brain is static, the motor manifestations are usually dynamic in nature, due to the fact that brain

---

- Cerebral palsy is a disorder of motor function with clinical manifestations that change with time.
- The damage happens to the motor areas of the developing brain (birth to five years).
- Most children are delayed in motor development.
- There are associated abnormalities including epilepsy, intellectual impairment, behavioural disorders, malnutrition, and language, visual and hearing problems.
- Intellectual impairment may not be present in all cerebral palsied children.
- Spasticity and mixed motor signs are common.
- Management requires a team approach consisting of physiotherapy, occupational therapy, speech therapy, a social worker, doctor, and special education and care.

---

maturation continues throughout childhood resulting in a changing clinical picture despite a static pathology.

There are a number of associated manifestations such as mental retardation, learning disabilities, epilepsy, language disorders, and behavioural problems.

Prevalence of cerebral palsy

The prevalence of cerebral palsy varies between 2 and 5 per 1 000 worldwide. The prevalence in South Africa is not known but is thought to be higher.

Aetiology

In developing countries, approximately 60 per cent are due to perinatal causes 20 per cent prenatal, 10 per cent postnatal, and 10 per cent unknown (*see* Table 26.19).

Types of cerebral palsy

There are four main clinical types of cerebral palsy (CP) depending, in most instances, on the areas of the brain that are damaged (*see* Table 26.20). These are the spastic group (motor cortex), dyskinetic (basal ganglia), hypotonic/ataxic (cerebellum), and a mixed group consisting of any combination of the other three types.

Spasticity

This group constitutes a large percentage of the cerebral palsy population. Spasticity is dependent on an intact muscle spindle system and reflex arc, which is normally controlled by the motor cortex, basal ganglia, cerebellum, and brainstem. In spastic cerebral palsy higher control has been interfered with which allows the reflex arc to run 'disinhibited'. There are two types of spasticity: phasic and tonic.

Phasic. An increase in muscle contraction (tone) will be produced by rapid stretching of the muscle. The type 2 muscle fibres are affected. Their contraction is dependent upon the velocity of stretch. (The so-called 'clasp knife' response is felt when the muscle is rapidly stretched from its shortest resting state and will not be felt if the limb or muscle is stretched slowly.) The clinical features include brisk tendon reflexes, clonus, and a clasp knife response on rapid stretch of

Table 26.19 Aetiology of cerebral palsy

Prenatal	Perinatal	Postnatal
▪ Toxaemia of pregnancy	▪ Prematurity	▪ Head injury
▪ Genetic factors	▪ SGA	▪ Infections (meningitis,
▪ Antenatal bleeding	▪ Birth asphyxia	encephalitis)
▪ Cerebral malformations	▪ Hypoxic/ischaemic	▪ Metabolic
▪ Hydrocephalus	encephalopathy	– hypoglycaemia
	▪ Cerebral birth trauma	– hypocalcaemia
	▪ Kernicterus	– hyponatraemia
	(hyperbilirubinaemia)	– hypernatraemia
	▪ Metabolic (e.g.	▪ Vascular
	hypoglycaemia)	– AVMs
	▪ Infections	– strokes
	▪ Cerebral haemorrhages (IVH)	– thrombosis
	▪ Perinatal strokes	– embolism
	▪ Hydrocephalus	▪ Toxins/drugs
		▪ Hydrocephalus

Table 26.20 Types of cerebral palsy

SPASTIC	Hemiplegia	One side of the body
	Diplegia	Legs > than arms
	Quadriplegia	All four limbs
	Double hemiplegia	Arms > legs
DYSKINETIC	Chorea	
	Athetosis	Alternating flexor/extensor dystonia
	Dystonia	May be transient
HYPOTONIC	With ataxia	
	Without ataxia	
MIXED		Combination of the above

the muscle. This is often seen in the quadriceps, calves, and biceps muscles and may be the first type of spasticity to appear in the young infant. There is no tendency towards contracture of the muscle.

Tonic. Type 1 muscle fibres are involved. The muscle is attempting to maintain its shortest possible length and is tonically (constantly) contracting. This tonic contraction will eventually result in contractures of the muscles and joints. Tonic spasticity causes reciprocal inhibition of the respective antagonistic muscle, resulting in weakness of that muscle. Phasic and tonic spasticity can coexist in the same muscle, but with time, tonic spasticity usually overrides the phasic component.

The spastic group is further classified into the various parts of the body that are involved.

Hemiplegia. In the congenital hemiplegias (80 per cent), the male-to-female ratio is 3:2. There is also a strong association with prematurity, birth asphyxia, and placental insufficiency. Although left hemiplegias are seen frequently in this group, language abnormalities are not common, as the neonatal and infant brain displays the phenomenon of plasticity, especially with language development. The hemiplegia is often not detected early in infancy, as the infant displays certain extrapyramidal progression movement patterns that may mask the weakness. In the established hemiplegia, the distribution of weakness and spasticity will affect the distal muscles more than the proximal, so that 99 per cent of hemiplegias should have the ability to walk.

Diplegia. The legs are more affected than the arms. Only fine motor movements may be abnormal or a mild form of athetosis, dyspraxia or spasticity may be present in the upper limbs. Diplegia that follows low birth weight or intra-partum asphyxia may present initially with dystonia, which often precedes the spasticity. It is important to differentiate paraplegia from diplegia. Paraplegia is due to a spinal cord lesion, whereas diplegia is of cerebral origin. The common causes of a spastic diplegia include low birth weight, prematurity, and birth asphyxia. In these conditions the developing leg areas of the fetal brain are in a selectively vulnerable stage of development and more susceptible to damage.

Dyskinesia

The basal ganglia and their pathways are involved, leading to involuntary movements in the form of chorea or athetosis, and abnormal muscle tone due to dystonia. The mature basal ganglia along with the motor cortex normally inhibit certain primitive brainstem reflexes (asymmetrical and symmetrical tonic neck reflex; primitive walking and swimming reflexes), and thus we see the retention of these reflexes when the basal ganglia and motor cortex fail to mature properly. In dystonia or rigidity, the body is in a state of hypertonia, which is constant throughout the range of the movement. The movements are slow and often laboured.

There are a number of types of dystonia: flexor, extensor, alternating and hemiplegic dystonia. The extensor type is most common in cerebral palsy. The arms are rigidly extended, internally rotated with the wrists flexed and the fingers extended. The extension of the legs is accompanied by an equinus deformity of the foot, which is inverted, and the big toe points upwards. Alternating dystonia (flexion and extension) is what constitutes athetosis. Dystonia is seldom seen before four months of age. Chorea and athetosis commonly occur in the same CP patient.

Hypotonia

This is due to the involvement of the cerebellum and its pathways. The cerebellum is involved in motor learning as well as in the coordination of movement, which includes judging the speed, force, and direction of the movement, stabilization of the limb or trunk, and the ability to rapidly start and stop a movement. The cerebellum matures postnatally therefore many cerebellar signs that would be regarded as abnormal in the adult, is normal in children at certain stages of development. In CP, hypotonia may occur with or without ataxia. During the first few months of life only hypotonia may be present but as the child begins to move more, the ataxia may become more evident. Although perinatal events may result in hypotonic CP, genetic factors appear to be important in the aetiology of cerebellar hypoplasia and certain syndromes associated with cerebellar malformations. The hypotonic CP child displays predominantly a truncal hypotonia and this very often evolves into a mixed form of CP with the limbs displaying spasticity at a later stage.

Mixed

The mixed group of CP may involve a combination of the other three groups, but the most common type is truncal hypotonia with either spastic or dystonic limbs. It is essential to remember that the clinical motor manifestations of cerebral palsy are **dynamic** and the clinical picture will change depending on the stage of development of the brain, the extent and severity of the insult to the developing motor brain, and the stage of development of the brain when it suffered the insult. Over time, different types of cerebral palsy may emerge, only to disappear when other areas of the brain reach a stage of maturation and exert their influence on a damaged, but developing brain. It is not unusual to find a child at three months of age who is hypotonic, then over the next few months displays dystonic posturing of one or more of the limbs and then at a year has spasticity of all four limbs. The same child may have dystonia and remain with dystonia for the next few years or the dystonia may melt away by the first year and the child may develop no further motor disabilities.

Diagnosis

Early warning signs of suspected cerebral palsy:

- Delay in motor milestones
- Persistence of certain postures or primitive reflexes (e.g. the asymmetrical tonic neck reflex)

• Hypertonia or hypotonia
• Clumsiness.

Very often the diagnosis is initially in doubt. These children should be regarded as being 'at risk' and followed up at regular intervals with possible referral to physiotherapy, speech and occupational therapy. With time, the clinical picture will become clearer.

Clinical features

These vary from patient to patient. The classical signs of hypertonus, whether due to spasticity or dystonia, may be present and can manifest as 'fisting' of the hands with the thumb adducted across the palm, scissoring of the legs, and equinus deformity of the feet giving rise to 'toe walking'. There may be truncal hypotonia with a marked head lag on pull to sit or neck retraction and opisthotonus due to excessive tone. Deep tendon reflexes may be brisk with ankle clonus and a Babinski reflex. The change in muscle tone may have affected the bulbar muscles due to a spastic, athetoid or ataxic dysarthria, leading to feeding problems and drooling.

Associated problems

The vast majority of children with cerebral palsy will have one or more associated abnormality of the central nervous system (*see* Table 26.21). The degree and variety of associated problems will depend on the extent of the damage to the rest of the brain.

There may be a whole spectrum of intellectual problems associated with cerebral palsy, ranging from normal intelligence, mild learning disabilities to severe mental retardation. Children with a spastic quadriparesis are more likely to have a severe form of mental retardation as opposed to the child with a dyskinesia (where the basal ganglia bears the brunt of the insult) or hemiple-

Table 26.21 Associated problems with cerebral palsy

Intellectual impairment
Language, vision, hearing abnormalities
Epilepsy
Behavioural problems
Malnutrition

gia and diplegia where the degree of intellectual impairment is usually not as severe. Language impairment may involve only the peripheral muscles of motor speech (dysarthria), or extend to involve the central receptive and/or expressive language areas.

It is important to realize the risk of malnutrition in children with cerebral palsy, resulting from feeding difficulties associated with abnormal bulbar tone or difficulties in the coordination of swallowing (very often complicated by abnormal posturing of the trunk, back, and spine due to deformities).

Management:

• **Prevention** relates to issues of antenatal care, avoidance of prematurity and asphyxia, good obstetrics, and postnatal care.
• **Early diagnosis and intervention**. The effectiveness of early intervention and therapy on those children diagnosed as having cerebral palsy is controversial, but much can be done in the prevention of positional deformities that may arise, either as a result of immobility or spasticity of the limb and trunk muscles

The main aim in the management of cerebral palsied children should be to make them as functional as possible without creating too much pressure on the child and parents or caregivers. Many children may become more functional with the use of certain aids such as a walker, rollator, splints, standing frame, or a wheelchair.

The management of cerebral palsy should involve a team of professionally trained people including physiotherapists, occupational therapists, speech therapists, social workers, dieticians, remedial teachers, paediatricians, paediatric neurologists, and at times, an orthopaedic surgeon. Physiotherapists and occupational therapists offer a wide range of different therapies in their management of cerebral palsy, which have been shown to reduce muscle tone and improve positions of posture and functionality. The speech therapist is not only invaluable in treating speech and language problems, but plays an important role in helping with feeding difficulties, particularly those due to pseudobulbar palsy, and athetoid or ataxic dysarthria.

The abnormal muscle tone may be reduced by drug therapy, such as diazepam or baclofen.

The intramuscular injection of small amounts of botulinum toxin is a relatively new form of therapy in cerebral palsy and can only be performed in competent and experienced hands.

The most common form of surgery is tendon lengthening, particularly the Achilles tendon. Posterior rhizotomy has been successful on selected children.

The management of educational, behavioural, language, emotional, and family and social problems as well as epilepsy, needs to be handled by the appropriate therapists and medical personnel.

Bacterial infections of the central nervous system

Infections may present with acute, insidious or chronic manifestations of a wide variety of CNS symptoms and signs.

Acute bacterial meningitis

Acute bacterial meningitis is the most common life-threatening bacterial infection affecting children in South Africa today. Current case fatality rates are 3–7 per cent in infants and children in good centres. If misdiagnosed, severe long-term neurological sequelae occur and therefore rapid diagnosis and treatment are essential. The initial clinical manifestations of meningitis in children are often not clear-cut or obvious and a high index of suspicion is necessary to ensure that the diagnosis is not missed.

The inflammation and damage that occurs in meningitis is more the result of host factors and the subsequent inflammatory cascade than of direct bacterial toxicity.

The host responds to bacterial invasion by producing cytokines such as tumour necrosis factor (TNF), interleukin-1, and other mediators of inflammatory responses, which result eventually in increased blood–brain barrier permeability (BBBP), hypercoagulability, raised intracranial pressure, vasogenic, cytotoxic and interstitial oedema, and reduced cerebral blood flow.

Clinical features

The clinical features of bacterial meningitis vary with the causal organism and the age of the child.

In the neonatal period, the signs are less specific and include signs of irritability, poor feeding, lethargy, a bulging fontanelle, and hypo/hyperthermia. One needs a high index of suspicion especially in the 'high risk' group where there has been premature rupture of membranes, low birth weight, male babies, and where there has been a difficult delivery with extensive manipulation.

The prevalence of the various organisms depends on the age of the child and varies also according to the area that the child comes from. Beyond the first year of life, the common organisms, in descending order of frequency in Johannesburg, are pneumococcal, meningococcal, and *H. influenzae* meningitis. (*See* Table 26.22.)

Aetiology

S. pneumoniae is a Gram-positive diplococcus. It should be particularly suspected in meningitis associated with a fracture of the skull, paranasal sinuses or frontal bones leading to a CSF leak, and otorrhoea. The risk of infection is also higher in children with sickle-cell disease because of the functional asplenia. Pneumococcal meningitis carries a very high morbidity and mortality rate. The onset is usually slow and insidious. One needs to be aware of multi-resistance of the organism, as in Johannesburg 50 per cent of isolates have been shown to be resistant to penicillin. Hopefully the new pneumococcal vaccine will reduce infection rates.

N. meningitidis is a Gram-negative intracellular organism, the epidemic forms being group A and C, although groups A, B, C, D, X, Y, Z and W135 have been identified as causing meningitis. Meningococcal meningitis is very rapid in onset (a few hours) and is characterized in the early stages by a petechial or purpuric rash that can evolve very quickly into purpura fulminans. The

---

The common clinical features of meningitis are:

- Signs of infection such as fever
- Signs of raised intracranial pressure such as headache and nausea/vomiting
- Signs of meningeal irritation such as neck stiffness or Kernig's and Brudzinski's sign and
- Signs of cortical involvement, such as encephalopathy and coma.

Table 26.22 Age-related meningitis

Neonate (0–28 days)	E. Coli Group B streptococcus L. Monocytogenes	Klebsiella Enterobacter
Infants (1 month–2 years)	Group b streptococcus H. influenzae type B S. pneumoniae	N. meningitidis Salmonella species
Childhood and adolescence	S. pneumoniae N. meningitidis	H. influenzae type B

organism can be found in the petechial rash and may be cultured after a scrape of the skin lesion. In some instances, the endotoxin of the organism induces shock, bilateral adrenal haemorrhages, and DIC. Pericarditis, arthritis and eye involvement are uncommon complications.

H. influenzae is a Gram-negative pleomorphic bacillus. The onset of haemophilus meningitis is also moderately slow. It is found in conditions of overcrowding and in children who have had splenectomies. It is primarily a disease of infants and pre-school children below the ages of two years. Haemophilus meningitis is often associated with sequelae such as subdural effusions, hearing loss, epileptic fits, mental retardation, and cerebral infarctions. It is largely prevented by HiB vaccination.

Diagnosis

A high index of suspicion must be maintained at all times, especially in the very young child.

The definitive diagnosis of meningitis can only be made on examination of the CSF, obtained by lumbar puncture (LP). It is essential to ensure that the child does not have a space-occupying lesion before proceeding with the LP. A comatose child presenting with signs of meningitis should have a CT/MRI scan performed before the LP. If meningitis is very likely in such a child, then treatment with a third generation cephalosporin should be started once blood cultures have been taken and while one is waiting for the CT/MRI scan.

The CSF is evaluated by Gram stain, cell count, biochemistry, and culture of the organism and the presence of certain bacterial antigens. A few drops of the CSF are dropped onto a labstix immediately to ascertain the CSF glucose, protein, and presence of leucocytes, so as to initiate therapy while still awaiting the laboratory report. The CSF opening pressure should also be measured at the time of the LP as this information may prove valuable at a later stage.

Table 26.23 Comparisons of CSF in viral and bacterial meningitis

Type	White cells (mm³)	Glucose (mmol/l)	Protein (gm/l)
Normal	0 Nentrophils 0–6 Lymphocytes	3.6–5.6	0.15–0.45
Bacterial	100–50 000 Nentrophils predominate	1.1–1.6 <0.5 = severe infection	Mild to moderately increased
Viral	25–500 Lymphocytes predominate	Within normal range	Mildly increased
TBM	25–100 (can go up to 500) Lymphocytes predominate but nentrophils predominate early on	Less than 2.2–2.7 Usually less than 0.5	Moderately increased

Typical CSF findings are illustrated in Table 26.23.

A CT/MRI scan of the brain is indicated in the following circumstances:

- Prolonged or persistent obtundation or coma;
- Persistent focal neurological signs
- Relapse after an initial response
- An enlarging head (hydrocephalus)
- Deteriorating level of consciousness
- Suspicion of a subdural effusion (focal neurological signs, re-emergence of a fever on day three to six)
- Change in mental status
- Associated purulent otitis media with the fear of a brain abscess.

Difficulties in diagnosis

There are a number of common problems that may be encountered when confirming the diagnosis of childhood meningitis.

Partially treated meningitis. Confusion may arise when children have received prior antibiotic therapy, either orally, intramuscularly or both, rendering the CSF sterile. However, CSF pleocytosis and neutrophil predominance, high protein and low glucose are usually present. The latex agglutination test is usually positive.

Early viral encephalitis. It is not uncommon for neutrophils to predominate in the CSF in the first 12 hours of the illness. The CSF protein and glucose concentrations are usually normal and there is often marked clinical improvement soon after the lumbar puncture. The exception to this is herpes encephalitis.

Tuberculous meningitis (TBM). The CSF in early TBM may have a neutrophil predominance with high protein and low glucose concentrations and occasionally a low concentration of CSF chloride. The neutrophil predominance will revert to a lymphocyte predominance over a few days but the abnormal CSF chemistry will remain for some time. A history of possible exposure to TB should be checked for and a chest radiograph and an appropriate TB skin test (Mantoux) should be performed.

Recurrent meningitis. This is an uncommon condition and one that is difficult to investigate for a possible cause. Recurrent purulent meningitis usually occurs in children with an underlying surgical, anatomical or medical disorder (immune deficiency) facilitating infection of the nervous system. The possible causes are listed in Table 26.24.

Complications of meningitis

Vasculitis causes thrombosis of veins and small arteries with resultant infarction and necrosis of cortical tissue and is the main cause of the focal neurological deficits seen in cases of bacterial meningitis.

Subdural effusions. The great majority of subdural effusions in children with meningitis will be due to *H. influenzae* infections, although *N. meningitidis* and *S. pneumoniae* can also cause subdural effusions. Diagnosis may be confirmed by CT scan. Small effusions do not need surgical intervention but large ones causing significant shift of the midline on a CT scan, persistent focal signs, depressed mental state, and the presence of an empyema (enhances with contrast) will need to be drained.

Epileptic fits. These are common in children with meningitis and may be focal or generalized in nature. Prompt treatment is vital, to prevent exacerbation of an already depressed mental state and the avoidance of status epilepticus. Beware of the combination of benzodiazepines and phenobarbitone as this combination can cause marked CNS and respiratory depression often necessitating assisted ventilation.

Table 26.24 Causes of recurrent meningitis

Organism
- Unusual organism (listeria, cryptococcus, TB, *S. aureus*)
- Organism unresponsive to antibiotic

Brain abscess, subdural empyema/effusion

Anatomical defect
- Fractured skull, paranasal sinuses, orbits, cribriform plate
- Meningomyelocoele, congenital dermal sinus (lumbosacral/cervico-occipital), neurenteric cyst

Defects of the middle ear

Immune deficiency
- Congenital hypogamma-globulinaemia
- Deficiency of the terminal components of complement (C5-C9)
- Splenectomy
- Sickle-cell anaemia

Cerebral oedema consists of both vasogenic and cytotoxic oedema, adding to the problems of raised ICP and poor cerebral perfusion.

Hydrocephalus is seen more frequently as a complication of neonatal meningitis and is uncommon following meningitis in older children. It may follow pneumococcal and TBM, as both these are prone to causing thick pus at the base of the brain, occluding outflow of CSF from the fourth ventricle. Arachnoiditis interferes with the reabsorption of the CSF from the subarachnoid granulations. Communicating hydrocephalus is the more common type seen after meningitis.

Syndrome of inappropriate ADH secretion (SIADH), with the resultant hyponatraemia, occurs in approximately 15–20 per cent of children with bacterial meningitis. Symptoms consist of those of water intoxication (irritability and convulsions).

Cranial nerve palsies, in which perhaps the most common cranial nerve damage is a sensorineural hearing loss, which may be either transient or permanent. This is seen in about 10 per cent of cases.

Hemiplegias and other forms of focal neurological deficit follow vasculitis with infarction of cortical neurons.

Brain abscess is an extremely uncommon entity after meningitis. A brain abscess, however, may give rise to meningitis as it breaks through to the meninges.

Treatment

Treatment is directed at eliminating the organism by the appropriate antibiotic, preventing and treating the potential and associated complications of meningitis, and the general care of the child with impaired consciousness. Antibiotic therapy is instituted according to a protocol depending on the child's age (*see* Tables 26.25 and 26.26). In the two-month and older age group, the antibiotics of choice are either one of the two third-generation cephalosporins, namely cefotaxime and ceftriaxone.

The third-generation cephalosporins are preferred because of the increasing emergence of resistant strains of *S. pneumoniae*. In areas where these antibiotics are not available, a combination of ampicillin/penicillin and chloramphenicol may be used, but one needs to be aware of the potential limitations of this combination.

There is compelling evidence that dexamethasone reduces the audiological and neurological sequelae of bacterial meningitis, as long as it is given 15–30 minutes before the initiation of the antibiotics. One of the mechanisms of action is thought to be inhibition of the inflammatory cascade before it is precipitated by the introduction of the antibiotics. The efficacy of dexamethasone in neonatal meningitis is unknown, but is presently being studied. Dexamethasone should not be used in neonatal meningitis before these reports have been verified.

Table 26.25 Management of bacterial meningitis in infants younger than two months

Initial therapy:
Cefotaxime 50 mg/kg 8-hourly (12-hourly <7 days old)
PLUS
Ampicillin 50 mg/kg 6-hourly (8-hourly if <7 days old)

When organism identified:

Group B streptococci	*Gram-negative enteric bacilli*	*Listeria*
Cefotaxime	Cefotaxime	Ampicillin alone
OR	PLUS	OR
Ampicillin alone or combined with an aminoglycoside	Aminoglycoside (1st 7 days)	Penicillin

Duration of therapy:
Listeria and group B streptococci–14 days
Gram-negative enteric bacilli–31 days

Table 26.26 Management of bacterial meningitis in infants and children older than two months

Initial therapy

Ceftriaxone 100 mg/kg immediately then
   80–100 mg/kg once daily or 40–50 mg/kg
   twice daily

OR

Cefotaxime 75 mg/kg 8-hourly

AND

Dexamethasone 0.6 mg/kg/d 8-hourly for 4 days,
   ideally given 15–30 minutes prior to initiating
   antibiotics

Duration of therapy:

H. influenzae: 7–10 days
S. pneumoniae: 10–14 days
N. meningitidis: 7 days

If penicillin-resistent pneumococcus is isolated and the child is not improving, then vancomycin should be added to the antibiotic regime.

Prognosis

This depends on a number of factors listed in the Herson-Todd scoring system, which is used at the time of admission of the child. A score of 4.5 or greater is usually associated with a poor prognosis. Pneumococcal meningitis is one of the more common types and carries the worst prognosis with a fatality rate of 10 per cent and long-term neurological sequelae occurring in up to 30 per cent of survivors.

Herson-Todd scoring system for prediction of morbidity

Factors on admission	Points
Severe coma	3
Hypothermia (<36.6 A1C)	2
Seizures	2
Shock (BP <60 mmHg systolic)	1
Age <12 months	1
CSF WBC <1 000/cu mm	1
Haemoglobin <11 g/100 ml	1
CSF Glucose <1 mmol/LLl	0.5
Symptoms for more than 3 days	0.5

Prophylaxis

Close contacts (immediate family members and nursery school friends) of patients with meningitis caused by *N. meningitidis* will need prophylaxis because they are at a substantially increased risk of contracting the disease. Only children younger than five years and who are immediate family members will need prophylaxis against *Haemophilus* meningitis.

Prophylactic drugs for bacterial meningitis (contacts):

* **Meningococcal disease:**
   - Rifampicin 10 mg/kg twice a day for 2 days. Less than 1 month 5 mg/kg twice a day for 2 days
   - Ceftriaxone 250 mg imi stat (adults) 125 mg IMI stat (children)
   - Ciprofloxacin 500 mg bd (adults only).
* ***H. influenzae* (family member 5 years and younger):**
   - Rifampicin 20 mg/kg twice a day for 4 days <1 month 10 mg/kg twice a day for 4 days.

Prevention

The introduction of the *H. influenzae* conjugated vaccine in the USA and Europe has dramatically reduced the incidence of *H. influenzae* infections and in particular meningitis. Hopefully the pneumococcal vaccine will have similar effects.

Brain abscess and empyema

Brain abscesses consist of localized suppuration within the brain tissues. The organisms can gain access to the brain either via the bloodstream or extension from a nearby focus such as the paranasal sinuses or middle ear. The most common organisms are streptococci, staphylococci, pneumococci, *H. influenzae* and bacteroides. Anaerobic organisms are found in about 25 per cent of cases. A major predisposing factor is cyanotic congenital heart disease with a right to left shunt, especially under two years of age. Purulent otitis media, mastoiditis and sinusitis, however, make up a large proportion of the cases seen in Johannesburg. Abscesses arising from a bacteraemia are more likely to be found in the central regions of the cerebral hemispheres, at the border between the white and grey matter. They often extend towards the ventricular cavities, into which they may rupture. Abscesses from focal lesions are more commonly found in the temporal and frontal lobes. The frontal lobes are known as the 'silent areas', where lesions can grow to considerable sizes before manifesting with neurological signs.

The diagnosis is confirmed by CT/MRI scan of the brain. This reveals a localized hypodensity, which may initially be ill-defined, and a mass effect with resulting shift of neural tissue due to the surrounding abscess and oedema. The abscess takes up contrast with ring enhancement, which will thicken with time and the oedema surrounding the mass may reach massive proportions. A lumbar puncture should not be attempted in such circumstances as it may lead to cerebral coning. However, in the early stages, the CSF will show evidence of a few polymorphonuclear cells (less than 100), a low CSF glucose content, and sterile fluid.

Management consists primarily of appropriate antibiotic therapy, usually a third-generation cephalosporin, for four to five weeks with repeated CT scan monitoring. If antibiotic therapy is not effective, then surgical drainage of the abscess is performed. Sequelae of brain abscesses include epilepsy, focal neurological deficits, hydrocephalus, and mental retardation.

Subdural empyema

The symptoms and signs of subdural empyemas are almost identical to brain abscesses. The common causes are sepsis from a meningitis, subdural haematoma, extension of infection from mastoiditis, sinusitis or a brain abscess. They are best diagnosed on CT scan where they show up as thin, lens-shaped lesions with enhancement of the medial membrane. If large enough, they will cause shift of the hemisphere to the opposite side and compress the ipsilateral

---

The clinical manifestations of brain abscesses consist of

- Raised intracranial pressure with headache, vomiting and often papilloedema
- Sepsis and fever, and
- Focal neurological signs with seizures.

In a minority of cases the clinical features may suggest a diagnosis of meningitis. This occurs when the abscess breaks through into the ventricular cavity.

---

lateral ventricle. Management usually combines antibiotic therapy with surgical drainage.

Viral infections

There is a wide spectrum of viral infections of the CNS ranging from mild to potentially lethal conditions. Some viruses show a predilection for specific areas of the CNS (e.g. polio virus – anterior horn cells; varicella – cerebellum; herpes virus – temporal lobe; rabies virus – cortex).

Human immunodeficiency virus (HIV)

There are a number of ways in which HIV infection can affect the CNS:

- Those indirectly related to the effects of HIV on the brain, such as **opportunistic infections** (CMV, herpes simplex virus, varicella-zoster); fungal infections (*Candida* and aspergillosis); cryptococcal meningitis; *Listeria monocytogenes* and toxoplasmosis. **Neoplasms** (CNS lymphoma). **Cerebrovascular disease**. Strokes are common in children with HIV, either due to ischaemia from emboli or infectious vasculitis, secondary to haemorrhage or as the result of an increased incidence of a hypercoagulable state. There is also an associated vasculopathy seen in many HIV infected children resulting in aneurysmal dilation of vessels around the circle of Willis.
- Those directly related to HIV brain infection The most common CNS presentation is a progressive encephalopathy, marked by loss of developmental milestones (motor and expressive language), intellectual fall-off and motor deficits consisting of spasticity, ataxia, and weakness. The introduction of appropriate and early antiretroviral medication has thankfully altered the initial relentless progression of the encephalopathy.

Viral meningitis

Viral meningitis is due to haematogenous spread of many different types of viruses such as HIV, mumps, coxsackie, echovirus, poliovirus, herpes simplex virus (HSV) types 1 and 2, adenovirus, varicella-zoster, Epstein-Barr, lymphocytic choriomeningitis, and certain undetermined viruses. Each virus produces certain specific features.

The clinical features of viral meningitis include fever, headache, vomiting, and neck stiffness. This may progress to include a depressed mental state ranging from confusion to frank delirium. There usually are no focal neurological signs to find on examination. The course of the illness is benign in the vast majority of cases. Lumbar puncture reveals a lymphocytic predominance with normal levels of glucose and a slightly raised protein. Often the release of pressure from the LP relieves the headache.

Encephalitis (meningoencephalitis, encephalomyelitis)

Encephalitis results from invasion of the CNS by virus. The inflammatory response may also be an indirect effect due to an immune reaction between the virus and the host (post-infectious meningoencephalitis or para-infectious demyelinating encephalomyelitis). There is often no clinical distinction between these various pathophysiological responses. The clinical features of acute meningoencephalitis and encephalomyelitis vary with the particular infecting virus. Seizures and disturbances of consciousness are the usual features. Neurological manifestations are more common than in viral meningitis and may affect any part of the CNS, from the cortex extending right down the spinal cord. The EEG invariably demonstrates generalized and diffuse slowing. The CSF shows similarities to that seen in viral meningitis. The CT scan and MRI are usually normal except in certain cases of herpes simplex encephalitis, which may show hypodensities, particularly in the temporal lobes. The course of the encephalitis is characteristically progressive over two to five days with new signs emerging daily. The primary encephalitides include HSV; rabies virus; varicella zoster virus; enterovirus; and arbovirus. The viruses involved in para-infectious encephalitis include measles; mumps; chickenpox; Epstein-Barr virus; rubella; adenovirus; influenza A; and para-influenza. In most cases, no virus can be isolated.

Herpes simplex virus (HSV)

HSV encephalitis is characterized by focal haemorrhagic necrotic lesions, which seem to have a predilection for the temporal and orbital areas of the brain, but can also affect a wide area including the brainstem. Most cases are due to reactivation of a latent virus, usually situated in the trigeminal ganglia from a previous primary infection. The virus may enter the brain by spreading along branches of the meningeal nerves, or from the nasal mucosa through the cribriform plate. Primary infection of the CNS is unusual except in the neonate and young infant in whom most of the infections are caused by HSV type 2 and tend to be more severe than the type 1 disease.

The clinical features of HSV encephalitis are commonly preceded by a prodrome of fever and malaise. Mucosal lesions of HSV infection may or may not be present. The prodrome is followed by disturbances of memory and behavioural changes. Focal fits are a common feature, and focal neurological signs appear in the form of hemiplegias and signs suggestive of temporal lobe involvement (disordered behaviour, olfactory and memory hallucinations, aphasia). Lethargy, obtundation, and coma are often accompanying features. The signs can be subtle and non-suggestive. Atypical forms have involved the brainstem with damage to cranial nerves and very rarely the spinal cord.

The EEG may be helpful in older children and may show very asymmetrical foci of spikes, especially over the temporal lobes, on an abnormally slow background. Periodic complexes, one to three seconds apart, are commonly seen in the same areas between the second and fifteenth days. A CT scan or MRI can be helpful in the diagnosis and shows attenuation in the temporal lobes. A few weeks later the temporal lobes may show large areas of atrophy and porencephalic cysts, evidence of severe necrosis and haemorrhagic lesions. Establishing a definitive diagnosis of HSV encephalitis is not easy in most cases. The virus is very seldom isolated from the CSF and attempts to isolate it from brain tissue are often met with similar results due to sampling errors. A rise of HSV antibodies (especially the IgM class) in the CSF may be helpful, but takes time to develop. They are usually accompanied by the presence of an oligoclonal protein pattern in the CSF. Measurement of interferon alpha (it represents the replication of virus in the CNS and is not specific to HSV) in the CSF and plasma can be performed in the first 48 to 72 hours of the illness. It is hoped that HSV may be detected a lot earlier in the course of the disease by means of immunofluorescent and polymerase chain reaction (PCR). Brain biopsy remains the definitive proof of diagnosis, but can be hazardous.

Treatment with acyclovir should be started as soon as possible in an attempt to reduce the mortality and morbidity and continued for at least 10 days. Steroids are not recommended in the treatment of HSV. The diagnosis is usually confirmed two weeks later with the results of the antibody and oligoclonal protein pattern.

The **chronic encephalitides** include the 'prions' (where the virus is thought not to have nucleic acid and relies on an aberrant protein from the host for survival and multiplication)– Creutzfeldt-Jakob disease, Kuru, and Gerstmann-Straussler disease.

Subacute sclerosing panencephalitis (SSPE)

SSPE is the most common of the chronic encephalitides. This disease is the result of a prior measles infection, usually one to three years or more previously. The illness begins with the slow onset of personality changes and intellectual deterioration, often resulting in a fall-off in schoolwork. There is also an aphasic-apraxic-agnostic predominance. The disease progresses within the next few months to involve involuntary movements in the form of 'metronomic' myoclonic jerks. This then progresses to pyramidal and extrapyramidal signs in the form of spasticity and dystonia. There is a progressive severe dementia leading to death in most cases. Treatment has been unsatisfactory.

Progressive rubella panencephalitis

This disease presents with progressive cerebellar dysfunction, dementia, myoclonic jerks and is fatal in most cases.

Human T-lymphocytotrophic virus type 1 (HLTV-1) infection

HLTV-1 causes a progressive spastic paraplegia and is mainly seen in adults. It is particularly common in KwaZulu-Natal and the Eastern Cape and is thought to be sexually transmitted.

Poliomyelitis

(*See the section under* 'The floppy infant', *earlier in this chapter.*)

Parasitic infections

Malaria

Malaria is common in the low-lying tropical northern and eastern parts of South Africa. Cerebral malaria is a severe complication of *Plasmodium falciparum* and manifests with disturbances of consciousness, often leading to coma and movement disorders. Focal neurological signs are uncommon but seizures are particularly common. Most cases need quinine in their management.

Neurocysticercosis

This is a common CNS infection in children predominantly from the Eastern Cape. It is caused by the ingestion of ova of *Taenia solium*, the pig tapeworm, when the human becomes the intermediate host. These hatch into the larval form and penetrate the intestinal mucosa and lodge in various parts of the body including the brain. The cysts can affect any area of the brain, but are more likely to be found in the vascular areas of the brain, particularly the grey matter. Viable cysts evoke an inflammatory response in the brain tissue, with surrounding oedema. A cyst usually survives for two to five years after infection. When it dies it causes a marked inflammatory response, which is thought to produce the neurological signs and symptoms.

The cysts may present as a single or multiple lesions. The most common clinical presentation is with focal seizures, but may also include headaches, focal neurological signs, and raised ICP. Heavy infestations are not infrequent and these children can present with focal fits and deterioration of consciousness ranging from a psychotic state to coma. Very occasionally a cyst occludes a ventricle, resulting in an obstructive hydrocephalus.

Investigations

Eosinophilia is non-specific. The CSF shows mild pleocytosis, a slightly elevated protein and antibodies that can be detected by complement fixation or ELISA tests. The CT/MRI scan is usually diagnostic, revealing either a solitary cyst or multiple cysts within the cerebral hemispheres as well as patches of hypodensity with ring enhancement, and single or multiple calcified lesions. These different appearances on CT represent the cysts in different stages of their life cycle. The cyst is often thin-walled and surrounded by oedema. Albendazole (15 mg/kg/d for 8 days) or praziquantel (50 mg/kg/d for 14 days) is the treatment of choice accompanied by steroids to prevent the Herxheimer reaction. However, this is controversial and some centres choose not to use anti-helminthic agents in the belief that neurocysticercosis is a self-limiting disease, which requires only symptomatic and supportive therapy. Appropriate anti-convulsants should be used in the presence of seizures.

Fungal infections of the CNS

The majority of children who develop a CNS fungal infection have a depressed immune system from whatever cause, including HIV/AIDS, or have been on antibiotics for a primary infection. The fungi that can infect the CNS include *Candida albicans*, *Cryptococcus neoformans*, *Coccidioides immitis*, *Histoplasma capsulatum*, mucormycosis, aspergillus, and blastomycosis.

Candida albicans

Candida albicans invades the meninges from the bloodstream in cases of disseminated candidiasis. Commonly affected are premature neonates who are on total parenteral nutrition and antibacterial drugs. CNS candidiasis results in widespread micro abscesses with granulomatous vasculitis and thrombi formation.

Cryptococcosis

This is the most common fungal infection of the CNS. The fungus is found in soil and often in pigeon droppings. Primary infection occurs via the respiratory system, spreading to the bloodstream and other organs including the CNS. It occurs more specifically in immune-compromised patients (HIV/AIDS), those with neoplasia, collagen disorders or on steroid therapy, but may also occur in well children. The organism produces a granulomatous arachnoiditis resembling a chronic basilar meningitis, similar to tubercu-

lous meningitis (TBM), and vasculitis of large vessels. The arachnoiditis may extend to involve the spine in a minority of cases. Headache and meningeal irritation are the main clinical presenting signs. Other neurological signs usually develop, including cranial nerve palsies, raised intracranial pressure with papilloedema, impairment of consciousness, and signs and symptoms of hydrocephalus. Involvement of skin, bone, joint, eye, kidney, or adrenal gland may occur.

The clinical diagnosis of cryptococcus is difficult, especially in immune-compromised patients. The CSF pressure is high and shows lymphocyte pleocytosis, increased protein and a low sugar, similar to that found in TBM. In over 60 per cent of cases the encapsulated organism can be demonstrated on Indian ink staining of the CSF. Culture of the organism in the CSF will confirm the diagnosis. Demonstration of the antigen in the CSF by latex agglutination test is both reliable and specific. The CT scan may show cerebral oedema, hydrocephalus, occasionally mass lesions (granulomas) and basilar enhancement.

Treatment is prolonged for at least six weeks and consists of a combination of amphotericin B (1 mg/kg/d) and 5-fluorocytosine (150 mg/kg/d divided into six-hourly doses). Relapses are not uncommon and may occur up to two to three years after completion of the treatment. Untreated cases will invariably result in death. HIV positive patients should subsequently receive life-long therapy with low dose fluconazole.

Brain tumours

Brain tumours in children usually present with cerebellar ataxia, pyramidal tract signs, and cranial nerve palsies due to the fact that most of them are found in the posterior fossa, i.e. brainstem and the cerebellum.

Brain tumours are the second most common neoplasms in children after childhood leukaemias. There are many ways in which CNS tumours may be classified. A commonly used classification is the WHO's system of grading tumours according to site, histological type, and degree of malignancy. The location of brain tumours varies with age (*see* Table 26.27).

In infants there is a predominance of supratentorial tumours, especially astrocytomas. Spanning the different age groups of childhood, infratentorial tumours are slightly more common than supratentorial tumours, astrocytomas being the most common (which include tumours such as cerebellar astrocytomas, brainstem gliomas, and high-grade and low-grade supratentorial astrocytomas), followed by medulloblastomas and ependymomas. There are well-known risk factors that are associated with the subsequent development of brain tumours.

Risk factors associated with the development of brain tumours:
- ◆ **Genetic syndromes**
  - – Neurofibromatosis
  - – Tuberous sclerosis
  - – Von Hippel-Lindau disease
  - – Basal cell nevus syndrome
- ◆ **Immunosuppression**
  - – Renal transplant suppression
  - – Ataxia telangiectasia
- ◆ **Environmental**
  - – Aromatic hydrocarbons
  - – Nitrosoureas
  - – Triazines
  - – System hydrazines
  - – Background radiation
  - – Maternal consumption of barbiturates.

An important point to note is that even malignant tumours rarely metastasize outside the CNS and most of them spread along CSF pathways, rather than by blood. Often a benign tumour located in a neurologically significant place and which cannot easily be removed, may present with more problems, because of its locality, than a very malignant tumour.

Clinical features of brain tumours are usually non-specific. Focal neurological signs will depend on the location of the lesion. Most of the signs and symptoms of brain tumours result from either increased ICP or focal effects of the tumour on surrounding neural tissue or a combination of the two. Supratentorial tumours may be large enough to cause shift of cerebral tissue with eventual herniation. Raised ICP is caused by the tumour mass, the associated cerebral oedema, or obstructive hydrocephalus. Features of raised ICP include headaches (especially on awakening or those that wake the child at night); vomiting, which is common and usually accompanied by headache; papilloedema, which is not always a

Table 26.27 Primary intracranial tumours according to location
Supratentorial
Cerebral hemisphere and meninges
▪ Astrocytoma
▪ Ependymoma
▪ Meningioma
Midline structures
▪ Pituitary adenoma
▪ Craniopharyngioma
▪ Colloid cyst
▪ Pineal parenchymal tumour
▪ Germ cell tumour
▪ Astrocytoma
▪ Optic nerve glioma
Infratentorial
Cerebellum and 4th ventricle
▪ Astrocytoma
▪ Medulloblastoma
▪ Ependymoma
Brainstem
▪ Astrocytoma

sign of raised ICP and is only present in 50 per cent of patients with brain tumours. Ataxia and to a lesser degree cranial nerve palsies, are very common features of posterior fossa tumours while visual disturbances are more commonly found in supratentorial tumours. Obstructive hydrocephalus due to blockage at the 4th ventricle is a common complication of infratentorial tumours.

Diagnostic evaluation includes skull X-ray (signs of raised ICP and calcification); CT scan with contrast for supratentorial and posterior fossa tumours, but is less accurate in evaluating brainstem tumours where MRI scans are more helpful. Cerebral angiography is useful in vascular tumours or vascular malformations.

Management requires adequate clinical evaluation of the child. Deteriorating levels of consciousness and neurological signs, failing vision, and neck stiffness require urgent attention to relieve raised ICP (*see* 'Coma', *earlier in this chapter*). Dexamethasone and mannitol may be used as an interim to neurosurgical decompression. Depending on the type of tumour, surgical removal, radiotherapy or chemotherapy may need to be considered.

Disorders of the spinal cord

Disorders of the spinal cord are usually complex and very varied and a detailed discussion of the various disorders is beyond the scope of this book. Some of the more common conditions are mentioned below.

Anatomically there are four main pathways in the spinal cord that one needs to consider when faced with a patient with an acute spinal cord disorder. These are the *descending cortico-spinal tracts* (pyramidal tracts; motor); *autonomic tracts* (in cervical and sacral segments–carrying sensation to and from bladder and bowel); *ascending spino-thalamic tracts* (carrying pain and temperature); and *posterior columns* (carrying proprioception, vibration, pressure).

Spinal cord compression syndromes

Children presenting with features of spinal cord compression must be regarded as a medical, and often surgical, emergency requiring a speedy diagnosis and prompt treatment. Clinically, these patients present with pyramidal tract signs (upper motor neuron signs) initially. If the compression progresses then sensory loss and autonomic impairment such as bladder and bowel incontinence follow.

The blood supply of the spinal cord consists of a single anterior spinal artery, which supplies most of the spinal cord and tracts, and two posterior spinal arteries, which supply the posterior columns. Most compressive lesions of the spinal cord will initially cause compression of the anterior spinal artery. This results in ischaemia to the watershed areas of the spinal cord, which are the cortico-spinal tracts. That is why motor symptoms and signs appear initially in most compressive spinal cord disorders. If the compression progresses then the other tracts (spino-thalamic and autonomic) will suffer ischaemia with resultant loss of sensation and bladder and bowel control. This is known as the anterior spinal artery syndrome. The order in which the tracts became involved needs to be carefully elucidated from the history. If the patient has normal proprioception and vibration sense then the posterior columns are intact and one is dealing with an anterior (compressive) spinal artery disorder. The more common causes in children are tuberculous spondylitis (anterior

erosion of adjacent vertebrae with anterior collapse and compression of the anterior spinal artery); spinal tumours (malignant or benign), tuberculous abscess, bilharzial granulomas, and trauma.

An intrinsic cord lesion is more likely to present with sensory loss as the initial physical sign and then progresses to involve the autonomic pathways before any motor signs and symptoms develop.

Transverse myelitis

This syndrome is characterized by the sudden onset of progressive weakness of the lower limbs, loss of bladder and bowel sphincter control, and sensory loss, often preceded by a respiratory infection. It is thought to be due to an acute occlusion of the anterior spinal artery caused by an auto-immune or post-infectious vasculitis. At first the weakness is flaccid but gradually evidence of pyramidal tract involvement is seen with spasticity, increased deep tendon reflexes, and a positive Babinski reflex. Posterior column function (proprioception, vibration sense) is usually spared. Most children affected have a pleocytosis and an elevated protein in the CSF. Prognosis is usually good, with 60 per cent of patients showing full recovery.

Neural tube defects (spinal dysraphism)

(*See also* Chapter 8, Surgical conditions of the newborn.)

These conditions present clinically as spina-bifida occulta, meningocele or myelomeningocele. These disorders are due to the failure of closure of the midline mesenchymal, bony and ectodermal neural structures that arise from the primitive neural tube.

The clinical manifestations of these neural tube defects will depend on the degree of involvement of the neural tissue. Some of the more common spinal dysraphic syndromes are listed below:

Spina bifida occulta where the dorsal spine has failed to close. Usually the underlying meninges and neural tissue are intact with no neurological deficit. Commonly picked up as an incidental finding on X-ray of the spine. A clinical clue may be a tuft of hair or dimple on the skin over the lower lumbo-sacral spine.

Meningocele. The dorsal spine is bifid and the meninges of the cord extend as a cystic swelling over the defect. Usually the underlying neural tissue of the cord is not involved.

Meningomyelocele. The neural tissue is exposed and very often damaged with resultant neurological deficits at the site of the lesion as well as the levels below. These children present with lower motor neuron weakness at the site of the lesion, usually with a flaccid paralysis, sensory loss as well as bladder and bowel incontinence. These babies need to be referred for surgical correction within the first 48 hours of delivery.

27

Renal and urinary tract disorders

A whole range of renal abnormalities can occur in the developing fetus, involving both embryological and functional development.

In recent years knowledge of genetic control of molecular biology in kidney development has increased remarkably, and so has the understanding of renal malformation syndromes with a genetic basis.

Functional development of the kidneys

Fetal renal function

With the development of the kidneys, renal blood flow increases from 20 ml/min at 25 weeks gestation to >60 ml/min at 40 weeks gestation. Likewise the urine production increases from 5 ml/hr at 20 weeks gestation to 50 ml/hr at 40 weeks gestation. With such significant urine flow during pregnancy, it is understandable that the excretory systems may be dilated at times. On ultrasound, pre-natal hydronephrosis is found in approximately 0.25 per cent of pregnancies, but 25–50 per cent of the dilated urinary tracts in the fetus seen on sonar, do not persist post-natally on follow-up.

Post-natal functional development

All normal neonates void within the first 24 hours, regardless of gestational age. After the first two days, oliguria is defined as <1 ml/kg/hr, but with restricted fluid intake, neonates can remain in balance with urine flow rates of 0.5 ml/kg/hr. Polyuria is defined as >2 000 ml/1.73 m² daily

(1 156 ml/m²/day) therefore a newborn with >230 ml/day = >3.2 ml/kg/hr would be polyuric.

Renal blood flow increases sharply at birth with a 5–18 fold rise. There is redistribution of flow from the inner to outer renal cortex. The glomerular filtration rate (GFR) doubles during the first week in term infants and the serum creatinine decreases by 50 per cent in the first week in term or near term infants. This is related to:

- Diminished renal vascular resistance
- Increasing perfusion pressure
- Increased glomerular permeability and
- Increasing filtration surface.

The GFR reaches adult levels at two years of age (*see* Table 27.1). Very low birth weight infants: GFR catches up to term infants of same conceptual age nine months or later after birth.

Tubular function

The neonate's tubular immaturity manifests by a limited concentrating capacity (600–700 mosm/l; premature 500 mosm/l), while achieving good diluting ability (25–35 mosm/l). Prematures <35 weeks have sodium wasting because of tubular immaturity.

Functional response of developing kidney to malformation or injury

If there is reduced functioning renal mass, compensatory renal growth can begin prenatally. Compensatory growth progressively declines from fetus to neonate to young child to adult. Fetal compensatory growth occurs by hyperplasia

Table 27.1 Glomerular filtration rate in children (adapted from C. Chantler with permission from Blackwell Science Ltd.)*

Age	Mean GFR (ml/min/1.73m²)	Range (± 2 SD)
Birth	20	
7 days	38	26–60
1 month	48	28–68
2 months	58	30–86
6 months	77	41–103
9 months	103	49–157
12 months	115	65–160
2 to 12 years	127	89–165

*Chantler C, The Kidney. In: Godfrey S and Baum JD, eds. Clinical Paediatric Physiology. Oxford: Blackwell Scientic Publications 1979, pp 356-98.

and hypertrophy, but only the latter occurs after birth except for tubules. Significant urinary obstruction hampers optimal renal development, and if left untreated, will cause progressive renal functional deterioration.

Clinical assessment and simple investigations

The assessment of renal problems and urinary tract disorders should, like other systems, begin with a thorough history (*see* Table 27.2) and examination and at least a dipstick examination of the urine.

In the clinical examination, take note of the following:

- Height, weight, head circumference: poor growth may indicate a chronic disorder.
- Pulses and blood pressure: Absent pulses/bruits suggest coarctation, vasculitis or thrombosis.
- Congenital or acquired infections may be accompanied by anaemia and hepatosplenomegaly, petechiae, jaundice or abnormal temperature control
- Features at birth suggestive of urinary tract anomalies. These include:
  - Oligohydramnios: absent or decreased renal function
  - Polyhydramnios: tubular problem
  - Large placenta: congenital nephrotic syndrome
  - Potter facies: bilateral renal agenesis
  - Absent abdominal muscles: prune-belly syndrome
  - Single umbilical artery: renal abnormalities
  - Abnormal and low set ears: renal abnormalities
  - VACTERL group of anomalies: unilateral agenesis
  - Myelomeningocele: neurogenic bladder
- Large kidneys at birth can be caused by the following:
  - Hydronephrosis due to urinary obstruction or reflux
  - Cystic disease: Unilateral: consider multicystic disease; Bilateral: consider autosomal recessive polycystic disease
  - Tumour: Congenital mesoblastic nephroma (primitive Wilms tumour)
  - Reno-vascular thrombosis. The kidneys are larger in venous thrombosis, but associated with less hypertension than in arterial thrombosis
- Abdominal distension: ascites or large bladder (obstructed or neurogenic)
- Back and urogenital examination: sacral sinus, patulous anus and impaired peri-anal sensation suggest spina bifida or tethered cord. Ambiguous genitalia or cryptorchidism may be associated with urinary tract anomalies.
- Abdominal wall defect or muscle deficiency is associated with triad (prune belly) syndrome.
- Eye abnormalities are often associated with renal problems. These include:
  - Coloboma–dysplastic kidneys.
  - Retinis pigmentosa–medullary cystic disease.
  - Peri-macular white spots (especially with high tone neural deafness) :
  - Alport's syndrome.
  - Corneal crystals (best on slit lamp examination) : cystinosis
- Rickets, especially when nutritional vitamin D deficiency is unlikely, may be related to chronic renal failure or a renal tubular problem.

Table 27.2 Important pointers in the history for possible renal disease

Timing	Pointer	Possible problem
Family history	Diabetes mellitus in mother	caudal regression syndrome renal vein thrombosis in the newborn
	Consanguinity	hereditary conditions, e.g. congenital nephrotic syndrome or polycystic kidneys
Antenatal period	Excessive maternal alcohol intake	small kidneys
	Fetal sonar	dilated urinary tract
	Maternal syphilis	congenital nephrotic syndrome
	Maternal HIV	enlarged kidneys with proteinuria in infant
Perinatal	Premature	immature renal function, e.g. tubular Na loss
	Low Apgar score at birth	hypoxic ischaemia and acute tubular necrosis
	Umbilical arterial catheter	renal artery thrombosis
	Nephrotoxic drugs	renal dysfunction
Postnatal	Prolonged conjugated hyperbilirubinaemia	urinary infection
	Urinary amount, stream,	renal failure, obstructive uropathy and urinary function
	Urine abnormalities on dipstick	renal disease, infection, calculi
	Abdominal pain, fever, dysuria, frequency	urinary infection
	Generalised oedema	nephrotic syndrome
	Failure to thrive, especially growth in height	chronic renal disease
	Rickets, pallor	renal tubular disease, chronic renal failure
	Environmental, eg exposure to bilharzia	urinary involvement

- Skin rashes : impetigo may precede glomerulonephritis, Henoch-Schönlein purpura and other vasculitides are associated with renal involvement

Calculated glomerular filtration rate

The previous method of estimating creatinine clearance using the urine and serum creatinine with a 24 hour urine collection is not recommended in children because of the difficulty of obtaining an accurate 24 hour collection in children, and the variability of results because of the additional tubular excretion of creatinine.

A calculated GFR can be ascertained using the height of the child in cm, the serum creatinine

Counahan-Barratt height formula for calculating creatinine clearance in children

$$\frac{\text{height (cm)} \times 40}{\text{serum creatinine (}\mu\text{mols/l)}} = \text{creatinine clearance}$$

$$(\text{ml/min/1.73 m}^2)$$

(in μmol/l) and a factor 'K' = 40 for most children above one year of age. In infancy, 'K' should be reduced to '10' in the first two weeks, '25' at three months, '30' at six months and '35' at nine months.

A urine dipstick examination is an essential initial screening test

- For infection: a fresh midstream or (in infants) a fresh bag specimen must be used: observe for a positive leukocyte esterase to indicate increased neutrophils in the urine, and a positive nitrite indicates sufficient bacteria with enzyme to break down nitrate to nitrite in urine
- An early morning specimen is used to screen for:
  - pH 5 indicates normal distal acidification
  - SG 1020 or more indicates reasonable concentration ability
  - Absent protein rules out significant pathological glomerular proteinuria
- Other dipstick tests include blood (haematuria), glucose (glycosuria) - if positive, do blood glucose to rule out diabetes mellitus

In the larger adolescent, after age 16 years, it may be more accurate to use the Cockroft-Gault equation for estimating creatinine clearance. With either method, normal renal function after nine months of age would be at least 80 ml/min/1.73 m². If an accurate GFR measurement is required, then chromium EDTA two blood sample method would be closest to the gold standard of inulin clearance.

Table 27.3 lists some features of glomerular and tubular pathology .

Congenital and inherited renal disorders

Few genetic renal disorders are confined to the kidneys and many malformation syndromes (e.g. Turner's syndrome) or genetic disorders

Table 27.3 Features of glomerular and renal tubular pathology

Glomerular pathology	Urine microscopy	Dysmorphic red cells Red cell casts Hyaline and mixed cellular casts may also be seen
	Proteinuria : monitor early morning protein/creatinine ratio (g/mmol)	<0.02 g/mmol is normal >0.2 g/mmol in nephrotic range
Renal tubular pathology	Fractional excretion of sodium *	FeNa <1% usually normal Na reabsorption or prerenal factors FeNa >2% abnormally reduced Na reabsorption, ? early acute tubular necrosis FeNa >6% highly suggestive of acute tubular necrosis or chronic renal failure
	ß2 microglobulin/creatinine ratio in urine	>0.052 mg/mmol abnormal. The greater it is, the more significant the tubulointerstitial pathology
	Specific tubular function disorders	
	Proximal tubule	Phosphoglucoaminoaciduria suggests Fanconi's syndrome
	Loop of Henle	Na, K, Cl loss often with metabolic alkalosis, eg Bartter's syndrome
	Distal tubule	Urine pH >5.5 with positive urine anion gap ** indicates distal renal tubular acidosis (RTA)

*Urine Na (mmol/l) X serum creatinine (μmol/l) X 100 / serum sodium (mmol/l) X urine creatinine (mmol/l) X 1000 = %
** Positive urine anion gap = Urine [Cl] < Urine [Na] + Urine [K]

may commonly have associated renal developmental defects. Variable expression of congenital renal defects may occur within a family, and among kindreds.

Minor and major malformations of the urogenital tract occur in up to 10 per cent of the population and account for one-third of all congenital malformations. Sporadic malformations were thought to be more common than inherited, but more predisposing genetic factors have been found over the past 20 years.

Duplications of the collecting system occur in 0.9 per cent of the population. Many are partial with no sequelae. If total duplication occurs and the upper moiety is dilated, then commonly the upper moiety's ectopic ureter is inserted into the bladder at a lower point than that of the lower moiety and is narrowed at the point of insertion. If the lower moiety is dilated, then association with reflux or pelvi-ureteric junction obstruction is likely.

Deficiency of renal tissue

Renal agenesis occurs unilaterally in 1 in 1 500 births and bilaterally in 1 in 4 000 births, when it results in Potter's syndrome.

Associated abnormalities of the urogenital system occur frequently

Renal hypoplasia refers to a decreased number of nephrons, which is most frequently unilateral, but in bilateral cases accounts for up to 20 per cent of chronic renal failure in children. It is more frequent in males

Abnormalities of renal location

A horse-shoe kidney is a sporadic disorder, occurring in 1 in 700 patients. 90 per cent have a fused lower pole.

Ectopic kidneys are displaced from the expected position. They may be solitary, and pelvic ectopic kidneys are commonly associated with abnormalities of the skeleton, gastrointestinal tract or heart.

Abnormalities of renal differentiation

Renal dysplasia refers to the presence of primitive tissue of mesenchymal origin including cartilage:

- ◆ Without cysts : If bilateral,chronic renal failure eventually occurs.
- ◆ With cysts : multicystic kidney: invariably unilateral,and associated with an atretic ureter. The other kidney is usually normal.. The multi-cystic kidney often involutes after a few years.

Cystic kidneys:
- ◆ Autosomal recessive polycystic kidney disease (ARPKD) – very large kidneys with small cysts present at birth. Invariably, there is associated hepatic fibrosis, portal hypertension, varices and hyperplenism Complications of portal hypertension and reduced hepatic reserve, may require both liver and kidney transplantation. Chronic renal failure commonly begins in the first decade. It is rare in black children, but more common in the Afrikaner due to a founder effect.
- ◆ Autosomal dominant polycystic kidney disease (ADPKD) – previously called adult type. This is more common than ARPKD, occurring in 1 in 3 000 deliveries. Only a few cysts are present in the neonatal period. Cysts occur in the liver in 30 per cent of ADPKD patients, but the liver is not fibrotic. Chronic renal failure is common in older adulthood.
- ◆ Nephronophthisis/medullary cystic kidney disease complex is an autosomal recessive condition and may be associated with extrarenal organ involvement.
- ◆ Medullary sponge kidney is rare in children but can present in the first decade.

Congenital renal neoplasms:
- ◆ Congenital mesoblastic nephroma is a variant of Wilms tumour but presents earlier and has a better prognosis.
- ◆ Nephroblastoma (Wilms tumour) (*see* Chapter 22, neoplastic disorders).

Vesico-ureteric reflux (VUR)

Vesico-ureteral reflux (VUR) is the backflow of urine from the bladder into the ureters. The reflux is related to a shorter intra-mural length of the ureter in the bladder wall, which is often more laterally placed than in the normal child. As the bladder matures the wall thickens and the natural tendency is for the reflux to lessen or stop.

Reflux is rare in black children, but common in Asians and Caucasians, occurring in 1 in 50–100 children. In males of all races reflux may be associated with a dysplastic kidney on one or both sides. Fifteen percent of reflux cases are familial with an autosomal dominant inheritance.Therefore siblings have a 30–50 per cent chance of also having VUR.

VUR is a risk factor for pyelonephritis. VUR alone does not cause renal damage, but in the presence of reflux, particularly grades IV and V, urinary tract infection with an invasive organism can cause scarring of the kidneys. This may be related to compound papillae, occurring more in the poles of the kidney, allowing intra-renal reflux that the usual simple papillae would not, but the vital factor is still the urinary tract infection. Even in the absence of reflux, certain virulent bacteria with better adherence to the uro-epithelium of the urinary tract, e.g. P-fimbriated *E. Coli* will gain access to the renal parenchyma and damage the tissue.

Eighty percent of grades I to III stop refluxing with time, as do 40 per cent of grades IV and V.

If the natural history is for the reflux to settle, then simply keeping the urine free of infection with prophylactic antibiotics would seem to be the most logical approach. Sub-mucosal injection of Teflon or Deflux at the ureteric opening to try to prevent reflux should not be used because of the natural history of less reflux with time, the development of complications and because it is less effective than surgical reimplantation. Re-implantation of the ureter to correct the reflux can be done surgically, but controlled trials of medical versus surgical treatment have shown no significant differences. Only with grades IV and V, where there is a greater chance of the VUR not settling, may re-implantation be preferable to the problem of potential secondary bladder dyssynergia. In these cases, the bladder loses synchronization and tends to empty up into the dilated ureters rather than down the urethra. This can cause dysfunctional obstructive uropathy.

Obstructive uropathies

Possible consequences of urinary tract obstruction during development include:

Figure 27.1 International classification of vesico-ureteric reflux

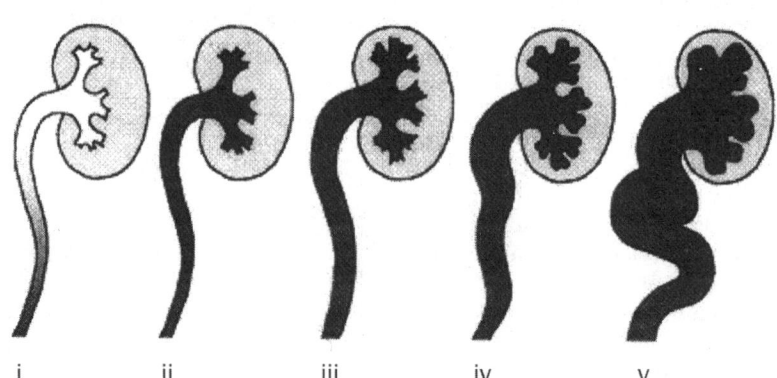

| i | ii | iii | iv | v |

Grade I: ureter only. Grade II: ureter, pelvis, calyces; no dilation, normal calyceal fornices. Grade III: mild or moderate dilation or tortuosity of the ureter, and mild or moderate dilation of the pelvis, but no or slight blunting of the fornices. Grade IV: moderate dilation or tortuosity of ureter and mild dilation of renal pelvis and calyces; complete obliteration of sharp angle of fornices but maintenance of papillary impressions in most calyces. Grade V: gross dilation and tortuosity of ureter; gross dilation of renal pervis and calyces; papillary impressions are no longer visible in most calyces.

(Modified from International Reflux Committee. Medical versus surgical treatment of primary vesico-ureteral reflux. With permission, Pediatrics 1981 67:392. Copyright American Academy of Pediatrics.)

- Oligohydramnios with development of the Potter sequence and pulmonary hypoplasia
- Renal insufficiency or failure
- Fluid and electrolyte abnormalities due to renal tubular sodium wasting and urinary concentrating defects, hyperkalaemia or renal tubular acidosis
- Hypertension
- Infection
- Growth failure.

Posterior urethral valves are abnormal mucosal folds that function as a valve to obstruct the flow of urine. They occur only in males, and are the commonest cause of obstructive uropathy in children. They must be suspected if the bladder is still palpable after micturition.

Ectopic ureters are more common in females, and often associated with ureteroceles.

Pelvi-ureteric obstruction is much more common in males, as is **ureterovesical** obstruction. In a third of cases, the obstruction is bilateral.

Timeous treatment of significant obstruction should be done prior to the development of irreparable damage, and therefore ultrasound, and if necessary diuretic MAG3, should be used to define the effect of the obstruction on kidney function.

Inherited tubular disorders

Most patients with genetic defects of tubular function present in the first years of life with non-specific symptoms. Although polyuria is a common sign, most children who 'drink too much' do not have a tubular disorder. Growth is usually affected. Patients with poor growth, polyuria, unexplained metabolic acidosis or rickets should be suspected of having a renal tubular disorder such as Fanconi's syndrome, renal tubular acidosis, nephrogenic diabetes insipidus or Bartter's syndrome. (*See* Table 27.3). The majority of cases are inherited as autosomal recessive conditions.

Hereditary glomerulopathies

A number of genetic conditions present with predominant glomerular involvement.

Predominant haematuria

Alport's syndrome is a genetically heterogenous disease arising from mutations in genes coding for type IV collagen, a major constituent of basement membranes. Patients usually present with persistent haematuria, often progressing to proteinuria, hypertension and renal failure, especially in males. High frequency sensori-neural deafness and ocular defects are often associated and may herald a worse renal prognosis.

Benign familial haematuria is usually due to Thin Basement Membrane disease. There is no associated deafness, and the condition is inherited as an autosomal dominant.

Haemolytic uraemic syndrome may occur as an autosomal dominant or autosomal recessive condition and may also be recurrent.

Predominant nephrotic syndrome

Congenital and inherited nephrotic syndrome. Several different conditions are described, including the congenital Finnish-type nephrotic syndrome, and autosomal recessive disorders (e.g. familial glomerulosclerosis, diffuse mesangial sclerosis, familial minimal change nephrotic syndrome).

Because podocyte effacement is the common initial abnormality of the glomerular filter, this group of conditions is now also labelled as podocytopathies. A large number of proteins show altered expression in the podocytopathies, as demonstrated in Figure 27.3. For orientation, *see* Figure 27.2 where the epithelial cell is in fact the podocyte.

Figure 27.2 Normal glomerulus on electron microscopy

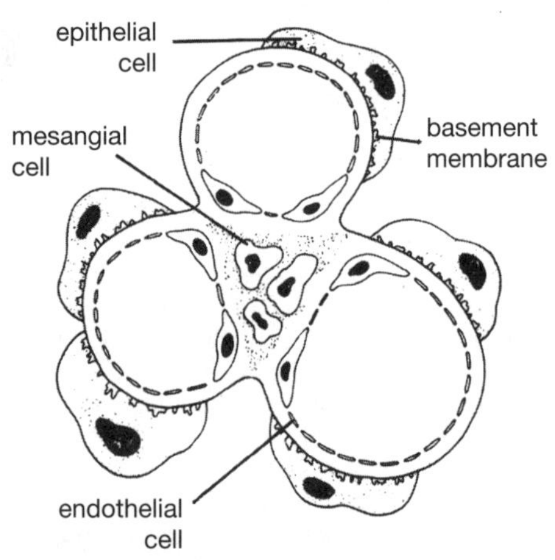

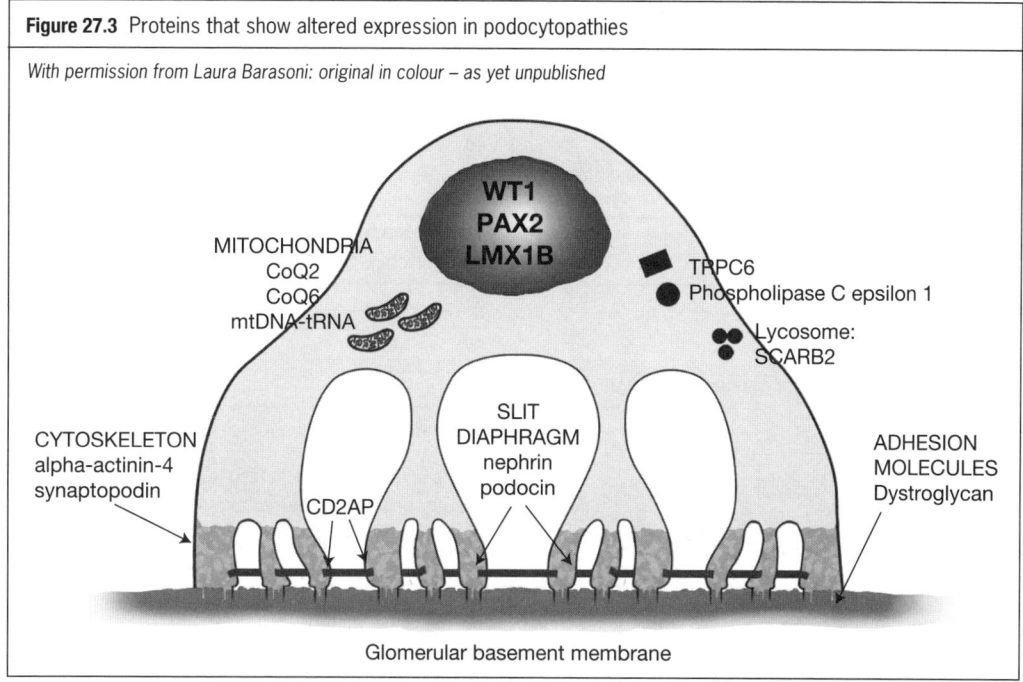

Figure 27.3 Proteins that show altered expression in podocytopathies

With permission from Laura Barasoni: original in colour – as yet unpublished

Urolithiasis (kidney stones)

Calculi are often associated with strong genetic factors in children, and include:

- **Familial urolithiasis**, with or without hypercalciuria – common. Usually inherited as an autosomal dominant condition.
- **Distal renal tubular acidosis** is also inherited as an autosomal dominant.
- **Dent's disease** is an X-linked recessive condition, with nephrocalcinosis and progressive renal failure, hypercalciuric rickets and low molecular weight proteinuria.
- **Lesch-Nyhan syndrome**. An X-linked recessive condition due to hypoxanthine–guanine phosphoribosyl transferase deficiency.
- **Autosomal recessive** diseases associated with hypercalciuria, hyperoxaluria or cystinuria.

An approach to haematuria in children

A number of conditions are associated with a red/pink discolouration of urine. *See* Table 27.4 A

Table 27.4 Causes of red/pink urine

Food, e.g. beetroot, blackberries, rhubarb, red dyes.

Drugs, e.g. chloroquine, phenolphthalein, sulfasalazine, rifampicin (more orange).

Physiological–urates (pink) in neonates: may stain nappy.

Beware false-positive with urine contaminated with household bleach.

Pathological–red cells, haemoglobinuria (more port wine colour), myoglobin, porphyrins.

urine dipstick test must be read before 60 seconds because this is a sensitive test and false positives are likely thereafter.

Further assessment is best made on microscopy. Haemoglobinuria often gives a portwine colour with no or few red cells on microscopy. This suggests a haemolytic problem, e.g. malaria, cold agglutinin haemolysis (most commonly mycoplasma), and enzyme deficiency, e.g. of glucose-6-phosphate dehydrogenase (G-6-PD).

If red cells are present (>10 per high power field = 50 per microlitre), then establish whether

Table 27.5 Haematuria	
Non-glomerular	**Glomerular**
Normal morphology of red cells Protein usually <2 + If lower urinary tract, terminal haematuria and blood clots more common Dysuria – if urethritis/cystitis	Dysmorphic red cells Red cell and other casts Often 2+ or >proteinuria Brown or cola-coloured urine If flow cytometry used–red cells smaller because of dysmorphism

Table 27.6 Non-glomerular causes of haematuria	
Causes	**Investigations/Comment**
Non-urinary regional bleeding ▪ anal fissure ▪ trauma – foreign body, masturbation, child abuse ▪ infection – vulvo-vaginitis	Vulva/anus often easier to inspect with child in kneeling, head down and bottom up position
Urinary tract infection ▪ bacterial urinary tract infection ▪ adenovirus haemorrhagic cystitis ▪ schistosomiasis	15% may have macroscopic haematuria, usually a severe infection. Haematuria may make nitrite strip difficult to read Especially terminal haematuria, If ova of *S. haematobium* (terminal spine) not seen on microscopy, bilharzial ELISA/rectal biopsy may be required
Sickle cell disease	Characteristic red cells on smear. Urinary concentrating defect early
Bleeding disorder	INR, PTT and platelets should be checked
Calculi/ hypercalciuria	Calcium/creatinine ratio is normally <0.7 mmol/mmol on 2nd urine specimen in morning
Hydronephrosis–reflux or obstruction.	
Renal cysts	
Tumours, e.g. Wilms, rhabdomyosarcoma	Rectal examination should be done to exclude local spread
Renal artery or renal vein thrombosis	In neonates, especially if umbilical catheterisation was used or if mother is diabetic

they are of glomerular or non-glomerular origin (*see* table 27.5). Note that flow cytometry only identifies 35 per cent of the casts seen on microscopy.

Non-glomerular causes of haematuria are listed in Table 27.6 Plain X-ray abdomen and ultrasound are done for kidney size, calcification, calculi, cysts, hydronephrosis and tumour. Further radiological investigations are done if indicated, but cystoscopy is seldom necessary unless a bladder problem requires better definition. In schistosomiasis, the major complication to exclude is obstructive uropathy. This is because of the swelling and scarring related to deposition of ova at the lower end of the ureters and the bladder wall. If the disease has been active for a a few months, the bladder may be calcified.

Glomerular causes of haematuria are listed in Table 27.7.

Glomerular haematuria is often associated with an acute nephritic syndrome, the features of which are illustrated in Figure 27.4, which shows a comparison of nephritic and nephrotic features in the spectrum of glomerular disease.

This highlights the dominant features of each syndrome, but also shows that there may well be overlapping features. Where there is more of a mixed picture, ie a nephritic-nephrotic presentation with ongoing proteinuria, particularly if it is associated with reduced function, this may well suggest a poorer prognosis.

Henoch-Schönlein nephritis/IgA nephropathy

Nephritis occurs in about half of children with Henoch-Schönlein (anaphylactoid) purpura. (*See* Chapter 21, Immune and connective tissue disorders.)

IgA nephropathy (Berger's disease) presents in the same way but without the rash. In both conditions, the haematuria follows an upper respiratory viral infection or strenuous exercise after two to three days, and can be recurrent. The typical kidney involvement in both conditions is of focal segmental glomerulonephritis with immunofluorescence showing particularly IgA in the glomerular mesangium.

Lupus nephritis

In children, nephritis may be one of the presenting features of systemic lupus erythematosus (*see* Chapter 21, Immune and connective tissue disorders). It occurs more frequently in girls, especially after puberty. The serum complement shows classical pathway activation: decreased C3 (especially if active focal segmental glomerulonephritis or diffuse proliferative glomerulonephritis) and C4. Adequate control of this disease is vital, and renal involvement should be managed and monitored by a paediatric nephrologist.

Acute post-streptococcal glomerulonephritis (APSGN)

This may present with purely haematuria or the full blown acute nephritic syndrome with the features as given in Figure 27.4. Some associated features, shown in Table 27.8, depend on whether the causative organism, group A β-haemolytic streptococcus, is from an impetiginous skin

Table 27.7 Glomerular causes of haematuria	
Typical picture that can often be diagnosed on examination	**Major clinical syndrome often without an obvious physical clue**
Henoch-Schönlein nephritis* Lupus nephritis* Alport syndrome* Nail Patella syndrome* Partial lipodystrophy* Infective endocarditis* Haemolytic uraemic syndrome*	Acute glomerulonephritis (GN) ▪ acute post-streptococcal GN ▪ IgA nephropathy* ▪ interstitial nephritis. Nephrotic syndrome*
*All of the above may have a significant nephrotic component	

lesion or from pharyngitis. Because of the longer incubation period with skin-derived streptococci, the initiating lesion/s may no longer be seen easily by the time the patient presents, and if only the ASO titre is used as a screen for streptococcal infection, the dominant rise of anti-DNase B titres (and the diagnosis) will be missed in skin induced nephritis.

As a consequence of streptococcal infection, there is predominantly alternate pathway activation of complement (decreased C3, normal to low normal C4) and immune complex formation.

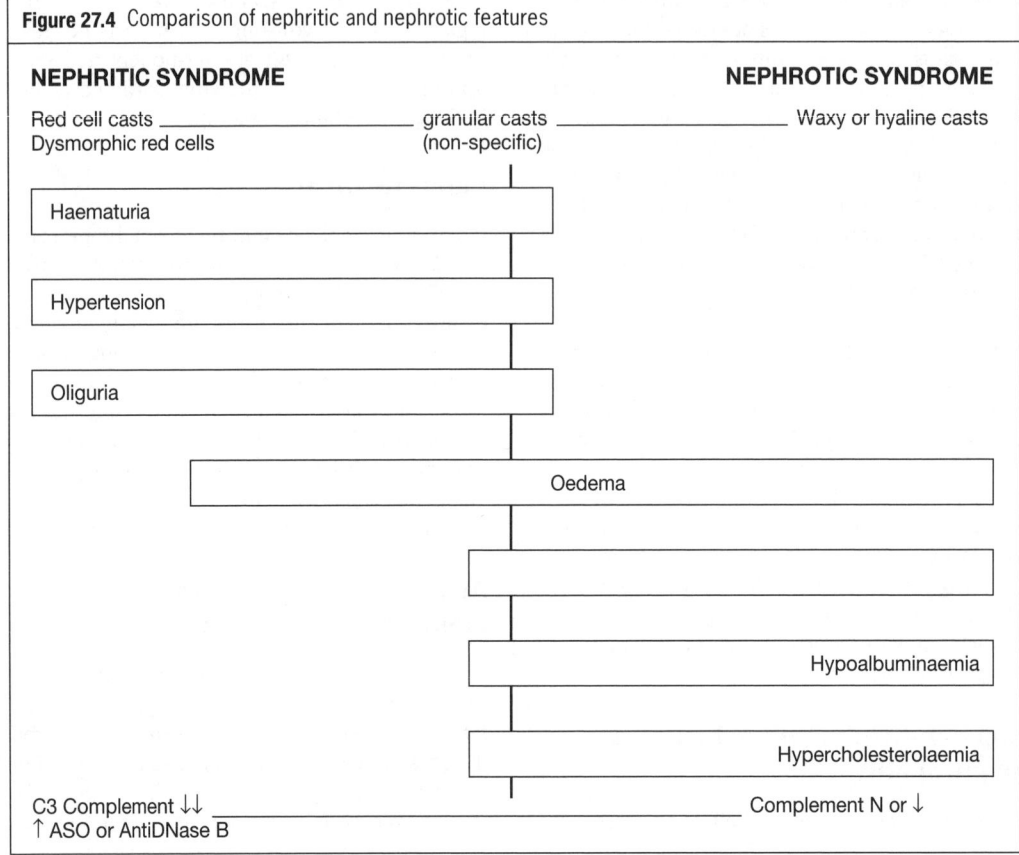

Figure 27.4 Comparison of nephritic and nephrotic features

Table 27.8 Glomerulonephritis according to infected site

	Skin	Throat
Country	Tropical, subtropical	Temperate
Season	Summer	Winter/spring
Age of onset	Pre-school and school-going children	Mainly schoolchildren
Sex distribution	M = F	M >F
Risk of developing nephritis	High	Low
Period from infection to nephritis	21 days	10 days
Antibodies	Anti-DNase B	ASOT
	Anti-hyaluronidase	Less antiDNase B

These immune complexes lodge as sub-epithelial bumps on the basement membrane, triggering the inflammatory response. This is highlighted histologically by the influx of polymorphs, which disrupt the integrity of the basement membrane, allowing escape of blood into the urine. Proliferation of endothelial and mesangial cells in the glomerulus, fibrin deposition and varying degrees of capillary narrowing, plus the attracted polymorpho-nuclear leucocytes give rise to diffuse generalized proliferative glomerulonephritis. Occasionally the reaction may be more severe with mesangial/monocytic cells traversing into Bowman's space and causing crescentic glomerulonephritis. The natural tendency in APSGN is towards healing, rather than scarring, with well over 90 per cent of patients recovering completely, although the haematuria may continue for months or even years in the face of progressive healing. Acute renal failure requiring dialysis is an unusual complication. Scarring with the development of chronic renal failure may be more common in black children.

The important complications of acute nephritis are given in Table 27.9

The possible pathogenetic mechanism for hypertension in APSGN is given in Figure 27.5.

Patients with acute post-streptococcal glomerulonephritis must be admitted to hospital if any of the following are present:

- Oliguria
- Hyperkalaemia
- Hypertension
- Seizures
- Congestive heart failure.

Fluid and salt balance differs in the acute nephritic and nephrotic syndromes, but this is not the full story, because a patient may be less overloaded but have more significant hypertension, and this may well be aggravated by increased endothelin and a decreased response to atrial natriuretic peptide.

Interstitial nephritis

About 50 per cent of patients with interstitial nephritis may show eosinophilia (best seen with Hensel's stain), but an increased β2 microglobulin/creatinine ratio may be more sensitive. This is usually induced by drugs or infection. Streptococci are common, but C3 of complement remains normal in cases of interstitial nephritis. Causative viruses include Ebstein-Barr virus and HIV. While the interstitial

---

Management and treatment of APSGN

- Penicillin is invariably given to eradicate the causative streptococcus, but this is 'after the event'.
- Restrict fluid and salt; weigh patient daily. Weight gain denotes fluid retention.
- Monitor urea, creatinine and electrolytes. Potassium may also require restriction.
- Provide adequate nutrition; only moderate protein restriction if severe oliguria and elevated urea.
- Furosemide to clear extra salt and water retention: this reduces hospital stay.
- Antihypertensives: control blood pressure within the normal range.
- Only consider steroids/cytostatics (e.g. cyclophosphamide) if rapidly progressive glomerulonephritis (this presumes an early renal biopsy).

Table 27.9 Important complications of acute nephritis

Fluid volume overload

Pulmonary oedema and congestive cardiac failure

Hypertension and hypertensive encephalopathy – may have seizures

Rapidly progressive glomerulonephritis (usually crescentic on biopsy)

Acute renal failure

Chronic renal failure

Posterior leuko-encephalopathy* – may have seizures

*Rapid changes of blood pressure and dysregulation of the blood-brain barrier may cause cerebral oedema

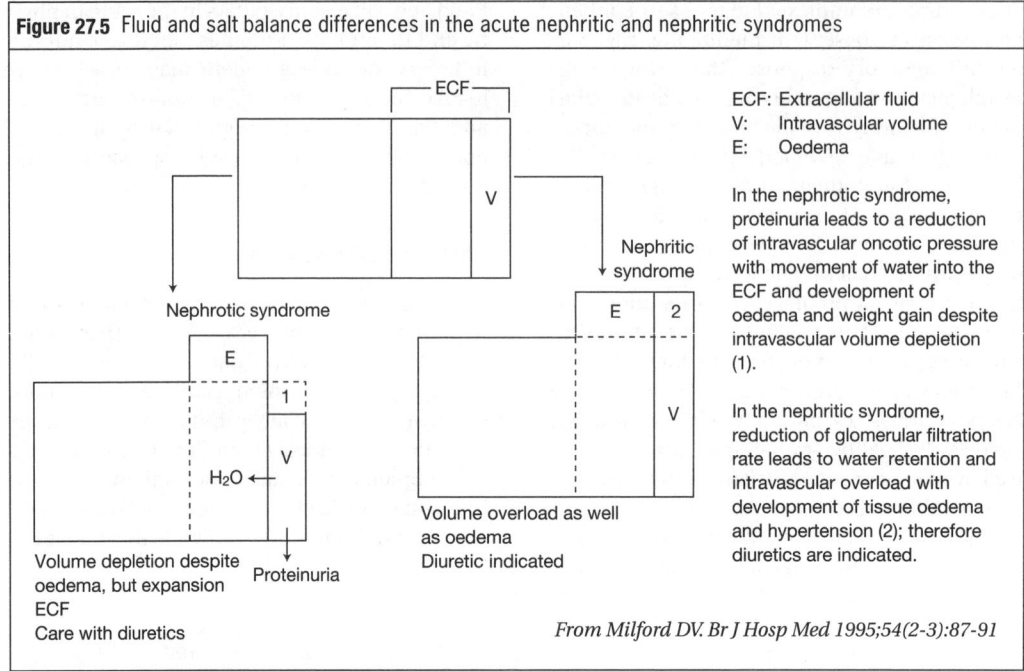

Figure 27.5 Fluid and salt balance differences in the acute nephritic and nephritic syndromes

ECF: Extracellular fluid
V: Intravascular volume
E: Oedema

In the nephrotic syndrome, proteinuria leads to a reduction of intravascular oncotic pressure with movement of water into the ECF and development of oedema and weight gain despite intravascular volume depletion (1).

In the nephritic syndrome, reduction of glomerular filtration rate leads to water retention and intravascular overload with development of tissue oedema and hypertension (2); therefore diuretics are indicated.

From Milford DV. Br J Hosp Med 1995;54(2-3):87-91

---

nephritis due to E-B virus usually settles, HIV-associated nephritis may progress to focal glomerulosclerosis or immune complex type.

Approach to proteinuria and the nephrotic syndrome

Lesser amounts of proteinuria are not specific and may occur with fever, infection or other inflammatory processes. If it is persistent, then one should rule out orthostatic proteinuria, which is postural, i.e. particularly in children without evidence of illness, the first urine of the morning shows no or very little protein, whereas later in the day with the child ambulant, greater amounts of protein may be passed.

Persistent proteinuria >0.02 g/mmol of creatinine in a first urine specimen in the morning should be investigated by doing at least a dipstick, urine microscopy and serum creatinine. Further workup is required if proteinuria is persistent or in the nephrotic range (on dipstick, 3 to 4+, or >0.2 g/mmol creatinine), particularly if there are other features of the nephrotic syndrome. The degree of proteinuria can be conveniently monitored with a urine dipstick (e.g. Albustix®)

Proteinuria with associated haematuria entails the investigation of haematuria as discussed above. Microscopic haematuria is present in 25 per cent of patients with nephrotic syndrome due to minimal change disease (but red cell casts are very unusual); more haematuria is found with other types of glomerular pathology, and if cellular casts are present, proliferative or scarring glomerular lesions are more likely.

The dominant features of the nephrotic syndrome, as seen in Figure 27.4, are significant proteinuria, hypo-albuminaemia (usually <25 g/l) and oedema. In this situation, the kidney tends to avidly absorb sodium, which aggravates the oedema. The different emphasis in fluid and salt balance was illustrated in Figure 27.5 above.

Additional investigations may be performed to exclude or confirm specific diagnoses.

The common causes of nephrotic syndrome in black South African children, as found at kidney biopsy in three centres, are given in Table 27.10. Minimal change disease is the commonest cause in Asians and Caucasians (about 80 per cent), whereas it accounts for only 20 per cent of black Africans with nephrotic syndrome. Focal glomerulosclerosis is the most common cause of nephrotic syndrome in South African black chil-

Basic investigations in a patient with suspected nephrotic syndrome include the following:

- Urine dipstick and microscopy
- Define degree of proteinuria with early morning urine protein/creatinine ratio
- Serum chemistry: creatinine, urea and electrolytes, serum albumin, cholesterol
- Serum complement C3 and C4
- Hepatitis B serology
- HIV PCR
- Tuberculin skin test.

dren (>30 per cent) and shows a more aggressive course if tuberculosis is associated. Membranous nephropathy is hepatitis B-induced and has become less common with routine hepatitis B vaccination. Congenital nephrotic syndrome occurs in association with infection, such as congenital syphilis or HIV. Treatment of the underlying infection can be expected to improve the renal outcome. Hereditary congenital nephrotic syndrome is usually an autosomal recessive condition, is often associated with pulmonary stenosis and has a poor outcome without renal transplantation.

Minimal change disease (MCNS) is the commonest glomerular disorder in South African

Asian and Caucasian children. The median age of presentation is four years and it is more common in boys (2:1). Over 90 per cent will respond to corticosteroid therapy but many (over 70 per cent) subsequently develop a relapsing course. Nevertheless, about 80 per cent will enter a long term remission during childhood. This is similar to experience reported from elsewhere.

At one stage, the impression was that South African black children with minimal change disease did not respond as well to steroids as Indians and Caucasians. However, this idea has not been upheld because many black children with a picture of minimal change on the initial biopsy, were found to have **focal glomerulosclerosis** on repeat biopsies. The age and pattern of presentation of the nephrotic syndrome in black South African children due to focal glomerulosclerosis, membranous nephropathy and mesangial proliferative glomerulonephritis is similar to that of MCNS.

Prior to biopsy and while responding to steroids, these patients could be labelled as steroid-responsive nephrotic syndrome and thought to have MCNS. The usual plan of therapy to try to keep them in remission is given in Table 27.11. Some have preferred to change to alternate day steroid therapy soon after the patient is in remission, but then also to wean slowly to prevent relapse.

In steroid-dependent or resistant cases,

Table 27.10 Common causes of nephrotic syndrome in black South African children as found at kidney biopsy in three centres

Diagnosis	Johannesburg/Pretoria N = 720	Durban N = 234	Total N = 954
Focal glomerulosclerosis FGS	31.3%	28.6%	30.5%
Minimal change nephrotic syndrome MCNS	24.4%	13.7%	20.7%
Membranous nephropathy (most hepatitis B associated)	13.5%	40.2%	20.0%
Mesangial proliferative and post-infectious	13.2%	7.3%	11.7%
Membranoproliferative	4.2%	5.1%	4.4%
Congenital nephrotic syndrome	6.5%	n/e*	6.0%
Lupus nephritis	5.0%	n/e*	4.6%
Others	1.9%	5.1%	2.1%

the management requires expert supervision by a paediatric nephrologist. The previous management scheme of the International Study of Kidney Disease in Children suggested the earlier use of levamisole, and if relapse occurs after cyclophosphamide, cyclosporine at a dose of up to 5 mg/kg/day was suggested for one year as a steroid sparer. Since then, low dose tacrolimus has often been used in preference to cyclosporine, because it is thought to be less nephrotoxic. Also, particularly if the patients have

been steroid dependent, cyclophosphamide or chlorambucil have been given for 12 weeks.

The earlier the patient presents the longer minimal change relapses tend to carry on, but renal function is maintained and mortality should be low. The prognosis in other cases depends on the cause. Hepatitis B-induced nephrotic syndrome tends to settle as the antigenaemia is cleared and generally has little long term renal sequelae. Focal glomerulosclerosis is invariably progressive, leading to end stage renal failure. Because of the lower prevalence of minimal change in black children, early biopsy may be preferable to a trial of steroids.

Where the patients are steroid-resistant (commoner in focal glomerulosclerosis or mesangial proliferative glomerulonephritis) more aggressive therapy has been tried, e,g. monthly intravenous injections of cyclophosphamide or daily tacrolimus. There has been some success, but with significant morbidity and mortality. It may be wiser to give less aggressive therapy and to do a renal transplant when required. The one positive feature in black South African children with FSGS requiring transplantation, is that recurrence of the original disease in the transplanted kidney is very unusual.

Hypovolaemia is associated with abdominal pain, low blood pressure and cold extremities. It is aggravated by fluid loss, including that induced by diuretics, therefore it is safer to give a diuretic such as furosemide, together with intravenous albumin if the serum albumin is critically low. Measuring haematocrit is an easy method of monitoring the degree of intravascular volume contraction.

If the haematocrit is monitored carefully, one may achieve a safe diuresis with amiloride

---

Table 27.11 Levels of management of steroid-sensitive nephrotic syndrome

Initial episode
Prednisone 60 mg/d/m^2 (max 60 mg/d) in divided doses for 4 weeks, followed by 40 mg/m^2 as a single dose on alternate days for 4 weeks. Reduced by 15 mg/m^2 per month over 2.5 months (Adapted from the International Study of Kidney Disease of Children)

↓

First two relapses
Prednisone 60 mg/m^2/d (maximum 60 mg/d) until remission, followed by 40 mg/m^2 (maximum 60 mg/d) on alternate days for 4 weeks

↓

Frequent relapses
Maintenance prednisone 0.1–0.5 mg/kg/alternate day for 3–6 months, then reduce

↓

Relapse on prednisone
>1.0 mg/kg/alternate days

↓

Cyclophosphamide 3 mg/kg/d orally for 8 weeks

↓

Post-cyclophosphamide relapses or steroid resistance

↓

BIOPSY

Complications of the nephrotic syndrome:

- Hypovolaemia
- Acute renal failure
- Thrombosis
- Infection
- Complications of drug therapy, especially steroids
- Malnutrition
- Hyperlipidaemia.

5 mg/m^2 (this is available with 50 mg of hydrochlorothiazide in one tablet : Adcoretic®). Daily weighing in hospital helps to monitor the fluid balance.

If hypovolaemia is severe enough, it may precipitate acute renal failure, which is uncommon.

Thrombosis is more prevalent than realized and can be catastrophic. The primed clotting mechanism in the nephrotic state is aggravated by haemoconcentration. Thrombosis may involve the pulmonary artery or deep vein thrombosis can lead to pulmonary emboli, and cerebral vein thrombosis can result in stroke. It is probably safer to use dipyridamole or low dose aspirin in an attempt to prevent thrombosis during nephrotic relapse.

Nephrotic patients in relapse are prone to infection with encapsulated organisms. Peritonitis, especially pneumococcal, is common and other bacterial infections, e.g. *E.coli* and *Haemophilus influenzae* are not unusual. If not already given, vaccination against pneumococci and *H. influenzae* is advisable. Measles and varicella vaccination is also advisable, and if the patient is on steroids, chickenpox must be treated early with acyclovir.

The gross oedema can 'hide' a poor nutritional state, and ongoing assessment of the latter is necessary. The diet must contain adequate protein and energy to also compensate for urinary losses. Strict salt restriction is necessary.

Hyperlipidaemia should only require statin prevention if the nephrotic state is intractable with long term hypercholesterolaemia.

Renal biopsy

In children with glomerulonephritis, renal biopsy may add in acute management or in the diagnosis. Indications are given Table 27.12.

Urinary tract infection (UTI)

This is a common infection, affecting about 5 per cent of girls up to the age of adolescence and 1 per cent of boys. It is more common in girls except in early infancy, where the increased prevalence in boys is probably related to more blood-borne infection. In girls the common pathogenesis is ascending infection, most commonly from faecal coliforms. Other common pathogens are *Proteus*, *Klebsiella*, *Pseudomonas* and enterococci (*S.*

Management of children with nephrotic syndrome:

- Weigh regularly; daily in hospital.
- Diet: adequate protein and energy but strict salt restriction.
- Critically low serum albumin and oedema causing symptoms: IV albumin 0.5–1 g/kg slowly, together with furosemide 0.5–1 mg/kg IV. Mannitol 0.5 g/kg slow infusion may improve diuresis.
- Maintenance diuretic with amiloride or spironolactone and hydrochlorothiazide may be given, but monitor haematocrit carefully to prevent haemoconcentration.
- ACE inhibitors, to reduce proteinuria, but monitor potassium levels and blood pressure.
- Hypertension, if present, should be controlled.
- Prednisone 2 mg/kg as single daily dose in morning, contraindicated in hepatitis B. If there is no response to steroids in up to 6 weeks, the patient is steroid resistant and should be referred. Focal glomerulosclerosis is often steroid resistant. Ongoing prednisone treatment: refer to Table 27.11.
- Once in remission, ensure full immunization against pneumococci and *Haemophilus influenzae*.
- Early antibiotic therapy for infections.
- Specialist paediatric nephrologist supervision is essential for additional therapy with:
  - Levamisole 2.5 mg/kg/day usually with tapering steroid therapy
  - Calcineurin therapy (cyclosporine and tacrolimus) to spare steroids which are nephrotoxic
  - Cyclophosphamide, 2.5–3 mg/kg/day, or chlorambucil 0.2 mg/kg/day as stabilizing medication: both for maximum of 8–12 weeks
  - In focal glomerulosclerosis, a combination of chlorambucil 0.2 mg/kg/day for maximum of 12 weeks and sirolimus 1 mg/m^2 daily may be efficacious.

---

faecalis). In older children, staphylococcus is prevalent. Girls, followed up for more than two years after the first infection, will have up to an 80 per cent chance of having another infection.

These may be associated with vulvo-vaginitis or balanitis, rather than UTI. Hence it is important to establish the diagnosis initially.

Table 27.12 Indications for renal biopsy in children

Urgent for appropriate treatment	Diagnostic
Rapidly progressive glomerulonephritis (including post-streptococcal)	Steroid resistant nephrotic syndrome (not responding within 4 weeks)
Potentially aggressive glomerulonephritis, e.g. lupus nephritis	Atypical hepatitis B nephropathy
Renal transplant rejection	Persistent hypo-complementaemia especially with proteinuria or renal dysfunction
	Family history of nephritis or congenital nephrotic syndrome (except congenital syphilis)

In infancy, symptoms of UTI are non-specific:

- Fever
- Poor feeding
- Vomiting
- Jaundice and septicaemia may develop rapidly.
- In older children, more specific symptoms occur commonly:
- Dysuria
- Frequency
- Loin pain.

Diagnosis of urinary infection

To screen, a fresh urine bag specimen in infants or a fresh midstream urine sample must be used. It is essential to emphasise aseptic techniques for the collection of urine samples (*See* Chapter 36, Procedures).

Leukocytes alone on dipstick cannot be used to diagnose UTI because there are many other causes of leukocyturia in children (*see* Table 27.13).

Urine culture

The following criteria are applied to identify significant urine culture in pure growth:

- in fresh midstream urine > 10^5 organisms/ml. (In younger children especially >10^4 to 10^5).
- Catheter specimen >10^4 organisms/ml.
- Supra-pubic aspiration of bladder: >10^3 organisms/ml.

A urine dipstick reading is a positive screen for UTI if both

- Positive nitrite present (i.e. sufficient organisms with enzyme to break down nitrate in urine to nitrite) *and*
- Positive leukocyte esterase indicates increased polymorphs, i.e. inflammatory response.

Table 27.13 Causes of leukocyturia in children, other than bacterial urinary tract infection

Fever
Dehydration
Vulvovaginitis
Balanitis
Traumatic urethritis
Viral cystitis
Bilharzia
Tuberculosis
Appendicitis
Glomerulonephritis
Chronic non-infective renal conditions eg autosomal recessive polycystic kidney disease

Asymptomatic bacteriuria alone, without leucocytes in the urine does not require treatment, but if the patient has had a renal transplant, it would be prudent to treat because of the immunosuppressives.

A urinary diagnosis of a UTI should be followed up with further investigations to identify whether there is renal involvement or systemic spread. Acute pyelonephritis is more likely if the serum creatinine is raised, temperature is 38 °C and CRP >20 mg/l (PCT >1 ng/ml). A positive blood culture would reinforce this diagnosis, as would an increase in kidney size on ultrasound compared to the expected size from height of child.

Management of UTI

General measures include:
- A liberal fluid intake to maintain a high urine output.
- Paracetamol® for fever and analgesia.

Specific measures depend in part on the presence of any predisposing conditions:
- Relieve obstruction to urinary flow if present, e.g. by catheterization.
- Specific antibiotic according to culture. If the patient is an infant or ill (especially if vomiting), start with empiric intravenous antibiotics, e.g. clavulenate/amoxycillin plus aminoglycoside (monitor level) or cephalosporin, e.g. cefotaxime. Once the temperature is under control and the child is tolerating oral fluids, the antibiotic may be changed to an oral preparation. In serious cases, antibiotics are given for a total of 7–10 days, but if the child is not ill, five days of oral antibiotics are usually adequate.
- Prophylactic antibiotics are used if there is ongoing reflux, an obstruction is not fully corrected or if scarring has already

occurred, e.g. trimethoprim (2 mg/kg as night-time dose–preferable to cotrimoxazole because of increased risk of reaction to sulphur), nitrofurantoin– 2 mg/kg as night-time dose, cephalexin or equivalent: 250 mg/m² as single night-time dose, clavulanate/amoxycillin 250 mg/m² at night. Continue prophylaxis until at least initial ultrasound done and shown to be normal, also for at least three months in infants. If no breakthrough infections occur, try changing to cranberry–preferably in tablet form 10 g/m², also given at night.
- If neuropathic bladder, clean intermittent catheterization would be most efficacious, and antibiotics should not be required if this is done four times a day.

Further investigations

Do not wait until a second infection before investigating, because the majority will have further infections and this may cause renal scarring if the underlying problem not corrected timeously, especially obstruction.

Ultrasound examination is requested acutely if the patient has pyelonephritis or a poor response to treatment. Otherwise it is performed within six weeks.

If abnormal dilatation of the urinary tract is found:
- Child under three years: MCUG, especially if the bladder is large or thick-walled, and then followed with a MAG3 scan with furosemide if the obstruction has not been defined
- Child over three years: MAG3 with furosemide, and as part of the test, an indirect radio-isotopic cystogram is done as well.

If no abnormality is found on the above investigations, urine is checked monthly by dipstick for three months, then once every three months or at any time if unexplained symptoms occur, for at least two years of follow up.

With abnormalities identified or with recurrent infection, a DMSA scan should be considered after at least six months of follow up to define the degree of scarring, if any. If that shows no major problems, a repeat ultrasound is done to ascertain renal growth after one or two years.

Table 27.14 Investigations in an ill or febrile child with a urinary diagnosis of UTI

1. Blood culture.
2. C reactive protein (CRP) and/or procalcitonin (PCT)
3. Serum creatinine, urea & electrolytes.
4. Urgent ultrasound if
   a Child toxic.
   b Any suggestion of obstruction/reflux, e.g. antenatally diagnosed renal abnormality, family history of renal disease, enlarged bladder, abdominal mass, spinal lesion.

Childhood wetting disorders

Bladder control during the day should be achieved between two and four years, and dryness at night by five years. This is related to bladder capacity, which increases with age. A rough guide to bladder capacity is the following formula: [age (in years) + 2] $\times$ 30 = bladder capacity in ml.

Nocturnal enuresis

This is defined as wet at night after five years of age. (*See* Chapter 6, Developmental, psychological and behavioural disorders).

Primary enuresis (never yet dry at night) is far more common than secondary enuresis (recurrence of bedwetting after having achieved bladder control for six months or longer). The high rate of spontaneous remission of 10–15 per cent per annum with no treatment is largely related to bladder maturation. The major factors causing enuresis are thought to be related to:

- Bladder instability or lower capacity
- Lack of arousal from sleep
- Nocturnal polyuria – often related to less vasopressin excretion at night.

This condition should not be over-investigated. A thorough evaluation should include a history of potential social and psychological problems and a detailed physical examination. The urine dipstick should be done on the first morning specimen when the specific gravity can also be obtained.

Behavioural measures such as 'star charts', night time lifting, increased fluid intake during the day and effective treatment of constipation may help. The alarm system is more effective than behavioural or drug therapy but usually takes three weeks to work. The latter should not be contemplated before seven years of age. Tricyclic antidepressant agents are best avoided because of their cardio-toxicity, and can be replaced with anti-cholinergic drugs, such as oxybutynin hydrochloride 2.5 mg–5 mg nocte, but given early with supper. Added desmopressin 200–400 micrograms orally at bed time may give added control, or be kept for special occasions when the child sleeps away from home. If desmopressin is used, there must not be excessive water intake towards evening.

Day-time incontinence

If this is present, one should exclude pathology more vigorously, e.g. ectopic ureteric insertion, posterior urethral valves and neuropathic bladders. If no obvious cause for the latter is found, a tethered cord should be considered.

Over-active bladder

These children often have frequency, urgency, wetting towards the end of the day, suprapubic or perineal pain and a strong stream and many have associated constipation and urinary tract infections. The condition was previously called 'unstable bladder', 'urge syndrome', 'urgency-frequency syndrome' or 'hypertonic bladder'.

Anti-cholinergic treatment is often more effective than it is with nocturnal enuresis, but has to be given twice or even three times a day.

Dysfunctional voiding

An overactive bladder may lead to a secondary overactive sphincter, which in turn may be followed by a lazy bladder (underactive detrusor). Such children may present with constipation or encopresis, recurrent urinary tract infections, stop-start flow and straining to pass urine. Management requires effective treatment of urinary tract infection and constipation, but sphincter relaxation training is often necessary. If the detrusor is overactive, anti-cholinergics may be helpful, but if other therapy is not effective in achieving sphincter relaxation, one may have to use alpha blockers and occasionally botox treatment. In this situation, referral to urological care with a reliable urodynamic service is required.

Acute renal failure

ARF is usually associated with oliguria (less than 300 ml per m^2/day i.e. <0.5 ml/hg/hr in the neonate or infant, or <0.3 ml/kg/hr in an older

Acute renal failure (ARF) is defined as a sudden inability of the kidneys to regulate water and solute balance, be that in the face of reduced, normal or high urine flow.

child). High output renal failure (as occurs, for example, in partial obstruction and interstitial nephritis) has normal urine volumes but decreased urine quality.

Pathogenesis

The following factors singly or in combination may lead to a decreased glomerular filtration rate (GFR) and oliguria:
- ◆ Vascular occlusion
- ◆ Severe glomerular disease and/or
- ◆ Hypoperfusion related to changes in renal blood flow:
  - – decreased glomerular capillary hydrostatic pressure
  - – increased hydrostatic pressure in Bowman's space
  - – hypoalbuminaemia
  - – dehydration, therefore increased oncotic pressure from more concentrated plasma proteins
  - – decrease in the ultrafiltration coefficient.
- ◆ Tubular dysfunction secondary to altered blood flow or toxins :
  - – ischaemia and nephrotoxins

- – hypoxia
- – decreased ATP levels
- – injury from reactive oxygen molecules especially if there is reperfusion.
- ◆ Vasoconstriction may impact on the above and be enhanced by the renin/angiotensin system:
  - – adenosine; catabolism of adenine nucleotides
  - – endothelin and
  - – prostaglandin inhibitors.

The toxic effect on cells is schematically represented in Figure 27.6.

Factors influencing recovery

Heat shock proteins are important in the restitution of function and growth factors (e.g. epidermal growth factor) govern regeneration.

Aetiology

The causes of ARF can be divided into pre-renal, renovascular, renal and post renal as shown in Table 27.15.

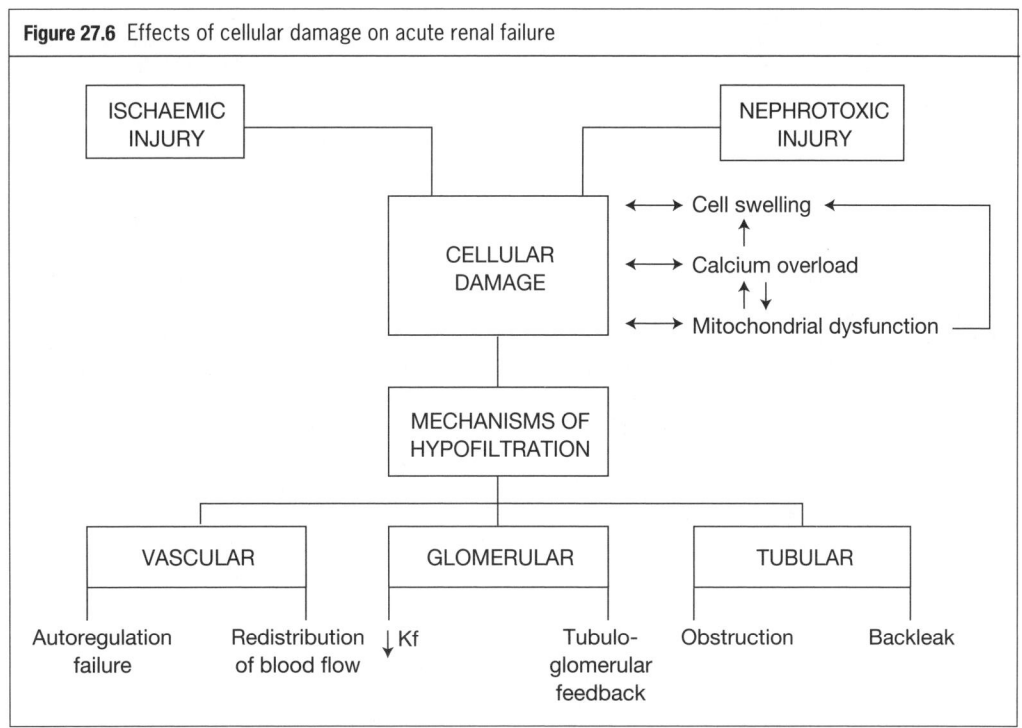

Figure 27.6 Effects of cellular damage on acute renal failure

Table 27.15 Causes of acute renal failure

Pre-renal
- Dehydration
- Hypotension
- Haemorrhage
- Major surgical procedures
- Hypoalbuminaemia

Renovascular
- If there is bilateral obstruction of renal arteries:
  - Neonates: renal arterial thrombosis.
  - Children and adolescents: Takayasu's arteritis.

Renal
- Haemolytic uraemic syndrome
- Glomerulonephritis, e.g. post-streptococcal
- Interstitial nephritis, e.g. infections or drug-induced
- Acute tubular necrosis, e.g. secondary to ongoing pre-renal factors, ischaemia, toxins or drugs.
- Congenital abnormalities, e.g. cystic disease–usually a chronic predisposing factor.

Post-renal
- Vesico-ureteric reflux (usually with infection)
- Obstructive uropathy, e.g.
  - Congenital anatomical factor such as posterior urethral valves
  - Calculi as with oxalosis (usually acute-on-chronic)
  - Tumour lysis syndrome.
  - Schistosomiasis.

Assessment

A thorough history must be taken, including an enquiry about possible exposure to traditional medicines (often given by enema). The examination must be complete. Do not forget to palpate for kidneys and to percuss the bladder.

Urinary obstruction must be excluded by means of the following:

- Straight X-ray abdomen and ultrasound
- Rectal examination if ultrasound is to be delayed
- Voiding cystourethrogram if infra-vesical or intra-vesical pathology suspected
- MAG3 radio-isotope study, usually with furosemide.

The Whitaker test is only done if a percutaneous catheter has been placed into a dilated system: pressures can be measured serially with a prograde volume challenge of 10 ml/minute. A posi-

tive test is indicated by a progressive increase in pressure once the system is full. This test is often done in conjunction with a prograde contrast study to demonstrate the point of obstruction or narrowing.

The following clinical questions must always be addressed:

- The state of hydration and blood pressure (also peripheral perfusion by capillary refill after blanching or by comparing core temperature with peripheral temperature).
- Look for cardiac failure. Do not keep on giving the patient volume expansion unless he is still dehydrated.
- Is any infection present? Severe infection may precipitate ARF or ARF can be complicated by infection.
- The general state of the patient, especially mental and gastrointestinal symptoms.
- Evidence of bleeding. Disseminated intravascular coagulation may precipitate

acute renal failure or, because of ARF, bleeding may occur more easily.

♦ Could it be acute-on-chronic renal failure? The patient may show signs of chronic renal failure eg, short stature (therefore measure length of patient while he is lying in the bed) or signs of rickets.

In assessing the clinical problem of oliguria, the following guidelines can be useful. (Table 27.16)

Urinalysis

Apart from dipstick examination of urine, microscopy is performed to identify renal tubular cells and granular casts, especially broad brown renal failure casts. Urine chemical analysis is essential, particularly fractional excretion of sodium (*see* Table 27.3). A urine/plasma creatinine ratio of <20 is suggestive of acute renal failure.

Management of ARF

Prevention

In a situation of increased risk of ARF, addressing the following points may prevent it from developing :

♦ Adequate hydration
♦ Administration of mannitol 0.5–1 g/kg prior to a major procedure, e.g. open heart surgery using bypass.

Treatment

As indicated in Table 27.16, management depends on the pathophysiological cause of the oliguria. The patients' weight should be carefully monitored and a central venous line should be used as an additional measure of fluid balance. If there is fluid depletion, rehydrate with normal saline, half normal saline or a colloid solution,

depending on the likely serum sodium and albumin levels.

If the patient remains oliguric, insensible fluid losses must be replaced, which is roughly equivalent to 300 ml/m²/24 hours. The smaller the child, the greater the replacement per kg body weight, i.e. at least 6–30 ml/kg/24 hours are given. If there is urine output, replace this loss with 0.45% saline in dextrose, particularly if there is a situation of higher urine sodium, e.g. post obstructive diuresis, such as with treated posterior urethral valves. If there is little urine output, it may be safer to give fluid as dextrose water.

For every 1 °C above 37.5 °C, increase the insensible fluid replacement by 18 per cent. Gastrointestinal losses should also be replaced as necessary. If there is a significant anaemia, e.g. <7 g/dl, and particularly if this has developed rapidly, one can give a blood transfusion (usually with packed cells), aiming to correct the Hb to 9–10 g/dl. The transfusion must be given slowly and the cardio-respiratory state watched carefully, with blood pressure controlled. One should also continue monitoring the weight, not allowing a significant increase after the patient is well hydrated.

At the initial assessment, urgent blood tests must include serum potassium. An ECG should also be done urgently, but do not rely on this alone because the serum potassium can be significantly increased without the obvious ECG effects such as peaking of the T waves, increased PR interval, widening of the QRS and eventually ventricular fibrillation.

The management of hyperkalaemia is given in Table 27.17, and it should be addressed if serum potassium >5.5 mmol/l. Active treatment is required if K >6.0 mmol/l, and urgent treatment if above 6.5 mmol/l. Furosemide, a powerful loop

Table 27.16 Guidelines in the management of oliguria				
BP	**CVP**	**Skin temp**	**Interpretation**	**Treatment**
Decreased	Decreased	Decreased	Hypovolaemia	Volume expansion
Decreased	Raised	Decreased	Cardiac	Inotropic support
Raised	N or Raised	Decreased	Vasoconstriction	Vasodilator
Normal or Raised	Normal or Raised	Normal	Renal	Diuretics/dialysis

diuretic, will help control hyperkalaemia as well if there is still urine output.

Other than adequate hydration, medications to help 'kick start' the ARF, are unproven.

Mannitol can be used prophylactically. Its renoprotective effects are thought to work through:

- Solute diuresis
- Decreasing cell swelling
- Prevention of tubular obstruction
- Renal vasodilatation and
- Scavenging of free hydroxyl radicals.

It can also prevent the disequilibrium syndrome. Should the patient be volume replete, then a test dose of mannitol of no more than 0.25 g/kg over 30 minutes, could be given. In the early stages of acute renal failure, it may have a beneficial effect and it will tend to have a central nervous system protective effect if given at a dose of 0.5 g/kg. The mannitol infusion is often followed by a loop diuretic, e.g. furosemide 2–4 mg/kg IV to try to convert the ARF from oliguric to high output renal failure. This will make fluid and energy management easier, although there is no evidence that it shortens the period of ARF.

Dopamine may increase urine flow and natriuresis through renal vasodilatation if given at the so-called 'renal dose' of 0.5–2 micrograms/kg/min, but this has not been proven to decrease the need for dialysis. At higher doses it is likely to cause vasoconstriction, and should only be used temporarily as a blood pressure maintaining agent, accepting that there is likely to be decreased blood flow to the kidney.

Table 27.17 Emergency management of hyperkalaemia

Way of lowering serum potassium	Treatment	Dose	Side effects
Reduces toxic effect of K by stabilizing the myocardium	10% calcium gluconate IV	0.5 to 1 mL/kg over 5 to 10 minutes	Bradycardia, hypercalcaemia
Shifts K into cells	Salbutamol nebulizer	2.5mg if <25kg 5.0mg if >25kg maximum 2 hourly	Tachycardia, hypertension
	Salbutamol IV	4 µg/kg over 10 mins	
	Sodium bicarbonate 8.4% IV	1–2mmol (mL)/kg over 10–30min	Hypernatraemia, reduces ionized calcium
	Glucose and insulin IV	0.5–1.0g/kg/hr dextrose (2.5–5.0mL/kg/hr 10% dextrose) and insulin 0.1–0.2 units/kg as a bolus or continuous infusion of 10% dextrose at 5mL/kg/hr (0.5g/kg/hr) with insulin 0.1 unit/kg/hour.	Hypoglycaemia, monitor blood glucose every 15 minutes during bolus then at least hourly
Removal of K from the body	Calcium resonium orally or per rectum with oral lactulose	1 g/kg every 4 hours	Effect is slow Large doses can become impacted in the gut if given orally
	Sodium resonium as above	2.5mL<1 year; 5 ml 1–5 years, 10 m>5years	

Theophylline at a dose of only 1 mg/kg/6 hrs as a constant infusion, or as a six hourly oral dose, may also improve urine output in ARF. It is thought to work by abrogating the vasoconstrictive effect of adenosine, and may enhance ATP energy recovery leading to a more functional renal tubular cell and improve recovery from acute tubular necrosis.

Nutrition should be optimized in ARF, and given parenterally if necessary. The aims of dietary management are to reduce the endogenous protein breakdown to a minimum, fulfil energy needs and avoid overloading the patient with fluid and electrolytes. Nutrition should attempt to supply the normal requirements of a child of that size. Therefore, dialysis should rather be started earlier than restricting nutrition, if adequate volumes of food cannot be given because of the oliguria. Hyperphosphataemia should be controlled with phosphate binders such as calcium carbonate (*see* management of chronic renal failure).

The type of dialysis used will depend upon the facilities available and the experience of the unit treating the patient. The choices are:
- Peritoneal dialysis
- Haemodialysis
- Haemofiltration
- Haemodiafiltration (dialysis added to haemofiltration).

The first two work by a combination of osmosis, diffusion and ultra-filtration across a semipermeable membrane (the peritoneal capillaries in the former and the synthetic membrane of the dialyzer in the latter). Haemofiltration works by ultra-filtration because of hydrostatic pressure across a highly permeable membrane.

The commonly used modality in developing countries is peritoneal dialysis. The surgical placement of a cuffed Tenckhoff catheter for peritoneal dialysis requires theatre and the surgeon often does a partial omentectomy of the greater omentum. Peritoneal dialysis may be able to be started more quickly if a Cooke catheter is used because it can be done in the ICU/ward with sedation and local anaesthetic. However it may not be as effective as the Tenckhoff catheter if larger fluid volumes are required to be removed by dialysis.

The mortality rate of children requiring dialysis has been minimized over many years, but

Indications for dialysis:

- Hyperkalaemia >6.5 mmol/l, not responding rapidly to other measures.
- Severe fluid overload with pulmonary oedema, not responding well to furosemide.
- Profound central nervous system changes, e.g. semi-coma.
- Continuing nausea and vomiting without another correctable cause.
- To achieve adequate nutrition because of continuing oliguria.

remains high in the presence of multiple organ failure (particularly in infants).

Haemolytic uraemic syndrome (HUS)

Mild causes of HUS (less than 24 hours oliguria) should recover well as long as they are carefully nursed and given packed cells slowly for the haemolytic anaemia (there is no relationship between the degree of renal failure and haemolysis/ thrombocytopenia).

The more severe cases (oligo-anuria >24 hours) are more of a problem the longer they remain oliguric.

Dialysis is best done earlier rather than later, and particularly if there is significant gut involvement, it would be safer to use haemodialysis rather than peritoneal dialysis. However, peritoneal dialysis is usually the initial choice, even in developed countries. Other treatment is generally that of acute renal failure but with meticulous control of blood pressure. Anticoagulants are not indicated, but neither is fresh frozen plasma. Antibiotic therapy is controversial, and may even aggravate the problem by increasing verocytotoxin release.

Mild cases should all recover well, but with severe cases the prognosis is poorer if there is prolonged oliguria (particularly >2 weeks), persistent proteinuria and ongoing hypertension. If on biopsy there is significant arteriolar involvement, chronic renal failure will result in the majority.

A number of conditions can present with features of acute renal failure and anaemia or throm-

HUS is a syndrome of a sudden haemolytic anaemia with fragmented cells on the blood smear, acute renal failure with oligo-anuria in the more severely affected patients, and thrombocytopaenia.

Poor prognostic factors in HUS include:

- Oligo-anuria of >2 weeks
- Neutrophilia of $>20 \times 10^9/l$
- Central nervous system involvement
- Cortical necrosis or thrombolic microangiopathy on biopsy
- Severe colitis
- Atypical HUS, e.g. idiopathic autosomal recessive, factor H deficiency or mutations, pneumococcal associated HUS.

Table 27.18 Aetiology of the haemolytic uraemic syndrome

Common

- Infection
  Diarrhoea related: verocytotoxin producing bacteria:
  a) Enterohaemorrhagic *E. Coli* e.g. *E. Coli* 0157:H7
  b) *Shigella dysenteriae* type 1.
  Non-diarrhoea related:
  Streptococcus pneumonia producing neuramidase (Thomson-Friedenreich (T) antigen).

Less common

- Other infections, e.g. HIV
- Inherited forms of HUS
  a) Complement abnormalities: factor H deficiency and factor H gene mutations
  b) Von Willebrand factor–cleaving protease deficiency
  c) Other familial causes
- Autosomal recessive – mainly in children – rare
- Autosomal dominant – mainly in adults – rare
- Drug associated
  Calcineurin inhibitors – cyclosporine, tacrolimus
- Secondary HUS
  a) Post renal transplantation.
  b) Systemic lupus erythematosis or antiphospholipid syndrome – rare

Chronic renal failure may be suspected in children if urine is tested routinely or on investigation of the following symptoms or signs:

- Polyuria and polydipsia
- Growth failure or signs of rickets
- Unexplained anaemia
- Complications of hypertension eg breathlessness, convulsions
- May just be feeling generally unwell and 'run down'.

On the other hand, a patient may also present critically ill due to acute on chronic renal failure.

CRF leads to the following disorders of function:

- Retention of toxic metabolites, such as urea, together with increased creatinine, uric acid, phosphate and hydrogen ions. This results in uraemia, acidosis, decreased bicarbonate (used in attempted buffering), decreased calcium (less absorbed, reciprocal fall as PO_4 increased, plus effect of changes in Vitamin D and parathormone).
- Loss of substances in the urine, e.g. red blood cells, white cells, salt, water, potassium and glucose, but the most prognostic is loss of protein.
- Failure to regulate electrolyte and water balance: large volumes of dilute urine plus osmotic diuresis.
- Disturbances of hormone secretion, e.g. increased renin, angiotensin and aldosterone. Erythropoietin decreases and 25-hydroxy Vitamin D not activated to 1,25 Vitamin D because of loss of functioning kidney tissue.

bocytopaenia and thus mimic HUS. Conditions that can mimic HUS are listed in Table 27.19.

Chronic renal failure (CRF)

CRF occurs when there is a progressive reduction in the number of working nephrons. The effect on the body is marked once 50 per cent of the function has been lost.

Table 27.19 Conditions that may mimic HUS

Condition	Haematological picture	Renal pathology
Plasmodium falciparum malaria	DIC, haemolysis	Acute tubular necrosis
Mycoplasma	Cold agglutinin haemolysis	Glomerulonephritis
Typhoid fever	DIC	Acute tubular necrosis
Infective endocarditis	Haemolysis, DIC	Mesangio-capillary glomerulonephritis
EBV, parvovirus	Aplastic or haemolytic anaemia	Interstitial nephritis
HIV	Aplastic or haemolytic anaemia	Interstitial nephritis, focal glomerulosclerosis with cystic dilatation of tubules or immune complex glomerulonephritis
Leptospirosis	DIC	Interstitial nephritis, occasionally vasculitis
Toxins, e.g. *Callilepsis laureola*	Anaemia	Acute renal failure
G-6-P-D deficiency	Haemolytic anaemia	Acute tubular necrosis
Sickle cell disease	Haemolytic anaemia	Papillary necrosis; later focal glomerulosclerosis
Systemic lupus erythematosus	Auto-immune haemolytic anaemia	Glomerulonephritis
Macrophage activation syndrome	Haemophagocytosis (markedly increased ferritin and LDH)	Acute renal failure

The prevalence of end stage renal failure (requiring replacement therapy in the form of dialysis or transplantation) is at least 10/100 000 population in children. The causes of end stage renal failure differ in different groups of South African children. In Caucasian children the predominant causes are reflux nephropathy, dysplastic kidneys, autosomal recessive polycystic kidneys, glomerulonephritis, obstructive uropathy, medullary cystic and the haemolytic uraemic syndrome.

In black South African children, the following renal diseases predominate (*See* Table 27.20).

Where children have a prior history of renal or urinary tract problems, it is mandatory that they should be followed up if there is any chance of chronicity or recurrence. At follow-up, in addition to examination and anthropometry, blood pressure measurement is mandatory (at least yearly).

The following test should also be done:
* Urine dipstick test on an early morning urine sample
* Serum creatinine.

Depending on the type of original disease, the following tests are indicated:
* Where there have been glomerular problems, an early morning urine for protein/creatinine ratio
* With previous tubulo-interstitial problems, urine for a β2 microglobulin/creatinine ratio.
* With insulin dependent diabetic children, an albumin/creatinine ratio on the early morning urine.

Other ongoing problems should be controlled or treated, e.g. hypertension, hyperlipidaemia, recurrent urinary tract infections in an already

Table 27.20 Renal disease in black South African children	
Common	**Rare or less common**

■ Focal glomerulosclerosis
■ Acute post-streptococcal glomerulo-nephritis (impetigo-induced)
■ Hepatitis B membranous nephropathy (now decreasing because of immunization).
■ Congenital nephrotic syndrome:
  Autosomal recessive
  Congenital syphilis
  HIV associated
■ Acute renal failure due to traditional healer 'medicines'
■ Obstructive uropathy due to
  Schistosomiasis
  Post-urethral valves in younger children
■ Oxalosis
■ Renovascular hypertension (Takayasu arteritis)
■ Family history of essential hypertension
	■ Minimal change nephrotic syndrome
	■ Henoch Schönlein/IgA nephropathy.
	■ Vesico-ureteric reflux
	■ Polycystic kidney disease–both autosomal dominant and recessive.
	■ Haemolytic uraemic syndrome, (but that induced by *S. dysenteriae type 1* has become more common since 1994)

scarred urinary tract and hypoplastic/dysplastic kidneys.

If there is ongoing proteinuria, ACE inhibitors and/or angiotensin receptor blockers may be indicated to control hypertension, lessen proteinuria, but most importantly, to try to prevent the expected fall-off in renal function. Should the child have any signs of chronic renal failure, then follow up by a paediatric nephrologist would be optimal, and mandatory if the calculated creatinine clearance was <60 ml/min/1.73 m². If the child had a clearance of <30 ml/min/1.73 m² workup towards dialysis, or even transplantation should be considered, particularly if the child was not growing well despite addressing other factors in the conservative treatment of chronic renal failure.

Chronic dialysis is now well established for children, usually as peritoneal dialysis (continuous ambulatory peritoneal dialysis (CAPD) or overnight cycling to allow more freedom during the day). Both require the placement of cuffed Tenckhoff catheters with meticulous care. The advantage of peritoneal dialysis is that many patients can be home based. Haemodialysis is done at least three times per week, usually in a renal unit with ongoing audit being important, so that optimal care is given.

The aim for the vast majority of patients is successful transplantation, either from a living donor or a deceased donor. The shortage of donors is still a major problem for South African children. Where successful transplants have been done, meticulous follow up is necessary, re-inforcing the need for compliance with the ongoing treatment.

Hypertension in childhood

Hypertension is a problem in children of all ages, which, although not common, is often undiagnosed because of the doctor's omission of routine blood pressure measurements in children even when they are ill. Furthermore, when the blood pressure is actually measured, the technique is often incorrect. The younger the patient and the more severe the hypertension, the more likely it will be due to a secondary cause. In this section, hypertension in children related to renal disease or renovascular problems will be highlighted.

Causes of hypertension

Renal diseases, renovascular hypertension and coarctation of the aorta, together make up over

Conservative management of chronic renal failure

Nutrition and diet:
- Maintain a high energy intake, particularly of carbohydrate and fat.
- Protein intake – aim for as close to normal requirements as possible; rather start dialysis if one cannot achieve >1 g/kg/day. Preferably use protein of high biological value, e.g. milk and egg.
- Vitamins – supply normal requirements except extra Vitamin D – *see below*. Do not give excessive vitamin A.
- May need extra iron; possibly zinc supplementation.

Water and electrolytes:
- Water – balance intake and output. There is a decreased concentrating ability, so the patient may need extra until the decrease in urine output of the end stage is reached. (Dialysis has been started too late if this situation develops).
- Sodium – may need extra if a tubulo-interstitial problem leads to sodium loss. Less sodium is needed if the patient has volume dependent hypertension.
- Potassium – only needs restriction when kidney function is poor. If K >5.5 mmol/l, partially correct acidosis if present. May need to stop ACE inhibitors or angiotensin receptor blockers

Acidosis:
- only partially correct if serum bicarbonate level <16 mmol/l. Sodium bicarbonate is used, preferably orally. Citrate is sometimes used, but aluminium absorption may increase.
- *Renal osteodystrophy:*
- Hyperphosphataemia – low phosphate diet. Phosphate binders, e.g. calcium carbonate with each meal. Keep PO^4 <1.8 mmol/l.
- Hypocalcaemia – calcium carbonate is better absorbed than calcium gluconate.
- Hyperparathyroidism – one alpha Vitamin D (1a hydroxycholecalfciferol) or Rocaltrol® (1.25–dihydroxy cholecalciferol) 0.25 micrograms daily is usually required as starting dose. This often needs to be increased, but monitor calcium, phosphate and PTH.

Anaemia:
- Hb <10 g/dl – folic acid 5 mg daily and check iron.
- Hb <9 g/dl – start erythropoietin (50–100 units/kg) subcutaneously 2–3 times/week, aiming at Hb of 9.5–11 g/dl.

- If Hb <6 g/dl (and patient symptomatic) consider washed or irradiated packed red cell transfusion.

Hypertension:
- Important to control hypertension (see below).

Infections:
- Treat vigorously but adjust antimicrobial dose if required for degree of renal dysfunction (monitor levels if nephrotoxic).

90 per cent of causes of sustained hypertension (*see* Table 27.21)

Noting the many causes of secondary hypertension in table 27.22, the majority are renal or renal-related.

The approach to renovascular hypertension depends on the age at presentation:

- ◆ In neonates:
  - Renal artery thrombosis (umbilical arterial catheters)
  - Rarely, the thrombosis may be related to a genetic thrombogenic factor
- ◆ In the infant:
  - Idiopathic arterial calcification of infancy (rare)
  - Williams syndrome
  - Congenital rubella
- ◆ In the child or adolescent:
  - Takayasu's arteritis (fibromuscular hyperplasia with or without associated neurofibromatosis being far less common).

Table 27.21 Causes of sustained hypertension

Renal		
Chronic glomerulonephritis	30%	
Chronic pyelonephritis/obstruction	20%	
Cystic disease of the kidneys	10%	72%
Haemolytic uraemic syndrome	8%	
Hypoplastic/dysplastic kidneys	4%	
Reno-vascular		
(including Takayasu arteritis, renal artery		
thrombosis, renal artery stenosis)		10%
Co-arctation of the aorta		10%
Essential and others, e.g. endocrine		8%

Table 27.22 Causes of secondary hypertension

Renal diseases

Glomerulonephritis (due to infections or auto-immune processes)
Interstitial nephritis
Reflux nephropathy (pyelonephritis)
Obstructive uropathy
Congenital abnormalities (dysplasias, polycystic disease)
Renin-secreting tumours

Vascular diseases

Coarctation of the aorta
Renal artery stenosis or thrombosis
Takayasu arteritis

Endocrine disorders

Adrenal disorders (adrenogenital syndrome, Cushing's disease, primary hyperaldosteronism, phaeochromocytoma, monogenic mineralocorticoid)
Neuroblastoma
Hyperthyroidism
Hyperparathyroidism
Diabetes mellitus

Miscellaneous causes

Poliomyelitis, Guillain-Barré syndrome, neurofibromatosis, hypercalcaemia, mercury poisoning, leg traction, raised intracranial pressure, administration of corticosteroids and other drugs
Excessive intake of liquorice

Secondary causes of hypertension are more common in all age groups, except in the adolescent where essential hypertension is likely to be apparent in 1–2 per cent of that age group. This is because even though 5 per cent could be labelled as being hypertensive (above the 95th percentile), the blood pressure tends to be labile in the adolescent, and only 20–40 per cent of these show persistent hypertension; hence 1–2 per cent of the total adolescent population.

In this adolescent group, an increasing BMI, frank obesity, diabetes and smoking have exaggerated the prevalence of hypertension, and careful assessment, initiation of non-pharmacological measures and long-term follow up with possible anti-hypertensive therapy is necessary.

However, in all age groups in children, secondary causes of hypertension should first be considered.

Measurement of blood pressure in children

Important points are listed in Table 27.23. Ambulatory blood pressure monitoring is worthwhile if the child remains anxious or if a more realistic measurement of blood pressure control is required.

Definition (*see* Table 27.24)
Following research in adult hypertension, the National High Blood Pressure Education Programme Working Group on High Blood Pressure in Children and Adolescents, in its fourth report on the diagnosis, evaluation, and treatment of high blood pressure in children and adolescents (Pediatrics 2004; 114 (2): 555-576), has defined three categories of high blood pressure in children:

  ◆ **Prehypertension** systolic or diastolic BP >90th to 95th percentile or if BP exceeds 120/80 mmHg even if <90th to 95th percentile.
  ◆ **Stage 1 hypertension** systolic or diastolic BP between 95th–99th percentile plus 5 mmHg.
  ◆ **Stage 2 hypertension** systolic or diastolic BP >99th percentile plus 5 mmHg.

Percentile is value for age, gender and height percentile measured on at least three separate occasions.

In an asymptomatic patient with essential hypertension it is reasonable to attend to non-

- Because renal causes form the bulk of these cases, examination of the urine is mandatory in all hypertensive children.
- Glomerular pathology is more likely to cause hypertension earlier, because in tubular pathology sodium loss may be protective of the blood pressure until renal function worsens considerably.

Table 27.23 Measurement of blood pressure in children

- Quiet and relaxed; repeat after a while if not sure
- Lying or sitting with arm extended at heart level
- Adequate cuff: length of cuff bladder should encompass at least 80% (preferably 100%) of circumference of upper arm and width of cuff should be at least 40% of circumference of upper arm (cuff can be folded if linen covered)
- Feel pulse to see when it disappears as one pumps up the pressure; this will take it above systolic but not too high. Release pressure slowly (2 mm/pulse beat)
- Infant: Doppler (preferably) or 'flush' technique
- Oscillometric easiest at all ages, giving more accurate systolic readings
- Do not press too firmly if stethoscope used

Table 27.24 Definition of hypertension in children

Systolic or diastolic greater than 2 standard deviations above the norm for age, gender and height percentile = >95th percentile.

A simple formula for systolic and diastolic pressures separately, gives a correlation very close to the 95th percentile of BP for the 50th percentile for height (i.e. average for any particular age) up to 16 years of age.

Systolic BP: $100 + (2.5 \times$ patient's age in years) mmHg

Diastolic BP: $60 + 2$ for each year until 11 years = 82 mmHg, then + 1 for each year thereafter.

drug factors of stage 1 hypertension, provided close follow up is ensured.

However, with secondary hypertension where the patient is usually symptomatic, it would be safer to start antihypertensive therapy once the blood pressure was at or above the 95th percentile (in children, the systolic pressure reading is more reliable and therefore best used).

In symptomatic children hypertensive urgency should be managed in a similar manner to hypertensive emergency because it is difficult to be sure whether there is end-organ damage or not, particularly of the brain (*see* Table 27.27).

Drug exposure can result in acute hypertension:

- Cold remedies (sympathomimetic)
- Liquorice (mineralocorticoid effect)
- Corticosteroids (salt and water retention)
- Calcineurin inhibitors (cycloporin and tacrolimus: arteriolar constriction, salt and water retension and in the longer term, structural changes, e.g. interstitial fibrosis if scarring persists)
- Contraceptives (oestrogen causes salt and water retention).

Presenting symptoms and signs

In taking the history of a hypertensive child, it is important to inquire about the family history in detail, including renal disease and hypertension. In addition, a thorough systematic history is indicated, not forgetting to ask about possible precipitating factors eg neonatal umbilical arterial catheterization (renal artery thrombosis) or exposure to medication that can cause hypertension.

Table 27.25 lists symptoms from many previous series of hypertension in children. It is noteworthy that a minority are asymptomatic, half have neurological symptoms, and the common other groups are renal, cardiac or gastrointestinal. Because many symptoms are non-specific, if the blood pressure is not taken by the doctor, hypertension may well be picked up too late.

Possible signs that can be identified on clinical examination and associated with hypertension are given in table 27.26. The majority are related to renal problems.

The blood pressure relates to the product of cardiac output and total peripheral resistance. Both are influenced by renal factors, as seen in Figure 27.7.

In the management of hypertension, it is therefore useful to consider the sites of action of potential antihypertensive medications. These are summarized in the box.

Sites of action of antihypertensives include:

Reduction of cardiac output

Decrease extracellular volume by promoting excretion of salt and water. Diuretic, e.g. thiazides, eplerenone, spironolactone, amiloride, and furosemide (latter in specific instances eg acute nephritis, acute renal failure and chronic renal failure).

Beta-adrenergic antagonist (β-blockers) also have a central effect and decrease renin secretion.

Reduction of total peripheral resistance

1 Vascular smooth muscle (direct action causing vasodilation) e.g.
   a Calcium channel blockers e.g. amlodipine – very long half-life.
   b Sodium nitroprusside (especially in ICU situation)
   c Hydralazine
   d Thiazides – minor dilatation effect
2 Alpha-1-blocker (peripheral) e.g. prazosin (short acting), doxazosin (longer acting).
3 Alpha-2-stimulation (central and peripheral) – secondary inhibition, e.g. clonidine – generally not used because of rebound hypertension and increased tachyarrhythmias
4 Alpha- and beta-blocker e.g. labetalol useful if given intravenously in controlling acute hypertension
5 Angiotensin converting enzyme inhibitors and angiotensin II receptor blockers.
ACE inhibitors may have added beneficial antihypertensive effect because the same inhibitor decreases the breakdown of bradykinin. ACE inhibitors are best known for their ability to decrease proteinuria and help maintain renal function. ARBs block the deleterious effects of the AT1 receptor, especially vasoconstriction and decreased renal blood flow.

Once control is reached, it is important to add the most appropriate combination or oral antihypertensives, depending upon the situation.

Investigations

In acute hypertension, the investigation will usually be related to the likely renal cause of the hypertension, as discussed above, therefore

Table 27.25 Symptoms in hypertensive children

	%
Previous diagnosed disease	50
Asymptomatic	20
Central nervous system:	
Headache	25
Convulsions	15
Coma	2
Tiredness, irritability	6
Visual problems	3
Facial palsy	2
Cardiovascular–renal:	
Cardiac murmur	10
Cardiac failure	5
Oedema	10
Haematuria	5
Polydipsia, polyuria	5
Enuresis	2
Gastrointestinal:	
Nausea, vomiting, anorexia	10
Abdominal pain	10
Miscellaneous:	
Weight loss or poor growth	5
Epistaxis	3

one will start with the examination of the urine with a dipstix and microscopy, then further investigations depending on the likely cause. It is often related to salt and water retention in both acute nephritis and in acute renal failure. In the HUS, micro-angiopathy is associated with hyperreninaemia.

In sustained hypertension, it would be advisable to consult with or refer the patient to a paediatric nephrologist or another paediatrician with an interest in hypertension.

Treatment of hypertension in children

This is divided into the treatment of acute hypertension, including hypertensive emergency/urgency, and that of chronic sustained hypertension.

Table 27.26 Possible clinical signs in hypertension

Organ		Feature	Association
General		Oedema	Nephritic/nephrotic Renal failure
		Excessive sweating, flushing, tachycardia	Phaeochromocytoma
Head & Neck	Eyes	Papilloedema alone With haemorrhages or exudates	Raised intracranial pressure Malignant hypertension
	Face	Butterfly rash Moon facies	Lupus nephritis Cushing's syndrome Steroid therapy
CNS		Coma	Hypertensive encephalopathy Chronic renal failure Precipitous fall in blood pressure HUS in infants
Thorax		Cardiomegaly, thrusting apex	Sustained hypertension
		Posterior thorax murmur/s	Coarctation
Abdomen		Loin masses	Hydronephrosis Wilms tumour or neuroblastoma Renal vein thrombosis
		If bilateral	Infantile polycystic kidneys
		Palpable bladder post-micturition	Posterior urethral valves Neurogenic bladder Functional hypertrophy All of these suggest obstructive uropathy
		Pregnancy in adolescent girl	Toxaemia of pregnancy
		Abdominal bruit	Renal artery stenosis Abdominal coarctation
Periphery		Decreased/absent femoral pulses; Decreased BP in lower limbs	Coarctation of aorta Takayasu arteritis
		Café-au-lait spots (2 cm × 5, or axillary)	Neurofibromatosis (renal artery stenosis or phaeochromocytoma)
		Purpura	Henoch-Schönlein purpura Haemolytic-uraemic syndrome Chronic renal failure Leukaemia

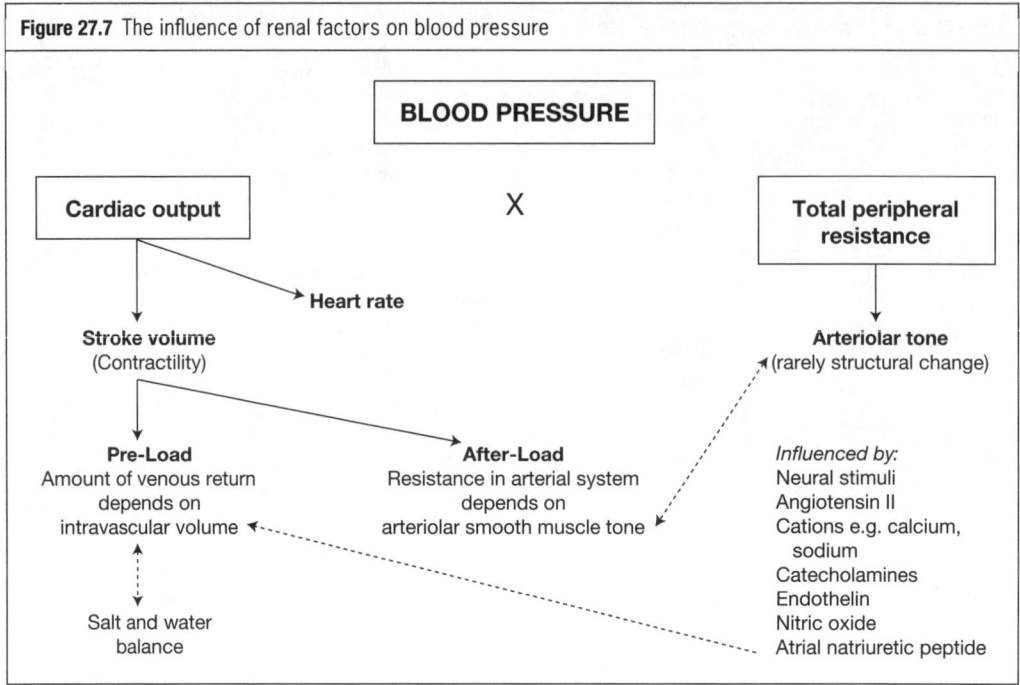

Figure 27.7 The influence of renal factors on blood pressure

Acute hypertension

Sustained hypertension

In sustained hypertension or if there is a central nervous system problem, the danger of precipitously dropping the blood pressure, and therefore disrupting the auto-regulation which may have been reset at a higher level, also requires a careful approach. The safest initial therapy would be either a long-acting calcium channel blocker such as amlodipine, or a long-acting β- (predominantly β1-) blocker such as atenolol. If one of these single agents cannot hold the blood pressure below the 90th percentile at all times then additions or changes should be made.

The single agent/combination will depend upon the pathogenesis of the hypertension e.g:

♦ Salt and water retension : diuretic plus β-blocker and β1-blocker

---

Table 27.27 Treatment of acute hypertension

To prevent cerebral ischaemia, it is best to use continuous infusion for a hypertensive crisis, and to lower the BP by up to 25% in the first 6–8 hours, then aim for further gradual reduction over the next 26 to 48 hours, only reaching the 95 th percentile by 48 hours.

IV infusion:
1 Furosemide 1–5 mg/kg/dose IV over 30 mins or longer.
   – associated acute renal failure
   – pulmonary oedema.
2 Sodium nitroprusside 0.5–8 micrograms/kg/minute.
3 Labetalol 0.25–4 mg/kg/hour.
4 Nicardipine 0.5 microgram/kg/minute starting, then 1–4 microgram/kg/min. depending upon response.

continued

Table 27.27 Treatment of acute hypertension *continued*

5 Esmolol hydrochloride: 500 micrograms/kg IV over 1 minute then 50 micrograms/kg/minute for 4 minutes, then increments of 50 microgram/kg/minute until maximum dose of 200 micrograms/kg/minute.
(Beware asthma or renal failure.)

Oral agents:
1 Amlodipine 0.2–0.4 mg/kg/dose 4–12 hourly.
2 Nifedipine 0.15–0.3 mg/kg dose 4–6 hourly.
   Amlodipine has a long half-life, but may take up to 2 hours to have an effect. Nifedipine acts more quickly but has a short half life. The danger of nifedipine is that it has a significant negative inotropic effect and may drop the blood pressure precipitously. Therefore safer to be used only in uncomplicated situations without possible end-organ risk.

- Hyper-reninaemia : ACE inhibitor/ARB as long as bilateral renal artery stenosis has been excluded
- Obstructive uropathy: relieve obstruction and particularly if proteinuria or tubulo-interstitial problem, ACE inhibitor/ARB. Likewise with reflux nephropathy, especially with ongoing proteinuria.

Many children with significant renal disease need multiple anti-hypertensives, but the care-giver should make sure that the patient is not retaining excess salt and water. Adequate volume control which includes improved dialysis, allows easier blood pressure control. However, if there is sufficient renal function, too aggressive diuretic therapy can lead to sodium depletion and a fall off in function.

Table 27.28 lists recommended anti-hypertensives for sustained hypertension with important side effects.

The suggested common groups of antihypertensives are:

A – ACE inhibitors/Angiotensin receptor blockers.
B – β-blockers.
C – Calcium channel blockers/other vasodilators, e.g. alpha-1-blocker.
D – Diuretics.

Table 27.28 Agents for sustained hypertension

	mg/kg/day (unless stated otherwise) dose			
	Starting	Max	Interval	Side effects
ACE Inhibitors				
Enalapril	0.1	05	Daily (night) or twice daily	Hyperkalaemia. Stop if patient volume depleted
Ramipril	0.1	0.4	Daily (night)	Cough
Captopril	0.5	5	6–8 hourly	Not very long term
Angiotensin receptor blockers				
Losartan	0.75	1.4	Daily (night)	As for ACE inhib. but no cough
Valsartan	4	6	Daily (night)	
α and β receptor blocker				
Carvedilol	0.1	0.75	Twice daily	More for cardiomyopathy
β adrenergic blockers				
Propranolol	2	12	Twice daily	Asthma precipitated
Metoprolol (more β1)	2	8	Twice daily	Not >100 mg bd
Atenolol (more β1)	0.5–1	2.5	Daily (best at night)	Max 100 mg. Beware >effect if poor renal function
Calcium channel blockers				
Amlodipine	0.1	0.6	Daily or twice daily	Oedema Gum hypertrophy
Other vasodilators α1 Blocker				
Prazosin	0.1	0.4	Twice daily	Beware 1st dose hypotension
Doxazosin XL	4 mg/m^2	4 mg/m^2	Daily (night)	
Hydralazine	0.5	5 mg	Twice daily	Tachycardia. Positive ANF
Diuretics				
Hydrochlorothiazide	0.5	3	Daily	Maximum of 50 mg/day Hypercalcaemia Hyperuricaemia
Furosemide	0.5	6	Twice daily or daily	Best in chronic renal failure. Low serum K
Spironolactone	1	3	Twice daily or daily	Hyperkalaemia
Eplerenone	0.5	1	Daily	Hyperkalaemia
Amiloride	0.1 mg/day	0.4 mg/day	Twice daily	Hyperkalaemia

28

Cardiovascular disorders

Congenital and rheumatic heart disease together account for the majority of cardiac problems in childhood. Congenital heart abnormalities occur with equal frequency among black and white children. On the other hand, rheumatic heart disease has a prevalence among black school children at least equal to that of congenital heart anomalies, but is rare in white children. Other important heart conditions that may be encountered are idiopathic congestive cardiomyopathy (more common among black children); infective endocarditis (either on a previous rheumatic valvular lesion or complicating a congenital heart abnormality); or cor pulmonale consequent upon upper airways obstruction – the result of enlarged adenoids and tonsils (very common in black infants and children). Pericardial disease is almost always infective, e.g. acute bacterial or tuberculous. It may be viral (coxsackie B), or the result of acute rheumatic fever. An arrhythmia is less likely to occur in children than is the case with adults. If it does, it will almost certainly be a supraventricular tachyarrhythmia.

Clinical approach to heart disease

The **diagnostic evaluation** should consist of a careful history, including family history, the clinical examination, a chest X-ray, and an electrocardiogram (ECG). With this information it should be possible to arrive at a diagnosis in at least 90 per cent of the patients. Echocardiography, which will be carried out at the tertiary

---

The following symptoms and signs may be suggestive of cardiac disease in children:

- Central cyanosis not responding to oxygen
- Pallor and sweatiness despite a good haemoglobin; consider heart failure
- Failure to feed and shortness of breath after feeding
- Tachypnoea and respiratory distress
- Failure to thrive and grow in a well cared-for child
- Sudden gain in weight or the development of oedema
- Unexplained hepatomegaly
- Heart murmurs
- Irregular or abnormally fast or slow pulse
- Apnoea or syncopal attacks.

---

centre, has proved to be an invaluable tool in the final assessment.

All neonates should be examined soon after birth for possible congenital heart disease and again at six weeks of age. This is because a significant murmur arising from a ventricular septal defect (VSD) may only become audible some time after birth, after the fall in pulmonary artery pressure and vascular resistance.

Central cyanosis

Cyanosis which does not respond to oxygen therapy is indicative of cyanotic congenital heart defect (CHD). Other causes of cyanosis must first be excluded, namely pulmonary conditions, cyanotic attacks in neonates (central nervous system problems, metabolic causes such as hypoglycaemia, hypocalcaemia).

The respiratory pattern of the child must be observed, while physical examination should particularly include the signs of congestive cardiac failure (CCF). Cyanosis in itself is not, however, a sign of heart failure *per se*. Thereafter, a chest radiograph is taken (antero-posterior and lateral) and an ECG performed. (*See* Table 28.1.)

- Administer oxygen. If there is no immediate improvement, and there are no other signs of respiratory disease or cerebral depression, the cause is probably cardiac.

If the cyanosis is of cardiac origin do not continue to give oxygen which may aggravate the situation by provoking closure of the ductus arteriosus.

- Maintain the infant's temperature.
- Give 5 per cent glucose solution IV.
- Give sodium bicarbonate IV to correct acidosis.
- Give oral prostaglandin E$_2$ 30–60 mcg/kg hourly. (Dissolve 500 mcg tablet in 10 ml sterile water. Each 1 ml = 50 mcg). Alternatively intravenous prostaglandin E1 0.05 – 0.1 mcg/kg/min can be given as a continuous infusion.

All cyanotic infants should be referred to a specialist unit as soon as possible. While many require prompt surgical intervention or atrial septostomy to survive, some do not require or are not suitable for immediate treatment. All these patients, as well as those who have had palliative procedures, remain cyanosed. With time, these patients all develop finger clubbing and polycythaemia.

Patients with complicated and multiple defects, e.g. transposition of the great vessels with single ventricle and subpulmonary stenosis, are cyanosed but may be haemodynamically balanced so that their lives and well-being are not immediately threatened. Patients with other conditions, e.g. Ebstein's anomaly, live into adult life without any surgical intervention.

The **long-term management** of these cyanosed children requires regular examination with particular reference to the following points:

- Serial measurements of height, weight, and skull circumference: their growth may be stunted, especially if they are in cardiac

failure, otherwise they should maintain a steady gain. If cyanosis is severe, there is a delay in closure of the anterior fontanelle.

- Estimation of the haemoglobin level and haematocrit: anaemic children do not look cyanosed. A raised haematocrit indicates severe cyanosis. Iron deficiency is common and must be corrected. If not, this may lead to cerebral thrombosis, especially below the age of two years.
- Septic skin lesions and dental caries should be avoided and must be treated promptly. The greatest danger to children with cyanotic heart defects is paradoxical embolization and the development of cerebral abscesses.
- A brain abscess should always be suspected in such children who develop intractable headache, unexplained fever, or neurological signs. This is more likely to occur above the age of two years.
- Early detection and management of cardiac failure. If complications occur, appropriate action must be taken, including referral for reappraisal.

Children with cyanotic heart defects are not athletic but should be allowed to exercise within their own limits. They should be encouraged to take an interest in non-athletic pursuits and require the support and encouragement of the whole family to enable them to develop their personalities and achieve intellectual satisfaction. Many have the ability to attain the highest intellectual levels. Children with uncorrected tetralogy of Fallot, who may develop hypercyanotic spells from infundibular spasm, should not be allowed to overexert themselves or become too excited. Generally, gentle exercise should be encouraged and competitive exercise excluded.

Heart failure

In **infancy**, cardiac failure presents with rapid breathing, poor colour, sweating, inability to complete feeds, failure to gain weight or sudden increase in weight (due to oedema), puffy eyes (early sign of oedema), hepatomegaly, and a palpable spleen. There is a tachycardia and the heart sounds may show a typical 'gallop rhythm'. It must be emphasized that infants can have cardiac failure without any evidence of dependant

Table 28.1 Distinguishing features of cyanotic conditions

Cardiac anomaly	Cyanosis	Pulse	Auscultation	Chest X-ray	ECG
Transposition	Within the first week of life. Increasing	Normal	Usually without murmur. May be precordial systolic murmur	Plethora	Right axis, RVH. Upright T wave in V4R, V1
Pulmonary atresia (+ intact ventricular septum)	From birth	Poor/normal	Pansystolic xiphisternum (TI). Single HS2	Oligaemia	Normal to left axis. Poor RV forces
Tricuspid atresia	From birth	Poor/normal	No murmur or soft systolic over precordium. Single HS2	Oligaemia	Left axis, poor RV forces, P pulmonale
Tetralogy	Variable. Often acyanotic in infancy, increases gradually. May have spells	Normal	Ejection systolic murmur at left sternal border. Single HS2	Oligaemia	Right axis, RVH
Ebstein	From birth. Tends to improve	Normal	Pansystolic murmur and diastolic scratch at xiphisternum	Oligaemia	Large RA, poor RV forces, right bundle branch block
Eisenmenger	Initially not cyanosed. Progressive	Normal	Ejection systolic click at left sternal border. Soft ejection systolic murmur. Very loud pulmonary HS2	Oligaemia	Right axis, RVH
Critical pulmonary stenosis	Mild to moderate	Normal	Ejection systolic murmur at 2nd left interspace. Soft pulmonary HS2	Oligaemia	Right axis, RVH, P pulmonale
Truncus arteriosus	Moderate	Collapsing	Systolic ejection click and long systolic murmur at left sternal border. May be early diastolic murmur as well	Plethora	Normal to right axis, biventricular hypertrophy
Total anomalous pulmonary venous connection	Mild to moderate	Small	Ejection systolic murmur at 2nd left space. Wide split of HS2. Mid-diastolic murmur at xiphisternum	Plethora	Right axis, RVH
AVCC	Variable	Normal	Precordial systolic murmur	Plethora	Left axis, biventricular hypertrophy. Prolonged PR
Hypoplastic left-heart syndrome	Mild to moderate	Very poor	Precordial systolic murmur. Ejection systolic click. Gallop	Plethora	Right axis, RVH. Poor LV forces

AVCC = Atrio-ventricular communis canal   HS2 = 2nd heartsound   LV = Left ventricle   RA = Right atrium   RV = Right ventricle   RVH = Right ventricular hypertrophy   TI = Tricuspid incompetence

oedema as it is a late sign. Hepatomegaly develops much earlier. Likewise one can not rely on the raised jugular venous pressure, as it is technically difficult to demonstrate in infants who have very short necks.

Causes of heart failure in infancy:
+ Acyanotic congenital heart disease
+ Cyanotic congenital heart disease with increased pulmonary blood flow
+ Myocarditis
+ Cardiomyopathy
+ Tachyarrhythmias.

In **childhood**, the features of cardiac failure are similar to those in adulthood, namely tachypnoea, inspiratory crepitations at the bases of the lungs, elevated jugular venous pressure, hepatomegaly, and dependent oedema.

Treatment of heart failure
+ Nurse the baby propped up at 60 degrees.
+ Administer oxygen by nasal prongs, mask or funnel.
+ Restrict fluid intake (60 ml/kg/d in neonates); preferably breast milk or low sodium milk.
+ Inotropes improve myocardial contractility. Digoxin is commonly used. Digoxin (elixir 0.05 mg/ml, tablets 0.125 and 0.0625 mg, or injection 0.25 mg/ml). *See* Table 28.2. Oral digoxin acts almost as quickly as an intramuscular injection and is preferred for infants who are not vomiting. Intravenous

digoxin is rarely indicated and must be given with care at three-quarters of the oral or intramuscular dosage under ECG control. An intravenous infusion of either isoprenaline at a rate of 0.05–0.10 mcg/kg/min or dopamine at a rate of 3–10 mcg/kg/min can be used in severe cardiac failure.
+ Diuretics decrease the preload. Furosemide (Lasix®) is the most effective diuretic for acute cardiac failure. It is best given intravenously initially and then by mouth for maintenance (1–6 mg/kg/d) (0.5–1 mg/kg/dose).
+ Spironolactone (Aldactone®) can be used as a potassium-sparing diuretic in a dose of 2–3mg/kg/d in two to three divided doses, given orally. This can be combined with furosemide.
+ Vasodilators will reduce the left ventricular after-load, and are particularly useful in cases of dilated cardiomyopathy. Captopril is used in a dose of 0.5–6 mg/kg/d divided into three to four doses.

The most important assessment of control of cardiac failure in infancy is the baby's ability to feed adequately by checking the gain in weight.

Heart murmurs
Careful, repeated auscultation of infants will reveal transient systolic murmurs in most normal infants. Fifty per cent of all children will have a functional murmur when febrile, excited, or after exercise. Significant systolic murmurs are usually loud, often associated with a thrill, and are heard maximally at one of the main auscultatory areas.

> For infants and children presenting with heart failure, treatment is aimed at reducing preload or volume overload (diuretics), improving myocardial contractility (digoxin) and afterload reduction (vasodilators), regardless of the diagnosis.

> *Note:* Potassium supplementation of 1–2 mmol/kg/d in divided doses is required if a diuretic is used which causes potassium loss.

Table 28.2 Digitalizing schedule for infants

Age of infant	Total digitalizing dose (TDD) divided into 4 doses, 6 hourly	Daily maintenance given in 1 or 2 doses
Pre-term	0.04–0.05 mg/kg	1/4 of TDD
2 months–2 years	0.06–0.08 mg/kg	1/4 of TDD
Over 2 years	0.04–0.06 mg/kg	0.01 mg/kg/d

Systolic murmurs which **persist** or which are **loud** or associated with **other signs of cardiac disorder** should be considered significant. Serious heart malformations may not have a murmur.

Diastolic murmurs are always significant, but are found in very few infants with congenital heart defects.

Functional systolic murmurs

These murmurs at the 4th left intercostal space (vibratory ejection) or at the 2nd left intercostal space (blowing ejection) must be differentiated from organic murmurs. They are very common in school children (60–70 per cent). The common features are:

- Usually grade 3/6 or less localized mid-systolic murmur
- Louder during fever
- Louder in supine, softer in erect position and may disappear with an valsalva manoeuvre
- Second sound splits normally, i.e. widens on inspiration
- Commonly a dull 3rd sound at the apex
- There may be associated venous hums (continuous) below both clavicles. These disappear with alteration of neck position or pressure over the external jugular veins at the root of the neck.

Chest deformity

This is not usually seen in early infancy as it takes time to develop, but in children the presence of a pectus carinatum with Harrison's sulci suggests intrathoracic airways obstruction. In the cardiac context, this is usually due to and associated pulmonary arterial hypertension. A left precordial bulge or chest asymmetry may also be evident.

Congenital heart disease (CHD)

Incidence and aetiology

Congenital heart malformations occur in at least 7/1 000 live births. If follow-up of every new-born were complete, it is probable that the figure would increase to 10/1 000 live births (i.e. 1 per cent).

The top congenital cardiac anomalies:	
Ventricular septal defect	38%
Patent ductus arteriosus	20%
Coarctation of the aorta	10%
Tetralogy of Fallot	6%
Aortic stenosis	4%
Atrial septal defect	3%
Isolated pulmonic stenosis	3%

In the majority of instances (85–90 per cent) the cause is not known. It is thought to be due to a multifactorial interaction between environmental factors and genetic predisposition. Known teratogenic agents include maternal alcohol and phenytoin ingestion during pregnancy, or exposure to rubella in the first trimester. Single gene abnormalities, e.g. Marfan's syndrome, may have associated congenital heart malformations. Similarly, congenital heart abnormalities may be found in children with chromosomal aberrations (e.g. 40 per cent chance in trisomy 21 or 45X0; 90 per cent chance in trisomy 13 or trisomy 18).

A positive family history of congenital heart disease may be found in at least 10 per cent of first-degree relatives. It should be noted that the following abnormalities account for over 80 per cent of all congenital heart disease.

Cardiovascular dynamics

The clinical identification of congenital heart defects requires a basic knowledge of the dynamics of the cardiovascular system (CVS). The normal heart consists of two pumps working simultaneously alongside each other (*see* Figure 28.1.)

The right side has a low pressure atrium receiving desaturated blood from the systemic circulation and a muscular pumping ventricle which propels the blood into the pulmonary circulation. The pressure which the right ventricle (RV) must generate depends on the resistance to flow in the sponge-like, pulmonary vascular bed. This is normally low, therefore the RV pressure does not need to be more than 15–25 mmHg in systole.

In the right atrium (RA) pressure is determined by the compliance of the RV which is normally

Figure 28.1 A normal heart

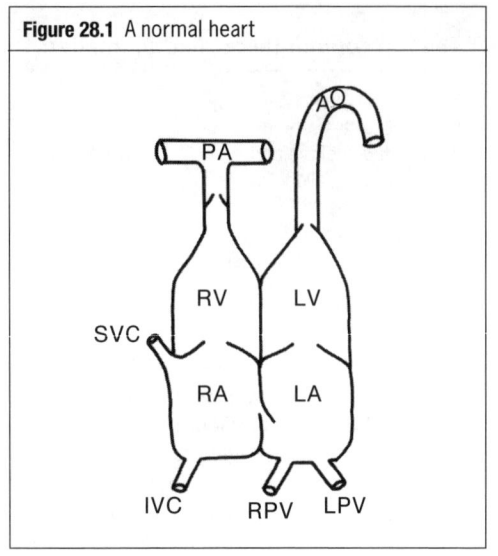

good and RA pressure does not rise above 5 mmHg.

On the left side of the heart the left atrium (LA) receives oxygenated blood from the pulmonary veins and the left ventricle (LV) has to generate enough pressure to ensure that the blood will circulate throughout the body. The systemic resistance is much higher than pulmonary resistance and therefore, LV pressure needs to be 60 mmHg systolic in an infant, rising to 120 mmHg in the normal adult. The LV is therefore a thick, muscled chamber which makes it relatively non-compliant and LA pressure needs to be greater than RA pressure to fill the LV (normal LA mean pressure is 5–10 mmHg).

In the normal situation, the mean pressure in the LA is always higher than RA pressure and the LV systolic pressure is always about four times greater than the RV pressure. In the same way,

Figure 28.2 Approach to CHD

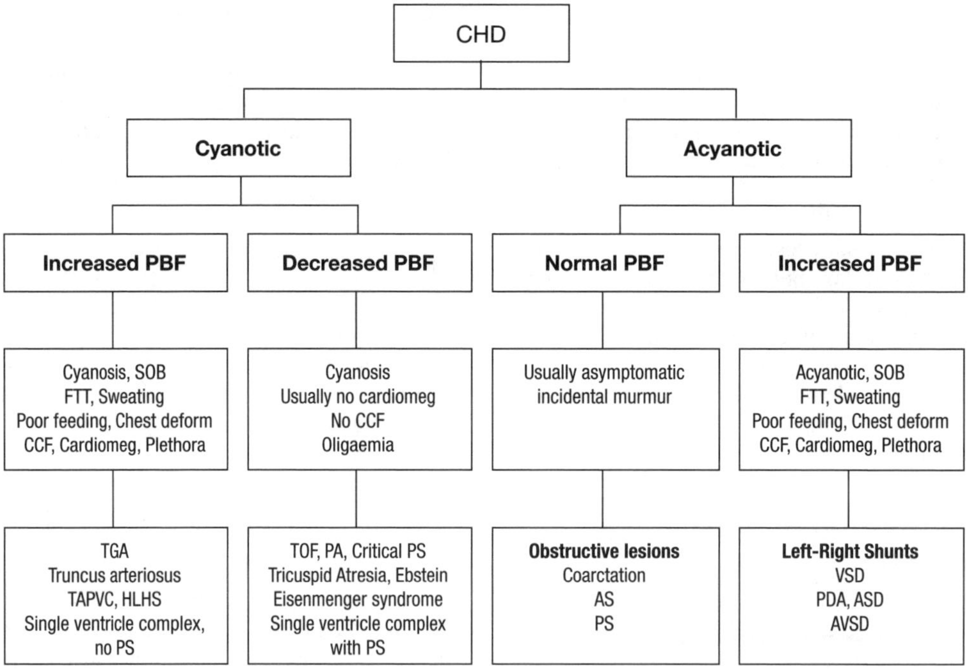

CHD

Cyanotic — Acyanotic

Increased PBF	Decreased PBF	Normal PBF	Increased PBF
Cyanosis, SOB FTT, Sweating Poor feeding, Chest deform CCF, Cardiomeg, Plethora	Cyanosis Usually no cardiomeg No CCF Oligaemia	Usually asymptomatic incidental murmur	Acyanotic, SOB FTT, Sweating Poor feeding, Chest deform CCF, Cardiomeg, Plethora
TGA Truncus arteriosus TAPVC, HLHS Single ventricle complex, no PS	TOF, PA, Critical PS Tricuspid Atresia, Ebstein Eisenmenger syndrome Single ventricle complex with PS	**Obstructive lesions** Coarctation AS PS	**Left-Right Shunts** VSD PDA, ASD AVSD

CHD: congenital heart disease; PBF: pulmonary blood flow; TGA: transposition of great arteries; TAPVC: total anomalous pulmonary venous connection; TOF: tetralogy of Fallot; PA: pulmonary atresia; PS: pulmonary stenosis; AS: aortic stenosis; Coarct: coarctation of the AO; VSD: ventricular septal defect; PDA: patent ductus arteriosus; ASD: atrial septal defect; AVSD:atrio-ventricular septal defect; SOB: shortness of breath; FTT: failure to thrive; CCF: congestive cardiac failure

the pulmonary artery systolic pressure, being that generated by the RV, is always lower than the aortic pressure generated by the LV.

It is obvious therefore, that if there is a simple defect connecting the two sides of the heart at any level, from the atrium to the great vessels, blood will only flow across the defect from left to right following the pressure gradient. Patients with such defects are not cyanosed.

Congenital heart defects are classified into those which cause **cyanosis,** and those which are **acyanotic**. *See* Figure 28.2.

Acyanotic congenital heart defects

Acyanotic conditions are divided into two groups:
- Acyanotic with increased pulmonary blood flow (left to right shunts).

These are defects connecting the systemic and pulmonary circulations and allow left to right shunting of blood to occur. These include ventricular septal defect (VSD), atrial septal defect (ASD), atrio-ventricular septal defect (AVSD) (or endocardial cushion defect (ECD)) and patent ductus arteriosus (PDA).

When significant, these lesions present with symptoms and signs of cardiac failure. These infants have excessive sweating during and interrupt feeds. As a result they fail to thrive. Recurrent lower respiratory tract Infections (LRTIs) are common in these infants. As they grow older chest deformities like pectus carinatum, Harrison's sulcus, precordial bulge and chest asymmetry develop. Small defects may be discovered because of a cardiac murmur being found at examination with no cardiac symptoms evident. Table 28.2 should be consulted for the distinguishing features of conditions discussed below.

Patent ductus arteriosus (PDA)

(*See* Figure 28.3.)

In infants born preterm, particularly those with respiratory distress, the ductus arteriosus often remains patent and a significant left to right shunt develops through it towards the end of the first week of life. These infants develop tachypnoea again and a systolic murmur becomes audible on the left just below the clavicle. In preterm infants, a PDA usually closes by the time the infant reaches its expected term. Non-

steroidal anti-inflammatory drugs (NSAIDS) eg indomethacin or ibubrofen may be administered to close the PDA in preterm neonates. They are, however, not effective in term neonates. If it does not close, surgical removal of the PDA will be necessary. PDA may also occur in term infants. This is characterized by a continuous (machinery) murmur just below the left clavicle. If there is a large flow through the PDA, a mid-diastolic murmur will be heard at the apex. The peripheral pulses are bounding or collapsing. The pulse pressure is wide and the dorsalis pedis is easily palpable.

Figure 28.3 Patent ductus arteriosus

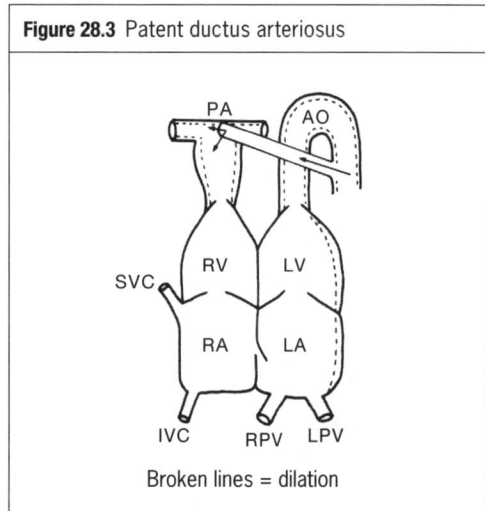

Broken lines = dilation

Figure 28.4 Ventricular septal defect

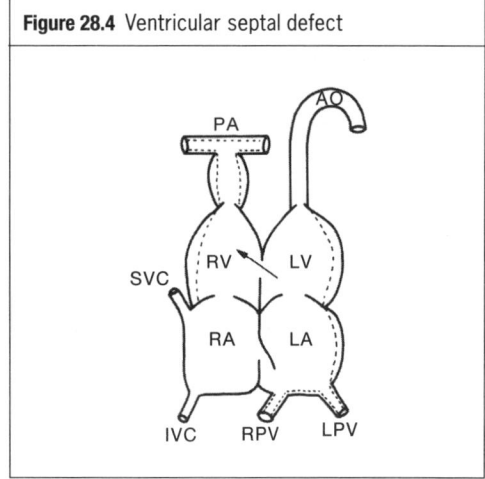

Table 28.3 Distinguishing features of acyanotic defects

Defect	Pulse	Systolic murmur	Diastolic murmur	2nd heart sound	Chest X-ray	ECG
Coarctation	Brachials bounding. Femorals absent (or delayed)	Ejection at back	Mid (33%) at apex	Normal	Large proximal aorta. 3 sign (in older children) descending aorta	Normal or LVH
Aortic stenosis	Small volume	Ejection at 2RS radiates to neck. Ejection systolic click if valvar. Thrill = severe	Early (20–25%)	Normal	Large proximal aorta	Normal axis. LVH if severe
Ventricular septal defect	Normal	Pan at 4LS Grade 3–5/6 (may be thrill)	Mid at apex = high flow	Loud P2 = pulmonary hypertension	Cardiomegaly. Pulmonary plethora	Biventricular enlargement
Endocardial cushion defect (ASD + MI)	Normal	Pan at apex. Ejection at 2LS	Mid at 4LS	Fixed split Loud P2 = pulmonary hypertension	Cardiomegaly. Pulmonary plethora	QRS axis–60° RsR in V1
Atrial defect (ostium secundum)	Normal	Ejection at 2LS	Mid at 4LS	Fixed split	RA and RV enlarged. Pulmonary plethora	Rt. axis RsR in V1
Patent ductus arteriosus	Collapsing	Ejection at 2LS in infants. Continuous machinery	Mid at apex	Loud P2	Cardiomegaly. Pulmonary plethora (normal in asymptomatic)	Normal or biventricular enlargement
Pulmonary stenosis	Normal	Ejection at 2LS. Ejection systolic click. Thrill = severe	Nil	Soft P2. Wide split	Large MPA, RV enlargement. Normal lung vascularity	Rt. axis, RVH

ASD = Atrial septal defect   LS = Left intercostal space   LVH = Left ventricular hypertrophy   MI = Mitral incompetence   MPA = Main pulmonary artery
P2 = 2nd pulmonic sound   RA = Right atrium   RS = Right intercostal space   RV = Right ventricle   RVH = Right ventricular hypertrophy

PDA in term infants very rarely closes spontaneously and always requires surgical removal or device closure before six months of age, even if it is asymptomatic.

Ventricular septal defect (VSD)
(*See* Figure 28.4.)

This is the most common form of CHD. Large defects present between two and six weeks of life (later at higher altitudes), when the pulmonary vascular resistance has decreased from the high fetal level. These infants become breathless on feeding and, as a result, fail to gain weight adequately, due to the large left to right shunt causing overloading and failure of the left ventricle. The typical loud pansystolic murmur is heard at the left lower sternal edge, below a line drawn through the nipples. If the left to right shunt is large, a mid-diastolic murmur will be heard at the apex. If there is pulmonary hypertension, the pulmonary component of the second sound (P2) will be loud.

If a child with the signs of a VSD fails to respond to anti-failure therapy, a coexistent defect must be suspected, e.g. PDA and/or coarctation of the aorta, when surgical intervention will be required sooner. The natural history for VSDs is that moderate sized defects may become smaller, small defects may close spontaneously and both may not require surgery. Large defects presenting with cardiac failure invariably require surgical closure.

Note: Small VSDs are asymptomatic. These children have a typical loud pansystolic murmur at the fourth left intercostal space due to a high velocity but low volume shunt from the LV to the low pressure RV. They will have neither symptoms nor the loud P2 or an apical mid-diastolic murmur. The ECG and chest X-ray are usually within normal limits. The majority will close spontaneously before adult life, particularly within the first two years after birth.

Prophylactic amoxicillin must always be given one hour before the extraction of teeth, to prevent infective endocarditis occurring in the right ventricle opposite the defect.

Atrial septal defect (ostium secundum and solitary ostium primum)

(*See* Figure 28.5.)

Children with these defects are usually asymptomatic, although they are not athletic

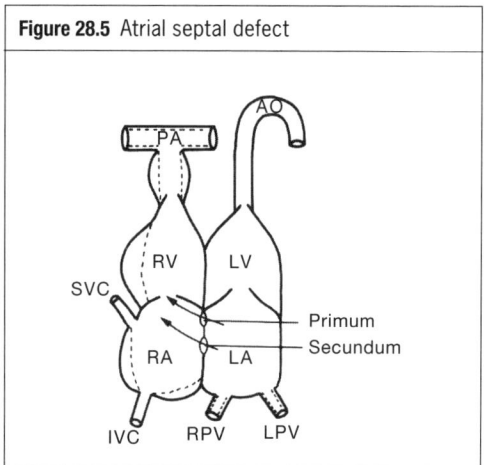

Figure 28.5 Atrial septal defect

and may suffer frequently from chest infections because of a large left to right shunt into the pulmonary circulation.

They show clinical signs of right ventricular hypertrophy, with a palpable lift over the pulmonary outflow tract. A grade 2/6 pulmonary ejection systolic murmur is heard at the second left intercostal space and there is fixed splitting of the second heart sound. A tricuspid diastolic murmur may be heard at the lower left sternal edge. The chest X-ray is typical, showing a large, main pulmonary artery and plethoric lung fields.

The ECG differentiates secundum from primum defects, there being right axis deviation in the former and left axis deviation in the latter. Both show an RsR pattern in V_1. Most patients with secundum defects require surgical or device closure of the defect during childhood, preferably prior to school-going age. Only large primum defects require closure.

Endocardial cushion defect (ECD) or atrio- ventricular septal defect (AVSD)

(*See* Figure 28.6.)

AVSD can either be complete or partial. A complete AVSD involves an ostium primum ASD and an inlet VSD with a common atrioventricular valve. A partial AVSD refers to an ostium primum ASD only, with no associated VSD. A common form of this abnormality is an ostium primum ASD, associated with a cleft in the mitral valve which allows a left to right shunt between the left ventricle and the right atrium. Such a shunt

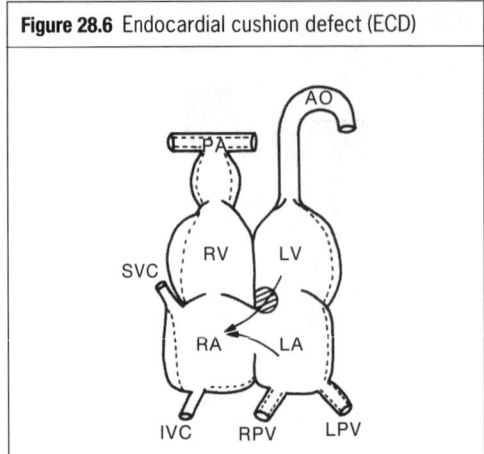

Figure 28.6 Endocardial cushion defect (ECD)

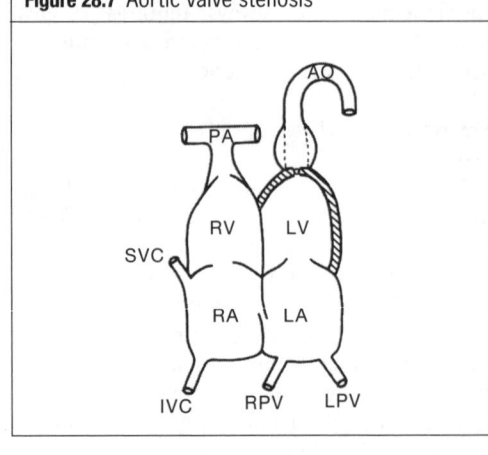

Figure 28.7 Aortic valve stenosis

may be very large and cause cardiac failure early in life. Half of the infants with this defect have Down's syndrome (*see* Chapter 3, Genetic and congenital disorders). On auscultation, a pansystolic murmur is heard at the apex due to mitral incompetence, and an ejection systolic murmur is heard at the left sternal border due to increased flow through the pulmonary valve. With a complete AVSD a pansystolic murmur may be heard in the left lower sternal edge or at the apex. Sometimes no murmur is audible due to the balanced pressures in large defects. The ECG usually shows left anterior hemiblock, with a QRS axis between –60 degrees and –90 degrees and an RsR pattern in lead V_1, indicating right ventricular hypertrophy due to the volume overload.

Acyanotic with normal pulmonary blood flow

These are obstructive defects which affect either the left or right side of the heart and cause hypertrophy of the chamber which is obstructed, e.g. aortic or pulmonary stenosis and coarctation of the aorta.

These are often discovered incidentally because of a cardiac murmur being found at examination. Rarely if the lesions are severe signs of heart failure may develop.

Aortic stenosis, valvar (rarely subvalvar or supravalvar)

(*See* Figure 28.7)

Aortic stenosis accounts for 4 per cent of congenital heart defects, with males predominating

4:1. Isolated aortic stenosis presenting in childhood is almost always congenital in origin. Rheumatic fever invariably causes incompetence as well as stenosis of the aortic valve and in these cases AS is rare before the third decade of life and thus is a disease of adulthood.

Aortic stenosis is usually asymptomatic in infancy, as it commonly develops later in an aortic valve which is often bicuspid. Significant aortic stenosis in the older child usually has a palpable thrill, as well as a loud and long ejection systolic murmur which radiates to the right side of the neck from the second intercostal space. The chest X-ray may look normal, but the proximal aorta is usually enlarged. A short, early diastolic murmur is audible in 20–25 per cent of cases, and there is an ejection click in valvar stenosis. Absence of a click suggests subvalvar or supravalvar stenosis. If severe, these may present in infancy with left heart failure, poor volume pulses and a narrow pulse pressure. Cardiomegaly may be evident on chest X-ray in this group.

Pulmonary valve stenosis (PS)

(*See* Figure 28.8)

This is a common congenital heart defect, but varies widely in its degree of severity. Most cases are mild and asymptomatic. The most severe cases may develop right heart failure. When there is critical PS they will present with cyanosis due to right to left shunting through a patent foramen ovale, because the right atrial pressure exceeds the left atrial pressure. Without right to left shunting, isolated PS remains an acyanotic

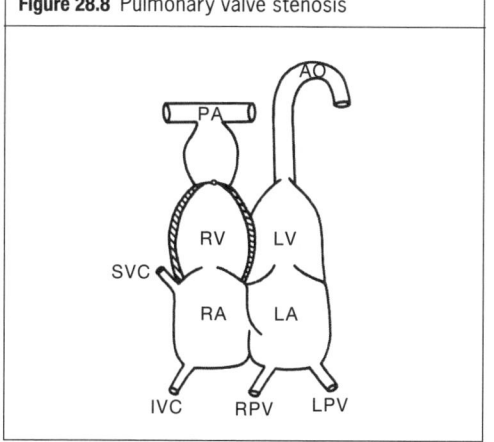

Figure 28.8 Pulmonary valve stenosis

Figure 28.9 Coarctation of the aorta

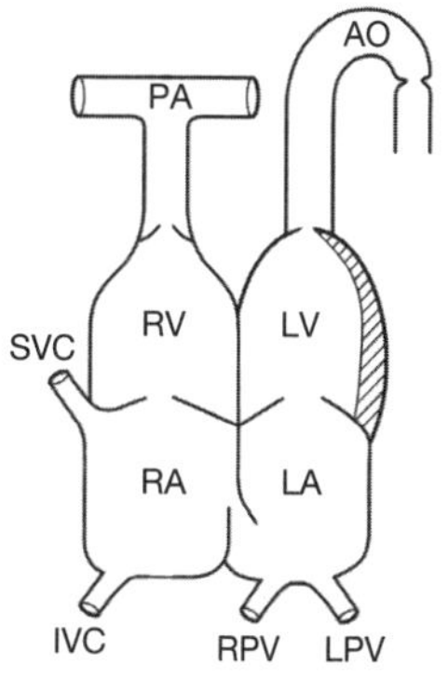

condition. An ejection systolic murmur is heard at the second left intercostal space and is often preceded by an ejection systolic click. In severe cases the murmur will be long, obscuring the aortic component of the second heart sound and a thrill will be palpable. The pulmonary component of the second heart sound is soft and delayed. Severe cases with a thrill and documented on echocardiography, should undergo cardiac catheterization during which a balloon valvuloplasty is performed. If this is not possible, then surgical treatment is indicated.

Coarctation of the aorta

(*See* Figure 28.9.)

This is a constriction in the thoracic aorta in the region of the ductus arteriosus (i.e juxtaductal). If severe, this causes left heart and, soon thereafter, right heart failure, usually in the second week of life after the ductus arteriosus closes. Diagnosis is made by palpating the pulses in the arms and legs. The arm pulses are easily felt, whereas the femoral pulses are impalpable. The difference in blood pressure by means of the flush technique is more than 20 mmHg. A systolic murmur is usually heard at the back between the left scapula and the spine. An apical mid-diastolic murmur is audible in about one-third of infants, and is due to mild mitral valve deformity. Two-thirds of these symptomatic babies have an associated major cardiac defect, e.g. VSD and/or PDA. The chest X-ray shows generalized cardiomegaly and congestion of the lung fields.

In older children and adults, coarctation may

be asymptomatic or present as hypertension with symptoms of headache, chest pain, or cerebro-vascular accidents. Some patients complain of claudication in their legs. The diagnosis is made by palpating the discrepancy between the pulses in the arms and legs. Because of the development of collateral circulation, the femoral pulses will be palpable, but weaker and delayed compared with the arm pulses. Recording the blood pressure in the arms and legs will confirm the discrepancy, with hypertension in the arms and relatively low pressure in the legs.

The right arm must always be used for blood pressure recordings, as the left subclavian artery may occasionally be involved in the coarctation.

A systolic thrill may be felt in the suprasternal notch and the typical, harsh, systolic murmur may be heard at the back at the angle of the left scapula, but often there is only a soft systolic murmur over the precordium.

In older children and adults, the chest X-ray shows slight enlargement of the left ventricle due to concentric hypertrophy. The proximal aorta is enlarged and an indentation may be seen in the descending aorta to the left of the vertebral column, making a figure '3' sign. A radiological feature of children of school-going age and older is notching of the inferior edges of the third to eighth ribs, caused by enlarged collateral inter-costal arteries. The ECG is usually normal in children, but may show left ventricular hyper-trophy in older patients.

Older asymptomatic infants and children require elective surgical repair to prevent the development of permanent hypertension. (Recommended age: two years.)

If a child older than one year presents with signs of coarctation and is in congestive cardiac failure (CCF), aortic arteritis (Takayasu's) should be suspected.

Cyanotic congenital heart defects

Congenital heart defects which cause central cyanosis can be divided into two groups:
- Cyanotic with decreased pulmonary blood flow
- Cyanotic with increased pulmonary blood flow.

Table 28.1 should be consulted for the distinguishing features of the conditions discussed below.

Cyanotic with decreased pulmonary blood flow

In these conditions desaturated, systemic, venous blood cannot adequately reach the pulmonary circulation to pick up oxygen. They include tetralogy of Fallot, pulmonary atresia, tricuspid atresia, Ebstein's anomaly, critical pulmonary valve stenosis, Eisenmengers syndrome and complex cardiac defects with associated PS.

These infants are often cyanosed, but appear comfortable with no respiratory distress. They usually do not develop symptoms and signs of cardiac failure. Chest deformities are not common in this group barring Eisenmengers syndrome. Except for Ebstein's anomaly, there is usually no cardiomegaly. Chest X-ray demonstrates oligaemic lung fields.

Tetralogy of Fallot
(*See* Figure 28.10.)

This is the most common cyanotic heart abnormality found in children. The clinical picture depends mainly on the degree of right ventricular outflow tract obstruction (pulmonary stenosis). The more severe the stenosis the sooner persistent central cyanosis will develop, with clubbing and polycythaemia to follow. Tetralogy of Fallot must be suspected in any child between six months and five years presenting with central cyanosis, right ventricular hypertrophy, a single second heart sound, and an ejection systolic

Figure 28.10 Cyanotic: tetralogy of Fallot

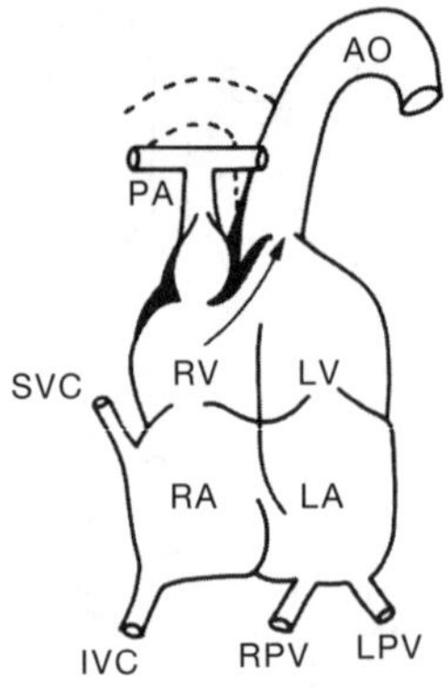

murmur over the pulmonary area radiating to the left clavicle.

Obstruction occurs mainly in the outflow tract of the right ventricle and is muscular and variable. A large VSD permits the obstructed desaturated blood to pass from the right ventricle into the overriding aorta. These children tend to get hypercyanotic attacks due to infundibular spasm or a drop in systemic vascular resistance. Emergency treatment for this is given below:
- Place infant in knee-chest or squatting position.
- Administer morphine 0.1–0.2 mg/kg IV or SC or IM.
- Administer propranolol 0.1 mg/kg IV and continue on propranolol by mouth 1–5 mg/kg/d in divided doses.
- Administer sodium bicarbonate 1 mEq/kg IV to counteract metabolic acidosis.
- Check haematocrit for hypochromic anaemia and treat accordingly.

Pulmonary valve atresia with a VSD
This is an extreme form of TOF. The only difference being the presence of complete pulmonary valve atresia instead of pulmonary stenosis. There is no prograde flow from the right ventricle to the pulmonary arteries. The source of pulmonary blood flow is a PDA or multiple systemic collaterals from the aorta. These children present with cyanosis in the early neonatal period. Usually no murmur is audible, but there may be

a soft continuous murmur present from the PDA or collaterals.

Tricuspid valve atresia (See Figure 28.11) and Pulmonary valve atresia with intact ventricular septum.

Both conditions are part of the hypoplastic right heart syndrome. In both cases, desaturated blood passes from the right atrium through the foramen ovale to the left atrium.

Ebstein's anomaly of the tricuspid valve
(See Figure 28.12.)

The tricuspid valve is displaced into the body of the right ventricle and is incompetent. Part of the right ventricle is above the valve (atrialized). A right-to-left shunt occurs through the foramen ovale. Chest radiography demonstrates a typical enlarged 'wall-to-wall' heart with oligaemic lung fields.

Critical pulmonary valve stenosis (trilogy)
(See Figure 28.13.)

If the stenosis is critical, the pressures in the right ventricle and right atrium may be greater than on the left, and a right-to-left shunt will occur through the foramen ovale or sometimes across a coexistent ASD.

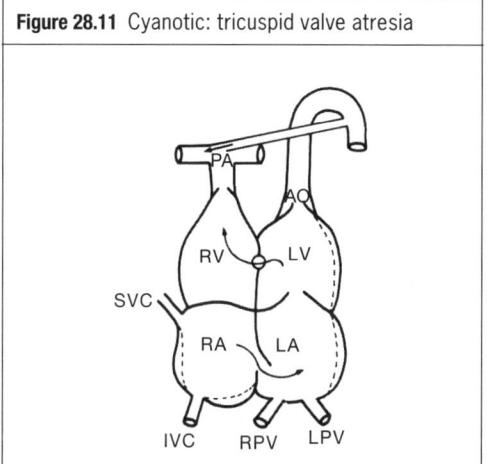

Figure **28.11** Cyanotic: tricuspid valve atresia

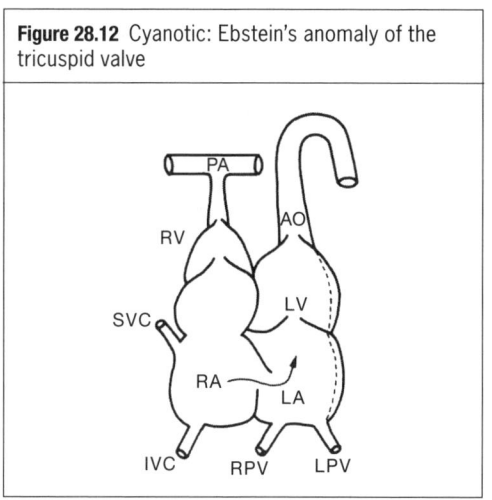

Figure **28.12** Cyanotic: Ebstein's anomaly of the tricuspid valve

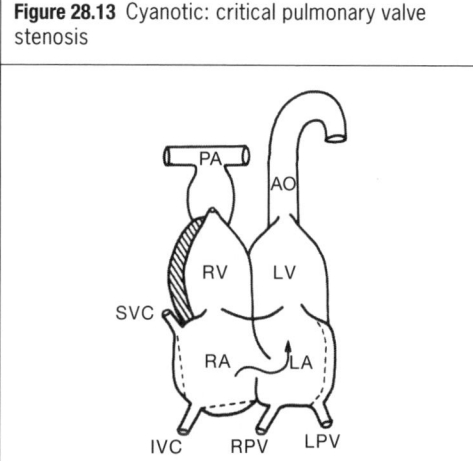

Figure **28.13** Cyanotic: critical pulmonary valve stenosis

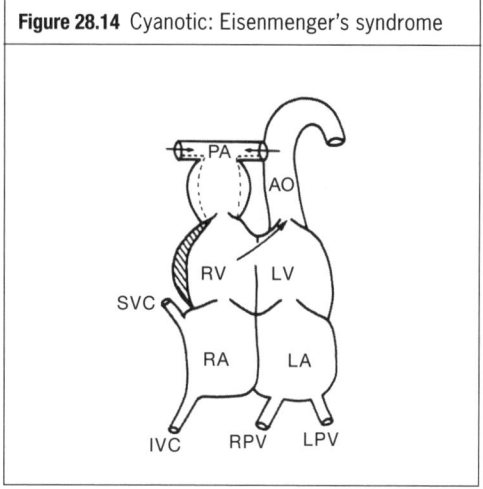

Figure **28.14** Cyanotic: Eisenmenger's syndrome

Eisenmenger's syndrome
(*See* Figure 28.14.)

Obstruction is due to pulmonary arteriolar disease causing severe pulmonary hypertension. A right-to-left shunt occurs through a VSD.

If severe pulmonary hypertension complicates an ASD or PDA there will also be a reversal of the shunt through these defects.

Complex lesions with associated PS
These include single ventricle complex and double outlet right ventricle with associated PS. There is common mixing and decreased pulmonary blood flow dependant on the severity of the PS.

Cyanotic with increased pulmonary blood flow

Those in which there is mixing of saturated and desaturated blood (common mixing situations). All of these have plethoric lung fields and are cyanosed. They often present in cardiac failure, have repeated chest infections and fail to thrive. Later in infancy chest deformities develop.

+ Transposition of great vessels (TGV)
+ Persistent truncus arteriosus (PTA)
+ Total anomalous pulmonary venous connection (TAPVC)
+ Hypoplastic left heart syndrome (HLHS)
  This usually comprises aortic valve atresia, mitral atresia, or hypoplasia, hypoplastic ascending aorta, and a diminutive left ventricle
+ Single ventricle complex with no PS
  This is usually associated with transposition of the great vessels.

Transposition of the great vessels (with VSD, PDA or intact ventricular septum)
(*See* Figure 28.15.)

The great arteries arise from the inappropriate ventricles. The aorta arises from the right ventricle and the pulmonary artery from the left ventricle. Desaturated blood from the systemic veins enters the right atrium, right ventricle and is then pumped into the aorta. Oxygenated pulmonary venous blood enters the left atrium, left ventricle and is pumped back into the pulmonary circulation. This results in two separate circulations in parallel, with hypoxaemic blood perfusing the body and highly oxygenated blood circulating in the lungs. Survival is dependant on the pres-

ence of a VSD, ASD or PDA for mixing of blood between the two circulations. Cyanosis is noted soon after birth. Precordial examination may be uneventful with no murmurs if there are no associated defects. An egg-on-side cardiac silhouette with a narrow pedicle and plethora is typical on chest X-ray. Plethora may not be evident in TGV with intact ventricular septum.

Persistent truncus arteriosus
(*See* Figure 28.16.)

In this condition a single common arterial trunk with one semilunar valve (truncal valve) arises from the heart and gives rise to the aorta

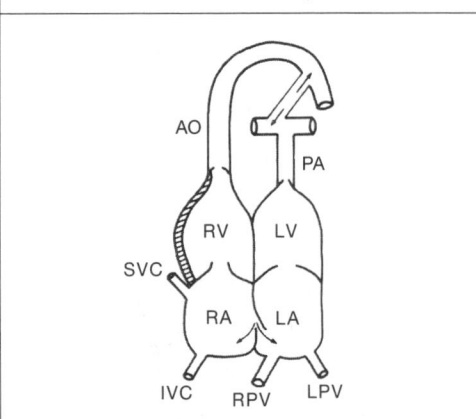

Figure 28.15 Cyanotic: transposition of the great vessels with intact ventricular septum

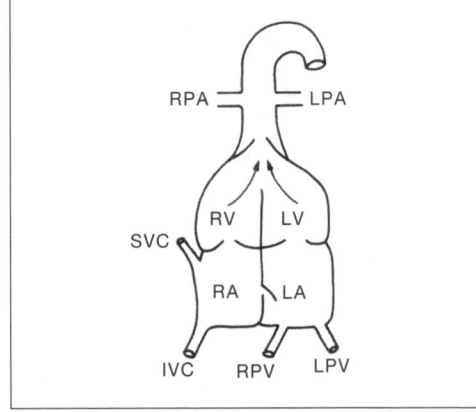

Figure 28.16 Cyanotic: persistent truncus arteriosus

and pulmonary arteries. A large VSD is present just below the valve allowing both ventricles to pump into the common trunk. The truncal valve is often abnormal with stenosis and regurgitation creating a to-and-fro murmur. Mild to moderate cyanosis and signs of CCF develop in early infancy. The peripheral pulses are bounding or collapsing with a wide pulse pressure. An ejection click with a loud and single 2nd heart sound is audible. Cardiomegaly with plethora is evident on chest radiography.

Total anomalous pulmonary venous connection (TAPVC)
(*See* Figure 28.17.)

In this condition all the pulmonary veins drain abnormally into the right atrium (RA). This can be

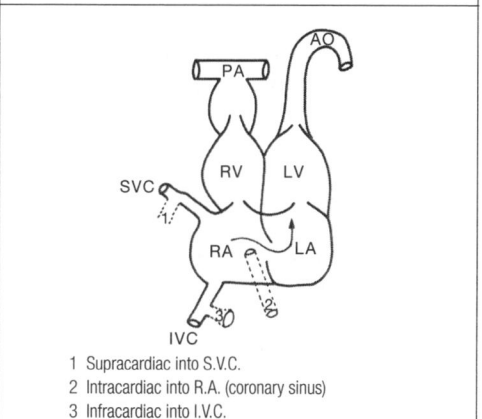

Figure 28.17 Cyanotic: total anomalous pulmonary venous connection (TAPVC)

1 Supracardiac into S.V.C.
2 Intracardiac into R.A. (coronary sinus)
3 Infracardiac into I.V.C.

Complications of cyanotic CHD and right to left shunting:

* Chronic hypoxia
* Myocardial and somatic tissue dysfunction
* Paradoxical emboli
* Neurological sequelae
* Hemiplegia or hemiparesis
* Cerebral abscess
* Polycythaemia and hyperuricacidaemia
* Thrombocytopaenia and bleeding tendencies
* Iron deficiency
* Exercise intolerance.

via the SVC (supracardiac), via the coronary sinus or direct into the RA (cardiac) or via the IVC and hepatic veins (infracardiac / infradiaphragmatic). There is obligatory right to left shunting across an ASD or foramen ovale, the only supply to systemic circulation. The left atrium and ventricle are smaller compared to the dilated right heart. Features of cardiac failure, recurrent chest infections and failure to thrive develop in infancy. Chest radiography shows a 'figure-of-8 or snowman' configuration with the commoner supracardiac type. The lung fields are plethoric.

Rheumatic fever

In Africa, Asia, and South America, rheumatic fever remains a common disease and is associated with significant morbidity and mortality rates, both in the acute phase of the disease and as a result of chronic, cardiac valvular sequelae. It remains the most common cause of acquired heart disease in children.

In most European and North American countries, the incidence of rheumatic fever declined in the 50 years preceding 1980. The reduction, both in incidence and severity, commenced before the advent of antibiotics and appears to have been related mainly to improvements in the general health and socio-economic standards of the populations in these countries.

However, since the mid-1980s, there has been an unexpected resurgence of rheumatic fever in the United States. This has occurred in middle-class families with ready access to medical care. The exact reasons are still unclear, but there has been the re-appearance of 'rheumatogenic' strains of Group A haemolytic streptococci (M-types 1, 3, 5, 6, and in particular 18) in the affected areas (*see below*).

Aetiology

In susceptible individuals (possibly with a specific class II HLA antigen) rheumatic fever is a sequel to a pharyngeal infection with one of the Group A beta-haemolytic streptococci. Specific 'rheumatogenic' strains of streptococci can now be identified and it is significant that these strains are rarely found today in populations where rheumatic fever has virtually disappeared.

Clinical features of acute rheumatic fever

In children between the ages of 5–15 years, the signs and symptoms of rheumatic fever occur two to three weeks after a pharyngeal infection. Very rarely it occurs in children as young as eighteen months.

A fairly wide spectrum of presenting features exists, from the unequivocal signs of fever associated with flitting polyarthritis, and obvious carditis causing signs of cardiac failure, to milder almost insignificant symptoms, where the diagnosis must be made on the evidence of a combination of factors. In 1944, Jones enumerated major and minor criteria which, with modifications in 1965 by a committee of the American Heart Association, have been accepted as indicators of probability in making the important diagnosis of acute rheumatic fever. The need to make an accurate diagnosis in all cases is emphasized, because serious involvement of heart valves may follow a relatively mild first attack and prevention of further attacks is imperative if the grave long-term cardiac complications are to be avoided.

Major criteria

(*See* Table 28.4.)

Carditis. Seventy per cent of hospitalized black children presenting with rheumatic fever have evidence of carditis on their first admission (elsewhere 40–75 per cent). The diagnosis of

Table 28.4 Diagnostic criteria of rheumatic fever

Major	Minor
1 Carditis	1 Prolonged PR interval on ECG
2 Polyarthritis	2 Arthralgia
3 Chorea	3 Previous history or evidence of rheumatic fever
4 Erythema	
5 Nodules	4 Fever marginatum
	5 Acute phase reactants

Note: Use 1 and 2 as either minor or major criteria but not as both.

carditis is made if one or more of the following signs is present:

- *Cardiac murmurs* indicate endocarditis. The most common of these is a high-pitched, blowing, pansystolic murmur heard at the apex and is due to mitral valve incompetence caused by distortion of the mitral valve cusps and mitral annular dilatation. Sometimes this is associated with a short, low-pitched mid-diastolic murmur at the apex, which disappears as the acute process resolves. Involvement of the aortic valve causes incompetence, which is recognized by a high-pitched, early diastolic murmur, heard best at the aortic area and down the left sternal edge when the patient is sitting up and leaning forward. If severe, a wide pulse pressure and collapsing pulses will also be present.
- *Cardiac enlargement* is most easily detected by X-ray examination of the chest. When this is associated with soft heart sounds, a diffuse apical impulse and tachycardia (out of keeping with the degree of fever), myocarditis must be suspected even if murmurs are absent. When the patient is asleep a record of the pulse will reveal a fast rate if the myocardium is involved. A rapid 'sleeping' pulse may be the only indication of carditis.
- A *friction rub* is usually heard early in the illness if there is pericarditis. This often disappears or may be absent if a pericardial effusion occurs. A large pericardial effusion may cause tamponade, distended neck veins, hepatomegaly and pulsus paradoxus, or may be suspected if there is a globular enlargement of the cardiac shadow on the chest X-ray and S-T elevation on the electrocardiogram. Pain in the chest or abdomen is often a presenting feature of rheumatic fever, with or without pericarditis. Careful repeated auscultation for a rub should be done if pain is a symptom.
- *Pancarditis*, with involvement of the endocardium, myocardium, and pericardium often presents with congestive cardiac failure.

Polyarthritis. The typical presentation is a flitting or migratory arthritis with red, hot, swollen, tender, large joints which become involved sequentially. As a new joint is involved, the arthritis in the previously affected joint subsides. It is important to consider rheumatic fever in the differential diagnosis of mono-arthritis in children.

Once the acute inflammation has settled, the joints recover completely.

Chorea. This occurs most often in girls between seven and fourteen years of age. There is a long latent period of weeks or months between the streptococcal infection and the onset of symptoms. In some cases, chorea may develop some weeks after joint symptoms, but often it occurs without any recognized symptoms or signs of rheumatic fever. Between 20–30 per cent of patients with chorea have, or develop, cardiac valvular disease. The onset is gradual over one or two weeks during which the child is scolded for being clumsy, spilling drinks, or dropping articles. Involuntary grimacing, accompanied by purposeless and asymmetrical, jerky, in coordinate movements which may be bilateral or unilateral, make writing impossible and managing buttons and shoelaces difficult. Emotional lability is striking: crying alternating with laughing. Speech may be affected. When asked to perform tasks, the involuntary movements become exaggerated and the hand grip cannot be sustained. When asked to extend their arms forward, their hands and wrists form a typical 'eating-fork' configuration. In the most severe cases, patients cannot even remain lying on a bed because of violent involuntary movements. Shining a light into the eye may produce hippus, i.e. alternating constriction and relaxation of the pupil. Chorea often runs a prolonged and relapsing course over weeks and months.

Erythema marginatum. This is a transient erythematous rash. When it fades it leaves irregular thin lines which make circular patterns on the trunk and occasionally the limbs, but never on the face. It is easily seen on light-skinned patients, but neither easily nor often seen on darkly pigmented skin.

Nodules. Subcutaneous, non-tender, small, mobile nodules are found over the extensor surfaces (around the elbows, wrists, knuckles, knees, ankles), over the spinous processes of the vertebrae, the occiput, and sometimes on the scalp and ears of patients who usually have or develop severe cardiac involvement.

Minor criteria

Previous history or **evidence of previous episode** of rheumatic fever.

Arthralgia. It is important to exclude vague limb pains due to myalgia. This should not be used as a criterion if arthritis is a major manifestation.

Fever. Temperature recordings are usually 38 °C or more in acute rheumatic fever.

Prolonged P-R interval on the electrocardiogram (ECG) to greater than 0.18 seconds. This should not be used as a criterion where carditis is a major criterion.

Raised acute phase reactants. These are not specific for rheumatic fever.

- Leucocytosis. This is usually between $12–15 \times 10^9$/l.
- Erythrocyte sedimentation rate (ESR). This is raised, but the level does not correlate with severity. It may, however, be normal in chorea.
- C-reactive protein (CRP). This is invariably found in the serum of almost all cases.

Invariably, the acute pharyngitis has resolved before the symptoms of rheumatic fever commence, but a throat swab should always be done as it may reveal streptococci. Indirect evidence of a preceding streptococcal infection may be obtained from an elevated antistreptolysin O titre (ASOT), or the finding of other streptococcal antibodies (anti-DNase B or anti-hyaluronidase) in high titre in the blood. These findings by themselves are not diagnostic of rheumatic fever, and not all streptococci cause elevation of the ASOT.

Treatment of rheumatic fever

Prevention

Rheumatic fever is rare where standards of living are good. A high incidence is associated with poor housing, overcrowding, and lack of primary health care facilities. Treatment of streptococcal throat infections with penicillin within one week of the onset of symptoms prevents the development of rheumatic fever, provided

> The presence of two major criteria, or one major and two minor criteria, together with evidence of a preceding streptococcal infection, makes the diagnosis of rheumatic fever probable.

the treatment is adequate. The recommended dosages are:

- One IM injection of benzathine penicillin G 600 000 units (below 30 kg body weight) or 1 200 000 units (over 30 kg); or
- Oral penicillin V 50 mg/kg/d, given three times a day for 10 days. It is important that oral penicillin is given before meals and the course completed.
- In patients sensitive to penicillin, treatment is with erythromycin 125–250 mg, four times daily for 10 days; or cephaloridine IM 30–50 mg/kg/d in divided doses, eight-hourly; or oral cephalexin, 25–100 mg/kg/d in divided doses, eight-hourly.

Ideally, all children complaining of a sore throat should have a throat swab cultured and, if Group A beta-haemolytic streptococci are found, the patient should be given penicillin treatment (or erythromycin, if they are penicillin-sensitive). As this is frequently not possible, the decision to give antibiotics depends on the likelihood of the pharyngitis being streptococcal. This can be extremely difficult to determine.

Acute rheumatic fever

Antibiotics. Once a throat swab has been taken, treatment with penicillin (or a substitute) must be started immediately. The first dose should be intramuscular and followed by intramuscular or oral administration for 10 days.

Rest. Children with painful joints and acute carditis invariably lie still. As they recover they may be allowed to move around in bed, but should not be allowed to walk until joint involvement has subsided, cardiac enlargement decreased, and the 'sleeping' pulse rate diminished. Thereafter they should be allowed progressively more activity; most children on adequate treatment should be back to normal, non-strenuous activity within three weeks. If there has been cardiac failure, convalescence may be prolonged and activity should be restricted until evidence of rheumatic activity has been absent for two weeks.

Anti-inflammatory treatment

- **Salicylates** are particularly useful in alleviating the pain of arthritis and the discomfort of fever. The ESR returns to normal more quickly, but salicylates do not have any effect on valvular damage.

Dosage. Sodium salicylate 40–60 mg/kg/d, or acetylsalicylic acid (aspirin), 80–120 mg/kg/d.

Treatment should continue until all signs of activity have subsided and then be gradually withdrawn over a two-week period. Recurrence of symptoms will require increasing the dosage until control is achieved.

Side-effects. Symptoms of salicylate toxicity (tinnitus, dizziness, nausea, and vomiting) are rarely seen at the recommended dosage. If they occur, treatment must be stopped for 48 hours and recommenced at a lower dosage. Gastric irritation with bleeding from the mucosa may occur and, therefore, stools should be examined for occult blood regularly while the patient is on treatment. Giving extra milk or using buffered aspirin may overcome this problem.

Contra-indications. Salicylates may precipitate pulmonary oedema in patients with acute carditis and are, therefore, best avoided in patients with obvious cardiac embarrassment.

- The value of **corticosteroids** in the treatment of children with carditis is controversial. They may possibly be life-saving in cases of pancarditis. Signs of acute rheumatic fever (e.g. fever, raised ESR, and arthritis) may respond rapidly to corticosteroid therapy but there is no effect on long-term valvular damage.

A recent double-blind placebo-controlled trial of prednisone failed to show any benefit either in the short-term clinical response or in the long-term follow-up of patients with active rheumatic carditis.

Dosage: Prednisone, 2 mg/kg/d in four divided doses.

Treatment should be continued at full dosage until the patient is symptomatically well and the acute phase reactants have been normal for one week. This usually takes two to three weeks. Thereafter the dosage should be reduced by 10 per cent every second day, until the daily dose is one-third of the initial dose. Thereafter the reduction should be by 5 per cent every second day. Regular assessment of the acute phase reactants should show a decline to normal levels. Should these become elevated again during the withdrawal period, the dosage should be increased to the previous level and maintained at that until signs of activity have subsided, before gradual withdrawal is recommenced.

Congestive cardiac failure

* Slow digitalization with digoxin, 0.04–0.06 mg/kg total in four equal doses at six-hourly intervals is recommended. The maintenance dose is 0.01 mg/kg/d in two divided doses. Large doses of digoxin are dangerous in children with myocarditis.
* Diuretics are indicated if there is pulmonary oedema or severe congestive failure. Hypokalaemia is particularly dangerous in children with myocarditis during digitalization and potassium supplements must be given if a diuretic which eliminates potassium is used. Hydrochlorothiazide, 0.5–2.0 mg/kg/d in two to three divided doses, is a safe diuretic. Furosemide, 1 mg/kg/dose IV, is used for pulmonary oedema. This can be repeated until improvement occurs. Potassium supplementation is essential when using furosemide.
* Spironolactone (Aldactone®), 2–3 mg/kg/d, divided in two to three doses, may be required when oedema is chronic and does not respond to the above-mentioned drugs.
* Captopril (a vasodilator) in a dose of 0.5–6.0 mg/kg/d, in four divided doses may be added to the anti-failure therapy, especially if there is significant mitral regurgitation.

Emergency surgery may be indicated in the acute phase of carditis, particularly with a rapid onset of pulmonary oedema. This indicates haemodynamic deterioration in the degree of mitral regurgitation.

Chorea. If involuntary movements are severe, haloperidol (Serenace®) 0.025 mg–0.05 mg/kg/d or sodium valproate (Epilim®), can be given orally in divided doses. In milder cases phenobarbitone 3–5 mg/kg/d may be used.

Chronic rheumatic heart disease

This refers to the heart damaged by previous rheumatic fever. The symptoms and signs of acute rheumatic fever subside, the joints recover completely and in those who have not had carditis, there is a return to complete normality. If there had been carditis during the first attack, subsequent attacks will involve the heart again, causing increasing damage to the valves. These become progressively more distorted and incompetent and/or adherent and stenotic.

Mitral valve disease

The mitral valve is the most commonly affected by rheumatic fever, either alone or in combination with the aortic valve and, occasionally, with the tricuspid valve.

By far the most common lesion is **mitral incompetence**. The apical pansystolic murmur radiating to the axilla, heard during the acute attack, may disappear within a few months, only to reappear and become harsher and louder as the valves contract. The haemodynamic effect of mitral incompetence depends on the amount of blood which regurgitates into the left atrium through the damaged valve during ventricular systole. A small amount has little effect, but large amounts of blood result in distension and increased pressure in the left atrium and pulmonary veins. The left ventricle becomes enlarged and hypertrophied and, if the load becomes too great, left heart failure and pulmonary oedema will occur.

In severe mitral incompetence there is displacement of the apex which is thrusting in character, and the pansystolic murmur will be loud and may be heard not only in the left axilla, but at the back as well. A mid-diastolic rumbling murmur is heard at the apex due to the large amount of blood passing across the damaged mitral valve in diastole. If a third heart sound is heard before the diastolic murmur, it indicates critical overloading of the left ventricle. Such patients are symptomatic, with poor effort tolerance, orthopnoea, and paroxysmal nocturnal dyspnoea, and require treatment with digoxin to prevent cardiac failure. In these cases a chest X-ray shows enlargement of both the left atrium and left ventricle. Only severe cases show ECG changes of left-atrial and left-ventricular hypertrophy.

Mitral stenosis usually takes some years to develop as the cusps of the damaged valve fuse together along their commissures. The author has, however, seen children as young as eight years old with tight mitral stenosis. When rheumatic fever occurs at a young age in impoverished children, the progression of the valvular disease to incompetence and/or stenosis appears to be more rapid. The obstruction of flow into the left ventricle causes enlargement and increased pressure in the left atrium and pulmonary veins, which leads to pulmonary arteriolar hypertension. When the overloading of the left atrium becomes critical, pulmonary oedema will occur.

Children with mitral stenosis have poor effort tolerance, dyspnoea and coughing, but haemoptysis is rare in childhood. Examination reveals a tapping apex and a rumbling diastolic murmur which increases in intensity just before a loud first heart sound. An opening snap may be heard if the valve cusps are mobile. A chest X-ray shows left-atrial enlargement and increased pulmonary vascular markings. Right ventricular enlargement is demonstrated on the ECG, which will also show wide bifid P waves, indicative of left-atrial enlargement.

Aortic valve disease

Involvement of the aortic valve may occur alone following rheumatic fever, but it is more often associated with mitral valve disease. Pure aortic stenosis is usually due to a congenital defect. Incompetence invariably occurs if the aortic valve is damaged by rheumatic fever and this may be associated with some degree of stenosis if the distorted cusps fuse together. The progression of aortic valve damage is much slower than mitral valve disease and rarely causes severe disability or symptoms during childhood, unless there is gross incompetence. In most cases of isolated aortic valve disease, left ventricular failure occurs only after many years.

There may be evidence of left ventricular enlargement, clinically detectable as a thrusting apical impulse. Significant aortic incompetence always causes a large pulse pressure with collapsing pulses. A 'pistol shot' is heard over the femoral arteries. In addition, there may be a positive Duroziez sign, i.e. both systolic and diastolic bruits will be heard with the stethoscope proximal to the site of gradual compression of the femoral pulse. The soft, early diastolic murmur, heard during the acute attack, often persists for many years before becoming longer

and louder, with wider radiation as the degree of incompetence increases. An ejection systolic murmur, which may be soft or loud, with a thrill if there is significant stenosis, is often heard at the aortic area as well.

In severe aortic incompetence, a mid-diastolic murmur is frequently heard at the apex (Austin Flint murmur). This is caused by the regurgitant flow striking the anterior mitral leaflet open in diastole which then shudders, thus setting up turbulence. This may lead to a mistaken diagnosis of coexistent mitral stenosis.

Tricuspid valve disease

Occasionally the tricuspid valve may be damaged by rheumatic fever. This usually causes incompetence, with or without some degree of stenosis. Usually the mitral valve, but occasionally the aortic valve, is also involved.

More often, tricuspid valve incompetence occurs as a functional complication of severe pulmonary hypertension associated with mitral valve disease, particularly tight mitral stenosis. The features of tricuspid incompetence are a pansystolic murmur (heard best at the xiphisternum and becoming louder during inspiration), systolic pulsation in the neck veins, and pulsation of the liver. A mid-diastolic murmur is heard over the xiphisternum on inspiration if the regurgitant flow is great or if there is stenosis of the valve.

Management of chronic rheumatic heart disease

Prevention of recurrent attacks

Once rheumatic fever has occurred, the most important aspect of treatment is to prevent recurrences, particularly if there has been any evidence of carditis, as each subsequent attack causes increasingly severe damage to the heart valves. This is achieved by preventing streptococcal infection by continuous prophylactic treatment with penicillin or, in those few patients who are allergic to penicillin, by sulphonamide or erythromycin therapy.

While it is rare for a patient to develop a recurrence of rheumatic fever after 10 years, adolescents and young adults in close communities, such as boarding-schools, army camps, or mine compounds, are at risk of developing streptococcal pharyngitis with rheumatogenic strains and recurrence of rheumatic fever. Prophylactic treatment should, therefore, be continued into adulthood in patients who are in these situations. When prophylactic treatment is uninterrupted, incompetent lesions have been found to improve in some patients.

Oral penicillin V 250 mg twice daily may be used but is less successful in achieving complete protection. Patients forget to take their pills before meals and absorption can be disturbed by enteral illness.

Oral sulphonamide 0.5–1 g twice daily, or erythromycin 250 mg twice daily, may be used as alternatives, but patient compliance must be ensured.

> The most effective prophylactic regime is achieved with an injection of long-acting benzathine penicillin (Bicillin LA®), 600 000 units IM for those under 30 kg, and 1.2 million units for bigger children and adults, administered every three weeks.

Surgical correction of valve defects

Patients who are incapacitated by damaged valves should be referred for detailed echocardiographic and catheterization studies so that surgical intervention or mitral balloon valvuloplasty can be planned.

Tight pliable mitral stenosis can be relieved either by balloon valvuloplasty (at catheterization) or by surgical commissurotomy with or without cardiopulmonary bypass support. Mitral stenosis, with significant subvalvar thickening, or incompetent valves can be repaired or replaced by prosthetic, homograft, or heterograft valves at open heart operations.

Occasionally, a child with established mitral incompetence and acute carditis, who fails to respond to anti-failure therapy, will require surgical correction of the mechanical defect.

> Unfortunately, no child who undergoes a surgical procedure for valves damaged by rheumatic fever ever ceases to be a patient and most require repeated operations.

Occasionally ruptured chordae are also in need of repair. Despite the presence of active carditis, such patients recover well in the short term.

In Africa, acute rheumatic fever still has a mortality of 2–3 per cent and there is a considerable morbidity. The life-span in those who have established heart disease has been prolonged by surgical intervention, but it is still limited and the quality of life is poor, with affected individuals being unable to undertake occupations requiring physical exertion.

Only through well-organized health programmes aimed at improved living standards (especially housing), early treatment of streptococcal infections, and persistent prophylaxis of affected individuals, can a reduction in this common and eminently preventable cause of serious cardiac disease be achieved.

Cardiomyopathy

The term cardiomyopathy is used to describe a variety of non-inflammatory conditions causing myocardial dysfunction and resulting in cardiac failure. These may present acutely, but all have the characteristic feature of chronic myocardial failure with a tendency to form intracardiac thromboses.

When faced with the problem of a child in cardiac failure it is important to look first for signs of a treatable cause. The diagnosis of cardiomyopathy is only made after treatment of heart failure and exclusion of all other causes. The definition of the type of cardiomyopathy usually requires investigation in a specialist cardiac unit.

Cardiomyopathy is a common disease in Africans; it is one of the most frequent causes of heart failure. In most cases an aetiological factor cannot be identified and prognosis is generally poor. The most common variety is dilated or congestive cardiomyopathy.

Clinical features of congestive cardiomyopathy

Most patients present with congestive cardiac failure and a history of effort dyspnoea, fatigue, and orthopnoea. Occasionally children present with syncope and sometimes with signs of systemic embolization from intracardiac mural thrombosis. Hemiplegia, loss of consciousness, or sudden death from cardiac arrhythmia or cerebral embolus occur.

Examination reveals distended neck veins (often with a large 'A' wave followed by a sharp 'Y' descent), peripheral oedema, hepatomegaly and in long-standing cases, ascites and pleural effusions. The pulse pressure is often reduced due to peripheral vasoconstriction raising the diastolic pressure. Pulsus alternans may be present, indicating a severely compromised myocardium or there may be atrial fibrillation. The apex is usually displaced towards the axilla and is left ventricular in type, but not over-active. The heart sounds are usually soft and a triple or gallop rhythm due to a third heart sound is common. Cardiac murmurs are usually absent, but in grossly enlarged hearts there may be dilatation of the mitral and/or tricuspid rings causing incompetence of the valves. Accordingly, pansystolic murmurs may be heard, which diminish or disappear with treatment of heart failure.

The ECG, although not specific, is always abnormal. There may be left axis deviation. T-wave inversion on the left-sided leads is common and there may be evidence of left ventricular hypertrophy. Large, wide P waves indicate biatrial enlargement. Arrhythmias may occur; atrial or ventricular ectopics and atrial fibrillation are not uncommon. Occasionally there may be evidence of the Wolff-Parkinson-White (W-P-W) syndrome, i.e. a short PR interval with a prolonged QRS complex due to a 'delta' wave. The chest X-ray usually shows a grossly enlarged heart with pulmonary congestion. Occasionally the heart is not markedly enlarged and the term 'restrictive cardiomyopathy' has been used to describe these cases.

Treatment of cardiac failure

(*See* Rheumatic heart disease: congestive cardiac failure, *above*)

Differential diagnosis

Acute myocarditis, pericarditis, and rheumatic fever can usually be excluded on clinical, ECG, and X-ray features, but echocardiography may be necessary to differentiate pericardial effusion from cardiomyopathy. Pericardial paracentesis to confirm an effusion should not be undertaken without ECG control.

Cardiac failure due to severe anaemia or acute glomerulonephritis must also be excluded by appropriate investigations. An aberrant, left coronary artery arising from the pulmonary artery causes left ventricular hypoxaemia and ischaemia leading to heart failure. Characteristic ECG changes assist in the diagnosis.

Specific types of cardiomyopathy

Familial and congenital

Familial cardiomyopathy. A family history of cardiomyopathy or sudden death identifies this rare condition. Bundle branch block is an ECG feature.

Hypertrophic obstructive cardiomyopathy (HOCM). A family history of heart disease and sudden death is usual. There is symmetrical or asymmetrical hypertrophy of the myocardium affecting, particularly, the ventricular septum and papillary muscles, causing obstruction of the outflow tract and distortion of valves, especially on the left side. Systolic murmurs may be present. The ECG shows septal hypertrophy, left axis deviation, and bundle-branch block patterns.

Treatment with a beta-blocking agent (propranolol), together with a calcium channel blocker (verapamil), is often successful, but surgical removal of the obstructing muscle is sometimes necessary. Digoxin should not be used as it increases myocardial contractility.

Asymmetrical septal hypertrophy (ASH) can occur in infants born to diabetic mothers, particularly if control of the diabetes has been poor. If the baby is symptomatic, treatment is the same as for HOCM. ASH usually resolves in about six months.

Cardiomyopathy may be associated with **inherited disorders of the muscles and nerves**, e.g. Duchenne's muscular dystrophy, myotonia atrophica, and Friedreich's ataxia, in all of which it is often the cause of death. It also occurs in **disorders with deposition of abnormal substances**, e.g. mucopolysaccharides in Hurler's and Hunter's syndromes, and glycogen in Pompe's Type 2 glycogen storage disease.

Primary endocardial fibroelastosis (EFE) presents within the first two years of life with congestive cardiac failure. The disorder is confined to a greatly thickened endocardium, particularly in the left ventricle, which restricts contraction of the heart. Left ventricular hypertrophy is striking on the ECG and the heart size does not diminish with treatment, even though failure may be controlled. If the mitral valve is involved the characteristic pansystolic murmur of mitral incompetence will be heard. The cause of EFE has not been identified, but it is probably the result of fetal myocarditis.

Acquired cardiomyopathy

Cardiomyopathy of unknown origin is the most usual variety found in children and adults in southern Africa. The clinical features are those of congestive cardiomyopathy, and the course is one of repeated episodes of cardiac failure and multiple embolic episodes resulting in early death. Postmortem examination of the heart shows dilatation and hypertrophy without fibrosis. Adherent thrombus may be present on the endocardium of the left ventricle.

Endomyocardial fibrosis is a common cause of heart failure in central Africa and sporadic cases have been described from other parts of the world. Incompetence of the mitral and tricuspid valves is more common in this type of cardiomyopathy, but emboli are rare. Fibrosis of the endocardium of both ventricles, with involvement of the valves, is the outstanding pathological feature. In some cases the cavity of the right ventricle is almost completely obliterated.

Beriberi due to thiamine deficiency causes a high output cardiac failure with tachycardia, a large pulse pressure, dilated pulsating forearm veins, and warm extremities (low output failure with orthopnoea and oliguria has also been described). Neurological signs of thiamine deficiency, peripheral neuropathy, nystagmus and encephalopathy, as well as signs of malnutrition will also be present. Beriberi is found in children fed exclusively on a diet of polished rice and the cardiac dysfunction is dramatically cured by treatment with thiamine 50 to 100 mg IM daily, together with digoxin and a diuretic.

Chagas' disease occurs in South and Central America where it is caused by the parasite *Trypanosoma cruzi*. Infestation of children, particularly in the first year of life, may cause an acute interstitial myocarditis which heals by fibrosis, causing chronic myocardial dysfunction associated with hypertrophy and arrhythmias. Effective treatment is not available and the prognosis in children is poor.

HIV cardiomyopathy. This can present in various ways, most commonly as a congestive cardiomyopathy. This may be evident clinically, or only discovered at autopsy. Damage to the cardiac conduction system has been reported, as well as the presence of pericardial effusions. An arteriopathy involving small- and medium-sized arteries (heart, lungs, kidneys, spleen, intestine, brain) has also been documented.

Infective endocarditis

This is a serious infection of the endocardium, usually caused by organisms lodging on previously abnormal valves. It is an uncommon disease and may be seen in about 1 out of 4 600 hospital in-patients.

Changing pattern of the disease

Since the classic accounts by Osler and Horder at the turn of the previous century, the pattern of this disease has altered among children in developed countries. The spectrum has been shifting from the subacute to the acute form. This has been attributed to the more frequent use of antibiotics. Whereas *Streptococcus viridans* used to be the cause in the vast majority of cases, its importance has decreased. Despite this, it is still the most frequently isolated organism in this disease. Congenital heart disease has replaced rheumatic fever as the main cause of susceptibility to endocarditis. Children who have undergone open-heart surgery are particularly at risk.

Aetiology

Staphylococci and streptococci account for more than 90 per cent of cases in most parts of the world. In South Africa, *Staphylococcus aureus* is the most common cause of infective endocarditis in black children. The source of staphylococci is probably the skin, but may occasionally be other sites. *S. viridans* infection follows dental extractions or other oropharyngeal surgery.

Underlying cardiac disease. In Africa, this infection occurs predominantly in valves damaged by rheumatic fever. This is not unexpected as rheumatic heart disease is widely prevalent, is severe, and requires cardiac surgery at a young age.

Occasionally there is no pre-existing heart lesion, with the infection occurring on a normal tricuspid or mitral valve.

Clinical features of infective endocarditis

The cardinal features are due to infection, cardiac abnormalities, and immune complexes/embolism. The full-blown picture, which is rarely seen, includes fever, anaemia, clubbing, murmurs, cardiac failure, splenomegaly, petechiae, purpura, Roth's spots (haemorrhagic areas with white centre in retina), absent pulses, splinter haemorrhages under the nails, Osler's nodes (tender red nodules in finger pulp), Janeway's lesions (painless haemorrhagic areas in palms and soles), and haematuria and proteinuria. Fever and anaemia occur early in the disease while splinter haemorrhages, Osler's nodes, and Janeway's lesions are late features.

Affected African children are usually seven to ten years old and the most frequent features are fever, murmurs, and anaemia. The remaining signs described above are uncommon. Glomerulonephritis is sometimes a serious problem in *S. aureus* endocarditis. Neurological complications can be severe, due to septic emboli in the brain.

Diagnosis

A high index of suspicion must be maintained in those with pyrexia of unknown origin and in patients with rheumatic or congenital heart disease who have fever and anaemia. Positive blood cultures confirm the diagnosis, but sometimes these can be negative. If in doubt, treat!

Prognosis

The mortality is lowest for *S. viridans* and greatest for *S. aureus*. Depending on which organism predominates, the average mortality is between 17 and 60 per cent.

Treatment

Preventive measures include attention to skin sepsis and antibiotic cover (penicillin) during surgery (especially to the oropharynx, ears, and nose) in children with any heart lesion. (*See* Table 27.5 for details.)

Choice of antibiotics for cure depends on sensitivity of the organism. Useful combinations (intravenous) are penicillin and gentamicin or amikacin (for *S. viridans*), and cloxacillin, together with gentamicin or amikacin, (for *S. aureus*). Minimum duration of treatment is six weeks.

Miscellaneous cardiac disorders

Myocarditis

Myocarditis can occur at any age and is caused by a variety of viral infections. A newborn infant may be infected if the mother has pleurodynia due to a coxsackie B virus and epidemics have occurred in nurseries when the infection has spread to other infants.

Infants present with cardiac failure, tachypnoea, and tachycardia being the earliest features. Older children may complain of precordial pain. A loud third heart sound is heard at the apex, there is generalized cardiomegaly on the chest X-ray, with pulmonary congestion, and the ECG shows inversion of T waves in leads 1, V5, and V6. Treatment aims at control of cardiac failure with digoxin and a diuretic.

Pericarditis

Three types of pericarditis are recognized in children.

Dry pericarditis

Here a fibrinous exudate involves both layers of the pericardium. This type often presents with pain in the epigastrium or over the lower chest. A squeaky friction rub is heard in about half the cases. This is best heard at the left sternal border when the child is sitting, and is accentuated by pressing on the chest with the stethoscope.

Pericardial effusion

This may be serous, haemorrhagic, or purulent. There may be epigastric pain and dyspnoea is common. A friction rub may be heard and the heart sounds are muffled. The area of cardiac dullness is increased. Cardiac tamponade occurs if an effusion collects rapidly, compressing the heart and obstructing diastolic filling. The pulse is rapid and there is a small pulse pressure with pulsus paradoxus. The jugular venous pressure is greatly elevated and the liver is distended and tender. Pleural effusions are commonly found in children with pericarditis.

Constrictive pericarditis

This usually follows a pericardial effusion with the heart shadow becoming smaller. There is distension of the neck veins and liver, often with ascites. A diastolic 'beat' is felt medial to the apex due to rapid filling of the constricted ventricle and there is pulsus paradoxus.

Causes of pericarditis

Rheumatic fever may cause either dry pericarditis or pericardial effusion when it is most often associated with a pancarditis. Other features of rheumatic fever will usually suggest the diagnosis. It does not cause constrictive pericarditis.

Tuberculosis is the most common cause of pericardial effusion in endemic areas, but it may also cause a dry pericarditis and become constrictive. The effusion may be straw-coloured or bloodstained. Diagnosis is made by aspiration of the fluid and tuberculin testing. (*See* Chapter 17, Tuberculosis.)

Viral infections may be associated with any type of pericarditis. The onset is abrupt, usually following an upper respiratory infection. There may be precordial or epigastric pain.

Bacterial infections with staphylococci, streptococci, pneumococci or *Haemophilus influenzae* can cause a purulent pericarditis. Other sites of infection, e.g. osteitis or trauma, are often present and are particularly associated with staphylococci.

Amoebic pericarditis results from rupture of a liver abscess into the pericardial sac.

Malignant lymphomas in the mediastinum may cause both pericardial and pleural effusions.

Treatment

This depends on the cause. Pericarditis due to rheumatic fever responds dramatically to treatment with prednisone and does not require aspiration. Effusions should be aspirated once to establish the diagnosis and tamponade must always be relieved by aspiration. Tuberculous pericarditis is treated with isoniazid, ethionamide, and/or rifampicin. Purulent pericarditis requires repeated aspiration or surgical drainage, as well as appropriate antibiotic treatment. Constrictive pericarditis may complicate tuberculous and amoebic pericarditis. In these cases surgical stripping of the pericardium is required.

Arteritis

Takayasu's disease (or pulseless disease)

(*See* Chapter 21, Immune and connective tissue disorders.)

Congenital coarctation of the aorta is relatively uncommon in African children and will be symptomatic within the first month of life. Thus aortic arteritis should be suspected in older infants and children presenting with upper limb hypertension and poor leg pulses, especially if they are in CCF.

Kawasaki disease

(*See* Chapter 21, Immune and connective tissue disorders.)

Aneurysms of the proximal portions of the coronary arteries may occur in 20–25 per cent of cases. Deaths are due to myocardial infarction or myocarditis in 2 per cent of patients.

Pulmonary hypertension

(Not due to congenital heart disease.)

Chronic upper airway obstruction

Severe upper airway obstruction may be caused by very large tonsils and adenoids, resulting in chronic hypoxaemia which causes reflex constriction of the pulmonary arterioles. These children present in right heart failure and are recognized by their noisy breathing. They also snore loudly when asleep.

Treatment of cardiac failure with digoxin, diuretics, and oxygen, followed by removal of the tonsils and adenoids results in complete cure.

Bilharzia

Schistosomal infestation of the bladder and/or bowel may be complicated by embolization of ova to the lungs, causing both obstructive and reactive pulmonary arteriolitis which proceeds to fibrosis. This cause of pulmonary hypertension produces unremitting right heart failure and death. The diagnosis is presumptive in a child with schistosomiasis, but can be confirmed by lung biopsy.

Cor pulmonale

(*See also* Chapter 25, Respiratory disorders.)
This can occur following on chronic lung damage secondary to measles and adenovirus infections, or with cystic fibrosis in Caucasians. It has also been recently described in children with HIV/AIDS who present with progressive nodular and interstitial pulmonary disease.

Persistent pulmonary hypertension of the newborn (persistent fetal circulation syndrome)

(*See also* Chapter 7, Care of the newborn.)
This problem usually occurs in full-term or post-date neonates appropriate for gestational age. There may be a history of meconium staining and/or birth asphyxia, as well as maternal risk factors such as increased maternal age, pre-eclampsia, Caesarian section, precipitous delivery, polyhydramnios, or diabetes.

The baby usually has signs of respiratory distress and is cyanosed soon after birth. The blood pressure may be normal or decreased. There is a right ventricular heave, and on auscultation there is a pansystolic murmur of tricuspid incompetence best heard at the fourth left interspace. There may even be signs of congestive cardiac failure. The ECG may display evidence of right ventricular and/or right atrial hypertrophy with ischaemic changes. A chest radiograph will show cardiomegaly.

These infants are often difficult to distinguish from those with cyanotic congenital heart disease. They should be referred to a specialist centre, where echocardiography will resolve the problem. Treatment includes hyperventilation with the aid of a ventilator, additional oxygen, and correction of metabolic acidosis to induce pulmonary arteriolar vasodilatation.

Arrhythmias

Paroxysmal supraventricular tachycardia

This is the most common arrhythmia. Infants present with pallor, diminished activity, and difficulty in finishing their feeds. Often there is a precipitating febrile illness, e.g. urinary tract infection. Older children complain of suddenly feeling their heart beat faster, together with weakness. Examination reveals a heart rate in excess of 240/min. Attacks may stop as abruptly as they start; without treatment. ECG will show tachycardia with P waves followed by normal QRS complexes.

Infants require digitalization and treatment of any precipitating causative illness.

In older children the tachycardia may be stopped as abruptly as it started by pressing on the right carotid artery or the eyeball, or by getting the child to perform the Valsalva manoeuvre. These manoeuvres are rarely successful in infants and eyeball pressure must never be used as it may result in detachment of the retina. A cold (ice) pack to the face can be tried in these babies.

If available, adenosine can be given IV starting at 50 mcg/kg and increasing by 50 mcg/kg increments every two minutes up to a maximum of 250 mcg/kg.

If medical treatment fails, electrical (DC) conversion is recommended: 2–4 J/kg.

Atrial flutter

Atrial flutter may be present at birth causing congestive cardiac failure. It has been diagnosed in utero by the finding of fetal tachycardia before labour commences. The ECG shows typical flutter waves instead of P waves. Treatment is with digoxin. If the flutter is resistant to medical therapy, electrical conversion is indicated: 2–4 J/kg.

Congenital heart block

This presents at birth and is suspected if an otherwise normal infant has bradycardia, i.e. less than 100/min. The diagnosis is confirmed by the ECG which shows an atrial rate faster than the ventricular rate. The QRS complexes are usually of normal duration (<0.10 sec). If Stokes-Adams attacks or severe congestive cardiac failure occur, an artificial pacemaker is required.

There is a frequent association between congenital heart block and maternal systemic lupus erythematous. Therefore the mothers of affected infants should be routinely checked for specific antibodies (Anti-Rho and Anti-La).

Cardiac arrest

Asystole accounts for 90 per cent of cases, the

other 10 per cent being caused by ventricular fibrillation. The only way to differentiate is by ECG.

Management

- Establish a clear airway and give artificial ventilation, 20–30 breaths a minute, with 100 per cent oxygen from a bag via a face mask or by endotracheal intubation (mouth-to-mouth ventilation if equipment is not available).
- Give external cardiac massage simultaneously. For infants, the operator's hands should be placed on either side of the chest and the infant's sternum compressed by both thumbs at a rate of 80–100/min.
- Give sodium bicarbonate, 2 mEq/kg body weight IV, to counteract metabolic acidosis.
- Check serum electrolytes and correct hypokalaemia and/or hypocalcaemia.
- If ECG reveals ventricular fibrillation, electrical defibrillation is necessary.

29

Hepatic disorders

The liver is the largest gland in the human body and plays a primary role in homeostasis.

- It stores nutrients and regulates levels of circulating nutrients (e.g. amino acids, glucose).
- It excretes waste products into the bile (e.g. bilirubin, drugs, toxins).
- It reduces circulating ammonia through production of urea.
- It produces a battery of important serum proteins (e.g. albumin, clotting factors).
- It produces bile acids required in digestion of lipids.
- It acts as the primary site of metabolic defence against carcinogens that enter through the gastrointestinal tract.

The clinical manifestations of liver dysfunction arise from cell damage and impairment of the normal liver functions. There may be acute disease with jaundice, enlargement of the liver, a change in stool or urine colour or features of liver failure with encephalopathy and bleeding diathesis. Chronic liver disease can manifest with failure to thrive, abdominal distension, hepatosplenomegaly and ascites or evidence of portal hypertension, or with non-specific signs such as oedema or finger clubbing.

Hepatomegaly and splenomegaly

The presence of a palpable liver does not always represent liver enlargement. Lung pathology such as asthma may displace the liver and spleen downwards without enlargement of the organs. Hepatomegaly is determined on the basis of liver span and the degree of extension below the right costal margin. The spleen is the largest separate lymphoid organ in the body. Splenomegaly is usually caused by systemic disease and not by primary splenic disease. There is a long list of possible causes of hepatosplenomegaly. (*see* Tables 29.1 and 29.2)

The history and clinical examination may suggest the possible cause of the enlarged liver and spleen. A history of maternal HIV, exposure to tuberculosis, familial inherited metabolic or haematological disorders raises suspicion of these conditions. Generalised lymphadenopathy may suggest reticuloendothelial hyperplasia as the cause of hepatosplenomegaly. In the inflammatory group, jaundice is often present. Examination of the cardiovascular system is essential to exclude the possibility of congestive cardiac failure or constrictive pericarditis resulting in venous congestion. The Budd-Chiari syndrome is characterized by marked ascites and the absence of filling of the jugular veins with pressure over the liver. A liver abscess is suggested by local tenderness and swelling in an acutely ill child. A bleeding tendency, lymphadenopathy, severe or unusual infections, and anaemia, may indicate an infiltrative process involving the liver and possibly the spleen. Storage diseases often are associated with an abnormal appearance, neurological signs, and marked firm enlargement of liver or spleen. The smooth, firm appearance of fatty infiltration of the liver is typical of kwashiorkor. Malnutrition is one of the most common causes of hepatomegaly in childhood in southern Africa.

Table 29.1 Causes of hepatomegaly

Inflammation	**Vascular congestion**
Infections	Congestive heart failure
Neonatal and congenital infection	Budd-Chiari syndrome
Viral infection involving the liver	Veno-occlusive disease
Bacterial infection and tuberculosis	
Parasitic infection	**Infiltration**
Immune and auto-immune liver disease	**Extramedullary haematopoiesis**
Drug and toxin mediated inflammation	Hepatoblastoma
	Haemangioendothelioma
Reticuloendothelial hyperplasia	Metastatic disease
HIV disease	Neuroblastoma
Septicaemia	Lymphoma
Granulomatous diseases	Leukaemia
	Histiocytosis
Storage and metabolic disorders	
Glycogen storage diseases	**Fat accumulation**
Lipid storage diseases	Malnutrition
Mucopolysaccharidoses	Hyperalimentation
Amyloidosis	Uncontrolled diabetes mellitus
Metals: Copper (Wilson's disease), iron (hemochromatosis)	Steatohepatitis
	Hepatotoxic drugs
Metabolic disorders, e.g. galactosaemia, tyrosinaemia	Reye's syndrome
	Fatty acid oxidation defects,
Biliary obstruction	
Biliary atresia	**Miscellaneous**
Alagille syndrome	Subcapsular haematoma
Cystic fibrosis	
Primary sclerosing cholangitis	
Inspissated bile syndrome	
Choledochal cyst	

Diagnosis

In many cases the diagnosis can be made clinically and confirmed by relatively simple, directed laboratory investigations.

Laboratory tests include haematological, biochemical, immunological, microbiological and serological investigations to identify dysfunction, aetiology and complications.

Imaging investigations include ultrasonography and Doppler flow ultrasound, chest radiographs, CT and nuclear scintigraphy to assess the anatomical and pathological status.

Bone marrow and liver biopsy are indicated for histological and occasionally microbiological diagnosis.

Cholestasis in infancy

Cholestasis occurs because of a reduction in canalicular bile flow and manifests as conjugated hyperbilirubinaemia. The differential diagnosis of an infant with cholestasis presents an interesting challenge to the physician (*see* Table 29.3).

Cholestasis is defined by a conjugated bilirubin fraction greater than 20 per cent of the total bilirubin. Prompt diagnosis enables early surgical intervention or specific medical therapy where available.

Table 29.2 Causes of splenomegaly

Spleen palpable in normal children 15–30% of neonates 10% of healthy children 5% of adolescents	**Haemolytic anaemias** Hereditary spherocytosis Haemoglobinopathies
Infection/inflammation Viral (Hepatitis A, B, C, EBV, CMV, HIV) Bacterial (SBE, tuberculosis, Salmonella) Protozoal infection (malaria and schistosomiasis)	**Extramedullary haematopoiesis** e.g. Thalassaemia major **Malignancy** Leukaemia Lymphoma
Congestive Chronic congestive heart failure Constrictive pericarditis Portal hypertension from chronic liver disease Portal or splenic venous thrombosis	**Storage/Infiltrative disorders** Histiocytosis Lipidoses (e.g., Niemann-Pick, Gaucher) Mucopolysaccharidoses (e.g., Hurler, Hunter)
Immune-mediated inflammation Rheumatoid arthritis Inflammatory bowel disease Coeliac disease	**Structural** Haematoma (trauma) Cysts or pseudocysts

Table 29.3 Causes of conjugated hyperbilirubinaemia in infants

Extrahepatic disorders ▪ Biliary atresia ▪ Choledochal cyst ▪ Mass (stone/neoplasia) ▪ Bile plug syndrome ▪ Neonatal sclerosing cholangitis	**Hepatitis from toxic exposure:** ▪ Parenteral nutrition-associated cholestasis ▪ Drug induced
Intrahepatic cholestatic disorders ▪ Idiopathic neonatal hepatitis ▪ Persistent intrahepatic cholestasis ▪ Syndromic or non-syndromic paucity of bile ducts **Anatomic** ▪ Congenital hepatic fibrosis ▪ Caroli's disease (cystic dilatation of intrahepatic ducts)	**Metabolic disorders** ▪ Disorders of amino acid metabolism, e.g. tyrosinaemia ▪ Storage disorders: neonatal haemochromatosis, infantile copper overload ▪ Disorders of metabolism, e.g. carbohydrate (galactosaemia, glycogen storage disease), lipids (Nieman Pick, Gaucher's disease) ▪ Cystic fibrosis ▪ α–1 antitrypsin deficiency
Hepatitis from infection: ▪ Viral: Cytomegalovirus, Herpes simplex virus, HIV, hepatitis virus, congenital rubella ▪ Bacterial: Urinary tract infection (especially *E.coli*), sepsis, congenital syphilis ▪ Protozoal: *Toxoplasma gondii*	**Miscellaneous** ▪ Hypothyroidism ▪ Shock/ hypoperfusion ▪ Chromosomal disorders, e.g. Trisomy 21

It is also important to institute effective nutritional and medical support as early as possible, to allow for optimal growth and development.

Clinical features

Infants present with jaundice, often present from the neonatal period. On examination there is usually hepatosplenomegaly. Infants with biliary atresia may be well nourished if they present early, whereas those with congenital infections tend to be growth retarded. Associated congenital heart disease or dysmorphic features suggests congenital infections, Alagille syndrome and biliary atresia. Eye examination is important to exclude cataracts, chorioretinitis, or posterior embryotoxon. Examination of the stool and urine will assist in differentiating the acholic, pale stool of biliary atresia from the yellow, pigmented stool found in conditions with patency of the extrahepatic biliary system. When presentation is delayed, the infant may not only demonstrate sequelae of cholestasis but also those of cirrhosis and portal hypertension (*see* Figure 29.1)

Diagnosis

The first priority is to identify treatable conditions. For this reason thyroid function tests, serology for syphilis, reducing substances in the urine for galactosaemia, and urine and blood cultures are a priority. After this, patients should be referred early to a specialist centre for a full diagnosis. The majority of infants fall into the diagnostic category of either biliary atresia or neonatal hepatitis. A number of investigations are available to help differentiate between these two main conditions (*see* Table 29.4)

Ultrasonography

This is essential to evaluate the liver and biliary tract. An inability to visualize the gall bladder is suggestive of biliary atresia. Dilated intra- and/or extra-hepatic ducts are suggestive of a choledochal cyst.

Hepatobiliary scintigraphy (HIDA)

Hepatic uptake and excretion of isotope into bile depends on the integrity of hepatocellular function and biliary tract patency. Hepatobiliary scintigraphy will document biliary patency and define any abnormal dilatation in the biliary tree.

Liver biopsy

This is the most reliable and definitive procedure in the evaluation of the cholestatic infant. The degree and pattern of fibrosis will identify incipient or established cirrhosis.

Biliary atresia

This accounts of about one third of cases of neonatal cholestasis and is caused by an idiopathic inflammatory process resulting in fibro-obliteration of the bile ducts. Aside from

Table 29.4 Approach to an infant with persistent jaundice

Step 1 Differentiate unconjugated or conjugated hyperbilirubinaemia as cause of jaundice
- Conjugated bilirubin >20% of total bilirubin – conjugated hyperbilirubinaemia
- Unconjugated hyperbilirubinaemia: Haemolysis or defective conjugation: Investigate further to determine aetiology

Step 2 Investigate conjugated hyperbilirubinaemia as follows:

	Idiopathic neonatal hepatitis	Biliary atresia
Stool collection	Yellow pigmented stools	White, acholic stools
Sonar	Gall bladder seen	Gall bladder absent
Laboratory investigations	AST, ALT raised	GGT, ALP raised
Step 3	Refer	Urgent referral required
HIDA scan	Excretion of tracer into gut	No excretion of tracer into gut
Liver biopsy	Giant cells	Bile duct proliferation

jaundice these infants do not appear ill. Laboratory tests show conjugated hyperbilirubinaemia and the enzymes alkaline phosphatase (ALP) and γ-glutamyltransferase (GGT) raised to more than five times normal with only mildly elevated transaminases. Liver biopsy reveals bile duct proliferation, bile plugs and in some cases already established biliary cirrhosis.

Untreated, the life expectancy is less than two years. Surgical management involves a Kasai porto-enterostomy, the success of which depends on age at presentation and the size of the bile duct remnants. The optimal age at surgery is under 60 days, with the success rate decreasing to less than 20 per cent in infants operated on after three months of age. Post-operative complications include ascending cholangitis. If surgical drainage is not performed successfully early, progression to cirrhosis and liver failure is inevitable. Despite surgery the majority will eventually require transplantation.

Idiopathic neonatal hepatitis

This makes up 30–35 per cent of neonatal cholestasis. The infants usually have low birth weight and more than 50 per cent present with jaundice in the first week of life. Hepatomegaly and/or splenomegaly may be present. The stools are usually pigmented. The serum transaminases are elevated 2 –10 times normal with normal or mildly elevated ALP and GGT. The presence of

multinucleated giant cells (fused hepatocytes) on liver biopsy is characteristic. Management involves nutritional support and vitamin supplementation. These infants have a good prognosis overall, with spontaneous resolution occurring in most cases. The rest progress to cirrhosis and portal hypertension.

Galactosaemia

This is an autosomal recessive condition caused by deficiency of the enzyme galactose-1-phosphate uridyl transferase (GALT) which is involved in the conversion of galactose to glucose. Common symptoms and signs include vomiting, poor weight gain, jaundice, cataracts, hypotonia and encephalopathy. Liver dysfunction and renal tubular dysfunction can be the presenting features. Diagnosis is made by identifying reducing substances in the urine and confirming with a GALT assay in the blood. Treatment involves lifelong exclusion of galactose in the diet.

Management of cholestatic jaundice of infancy

Treatable causes such as syphilis and urinary tract infection are managed appropriately. In some cases no definite cause for the hepatitis will be determined and management will be supportive, e.g. vitamin and mineral supplements.

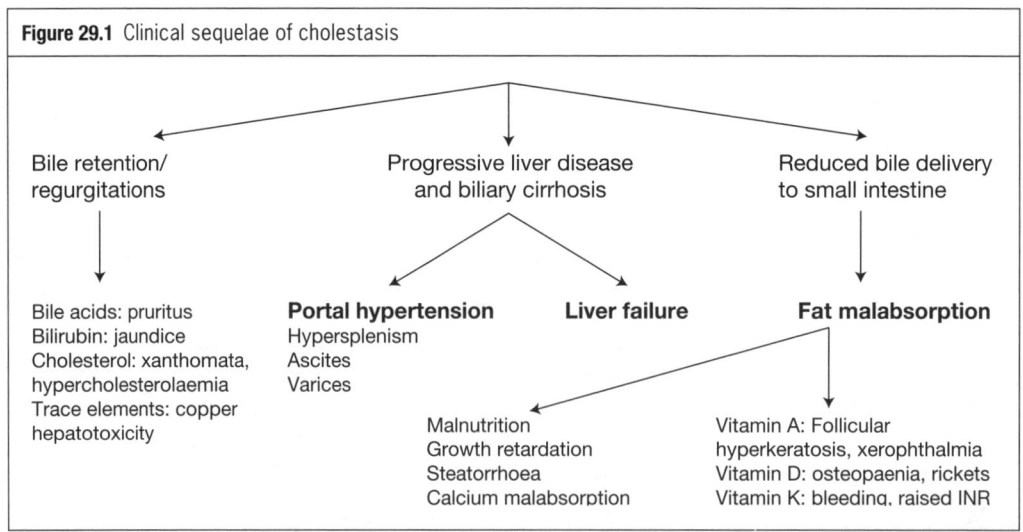

Figure 29.1 Clinical sequelae of cholestasis

The aim of medical management of cholestasis is to prevent nutritional deficiencies accompanying intraluminal bile salt insufficiency, to enhance or stimulate bile flow, to treat complications of disease such as ascites and to treat infections promptly with broad spectrum antibiotics.

Energy intake should be 150 per cent of the recommended daily allowance for height and age, to allow for catch-up growth. A diet containing fat with more than 40 per cent medium chain triglycerides should be used to maximize fat absorption in the face of cholestasis. Protein intake is only restricted in hepatic encephalopathy. Fat soluble vitamins A, D E and K must be given in high doses, and water soluble vitamins are given at twice the recommended doses. Minerals such as zinc and phosphate are also supplemented. Choleretic agents such as rifampicin, phenobarb and ursodeoxycholic acid are used to manage the pruritus.

The child and adolescent with acute-onset jaundice

The aetiology of acute jaundice in the older child and adolescent is different to that discussed in the infant and neonate. In most cases the history will be non-contributory but the following may give a clue to the possible aetiology. Exposure to blood transfusion and blood products or recent contact with Hepatitis A or B is suggestive of viral hepatitis. Exposure to drugs for the treatment of tuberculosis, epilepsy or HIV may be significant. Herbal medication taken either orally or in the form of an enema may be responsible for the acute onset of jaundice. A previous history of jaundice and liver disease suggests pre-existing chronic disease.

Clinical features

Differentiate between the acutely ill jaundiced child and the jaundiced child who appears well. The acutely ill child may have fulminant hepatic failure, sepsis, acute cholangitis, metabolic or toxic liver disease. The child who looks well will often have acute infectious hepatitis as a result of hepatitis A. Sore throat, fever and lymphadenopathy suggest infectious mononucleosis. Growth retardation and de-layed onset of puberty is often an indication of cryptogenic cirrhosis. Hepatosplenomegaly is relatively non-specific. Hard hepatomegaly and clubbing suggest the presence of underlying cirrhosis. Massive hepatomegaly suggests Budd-Chiari syndrome, severe right-sided heart failure, or neoplasm of the liver.

Diagnosis

The child who appears healthy with jaundice should have limited special investigations initially including full blood count, liver function tests, INR and hepatitis A and B serology. Unconjugated hyperbilirubinaemia indicates possibilities such as haemolysis or Gilbert's disease. Conjugated hyperbilirubinaemia is, in most cases, due to hepatitis A, or less commonly B. Other possibilities include viruses such as Epstein-Bar virus or cytomegalovirus, autoimmune hepatitis, gall stones, toxic substances, including drugs, and metabolic disorders (*see* Table 29.5)

Management

If the initial blood investigations do not indicate an aetiology and the jaundice persists, the patient should be referred for further investigations. The child who appears ill and encephalopathic, or has a bleeding tendency together with jaundice, is a medical emergency and should be admitted for management of the liver failure and investigation of the underlying condition.

Gallstones

Cholelithiasis is uncommon in infancy and childhood. Pigment stones and cholesterol stones are the predominant types of gall stones. Risk factors include underlying conditions such as haemolytic anaemias, haemoglobinopathies, congenital anomalies of the biliary tract, defects in bile salt synthesis, hypercholesterolaemia, cystic fibrosis, total parenteral nutrition, ileal disease or resection and Crohn's disease. Gall stones may be asymptomatic or present with biliary colic or acute cholecystitis. Most stones in children are radiolucent. Ultrasonography is the most sensitive and specific method to detect gall stones. Complicated gall stones require cholecystectomy.

Table 29.5 Causes of hepatitis in childhood

Infection	Drugs and Toxins
Viral	Toxins
Hepatitis A, B, C, D, E, G	Senecio alkaloids
Infectious mononucleosis (EBV*)	Aflatoxins
Cytomegalovirus	Amanita mushrooms
Herpes simplex	Organic solvents
Human immunodeficiency virus	Drugs
Parasitic	*Antimicrobials, e.g.*
Toxoplasma gondii	tetracyclines
Entamoeba histolytica	erythromycin
Schistosoma mansoni (bilharziasis)	ampicillin
Bacterial	sulphonamides
Leptospirosis	*Anti-tuberculous drugs*
Pyogenic bacteria	isoniazid
	rifampicin
	pyrazinamide
Physical agents	ethionamide
Burns	*Antiretroviral therapy e.g.*
Irradiation	nevirapine (NNRTI)*
Hypothermia	zidovudine (NRTI)*
	Cytotoxic and immunosuppressives
Metabolic disorders	methotrexate
Wilson's disease	azathioprine
Non-alcoholic steatohepatitis	cyclophosphamide
	Anticonvulsants
Miscellaneous	sodium valproate
Autoimmune hepatitis	carbamazepine
Reye's syndrome	*Analgesics and anti-inflammatory agents*
Ischaemic hepatitis	paracetamol
Cholangitis	salicylates
	phenylbutazone
	indomethacin
	Anaesthetic agents
	halothane

* EBV: Epstein-Barr virus; NNRTI: non-nucleoside reverse transcriptase inhibitor; NRTI: nucleoside reverse transcriptase inhibitor.

Hepatitis

The term hepatitis implies an inflammatory process of the liver. Histologically there is an inflammatory mononuclear cell infiltrate and varying degrees of damage to the hepatocytes. The latter may result in swollen hepatocytes with a granular appearance, shrinkage or loss of hepatocytes as indicated by disruption of the normal reticulin network. The overwhelming majority of children develop hepatitis as a result of infection with hepatitis A or B viruses.

Hepatitis A (HAV)

HAV is a small 27 nm cubic ribonucleic acid (RNA) virus classified as a picornavirus (*see* Figure 29.2). The liver is the principal site of viral replication.

HAV is spread by faecal-oral transmission via

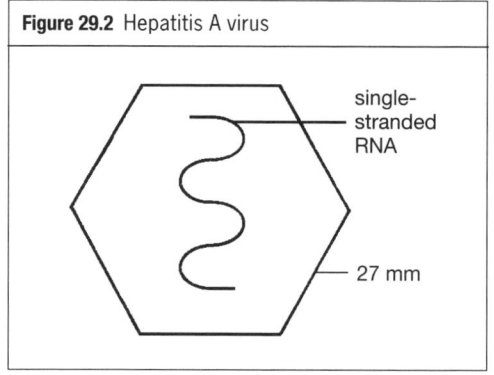

Figure 29.2 Hepatitis A virus

single-
stranded
RNA

27 mm

contaminated water supplies and foodstuffs. For this reason HAV infection is common among children in developing areas where there is inadequate sewerage disposal. By the age of six, 95 per cent of children in Africa have antibodies, as compared to less than 10 per cent of children in developed countries. The incubation period is usually two to four weeks. The virus multiplies in the liver and is shed via the bile into the stools within one to two weeks of exposure. Infectivity is maximal at the onset of the non-specific prodromal symptoms and before there is biochemical evidence of hepatitis. Hepatitis A IgM antibodies appear in the serum at this stage and result in a rapid fall in the concentration of the virus in the stool. IgG antibodies, which

Figure 29.3 Hepatitis A infection

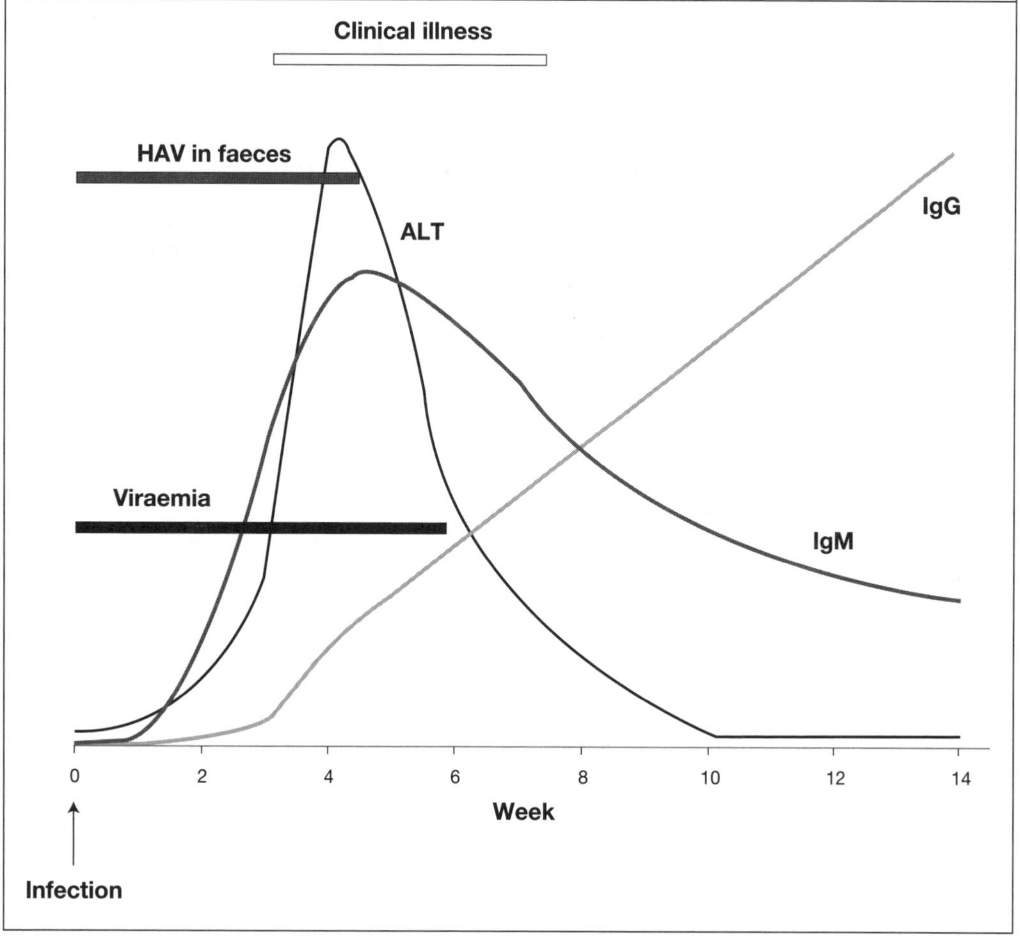

Clinical illness

HAV in faeces

ALT

IgG

Viraemia

IgM

0   2   4   6   8   10   12   14

Week

Infection

persist for many years, result in permanent immunity (*see* Figure 29.3)

Clinical features

The illness is usually mild, often anicteric and in young children is frequently asymptomatic. Prodromal symptoms include nausea, vomiting, diarrhoea, fever, and at times right upper quadrant abdominal pain. These are followed within a few days by the onset of jaundice. Symptoms tend to diminish as the jaundice peaks , heralding recovery. On examination there is a tender hepatomegaly in most patients and splenomegaly in about 30 per cent of patients. The urine is dark and the stools are pale if there is significant cholestasis. In the majority of cases jaundice resolves within two weeks. Only 10 per cent require hospitalization. Complications are rare, but fulminant hepatic failure is the most serious complication and has an incidence of about five per 1 000 cases. There is no chronic carrier state and immunity is lifelong.

Investigations

Liver function tests show a rise in serum transaminases a few days before the onset of jaundice and peak shortly afterwards 10–30 times above the normal levels. The serum alkaline phosphatase is usually only moderately elevated. Bilirubin levels rise and peak several days after the transaminases. The INR is usually normal and abnormality may indicate significant liver necrosis. The diagnosis is confirmed by the presence of IgM antibodies to HAV.

Management

As there is no specific treatment the management is supportive. Uncomplicated cases are best managed at home. The diet should be tailored to the child's own preferences to ensure an adequate intake of fluids and energy. Hepatitis A is a notifiable condition in South Africa.

Prevention

Since the majority of cases are asymptomatic and those that develop symptomatic hepatitis are most infective in the prodromal phase, it is impossible to identify and isolate all cases from the general population. For this reason it is imperative to ensure adequate sewage disposal, safe drinking water, and to encourage basic personal hygiene such as hand washing after defaecation and before handling food. School avoidance is advised during the period of infectivity. Travellers to endemic areas are advised to avoid drinking local water and improperly cooked food such as shellfish, fruit, salads.

Immunization

Passive immunization uses human immunoglobulin, which contains sufficient antibodies to HAV to give passive immunity for about three months, at a dose of 0.02–0.04 ml/kg. It is recommended for pre-exposure prophylaxis in travellers or for post-exposure prophylaxis in staff of day-care centres, prisons or army barracks. The immunoglobulin has to be given within two weeks of exposure; the earlier it is given the greater the efficacy.

Active immunization uses HAV vaccines. These vaccines are highly effective and are given as two doses six months apart in children over two years of age who are considered at increased risk from the infection, such as those with other chronic liver disease. The immunity is thought to last 10–20 years.

Hepatitis B (HBV)

Hepatitis B is a 42 nm spherical deoxyribonucleic acid (DNA) virus occurring primarily in humans. (Figure 29.4).The whole virus or Dane particle consists of an outer lipoprotein coat (hepatitis B surface antigen, HBsAg) and an inner nucleocapsid core (hepatitis B core antigen, HBcAg) which contains the viral DNA and a HBV-specific

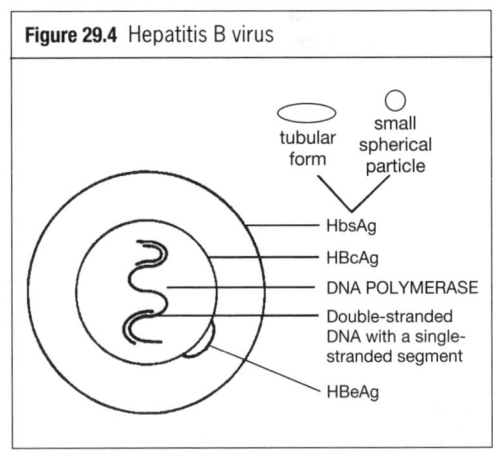

Figure 29.4 Hepatitis B virus

tubular form

small spherical particle

HbsAg

HBcAg

DNA POLYMERASE

Double-stranded DNA with a single-stranded segment

HBeAg

DNA polymerase. A soluble protein, hepatitis B 'e' antigen (HBeAg), is expressed during viral replication and is a marker of infectivity.

Epidemiology

Prior to the introduction of routine HBV vaccination, the disease was highly endemic in South Africa with 10–20 per cent of the population being chronic carriers. This is in contrast to first world countries such as the United Kingdom where the prevalence is 0.2 per cent. Routes of transmission in children include perinatal, parenteral, sexual and horizontal. Vertical transmission of HBV from an infected mother to her baby does occur, but horizontal transmission (e.g. child to child) is more important in South Africa. Dental work, ear piercing, tattooing and traditional healer scarification are other ways that people can acquire hepatitis B. The role of blood sucking insects such as mosquitoes in the transmission of HBV remains controversial. HBV can also be transmitted via other bodily secretions such as tears, saliva and breast milk. The peak incidence of HBV infection in African children is between the ages of two and eleven years. The incidence of hepatitis B among urban black children in Soweto, Johannesburg, has shown a decline, indicating the positive effect of urbanization and immunization. The fact that HBV produces chronic carriers results in a pool of infectious individuals who can infect the rest of the community.

Clinical features

The clinical features of the infection depend to a large extent on the immune response of the patient. The incubation period varies between 60 and 180 days. The majority of acute infections in children are asymptomatic. There may only be symptoms suggestive of a minor 'flu'-like illness, or the infection may present as an acute hepatitis with jaundice or in 1 per cent of cases as acute fulminant hepatitis with liver failure. Five to 10 percent will go on to develop cirrhosis. Clinical features found in adults, such as arthralgia and skin rashes are not commonly associated with HBV infection in children.

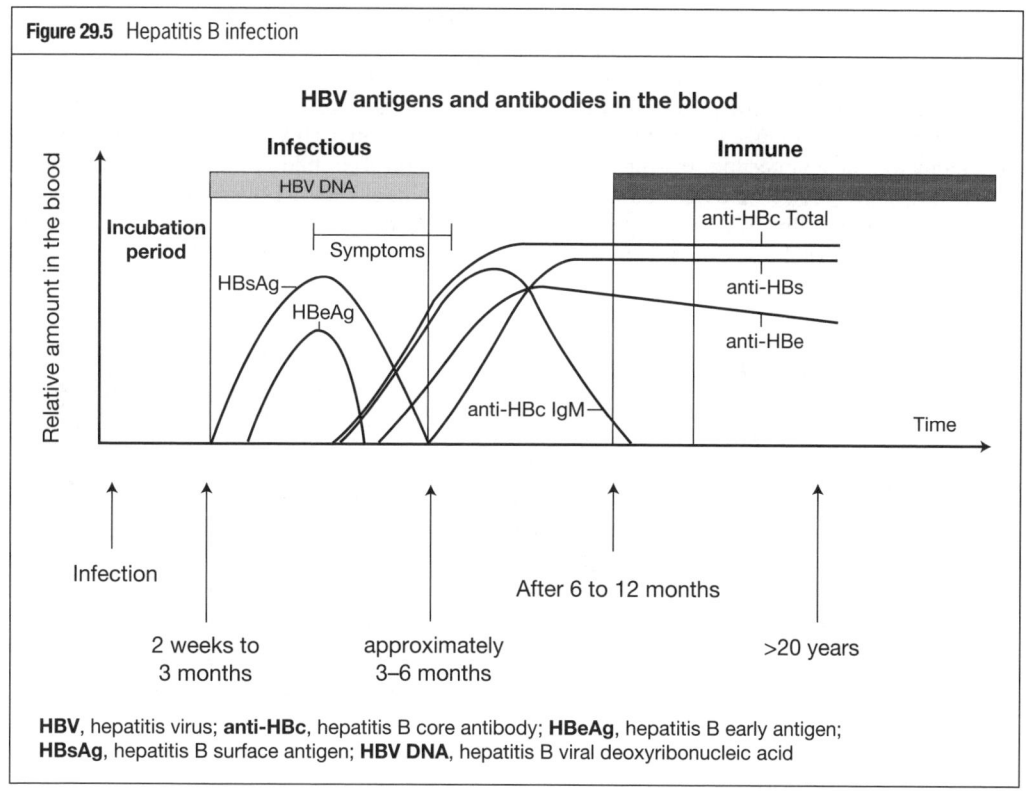

Figure 29.5 Hepatitis B infection

HBV, hepatitis virus; **anti-HBc**, hepatitis B core antibody; **HBeAg**, hepatitis B early antigen; **HBsAg**, hepatitis B surface antigen; **HBV DNA**, hepatitis B viral deoxyribonucleic acid

Complications

Numerous complications include a chronic carrier state, with 20–30 per cent at risk of developing hepatocellular carcinoma. The tumour does occur in childhood but is unusual.

Chronic hepatitis may follow an acute episode, but often is detected incidentally due to the presence of HBsAg in the blood. Infection at an early age is more likely to result in chronic disease. Clinically the patient may be asymptomatic, or present with fatigue, failure to thrive, cirrhosis or portal hypertension.

Extra-hepatic manifestations such as glomerulonephritis may result from HBV-circulating immune complexes. These children develop a membranous glomerulonephritis and present with nephrotic syndrome. Arthritis and pericarditis may also result from circulating immune complexes. Aplastic anaemia is a rare but often fatal complication.

Investigations

Liver function tests show raised tranasaminases and bilirubin. The relationship of these parameters to the clinical course is shown in Figure 29.5.

The INR is usually normal and abnormality indicates significant liver necrosis. The diagnosis of HBV infection is confirmed by the presence of HBV-related antigens and antibodies (*see* Table 29.6). In patients with acute infection, HBsAg, HBeAg, HBc IgM Ab, and HBV-specific DNA polymerase are present in the serum. The latter is the most sensitive marker of viral replication. HBeAb and HBsAb develop in those patients who overcome the infection and acquire permanent immunity to the virus. In certain individuals HBsAg, HBeAg, and HBV DNA polymerase activity persists in the serum and these patients are hepatitis B carriers. If a child remains HBsAg positive for six months, a liver biopsy is indicated. The histology may show features of chronic persistent hepatitis, chronic active hepatitis, or established cirrhosis.

Management

Acute infection with HBV is generally self-limiting and management is supportive. The risk of horizontal transmission is quite high in Africa and it is standard practice to isolate patients with acute hepatitis B. Currently available treatments for chronic infection include interferon alpha and the DNA polymerase-inhibiting agents, lamivudine and adefovir. The immediate goals of therapy are to suppress viral reproduction (eliminate HBeAg and HBV DNA in the blood) and improve liver tests (serum aminotransferases become normal). The ultimate goals are to prevent further liver injury, the progression towards cirrhosis, and thereby prevent the complications of cirrhosis, including liver carcinoma.

Prevention

Active immunization with a safe and effective vaccine against HBV is recommended for the protection of all children and newborns as well as for groups at high risk of acquiring the infection, such as those with occupational exposure to HBV, patients on haemodialysis, recipients of

Table 29.6 Markers of HBV infection and infectivity

Marker	Acute infection	Past infection	Carrier *High risk*	Carrier *Low risk*
HBsAg	Present	Absent	Present	Present
HBsAb	Absent	Present	Absent	Absent
HBeAg	Present	Absent	Present	Absent
HBeAb	Absent	Present	Absent	Present
HBcAb IgM+	Present	Absent	Absent	Absent
HbcAb IgG	Absent	Present	Present	Present
Liver enzymes	Increased	Normal	Mildly increased	Normal

+*Marker of active infection*
Refers to likelihood of transmitting the virus

blood or blood products, intravenous drug users and household members and sexual contacts of HBV carriers. Pre-natal screening of all pregnant women identifies HBV-positive mothers and enables preventive measures to be taken to protect their offspring. Both passive and active immunization are given to babies born to HBsAg positive mothers.

Vaccination of all newborns has been implemented in South Africa, as part of the routine immunization schedule since 1995, but at present high risk groups should also be targeted for immunization. Carriers pose a major problem for health professionals in southern Africa and all blood products and bodily secretions must be handled with utmost care. Improvement of general standards of hygiene will also serve to reduce the number of carriers in the community.

Immunization

Passive immunization with hepatitis B immune globulin, which contains high titres of HBsAb, is advised within hours of exposure to HBV. This is indicated in babies born to carrier mothers and after accidental needle prick or contamination of a wound or mucous membranes with infected material.

Hepatitis C (HCV)

Hepatitis C (HCV) is a single stranded RNA virus, which was first cloned in 1989 when it was identified as the major cause of post-transfusion hepatitis in adults and children. Currently only 0.5–1.5 per cent of cases are transfusion-related because of routine screening of all blood donors. Other modes of transmission include intravenous drug abuse, sexual, sporadic and vertical from infected mother to newborn baby. The risk of vertical transmission of HCV varies from 5–12 per cent. Transmission is higher in mothers with high titres of HCV RNA and in those who are HIV positive. Acute HCV infection is not seen and chronic HCV infection is uncommon in children.

The incubation period is between six and 12 weeks. Six genotypes are identified, of which subtypes 1b and 5a are prevalent in South Africa. The most useful screening test is the detection of anti-HCV IgG in the serum. HCV RNA identifies patients with persistent viraemia and is a reliable guide to infectivity at any age. It is also useful in determining response to therapy.

Adult studies indicate a high degree of chronicity, with up to 50 per cent developing progressive liver disease and 20 per cent developing cirrhosis 20–30 years after infection. In South Africa 12–15 per cent of hepatocellular carcinoma is associated with chronic hepatitis C infection. Most chronically infected children are asymptomatic with normal growth and development. There is usually little biochemical evidence of liver disease, but the majority will have chronic hepatic inflammation and progression to cirrhosis in later life.

A combination therapy of alpha interferon and ribavirin is currently available. The response corresponds to the viral genotype, with type 1b associated with poor results.

Hepatitis D or delta agent (HDV)

This is a small, incomplete RNA-containing virus, which requires HBV for infectivity and replication. It is transmitted parenterally. Children are susceptible, but infection is more common in adults. The diagnosis of HDV is based on the detection of HDV antigen or serology. HDV should be measured in known carriers of hepatitis B, as co-infection may lead to acute or fulminant hepatitis, or a more rapid progression of chronic hepatitis. Interferon therapy for chronic hepatitis B is also effective for HDV co-infection, but eradication of the disease is dependent on successful vaccination and prevention of hepatitis B worldwide.

Hepatitis E (HEV)

HEV is a RNA virus and is transmitted by the faecal-oral route. HEV is commonest in the 15–40 age group and can be a significant cause of fulminant hepatitis in endemic areas. Mortality is low except in pregnant women. Persistent viraemia and chronic hepatitis have not been reported. There is no specific treatment. Hepatitis E infection can be documented by PCR or serology. Anti-HEV seroprevalence in black South African adults ranges from 6.6 per cent in urban areas to 15.3 per cent in rural areas. Contaminated water plays a major role in HEV spread in South Africa.

Hepatitis G (HGV)

HGV is a single stranded RNA virus belonging

to the Flaviviridae family. It was first described in 1995–96 and is a cause of giant cell hepatitis. It is frequently found in co-infections with other viruses, such as HCV, HBV and HIV but is also found in normal children. There is currently no recommended treatment for Hepatitis G.

Chronic liver disease

Chronic hepatitis is a continuous inflammatory disease capable of progression to cirrhosis and liver failure. In children this is generally defined as lasting more than three months. Not all patients have a recognized initial acute episode, as many present for the first time with symptoms and signs of chronic liver disease.

Histologically, chronic hepatitis can be classified into chronic persistent and chronic active hepatitis. In chronic persistent hepatitis there is limitation of the inflammatory round cell infiltrate to the portal tract with no or minimal periportal necrosis. In chronic active hepatitis there is moderate to severe periportal necrosis with portoportal bridging fibrosis.

HBV is the major cause of chronic liver disease in most parts of the world. Other infections include HCV and CMV. Biliary atresia is a major cause in younger children. Other conditions include autoimmune hepatitis and steatohepatitis. Metabolic conditions include Wilson's disease, alpha-1-antitrypsin deficiency and cystic fibrosis. Certain drugs can also induce chronic hepatitis.

Autoimmune hepatitis

This is an inflammatory liver disease character-ized by the absence of a known aetiology and by the presence of a variety of tissue autoantibodies and increased concentrations of IgG. The disease is associated with the HLA B8-DR3 haplotype and notably responds to immunosuppressive therapy. The disease has two peaks of onset, peripubertally and between the fourth and sixth decades of life.

Clinical features

Clinical features can vary from asymptomatic or non-specific complaints such as weight loss, to acute hepatitis with liver failure or chronic disease with portal hypertension. At presen-tation most patients have jaundice, hepato-splenomegaly, and cutaneous features of chronic liver disease, such as spider angiomata, striae, acne, and palmar erythema. Extrahepatic mani-festations of the auto-immune process such as arthritis, glomerulonephritis or inflammatory bowel disease may be present.

Investigations

The bilirubin and liver transaminases are raised while there is hypoalbuminaemia and abnormal coagulation studies. The immunoglobulin frac-tion, particularly IgG, is raised. Auto-antibodies, such as smooth muscle antibody, liver kidney microsomal antibody, mitochondrial antibody and antinuclear antibody are often positive. Liver biopsy shows the presence of a plasma cell rich infiltrate extending from the portal tracts into the liver parenchyma, with piecemeal necrosis and portoportal bridging fibrosis.

Management

Initially steroids are commenced and the response is monitored by regular liver function tests. Immunosuppresants such as azathioprine are added if the response to steroids is inadequate or there is relapse on weaning the steroids. The aim is to control the inflammatory process with a minimum of side-effects. In a small percentage of patients treatment can be stopped after three to five years. However a significant number will eventually develop cirrhosis.

Cirrhosis

In patients with cirrhosis the normal liver architecture is destroyed and replaced by nodules of regenerating tissue surrounded by prominent fibrous tissue. The fibrosis and abnormal porto-systemic vascular connections that result cause ongoing damage.

Clinical features

The most simple and practical classification of the causes of cirrhosis is a division into biliary cirrhosis due to bile duct obstruction, and post-necrotic cirrhosis where the lesion is primarily hepatocellular (*see* Table 29.7). The clinical features may be those of the underlying condition, e.g. Wilson's disease, or nonspecific signs of chronic liver disease, portal hypertension and liver failure. Despite significant cirrhosis there may be no physical signs on examination.

Table 29.7 Causes of childhood cirrhosis
Biliary cirrhosis
Biliary atresia or hypoplasia
Choledochal cyst
Cystic fibrosis
Bile duct stenosis or obstruction
Ascending cholangitis
Post-necrotic cirrhosis
Post-hepatitis
Neonatal hepatitis
Viral hepatitis
Chronic hepatitis
Drugs, toxins, or poisons
Venous congestion
Constrictive pericarditis
Congestive heart failure
Budd-Chiari syndrome
Veno-occlusive disease
Genetic causes
Wilson's disease
Galactosaemia
Alpha-1-antitrypsin deficiency
Glycogen storage disease

Table 29.8 Causes of portal hypertension in childhood
Extrahepatic
Presinusoidal
Portal or splenic vein obstruction
Post-sinusoidal
Budd-Chiari syndrome
Inferior vena caval obstruction
Pericarditis or heart failure
Intrahepatic pre- and post-sinusoidal
Cirrhosis
Schistosomiasis
Congenital hepatic fibrosis
Acute or chronic hepatitis
Veno-occlusive disease

Investigations

The serum albumin is low, while liver enzymes are raised. The clotting profile may be abnormal. Hypergammaglobulinaemia is a common feature in autoimmune hepatitis. Alkaline phosphatase, gamma-glutamyltransferase and serum cholesterol are characteristically raised in biliary cirrhosis. A liver biopsy should be done to confirm the diagnosis of cirrhosis and may identify the underlying cause, such as autoimmune hepatitis. However cirrhosis is the end stage of many conditions and once established it may be impossible to determine the original cause.

Management

The management is essentially supportive. Maintenance of general nutrition is important. When possible, the underlying condition should be addressed. In biliary cirrhosis complications such as fat malabsorption and fat soluble vitamin deficiencies should be prevented. Ascites and oesophageal varices require attention. Liver transplantation can be offered where health budgets provide for such services.

Portal hypertension

The aetiology of portal hypertension in childhood is categorized into extrahepatic (pre-and post-hepatic) and intrahepatic (*see* Table 29.8). Extrahepatic portal hypertension is primarily due to portal vein thrombosis whereas intrahepatic portal hypertension is primarily due to parenchymal liver disease such as cirrhosis.

Clinical features

These children may present with a gastrointestinal haemorrhage from oesophageal varices, hypersplenism manifested by thrombocytopaenia, anaemia and neutropaenia, abdominal distension and ascites, or asymptomatic splenomegaly. In patients with portal vein thrombosis the liver is normal, but enlargement of the liver is mainly seen along with intrahepatic portal hypertension. At a late stage there may be hepatic decompensation and encephalopathy.

Investigations

Where possible, the primary cause of the portal hypertension is determined by serology, specific biochemical tests, liver scan or biopsy. Liver function tests and a clotting profile are indicated. A full blood count serves to identify evidence of hypersplenism. Patients with cirrhosis tend to have disordered coagulation, electrolyte disturbances, and varying abnormalities of the liver function tests. In contrast, the child with portal vein thrombosis has normal liver function tests and coagulation studies and mild manifestations of hypersplenism. Doppler ultrasound studies of the portal vein and splenic vein will confirm thrombosis. Oesophageal varices are best identified by endoscopic examination.

Management

The management of portal hypertension in childhood is essentially symptomatic. Ascites can be effectively controlled by sodium restriction, use of diuretics and, if necessary, albumin infusions. Despite the fact that massive splenomegaly may occur, there is very little place for splenectomy. Prevention of bleeding of oesophageal varices is achieved by the use of a nonselective beta-blocker (propranolol) to reduce portal pressure. If haematemesis and melaena occur the patient should be referred as an emergency to a centre capable of managing the complication. Patients are covered with antibiotics, and given acid-blocker therapy. Bleeding is controlled medically by using somatostatin (octreotide) infusion, a selective vasoconstrictor which decreases portal blood flow. Endoscopic injection sclerotherapy or banding of varices should be performed once stabilized. In the event of a catastrophic haemorrhage surgical shunts may be necessary.

Ascites

Ascites is an abnormal accumulation of fluid in the peritoneal cavity, indicated clinically by abdominal distension, shifting dullness to percussion, and the presence of a fluid thrill when considerable fluid is present.

Diagnosis

The approach to a child with ascites is determined by the type of fluid present in the peritoneal cavity and the underlying pathology. A diagnostic paracentesis is done to determine the serum-ascitic albumin gradient (SAAG), which is a better discriminant than older measures (transudate versus exudate) for the causes of ascites (see Table 29.9) It correlates directly with portal pressure and can classify ascites into portal hypertensive (SAAG >1.1 g/dL) and non–portal hypertensive (SAAG <1.1 g/dL) causes.

Management

General management includes bed rest, fluid restriction and salt restriction. This in combination with potassium-sparing diuretics (spironolactone) will be able to control most cases of ascites. Loop diuretics should not be used alone but may be added to spironolactone if the ascites is refractory. Daily albumin infusions will improve the ascites by correcting the hypoalbuminaemia. Oedema is rarely dangerous in its own right and attempts to clear it rapidly may create problems. Therapeutic paracentesis should be reserved for cases with severe respiratory distress, or imminent umbilical hernia rupture. The procedure carries a high risk of infection, leads to significant loss of protein and the relief is only transient. Spontaneous bacterial peritonitis is a well-known complication in patients with ascites and contributes to acute liver decompensation. Antibiotics are therefore indicated. Management of the underlying disease is imperative in conditions such as tuberculous peritonitis.

Hepatic schistosomiasis (bilharzia)

Infestation with *Schistosoma mansoni* occurs frequently among school-going children in the provinces of Limpopo, Mpumalanga and Kwa-Zulu-Natal. The intermediate host is a freshwater snail. Cercaria released from the snail penetrate the skin of humans exposed to infected water. As a result of deposition of eggs there is an intense inflammatory response and healing by fibrosis. In the liver the lesions involve the portal tract and result in marked peri-portal fibrosis.

Clinical features

Liver enlargement and portal hypertension may occur. Hepatic decompensation, ascites and signs of liver failure, are rare because liver synthetic function is preserved. Splenomegaly may be an incidental finding in an apparently well child. Gastrointestinal bleeding from oesophageal varices may be the first presentation of schistosomiasis.

Diagnosis

The diagnosis is made by identifying ova in the stool and rectal biopsy. Liver biopsy will identify ova and confirm periportal (pipestem) fibrosis. Serological tests may facilitate the diagnosis. Liver function tests remain normal or minimally deranged until late in the course of the disease.

Table 29.9 Approach to ascites

Mechanism	Aetiology	Ascitic fluid	Diagnosis
Increased vascular permeability and inflammation	All causes of acute and chronic peritonitis, e.g. tuberculous peritonitis	Exudate	• Cloudy or dark yellow fluid • Protein >30 g/l • Low albumin gradient • Fluid LDH > 200 U/l • Fluid to serum LDH ratio > 0.6 • ADA may be raised • pH<7 • Low glucose • WCC high, neutrophil predominant if bacterial, lymphocyte if tuberculous • Culture/gram stain may be positive
Increased intra-vascular hydrostatic pressure	All causes of portal hypertension, e.g. cirrhosis	Transudate	• Clear fluid • Protein <30 g/l • High albumin gradient >1.1 g/dL
Decreased intra-vascular oncotic pressure	Hypoproteinaemia, e.g. nephrotic syndrome	Transudate	• Clear fluid • Protein <30 g/l • Low serum albumin • Low albumin gradient
Lymphatic blockage	Congenital or neoplastic	Lymph	• Chylous fluid • Milky with fat globules • Many lymphocytes • Triglycerides high

LDH, *lactate dehydrogenase;* **ADA**, *adenosine deaminase;* **WCC**, *white cell count.*

Management

Prevention of the disease is important in the light of potentially serious hepatic involvement. Prevention is best accomplished by eliminating the water-dwelling snails which are the natural reservoir of the disease. Individuals can also guard against schistosomiasis infection by avoiding bodies of water likely to harbor the carrier snails. The recommended treatment is a single dose of praziquantel (40 mg/kg). The efficacy of treatment depends on the degree and duration of infection as well as the severity of complications. Many children improve gradually with time.

Veno-occlusive disease

In southern Africa the disease follows the ingestion of pyrrolizidine alkaloids derived from plants of the genus *Senecio*. These plants are found growing wild in many parts of Africa and are used in traditional medications administered either orally or by enema. Veno-occlusive disease is also found in association with bone marrow transplantation and administration of certain chemotherapeutic agents. It occurs more frequently in children than in adults, especially children younger than six years. The onset is sudden with hepatomegaly and severe ascites in the absence of significant jaundice.

Liver biopsy confirms the diagnosis. Venous congestion around the central vein and necrosis of hepatocytes occur. Initial oedema of the intima of the terminal hepatic venules is followed by fibroblastic obliteration of the vessels and eventually cirrhosis.

There is no specific treatment, and management is directed toward controlling the ascites. Some patients die during the acute phase. Those that survive, may recover completely or progress to cirrhosis with portal hypertension. Education of the population regarding the risks of herbal enemas and traditional medicines is essential for the prevention of this condition.

Acute liver failure

Acute liver failure is a rare complication in childhood and is associated with a high mortality. Without supportive management or liver transplantation mortality is in excess of 70 per cent. It is characterized by critical impairment of the functions of the liver: synthesis, detoxification, and excretion.

The causes of acute liver failure in children are varied and may be categorized as infectious (mainly viral), metabolic, toxic, or immune mediated. The aetiology of acute liver failure varies according to the age at presentation. In neonates infection or an inborn error of metabolism are common while viral hepatitis, drug induced liver failure or autoimmune hepatitis are more likely in older children. Drug induced hepatotoxicity may be due to herbal or traditional remedies, drug overdose, or idiosyncratic reactions. If the patient is anicteric with encephalopathy, the possibility of Reye's syndrome should be considered. In South Africa, hepatitis A is the commonest cause of liver failure in acute liver disease.

The clinical features are those caused by the underlying liver disease and those caused by the complications of acute liver failure. Liver disease may present with jaundice, ascites, an enlarged or shrinking liver, foetor hepaticus and hypoglycaemia. Complications of acute liver failure include encephalopathy, cerebral oedema, coagulopathy, gastrointestinal bleeding, sepsis, renal failure and multi-organ failure.

Management

It is important to determine the cause, as specific therapy may be available or there may be genetic or epidemiological implications. Medical support is provided to allow for recovery of the hepatic lesion (*see* Table 29.10) In recent years the administration of N-acetylcysteine has been reported to decrease mortality in patients with fulminant hepatic failure even in non-paracetamol poisoning. The prognosis of acute liver failure has been improved by the development of effective medical therapy and success of liver transplantation, but is ultimately dependent on the presence of multisystem disease and reversible cerebral damage.

Liver transplantation

This offers children a chance for long term survival. In South Africa, liver transplantation for public patients is centralized in the Western Cape. Since 2004 a private facility in Gauteng has also been successfully providing liver transplantation. Careful selection of families and candidates is critical as regular follow-up and compliance with immunosuppressive regimens is essential for long-term success. Budget restraints also determine or limit selection policies. An experienced team of transplant surgeons, paediatricians, intensive care specialists, radiologists, pharmacists, psychologists and social workers is a critical requirement for successful intervention.

In children, the most common disease requiring liver transplantation is biliary atresia (70 per cent). Others include chronic active hepatitis and cirrhosis. Acute fulminant liver failure (viral, toxin or drug induced) is also an indication. Metabolic, neoplastic (rarely) or haematological conditions may also require liver transplantation. The current contra-indications in South Africa include hepatitis B e-antigen positivity, hepatitis C, HIV, TB (until treated for six months), malignancy outside the liver, irreversible disease or damage of other organs, and psychosocial factors.

Immunosuppressive drug combinations include steroids, azothiaprine, mycophenolate mofetil , cyclosporin, and tacrolimus. Long-term problems include growth retardation, cosmetic effects, infection, and malignancy. Some 85–90 per cent of children transplanted are likely to survive one year, and 70–80 per cent survive five years. In the South African context, limited organ donation and funding, as well as limited expertise in liver transplantation are still major factors curtailing this important therapeutic option.

Table 29.10 Management of liver failure

Monitor	**Coagulopathy**
Neurological observations	FFP only required if active bleeding or for procedures
Gastric pH	Platelet transfusions as required
Blood glucose	Vitamin K
Acid-base/electrolytes	Antacids – keep gastric pH >5
INR	
	Hypoglycaemia
Hepatic encephalopathy	IV glucose (10% solution)
No sedation except for procedures	
Lactulose via nasogastric tube, cleansing enemas	**Tissue hypoxia**
Oral neomycin	N-acetylcysteine
Restrict dietary protein	
Intubate to protect airway, if necessary	**Sepsis**
	Broad spectrum antibiotics and antifungals
Cerebral oedema	
Fluid restriction	**Renal failure**
Intravenous mannitol	Maintain intravascular volume
Treat seizures	Diuretics
Intubation and hyperventilation	Dialysis
Fluid	**Nutrition**
Fluid 75% of maintenance	Low protein diet
Balance	Enteral feeding (0.5-1g protein/day)
Maintain circulating volume with colloid/ FFP	Parenteral nutrition if ventilated

FFP, *fresh frozen plasma;* **INR**, *international normalized ratio.*

PART 8

Specialty disorders

Paediatric surgical disorders

Children's illnesses and infections evolve more rapidly than those of adults. In order to avoid unnecessary operations and costly delays in operating on those who need it, there must be a close and continuing working relationship between paediatricians and surgeons. The paediatric surgeon should be consulted early in the following cases:

+ Accidents, trauma and snake bite
+ Burns
+ Severe infections with possible collections of pus
+ Possible obstruction or perforation of a hollow viscus
+ Anatomical and functional disturbances amenable to mechanical correction
+ Mass lesions and adenopathy.

HIV/AIDS and the paediatric surgeon

Occupational infection with HIV is rare among health workers. Some workers such as surgeons, dentists, and operating theatre staff are at greater risk but even following documented needle stick injury and exposure to blood from HIV positive patients this risk is small. However,

- All patients, irrespective of age or clinical diagnosis, should be regarded as HIV infected.
- All staff, including medical students, should be aware of the local policy for post-exposure prophylaxis, and report all injuries.

sensible precautions should still be taken. The risk of seroconversion can be minimized by post-exposure prophylaxis with zidovudine.

Surgical approach

The paediatric surgeon may encounter HIV-infected patients in a number of scenarios:

+ The patient may present with an unrelated pathology, e.g. inguinal hernia, and may be coincidentally HIV infected.
+ The patient may present for management of a disorder that is likely to be HIV related, e.g. tuberculosis or fasciitis.
+ The patient may be referred for assistance in diagnosis of lymph node enlargement, particularly the differentiation between lymphoma and tuberculosis in an HIV infected individual.
+ The patient may present with an AIDS-defining pathology such as spontaneous recto-vaginal fistula or neonatal CMV enteritis.
+ The patient may present with an emergency condition, in whom the HIV status cannot be rapidly determined.

Asymptomatic HIV-infected individuals carry no greater surgical risk than non-infected patients, either in the general ward or the ICU. Other than subsequent referral for antiretroviral treatment no modification of surgical protocol is required.

In symptomatic patients it is important to remember that it is the patient that requires treatment, not merely the surgical pathology. Any treatment plan must accommodate the clinical and haematological status of the patient, but it is the clinical status of the patient that determines the management approach, not the patient's HIV status. Patients in a poor clinical condition should not undergo elective surgery no matter what their HIV status. Patients who are well should be offered surgery as needed, no matter what their HIV status.

Symptomatic HIV-infected patients exhibit a spectrum of clinical conditions from apparently well to moribund. Generally speaking the least possible surgical intervention should be performed that buys time for the patient's general condition to be improved by medical interventions. Untreated AIDS remains a lethal disease.

Thus an asymptomatic HIV-infected individual with an uncomplicated inguinal hernia would be a candidate for an immediate herniotomy. A similar patient who has AIDS, severe wasting, candidiasis, encephalopathy and any other co-morbidity might be better served by a period of medical treatment that may include antiretroviral treatment.

General trauma

By virtue of their natural curiosity, inexperience, and incomplete physical development, children of all ages are particularly prone to trauma. While it may be trite to repeat that children are not merely small adults, nowhere is this better demonstrated than in consideration of trauma. As children's bones bend rather than break, a normal X-ray at presentation may misrepresent the considerable bony and soft tissue deformity which occurred at the moment of impact. Conversely, bones that do break suggest major distortion at injury.

Children's heads are proportionately larger than those of adults and are supported by less well-developed neck muscles. In infants with open sutures, the skull can expand to accommodate increasing intracranial pressure, therefore neurological signs of a space-occupying lesion develop late.

The relatively small blood volume of the child exposes him to risks of hypovolaemia after apparently trivial bleeding. The relatively large and unprotected upper abdominal viscera are prone to both blunt and penetrating injury. Injured children tend to swallow air, causing significant gastric dilatation, necessitating naso-gastric decompression. Due to their large surface area they rapidly become hypothermic.

Remember the need for adequate tetanus immunization and for emotional and psychological support of the injured child.

The professional caring for paediatric trauma victims must be aware of the possibility of non-accidental injury which introduces ethical dilemmas onto an already crowded stage.

Mechanisms of injury

Children are exposed to blunt injuries from falls, blows, or motor vehicle accidents. Penetrating injuries result from civil violence including gunshots, dangerous play-acting or fighting, and falls onto sharp objects. Patterns of injury characteristic of non-accidental injury are described in Chapter 5, Social paediatrics. However, recurrent injury and/or delay in seeking professional help should increase suspicion.

Significant trauma in childhood frequently results in multiple injuries with more than one organ system affected. In major trauma head injury is an invariable associate.

Burns, drowning, electrical shock, and ingestion of foreign bodies or corrosives are common among children, and are important causes of morbidity and mortality.

Burn injury

Mechanisms

Burns commonly occur in the home where hot liquids may fall over a child (e.g. by pulling over a kettle or cup of beverage) or spill onto a floor where a child is sitting. Occasionally, burns result from such accidents as failure to test the temperature of bath water. Houses may be set alight resulting in flame burns in addition to the inhalation of smoke particles and noxious gases. Open-fire cooking carries similar risks. In fair-skinned babies overlong exposure to the sun can result in significant injury.

Chemical burns may result from contact with acids, alkalis, or petroleum products.

Pathology. Dermal injury in a burn is characterized by a central zone of maximum damage and concentric zones of lesser damage until uninjured skin is reached. Burns are classified according to the surface area affected and the depth of burn in the zone of maximum necrosis.

Superficial burns. There is no dermal involvement. The burn is characterized by erythema and blistering. Sensation is intact and spontaneous healing expected.

Partial thickness burns. Superficial layers of dermis are involved. Deeper structures (e.g. sweat glands, hair follicles) are unaffected and represent a source of new epithelial cells. Spontaneous healing is possible if infection is prevented.

Full thickness burns. Full depth of skin and appendages are burned. Clinically the burn may be charred or dead white. Sensation is absent. It is characterized by the development of slough, which separates after two to three weeks, leaving granulation tissue. Skin grafting is inevitable.

Body surface area (BSA). Children's body proportions vary with age (*see* Figure 30.1).

As a rule the area of the palmar surface of the hand represents 1 per cent of total surface area.

Management

At the scene. The immediate need is to minimize

Figure 30.1 Body surface proportion and relative change with growth

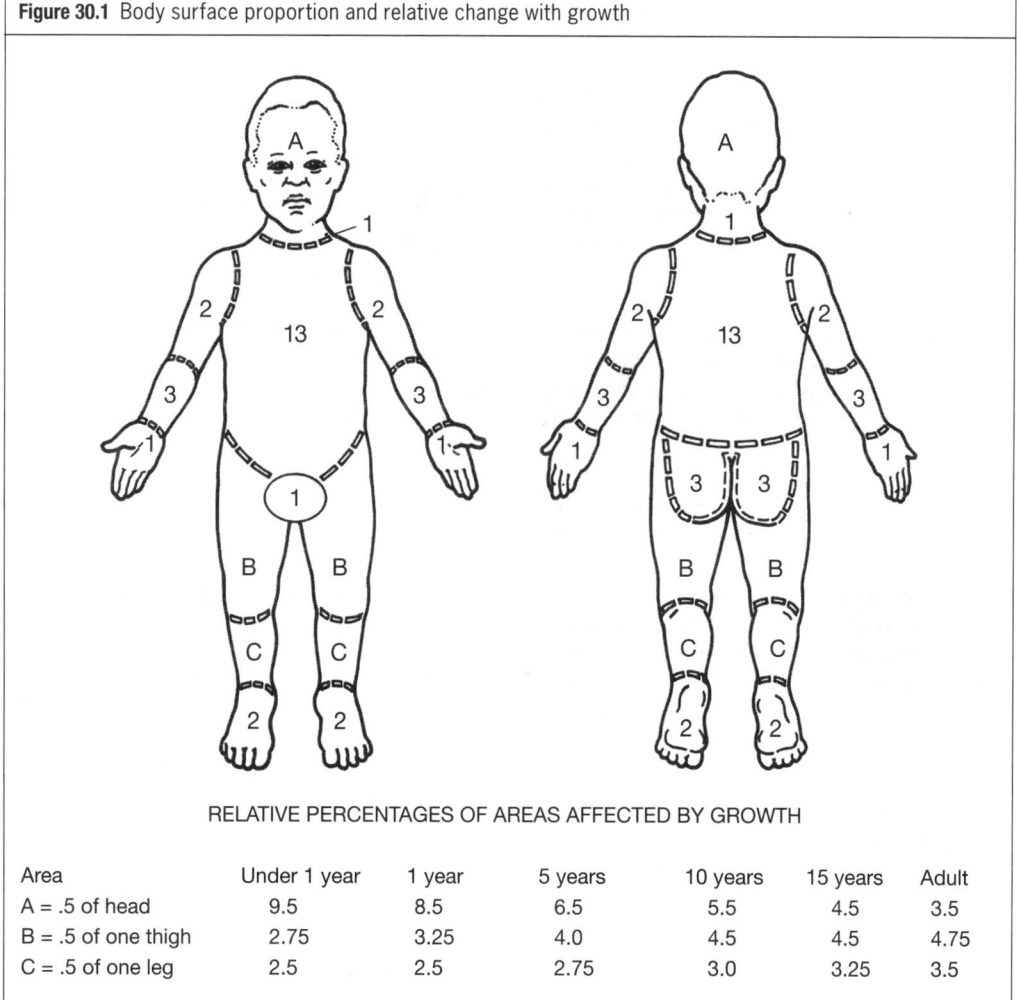

RELATIVE PERCENTAGES OF AREAS AFFECTED BY GROWTH

Area	Under 1 year	1 year	5 years	10 years	15 years	Adult
A = .5 of head	9.5	8.5	6.5	5.5	4.5	3.5
B = .5 of one thigh	2.75	3.25	4.0	4.5	4.5	4.75
C = .5 of one leg	2.5	2.5	2.75	3.0	3.25	3.5

the extent of the injury. Obviously it is important to remove the patient from the fire or hot liquid. However, burn injury continues for some time after removal of the exogenous source, and generous soaking or immersion in cold water is beneficial up to one hour after injury. The burned area should then be dressed in any clean cloth and the patient taken to a health facility.

Health professional. Burn injury assessment must include a search for other injuries and exclude inhalation injury. The burn depth and surface area are estimated.

Systemic care. Intravenous fluid replacement is urgent, as fluid loss starts at the time of injury and may precede arrival at hospital by several hours. The volume required can be estimated from the formula provided in Figure 30.2.

Regular clinical assessment of the patient, including urine output and haematocrit, is essential.

Analgesia and tetanus prophylaxis must not be forgotten. Prophylactic antibiotics are probably unhelpful but they may be indicated for associated problems. Ileus accompanies any major burn, and nasogastric decompression is important. Antacids, and early feeding, minimize stress ulceration.

A common gastrointestinal complication of burn injury is asphyxiation by ascaris worms, particularly if occlusive dressings around the chest and upper arm prevent infants from turning over or getting their hands to their mouths. Prophylactic vermifuge should be considered when ileus resolves.

Local care. The ideal is to provide a clean atraumatic environment for burn healing. *Infection effectively deepens the extent of a burn.* Many efficacious creams, impregnated tulle gras, and ointments are available. Where facilities exist, early tangential excision of deep burns, effectively cutting out the burn, is desirable. Few centres in the developing world enjoy such luxury. Skin-grafting usually follows the separation of slough at about 21 days.

Psychological care. All burns cause scars. Some scar the body as well as the mind, others just the mind. The sequelae of pain, separation from family, altered body image, and effects of visible scarring can be minimized by starting support early. The family may equally deserve consideration as guilt feelings may arise.

Ingestion of foreign bodies and corrosives

Foreign bodies

Infants will put any interesting object into their mouths as part of their exploration of the environment. Older children contrive to ingest a variety of objects, the most common being coins, razor blades, needles, safety pins, broken glass, and fish bones.

Oesophageal foreign bodies

Three physiologically 'narrow' areas in the oesophagus are the common sites of foreign body impaction, namely cricopharyngeus, level of aortic arch, and oesophageal hiatus.

If a foreign body is allowed to remain impacted, ulceration and perforation will ensue, hence removal should be arranged urgently. Smooth objects (e.g. coins) that have been impacted for less than 24–48 hours are conveniently removed using a Foley catheter. Under X-ray control the persistence of the coin is confirmed. A suitably sized, lubricated Foley catheter (usually size 8–10) is passed like a nasogastric tube. Once it has passed the impacted object the balloon is inflated and under an X-ray screen the catheter is pulled back to engage the coin. The patient is turned prone and the coin and catheter withdrawn together. Ideally oesophageal in tegrity is confirmed at the same sitting by performing a limited barium swallow.

Indications for hospital admission of a child with burns:

- Burn in any child younger than three months
- More than 8 per cent BSA burned
- Involvement of hand, face, or perineum
- Circumferential limb burn.

- If a foreign body sticks in the oesophagus it should be removed urgently.
- If a foreign body reaches the stomach it is likely to pass uneventfully.

Figure 30.2 Burn management chart

Name: .... Age: .... Weight: ....

Date of Admission: .... IP Number:...

Burn: Date: .... Time .... Time first seen: ....

      Cause:.............................. Area: .... %   Clean/Septic

Measles prophylaxis: Measles vaccine/immunoglobulin/nil   (delete those not applicable)

FLUID REPLACEMENT during first 36 hours

a) Basic requirement: Weight.................................. kg x Area: .... % (max 30%) = ... ml (a)

b) Supplement for raised PCV: (Actual PCV–Normal PCV*) x 5 x (age+1) = ... (b) .... ml

              This supplement is adjusted and added at 0, 8, and 18 hours, and
              may be necessary more frequently depending on severity of burn and
              response to fluid replacement.

From 0 hours–88 hours give (a).................... ml + (b) .... ml = ... ml plasma

      8 hours–18 hours give (a).................... ml + (b) .... ml = ... ml plasma

    18 hours–36 hours give (a)................. ml + (b) .... ml = ... ml plasma/blood

Use blood instead of plasma during third period if Hb below 12 g/100 ml.

MAINTENANCE FLUID required in addition to replacement fluid

For each kg up to 10 kg   give 100 ml = ... ml

+

For each kg from 11–20 kg give 050 ml = ... ml

+

For each kg over 20 kg   give 020 ml = ... ml

Total maintenance fluid requirement   = ... ml/24 hours IN ADDITION TO

                                              REPLACEMENT FLUID

Give IV for large burns: i.e over   8% if under 1 year of age

                           over 10% for children

                           over 15% for adults

Recommended fluid: Electrolyte No 2 (depending on serum electrolytes).

INVESTIGATIONS

	Admission	8 hours	12 hours	18 hours	24 hours	36 hours
Hb	....	....	....	....	....	....
PCV	....	....	....	....	....	....
Urea	....	....	....	....	....	....

*Guide to adequacy of fluid administration
i) Urine output. Minimum = 1 ml/kg/hour.
ii) PCV (haematocrit). Normal PCV: Neonate 60%, Child 38%, Adult 42%.

Sharp objects or pins and chronically impacted coins should be removed under general anaesthesia using a rigid oesophagoscope.

Gastric or more distal foreign bodies

Once an object reaches the stomach, or has negotiated the pylorus, it will pass atraumatically. The author has observed double-edged razor blades and broken glass pass without comment, and the patient has been totally unaware of their eventual elimination. There is no need to hospitalize such patients. An X-ray check in two to three days to confirm progress or evacuation is all that is required. Rarely abdominal symptoms develop or progress is halted where referral for surgery may be appropriate.

Fish bones. Fish bones may stick into or through the oesophageal wall and are usually not visible on plain X-rays. Diagnosis can be achieved by contrast swallow or oesophagoscopy. The history is usually diagnostic.

Strictures. It should be remembered that in patients with pre-existing oesophageal strictures, an unchewed food bolus may impact. Such patients clearly need further evaluation when the obstruction has been relieved.

Corrosives

Proprietary drain cleaners, pool acids, bleach, etc. are freely available and represent a continual hazard to a child. Storing acids or alkalis in containers that are attractive to children, within reach of children, and which can be opened by children, contributes significantly to this hazard. Strong alkalis cause more damage than acids as they tend to stick to mucosae. For this reason solid particles or granules tend to cause more significant, though more focal, damage than liquids.

Presentation. Rarely, if ever, is ingestion witnessed by an adult. Any suggestion of corrosive ingestion must therefore be taken seriously. In florid cases there may be burns of the lips and chin, salivation, and obvious mouth ulceration. Similarly, the oral mucosa may escape un scathed while the oesophagus or stomach is severely injured.

Management. All patients are admitted to hospital. Oesophagoscopy is the only way of diagnosing oesophageal injury and this should

be done as early as possible. Pending oesophagoscopy, antibiotics and fasting are advised. In those patients where oesophagoscopy reveals no injury these measures are discontinued and the patient discharged. Where injury is present they are continued and although the role of steroids remains debatable their use may be of value. Feeding may continue via a fine-bore tube.

Some patients will develop oesophageal scarring and stenosis requiring dilatation; rarely late oesophagectomy may be necessary. Immediate surgery may be required in patients with oeso phageal perforation manifested by mediastinitis, toxaemia, and pleural effusion.

Prevention is much easier than cure, and simple education campaigns have worked wonders in the United States and United Kingdom.

Blunt abdominal injury

The realization that there are no disposable abdominal organs, and particularly that splenectomy creates a state of life-threatening immunodeficiency, has revolutionized attitudes to trauma management in children. Viscera may be divided into:

- *Solid viscera*: liver, spleen, pancreas, kidneys.
- *Hollow viscera*: alimentary tract, urinary tract, biliary tree.
- *Diaphragm*.

The principal morbidity of trauma to solid viscera stems from blood loss and in the case of hollow viscera, from peritonitis.

Solid viscera

Bleeding usually stops spontaneously. Man agement depends entirely upon the patient's clinical status. Instability that fails to respond to resuscitation, is the only indication for intervention. When surgery is indicated every effort is made to prevent organ resection (particularly of the spleen), and many techniques have evolved to assist the surgeon.

Hollow viscera

Injury to hollow viscera can lead to peritonitis. The early detection of clinical signs forms the rationale for the frequent re-evaluation of the trauma victim by a single observer.

A confident diagnosis, or strong clinical suspicion, justifies laparotomy as delay is associated with significant morbidity.

Diaphragm

Injuries of the diaphragm are frequently missed, both clinically and radiologically. However, blunt injury often causes massive disruption with clinical features of herniation of abdominal viscera into the thorax. Diaphragmatic injuries require immediate repair through a transabdominal approach.

Multiple trauma

The child with multiple injuries creates major diagnostic and therapeutic challenges. Invariably a head injury coexists and response to painful stimuli may be depressed. Abdominal examination may be difficult in the presence of pelvic or rib fractures. Multiple sites of bleeding may conceal bleeding at one particular site.

Management

Evaluation may involve the adjunctive use of radiology, sonography, or radio-isotopes. Where staff shortages and lack of facilities make observation hazardous, consideration must be given to early surgery to diagnose and manage intra-abdominal injuries. Successful management may depend upon the input of specific surgical disciplines (e.g. facio-maxillary surgeons) but the child with multiple injuries should remain under the care of the general surgeon or paediatric surgeon whether in a district hospital or trauma centre.

Snake bite

Few species of snake are aggressive towards prey as large as a human, and unless provoked or cornered, are inclined to withdraw strategically. Furthermore, of all the world's snakes, less than 20 per cent are even mildly venomous, and of these, few are life-threatening to humans. Even bites by venomous species do not always lead to envenomation of the victim, or to the injection of lethal doses.

> ### The principles of trauma management are based on:
>
> - Resuscitation
> - Evaluation
> - Observation
> - Operation.

Small children are doubly at risk by virtue of their insatiable curiosity and small size. In areas where young boys are employed as herdsmen, especially when barefoot, the risks are increased. They should be warned of the dangers of probing crevasses in rocks or tree-stumps, termitaria, etc. with bare hands. Many bites occur at night when barefoot individuals tread on or near an unseen snake. This is particularly common with regard to the puffadder, *Bitis arietans*, whose reluctance to move until trodden on, is characteristic. Regular paths around dwellings or villages should be illuminated if possible. Most importantly, people must be educated not to chase and kill snakes on sight. Children are again at increased risk as their often playful aggression is likely to be misunderstood by the reptile. Slow withdrawal will allow the snake to move off. Many snakes feign death convincingly, therefore one should approach apparently dead snakes with reserve.

Mechanisms. Snakes 'bite' by ejecting a viscous salivary secretion, which is stored in venom sacs, through hollow fangs into the victim. This secretion is species-specific but contains a variety of enzymes and toxins. Certain species, notably the cobras, may also 'spit' venom onto an epithelial surface where it may be locally irritating or absorbed.

The effect of a standard injected venom dose is related to the mass of the victim. Small snakes, injecting a lower volume, are generally less dangerous than large snakes. Small victims, however, exhibit toxic effects earlier and these are more serious than in larger individuals.

Snake identification

Due to similarities in size and colouring between quite unrelated species, accurate identification can only be assured if the snake, complete with head, is brought with the victim.

Venomous snakes have fangs, situated either at

the front of the mouth or towards the back of the jaw, below the eye (*see* Figure 30.3).

Fangs may be 'fixed' or 'hinged'. The latter variety are not obvious to inspection but can be 'unhinged' by drawing a thin stick from the angle of the mouth forwards. Do not look for fangs with unclad fingers; envenomation can occur even when the snake is dead. 'Back-fanged' snakes tend to cling after striking, and a history of difficulty in removing the assailant is typical of this variety. Non-venomous snakes have numerous small teeth but lack fangs.

Clinical features of snake bite

While nearly all victims are able to give a history of snake attack, it is as well to recognize objective signs of injury to assist in the assessment of preverbal children, the comatose, and inaccurate historians.

Non-venomous snakes, lacking fangs, truly 'bite'. They leave a ragged wound in which their teeth may be shed. The effects of such a bite are entirely non-specific. Local tenderness and cellulitis may be present by the time of presentation, but there are no symptoms suggestive of envenomation. Non-specific signs such as nausea and vomiting may be present.

Paired fang marks are the hallmark of assault by a venomous species. In swollen tissue a magnifying glass may be needed to demonstrate the lesion. Single or paired 'scratch' marks may result from a 'side-swipe' strike.

The majority of bites occur on the foot or ankle, with the hand and arm next in order of frequency. Since back-fanged species need to draw the affected part into their mouths in order to strike, they rarely, if ever, bite more proximally than the wrist or ankle. Bites over the head and neck and trunk are sufficiently uncommon to raise clinical suspicion. In these circumstances, bites by a spider or scorpion should be considered.

Anxiety is an almost universal response to snake attack in adults, but small children may be deceptively calm about their experience.

Venomous snakes

In order to cause any significant effects, venomous snakes have to inject an adequate dose of venom into the victim. Protective clothing, an abrading strike, immature snake, broken fangs, or recently emptied venom sacs, all compromise the snake's ability to inject adequate volumes of venom. Thus a snake attack does not necessarily imply envenomation.

While snake venoms are all chemically highly complex, a broad division is possible depending on the principal system affected, namely cytotoxic, neurotoxic, and haemotoxic.

All snakes have each element represented in their venom, but the overall effect depends upon the proportion of each component:

- **Cytotoxic venom** fixes locally at the site of injury, causing swelling and local tissue necrosis, and often intense pain.
- **Neurotoxic venom** is disseminated along venous and lymphatic channels, causing a

> As aggressive treatment for envenomation is hazardous and occasionally lethal, there must be objective evidence of envenomation before such treatment.

Figure 30.3 Snake fangs

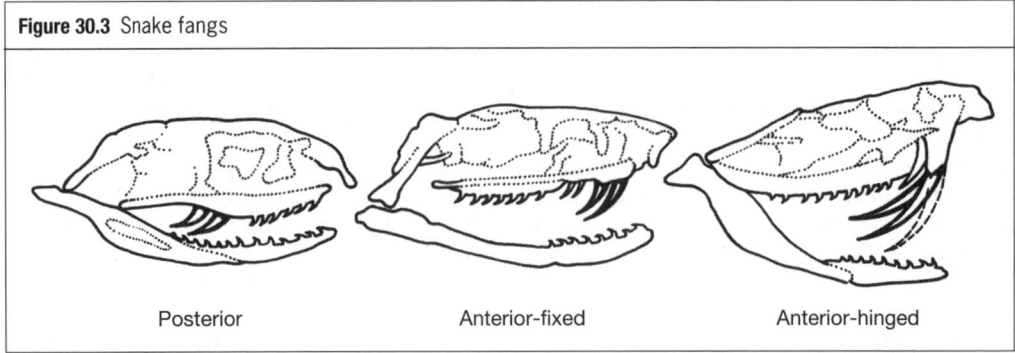

| Posterior | Anterior-fixed | Anterior-hinged |

non-depolarizing neuromuscular blockade. These effects may be relatively mild, e.g. transient ophthalmoplegia, or potentially lethal, e.g. respiratory paralysis.

- **Haemotoxic venom** may cause red cell destruction by phosphatases, resulting in haemolysis, jaundice, and thrombosis, or interfere with clotting mechanisms resulting in clot instability or frank bleeding from mucous membranes.

In all cases, secondary effects due to the liberation of chemical fractions such as histamine, kinins, and prostaglandins add to the clinical picture. The presence of this fraction means that the thromboelastogram may be used as an objective sign of envenomation.

The three important groups of venomous snakes are:

- **Viperidae** – vipers, adders
- **Elapidae** – cobras, mambas
- **Colubridae** – boomslang, bird (vine) snakes.

This classification is along anatomical lines and there is overlap of toxin secretion patterns between the groups.

Primary management

The aims of 'first aid' are to preserve the patient's life, minimize morbidity, and avoid the use of potentially lethal treatment methods. The absorption of toxins via lymphatics and veins is increased by exercising the affected limb.

- Immobilization delays the onset of symptoms. Ideally, the limb should be immobilized on a splint and firmly bandaged with crepe or similar material.
- Tourniquets should never be used. They increase the effects of cytotoxic venom by concentrating it at the site of injury; and there are safer ways of diminishing venous and lymphatic drainage in situations such as elapid bites, where these effects may be desirable.
- There is no place for incising, sucking, cauterizing, or bleeding the site of injury. The risk of local and systemic sepsis, injury to a major nerve, vessel, or tendon, or the absorption of venom, is increased by such manoeuvres.

Antivenom should only be administered in the field if:

- Accurate identification shows the snake to be venomous.
- The afflicted person is showing signs of envenomation.
- The offending snake's venom is known to be included in the antivenom.
- The antivenom has been correctly stored and transported (which usually implies refrigeration).
- The patient is known not to be sensitive to horse serum.

Antivenom should be injected intravenously, preceded by a test dose. Local injections have little effect on already fixed cytotoxic venom, and absorption of systemically active venom occurs rapidly, requiring systemic antivenom for its effective eradication. Thereafter transportation to a medical facility should be expedited.

Hospital management

All patients referred with snake bites should be detained for no less than 48 hours, as late manifestation of injury is common, particularly by colubrid snakes. Confirmation of injury is obtained by history-taking and examination. Envenomation may be confirmed by thromboelastography. Depending upon the delay in referral and snake identification, antivenom administration may be appropriate. Facilities for managing anaphylaxis should be available, and antivenom injected only after the response to a test dose has been assessed. Antivenom is rarely necessary in cases of adder bites where the local cytotoxic damage is already established, but may be indicated in elapid and colubrid bites. Supportive measures, ventilation, transfusion, and nutrition are provided as necessary. Fasciotomy may be necessary where venom has been injected deep to fascia or where a tourniquet has been applied. Children, particularly if hypovolaemic, develop compartment syndromes at low tissue pressures. The surgical management of necrosis and ulceration will proceed when the risk to life by the original envenomation has passed. However, joint mobility should be maintained by passive, then active physiotherapy.

Cardiac depressant effects are seen in some of the more dangerous elapid bites and monitoring is essential. It is important to recognize apparent 'relapses' after clinical improvement; therefore vigilance should be maintained for 24 to 48 hours after the restoration of normal functions. Simple measures such as tetanus prophylaxis, wound management, and antibiotics where appropriate, should not be forgotten.

Infections

Much of developing world surgical practice involves the management of patients with infection. The surgeon's contribution to such management lies in the drainage of pus and excision of necrotic tissue.

Soft-tissue abscesses

An abscess is a localized collection of pus within the tissues and may occur at any site and be due to any organism or combination of organisms. Common sites for abscess formation:

+ Skin and dermal appendages – furunculosis
+ Regional nodes – suppurating lymphadenitis
+ Muscles – pyomyositis.

Visceral abscesses are discussed under the appropriate organ system elsewhere.

Clinical signs. The classical signs of inflammation may be readily appreciated in superficial abscesses. However, deep-seated abscesses may be associated with only pain and loss of function. Pain is typically throbbing and disturbs or prevents sleep. The sign of fluctuation is difficult to elicit in these exquisitely tender lesions and in any case is superfluous to the diagnosis. Similarly, diagnostic 'aspiration' is rarely indicated and can be misleading as a negative aspiration cannot be held to mean an absence of pus. Aspiration of tender inflammatory lesions, with the necessarily wide bore needle, in unanaesthe-

Soft-tissue abscesses are the most common cause of surgical admission in paediatric practice. The majority are due to *Staphylococcus aureus*.

tized children is not conducive to good doctor-patient relationships.

Patients may be well, apart from the local lesion, suggesting adequate localization. However, many patients will be unwell, with fever, malaise, and cellulitis. Such signs suggest poor localization and continuing bacteraemia.

Management principles. The treatment of an abscess is surgical drainage and this should be performed as soon as possible. Antibiotics play an adjunctive role and are indicated in patients in whom signs of poor localization are present and in immunosuppressed patients, including neonates, the malnourished and diabetics. Their use is also justified in abscesses affecting the face, to minimize the risk of cavernous sinus thrombosis. An antibiotic effective against community strains of staphylococcus should be selected. Analgesia is important.

Suppurating lymphadenitis. Abscesses within lymph nodes are commonly seen in the inguinal, axillary, occipital, and submental groups. Invariably a portal of entry is evident. The causative lesion should be addressed. Inguinal nodes drain the lower anal canal and perineum in addition to the lower limbs, and a primary lesion should be sought at these sites.

Pyomyositis. It is believed that most intramuscular abscesses result from minor trauma, which leaves a haematoma within the muscle; this becomes infected thereafter during a transient bacteraemia. Muscles commonly affected include quadratus femoris, anterior abdominal wall muscles, and ilio-psoas. Diagnostic difficulty occurs frequently in abdominal wall abscesses where intra-abdominal pathology may be at first suspected, and in ilio-psoas abscesses where hip pathology is often the admission diagnosis. Spasm of the psoas causes the adoption of the classical position of flexion, adduction, and internal rotation. All movement, active or passive, is resisted, as any stretching of the psoas causes severe pain. Sonography is usually diagnostic. Drainage is performed via the most direct route. Psoas is reached via an extraperitoneal approach which allows additional access to iliacus.

Post-operative treatment. With adequate drainage an abscess cavity will heal by granulation. Dressings and drains are used to prevent the skin wound from healing before the cavity is obliterated and to contain any exudate. Packing the cavity is counterproductive and is used only to control bleeding from the abscess wall. A host of proprietary and non-proprietary dressings are available.

Unusual abscesses

From time to time abscesses may be encountered that do not follow the rules. Non-tender abscesses should provoke suspicion of tuberculosis (TB). Non-healing abscesses may be due to tuberculosis or perhaps a foreign body. Recurrent abscesses may be a manifestation of a specific immunological deficit. An unusual odour or character of pus may suggest an exotic organism. Whenever an unusual abscess is encountered, the pus must be sent for culture and the abscess wall must be biopsied.

Cellulitis

Cellulitis represents a spreading infection of the skin and subcutaneous tissue and is clinically associated with local erythema, pain and tenderness, and frequently with fever, malaise, and non-specific nausea and vomiting. Any area may be affected and the condition is classically associated with penicillin-sensitive streptococci but may be due to *Staphylococcus aureus*.

As the clinical features of cellulitis and osteitis are identical it is wiser to treat all such patients as if the pathology were osteomyelitis (*see* Chapter 31, Orthopaedic disorders).

Peritonitis

Inflammation of the peritoneum may be due to a primary infection but more commonly is secondary to pathology of the bowel or female genital tract. Non-bacterial peritonitis is much less common but may be due to the presence of urine in the peritoneal cavity following rupture of the bladder, the presence of CSF secondary to ventriculo-peritoneal shunting, or intraperitoneal bleeding.

Clinical presentation. Bacterial peritonitis, whether primary or secondary, presents with signs and symptoms colloquially known as 'acute abdomen'.

Tenderness on rectal examination is present when the pelvic peritoneum is inflamed. There is rarely sufficient free fluid to be clinically

> ### The signs of an 'acute abdomen' include:
>
> - Acutely ill with prostration
> - Marked abdominal tenderness (generalized or maximal over the affected quadrant)
> - Involuntary spasm of the abdominal wall muscles (guarding)
> - Rebound tenderness or percussion tenderness
> - Abdominal fullness secondary to bowel stasis and dilatation.

appreciated. Umbilical herniae are good sites for the assessment of peritoneal tenderness, as skin and peritoneum are closely associated at the umbilicus. In patients with a patent processus vaginalis, pus or inflammatory exudate may present in the scrotum as an acute hydrocele.

In the neonate, signs of peritonitis may be obscured and diagnosis is often delayed until features such as abdominal wall oedema or erythema appear. The diagnosis may also be delayed in children with spina bifida, in paraplegics, and following trauma, particularly if a head injury coexists.

Differential diagnosis. The differential diagnosis of the acute abdomen is broad and includes extra-abdominal as well as intra-abdominal pathology. However, the presence of peritonitis, with very rare exceptions, is an indication for laparotomy. Pre-operative preparation must cater for commonly occurring pathologies; appendicitis, typhoid, amoebiasis, ascariasis, intussusception, and trauma.

Pathophysiology. With peritoneal inflammation, there is massive fluid exudate into the peritoneal cavity with proliferation of organisms, usually of bowel or female genital tract origin; these include both Gram-positive and Gram-negative aerobic and anaerobic bacteria. The faeculent aroma of the peritonitic abdomen signifies the presence of anaerobes, among which will be penicillin-resistant bacteroides species. The omentum, appendices epiploicae and loops of the small bowel become oedematous and matted, creating intraperitoneal abscesses. Intraperitoneal fluid loss is sufficient to cause shock and requires urgent replacement. As the volume lost cannot be directly measured, replacement is effected using clinical signs as a guide.

Serosal inflammation of the bowel provokes an ileus with further concealed fluid losses within the lumen. This ileus contributes to the abdominal distension and is responsible for associated vomiting.

The massive absorptive area of the peritoneum facilitates absorption of toxins and organisms, leading to septicaemia and its sequelae.

Primary management. Patients in whom peritonitis is diagnosed should without exception be prepared for theatre. Such preparation should include:

* *Intravenous fluid replacement*. In shocked patients an initial plasma bolus should be followed by a balanced electrolyte solution to restore pulse, blood pressure, and an urine output of at least 1 ml/kg/hr.
* *Intravenous antibiotics*. Peritonitis is a mixed infection and antibiotics effective against aerobes and anaerobes are necessary. Where metronidazole is available this is an ideal anti-anaerobic agent. Elsewhere chloramphenicol is useful. Gram-negative cover can be provided by an aminoglycoside; ampicillin covers a wide range of Gram-positive organisms and is effective against *Salmonella typhi*.
* *Analgesia*. Once peritonitis is diagnosed, no useful purpose is served by leaving a child in pain. Indeed, relief of pain may have important therapeutic benefit. As the pain is severe, opiates are frequently employed. All drugs should be given intravenously, never intramuscularly, to ensure absorption and bioavailability.
* *Nasogastric decompression*. Ileus secondary to peritonitis will lead to vomiting which is distressing and particularly painful in children with peritonitis. Nasogastric drainage further relieves abdominal distension.

Primary peritonitis

In developed communities primary peritonitis has been virtually eliminated by the widespread use of antibiotics for respiratory and other infections. In the developing world primary peritonitis remains a significant problem and is seen in otherwise healthy children (especially females) and immunosuppressed children, typically with nephrotic syndrome.

Primary peritonitis is usually due to a single organism, particularly *Streptococcus pneumoniae* or *Haemophilus influenzae* and may be associated with a previous respiratory tract infection. In girls, organisms may ascend via the Fallopian tubes, and *Escherichia coli* or other Gram-negatives may be encountered. The pus of primary peritonitis never smells faeculent.

Management. Many patients are diagnosed at operation by the findings of thin, non-odorous pus with no other intraperitoneal pathology. Where clinical suspicion is aroused pre-operatively (for example in renal units) a short trial of high-dose penicillin is justifiable. Should no clinical response be evident in six to twelve hours, surgery should be advised.

Typhoid

Typhoid fever is fully discussed in Chapter 15, Systemic infections. Surgical interest in typhoid relates to the complications of ileal perforation and bleeding.

Typhoid perforation

Aggressive resuscitation and surgery for typhoid perforation have seen mortality rates drop from over 60 per cent to less than 10 per cent over the last 20 years. Clinical deterioration in a patient being treated for typhoid with onset of abdominal pain and peritonitis is sufficient to justify surgery. Non-operative management carries a prohibitive mortality. Peritonitis may be the presenting feature of typhoid.

Investigations. Half of the patients with perforation show evidence of pneumoperitoneum on X-ray. Similarly, while a relative leucopenia may be suggestive of typhoid any white cell count is compatible with perforation. Anaemia is found in half of the patients.

Pre-operative treatment. Resuscitation is the key to operative success. Antibiotic cover must be extended to encompass not only *Salmonella typhi* but also enteric organisms, which are now released into the peritoneal cavity. Fluid, electrolyte, and acid base balance should be corrected.

Surgery. Excision of the affected lymphoid patch, or patches, with repair of the bowel is required. Thorough peritoneal lavage is performed to remove pus and debris. 'Near' perforations are oversewn.

Post-operative care. Complications are frequent, including chest and wound infections. Recurrence or relapse of typhoid may be seen in 5 per cent of patients.

Typhoid bleeding

Bleeding from typhoid ulcers in the ileum or caecum may be torrential. Many patients with typhoid have a clotting disorder. Before surgery, correction of clotting defects using vitamin K, plasma or platelet infusion is mandatory. Blood transfusion is required to correct anaemia and hypovolaemia. At operation, localization of a bleeding site may be difficult and it may be necessary to perform a right hemicolectomy to be sure of resecting the causative lesion.

Appendicitis

Appendicitis can no longer be regarded as a rare disease in the developing world, but recognition is often delayed. While any age may be affected, the disease is typically seen in the older child from six years to adolescence. Inflammation of the appendix follows luminal obstruction, which may be due to lymphoid hypertrophy secondary to viral infection or to a faecalith. In the developing world additional obstructive factors include pin worms, round worms, bilharzia, and amoebae. Luminal obstruction is followed by progressive necrosis of the appendix wall, perforation, and peritonitis. Initially a perforation may be locally contained by loops of bowel and omentum so that an appendix mass or abscess develops. Small children localize intraperitoneal sepsis poorly and general peritonitis frequently arises with a marked deterioration in the prognosis.

Presentation. The great variation in signs and symptoms is partly responsible for the high rate of diagnostic error. This variation may be due to some extent to the highly variable position of the appendix and contiguous inflammation of a number of possible organs. Late presentation, whereby the symptoms of appendicitis are superseded by the signs of generalized peritonitis, is common and under such circumstances accurate pre-operative diagnosis may be impossible and is largely academic. During the early phase of luminal obstruction the visceral pain of appendiceal distension is appreciated at the umbilicus. As transmural inflammation reaches the serosal surface, which is somatically innervated, the pain is felt at the site of inflammation, usually the right lower abdomen. Thus the pain appears to move from the umbilicus to the iliac fossa.

With the onset of pain, nausea and vomiting are common. Loss of appetite is an almost constant symptom, and mucoid diarrhoea may occur, particularly if the rectum is secondarily inflamed. Other features are those of cystitis, and apparent hip irritability. Fever is frequent but rarely above 38.5 °C.

Examination may reveal a furred tongue and foetor but more specific signs include localized iliac fossa tenderness and involuntary guarding. Percussion tenderness over McBurney's point is a convincing finding, but the site of maximal tenderness will vary with the position of the appendix. Rectal examination will reveal tenderness on the right when the appendix is adjacent or the pelvic peritoneum inflamed. Without treatment the pain worsens until the appendix ruptures, when temporary relief may occur before the pain of peritonitis supervenes.

No objective investigations are available to confirm a diagnosis of appendicitis. Although both ultrasound and CT scanning have been advocated in difficult cases, the diagnosis remains principally a clinical responsibility.

Treatment. All patients in whom appendicitis is seriously considered should be admitted and watched for progression or regression of symptoms and signs. In many patients iliac fossa pain disappears rapidly and a formal diagnosis is never achieved. For those with convincing signs at admission or who deteriorate during observation appendicectomy is appropriate treatment. The patient is prepared for surgery as for peritonitis. Surgery through an iliac fossa incision is acceptable where a confident diagnosis has been made and signs are localized. Where the skills and facilities are available appendicectomy can safely be performed laparoscopically.

Post-operative care. Potential complications are numerous but uncommon, other than wound infection and intraperitoneal abscesses. Deaths are related not to appendicitis *per se* but to the sequelae of peritonitis and septicaemia.

Motility disorders

Intussusception

Intussusception occurs when proximal bowel (the intussusceptum) invaginates into the bowel immediately distal to it (the intussuscepiens). In the industrialized world this is almost exclusively a disorder of infants under one year of age and may be associated with viral respiratory tract disease or a weaning diet. In the developing world the condition is seen at any age with at least 50 per cent of patients being over the age of two years, and is frequently associated with non-specific diarrhoeal illness. Late presentation, which further alters management, is a feature of tropical intussusception.

Pathophysiology. As the proximal bowel passes within the distal bowel the mesentery becomes compressed. Initially lymphatic, then venous obstruction occurs causing oedema and congestion of the mucosa with bleeding into the distal lumen. This blood and mucus are passed as a typical 'redcurrant jelly' stool. Ultimately arterial occlusion leads to gangrene of the intussusceptum. Very rarely is there a pathological mural lesion which acts as a lead point and most cases are 'idiopathic'. The intussusceptum may start at any point in the bowel – most usually the ileocaecal region (but in children over two the transverse colon is commonly implicated) (*see* Table 30.1) and may pass a variable distance along the bowel, even prolapsing through the anus. The distinction between prolapsing intussusception and rectal prolapse is vital and discussed below (*see under* Rectal prolapse, *below*).

Clinical presentation. Symptoms begin during, or soon after, an acute diarrhoeal illness in approximately 30 per cent of patients. Initially, intestinal colic and reflex vomiting are seen in association with a somewhat tender sausage-shaped mass. As the pathology progresses, bloody mucoid stools are passed and pain becomes continuous. Ultimately bowel perforation with peritonitis occurs. In 25 per cent of patients the apex of the intussusceptum is palpable on rectal examination.

Differential diagnosis. In the developing world, because of the association with diarrhoea, intussusception must be differentiated from intestinal ascariasis, amoebiasis, and dysenteric illness.

Investigation. Clinical suspicion may be confirmed by:

- *Ultrasound*, which shows a characteristic bull's eye appearance of the bowel on transverse section.
- *Barium enema*, demonstrating a mass effect within the colon and the 'coil spring'of barium between mucosal folds.
- *Laparotomy* in those patients presenting with peritonitis.

Management. In the industrialized world many patients may be treated non-operatively by reducing the intussusception with a barium or air column at the diagnostic barium enema investigation. We have adopted a policy of attempting air reduction under general anaesthetic, in theatre, so that failure or any complication can be managed by an immediate laparotomy. Resection of gangrenous bowel will be required in up to 30 per cent of cases.

Post-operative care may be complicated by endotoxaemia, which results from flooding the portal circulation with bacteria and toxins which had previously been confined within the intussuscepted loop. Pre-operative use of anti-endotoxins or plasma may reduce the associated morbidity.

Special intussusceptions

Post-operative intussusception. This may follow any operative procedure and diagnosis is often delayed as usually only the small bowel is involved.

Chronic intussusception. Intussusception may rarely be present for several days without signs of intestinal obstruction or progression to intestinal necrosis. In such cases there is a higher than usual incidence of lead points.

Recurrent intussusception. Following non-operative or operative treatment, intussusception may recur in 1–2 per cent of patients, either

Table 30.1 Site of intussusception in 77 children			
	Under 2 yrs	**Over 2 yrs**	**Total**
Ileocolic	37 (80%)	11 (35%)	48 (62%)
Colocolic	5 (11%)	17 (55%)	22 (29%)
Entero-enteric	4 (9%)	3 (10%)	7 (9%)

because a lead point has been overlooked or the original reduction had been incomplete. Treatment of the recurrence is the same as for primary intussusception.

Rectal prolapse

'Something coming down' during defaecation or other straining, or 'something' persisting independently of bowel function is a distressing symptom. Rectal prolapse must be differentiated from prolapsing intussusception and prolapsing polyp. In prolapsing intussusception it is possible to pass the examining finger alongside the protruding mass into the rectum. Prolapsing polyps may be palpable and hooked down by the examining finger. Histologically they are usually benign juvenile polyps.

True rectal prolapse is a symptom of an underlying disorder, not a disease in its own right. The causes are shown in Table 30.2.

Management. The management of the prolapse is based primarily on the recognition and management of the underlying disease. In a developing world environment, non-specific diarrhoeal diseases and parasites predominate in malnourished children. Surgery is reserved for the correction of anatomical abnormalities. Conservative measures, pending primary disease control, may include raising the foot of the cot, sedation, and manual reduction. Gallow's traction, buttock strapping, and encircling peri-anal sutures are unlikely to be sufficiently secure to resist the *vis a tergo* of intra-abdominal pressure and may complicate any subsequent

Table 30.2 Causes of rectal prolapse	
Functional	Diarrhoea
	Parasites
Anatomical	Malnutrition with loss of supporting ischiorectal fat pad
	Pelvic floor paralysis, e.g. myelomeningocele
	Congenital anomalies
Others	Cystic fibrosis (5–10% of children with cystic fibrosis will develop rectal prolapse at some stage)
	Idiopathic

prolapse. Recurrent or resistant idiopathic prolapse may justify some intervention, be it submucosal injection or other manoeuvre, but such instances are extremely uncommon.

Gastro-oesophageal reflux

(*See* Chapter 24, Gastrointestinal disorders.)

Clinical presentation. Gastro-oesophageal reflux may present at any age and is certainly underdiagnosed in a developing world environment. This is due firstly to a non-specific symptomatology and secondly to the difficulty of confirming a clinical suspicion.

Diagnosis. Oesophagoscopy may reveal oesophagitis, which can be histologically confirmed and graded. Barium meal may reveal an associated hiatal hernia but unfortunately reflux can be provoked in many normal children and the demonstration of reflux under the artificial conditions of the X-ray suite is unreliable. Radioisotopes instilled directly into the stomach via a nasogastric tube may be picked up later in the lung fields confirming aspiration. The gold standard, however, is 24-hour pH monitoring using an intra-oesophageal electrode.

Management. Medical management is instituted on clinical suspicion. Surgery is necessary to deal with oesophageal strictures and patients with life-threatening complications, e.g. aspiration. Medical management failures, and neurologically impaired children should also be offered surgery in the form of a trans-abdominal fundoplication. Where the skills and facilities are available this can be achieved laparoscopically.

Paralytic (adynamic) ileus

Many insults, particularly inflammation, hypokalaemia, prolonged obstruction, and surgery provoke the intestine into a state of hypotonic inertia.

Pathophysiology. Generally the whole bowel is affected. Fluid loss into the bowel lumen may be considerable. Abdominal distension, vomiting, and hypovolaemia result. Bowel sounds are usually absent.

Clinical presentation. The presentation is usually that of the underlying pathology with the onset of the signs and symptoms of intestinal obstruction. A particular dilemma arises in the small child with severe gastroenteritis who after some days of profuse diarrhoea ceases to pass stool and develops abdominal distension. The distinction between mechanical and paralytic ileus in such patients may be clinically impossible. Following correction of any electrolyte deficit, further investigation is justified.

Diagnosis. As in mechanical obstruction (*see above*), air-fluid levels within distended bowel loops are seen on X-ray. Such air-fluid levels tend to occur at one level within the abdomen rather than in a stepladder pattern, and are all much the same length with no disproportionately dilated loops. In some individuals contrast enema may be required to exclude intussusception.

Management. The underlying pathology must be aggressively treated. Post-operative ileus can be expected to resolve in 24–48 hours. Persistent ileus should prompt consideration of a 'relook' laparotomy. In all patients, intravenous fluids and nasogastric drainage are indicated.

Genito-urinary tract

Testicular maldescent

It is believed that spermatogenesis is greatest at temperatures lower than core temperature. The testis, having developed in the retroperitoneum, is forced into the scrotum through the inguinal canal by abdominal pressure transmitted to the upper pole of the testis via the processus vaginalis. Should the testis fail to descend the processus persists and then constitutes a patent processus vaginalis or potential inguinal hernia.

The empty scrotum, unilaterally or bilaterally may be due to primary anorchia, antenatal catastrophe such as torsion, abdominal wall paralysis, or obstruction to the neck of the scrotum causing the testis to divert to an ectopic (usually inguinal) site. If clinical examination reveals testes, even if they cannot be induced to enter the scrotum, the prognosis is good. If no testes are palpable even in ectopic sites, the prognosis must be guarded pending the results of exploration.

Malignancy and maldescent

There is a higher than normal risk of testicular malignancy in the undescended testis, as well as the normally situated contralateral testis. Placing the testis surgically in the scrotum does not diminish the risk of malignancy, but may make surveillance easier. These risks justify removal of an intra-abdominal gonad which cannot be brought into the scrotum.

Management. Surgery is generally deferred until two years of age. The operation performed is an orchidopexy, part of which is a herniotomy of the inevitably accompanying hernia.

The prognosis for fertility in bilateral undescended testis is poor. In unilateral cases fertility may be slightly reduced or normal.

The retractile testis

An apparently undescended testis that can be coaxed into the scrotum is termed 'retractile'. Clinically the empty scrotum looks well developed, unlike the flat hypoplastic scrotum of genuine maldescent. The retractile testis is normal in all respects and has simply been drawn up by a strong cremaster muscle. No treatment is indicated.

Testicular torsion

Torsion of the testis is usually in fact torsion of the spermatic cord in patients in whom the tunica vaginalis invests the lower part of the cord, leaving the testis hanging freely and aptly described as a 'bell clapper'. Occasionally torsion of the testis proper on a long mesorchium occurs. The diagnosis must be firmly established as any anatomical abnormality allowing torsion will be bilateral and both testes are at risk. Thus, while early operation is desirable to salvage the affected testis, even when this opportunity has passed, late operation is justifiable to protect the remaining testis.

Clinical presentation. Torsion may occur at any age – even antenatally – but is usually associated with adolescence. Acute onset of loin or inguinal pain is frequently associated with vomiting. A mild pyrexia may suggest an inflammatory lesion, while tenderness, swelling, and erythema of the affected hemiscrotum may mimic orchitis.

Management. The scrotum must be explored. If the history is short, detorsion may salvage at least some testicular function. A gangrenous testis should be removed. In any event the contralateral side must be explored and the testis anchored to prevent torsion of the remaining gonad.

> No sexually inactive male should be diagnosed as having epididymo-orchitis without operative exclusion of torsion.

Paraphimosis

In this condition a retracted prepuce is prevented from returning to its normal position by an often mild stenosis of the preputial orifice. Oedema of the distal prepuce results in an alarming ring of swollen tissue at the base of the glans. The constricting ring can be identified proximal to this on the penile shaft. The glans itself is quite unaffected.

Management. Under local penile block anaesthesia the swollen prepuce can be so compressed that the oedema is forced under the constricting band and dispersed. This takes time and patience, but once achieved allows the constricting ring to slip distally over the glans into its normal position. Should this manoeuvre prove unsuccessful, incision of the constricting band in the midline dorsally may be necessary. Following reduction, the prepuce is inevitably swollen and oedematous for some time. Any decision with regard to future management should be deferred until all swelling has disappeared and a full assessment of any causative or provocative lesion can be made. Circumcision is not always necessary.

Balanitis

Inflammation of the preputial sac results in oedema of the prepuce and dysuria with a purulent discharge. Retraction of the prepuce is impossible. Antibiotics and local toilet are prescribed. Recurrent attacks may lead to preputial scarring and the need for circumcision.

Hypospadias

In hypospadias the urethral meatus may be situated at any site from the perineum to the penile tip. There is usually an abnormal hooded prepuce with chordee, i.e. ventral flexion of the penile shaft. In perineal or peno-scrotal hypospadias the bifid scrotum may be associated with genital ambiguity. In patients with hypospadias other genito-urinary abnormalities are more common than in the normal population and full evaluation is indicated. The hypospadic orifice may be narrow and its adequacy must be reviewed. Surgical correction begins at age three to four years and may involve a number of procedures. As the prepuce is essential to the reconstruction of the distal urethra these patients should not be circumcised.

Prune belly (abdominal muscle deficiency) syndrome

This peculiar disorder is aptly named as the wrinkled skin of the abdomen is draped over the subjacent viscera with no muscle intervening. The classical case is unmistakable, but occasionally only a single abdominal quadrant is affected, altering the clinical appearance. The condition is almost exclusively seen in males and the deficient abdominal wall results in undescended testes, broad substernal angle, and poor cough, predisposing to chest infections. The sinister effects of the syndrome are found in the urinary tract where megacystis, ectatic ureters, and hydronephrosis are seen, often with urethral atresia and patent urachus. Prognosis depends upon residual respiratory and renal function.

Parasites

Amoebiasis

(*See* Chapter 16, Parasitic and fungal diseases.)

Clinical presentation. Amoebic colitis must be suspected in any malnourished toxic child with a current or recent history of profuse diarrhoea with bloodstained stools and abdominal distension and tenderness on deep palpation. Procto-sigmoidoscopy will show typical ulcers with slough.

Management. Before peritonitis develops, surgery may be avoided in some patients by aggressive non-operative management. Thus, all patients are given amoebicidal drugs and antibiotics against coliform aerobes and anaerobes. Full supportive care, including transfusion of blood, plasma, or albumin, is instituted. Only if symptoms abate is surgery is deferred.

Surgery. Resection of the entire colon in these children carries a high mortality and recent experiences suggest that pancolonic disease is well managed by ileostomy diversion and pro-grade colonic lavage. Localized disease can be treated by a limited resection. The bowel ends are exteriorized rather than risk an anastomosis in such depleted patients.

Post-operative care. These patients need intensive nursing and medical care, particularly to prevent intractable pulmonary oedema. Late colonic strictures may occur at sites where affected areas have been left unresected.

Ascaris lumbricoides

(*See* Chapter 16, Parasitic and fungal diseases.)

Large numbers of adult worms may be present and stool ova counts of more than 50 000 ova/gram of stool are not unusual. Ascariasis may present as:

+ **Asymptomatic carriers.** Patients with quite unrelated pathology may be found to harbour ascaris worms. Their presence does not always mean that they are the cause of disease, and the vomiting of worms or rectal passage of worms should be viewed with circumspection.
+ **Subacute intestinal obstruction (worm colic)**. A large entangled bolus of worms may impact, commonly in the distal ileum, causing an incomplete obstruction. Clinically, abdominal colic with vomiting (often containing worms) and a palpable mass are present. The condition can be distinguished from intussusception if:
  – More than one mass is present
  – The palpable mass coincides with a radiologically evident mass of worms
  – The mass is seen on ultrasound to be composed of worms.

It may occasionally be necessary to perform a barium enema to exclude intussusception.

Management. Left alone, the worms will disentangle themselves and distribute themselves evenly along the bowel. Conservative management includes nasogastric drainage if vomiting is significant. Intravenous fluid replacement and antispasmodics must be given. Usually symptoms abate overnight and oral intake can be resumed.

Stool examination will reveal any co-habitors so that complete eradication of parasites can be achieved when all symptoms have settled.

Small bowel volvulus

A bolus of worms in the small bowel may act as the apex of a volvulus. Early recognition of this complication as well as surgical detorsion before intestinal necrosis occurs is an important aim of the observation of patients with worm colic. All patients with worm colic in whom obstructive symptoms persist after 12–24 hours should be re-evaluated radiologically to exclude volvulus.

Hepato-biliary ascariasis

A worm may enter the ampulla of Vater. A single worm will dilate the ampulla so that the likelihood of more worms finding access to the biliary tree is increased. Within the biliary tree worms ascend into hepatic radicles where they form 'nests' or abscesses. Surprisingly, biliary worms may be entirely asymptomatic and discovered only on sonography. More often hepatic tenderness and fever present in a patient with known intestinal ascariasis, suggesting a degree of hepatocholangitis.

Operative intervention is indicated for:
+ Intractable pain
+ Cholangitis persisting despite antibiotics
+ Obstructive jaundice
+ Pancreatitis
+ Persistence of intrabiliary worms on sequential sonographic examination over an empiric four- to six-week period.

Pancreatitis

A worm passing through the ampulla into the biliary tree may cause a transient hyper-amylasaemia, probably due to oedema of the ampulla. There is rarely clinically significant evidence of pancreatitis. Occasionally a worm will impact in the pancreatic duct with resulting acute pancreatitis with compelling symptoms justifying laparotomy. Pancreatic resection may be required.

All patients, once admitted for complications of ascariasis, must be advised to take regular vermifuge while asymptomatic in order to minimize the worm load. Appropriate measures to improve sanitation must be advocated.

Abdominal pain

Pain is a common indicator of surgical pathology but may also occur in syndromes for which operative treatment is inappropriate. As such disorders form part of the differential diagnosis of intra-abdominal surgical pathology, syndromes of abdominal pain without physical signs other than mild tenderness are briefly discussed here.

It must be clear that nearly all children suffer from abdominal pain at some time. Rarely is pain sufficiently severe or persistent to warrant medical attention. Pain that is of sufficient intensity or of such a character as to prompt hospital admission may similarly remain undiagnosed in 10–20 per cent of patients. Adding a speculative label to such patients is unhelpful and may inhibit the investigation of recurrent attacks.

Investigations

It may be difficult to decide how much investigation is justified in a given setting, particularly as the yield is extremely low. A complete physical examination is the minimum. Depending upon clinical findings a full blood count, stool parasitology, urinalysis, and occasionally abdominal ultrasound may be worthwhile.

Acute non-specific pain. This diagnostic category can include all pain that settles without specific treatment, and is typical of patients who are admitted for observation. Pain may be severe, is usually central, and may be associated with vomiting. Most importantly it disappears rapidly. The cause or causes are unknown.

Cyclical abdominal pain (recurrent non-specific abdominal pain). (*See also* Chapter 24, Gastrointestinal disorders.) Recurrent pain is not unusual, and if it results in disruption of school or social activities may present to the clinician. Although any age may be affected, it is common among girls aged between eight and twelve years.

The aetiology is unknown but may be indirectly related to migraine or may have a hormonal basis. Attacks settle spontaneously and treatment is purely symptomatic. Investigations are negative. Children inevitably 'grow out' of the condition.

Psycho-social pain. In many children pain is a response to stress, either at home or in school. Such pain may in fact be recurrent but lacks the periodicity of cyclical pain. Although presumably non-organic in origin, pain is nonetheless real, and may justify symptomatic treatment. If the social milieu of the child is known, a correct diagnosis may be possible. It must be remembered, however, that children in stressful environments can also develop appendicitis and clinicians should be reticent to ascribe symptoms to non-organic causes unless the evidence is incontrovertible. Thus, the diagnosis is frequently made in retrospect.

Referred pain. Pain originating in organs of foregut origin will be referred to the epigastrium, thus oesophageal, pulmonary, and occasionally cardiac pain may present as abdominal pain. Frequently lower lobe pneumonia causing pleuritis is referred to the upper abdomen. The paucity of objective signs will stimulate enquiry beyond the abdomen.

Miscellaneous causes of abdominal pain

A wide variety of conditions may occasionally present with abdominal pain:

- Juvenile diabetes
- Meningitis
- Tetanus
- Ovulation
- Viral respiratory infection (mesenteric adenitis).

In many instances the diagnosis is only made clear by the natural evolution of the disease. Diabetes occurs with sufficient frequency to justify urine testing for glucose on all patients admitted with abdominal pain.

Gastrointestinal bleeding

Gastrointestinal (GI) bleeding in older children may be acute or chronic and present as upper gastrointestinal haemorrhage with haematemesis and melaena, or as lower tract haemorrhage with haematochezia.

Chronic GI bleeding

By its very nature, chronic gastrointestinal bleeding is never massive and secondary symptoms such as anaemia predominate. Anaemia is usually of an iron-deficiency type.

Important causes include intestinal parasites, e.g. ankylostomes, gastro-oesophageal reflux (*see above*), and gastrointestinal polypi. While symptoms suggestive of gastrointestinal disease are often present, screening of anaemic patients for the presence of occult faecal blood has an acceptable yield. Investigation may include endoscopy once the secondary symptoms are controlled.

Acute GI bleeding

Bleeding above the duodeno-jejunal flexure may present as haematemesis often resembling coffee grounds. Melaena represents blood which has been partially 'digested' during its passage through the bowel and has a characteristic tarry appearance and consistency as well as a distinctive odour.

In any bleeding situation the priorities are:

- Patient resuscitation
- Excluding a bleeding diathesis
- Making a precise diagnosis
- Planning definitive treatment.

Endoscopy. Making a precise diagnosis is to a large extent dependent upon upper GI endoscopy. When the patient has been stabilized and circulating volume restored, endoscopy should be performed. Children over the age of seven or eight years tolerate endoscopy under sedation and mucosal anaesthesia. Younger children are best examined under general anaesthetic.

Radiology. Plain radiographs and barium studies are unhelpful other than in portal hypertension.

HIV and GI bleeding

Haematemesis is not uncommon in HIV-infected children although it is rarely catastrophic. Generally these patients are poor anaesthetic risks and investigation must be tailored to the patients' clinical status. Empiric treatment for oesophageal candidiasis is reasonable for patients in whom endoscopy under anaesthesia would be dangerous, particularly if there is evidence of oral fungal infection. It is not unreasonable to add a proton pump inhibitor. Endoscopy itself is rarely rewarding with mild gastritis or distal oesophagitis being the commonest endoscopic diagnosis.

Peptic ulcers

Acute ulcers are associated with head injuries and burns or any severe stress. Chronic ulcers are uncommon.

Antacids given regularly to patients at risk minimize the incidence. Treatment must include relief of the stress, be it sepsis, hypovolaemia, etc. Surgery is occasionally necessary if bleeding continues.

Mallory-Weiss tear

A gastro-oesophageal mucosal tear can be produced during vomiting. The diagnosis can only be confirmed endoscopically and this must be performed early. Conservative measures are usually successful.

Portal hypertension

Surgical treatment may be indicated for the sequelae of portal hypertension, namely oesophagogastric varices (often), hypersplenism (occasionally), and ascites (rarely).

Clinical presentation. Haematemesis may be the presenting complaint. Stigmata of portal hypertension, notably splenomegaly, ascites or abdominal wall collaterals may be present. Endoscopy will confirm variceal bleeding. Barium swallow will demonstrate the varices but cannot confirm them as the site of bleeding.

Management. The patient is resuscitated and early endoscopy performed. A bleeding varix may be sclerosed by injecting an irritant such as ethanolamine oleate into the lumen. Definitive management may include further sclerotherapy or some form of porto-systemic shunt surgery.

Gastritis/oesophagitis

Mucosal damage may result from drugs (particularly aspirin), inflammation, trauma, particularly from poorly managed gastric tubes, or acid injury to the oesophagus. While haematemesis is not common, such mucosal injury must always be considered in the differential diagnosis and a history of recent aspirin ingestion sought. Endoscopy is essential to the diagnosis. Rarely is surgery necessary to control bleeding.

Lower GI bleeding

Blood *in* the stool is indicative of colonic or lower small bowel pathology. Blood on the stool suggests rectal or anal blood loss. Enterocolonic disorders presenting with bleeding include inflammatory conditions; mechanical disorders such as intussusception; and neoplastic disease, particularly colonic polypi.

Anal bleeding may be painless, suggesting polypi, or painful suggesting fissures or haemorrhoids.

Rectal examination and sigmoidoscopy are pivotal investigations. All polypi must therefore be histologically evaluated.

Jaundice

Prolonged neonatal jaundice

A comprehensive account of neonatal jaundice is given in Chapter 7, Care of the newborn, and Chapter 29, Hepatic disorders. The need for surgical intervention should be determined before eight weeks of age. Delay reduces the chances of success proportionately.

Biliary atresia

The term biliary atresia is a misnomer as it is now believed that the biliary system scleroses perinatally in response to an agent presumed to be viral. Thus sclerosing cholangio-hepatitis would more accurately describe the pathology. Both the intra-hepatic and extra-hepatic biliary tree may be affected and usually the entire ductal system and gall bladder are sclerotic. In addition there is an associated hepatitis with progression to cirrhosis and liver failure.

Jaundice is late in onset and prolonged beyond the physiological period. Untreated the condition rapidly results in cirrhosis with portal hypertension, ascites, and progressive liver dysfunction, although death may be delayed for two to three years.

Diagnosis. Investigations cannot reliably distinguish neonatal hepatitis from biliary atresia as they are expressions of the same disease process. A patient with prolonged jaundice requires ultrasound examination (to exclude choledochal cyst) and other special investigations at a tertiary centre. Operative cholangiography must be planned with a view to a Kasai hepatoporto-enterostomy if biliary atresia is confirmed, before the tenth week of life.

Progressive liver disease is not halted by biliary drainage. Even where a Kasai procedure has been successful, there may still be an indication later for liver transplantation, which currently offers the best chance of longevity to these children.

Choledochal cyst

Cystic dilatation of the extra-hepatic bile ducts with loss of the normal epithelium must be suspected in any jaundiced infant. In the developing world most patients present under six months of age. Recognition is important as the lesion is eminently correctable by surgery before biliary cirrhosis develops. Cardinal symptoms are obstructive jaundice with a subhepatic mass lesion.

Mass lesions and lymph nodes

Indications for operation or biopsy

Enlargement of regional lymph nodes is part of the body's normal defence against acute infection. Enlargement is also seen in several haematological and other malignancies, and is also characteristic of tuberculosis. It is important to diagnose these pathologies as soon as possible so that effective treatment can be started, and the most important investigation is a lymph node biopsy. To avoid subjecting crowds of children with acute lymphadenitis to surgery, sensible clinical assessment should be peformed. Most benign nodes respond to treatment of the primary source of infection.

Nodes that enlarge, have a firm consistency and fail to respond to appropriate antibiotic treatment should be classed as suspicious and a biopsy planned. Fine needle aspiration cytology can be helpful in tuberculosis and does not require a general anaesthetic, but for accurate diagnosis of lymphoma a complete node is required.

Other surgical disorders

Tongue tie

The lingual frenulum is a normal structure, which secures the mobile tongue to the floor of the mouth. It is not necessary to protrude the tongue in order to speak normally or to suck. If it is considered that lingual mobility is seriously impaired, the frenulum may be divided. As the frenulum is avascular save a clearly visible vessel at its base, it is safely divided in the clinic using sharp scissors.

Parents must not be allowed to expect that such 'surgery' will improve diction, or compensate for delayed vocal milestones.

31

Orthopaedic disorders

The management of musculoskeletal disorders in children is dominated by concern for adverse effects on growth and development. The evaluation of the child may be for screening (such as for hip dislocation in the newborn), or may be focused towards a specific complaint. The complaint is often ascribed to trauma, but it may in fact be due to more serious disorder such as infection. Likewise, the clinician must be wary of diagnosing 'growing pains' as life threatening illness such as leukaemia could be missed. A history of the mother's pregnancy, the neonatal period, the child's developmental milestones, and the family history are of importance.

The limping child

Abnormalities of gait are often specifically diagnostic and are best analysed by observing the point in the gait cycle at which the abnormality occurs. A limp may be caused by:
- Pain
- Structural deformity of bones and joints
- Muscle weakness
- Neurological disorders.

It is important to identify the patient that needs urgent treatment (such as trauma, septic arthritis, osteomyelitis, neoplasm, haemophilia or slipped upper femoral epiphysis). Of particular concern is:
- A painful limp, especially of recent onset
- The systemically ill child
- Associated swelling.

Important gait patterns that help suggest the majority of causes of limping in a child are:
- **Antalgic gait**: due to pain in the lower limb, e.g. a thorn in the foot. The patient will be reluctant to bear weight on the painful limb and when walking will take a quick soft step on the painful side.
- **Short-limb gait**: due to a discrepancy in leg length. The body will rise up and down as the child walks. The discrepancy may be due to a true difference in leg length, e.g. after malunion of a fracture, or it may be an apparent difference due to a fixed hip deformity or pelvic tilt. A child can mask a discrepancy in leg length by walking on the toes (in equinus) on the short side or by flexing the knee on the longer side, or by tilting the pelvis.
- **Trendelenburg gait**: due to dysfunction of the hip abductor mechanism, e.g. in developmental dysplasia of the hip. During the stance phase of gait the pelvis cannot be stabilized and so the child compensates by leaning over the affected hip.
- **Other**: such as in neurological disorders (e.g. spastic hemiplegic gait, diplegic gait, or ataxic gait), or isolated muscle weakness or paralysis of muscles (e.g. polio), and in muscle dystrophies (e.g. Duchenne).

A history of trauma is important but is often a red herring, especially when the X-rays are normal. The clinician must beware of referred pain: anterior thigh pain or knee pain frequently arises from pathology in the hip, or even the spine.

The age of the child is useful in the differential diagnosis.

In the hip the most probable pathology is:
- 0–4 years: Developmental dysplasia of the hip
- 4–10 years: Transient synovitis, Perthes' disease
- 10–15 years: Slipped upper femoral epiphysis
- At any age: Infection–acute or chronic.

By carefully observing the abnormal gait pattern, the focused examination is directed towards the limb, the hip, the spine or the CNS. Special investigations are performed according to the clinical suspicion.

The swollen knee

The duration and progression of the swelling, presence and nature of pain or loss of function, and signs of local inflammation and systemic illness are important. The focused examination should consider:

Swelling of the entire joint (may be due to blood, effusion or synovitis):
- Post-traumatic haemarthrosis–fracture, avulsion of tibial spine, meniscal or ligament injury
- Bleeding disorder
- Acute septic arthritis
- Tuberculosis
- Juvenile rheumatoid arthritis.

Swelling in front of the knee:
- Prepatellar bursitis.

Swelling behind the knee:
- Popliteal cyst.

Bony swellings:
- Cartilage-capped exostoses
- Apophysitis of tibial tubercle (Osgood-Schlatter's disease)
- Primary malignant bone tumours.

Bone and joint infection

Acute bone or joint infection is an orthopaedic emergency. Failure to treat promptly and aggressively will lead to debilitating sequelae or even septicaemia and death. Underlying osteomyelitis should be excluded in any child presenting with cellulitis.

Acute haematogenous osteomyelitis

Pathology

Acute pyogenic infections of bone arise when bacteria (most commonly *Staphylococcus aureus*) colonise the metaphysis of a bone during a bacteraemia. Pus forms, and under pressure it spreads into the marrow cavity and to the surface of the bone. The pus elevates and strips the periosteum. If the pressure is not relieved, the blood supply to the bone is compromised and bone necrosis results. This devascularised, dead bone will form a sequestrum. The elevated periosteum lays down new bone, which is called the involucrum. The presence of a sequestrum or an involucrum indicates progression to chronic haematogenous osteomyelitis, with sinuses that chronically discharge pus. The infective process may also permanently damage the adjacent growth plate.

Clinical features

The child presents with a history of:
- Pain, usually severe and of recent onset, often ascribed to trauma
- Fever, malaise
- A limp, reluctance to bear weight, or in the neonate a pseudoparalysis of the limb
- A recent infection (such as a septic toe or discharging ear).

On examination:
- The child looks ill.
- The temperature and pulse rate are raised.
- The affected limb is held still.
- There is metaphyseal tenderness to palpation (often exquisite).
- The neighbouring joint is swollen, but not tense.
- Late in the process there is local oedema, cellulitis or even fluctuation.
- The child may be dehydrated with a decreased level of consciousness if septicaemic.

Investigations
- The white cell count, ESR and CRP are elevated.
- Blood cultures are taken to isolate the infecting organism.
- The U&E is done to assess hydration.

- An HIV test is done with consent, in case of immune compromise.
- X-rays are normal in the first 10 days. Later soft tissue swelling and a periosteal reaction may be seen.
- A technetium bone scan can help to localize the focus when the examination is equivocal and will demonstrate multifocal infection.

Treatment

- Supportive measures–intravenous replacement of fluids and electrolytes must be commenced immediately, together with analgesia. The limb is splinted.
- Intravenous antibiotics are commenced–an initial 'best guess' would be cloxacillin 200 mg/kg in four divided doses for staphylococcal infections.
- Surgical drainage and decompression of the bone follows promptly, once the patient is stable, to prevent further periosteal stripping. Pus is sent for culture. The choice of antibiotic may be modified later according to culture results. Post-operatively the limb is splinted.
- Oral antibiotics are continued for six weeks, while the limb remains protected with a splint or crutches.
- In instances where the child presents early and there is a dramatic response to intravenous antibiotics, surgery may not be indicated.

Acute septic arthritis

Pathology

A joint becomes infected via a penetrating wound, from an adjacent osteomyelitis, or by haematogenous spread from a distant site. The infecting organism is commonly *S. aureus*. As pus is formed, proteolytic enzymes are released that destroy articular cartilage. If left untreated, the process progresses to fibrosis or bony ankylosis of the joint and there may be destruction of bone. Permanent deformity and stiffness of the joint results. In the hip, increased pressure in the joint may lead to avascular necrosis of the femoral epiphysis (*see* Figure 31.1).

Clinical features

The presenting symptoms, signs and investi-

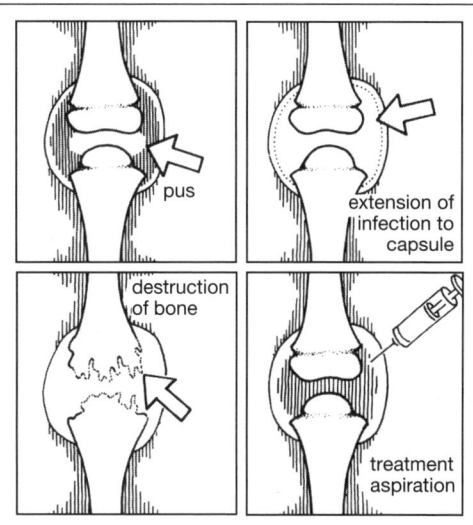

Figure 31.1 Pathology and treatment of pyogenic arthritis

gations are similar to those of acute haematogenous osteomyelitis:

- In superficial joints, such as the knee, there is tense swelling of the joint and the joint feels hot.
- Movements of the joint are markedly restricted, due to protective muscle spasm.
- In the hip, the joint is typically held in flexion and external rotation.
- X-rays (particularly in the hip) may show widening of the joint space, or even subluxation or dislocation of the joint.

Treatment

The treatment is similar to that of acute haematogenous osteomyelitis:

- Surgical drainage of the joint is by arthrotomy. It is imperative to promptly decompress the joint once the patient is stable and to irrigate the joint to remove all pus to prevent further cartilage damage.
- Post-operatively the joint is splinted in a position of function. In the hip, the limb must be splinted in abduction to prevent subluxation or dislocation.

Tuberculosis (TB)

The most commonly affected skeletal sites are the spine, hip and knee.

Tuberculous arthritis

Pathology

Mycobacterium tuberculosis infection of a bone or joint elicits a chronic inflammatory reaction. Destruction of bone occurs as a result of caseous necrosis. Caseation may extend into the soft tissues to form a 'cold abscess' and eventual sinus formation. Involvement of a joint results in the synovium becoming thick and oedematous. A pannus of granulation tissue spreads across the joint, which gradually destroys the articular cartilage. If treatment is commenced early, the disease can be cured medically without sequelae. However, once articular cartilage is damaged, healing by fibrosis results in ankylosis with permanent joint deformity and stiffness.

Clinical features

- Symptoms are present for a long time and are of gradual onset. Pain is usually not severe.
- The major features are swelling, stiffness and deformity. Swelling is due to synovial thickening rather than effusion and is therefore not fluctuant.
- Muscles around the joint are wasted. The joint feels warm.
- Movements are restricted in all directions.
- In patients presenting very late there may be evidence of a cold abscess or even a discharging sinus.

Investigations

- X-rays show soft tissue swelling and periarticular rarefaction of bone. The joint space may be narrowed and erosion of bone may be seen on both sides of the joint. Cystic bone lesions may be present, with little or no periosteal reaction. The joint may be subluxed or dislocated.
- A chest X-ray should be done to exclude concurrent pulmonary TB.
- The ESR and CRP are raised. There may be a relative lymphocytosis and the patient may be anaemic.
- The PPD may be done but is not reliable.
- An HIV test is done with consent, in case of immune compromise.
- Synovial biopsy may show histological features characteristic of TB, but frequently it only shows non-specific chronic inflammation.

- The diagnosis is sometimes not firmly established; the patient is nevertheless treated as TB on clinical suspicion.

Treatment

- The mainstay of treatment is medical, with appropriate antituberculous drugs. Treatment is continued for 9–12 months.
- The diseased joint is splinted in a position of function until symptoms subside, and then protected active movement is encouraged.
- If the joint remains painful or becomes stiff in a non-functional position, arthrodesis may be indicated when the underlying disease is controlled.

Spinal tuberculosis

Pathology

The infection begins in the vertebral body. With caseation the infection spreads to adjacent vertebrae and bone destruction results in collapse of adjacent vertebrae. This causes sharp angulation of the spine (kyphos or gibbus), which is most obvious in the thoracic spine. Caseous material or bone may compress the cord with resultant neurology. Caseous material may track through soft tissue planes and appear at a site remote to the site of original infection. Thus a lumbar spinal lesion could present as a psoas abscess in the groin.

Clinical features

There is usually a gradual onset of ill health. The most frequent presenting complaints are:

- Back pain which is gradual in onset
- Deformity, such as a gibbus, which is often the first observation by the mother in a younger child
- Weakness or paralysis (sometimes called Pott's paraplegia).

There is local tenderness and spinal movements are restricted due to protective muscle spasm.

X-rays:

- The soft tissues are examined on the AP X-ray for the presence of a paraspinal cold abscess.
- The vertebrae in the region appear osteoporotic and the intervertebral disc space becomes narrowed.

Figure 31.2 Tuberculosis of the spine: cold abscess formation

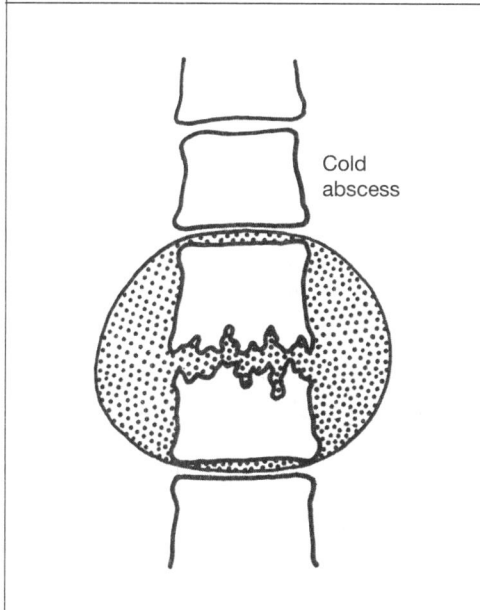

Cold abscess

Figure 31.3 Tuberculosis of the spine: destruction of the vertebrae and joints

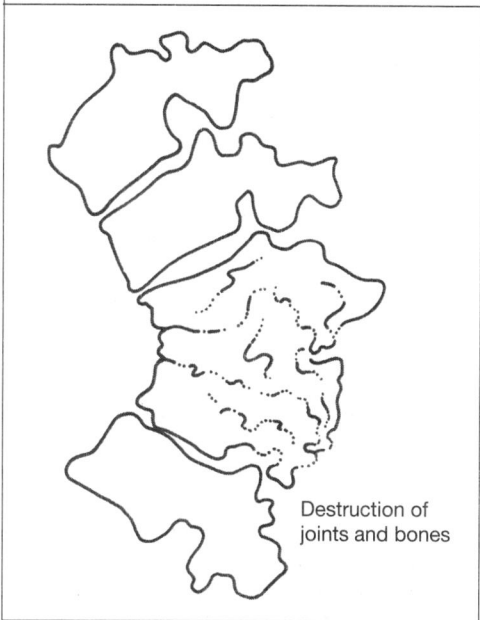

Destruction of joints and bones

♦ Later there is destruction of bone with collapse of adjacent vertebrae.

Treatment

♦ Eradicate the infection by the use of antituberculous drugs.
♦ Prevent or correct deformity by bracing or spinal fusion.

Paraplegia in children usually responds to conservative treatment. However, surgical decompression is indicated if there is no improvement with chemotherapy or if there is progressively deteriorating neurology.

Tumours

A bone tumour may be misdiagnosed both clinically and radiologically as a bone infection.

Benign bone lesions and cysts are fairly common in children, whereas primary malignant bone tumours are rare. Benign lesions often present as incidental findings on an X-ray or as a pathological fracture through the weakened bone. Pain or a gradually enlarging mass is the most common presenting complaint of a patient

with a primary bone malignancy. Progressive unremitting pain and night pain is of particular concern.

X-rays are the most useful first investigation: benign lesions usually have sharply defined boundaries, whereas a hazy or diffuse margin suggests an invasive tumour. A periosteal reaction, particularly a 'sunburst' appearance, a 'Codman's triangle' or an 'onion-peel' effect are suggestive of malignancy. (*See also* Chapter 22, Neoplastic disorders).

Juvenile chronic arthritis (JCA)

(*See also* Chapter 21, Immune and connective tissue disorders).

JCA should be considered in the differential diagnosis of any child presenting with a swollen or painful joint, a limp, or with early morning stiffness. In the pauciarticular form the degree of swelling is often out of proportion to the relatively minimal amount of pain and tenderness. The swelling is a combination of synovial thickening and effusion. The joint is warm and has some loss of motion.

Haemophilia

(*See also* Chapter 23, Disorders of the blood).

In this disease, bleeding into the joints is a common manifestation and may cause:

◆ Acute haemarthrosis: with severe pain and swelling in a boy, particularly affecting the hinge joints such as the knee, elbow and ankle. This may resemble an acute septic arthritis, but the systemic signs of infection are absent. It is important to be aware of the condition, even though it is uncommon, because aspiration of the joint would be dangerous. The diagnosis rests on the history of bleeding disorders in the family, minor trauma followed by severe symptoms, and laboratory assay of the clotting factors.

◆ Subacute haemarthrosis: after several episodes of bleeding into the joint, with synovial hypertrophy and persistent effusion. Clinically this may resemble tuberculous arthritis or rheumatoid disease.

◆ Chronic arthropathy: with progressive destruction and stiffness of the joint.

Treatment of acute haemophilic haemarthrosis

The clotting defect is corrected in consultation with a haematologist. The affected joint is gently compressed and immobilized in a position of rest, but a circular cast is never used. The limb is elevated and cold compresses (ice packs wrapped in a towel) are applied. Distal circulation must be closely monitored. Analgesics are given when necessary, but these must not inhibit platelet function. Factor administration is continued for three to seven days after cessation of bleeding. Physiotherapy is begun to gradually rehabilitate the muscle strength and joint movement. The need for joint aspiration (under sterile conditions) is debatable.

Developmental dysplasia of the hip (DDH)

The older terminology for this condition was congenital dislocation of the hip. The term DDH highlights that this is actually a spectrum of disorders of hip development. In the newborn it consists of instability of the hip, which may progress to a persistent dislocation. Girls are more commonly affected and there are geographic and racial variations in the incidence of DDH. When an unstable hip is diagnosed early the treatment is simple and effective, but when diagnosed late the treatment is complex with significant complications.

Risk factors for DDH:

◆ A positive family history of DDH
◆ Breech presentation during pregnancy
◆ Oligohydramnios
◆ Presence of other congenital deformities (such as foot deformities).

Clinical presentation and diagnosis depends on the age of the child. Every newborn child should have a screening examination at birth for clinical signs of hip instability by performing the Barlow and Ortolani tests:

◆ In the *Barlow test* an attempt is made to dislocate an unstable hip. The examiner holds the thigh with the thumb medially and fingers laterally over the greater trochanter. The hip is flexed and then adducted, while gentle backward pressure is applied. In an unstable hip, the hip will be felt to slide out of the acetabulum.

◆ In the *Ortolani test* an attempt is made to reduce a dislocated hip. The thigh is held in a similar manner and the hip is abducted and lifted forwards. A dislocated hip will be felt to slide back into the acetabulum.

X-rays in the newborn are misleading. If available, an ultrasound examination would confirm the diagnosis. However, when ultrasound is not available and clinical findings are doubtful, the baby should be re-examined at each well baby visit. Meaningful X-rays should then be done at three to six months of age.

In the infant the diagnosis of a dislocated hip is made by observing asymmetrical thigh skin creases, the leg is slightly short and externally rotated, and abduction of the affected hip is decreased. In addition, in the walking child the affected limb is shortened and the child may toe-walk to compensate for this. There will be a Trendelenburg gait.

DDH in childhood is painless. A painful dislocation would suggest another cause, such as septic arthritis. DDH does not cause any significant delay in motor milestones of development.

Treatment

When diagnosed in the first six months, the dislocated hip is treated in a simple harness for 12 weeks. After this, and up to walking age, treatment is by closed reduction and immobilization in a hip spica for six months. After walking age an open reduction is usually necessary, followed by a hip spica.

Transient synovitis of the hip

This is one of the commonest causes of hip pain in childhood. It occurs most frequently in boys aged 3–10 years. Transient synovitis of the hip is characterized by a sudden onset of hip pain and a limp, with restricted movement of the hip. The child is otherwise well. There is often a history of a recent upper respiratory tract infection, tonsillitis or ear infection. Clinical examination is aimed at excluding other more serious pathology. Laboratory investigations are non-specific and X-rays are normal. As the name suggests, the condition settles spontaneously within a few days. Treatment is by bed rest and analgesia.

Perthes' disease

Perthes' disease is due to an idiopathic avascular necrosis of the femoral head. Abnormal growth and remodelling of the femoral head may ensue, resulting in permanent deformity of the femoral head and osteoarthritis early in adult life. It is important to diagnose the condition and refer the patient early, as a golden opportunity to treat before the femoral head becomes deformed is otherwise missed.

Clinical features

* Perthes' occurs particularly in boys from 4–10 years of age.
* There is an insidious onset of hip, knee or anterior thigh pain.
* The patient walks with an antalgic limp.
* The thigh muscles are wasted.
* There is limited abduction and internal rotation of the hip.
* The child is otherwise well.

X-rays:
* Early: There is widening of the medial joint space, the femoral head appears smaller and more dense.
* Later: There is fragmentation of femoral head.

Investigations

* Blood tests are all normal.

TB of the hip is the main differential diagnosis, as this can have a similar clinical presentation and radiological appearance. Blood investigations are useful to differentiate the two. Occasionally a synovial biopsy is necessary.

Treatment

The principles of treatment are to identify those patients whose hips are at risk of healing with deformity of the femoral head, based largely on X-ray features. In these patients surgery may be advised.

Slipped upper femoral epiphysis (SUFE)

SUFE is characterized by displacement of the femoral epiphysis from the femoral neck through the growth plate. Consequent deformity of the hip joint results in osteoarthritis later in life, depending on the severity of the slip. It is important to diagnose and treat the condition as early as possible to prevent progressive displacement of the femoral head.

Clinical features

* SUFE occurs typically in adolescence. Boys are more frequently affected.
* The patient complains of hip, knee or thigh pain. This may be present for a few weeks and has suddenly become aggravated.
* Often the patient is either fat and sexually immature or very tall and thin.
* There is an antalgic gait. The leg is externally rotated and there is increasing external rotation as the hip is flexed.

X-rays:
* Early: The growth plate looks fuzzy.
* Late: A line drawn along the superior part of the femoral neck does not pass through the epiphysis as it normally should.

Investigations

- Further investigations are indicated if an underlying metabolic or endocrine abnormality is suspected.

Treatment

The patient is admitted on skin traction. Definitive treatment is by *in-situ* pinning of the hip with a single screw across the growth plate.

Back pain

Unremitting back pain, night pain and constitutional symptoms are all red flags for tumours and infections of the spine. Back pain in children less than 10 years of age is most likely to be caused by infection or neoplasm and needs urgent investigation. Children over 10 years are more likely to have back pain due to trauma, sport overuse injuries, spondylolisthesis or Scheuermann's disease. Pain in idiopathic scoliosis is not usual and may rather suggest the presence of a neural tumour as an underlying cause. Back pain may radiate to the leg and the child may present with a limp. X-rays are the most useful first investigation for children with back pain.

Deformities of the lower limbs

Genu varum (bow legs) and genu valgum (knock knees)

In the normal growth pattern of the lower limbs, the newborn baby has genu varum. The limbs are in neutral alignment at about 18 months, but progress to maximum genu valgum at three to four years. The legs then finally correct to almost neutral alignment by six years. There is a wide spectrum of normality for these physiological variations. Physiological conditions are bilateral and symmetrical.

Most bow legs and knock knees are physiological and even when severe do not need treatment other than reassurance to the parents that they will spontaneously correct with growth. However, possible underlying pathology must be excluded as this may require treatment:

- Metabolic causes, such as rickets
- Growth plate damage, such as after trauma or infection

- Skeletal dysplasias
- Blount's disease: In this condition there is disturbance of growth of the upper medial tibial growth plate, resulting in acute varus deformity at the knee. The condition may be unilateral or bilateral and has distinct X-ray features.

Warning signs that the condition may not be physiologic are:

- Severe deformity (greater than 20°)
- Unilateral or asymmetrical deformity
- Presence of other swollen joints, other deformities or other abnormal features on general examination
- Abnormally short stature
- Deformity that is getting worse or not correcting with growth.

In patients with any of the above features, X-rays and further investigations are indicated.

Club foot

All newborn babies should have a screening examination for congenital foot deformities, as these are common. A club foot requires early diagnosis and referral so that treatment can be initiated promptly. Most club feet are idiopathic,

Figure 31.4 Physiological bow-legs and Blount's disease. Note the sharp medial angle and lip

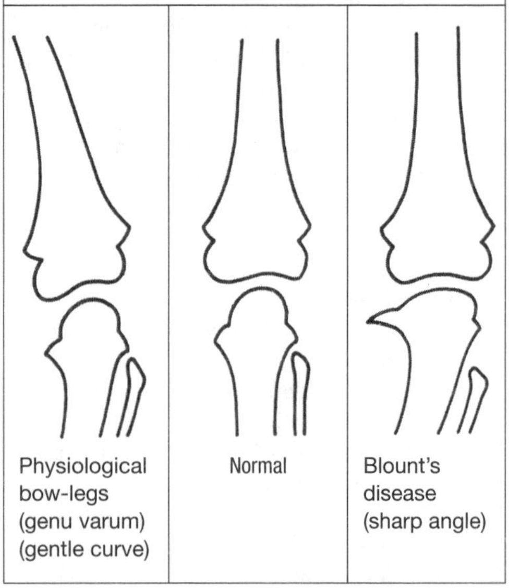

Physiological bow-legs (genu varum) (gentle curve)

Normal

Blount's disease (sharp angle)

but the baby must be examined to exclude other associated disorders such as spinal dysraphism (spina bifida), arthrogryposis (stiff joints), amniotic band syndrome, and DDH.

Clinically the club foot has the following features:

- The hindfoot (heel) is in equinus (high) and is in varus.
- The forefoot is adducted and supinated.
- There is a high medial arch (cavus).

In a normal baby the foot can be dorsiflexed so that the toes touch the front of the leg. In a club foot this is not possible, and the foot is twisted inwards and the sole faces the perineum.

Treatment

This should be initiated early once the baby is stable. The Ponseti method of weekly manipulations and casting, followed at about six weeks by a percutaneous Achilles tendon tenotomy and then long-term bracing in night splints is the treatment of choice. If treatment by this method is initiated within the first few weeks of life, the prognosis is good and more radical surgery is rarely indicated.

32

Skin disorders

When a child is examined for a rash, the whole skin surface should be inspected in a good light. Skin lesions evolve with time – for example blisters may rupture or initial lesions may heal with hyperpigmentation. Sometimes examination reveals different lesions at various stages of development which may make deciding on a diagnosis difficult.

It is essential to always determine the earliest (primary) lesions as these contribute significantly to the differential diagnosis.

Secondary effects, lesion arrangement, morphological pattern, anatomical distribution, age of patient and history are also useful clues.

Primary lesions include the following:
- Macule: flat lesion <1 cm
- Patch: flat lesion >1 cm
- Papule: raised lesion <1 cm
- Plaque: raised lesion >1 cm, may be a group of papules
- Vesicle: lesion <1 cm contains clear fluid
- Blister: lesion >1 cm, may contain clear or blood stained fluid
- Pustule: contains pus
- Scale: piled-up epidermal cells
- Nodule: a lump–may be under normal or part of raised skin

Secondary effects include:
- Scratch marks – excoriations
- Crusts – dried up fluid (serum, blood or pus)
- Scale – piled up epidermal cells (can also be primary)

- Thickening leathery skin due to rubbing
- Infection – pus, yellow crusts
- Pigmentary changes (i.e. post Inflammatory hyper or hypopigmentation).

Lesion arrangements include:
- Annular – e.g. tinea corporis
- Grouped – e.g. herpes simplex
- Linear – e.g. herpes zoster

Pattern recognition – decide which morphological pattern best fits the patient, these include:
Simple patterns:
- Blistering diseases – e.g. herpes, bullous pemphigoid
- Peeling or scaly (papulosquamous) – e.g. psoriasis
- Papules and nodules – e.g. acne
Altered colour:
- Erythematous (red)/pink – e.g. urticaria
- Purple lesions – e.g. lichen planus, drug reactions
- Brown/black pigmentary – increased melanin e.g. melanocytic naevus (mole), no melanin, e.g. albinism, vitiligo (NB: must distinguish from post inflammatory colour change).
Complex patterns:
Eczema can have a combination of features from more than one pattern and can be:
- acute (red, vesicles, weepy with crusts)
- subacute (some features of both) or
- chronic (thick leathery, pigment change and prominent skin markings = lichenification)

Anatomical distribution Although most diseases can affect various body surfaces it is useful to note the distribution of the lesions because some diseases are influenced by anatomical variation, e.g. the face and chest have more sebaceous glands and are more likely to be involved in acne vulgaris.

The mouth, throat, ears, perineum and organ systems (as indicated by history and general assessment) must also be examined. Underlying infections such as tonsillitis or gastrointestinal candidiasis may be the cause of seemingly unrelated skin rashes.

The **history** of symptoms (e.g. itch in eczema and pain in herpes) in the patient and of skin disease in the family or other contacts may give a clue on the condition and on whether it is contagious or inherited.

Bacterial and viral infections, eczema, and scabies are the most common causes of rashes in children and should always be considered in the differential diagnosis of any skin disorder (*see* Table 32.1).

Common disorders

Eczema

Eczema is the most common skin disease and occurs with equal frequency in all races. The term dermatitis is synonymous but is usually used

for eczema due to contact (irritant or allergic reactions).

Definition. Eczema is an inflammatory skin disease which affects mainly the epidermis, resulting in the formation of an intra–epidermal vesicle in the acute stage.

Most important features consist of itching, dryness, scaling, and thickening of the skin; or vesicles and secondary infection.

Most important aspects of treatment are:
* Avoid potential irritants (bath additives and soaps).
* Instead use bland liquid paraffin in bath and aqueous cream as soap.
* Apply bland moisturizers (the drier the skin the greasier).
* Treat the eczema lesions with corticosteroid creams.
* Treat infection with antibiotics.

Common types of eczema in babies:

* Xerosis – dryness of skin
* Atopic eczema
* Seborrhoeic eczema
* Napkin dermatitis ('nappy rash').

The differential diagnosis rests on a careful description of the primary lesions, their distribution, secondary effects, and any associated features.

Table 32.1 Skin disorders in children: approximate percentages of common conditions

Eczema	20
Staphylococcus and streptococcus infections	20
Scabies	15
Insect bites and papular urticaria	5
Warts	5
Fungal infections	5
Other	30

Table 32.2 Clinical presentation of atopic eczema

Acute	Chronic
Swelling (oedema)	Papules
Erythema	Lichenification
Vesicles	Scaling
'Weeping'	
Subacute	**Secondary changes**
Mild erythema	Excoriations
Scaling	Hyper- or hypopigmentation
	Secondary infection
Predominant anatomical distribution	
Babies	head and neck
Children	antecubital and popliteal fossae
Adults	
Any age	Localized (hands, feets, vulva etc)
	Severe disease can be extensive

◆ Use sedating antihistamines to reduce scratching.

Clinical features

(*See* Tables 32.2.and 32.3)

Eczema has many different causes, but the lesions are similar in all types. Itch is a common symptom. The clinical features of eczema can be divided into three stages, any of which may be present at the same time or at different times in the same patient.

Acute. The skin is red and swollen. Vesicles may be visible on the surface and may ooze to discharge a clear, serous fluid – so-called weeping eczema. The fluid dries up to form pale crusts. This vesicular stage may be followed by scaling or the formation of pustules if secondary infection occurs.

Subacute. Primary lesions consist of slight erythema, with or without scaling.

Chronic. The epidermis is thickened (leathery), hyperpigmented (sometimes hypopigmented) and the normal skin furrows (lines) are prominent, referred to as lichenification. Papules, nodules, and scaling may also be found.

Secondary changes. Because of the itch, excoriations are common and may lead to secondary infection. Constant rubbing of the skin causes it to thicken and increases the itch. Pigmentary changes consisting of hyper- or hypopigmentation may be prominent, particularly in dark-skinned patients. Once the eczema has healed, the skin colour and texture gradually return to normal.

Causes of eczema in children

Dryness of the skin

This is perhaps the most common cause of eczema in infants, in whom dryness is often aggravated by too much bathing, soaps, and powders. It is worse in dry winter months.

Pityriasis alba is a form of dry eczema which occurs commonly on the faces of children of all races. It results in hypopigmented, scaling patches which are cosmetically disturbing. It is often mistakenly ascribed to a fungal infection. It is common in children with atopic eczema or other atopic features (asthma, hayfever or family history of atopy).

Infection

Infections causing damage to the epidermis may result in a secondary eczematous rash, for example around the ear in a case of purulent otitis media. Secondary eczematization may occur around the lesions of scabies and molluscum contagiosum. Eczema following trauma of various kinds, including burns, is usually also due to secondary infection.

Atopic eczema

This is a constitutional form of eczema in which there may be a personal or family history of hay fever (allergic rhinitis), allergic conjunctivitis and asthma. In the infant with atopic eczema, a red, wet and/or scaling eruption usually starts on the cheeks and extensor parts of the limbs, but may become generalized (*see* Figure 32.1).

Itch is usually severe and excoriations and secondary infection are common. Atopic eczema commonly starts at about the age of three months and recurs in a fluctuating manner. In older children the eczema tends to become localized in the flexures of limbs (antecubital and popliteal fossae) and other joints (wrists and ankles).

Atopic eczema in babies is often wrongly ascribed to an allergy to cow's milk. In the small number of cases where milk allergy does play a role, gastro-intestinal signs such as vomiting and diarrhoea are also present.

Older children may be allergic to other foods such as eggs and fish, but it is important to

Table 32.3 Clinical signs of atopy
Face
Infraorbital fold (Danny Morgan lines) – prominent lines under eyes
Periorbital hyperpigmentation
Muddy discoloration of sclera – brownish stain (chronic rubbing of eyes)
Head lamp sign – the nose area is spared (looks normal compared to eczema changes on the rest of the face)
Salute sign – a crease across bridge of nose (chronic rubbing of the itchy nose)
Fissure below ear – more common in infants
Hands
Hyperlinearity of the palms

Infants with eczema should be allowed to continue breastfeeding.

remember that the typical skin manifestation caused by food allergy is urticaria, not eczema. Food allergy does not cause eczema but may make it worse in a minority of patients. Foods suspected of aggravating eczema should be temporarily avoided (one at a time for 3-4 weeks) and re-introduced if the eczema does not improve.

The fluctuating nature of atopic eczema must be explained to the parents, who should be warned that the rash is likely to recur until the child outgrows it, which occurs in about 50% by school going age. Most of those with persistent eczema have manageable mild localized disease (flexures, hands, foot, genital etc) although a few may continue to have life long severe disease.

Nummular or discoid eczema is the name given to round or coin-shaped patches of eczema which may occur in patients with or without atopic eczema.

Hand and foot eczema. In older children with atopic eczema, the lesions are often confined to the hands and feet, particularly the palms and soles. In some children the skin is very dry and cracked and this is called hyperkeratotic eczema. In others, the eczema consists of vesicles and pustules which may recur at intervals for years.

Papular eczema. Toddlers with a background of atopy may sometimes develop a fine papular eczematous rash.

Seborrhoeic eczema

This condition is considered to be one of the inborn or constitutional types of eczema. The characteristic lesions consist of yellowish scales on the scalp, so-called cradle cap. The flexural areas such as the groin, perineum, folds in the neck and behind the ears are commonly affected, and the distribution is thus similar to that seen in immune suppressed adults. The lesions often become moist and in severe cases the rash may become generalized. It usually starts during the first few weeks of life and may recur for several months but seldom persists beyond the first year (see Figure 32.2).

Seborrhoeic eczema is easier to treat and not

as persistent as atopic eczema. However, it is not always possible to differentiate between atopic and seborrhoeic eczema in a young infant. Seborrheoeic eczema in HIV positive children responds poorly to usual treatment, but tends to resolve with antiretroviral treatment.

Contact dermatitis

Objects such as school benches, car seats, and shoes are sometimes suspected of causing contact dermatitis in children. It may be difficult to decide whether the rash is due to an allergy or to mechanical irritation in a patient with atopic dermatitis. Patch tests may be helpful in the diagnosis. Contact dermatitis due to plants is seen in children of the older age group. The lesions of plant dermatitis are characteristically linear in shape and may be intensely irritating. More common causes of contact dermatitis include cosmetics (e.g. nail polish, hair dye), creams (e.g. topical antihistamines), jewelry (nickel - in earrings and jean stubs), rubber (e.g. foot dermatitis due to black rubber in shoes). The localized nature of the lesions and compatible history may be useful clues to the diagnosis.

Napkin dermatitis ('nappy rash')

Irritant or eczematous rashes due to soap powders, rinses, or infrequent changing of soiled nappies are easily recognized if it is remembered that the affected skin corresponds to the area in contact with the nappy and the folds in the groins and perineum are spared. The affected skin may be red, glazed, and shiny, or have an eczematous appearance. In severe cases, erosions, ulcers, and nodular lesions may occur. The condition

---

Common causes of dermatitis in the napkin area

- Napkin (contact) dermatitis usually spares the groin folds.
- Seborrhoeic eczema may be associated with greasy scale on scalp ('cradle cap').
- Candidiasis may be associated with papules/pustules scattered beyond the margin of skin involvement ('satellite lesions').
- Inverse psoriasis involves groin, axillae: when scratched the margin may reveal silvery white scale.

Figure 32.1 Atopic infantile eczema: lichenification and scaling (trunk), secondary infection with oozing and crusting (arm)

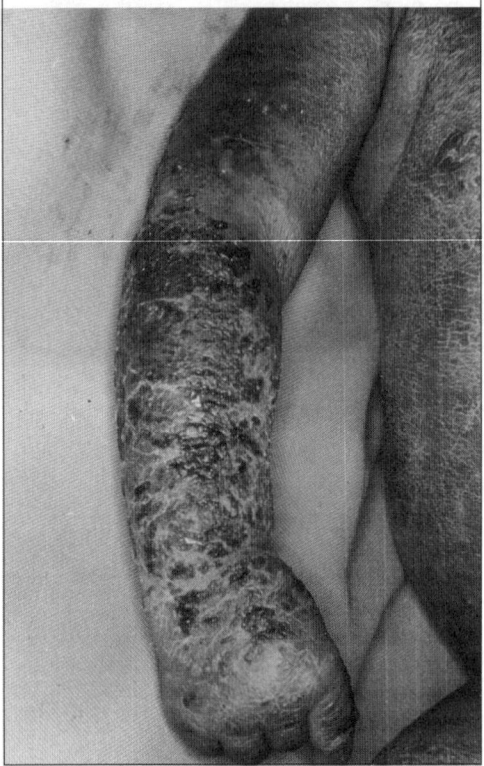

Figure 32.2 Seborrhoeic infantile eczema: erythema, scaling, and depigmentation in flexures, and involvement of scalp

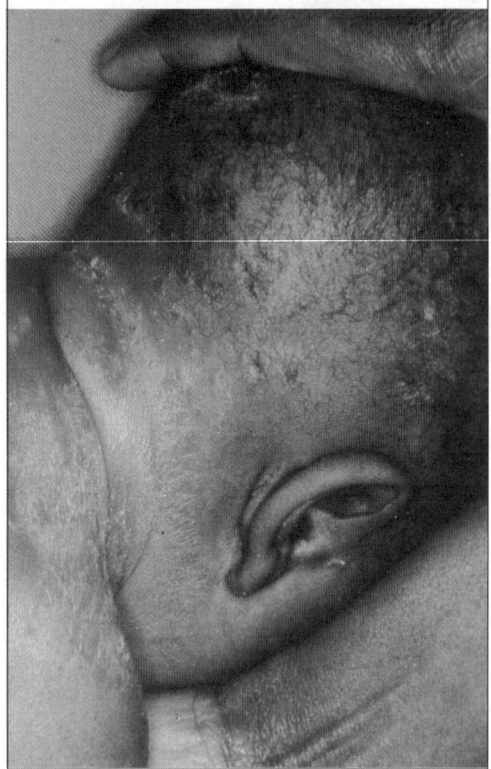

must be differentiated from seborrhoeic eczema, candidiasis, and bacterial infection. Maximal involvement is seen in the inguinal and intergluteal folds in seborrhoeic dermatitis and around the anus in candidiasis. Perineal cellulitis due to streptococcal infections is characterized by redness and pain. The term 'napkin psoriasis' is used to describe well-circumscribed, erythematous, smooth or scaling patches which may prove to be an early manifestation of psoriasis in some cases.

Treatment of eczema

Any patch of eczema should receive attention; if left in a state of activity, the eczema is likely to spread to other parts of the body and even become generalized.

  ♦ *Avoid potential irritants* in bath additives (as in bubble bath, bath crystals, bath

salts). Anything that foams dries out the skin! Replace soap with a bland cream (no colour or smell) e.g. aqueous cream or ung. emulsificans BP which contains white Vaseline®, liquid paraffin, and emulsifying waxes. It may be rubbed into the skin or used in bath water instead of bath oil .
  ♦ *Relieve dryness* of the skin by liberal use of bland moisturizers. Aqueous cream (ung.

Table 32.4 Treatment of atopic eczema

Avoid potential irritants
Replace soap with a bland cream
Liberal use of bland moisturizers
Use topical corticosteroids only when there is active eczema
Use sedating antihistamines to break the itch-scratch-cycle

emulsificans aqueosum UEA) is usually not very effective as it is made up of mostly water, which evaporates. Choose one as oily as can be tolerated. Emulsifying ointment (HEB) and vaseline are oily and ideal for dry skin, but cetamacrogol (often preferred by patients) is oilier than UEA but less than HEB.

♦ Oral steroids are best avoided, and *topical corticosteroids* should be used when there is active eczema. In the face, a hydrocortisone ointment is chosen, but on the body, betamethasone ointment is appropriate. Use undiluted corticosteroid preparations intermittently on localized and lichenified plaques and on extensive severe disease. In infants with large areas of eczema, the steroid should be diluted in order to minimize side-effects through absorption, and also to make the ointment or cream go further. A corticosteroid preparation such as betamethasone valerate may be diluted up to 10 times in ung. emulsificans if a greasy preparation is required; or in ung. emulsificans aqueosum if a cream base is preferred.

♦ Choose the *most suitable topical cortico-steroid preparation*. In general, ointments are preferred to creams. If the skin is dry, a greasy ointment should be used; if the skin is not dry and particularly under hot humid conditions or for very wet eczema, a cream may be better tolerated. If necessary a trial of each separately may be helpful.

The above steps should be continued during remissions to reduce chances of acute episodes.

♦ Any *secondary infection* always retards healing of the eczema and should be treated. For small areas of infected eczema, a combined antibiotic-steroid cream should be used. If there are hard crusts which need to be removed, a greasy ointment will do this more effectively than a cream. If the infection is widespread or severe, a systemic antibiotic such as erythromycin or cloxacillin should be given in addition.

♦ *Sedating antihistamines* are used for their sedative effect, as part of breaking the itch-scratch-cycle. If eczema were not scratched, secondary infection and lichenification would not occur!

♦ *Moist, weeping areas of eczema* should be treated with lotions, or wet dressings where bandaging is easy. Intermittent applications of 'wet wraps' are reserved for severe and/or extensive disease or thick lichenified areas. It is seldom necessary to use a wet dressing for more than a few days. The cream or ointment is covered with plastic or damp saline bandages (wet wraps) overnight and left open during the day. This method is particularly useful for keratotic eczema on the palms and soles. Occlusive dressings should not be used if there is any sign of infection, as they will cause it to spread. If an area of weeping eczema looks infected, weak potassium permanganate solution, or diluted eusol may be used instead of saline.

Bacterial diseases involving the skin

Staphylococcal and streptococcal infections

Staphylococci and streptococci commonly cause primary and secondary skin infections in children, particularly if they are malnourished and live in overcrowded conditions.

Staphylococcal infections result in the formation of pus and tend to be localized. Neonates are, however, particularly susceptible to *Staphylococcus aureus* and easily develop generalized infections (*see* Figure 32.3).

Streptococcal infections tend to spread diffusely with very little, if any, suppuration. In the newborn, infection by group B β–haemolytic streptococci may cause a bacteraemia, which may present in the skin as cellulitis or a purpuric rash. In older children, skin infections are caused by group A β–haemolytic streptococci and may be followed by glomerulonephritis. Infections with strains of streptococci and staphylococci which produce an erythrogenic toxin may result in widespread or localized erythema, followed by desquamation (peeling).

Treatment

Antibiotic ointments are usually sufficient for localized superficial infections. In widespread staphylococcal infections and for most strepto-coccal infections, a systemic antibiotic should be

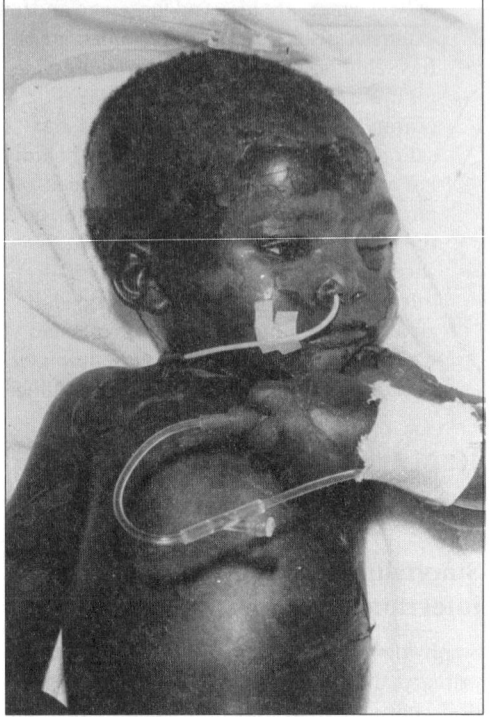

Figure 32.3 Staphylococcal scalded skin syndrome. Note abscess in left orbital region, the focus of infection

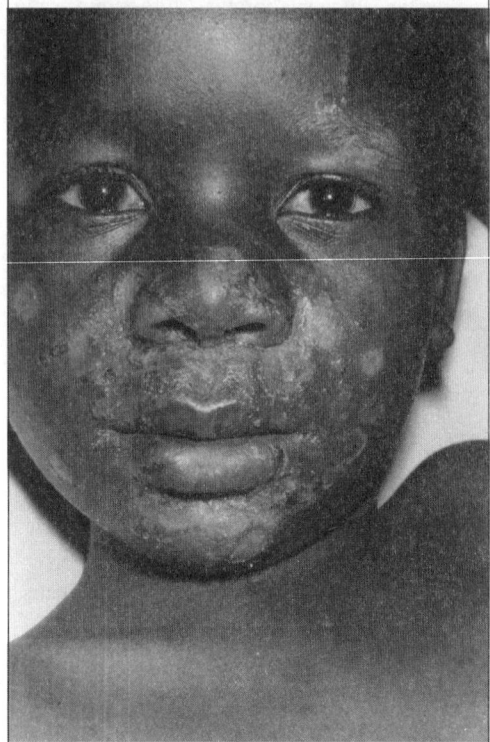

Figure 32.4 Impetigo: round, confluent, oozing, and crusted lesions extending into nostrils

given in addition. Erythromycin and cloxacillin are usually safe and effective where sensitivity tests are not available.

Impetigo

(*See* Figure 32.4)
Most important features are round, confluent, superficial blisters which rupture early and form yellow crusts.

Most important causes are staphylococcal and streptococcal infection from the patient's nose or from other children.

Treatment is by topical antibiotics and antiseptics, together with systemic antibiotics in severe or widespread infections.

Skin eruptions secondary to streptococcal infection elsewhere (e.g. tonsillitis)

Desquamation of the skin, particularly the palms and soles, may be the only complaint in a patient who is otherwise well and has not had scarlet fever. It is thought to be due to a previous asymptomatic infection with streptococci which produce an erythrogenic toxin. A fine rash, consisting of very small, diffuse, superficial papules, occurring in children with a fever, may be due to streptococcal tonsillitis (*see* Figure 32.5).

The rash and fever respond rapidly to an oral antibiotic. Streptococcal tonsillitis may precipitate an attack of guttate psoriasis.

Disseminated intravascular coagulation (DIC)

Gram-negative septicaemia is the most common cause of DIC in infants, but it may also follow septicaemia due to streptococcal and staphylococcal infections. Skin lesions in DIC are characteristic and consist of angulated purpuric macules which may be followed by the formation of large blisters and skin infarcts (*see* Figure 32.6).

Biopsy of these lesions shows necrosis of the

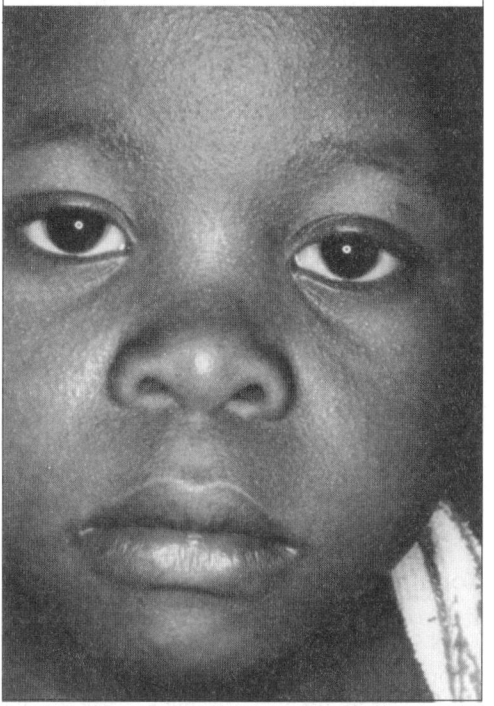

Figure 32.5 Streptococcal eruption: fine follicular rash associated with streptococcal tonsillitis

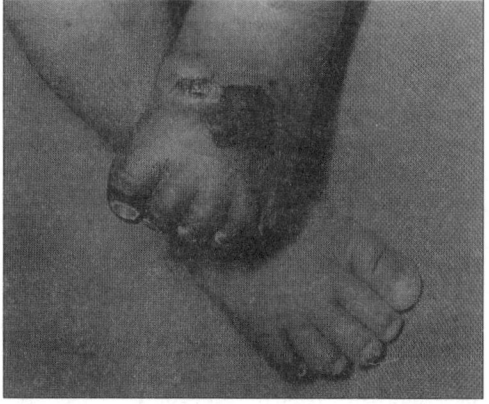

Figure 32.6 Disseminated intravascular coagulation: angulated skin infarct and gangrene of toes

Syphilis

Congenital syphilis

Widespread, scaling, red papular eruptions, mucous patches in the mouth, and moist condylomas in the perineum resemble those of early adult secondary syphilis (*see* Figures 32.7 and 32.8). The rash is usually non specific but involvement of palms and soles may be a clue.

Late congenital syphilis is rarely, if ever, seen, but the possibility of a gumma should be borne in mind in any older patient with a chronic ulcer of unknown cause.

Venereal syphilis

Primary chancres may occur as a result of sexual abuse of infants and young children. The

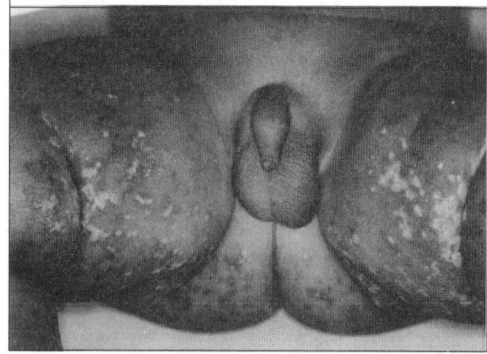

Figure 32.7 Congenital syphilis: scaling, pigmented maculo-papules

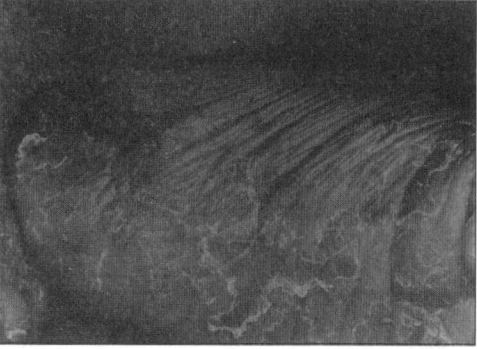

Figure 32.8 Congenital syphilis: confluent scaling macules on soles of feet

epidermis and multiple fibrin thrombi in the dermal vessels. Occlusion of deeper vessels may cause gangrene of larger areas such as the ears or digits.

characteristic firmness of the non tender ulcer and enlarged, rubbery, regional lymph nodes suggest the diagnosis. Serological tests may be negative in the early stage and should be repeated after three months. Secondary syphilis, although rare in children, should be considered in any infiltrated, papular rash involving the palms and/or soles of unknown cause.

Serological tests (VDRL, FTA) are needed to confirm the diagnosis. (*see* Chapter 7, Care of the newborn)

The treatment of choice is penicillin.

Tuberculosis

(*See also* Chapter 17, Tuberculosis.)

Skin lesions may be due to direct infection with *Mycobacterium tuberculosis* or to hypersensitivity reactions called tuberculides. Biopsy and a tuberculin test are needed to confirm the diagnosis.

Tuberculous chancre

This is extremely rare. Primary inoculation of the skin results in a nodule which soon ulcerates. The important feature is enlargement of the regional lymph glands.

Lupus vulgaris

This is the most common type of tuberculous skin infection, occurring in a partially immune patient who has previously been vaccinated or had tuberculosis elsewhere. Lesions may be single or multiple and occur on any part of the body. They may present as soft, flat, or warty plaques or raised spongy nodules. The most common type occurs around the nose and has a raised, slowly advancing edge and ulcerating centre. Destruction of the nasal cartilage may result in severe deformity. Patients should be investigated for other foci of tuberculosis.

Scrofuloderma

This represents direct spread of tuberculosis, e.g. from infected lymph nodes to overlying skin.

Tuberculides

These are multiple disseminated lesions resulting from an underlying tuberculous focus which is not always demonstrable. They are thought to be due to hypersensitivity reactions to *M. tuberculosis*

although recent studies have demonstrated the presence of viral DNA by PCR in the lesions. The tuberculin test is usually strongly positive. There are three clinical types which may occur singly or together in the same patient:

Papulonecrotic tuberculides

Lesions consist of papules and pustules which ulcerate, and heal to form oval to round depressed scars. They are symmetrically distributed and occur mainly over the extensor aspects of the limbs, particularly the elbows and knees, and on the buttocks. Biopsy shows a vasculitis due to a type III (Arthus) hypersensitivity reaction.

Lichen scrofulosorum

Lesions consist of small, firm papules which may be grouped together in round patches or diffuse and widespread. Biopsy shows tuberculoid granulomas which are due to a cell-mediated immune response.

Nodular tuberculides

Lesions occur mainly on the lower legs. In the acute form, known as erythema nodosum the lesions are usually on the shins. Chronic forms are known as nodular vasculitis, or erythema induratum. These lesions are predominantly at the back of the legs and tend to ulcerate. They tend to recur until the underlying tuberculous infection is treated. Erythma nodosum is not specific and may be associated with other infections (e.g. streptococcal) and inflammatory disorders (e.g. sarcoidosis).

Leprosy

(*See* Chapter 15, Systemic infections)

Viral infections

Herpes simplex

(*See* Chapter 15, Systemic infections.)

Primary infection in infants usually results in gingivo-stomatitis. In older children, herpes simplex takes the form of 'fever blisters', with clusters of vesicles grouped together on a red base.

Herpes simplex infection is sometimes followed after one to two weeks by erythema multiforme. Disseminated cutaneous herpes simplex consists of a few to many scattered vesicles with or without any herpetiform grouping and may be a complication of atopic eczema (referred to as eczema herpeticum). Herpes simplex infection should be considered in any vesicular rash of unknown cause.

Treatment of skin lesions consists of drying antiseptic applications such as calamine lotion. Antibiotics are indicated only if secondary infection is present. Severe and generalized infections should be treated with oral or intravenous acyclovir particularly in immunocompromised patients.

Herpes zoster

(*See* Chapter 15, Systemic infections)

The lesions of herpes zoster consist of grouped vesicles arranged along the cutaneous distribution of a spinal nerve (dermatome); they heal within two to three weeks in immune competent patients. In patients infected with HIV the eruption may involve more than one dermatome or be disseminated; the lesions may ulcerate and persist for months. Severe and generalized infections should be treated with acyclovir. Healed zoster may recur after starting antiretroviral treatment as part of the immune reconstitution syndrome.

Hand, foot, and mouth disease

This infection, due to a coxsackie virus type A, usually occurs in toddlers who have few systemic symptoms. The lesions consist of round or oval vesicles which heal within two weeks. The lesions are found commonly, but not exclusively, in the mouth and on the palms and soles. Symptomatic treatment suffices for this self-limiting condition.

Molluscum contagiosum

Caused by a pox virus, the lesions may be numerous. They consist of slightly shiny (pearly) papules which have an umbilicated dome-shaped centre and contain a whitish or cheesy material. Wart treatment should be avoided because that is designed to remove thick skin – the skin around mollusca is not thick and more likely to be eroded. Freezing with liquid nitrogen, if available, is effective but may cause post inflammatory hypopigmentation especially in dark skin. Acne creams are safer and can be applied to individual lesions for their potential to cause dryness and slight peeling enough to remove the virus-containing white core, e.g. tretinoin (Airol®, Retin-A®) or benzyl peroxide. The lesions become inflamed and then disappear. It is important to note that all treatments have the potential to cause scarring. In healthy children, this benign childhood ailment eventually resolves spontaneously without scarring.

Warts

Warts are caused by the human papilloma virus and are extremely common in children of school-going age. The ordinary wart (verruca vulgaris) may be single or multiple and is recognizable by its papillomatous surface. *Plane warts* are small, flat warts that occur in large numbers on the face and limbs (*see* Figure 32.9)

The tendency of these to grow in lines usually from scratch marks (so called Koebner phenomena) is a useful clue to diagnosis. Condylomata accuminata or genital warts, which occur on the genitalia or around the anus, have a moist, vegetating papillomatous surface. The possibility of sexual abuse must be considered; however, warts on the genitalia and perineum are often acquired non-venereally and are more common in immune suppressed patients.

Treatment

Until children develop immunity against the virus, warts are likely to spread and recur after any form of treatment. Most warts will, however, eventually undergo spontaneous healing, which may be preceded by inflammation (redness which is often misdiagnosed as infection).

In the treatment of warts in children, unnecessary pain and scarring must be avoided. The aim of conservative treatment is to cause irritation of the wart. The resultant inflammatory reaction is usually followed by disappearance of the wart.

Many topical treatments are available including wart paint, corn plasters (these contain the keratolytic salicylic acid which peels skin; the plaster can be left in place until it falls off and the softened skin is filed down) can be repeated until irritation develops after which the wart usu-

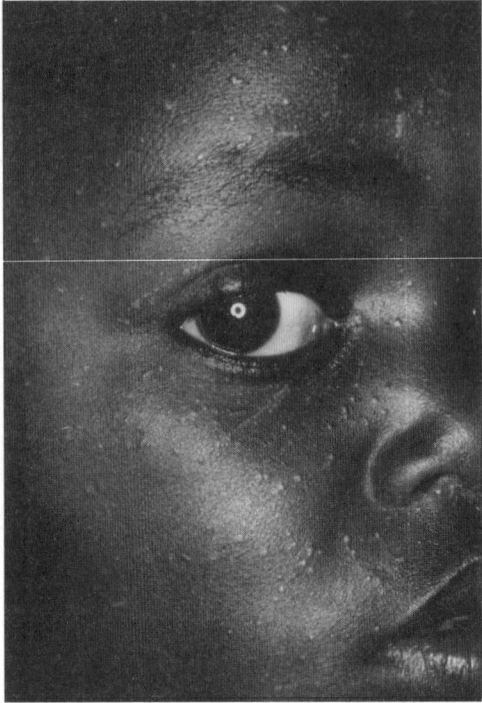

Figure 32.9 Plane warts: multiple small papules, some in lines along scratch marks

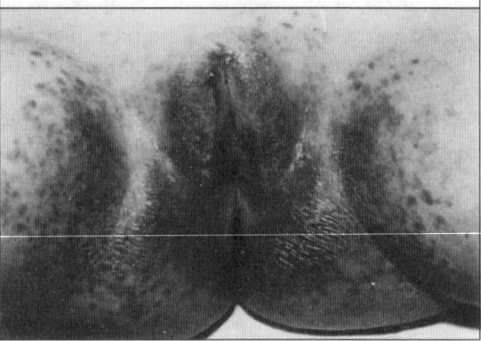

Figure 32.10 Candidiasis: perineal involvement in gastro-intestinal candidiasis. Note outlying pustules and scaly macules

ally disappears. Liquid nitrogen can also be used if available.

Condylomata acuminata are painted with 20 per cent podophyllin in tincture of benzoin and dusted with talc powder to protect surrounding skin, and washed off after six hours, or earlier if painful. Treatment may be repeated at weekly intervals if necessary. In non responsive patients imiquimod (Aldara®) a new immune modulator has potent antiviral activity.

In general, warts should never be excised, but curettage, with or without preceding light electro-desiccation, is at times justified.

Fungal infections of skin

The yeast *Candida albicans* and many of the dermatophytic fungi which grow in the horny layer of the epidermis, are common causes of infection in children. In all of these the diagnosis may be confirmed by microscopical examination. Skin, hair, and nail scrapings are covered with 30%

potassium hydroxide. The specimen should be re-examined after a few minutes if nothing is seen initially.

Candidiasis

Most important features are small, outlying pustules or macules with a peripheral scale surrounding red, glazed, or moist skin.

The most important cause in babies is immune immaturity. In older healthy children, candida overgrowth may occur after systemic antibiotics, usually presenting with 'thrush' in the mouth and gastrointestinal tract. In the absence of such a history, consider HIV infection.

Eruptions due to *Candida albicans* are common in babies. Apart from oral thrush, the skin rash usually starts around the anus and spreads to the perineum, groin, and intergluteal fold. Other moist, flexural areas such as the axillae and neck folds may also be involved. The rash is well circumscribed with a moist eroded surface and brick-red colour. Small, discrete, outlying papules and pustules (satellite lesions) are a characteristic finding (*see* Figure 32.10).

The pustules contain a whitish exudate and being very superficial, soon break to form erosions surrounded by a small peripheral scale. Occasionally a widespread secondary rash consisting of scaling papules occurs on the trunk and limbs.

Treatment

Topical applications of antifungal creams such as clotrimazole, nystatin (Mycostatin®) or one of the imidazole preparations (Daktarin®, Canesten®, Pevaryl®) soon clear any skin lesions, but these may recur if oral thrush is not treated simultaneously with an oral suspension of nystatin.

Ringworm (tinea)

Ringworm infections in children are caused by members of the *Microsporum* and *Trichophyton* species. As a general rule, scalp ringworm occurs before puberty and 'athlete's foot' usually after.

The most important causes of ringworm in children are *T. violaceum* infections acquired from other children and *M. canis* infections acquired from cats and dogs.

Scalp ringworm (tinea capitis)

Fungal carriage in children without clinical disease is relatively common.

T. violaceum, the most common cause of ringworm in disadvantaged communities, spreads easily among household contacts. (*See* Figure 32.11.) *M. canis* infections are more common in affluent children who own (and live in close contact with pets).

The typical presentation is with patchy or diffuse areas of scaling and hair loss, which may be mild and hardly visible. There may also be erythema, papules and pustules. Mild infections may heal spontaneously without leaving a trace but in some children secondary bacterial infection results in scarring and patchy permanent hair loss. Close inspection of a scalp affected with ringworm reveals thickened, white, opaque hair stumps in which the fungus is easily seen in scrapings taken for microscopic examination.

Occasionally a lesion may undergo an inflammatory reaction with the formation of a boggy swelling studded with pustules which is known as a kerion. These are often misdiagnosed as abscesses (and should be suspected if an apparent abscess coexists with scaly areas of hair loss). A kerion is due to a hypersensitivity reaction to the fungus and should not be incised.

Body ringworm (tinea corporis)

The lesions are characteristically ring-shaped, with active, raised, scaly margins which spread outwards. If not apparent, the scale may become

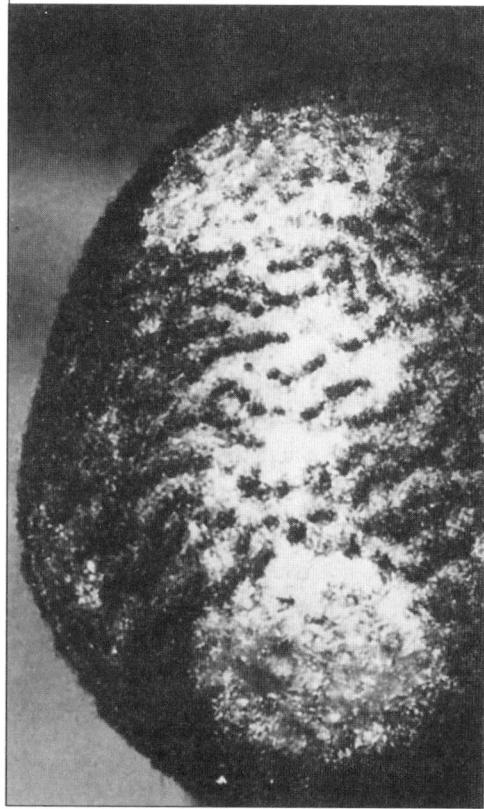

Figure 32.11 Scalp ringworm: broken-off white hair stumps in scaling patches of hair loss

prominent by scraping the margin. Sometimes more than one advancing edge is present and concentric rings are formed.

Nail ringworm is rare in children, and thickened, irregular or crumbly nails are more likely to be due to diseases such as eczema or psoriasis.

Treatment

Many topical antifungal preparations are available. Whitfield's ointment is cheap and worth trying in lesions of the skin (useless on the scalp). Topical antifungals such as Canesten® (clotrimazole) have a broad-spectrum antifungal effect and are effective in isolated or few lesions on the skin. For multiple skin lesions or involvement of the scalp or nails, systemic treatment is required. Nystatin, useful for candida infections, is not effective against dermatophytes. Griseofulvin (Grisovin®, Fulcin®, Microcidal®), is specific for dermatophyte infections; it is given by mouth at a dose of 10–20mg/day (for four weeks in extensive skin involvement, for six weeks for scalp infection, three months for finger nails and at least six months for toenail involvement). Griseofulvin should be given after a meal preferable with milk to prevent malabsorption (which together with underdosing is a common cause of treatment failure). Newer antifungals are particularly useful for the treatment of nail disease because they significantly shorten the treatment duration.

Sporotrichosis

This deep fungal infection should be suspected in any chronic purulent, ulcerative or granulomatous skin lesions which occur in a row and do not respond to antibiotic therapy. Lymphatic spread often results in a centrally extending row of nodules which may ulcerate. The diagnosis may be confirmed by culture and biopsy. Response to potassium iodide, given by mouth, is specific and may be used as a therapeutic test. Marked improvement is evident within one to two weeks, but treatment must be continued for two to three months, until the lesions are quite inactive. Itraconazole (Sporanox®) is an easier treatment alternative.

Infestations

Scabies

The most important features of scabies are a history of contact, severe itch, and small scratched papules and vescicles between fingers, on wrists, the trunk and limbs. The cause is direct skin-to-skin transmission of the mite from an infected person.

The mite *Sarcoptes scabiei* causes periodic epidemics of an intensely itchy rash. The characteristic lesions consist of small vesicles and short, superficial burrows, often seen between the fingers. Skin scrapings to demonstrate mites are best taken from these sites. The most common lesions, however, are small superficial papules which may be widespread on the trunk and limbs but tend to cluster around the axillae and on the buttocks. The papules may be few or numerous and invariably show evidence of scratching. They

heal to leave small white spots with a dark rim, which take several months to fade. Larger nodular lesions, so-called persistent scabies nodules, are sometimes found in the axillae and groins and on the genitalia. Often the diagnosis is suggested when one or more household contacts have a similar itching rash.

Treatment

The most important aspect of treatment is to apply the scabicide over the whole skin surface from the neck to the toes.

Three preparations are available and each is curative, provided it is applied over the entire skin surface. An ointment containing 2–5% sulphur is the safest for infants. It should be applied for three consecutive nights and include the head if this is involved. Ascabiol® (25 per cent benzyl benzoate emulsion), applied overnight and up to 24 seven days apart, can be diluted 1:1 with water to reduce irritation in babies (older than six months). Gamma benzene hexachloride (Quellada®, Gambex®) requires only one application, but is toxic and not recommended for babies nor for young children with many excoriated lesions. To avoid re-infection, close household contacts should be treated at the same time. Scabicidal soaps alone are not effective as treatment. Clothes and bed-linen are laundered in order for patients to change into clean clothes and linen at the end of treatment.

Skin lesions and itch decrease immediately, but take three to four weeks to clear completely. Persistence of itch after proper treatment is likely to be due to dryness and even eczema resulting from the topical applications; a bland moisturizer and topical steroid may be useful.

Insect bites

Insect bites cause itchy papules, in the centre of which a small punctum (the bite) can sometimes be seen. Vesicles or large blisters may form on some of them. Insect bites are invariably scratched and may be secondarily infected. Flea bites tend to be small, are often grouped in short lines and, although they occur mainly on exposed parts of the limbs, are often found around the waist. Mosquito and bedbug bites are larger and the latter usually have a prominent, haemorrhagic punctum. Jassids, small, hard, green flying insects found on grass, are an often unrecognized source of insect bites. Insect bites-related true urticaria is transient; the bite induces mast cell degranulation and histamin release. The latter is responsible for the redness (vasodilatation) and swelling (increased vascular permeability). Spontaneous resolution (or from antihistamine use) results in vasoconstriction and interstitial fluid removal (via lymphatics); this usually leaves behind completely normal skin.

Papular urticaria (lichen urticatus)

In some children who are hypersensitive to insect bites, numerous intensely itchy papules occur on the limbs, particularly during the months when insects abound. In addition to the histamin mediated initial response to the bite, patients with papular urticaria also have type IV (delayed) hypersensitivity. The lesions go on for longer, are more symptomatic, fixed, often scratched and secondarily infected. This results in limbs (and trunk) with a spotty appearance (i.e. lesions of various shades of brown – indicating chronicity and different stage of development). In addition there may be occasional red lesions (new bites). If the child still wears a nappy there is usually striking sparing of the nappy area (less so in older children who wear loose underwear). Children between the ages of two and six years are more commonly affected and attacks may recur during several successive summers.

This can worsen after starting antiretroviral retreatment and is part of the immune reconstitution inflammatory syndrome (IRIS); the pathogenesis is thought to be multifactorial (possibly including insect bite allergy, eosinophilic folliculitis, ptyrosporum folliculitis).

Treatment

Prevention of insect bites is difficult. Pets should be treated for fleas; insect repellents and mosquito nets could help. In mild cases, calamine lotion may suffice. Corticosteroid creams are preferred for new and itchy lesions to reduce

A similar spotty clinical picture is seen in HIV-positive children and adults, where it is referred to as papular pruritic eruption (PPE) of HIV or locally as 'itchy bumps disease'.

scarring. Combination of steroids and tar are also useful. The smell of tar is thought to act as an insect repellent. An antibiotic ointment should be prescribed if there is any sign of infection.

Sandworm (larva migrans, creeping eruption)

Larvae of the cat and dog hookworm (*Ankylostoma braziliense*) penetrate any part of the skin which comes into contact with soil contaminated with the eggs. The characteristic lesions are severely itchy, superficial, relatively large, winding burrows. Secondary infection is common. Albendazole (Zentel®) 400 mg daily for three consecutive days is curative.

Myiasis

The fly *Cordylobia anthropophaga* lays her eggs on clothing hung out to dry. Larvae burrow into the skin from infected clothing, causing red painful nodules. These are mistaken for boils until the larvae are seen moving in the central opening. Application of Vaseline® cuts off their air supply and causes them to wriggle outwards. Once the larvae have been removed, the lesions heal quickly, but secondary infection may need antibiotic treatment. Infestation can be prevented by ironing clothes before they are worn.

Lice

Head lice cause periodic epidemics usually among white and Indian schoolchildren. The easiest form of treatment is to shampoo with gamma benzene hexachloride (Quellada®, Gambex®). Resistance to treatment is increasing; physical removal of nits and lice with fine tooth combing is a useful adjunct to treatment.

Immunologically mediated skin disorders

Urticaria

Skin lesions appear within minutes, are intensely itchy, and disappear within hours without leaving a trace. They may be few or numerous and consist of flat red papules or large confluent plaques or rings. Crops of new lesions may continue to appear for days, months, or years. Recurrent urticaria lasting more than six weeks is referred to as chronic urticaria.

The lesions are red due to vasodilatation; oedema results from increased permeability of blood-vessels following the release of histamine and other substances in the skin. When deeper vessels are involved, diffuse, ill-defined swellings result. These are known as angio-oedema and often affect the eyelids or lips. Involvement of the larynx may be a life-threatening complication.

The term *dermographism* is used to describe the production of raised wheals by firm stroking of the skin. It is often found in patients with urticaria, but may occur as an isolated finding in perfectly normal individuals.

Causes of urticaria may be varied and can include physical factors such as cold, heat, pressure on the skin and even contact with water. More common causes include parasites, infections, foods or drugs; but the aetiology is often unknown. Investigations in chronic and recurrent urticaria maybe unnecessary, should be guided by the individual's clinical features could include blood count – a raised eosinophil count may suggest worm infestation, bilharzia serology, examination of urine and stools for infections and parasites, and X-rays of the chest, teeth and/or sinuses where necessary.

Treatment

An antihistamine by mouth is all that is needed in a mild attack of unknown cause. A systemic antibiotic should be given in addition if an underlying infection is suspected. Severe attacks of urticaria may require systemic corticosteroids as well. If laryngeal oedema threatens, adrenalin should be given subcutaneously and the antihistamines by IM or IV injection. Corticosteroids have a more delayed action.

Allergic vasculitis

(*See* Chapter 20, Allergic disorders)

Erythema multiforme

Lesions consist of small papules or vesicles which spread outward to form concentric rings with dark centres, the so-called target or iris lesions. They vary in appearance from small, flat papules with raised edges and a dark central crust, to large haemorrhagic bullae. The rash is symmetrical and occurs mainly on the face and extensor surfaces of the limbs and typically involves the palms.

Stevens-Johnson syndrome is a severe form of erythema multiforme, in which the lesions are large, bullous, and crusted and the mucous membranes of the mouth, genitalia, and eyes are involved (*see* Figure 32.12).

Some cases of Stevens-Johnson syndrome are due to infections such as *Mycoplasma pneumoniae*, others to drugs such as sulphonamides or phenolphthalein, but the cause is often unknown.

Toxic epidermal necrolysis is a severe form of erythema multiforme in which blistering of the skin resembles burns. It may be found in association with other forms of erythema multiforme. The epidermal blister is deeper than in staphylococcal scalded skin syndrome from which it should be distinguished, if necessary by biopsy.

Treatment

Erythema multiforme takes about three weeks to clear and no specific treatment is required for most cases. The frequency of recurrent attacks that following cold sores (herpes simplex) may reduce with antiviral treatment such as acyclovir.

Some causes of urticaria in children:

Infections	Tonsillitis
	Urinary tract infection
	Sinusitis
	Dental sepsis
Parasites	Worms
	Schistosomiasis
Drugs	Aspirin
	Penicillin
Foods	Eggs
	Fish
	Preservatives

It is often impossible to decide whether a drug, or the infection for which it is given, is the offender.

Drugs, bacterial and viral infections, notably herpes simplex, are known causes of erythema multiforme, but often the aetiology is obscure.

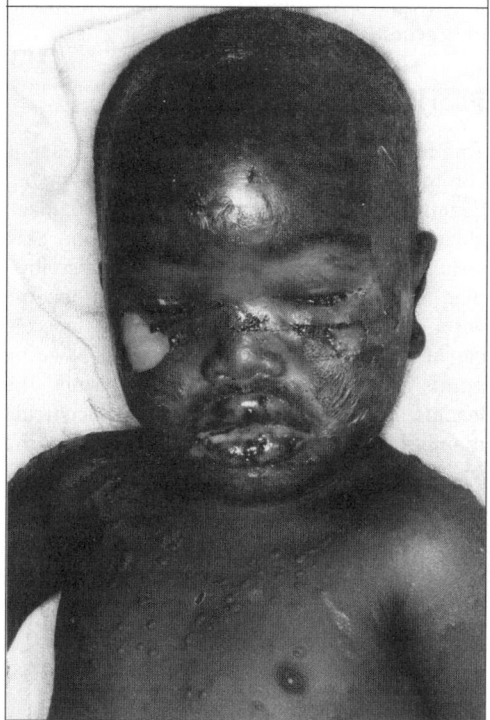

Figure 32.12 Stevens-Johnson syndrome: erosion of mucous membranes (mouth and eyes), erythema multiforme with target lesions (chest), and toxic epidermal necrolysis (cheeks)

Calamine lotion maybe used for symptomatic treatment. Lesions close to the eyes may be treated with an ointment soften crusts and a topical antibiotic used to prevent infection.

Erythema nodosum

Lesions consist of painful, deep nodules on the lower legs, mainly over the shins. They are usually bilateral and tend to recur for two to three months. The overlying skin may be red and oedematous and the condition is often misdiagnosed as cellulitis. Involvement of both legs aids in the diagnosis. Children should be examined for possible tonsillitis, sinusitis, and dental infection, as streptococcal infections are a common cause. Tuberculosis and sarcoidosis should be excluded. Often no cause is found and a viral infection suspected.

Vitiligo

Lesions consist of well-circumscribed symmetrical white patches which tend to spread progressively. The skin is otherwise normal. The loss of pigment is due to destruction of melanocytes, probably an auto-immune phenomenon. An association with other auto-immune diseases such as thyroiditis and diabetes has been described in adults, but children with vitiligo are invariably healthy. There is a family history of vitiligo in about one-third of patients. Vitiligo-like depigmentation may follow trauma and inflammatory skin diseases.

Treatment

Corticosteroid creams may be tried for three months and sunscreens should be used for large areas of depigmentation. The prognosis is good in children with limited disease, lesions may also repigment spontaneously. In extensive disease ultraviolet light treatment may be effective; however repigmentation is rarely achieved on the hands.

Alopecia areata

Like vitiligo, with which it is sometimes associated, alopecia areata is thought to be auto-immune in origin. It is characterized by round well-circumscribed areas of hair loss, which occur most commonly on the scalp and in which the skin is smooth and healthy. Sometimes the eyebrows or eyelashes are affected, with or without scalp involvement. In most patients the hair regrows within a few months, but in some, the patches of alopecia may recur and spread. Usually no cause is found. The prognosis is best with localized patches within the scalp, progressively worsens if the hair-line, entire scalp and body hair are involved.

Treatment

Corticosteroid creams are useless and should not be used; however long acting intralesional steroid injections to localized areas may be useful. Preparations that cause inflammation of the skin such as dithranol are effective but education on their use to avoid side effects is important. Systemic corticosteroids should only be prescribed to patients during active shedding of hair. They are used at an initial dose of 1mg/kg reduced every three days; the course lasting less than three weeks. There is no place for long-term use of systemic steroids in alopecia areata.

Miscellaneous skin disorders

Erythema toxicum

Lesions appear within the first few days of life and clear spontaneously within three days. They consist of small pustules on an erythematous base and occur on any part of the body, but mainly on the trunk and proximal parts of the limbs. The child is well and apyrexial. The cause is unknown and no treatment is required.

Pityriasis rosea

The cause is unknown but suspected to be due to a viral infection. It occurs sporadically or in small epidemics, affecting mainly children and young adults. The rash is usually confined to the trunk and proximal parts of the limbs, but in younger children may be more widespread, involving even the face and scalp. The lesions start as small papules, which soon enlarge to form oval macules covered with fine, superficial scales. On the back and chest they are arranged in lines which follow the direction of the ribs (see Figure 32.13).

The generalized rash may be preceded by a large, round, scaling lesion, the so-called herald patch, which is usually misdiagnosed as ringworm. The rash clears spontaneously within two

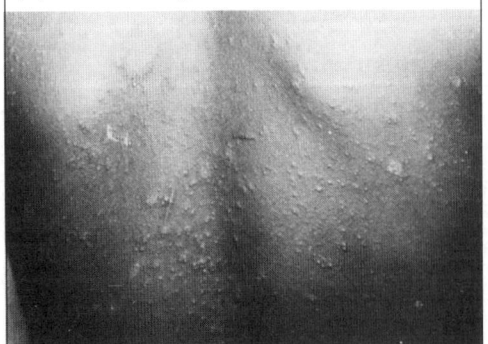

Figure 32.13 Pityriasis rosea: herald patch, papular and scaling lesions on back

months. Treatment consists of a bland cream such as ung. emulsificans aqueosum, a corticosteroid diluted to 10 per cent may be given if itchy. Atypical forms may need to be differentiated from seborrhoeic dermatitis and secondary syphilis.

Psoriasis

This chronic, usually recurrent, skin disease is common in all races. The cause is unknown, but genetic factors play a major role, and recognized eliciting factors include stress and infection. Skin lesions consist of raised, well-circumscribed plaques with rather shiny scales which become white and opaque on being scratched. The scale can often be scraped off, revealing small bleeding points on the exposed underlying dermis. The lesions are usually large and round, occurring mainly over the knees and elbows and on the scalp; but they may vary in size and shape and occur on any part of the body. Involvement of the nail bed results in pitting, thickening, and friability of the nail plate.

Guttate psoriasis consists of a widespread eruption of small (rain drop like) lesions which may appear rather suddenly on the trunk. It may occur after an acute infection, particularly streptococcal tonsillitis.

Treatment

Treatment of psoriasis remains a problem. Guttate psoriasis may clear after the precipitating infection is treated, but the disease usually recurs later in a chronic form. Psoriasis may respond temporarily to corticosteroid ointments, but they are best avoided as lesions tend to recur and even worsen. Ointments containing coal (e.g. 5 per cent coal tar and 10 per cent salicylic acid in ung. emulsificans) usually give better results and longer remissions. Other treatments include topical and systemic retinoids, methotrexate and ultraviolet light treatment.

Lichen planus

This disease of unknown cause is more common in adults than in children. Characteristic lesions consist of purplish, well-demarcated, polygonal flat-topped papules with a shining scaly surface. The lesions typically involve the flexor surfaces of the forearms but may be extensive. They are very itchy and sometimes spread along scratch marks – the so-called Koebner or isomorphic phenomenon. Less commonly, small superficial papules, larger ring-shaped lesions, or warty nodules are seen. Very itchy frequently scratched areas can be thick, leathery, develop pigment change and prominent skin markings (i.e. lichenification). Lichen planus in the mouth appears as lacy white lines or spots (most commonly seen in the inner cheek). Involvement of the nail bed may cause permanent loss of the nail plate. New crops of lesions usually appear for many months and further attacks are common. When healing, lesions develop a slate-coloured hyperpigmentation and itching subsides.

Treatment

Treatment consists of corticosteroid creams, full strength or diluted, depending on the size of the area involved. Occlusive dressings greatly enhance their effect and could be used on the limbs. Systemic corticosteroids are reserved for widespread lesions which are unresponsive to topical treatment.

Chronic bullous dermatosis of childhood

This chronic disease of unknown cause is usually misdiagnosed as impetigo or bullous insect bites in its initial stages. Skin lesions consist of itchy subepidermal bullae, symmetrically distributed on the trunk and limbs. Crops of new blisters may continue to erupt for many years and tend to be arranged in an annular pattern. Biopsy and histological examination is usually diagnostic. The disease responds well to treatment with dapsone.

Acne

Although this common condition is seldom a problem before puberty, some children with large sebaceous glands and an inherited tendency to acne may develop blackheads as early as the age of 10 years. The face can be washed twice daily with a mild toilet soap. The application of thick creams and ointments on the face and scalp should be avoided. Drying agents bought over the counter such as 2% sulphur in calamine lotion and benzyl peroxide may be

useful. Prescription of a topical retinoid and/or antibiotic may control flare-ups in patients. If the response is not satisfactory after a three-month trial, oral antibiotics maybe added. Doxycycline has the advantage of fewer adverse effects and a once daily dose, but erythromycin and cotrimoxazole may also be used. If necessary an anti-androgen (cyproterone acetate) containing contraceptive may be used in females and the systemic retinoid isotetrinoin has been found to be very effective in patients with severe or scarring acne. It is most important to remember that the latter is teratogenic. Pregnancy should be excluded and extensive counselling given prior to its use.

Genetic disorders

Ichthyosis

The term *ichthyosis* is used for a group of inherited disorders of the epidermis which are characterized by dryness and scaliness. The degree of skin changes varies from a mild superficial desquamation to an appearance resembling fish scales (it has also been compared to crazy paving and a dry river bed).

The term *collodion baby* is used to describe a neonate covered with a shiny, glazed membrane, which cracks and peels off within a few days. This may be an early manifestation of one of the persistent forms of ichthyosis.

Harlequin fetus is the most severe form of ichthyosis, in which marked hyperkeratosis and rigidity of the skin over the whole body results in the formation of deep fissures. It is rare, recessively inherited, and usually results in death before or shortly after birth.

Icthyosis vulgaris is the commonest type. It usually presents with dry fish scale-like skin on the shins. It is common in patients with atopic features and may co-exist with atopic eczema.

Treatment

Treatment of ichthyosis consists of the regular use of greasy ointments such as ung. emulsificans BP. But the most useful moisturizers are those that contain urea or lactic acid. Topical and systemic retinoic acid derivatives result in improvement while in use.

Epidermolysis bullosa (EB)

This is a group of inherited disorders of varying age of onset and severity in which recurrent blisters form because skin fragility. The genetic abnormality causes impaired attachment of the epidermis to the dermis. The result is three levels of blister formation: within the epidermis, at the junction of the two layers or below the epidermis referred to EB Simplex, Junctional EB and Dystrophic EB respectively. The latter is the most severe; often associated with scarring and loss of nails and hair. At, or soon after birth, blisters appear on any part of the skin and in the mouth. Some blisters heal, as new ones appear. Disease severity varies within subtype of the three groups; some are lethal, others lifelong or improve with age.

33

Disorders of the eye

Every paediatric examination should include an age appropriate visual assessment. For example, at around six weeks of age, a baby's vision has developed sufficiently for him to recognise his mother's face and smile at her. At around three months he should show purposeful, visually directed reaching. Failure to achieve these visual milestones implies either a serious eye defect or a serious brain deficit.

Although modern eye care, particularly eye surgery, is becoming increasingly sophisticated, relying on high technology equipment, a surprisingly large amount can be achieved by careful examination with basic tools such as a penlight torch. This simple fact is frequently forgotten. One of the simplest and most successful treatments of all is the reversal of visual loss from amblyopia by occlusion of the sound eye.

The commonest reasons for parents consulting a doctor about their child's eyes are pain and redness or visual difficulties.

Clinical examination

Every effort should be made to put the child at ease. Small children are best examined on their mother's lap. Visual alertness should be noted together with any obvious abnormalities such as proptosis, ptosis, abnormal head posture, squint or nystagmus. A finger puppet or toy is a better target than a penlight torch when determining central fixation and following. Each eye should be assessed separately using the examiner's thumb as an occluder. Visual acuity in pre-school children may be assessed with picture charts or by matching letters, particularly ones not subject to perceptive reversal problems like H, O, T and V. This can be done with an ordinary Snellen chart although a special paediatric Sheridan Gardiner test, which presents the letters singly, is better for younger children and the test can be done easily by an intelligent three-year old. The child is given a white card with seven different letters. She is then shown a single letter at either three meters or six meters and asked to 'find the letter on the card'. This should be presented as something that is fun – the letter game – with lots of praise and encouragement. Frequently the only available test at primary level is the illiterate E test better suited to illiterate adults than small children (see Figure 33.1).

The external eye should be examined carefully using a penlight torch and, when necessary, a loupe. A slit lamp microscope examination is the best method but availability is usually confined to specialised eye units. Fluorescein strips or single dose fluorescein eye drops (Minims®) should be used for staining the cornea. Multi-dose bottles of diagnostic eye drops, especially fluorescein, may become contaminated with pseudomonas and should be avoided. A lid speculum may be necessary, but requires local anaesthetic eye drops first. The pupil can be dilated safely with tropicamide 1% (single dose Minims®) which works quickly and is short acting, or cyclopentolate 1%. The fundus can then be examined with the direct ophthalmoscope noting particularly the optic disc and the macula. Abnormalities merit specialist examination.

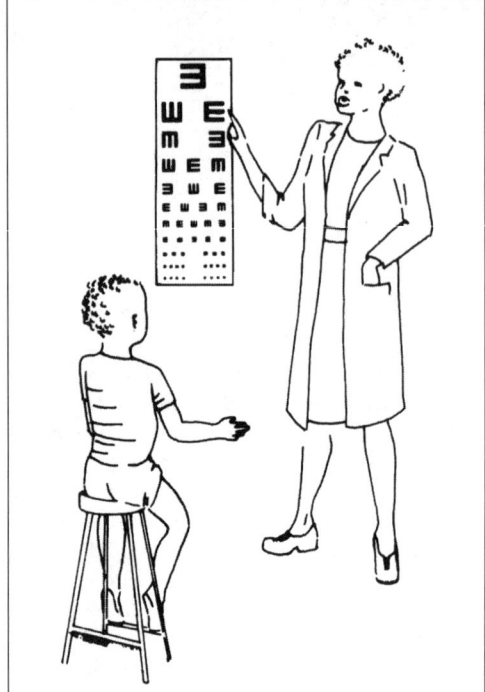

Figure 33.1 Testing acuity of a non-literate child: The child is taught to point his finger in the same direction as the horizontals of the E

External deformity

Coloboma of the eyelids

Various congenital anomalies may affect the eyelids. In particular, coloboma (absence of a portion of the lid) may give rise to corneal exposure, desiccation, ulceration and scarring. The cornea should be protected with ointment and the baby referred urgently for closure of the defect.

Ptosis

This refers to drooping of the eyelids and may be unilateral or bilateral.

Congenital ptosis is the commonest form and is occasionally associated with other abnormalities such as blepharophimosis (small interpalpebral fissures and a broad nasal bridge). It is important to ascertain whether the visual axes are obscured, particularly in the case of

unilateral ptosis when it will lead to amblyopia. Over action of the frontalis muscle and elevation of the chin are common in bilateral ptosis. Where the ptosis is unilateral and the visual axis is obscured, surgery to prevent amblyopia is urgent. Usually however, surgery for cosmetic effect and to prevent abnormal chin tilt is best deferred until the child is older.

Haemangioma of the lid may grow with alarming rapidity in infancy and may give rise to a mechanical ptosis with occlusion of the visual axis and resultant amblyopia. In this case, corticosteroid or bleomycin injection may be helpful in inducing regression. Most haemangiomata resolve spontaneously before five years of age.

Myasthenia gravis falls into the differential diagnosis but is not common in children.

Horner's syndrome (a lesion of the sympathetic pathway) gives rise to a mild ptosis with a small pupil on the same side. In congenital cases the affected iris may be paler than that on the other side. An acquired Horner's syndrome without obvious cause, such as recent cardiac surgery, requires investigation

Third cranial nerve (oculomotor) palsy causes ptosis but there are almost always much more obvious signs of extraocular muscle weakness. If the pupil is involved the lesion is likely to be traumatic, compressive or congenital.

Inflammatory conditions of the eyelids

Hordeolum (external stye). This is infective inflammation of the lash follicle usually due to staphylococci. The pus points at the eyelash, which should be removed. Hot compresses and antibiotic ointment aid recovery.

Meibomian cyst (chalazion or internal stye). This is due to infection/inflammation of a meibomian gland. In the acute phase it often resolves with antibiotic ointment and warm compresses. However, a small proportion goes on to a chronic lipogranulomatous inflammation of the meibomian gland known as a chalazion or meibomian cyst. This is a lump in the lid the size of a pea. On everting the eyelid a dark, or yellow lesion is seen on the tarsal surface. An incision along the meibomian duct at right angles to the lid margin on the tarsal surface with curettage of the cyst is curative. Unfortunately, in children this usually requires a general anaesthetic. A meibomian abscess occasionally occurs and should be incised and drained immediately.

Proptosis

Proptosis implies forward displacement of the globe and is not common. It may be congenital and bilateral, occurring with shallow orbits or in association with craniofacial abnormalities. Sinus pathology, orbital abscess and tumours such as rhabdomyosarcoma, should all be considered in the differential diagnosis of an acquired proptosis. Signs of inflammation, presence or absence of normal ocular movements, and the presence of masses palpated through the lids are all helpful in making the diagnosis. Any sudden onset of proptosis, particularly if unilateral and associated with pain and loss of vision or eye movements, should be referred for urgent assessment. A CT or MRI scan is almost always necessary. All patients with proptosis require referral to the ophthalmologist. Surgery will probably be required followed by chemotherapy and radiotherapy in the case of a tumour.

The red eye with discharge

The red eye with a purulent or watery discharge needs careful examination to differentiate conjunctival from ciliary injection. Ciliary injection indicates deeper more serious pathology. (*see* Figures 33.2a and 33.2b).

Conjunctivitis

This is an acute inflammation of the conjunctiva which is usually due to infection.

Bacterial conjunctivitis. This is an eye with purulent discharge. Common causative organisms are, *Staphylococcus aureus, Staphylococcus epidermidis,* haemophilus and streptococcus. The eyes are diffusely red with dilatation of the superficial vessels. There is a purulent discharge and the eyes may be stuck together in the morning. The cornea is clear, the iris should be clearly seen and the vision should be good. Frequent treatment with chloramphenicol eye ointment, two to three hourly at first and decreasing to four times per day, usually results in rapid cure. Quinolone eye drops, which are extremely effective, should not be used as first line drugs to prevent development of resistant strains. Patients who show no improvement within two to three days, or in whom the cornea develops an ulcer (a yellow or greyish spot) or in whom the vision deteriorates, should be referred for specialist treatment. A neglected ulcer leads to perforation of the globe and potentially loss of all useful vision.

Viral conjunctivitis (pink eye). This is an eye with a watery discharge. Adenovirus infection is the commonest cause of viral conjunctivitis, a follicular conjunctivitis, which is usually self limiting. However occasionally the child can be pyrexial and sick. Pharyngo-conjunctival fever (PCF) is due to adenoviruses and children have a simultaneous upper respiratory tract infection. Other adenoviruses produce epidemic kerato-conjunctivitis (EKC) when there is an associated keratitis and sometimes enlarged pre-auricular

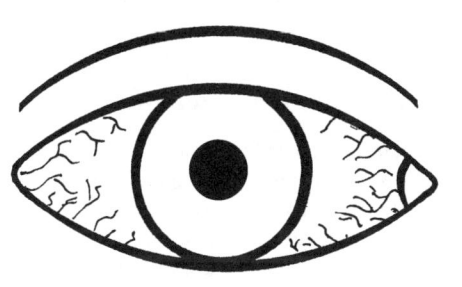

Figure 33.2a Conjunctival infection: The blood vessels are large, superficial, and emanate from the periphery

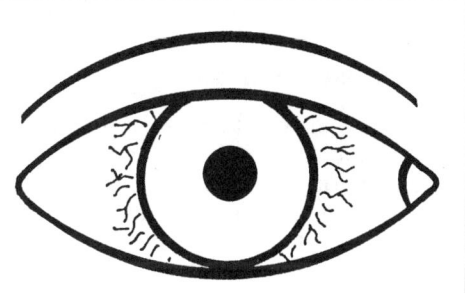

Figure 33.2b Ciliary infection as seen in keratitis, uveitis, etc.

nodes. Both viral conditions are highly contagious and spread rapidly via infected tears in places where a lot of children are gathered together as schools and crèches. It is very important to avoid hand-eye contact after touching something (e.g. a toy) contaminated with the virus. Hand washing by health care professionals between cases is essential. Treatment is supportive. A combined antihistamine and vasoconstrictor eye drop (e.g. Spersallerg®) can be very soothing. Anti-viral agents and corticosteroid eye drops should not be used. Mothers must be strongly discouraged from the practice of washing affected eyes with urine as this is the usual source of secondary bacterial infection which can be devastating in the case of gonococcal infection.

Ophthalmia neonatorum

This refers to purulent conjunctivitis, acquired from the mother's birth canal, occurring in the neonatal period.

Gonococcal infection causes a severe purulent conjunctivitis presenting around day two after birth. Uncontrolled gonococcal infection leads to corneal ulceration, scarring and blindness. The child should be admitted for saline washes of the conjunctival sac and given treatment with one intramuscular dose of ceftriaxone 62.5 mg. It is usually prudent to treat prophyllactically for chlamydial infection too.

Chlamydia trachomatis is the commonest cause of ophthalmia neonatorum, presenting around week two after birth. It is a mucopurulent conjunctivitis that is much less dramatic than gonococcal infection. Treatment is with oral erythromycin for 14 days (50 mg/kg/d) in four divided doses. Gonococcal or chlamydial conjunctivitis in an older child should give rise to suspicion of sexual abuse but is often simply due to the washing of the eyes with infected urine.

Allergic conjunctivitis

This is the commonest reason for red eyes not responsive to chloramphenicol ointment given at primary healthcare level.

Seasonal allergic conjunctivitis ('hay fever in the eye') is an IgE mediated follicular conjunctivitis with itchiness and watering. It characteristically lasts for about six weeks in the springtime.

Topical antihistamine and vasoconstrictor eye drops are often effective but stubborn cases respond well to olopatadine or ketotifen eye drops twice a day.

Vernal conjunctivitis has a much longer season, usually lasting about six months and is due to a cell mediated response. The eyes are chronically red and very itchy with copious lardaceous discharge. In pigmented people raised grey gelatinous infiltrates with associated pigmentation develop at the limbus. Non-pigmented people develop tarsal cobblestone infiltrates, which are more likely to be associated with corneal ulceration. Mild cases can be controlled with cromoglycate drops four times a day on a long term basis, but some topical steroid eye drops are usually necessary and this should only be given under the supervision of an ophthalmologist. Topical steroid eye drops on a long term basis can produce optic nerve damage due to raised intraocular pressure which is asymptomatic. Olopatadine and ketotifen eye drops can also be very effective and are very safe.

Atopic conjunctivitis can have both limbal and tarsal elements and is treated in the same way with mast cell stabilising and steroid eye drops. Occasionally it can be very severe, leading to visual loss from corneal scarring.

The red eye with corneal involvement (keratitis)

Vitamin A deficiency

(*See* Chapter 13, Nutritional disorders.)

Prophylactic vitamin A supplementation in South Africa has virtually eliminated the 'spontaneous' corneal ulceration and perforation that used to be a major cause of childhood blindness. It was often precipitated by measles or diarrhoea.

Phlyctenular conjunctivitis

A phlycten is caused by a delayed hypersensitivity reaction to bacterial antigens, usually the tubercle bacillus but possibly staphylococci. The condition presents as a nodule or nodules on the conjunctiva, most often near or astride the limbus. The child does not necessarily have active tuberculosis, although this must always be excluded. The phlycten may be the result of droplet infection of the conjunctival sac in a child previously immunised against tuberculosis. Treatment is with combination steroid and antibiotic eye drops or ointment. A phlycten heals leaving a triangular scar with its base at the limbus.

Herpes simplex keratitis

Herpes simplex is a common cause of viral conjunctivitis, which may lead to corneal ulceration which is often unrecognized. Corneal involvement starts with a classical epithelial dendritic ulcer that stains well with fluorescein. Left untreated this will often progress into a large amoeboid ulcer with stromal involvement and inevitable scarring.

Recurrent episodes lead to increased stromal involvement, scarring and visual loss. Precipitating factors include ultraviolet light and fever, hence the common occurrence in children with malaria or measles. Symptoms include pain, photophobia and tearing. *The diagnosis should be suspected in every red eye without purulent discharge.* Such eyes should always be examined with fluorescein. Treatment is with acyclovir eye ointment five times a day until the ulcer has healed.

Disciform keratitis, a grey cloudy patch in the cornea due to an immune response to the viral antigen within the corneal stroma, may occur even without a previous history of herpetic ulceration. It is usually unilateral and requires steroid and antiviral treatment under the supervision of an ophthalmologist.

> The use of combination steroid and antibiotic eye drops in a red eye due to unsuspected herpes simplex will cause rapid progression to the amoeboid stage with inevitable scarring and possible perforation.

Trachoma

South Africa is now trachoma free but the disease still exists in other developing countries. It is caused by chlamydia and spread mainly by flies and direct contact. In the early stages of the disease there is an acute inflammation of the lid conjunctiva which progresses to mature follicles on the lids and subsequently results in scarring and entropion (inturned eyelids.) Scarring of the cornea is caused by constant corneal abrasion from the inturned eyelids and lashes. The main thrust of treatment should be prevention. Improved sanitation and fly-control are very important. Daily face washing leads to a marked decrease in the incidence of the disease but can be difficult to achieve in arid places where every drop is for drinking. 'Every child should have a clean face every day.' Sharing face-cloths and towels must be discouraged in endemic areas.

A single dose of azithromycin is very effective treatment.

Alternatively, children require tetracycline eye ointment three times a day for six weeks and systemic erythromycin for three weeks.

Entropion must be corrected with lid surgery.

The red eye without discharge

Uveitis

This is intraocular inflammation, which may affect any portion of the uveal tract namely the iris, the ciliary body or the choroid. Generally, though, one speaks of an anterior, posterior or panuveitis (i.e. involvement of the whole uveal tract).

Symptoms include pain, redness, photophobia, and blurred vision. Injection is usually more prominent in the area of the limbus, giving rise to the so-called 'ciliary flush' as opposed to the diffuse redness of conjunctivitis (*see* Figure 33.2b). Careful examination with a bright penlight and the loupe may reveal clumps of inflammatory cells, keratic precipitates (KPs), on the endothelial surface of the cornea. Iris nodules might also be present. Uveitis is an uncommon paediatric diagnosis for which a cause should always be sought. Causes include:

- Blunt trauma is the commonest cause of unilateral uveitis.
- Tuberculosis should always be excluded particularly in bilateral cases.
- Previous streptococcal infection is commoner than previously thought in bilateral uveitis.
- Toxocara larval infestation a common cause of unilateral posterior uveitis and is due to

ingesting the faeces of puppies that have not been de-wormed. Ocular larvae migrans produce an inflammatory reaction when they die in the eye leading to uveitis and a big chorioretinal granuloma. The problem can be precipitated by thiabendazole treatment. Vitreous traction bands may lead to blindness from retinal detachment. This can be prevented by sophisticated vitreous surgery only available in specialised centres. The chorioretinal granuloma can be difficult to differentiate from retinoblastoma.

- Juvenile idiopathic arthritis, usually of the pauciarticular onset type can lead to a very destructive chronic uveitis in a white asymptomatic eye. Such children should be screened regularly from the onset of the disease.
- Cysticercosis, the encysted form of *Taenia solium* and other parasites may very occasionally cause posterior uveitis.
- Onchocerciasis (river blindness) is a chronic parasitic infection due to the microfilariae of *Onchocerca volvulus* with the black fly as the vector. The disease may give rise to chronic uveitis associated with corneal and retinal scarring. Secondary cataract, glaucoma and phthisis bulbi (shrinkage of the eyeball) may occur. The World Health Organization (WHO) has a long-term black fly control programme in affected West African countries. Affected patients have been treated with diethylcarbamazine with some success but only in experienced specialist hands. Ivermectin, safely and dramatically reduces the number of viable microfilariae after a single tablet, but it does not kill adult filariae. One tablet once or twice a year is all that is needed to control the disease. However, there is limited experience in treating children under the age of five years and breast feeding mothers should not be treated until the infant is at least one week old.

Episcleritis

This is a mild, self-limiting condition, usually in young adults, but it may occur in older children. There is segmental or diffuse redness without discharge, but sometimes a nodule may be present. It usually responds to topical nonsteroidal anti-inflammatory eye drops or topical steroids.

White pupil (leucocoria)

Cataract

Cataract occurs when the lens of the eye becomes cloudy and presents as a grey or white appearance in the pupil. The fundal 'red reflex' obtained with the direct ophthalmoscope may be poor or absent. Cataract may be unilateral or bilateral and present in varying degrees from birth and during childhood. The cause is often not found (*see* Table 33.1).

Management may be difficult in poor populations. Patients with dense bilateral cataracts from birth should be referred for surgery as soon as possible, ideally before six weeks of age. With a lot of parental co-operation a good visual outcome can be achieved with early surgery in congenital cases. Sadly this does not always happen in poor socioeconomic circumstances. Where congenital cataracts are bilateral and incomplete, surgery may be postponed until vision deteriorates to an impractical level. Unilateral congenital cataracts are more likely to be treated with intraocular lenses at an early stage but still have a very poor prognosis due to amblyopia. In some unilateral cases, especially after minor trauma in older children, cataract extraction with the insertion of an intraocular lens can have a very good visual outcome.

It is most important to differentiate cataracts from the leucocoria of retinoblastoma.

Table 33.1 Causes of cataract in childhood
• Hereditary
• Congenital rubella (may be associated with microphthalmia and/or retinopathy)
• General conditions, e.g. atopic dermatitis, diabetes, galactosaemia, and Down's syndrome
• Trauma (sudden, usually unilateral development of cataract)

Retinoblastoma

Retinoblastoma is a primary malignant neoplasm of the retina and is the commonest intraocular malignancy of children usually presenting in the second year of life. It is a dominantly inherited affliction, although most cases arise as a new mutation. About a third of cases are bilateral. A small percentage have a positive family history. The commonest presenting sign is a white pupil (leucocoria).In the early stages this is just an odd 'cats eye white reflex' seen by the mother in the twilight when the pupil is semi-dilated. At this stage it is missed by the paediatrician who examines the child in daylight with a small pupil. Such a history mandates a dilated fundal examination, preferably by an ophthalmologist. A tumour causing an obviously white pupil is already advanced. Careful examination will often reveal small blood vessels on the white surface, which is never the case with uncomplicated cataracts. Another frequent presenting sign is an acquired esotropia (convergent squint) in a previously normal infant. Advanced tumours produce painful, red, glaucomatous eyes and ultimately proptosis as the tumour spreads into the orbit. Spread into the central nervous system has often preceded this. Urgent referral to the nearest eye unit is mandatory. Advanced pathology is seen when there has been a delay in identification of the problem at primary level. Small tumours are amenable to local therapy with preservation of vision. Large ones require enucleation often with adjunctive radiotherapy and/or chemotherapy. No treatment results in a long and terrible death from widespread metastases.

Retinopathy of prematurity (formerly retrolental fibroplasia)

This is an iatrogenic disease caused by overzealous oxygenation of premature infants. (*See* Chapter 7, Care of the newborn). By the time that the pupil has turned white the baby is irrevocably blind.

The watering eye

Nasolacrimal duct obstruction

The tear drainage system is frequently not patent at birth. Watering eyes are a very common complaint in infancy and the problem usually resolves spontaneously. The slowest part to canalise is the nasolacrimal duct, which runs through the bone from the lacrimal sac to open under the inferior turbinate in the nose. Stagnant tears are prone to infection and the mother must be instructed to express the contents of the lacrimal sac into the conjunctival sac by firm pressure at least twice a day. A brief course of topical antibiotics may be necessary.

If the watering persists beyond the age of a year, it is usually due to a membranous block at the lower end of the nasolacrimal duct and can be solved with a simple probing. The snag is that this requires a general anaesthetic. Probing a child who has merely been restrained is painful and likely to be traumatic, causing scarring and permanent obstruction.

A lacrimal abscess occurs rarely but requires incision and drainage. Spontaneous perforation is often followed by a lacrimal fistula.

A very small proportion of cases require definitive lacrimal duct surgery currently best performed endoscopically by a suitably trained ENT surgeon.

Glaucoma

This often presents as a watering eye *with photophobia*.

Glaucoma occurs when the intraocular pressure is raised. A normal baby has an intraocular pressure around 12 mmHg. The baby sclera is very soft. Raised intraocular pressure makes it stretch so that the eye gets bigger. Only when it can no longer stretch fast enough does the intraocular pressure rise to the point where it produces corneal oedema. The hazy cornea with watering and photophobia is the usual presenting sign.

Primary congenital glaucoma is the commonest cause of glaucoma in infancy. The drainage angle of the area where the aqueous humor exits the eye is congenitally malformed. An enlarged cornea (buphthalmos = ox-eye) during the first three years of life should always raise the suspicion of glaucoma. This can be difficult to spot when the condition is bilateral and the cornea not yet oedematous. Uncontrolled intraocular pressure destroys the optic nerve, ultimately leading to irretrievable blindness. A corneal diameter greater than 11 mm in a term infant or greater than 12 mm in a one-year old child is highly suspicious. In a toddler, sudden onset of decompensated glaucoma might cause pain and vomiting together with loss of vision. Be very suspicious about the child with big eyes who hangs his head in the light.

Any child suspected of having glaucoma should be immediately referred to an ophthalmic centre. Surgery is urgently required to control the intra-ocular pressure and with early referral the outcome can be very good. The problem usually relates to late referral with optic nerve damage, and congenital glaucoma remains a significant cause of childhood blindness in developing countries.

In a minority of cases, the aqueous drainage problem is associated with some other syndrome, e.g. neurofibromatosis type 1 or Sturge Weber. Such children should be screened for glaucoma regularly but their surgical management is often much more difficult.

Squint (strabismus)

This occurs when the visual axes of the eyes are not aligned. Eyes which turn inwards are said to have a convergent squint (**esotropia**). Eyes which turn outwards have divergent squints (**exotropia**).The problem is that in the visually immature infant or toddler, the brain suppresses the diplopia produced by non aligned visual axes very quickly. This results in the central suppression of the image from the squinting eye so that an eye which is structurally completely normal, does not see (**amblyopia or lazy eye**). If this situation is not reversed promptly (usually by occlusion of the sound eye) the situation becomes irretrievable.

Thus, there is a big difference between whether the squint affects one eye constantly, when poor vision in that eye can be expected, or when the squint shifts from one to the other eye, a situation described as an alternating squint, which does not imply amblyopia.

The treatment of amblyopia is urgent.

Children who squint from an early age almost never achieve completely normal binocular vision but can be very successfully aligned surgically with two good seeing eyes and a normal appearance.

The child who presents with an *acquired* squint requires urgent referral to an ophthalmologist. Occasionally it is the presenting sign of a retinoblastoma or toxocara infection, which is why fundoscopy is mandatory. More usually it is a sign of decompensated hypermetropia which, when promptly corrected with glasses, will restore visual alignment and binocularity.

Examination of the ocular movements will establish whether there is a paralytic cause of the squint, another cause for concern and a sign of a problem within the central nervous system.

An *intermittent squint*, particularly if convergent at around the age of two or three years, is a warning that the child probably has uncorrected hypermetropia which will lead to a constant squint with amblyopia if not addressed.

An intermittent divergent squint, usually described as an 'eye standing still' is less likely to lead to amblyopia but still requires specialist treatment, (usually surgery) if binocularity is to be preserved.

Testing for a squint: the cover test

Shine the focused beam of a penlight torch onto the child's eyes from a short distance (around 30 cm).

The light reflex from the cornea should be centrally placed in each pupil if the child is fixating correctly.

Any deviation of the light reflex from the centre of the pupil will signify a squint.

Occasionally broad epicanthic folds in young children will simulate a squint which is shown not to exist on careful inspection. (*see* Figures 33.3 and 33.4).

Table 33.3 Causes of squint in childhood
• Congenital deviations, e.g. esotropia
• Hypermetropia (far-sightedness)
• Paralytic squints (exclude intracranial pathology)
• Special syndromes, e.g. Duane's syndrome
• Retinoblastoma or other serious ocular pathology

Figure 33.3 Left esotropia of 45° with the light reflex at limbus

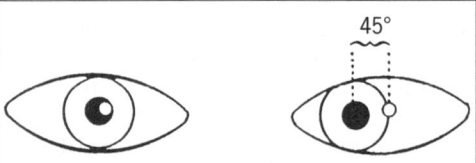

45°

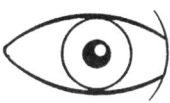 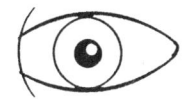

Figure 33.4 Large epicanthic folds cause pseudo-strabismus. Light reflexes central in both eyes

If a squint is suspected, cover the visual axis of the fixating eye with the thumb.

If the other eye was squinting it will now be forced to move, in or out, to take up fixation and that movement can easily be seen with careful observation.

A practised observer can even get a very good idea of probable visual acuity by observing the fixation pattern in preverbal children.

The child with acquired immune deficiency syndrome (AIDS)

Molluscum contagiosum

The umbilicated nodules of molluscum conta-giosum may be multiple and numerous on the eyelids of these patients.

Herpes zoster ophthalmicus

If this occurs in a child, the suspicion of HIV/AIDS should be raised. However, it is a more usual presentation in the young adult. Vesicles are strictly unilateral, involving the forehead and eyelids in the distribution of the first (ophthalmic) division of the trigeminal nerve. The tip of the nose may also be affected and in these cases the eye is more likely to be involved.

Cytomegalovirus retinitis

A severe retinitis occurs in the advanced stage of the disease. Various patterns of haemorrhage, exudates, and vasculitis are seen with a usual outcome of blindness in that eye. Intra-vitreal gancyclovir injections are an effective method of control when dealing with the preservation of vision in the single remaining seeing eye of a young adult but are not usually practical in babies and small children. HIV positive babies who are seropositive for CMV and who have signs of retinitis are best treated with systemic gancyiclovir and antiretrovirals.

Trauma

When assessing the child with an injured eye the history is of paramount importance. Examination can be extremely difficult requiring a lot of patience and sympathetic handling.

Corneal foreign body

In a paediatric situation these are often superficial and can be removed with local anaesthetic eye drops and a cotton bud. Antibiotic eye ointment and a firm eye pad should be applied afterwards. Deeply embedded foreign bodies will require a general anaesthetic and often a microscope.

Chemical burns

This is a dire emergency, especially if alkali burn is suspected. Alkalis such as household ammonia rapidly penetrate the cornea and involve the anterior chamber, iris, and lens. Copious washing with water or saline, if available, should be commenced immediately and in the case of alkaline burns should be continued for several hours while the child is being transported to hospital for specialised treatment. Local anaesthetic eye drops make the washing process much easier.

Thermal burns

These are usually accidental, caused by a careless adult's cigarette or the spark from a fire. Reflex blepharospasm means that they are usually superficial despite the alarming patch of white burnt corneal epithelium. Ash should be washed out after the instillation of anaesthetic eye drops, and then antibiotic ointment and a cycloplegic eye drop should be applied. The cornea usually heals within 24 hours, (check with fluorescein) but if not, the child should be referred to a specialised eye centre.

Blunt trauma

The eye should be carefully inspected. Internal bleeding into the anterior chamber (hyphaema) will present as a level of blood behind the cornea. Problems arise often with the secondary haemorrhage which happens about five days later. Large amounts of blood frequently lead to secondary glaucoma. The child with a hyphaema must rest until the blood has gone and the five day danger period is over. Strenuous activity and further eye injury must be avoided. Cycloplegic eye drops (e.g. atropine1%) and steroid eye drops reduce the incidence of secondary haemorrhage. Ideally these children should be managed in a specialised eye centre because raised intraocular pressure may require surgical evacuation of the blood. Small hyphaemas can resolve without permanent ocular damage but severe blunt injuries will cause a wide variety of problems ranging from dislocation of the lens through to permanent retinal scarring.

Penetrating injuries

These must be repaired surgically as soon as possible.

Laceration of the cornea is usually obvious, sometimes with a presenting knuckle of iris. Obscure penetrating injury may be suspected when the eye is very soft to digital palpation. This can be done by very, very gently alternating pressure on the upper lid, using both index fingers and with the eye in a downward gaze. A CT scan of the orbit is mandatory where intra-ocular foreign body is suspected.

34

Disorders of ear, nose and throat

Because upper respiratory infections are extremely common, symptoms involving the ear, nose, and throat are often treated and over-treated without proper diagnosis. Furthermore, symptoms are often non-specific, overlapping and poorly defined by young children. A sore mouth may be manifest by feed refusal or excessive salivation, and painful ears may give rise only to irritability.

The ear, nose and throat together form part of the upper respiratory tract and are therefore commonly affected together in acute illness.

Head and neck manifestations of disease involving the ear, nose and throat

Cervical lymphadenopathy

Lymph nodes are evaluated according to their position. Thus, the jugulodigastric node is also called the tonsillar node because it is commonly enlarged in conditions affecting the tonsils. The mouth and throat are drained by the lymph nodes in the anterior triangle of the neck and the preauricular node drains the parotid. Where such single groups of nodes are enlarged, the relevant anatomical drainage areas must be carefully inspected for pathology.

> A careful inspection of mouth and pharynx, and of the ear canals and tympanic membranes is a mandatory component of the clinical examination of each child.

Enlargement of lymph nodes may be caused by infections (viral, bacterial, tuberculous), by reactive lymphoid hyperplasia in circumstances of immune activation (HIV infection, auto-immune conditions) or by neoplasia (lymphoma).

Poor sensitivity of many tests and clinical findings makes it necessary to perform microbiologic and histologic evaluations of lymph node tissue in many cases.

The ear

Pain in or around the ear (otalgia)

(*See* Table 34.1)

Acute otitis media

Acute otitis media is caused by inflammation of the mucoperiosteal lining of the middle ear cleft, i.e. the eustachian tube, tympanic cavity, attic, mastoid antrum, and mastoid air cells. When inflammation affects the bony wall or spreads beyond the walls into the adjacent area, it is referred to as a complication of otitis media, e.g. otitis media with meningitis or otitis media with facial palsy. Otitis media is common in children. The peak age incidence is at one to two years. The offending organism is usually *Haemophilus influenzae*. Others include *Streptococcus pneumoniae* and staphylococcus. Otitis media usually follows an upper respiratory tract infection. The infection spreads to the middle ear via the eustachian tube.

Patients may present during one of four recognizable stages of acute otitis media:

Table 34.1 Earache

Diagnosis	Clinical Sign	Management
Perichondritis	Inflammation of the pinna	Antibiotics
Furunculosis	Very tender swelling at the entrance of the ear canal	Incision and drainage and antibiotics
Keratosis obturans	White debris in external auditory canal	Analgesia and refer
Acute otitis media	Inflamed tympanic membrane and fever	Antibiotics and analgesia
Referred pain	Normal ear canal and tympanic membrane	Exclude dental caries and tonsillitis. Refer the others

- **Stage of tubal occlusion** is characterized by negative middle ear pressure with an effusion. The patient complains of a blocked ear and autophonia (echoing of one's own voice). The ear drum is retracted and light reflex is absent. There may be clinical evidence of middle ear effusion, for example air bubbles in the middle ear.
- **Stage of presuppuration**. The middle ear effusion becomes infected and increases. Patients complain of fever and throbbing pain. Vomiting often occurs in children. The tympanic membrane is inflamed and bulges outwards.
- **Stage of suppuration**. The high intratympanic pressure occludes the blood supply to the tympanic membrane, resulting in necrosis and rupture. The typical history is excruciating pain followed by a 'pop' and discharge with immediate relief of pain. The tympanic membrane is perforated and there is pus in the ear canal.
- **Stage of resolution**. In 80 per cent of patients complete resolution occurs, the otorrhoea subsides after a week and the perforation heals spontaneously. In 20 per cent of patients, incomplete resolution occurs; the perforation and otorrhoea persist or the perforation heals with middle ear effusion.

Treatment of acute otitis media is by oral amoxycillin 90 mg/kg/d, given in three divided doses for five days. Analgesics are prescribed for pain. In areas where *H. influenzae* is resistant to amoxycillin, the recommended treatment is Augmentin® or cefuroxime.

Foreign body

A foreign body in the ear is a common problem in children. Foreign bodies include beads, stones, tips of cotton buds, tissue paper, insects, peas, and beans.

One needs proper experience, instruments and a cooperative child, otherwise refer to a specialist unit to avoid injuries. Forceps must be used for tissue paper and tips of cotton buds, and a Jobson Horne probe for the others. Most foreign bodies can also be removed by suction under a microscope.

If the foreign body lies in the deep bony portion of the ear canal, no attempt must be made to remove it with instruments. Organic foreign bodies (e.g. a bean or pea) are hydroscopic; they swell and impact in the ear canal. For this reason, they are regarded as emergencies requiring immediate medical attention and should be referred to an ear, nose and throat specialist for removal. Syringing should not be attempted if the

Removal of a foreign body with instruments should only be undertaken if the foreign body lies in the outer cartilaginous portion of the ear canal (see Figure 34.1)

Figure 34.1 Removal of a foreign body from the ear

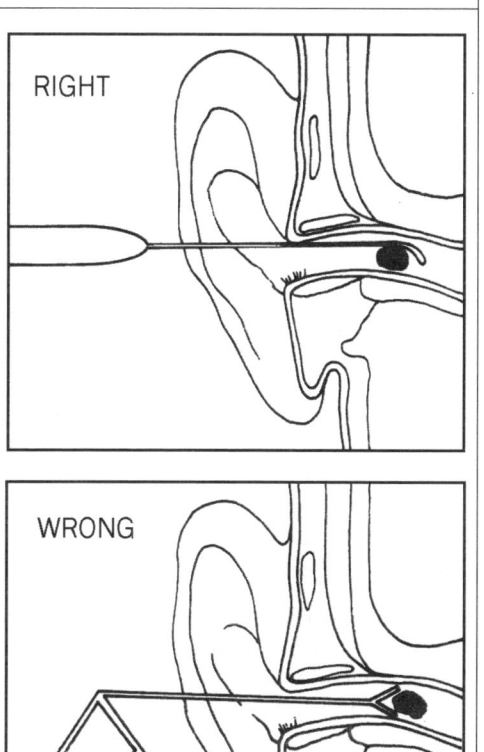

RIGHT

WRONG

foreign body occludes the ear canal completely. Insects may be 'drowned' with oil and then removed by syringing, suction or forceps.

Otitis externa

Patients with *mild otitis externa* present with itching of the external ear canal. On examination, the external ear canal is normal and the striking feature is an absence of wax. The treatment is application of steroid and antibiotic combination ear drops, twice daily for approximately five to seven days. Importantly, instruct the patient not to use paper clips, tooth picks, keys feathers, or cotton buds to scratch or remove wax in the ear. Avoid getting water in the ear from bathing or swimming.

A *moderate degree of otitis externa* is characterized by pain, itching and mild hearing loss. The external ear canal is inflamed and the eardrum is obscured by debris, which is similar in consistency to blotting paper. It may be either black or white. The treatment is removal of the debris by syringing and application of antifungal/antibiotic/steroid ointment (Quadriderm®). Pack the ear canal with 1 cm thick ribbon gauze impregnated with quadriderm® ointment. Change every 48 hours until the inflammation subsides. The technique of packing the ear canal is very important. The tip of the forceps must not pass beyond the outer cartilaginous portion of the external ear canal.

Severe otitis externa (folliculitis) is characterized by severe throbbing otalgia, with gross oedema, tenderness and complete occlusion of the ear canal. It commonly occurs after swimming, hence the term 'swimmer's ear'. The treatment entails packing the ear canal with 1 cm thick ribbon gauze impregnated with glycerine and ichthammol or quadriderm® and antibiotics (amoxicillin or Augmentin®) for five days. The pack must be changed every 72 hours until the oedema subsides.

Keratosis obturans

Keratosis obturans is a mass of desquamated squamous epithelium filling the ear canal. Typically the mass has a pearly white surface, which may be obscured by overlying wax. It is common in children and young adults and is thought to be due to failure of migration of squamous epithelium from the deep meatus. The tympanic membrane is intact. It is aggravated by attempted removal of wax with earbuds and other irritants as well as by secondary infection.

The patients present with severe otalgia and mild hearing loss. Diagnosis is made on otoscopy. A mass of desquamated debris (cholesteatoma), mixed with wax, is seen in the ear canal.

Keratosis obturans cannot be removed by syringing. The best method is manual removal piecemeal under microscopic vision with the aid of a Jobson Horne probe, cup forceps, and suction, either under local or general anaesthesia. The key to removal is to separate the mass from the wall of the external ear canal with the application of turpentine ear drops.

After complete removal, apply 1 cm thick

ribbon gauze, impregnated with Quadriderm® (antibiotic, antifungal, steroid) ointment to the external ear canal for five days.

Perichondritis

Perichondritis is inflammation of the cartilage of the auricle. It is a serious condition and if not appropriately treated, can lead to cartilage necrosis with permanent deformity. Two types are recognized: infective and auto-immune. In both types the patients present with sudden onset of pain and swelling of the auricle. The offending organism in the infective type is *Pseudomonas aeruginosa*.

The recommended treatment for this condition is intravenous piperacillin (30 mg/kg/d), amikacin (15 mg/kg/d), and metronidazole (20 mg/kg/d) for 48 hours, if the inflammation is subsiding, continue the treatment for another 72 hours. If not, then the diagnosis is relapsing polychondritis. Stop the antibiotics and prescribe prednisone 10 mg/kg/d for 10 days.

Furunculosis of the ear canal

The entrance of the external ear canal is the most common site for furunculosis. The furuncles are almost always situated inferiorly, and completely occlude the external ear canal. They are very painful and the patient may be pyrexial. The treatment is incision and drainage under local anaesthesia and antibiotics.

Haematoma of the auricle

Haematoma usually follows blunt trauma (sports) to the auricle. If left unattended, cartilage necrosis and permanent deformity of the auricle follow (cauliflower ear). The treatment is incision

and drainage of the haematoma, placement of a corrugated drain, and application of a pressure dressing for 48 hours.

Discharging ear (otorrhoea)
(*See* Table 34.2.)

Chronic suppurative otitis media

Chronic otitis media is characterized by persistent otorrhoea and tympanic membrane perforation. Two types are recognized, non-cholesteatomatous and cholesteatomatous chronic otitis media. The former is usually associated with central perforation and the latter with posterior superior marginal perforation (*see* Figure 34.2). It is important to make the distinction at the initial visit, so that appropriate treatment can be instituted immediately.

Non-cholesteatomatous discharging ear

(Central perforation.) The aim of treatment is to dry the ear so that spontaneous healing of the tympanic membrane can take place. There are four sequential steps to achieve a dry ear:

Step 1. Treatment is by means of antibiotics, aural toilet, and application of ear drops. The five-day antibiotic treatment consists of amoxycillin or Augmentin®. Aural toilet is performed twice daily with cotton wool sticks; commercially manufactured cotton wool buds are not recommended. Immediately after aural toilet ear drops containing 0.5% phenol are applied. Treatment period is for one month. Failures are moved to the next step.

Step 2. Removal of possible predisposing factors: this entails tonsillectomy, adenoidectomy, and bilateral antral wash-out. Radiograph of

Table 34.2 Discharging ear		
Diagnosis	**Type of discharge**	**Management**
Acute suppurative otitis media	Purulent	Antibiotics, aural toilet, analgesia
Chronic otitis media	Mucopurulent/ purulent	Aural toilet and ear drops
CSF otorrhoea	Clear, with dipstix test positive for glucose	Refer to ENT specialist

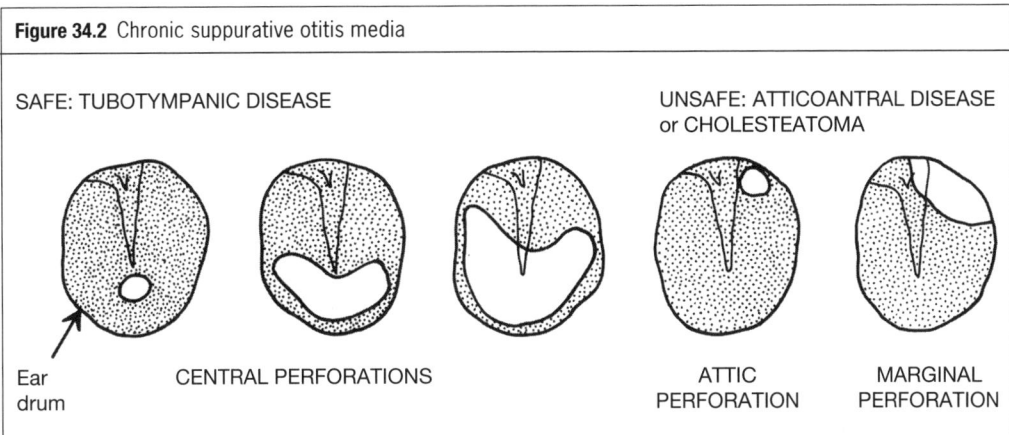

Figure 34.2 Chronic suppurative otitis media

SAFE: TUBOTYMPANIC DISEASE

UNSAFE: ATTICOANTRAL DISEASE or CHOLESTEATOMA

Ear drum   CENTRAL PERFORATIONS   ATTIC PERFORATION   MARGINAL PERFORATION

the paranasal sinuses and lateral neck may be requested to confirm or exclude sinusitis and/or enlarged adenoid glands. Radiological absence of adenoid gland hypertrophy does not exclude chronic adenoiditis. After removal of predisposing factors, continue with aural toilet and application of ear drops for one month. If otorrhoea fails to subside, then move to the next step.

Step 3. Intravenous antibiotic therapy. A pus swab is taken. Ampicillin (90 mg/kg/d) is administered intravenously for 48 hours. Thereafter, the response is reviewed. If the otorrhoea is subsiding, then the treatment is continued for another 72 hours. If the otorrhoea remains unchanged, then the culture and sensitivity results are checked and the appropriate antibiotic is selected and added to the treatment. Those who fail on this or in whom the otorrhoea recurs, move to the next step.

The success in drying the ear with Steps 1, 2, and 3 is in the region of 90 per cent.

Step 4. Surgery. Mastoidectomy is the surgical procedure to eradicate disease from the mastoid bone. It involves exenterating all the diseased mastoid air cells with a microsurgical drill, and removal of infected granulation tissue from the middle ear, attic, and mastoid cavity. Simple or cortical mastoidectomy is recommended for a non-cholesteatomatous ear.

Cholesteatoma

This consists of desquamated squamous epithelium in the middle ear cleft. In normal circumstances squamous epithelium is present only in the outer layer of the tympanic membrane and the skin of the external ear canal.

The underlying pathophysiology in cholesteatoma formation is eustachian tube dysfunction. With tubal occlusion a negative pressure is created within the middle ear cleft, resulting in invagination of the superior part of the tympanic membrane (pars flaccida) into the epitympanum (attic). The squamous epithelium in the retraction pocket desquamates continuously. Accumulated squamous epithelium in the retraction pocket is referred to as cholesteatoma. As more desquamated epithelium accumulates, the cholesteatoma pocket expands and extends into the attic and mastoid antrum.

The *diagnosis* of cholesteatoma is clinical, the presence of whitish material with the consistency of cheese is diagnostic. The most common site is the attic. A polyp in the ear canal often heralds the presence of cholesteatoma.

The *treatment of choice* for cholesteatoma is complete excision of the cholesteatomatous sac. This is best achieved with the modified radical mastoidectomy approach. Unless the patient

> Cholesteatoma is considered a serious condition because it favours growth of bacteria and it releases proteolytic enzymes, which destroy bone. Both factors are responsible for the spread of the infection within and outside the temporal bone, resulting in complications such as post-auricular subperiosteal abscess, facial palsy, labyrinthitis, and intracranial lesions.

is not fit for anaesthesia there is no place for conservative treatment because cholesteatoma never regresses spontaneously but continues to expand and destroy bone, and produce intra- and extracranial complications.

Complications of otitis media

Complications are commonly associated with chronic rather than acute otitis media. They can be divided into extracranial and intracranial complications (*see* Table 34.3).

The most common extracranial complication is post-auricular subperiosteal abscess (**mastoiditis**). Facial palsy is a rare complication of chronic suppurative otitis media and suspicious of tuberculous mastoiditis if present. The treatment for all extracranial complications is urgent intravenous antibiotic therapy, consisting of ampicillin 90 mg/kg/d and metronidazole 20 mg/kg/d. Mastoidectomy is performed as soon as possible, preferably within 12 hours of presentation.

Intracranial complications must be suspected in all patients presenting with severe headaches, nuchal rigidity or localizing neurological signs with chronic discharging ears. A brain computerized tomography (CT) scan is indicated.

The treatment of all otogenic intracranial complications is intravenous antibiotics, mastoidectomy and surgical drainage of the intracranial collection of pus if present. The neurosurgical procedure and mastoidectomy must be performed under the same anaesthesia with the neurosurgical procedure always preceding the mastoidectomy. Surgery must be undertaken as soon as possible, no later than 12 hours of presentation.

Otogenic intracranial complication is a serious condition with a mortality of about 10 to 30 per cent.

Tuberculous mastoiditis

Tuberculous mastoiditis is a disease of children, 80 per cent of whom are younger than 10 years of age. The typical clinical features include painless and profuse otorrhoea, multiple tympanic membrane perforations, pale granulation tissue, lower motor neuron facial palsy (40 per cent incidence), disproportionate hearing loss, and bone necrosis with sequestrum formation.

Table 34.3 Complications of otitis media

Extracranial complications		Intracranial complications	
Symptoms and signs	Consider	Symptoms and signs	Consider
Post-auricular swelling	Post-auricular abscess (mastoiditis)	Neck stiffness and fever with or without localising signs	Meningitis
Swelling of the mastoid tip	Bezold's abscess	Headache, pyrexia, hemiparesis, ataxia	Extradural empyaema
Drooling of saliva from angle of mouth and inability to close the eye on the same side	Facial palsy		Subdural empyaema
Dizziness with nausea and vomiting	Labyrinthitis		Lateral sinus thrombosis
Ipsilateral otorrhoea, 6th cranial nerve palsy, and facial pain	Petrous apicitis		Brain abscess

Evidence of tuberculosis (TB) in other sites reinforces the diagnosis, for example pulmonary TB (95 per cent) and pre-auricular lymphadenopathy (23 per cent).

The *diagnosis* is confirmed on histology of granulation tissue biopsied from the middle ear or mastoid cavity. The treatment is antituberculosis therapy for a minimum period of six months.

The role of surgery is to obtain tissue for diagnosis, decompress a posterior auricular abscess, and remove sequestra, if present.

Hearing impairment in children

Normal hearing is a fundamental requirement for the development of speech and language and hence for communication. Speech develops by repeating sounds that are heard. Hearing is essential for the acquisition of vocabulary since we learn the words first and then give them meaning. Vocabulary is the basis for all learning and, because we think in words, for intellectual development. (*See* Table 34.4.)

Hearing loss must be detected as soon as possible, preferably before the age of one, so that a rehabilitation programme can be commenced early. All high-risk babies must be screened, especially those with a family history of deafness, or intra-uterine rubella infection, low Apgar score, low birth weight, congenital deformities, neonatal jaundice, and meningitis. The mother may not yet be aware of the hearing problem. It is important that any complaints are heeded and the child's hearing assessed.

In childhood conductive hearing loss due to middle ear effusions is common. The hearing loss

> Mild hearing impairment causes both delay in speech development and distortion of the quality of speech. If there is severe sensorineural hearing loss it means that speech cannot develop. There is a limited period for the development of speech, the most critical period being the first two years of life. If a child is not speaking by the age of five, it is unlikely that intelligible speech will develop thereafter.

Table 34.4 Hearing impairment in infancy and childhood

	Mild conductive hearing loss	**Severe sensorineural deafness**
Aetiology	SOM and CSOM	Congenital: genetic or acquired (rubella)
Age of presentation	1–3 years	Birth
Site of lesion	Middle ear	Cochlea + 8th CN
Type of hearing loss	Mild conductive HL	Severe sensorineural HL
Presentation	Learning difficulty and delayed speech development	No speech
Investigation	Tympanogram	BERA
Diagnosis	Type B or C curve	Waves IV + V complex not identified
Treatment	SOM–myringotomy + VT CSOM–tympanoplasty	Hearing aid
School	Normal school	Special school

HL: hearing loss SOM: Secretory otitis media CSOM: Chronic suppurative otitis media
SND: Sensorineural deafness BERA: Brain-stem evoked response audiometry
VT: Ventilation tube (grommet) CN: Cranial nerve

is mild, but persistent loss over several months will impair speech quality and vocabulary development. Behaviour problems may occur. The treatment of choice is myringostomy and ventilation tube insertion.

Before any child is labelled as having mental retardation, autism, or speech developmental delay, the hearing must be evaluated. It must be emphasized that unilateral hearing impairment does not cause any hearing disability, apart from inability to localize the source of sound. In short, we need only one ear to hear.

Secretory otitis media

Secretory otitis media is characterized by the presence of non-purulent fluid in the middle ear space. The fluid may be serous or mucoid. In children it is predominantly mucoid with high viscosity, hence the term 'glue ear'. There are two types: acute adult type, and the chronic paediatric type.

Chronic secretory otitis media

This is a condition that predominantly affects children between six months and six years. The incidence is approximately 10 per cent. A higher incidence is reported in children attending day-care centres and in winter. The incidence is low in breastfed children.

The underlying pathophysiology in secretory otitis media is eustachian tube dysfunction, the exact cause of which is unknown. Infections of the throat, adenoids, tonsils and sinuses, and allergy, cleft palate, and nasopharyngeal tumors have been implicated.

The history from the mother is that the child is disobedient, turns up the volume of the radio or television, and performs poorly in school. On examination, the tympanic membrane is dull and prominent vessels are seen running radially from the centre. Under normal circumstances, blood vessels are not visible. The light reflex is lost and the tympanic membrane is retracted. Clinical testing with tuning forks confirms a mild conductive hearing loss with Rinne test negative for C_0 and C_1, and the Weber test showing a response lateralizing to the ear with greater degree of conductive hearing loss.

Pure tone audiogram confirms 10-30 dB conductive hearing loss. The tympanogram confirms the presence of a negative middle ear pressure by

recording either a type B or C curve. If the condition is unilateral, the disability is negligible but if bilateral, then the patient will not be able to hear normal speech beyond four metres.

The initial treatment consists of antibiotics, amoxycillin for one week, and antihistamine (Actifed syrup®) 5 ml nocte for one month. If there is no improvement, then myringotomy and ventilation tube insertion are indicated. Adenoidectomy is performed at the same time with the hope of improving eustachian tube function and removing the focus of infection.

It is important not to delay myringotomy and ventilation tube insertion because the prolonged negative pressure results in loss of tympanic membrane elasticity and the development of a retraction pocket predisposing to cholesteatoma formation. In the majority of patients, the ventilation tube is spontaneously extruded within six months. Recurrence is usually treated with repeat myringotomy and ventilation tube insertion.

Impacted wax

Wax is produced by ceruminous glands present in the outer third cartilaginous part of the external ear canal. Wax offers natural protection, the acid pH inhibits growth of bacteria and fungi, and the lipid content makes it impervious to water. Wax must not be removed unless it is impacted and producing hearing loss. The recommended method is to soften the wax with the application of turpentine and ear drops, and then syringe the ear. Failures must be referred to an ENT specialist for manual removal.

The nose

(*See* Table 34.5.)

Acute viral rhinitis (coryza)

The common cold is the most frequent infectious human disease, with its highest incidence in early childhood. The condition is caused by infection with rhinovirus and must be differentiated from acute hay fever. There is an acute onset of nasal congestion and a profuse clear nasal discharge. A short-lived fever is also common. The child has difficulty sleeping flat because of the nasal congestion. It is conveyed by contact or airborne droplets, and may be complicated by secondary

Table 34.5 Nasal and sinus disorders

Symptoms and signs	Diagnosis	Management
Failure to breathe through the nose at birth	Choanal atresia	Place oral airway and strap with tape. Pass orogastric tube for feeding and refer to specialist
Rhinitis and nasal blockage with fever and hyperaemic mucosa	Acute viral rhinitis	Antihistamine and paracetamol
Rhinitis, nasal blockage, sneezing with bluish nasal mucosa, no fever	Allergic rhinitis	Mild degree – antihistamine and topical steroid nasal spray
Bleeding from the nose	Epistaxis	Exclude haematological disorder, local plugging
Purulent nasal discharge with headache	Acute sinusitis	Antibiotics
Purulent nasal discharge with orbital cellulitis	Complication of sinusitis	Antibiotics (IV) and refer immediately
Purulent nasal discharge with neck stiffness and headache	Intracranial complication of sinusitis	Antibiotics (IV). Urgent CT scan of brain and sinuses, refer immediately
Purulent nasal discharge with nasal blockage	Chronic sinusitis or adenoiditis	Antibiotics

bacterial infection. Symptomatic therapy is recommended with ample fluids, elevation of the head end of the bed for sleeping, and oral antihistaminic decongestants.

Upper respiratory infection and nasopharyngitis

The combination of runny nose with fever and a sore throat is a common feature of upper respiratory infection that may precede or develop into a more significant illness with cough. The infection may spread through the mucosal lymphatics to the whole of the respiratory tract, resulting in otitis media, sinusitis, or bronchitis. Lower respiratory infections are thus common complications of acute viral rhinitis. This is also the first manifestation of many viral infections including measles. On examination there is a clear nasal discharge, the patient may have soft cervical adenopathy, and on inspection of the mouth and throat there is hyperaemia of the pharynx and

tonsillar region. Examination should include inspection of the buccal mucosa for Koplik's spots or other viral enanthems. Treatment is symptomatic including an antipyretic for fever.

Chronic recurrent viral rhinitis

Chronic rhinitis is very common among children in day-care centres, crèches, and nursery schools. The close proximity of children to one another in such centres results in continuous re-infection with a large number of viruses which cause infective rhinitis, rhinoviruses being the most common. Adenovirus may chronically infect lymphoid tissue and explain the persistence of symptoms. This condition must be differentiated from allergic rhinitis. (*See* Chapter 20, Allergic disorders.) Treatment is symptomatic, but secondary bacterial infection often supervenes and requires appropriate antibiotics. Prevention of repeated infection can be attained by removing the child from the group temporarily.

Choanal atresia

Choanal atresia is the most common congenital malformation of the nose. The atresia can be membranous, cartilaginous, or bony. It is thought to be due to the persistence of bucconasal membrane. It can be bilateral or unilateral.

Bilateral atresia is common and is evident at birth. Babies are obligatory nose breathers; attempting to breathe through a completely obstructed nose produces asphyxia and cyanosis. The immediate response is crying and when the mouth opens, air is drawn into the lungs and the pink colour returns. The treatment is to encourage the child to breathe through the mouth by placing an oral airway and securing it with tape. The diagnosis can be established clinically by attempting to pass a nasogastric tube through the nostrils to check the patency of the posterior choanae. The diagnosis is confirmed with contrast radiography, or a CT scan.

Surgical correction of the atresia must be undertaken as soon as possible, to establish nasal breathing, so that the child can feed orally.

Unilateral choanal atresia is less common and presents later in life with nasal obstruction and discharge. Surgical correction is undertaken once the diagnosis is confirmed.

Persistent rhinitis in the newborn

Persistent noisy breathing in the newborn may be obstructive in origin due to choanal atresia or rhinitis. Transient, idiopathic, stuffy nose of the newborn is a common condition characterized by a mucoid or clear nasal discharge, which lasts about three weeks. Nasal stuffiness with obstruction can also occur if the breastfeeding mother is taking drugs such as beta blockers.

When there is nasal congestion, babies become irritable and dyspnoeic. Babies only gradually learn to become mouth breathers by five to six months of age. A head-end-up position during sleep may help, or otherwise apply normal saline nose drops before feeding and sleeping.

Mouth-breathing and snoring

Children are often brought in with the complaint that they snore and sleep restlessly. The enlarged adenoid gland is the cause of the upper airway obstruction and a lateral X-ray will confirm the diagnosis. Snoring with obstructive sleep apnoea is a serious condition. Adenoidectomy must be undertaken as soon as possible, irrespective of the age of the child. Unattended chronic obstructive apnoea leads to hypoxia, pulmonary hypertension, right ventricular hypertrophy, and cardiac failure.

Foreign body

A foreign body in the nose is not an uncommon problem in children. Any child who presents with a unilateral, offensive, purulent nasal discharge has a foreign body stuck in their nose until proved otherwise. The common foreign bodies are sponge, tissue paper, beads, stone, and crayons. Sponge and tissue paper can be easily removed with a pair of forceps. The other foreign bodies, which can easily dislodge into the postnasal space and be aspirated, must be removed with a Jobson Horne probe.

Nasal trauma

The presenting symptoms are swelling and epistaxis. It is important to assess for cosmetic deformity and the presence of septal haematoma. Patients with cosmetic deformity must be referred immediately to an ENT specialist for correction, as delay can lead to permanent nasal deformity.

Septal haematoma is easily diagnosed on anterior rhinoscopy, the septum bulges and completely occludes the nostril on the affected side. Urgent intervention is necessary to prevent cartilage necrosis and nasal collapse. The treatment is to incise the mucoperichondrium on the fluctuant side under local anaesthesia, drain the haematoma, pack the nostrils with a 2.5-cm thick ribbon gauze impregnated with BIPP (bismuth, iodioform paraffin paste), prescribe erythromycin, and refer the patient to an ENT specialist.

Furunculosis

Furunculosis develops in the hair-bearing region of the nose, referred to as the vestibule. The patients present with painful swelling of the tip of the nose. On examination, the nasal tip is inflamed and tender. The furuncle will be noticed on the undersurface. Treatment is to puncture the furuncle with a hypodermic needle and prescribe erythromycin for five days. To prevent recurrence, recommend the application of antiseptic nasal cream to the vestibule of the nose, daily for one month.

Epistaxis

Epistaxis is very common in children. The majority have a few isolated nosebleeds, and do not seek medical assistance. Those with recurrent nose bleeding usually present to the family practitioner. The bleeding is from Little's area, the caudal end of the nasal septum, where all the arteries of the nose anastomose. The blood loss during each episode is minimal, less than 10 ml. Severe epistaxis is rare in children.

Although the cause is unknown, blood samples must be sent for full blood count, platelet count, prothrombin index, and partial thromboplastin time, to exclude bleeding disorders.

The first-aid treatment for epistaxis must be explained and demonstrated to the parent. Sit the child upright, bend the head forwards, and apply pressure to Little's area by compression of the ala of the nose, for 10 minutes. If the bleeding persists, reapply pressure for another 10 minutes. Continue in this manner until the bleeding stops.

The definitive treatment is either cauterization of the vessels in Little's area with electrical or chemical cautery, or packing of the nasal vestibule with a 2.5-cm thick ribbon gauze, impregnated with Kenacomb® ointment for 48 hours. To prevent aspiration of the packs, suture them together with 'O' silk thread and tape it to the nasal dorsum.

Once bleeding has ceased, recommend the application of antiseptic nasal cream to Little's area once daily for a month.

The paranasal sinuses

Acute sinusitis

Acute ethmoidal and maxillary sinusitis are common in children and are nearly always precipitated by viral rhinitis. A less common precipitating factor is swimming or diving, especially in the presence of an upper respiratory tract infection.

The causative organisms are pneumococci, streptococci, staphylococci, and *H. influenzae*.

Clinical features include:
- Headache
- Pain over the affected sinuses
- Periorbital cellulitis
- Nasal obstruction
- Percussion tenderness over the sinus
- Purulent nasal discharge.

The diagnosis is confirmed on CT scan of the para nasal sinuses.

Complications arise when the infection spreads beyond the confines of the sinus to either the orbit or intracranially. The orbital complications include periorbital oedema, lid abscess, chemosis, proptosis, ophthalmoplegia, and blindness. The intracranial complications include extradural abscess, subdural abscess, meningitis, brain abscess, and cavernous sinus thrombosis.

When treating acute sinusitis, all sinuses should be viewed as individual cavities which, when full of pus, can be regarded as abscesses. The basic principle involved in the management of any abscess is drainage, antibiotics, and analgesics.

In the absence of orbital and intracranial complications, the sinusitis should be treated conservatively with antral lavage and amoxycillin. Complicated sinusitis is a serious condition. The patient must be admitted and given intravenous antibiotics, ampicillin 150 mg/kg/d and metronidazole 20 mg/kg/d, and the sinus drained externally as soon as possible.

Chronic sinusitis

Chronic, non-specific, purulent sinusitis may follow after one or repeated attacks of acute sinusitis, or it may be associated with allergic rhinitis. Clinical features include a purulent postnasal drip, chronic nasal obstruction, and headache (especially frontal and periorbital). Anosmia may be present. Oedema of the tissues may be present and may be mild or severe, leading to nasal polyposis. All stages of mucosal inflammation, ranging from hypertrophy to atrophymay be found at the same time. Fibrosis of the mucosal lining renders the condition incurable.

The causative organisms are mixed, with streptococci, pneumococci, and anaerobes being the most common. Gram-negative organisms are often secondary invaders.

Coronal CT scan of the paranasal sinuses is the investigation of choice in patients with chronic sinusitis. It assists in locating the exact site and nature of the disease.

The treatment of chronic sinusitis in children is conservative. Endoscopic sinus surgery or any other form of sinus surgery must be considered only after excluding allergy and chronic ade-noiditis. Further, no surgery must be undertaken without a trial of intensive medical therapy con-sisting of amoxycillin and metronidazole for five days and an antihistamine for one month.

Throat

Acute tonsillitis

Tonsils are aggregates of lymphoid tissue, grouped in the nasopharynx (adenoids), the base of the tongue (lingual tonsils), and the lateral wall of the oropharynx (palatine tonsil).

Patients present with sore throat, fever, and pain on swallowing. On examination the tonsils are inflamed, and the jugulo-digastric lymph nodes are enlarged and tender. The initial inflam-mation produced by virus infection is followed by secondary bacterial invasion; the most common organism being *Streptococcus pyogenes*.

Three stages of inflammation are recognized in tonsillitis:

+ **Parenchymatous stage**: the tonsils are uniformly inflamed and appear hyperaemic.
+ **Follicular stage**: the tonsils are uniformly inflamed but, in addition, there is yellow exudate in the tonsillar crypts.
+ **Membranous stage**: the exudate coalesces to form a membrane over the tonsils.

The treatment is penicillin or amoxycillin for seven to ten days.

The complications of tonsillitis are chronic tonsillitis, peritonsillar abscess (quinsy), and parapharyngeal abscess.

Chronic tonsillitis

Chronic tonsillitis usually follows follicular ton-sillitis. The micro-abscesses that form in the tonsillar follicles become walled off by fibrous tissue. This produces a chronic sore throat. The treatment is tonsillectomy.

Peritonsillar abscess (quinsy)

The infection spreads from the tonsil into the peritonsillar space. The condition is rare in children. There is pain on swallowing, marked trismus, and drooling of saliva. On examination, there is inflammation of the tonsils and bulging of the soft palate above the tonsil on the affected side (*see* Figure 34.3). The treatment for the older child is incision and drainage of the abscess under local anaesthesia, procaine penicillin injections daily for three days, and amoxycillin for five days. Younger children must be admitted and given intravenous penicillin G and intravenous fluids.

Retropharyngeal abscess

Retropharyngeal abscess commonly occurs in children, 50 per cent of whom are under two years of age. It is due to inflammation and breakdown of the retropharyngeal lymph nodes, leading to unilateral swelling of the posterior pharyngeal wall. Infection spreads to the nodes from the adenoid.

The patients present with fever, torticollis, drooling of saliva, and swelling on the posterior

Figure 34.3 Peritonsillar abscess (quinsy)

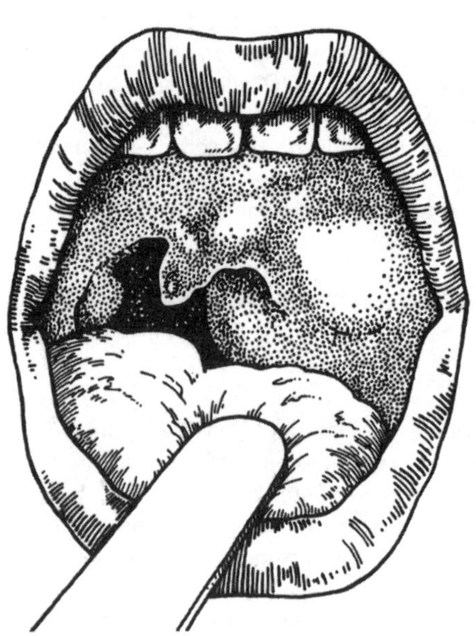

wall of the oropharynx, lateral to the midline. Diagnosis is made on soft tissue lateral neck radio graph. Enlargement of prevertebral soft tissue shadow, greater than twice the width of the body of the vertebra is diagnostic of a retropharyngeal abscess. The treatment is intravenous antibiotics and incision and drainage under general anaesthesia.

Parapharyngeal abscess

Parapharyngeal abscess is a very rare complication of tonsillitis. It occurs when infection spreads from the tonsil into the peritonsillar space, across the superior constrictor muscle of the pharynx, into the parapharyngeal space. The clinical presentation is painful swelling over the parotid gland region. The treatment is incision and drainage, and intravenous antibiotics.

Indications for tonsillectomy

- Recurrent tonsillitis – most common indication
- Chronic tonsillitis
- Tonsillolith – secretions from the tonsillar crypts solidify to form a tonsillolith, which is similar in appearance to a rice grain. It is one of the causes of halitosis
- Peritonsillar abscess
- Chronic suppurative otitis media
- Enlarged tonsils producing airway obstruction (either stridor or obstructive sleep apnoea syndrome), swallowing difficulty, or altered speech
- Tonsillar tumour.

Complications of tonsillectomy

Haemorrhage. Primary haemorrhage occurs within 24 hours and secondary haemorrhage, which is usually due to infection, around day 10. Post-tonsillectomy haemorrhage can be a life-threatening condition and must be attended to immediately.

Altered speech occurs in some patients but usually settles after one to two weeks.

Death occurs in 1 in 20 000 tonsillectomies.

Stridor

Stridor is noisy respiration due to incomplete airway obstruction; it can be inspiratory, expira-tory, or both. (*See also* Chapter 25, Respiratory tract disorders.)

Neonatal stridor

Laryngomalacia is the most common congenital abnormality affecting the larynx. There is excessive flaccidity of the supraglottic region of the larynx and during inspiration the supraglottis is sucked into the laryngeal inlet, resulting in obstruction and stridor. The stridor is present from birth, it is inspiratory and disappears in the prone position. It is usually absent when the infant is asleep. The cry is normal. The diagnosis is made clinically with the aid of the flexible pharyngolaryngoscope. On inspiration, the supraglottic tissue prolapses into the laryngeal lumen.

In the majority of cases the stridor is mild. Reassure the mother that the stridor will improve with increasing age and completely disappear by one to two years of age, but warn her that during episodes of upper respiratory tract infection the stridor may become worse and the child must be taken to a hospital.

Moderate to severe degree stridor usually occurs with a superimposed upper respiratory tract infection. Admit and nurse under humidified oxygen with frequent adrenalin nebulization. Intubate those with impending total airway obstruction.

Vocal fold palsy. Unilateral vocal fold palsy occurs in neonates after difficult labour, especially where instruments have been used to assist with delivery. The stridor is due to recurrent laryngeal nerve injury. It is present at birth, and is worse on physical effort, e.g. when the child cries. The cry is abnormal. The diagnosis is confirmed with the aid of a flexible pharyngolaryngoscope. Management is conservative as almost all recover within a few months.

The most common cause of bilateral vocal fold palsy is hydrocephalus. The stridor is severe, requiring tracheostomy.

Laryngeal webs. The webs are usually anterior. Stridor is present at birth. It is aggravated by effort. The cry is abnormal. Treatment is to divide the web.

Bifid epiglottis. The epiglottis is divided into equal and symmetrical halves, which are flaccid and prolapse into the inlet of the glottis. Stridor is inspiratory and present at birth.

Treatment is to amputate the flaccid portions of the epiglottis.

Laryngeal cysts. Vallecula cyst is a common cause of stridor in black neonates. Stridor is present at birth. Soft tissue lateral neck radiographs clearly show the cyst in the vallecula (i.e. the space between the base of the tongue and the epiglottis). Treatment is excision. Lymphangioma can produce airway obstruction.

Tumours. The most common tumour is haemangioma. It typically occurs in the subglottic region. Stridor may be present at birth, or develop later. Diagnosis must be suspected in infants with haemangioma elsewhere in the body. If the stridor is mild, the treatment is conservative as the majority regress spontaneously by one year. If stridor is severe, tracheostomy with excision of the haemangioma is indicated.

Micrognathia and glossoptosis are responsible for respiratory obstruction in some infants. When they are associated with a cleft palate, the entity is referred to as Pierre Robin syndrome. The small jaw and relatively large tongue are responsible for airway obstruction. Treatment depends on the degree of respiratory obstruction. Minor degrees of obstruction can be overcome by keeping the infant in a prone position. For severe obstruction, surgery is indicated.

Stridor in infancy

Acute laryngotracheobronchitis (LTB)

(*See* chapter 25, Respiratory tract disorders.)

Subglottic stenosis is the second most common cause of stridor in infancy. The stridor is not present at birth but comes on during upper respiratory tract infection. Stridor is expiratory, without any relieving factors. The cry is normal. Plain radiographs of the neck will reveal a smooth, usually symmetrical narrowing at 2–3 mm below the free edge of the vocal folds. The airway narrowing is at the level of the cricoid cartilage. Diagnosis is confirmed by direct laryngoscopy and bronchoscopy.

The treatment of mild and moderate degree stridor is conservative – admit to respiratory unit and nurse under humidified oxygen with regular adrenalin nebulization. Those with severe stridor must be intubated for 48–72 hours. Thereafter if the stridor is still severe, refer for specialist evaluation.

Epiglottitis

(*See* Chapter 25, Respiratory tract disorders.)

Mouth conditions

Aphthous ulcers

(*See* Chapter 35, Oral and dental disorders.)

Ranula

(*See* Chapter 35, Oral and dental disorders.)

A ranula is a retention cyst of the sublingual salivary gland. It is a thin-walled bluish cyst found in the floor of the mouth, to one side of the frenulum. Treatment is excision of the cyst, together with the sublingual gland.

Stomatitis

(*See* Chapter 35, Oral and dental disorders.)

A sore mouth must be distinguished from a sore throat. When the anterior part of the mouth is involved in a pathological process, this leads to a sore mouth. Feed refusal and excessive salivation and drooling are the common complaints. One of the most common conditions is oral candidiasis (thrush), seen especially often in patients with HIV infection.

Ear, nose and throat manifestations of HIV infection

The following features are commonly found in children with HIV infection:

- Cervical lymphadenopathy as part of generalized lymphadenopathy, or as a result of local mouth and throat conditions.
- Parotid enlargement: This is found commonly in association with lymphocytic interstitial pneumonitis and may be both uni and bilateral. In doubtful cases a fine needle aspiration may help to diagnose benign lymphoepithelial cysts, tuberculous or other infection and tumours.
- Pharyngeal lymphoid enlargement and 'cobblestone' mucosa from pharyngeal wall hypertrophy, adenoidal hypertrophy

leading to nasal blockage, tonsillar hypertrophy, tonsillitis and peritonsillar abscess (quinsy).

Mouth ulcers are seen in:

- Apthous ulceration
- Stomatitis (cheilitis)–Herpes and other viruses
- Oral candidiasis
  - Pseudo-membranous candiasis–smooth white or cottage cheese like plaques, when wiped off a bleeding erythemous base remains
  - Atrophic candidiasis–Zones of hyperaemia and tenderness on the dorsum of the tongue or hard palate
  - Hyperplastic candidiasis–white plaques on buccal mucosa that cannot be scraped off (leukoplakia)
  - Angular cheilitis–tender erythematous fissures and ulceration at the oral commissure
- Oropharyngeal sepsis
  - Ludwig's angina/quinsy
  - Tonsillitis
- Gingival and periodontal disease
  - Acute necrotizing ulcerative gingivitis
  - Necrotizing stomatitis

- Suppurative otitis media
- Oral ulceration and stomatitis
- Gingival and periodontal disease
- Rhinosinusitis and mastoiditis.

Recurrent parotitis

Some children experience repeated episodes of parotid gland swelling and pain. The cause is often unknown. The condition may be unilateral and may alternate sides. Sialectasia may be present. The treatment is analgesia and the use of a sialogogue such as lemon juice. Sialography should be performed if sialectasia is suspected. The dilatation produced by the sialogram often cures the condition and may prevent recurrences. Those who do not settle require antibiotics. If no improvement is noted, then superficial parotidectomy is indicated.

Tumours of the parotid gland

Mesothelial tumours, i.e. haemangiomas and lymphangiomas, are the most common tumours of the parotid gland in the paediatric age group. Hard or persistent masses are suggestive of a glandular or epithelial origin and are often (in 50 per cent of cases) malignant.

Oral and dental disorders

The mouth contains highly specialised structures not found anywhere else in the human body, all of which have their own types of pathology. Disorders of the structures and tissues of the oral cavity manifest as problems of teething and dentition, dental caries and toothache, gingival and periodontal conditions, as well as a variety of swellings and tumours. The reader is referred to more specialised oral pathology textbooks and literature should he or she want to learn more on any given topic concerning this highly specialised area.

Normal anatomy of the oral cavity and teeth

Teeth

Anatomically, each tooth has a crown, the visible part, and a root, which is normally situated in and anchored to the alveolar bone of the jaws by connective tissues consisting of the cementum which is firmly interlocked with the root dentin, and the periodontal ligament. (*See* Figure 35.1.)

The tooth consists of a hard, non-vital, insensitive outer layer of enamel, which is supported by less mineralized, more resilient bulk connective tissue, the dentin. Dentin is supported by the dental pulp, a soft connective tissue that contains the neurovascular plexuses, differentiated and non-differentiated cells. The small face and jaws of a child can only carry a few teeth of small size. As the face and jaws grow, the small deciduous teeth become inadequate and are replaced by the permanent or secondary dentition consisting of more and larger teeth.

Oral mucosa

The mucosa of the oral cavity is divided into various anatomical regions (*see* Figure 35.2).

Sixty per cent of the oral mucosa is made up of the non-keratinised lining mucosa of the cheeks, lips, floor of the mouth, ventral surface of the tongue and soft palate. The masticatory mucosa or mucoperiosteum is a firm and immobile keratinized type of mucosa that is directly attached to the underlying bone. It is found

Figure 35.1 Structure of a normal incisor tooth, longitudinal section

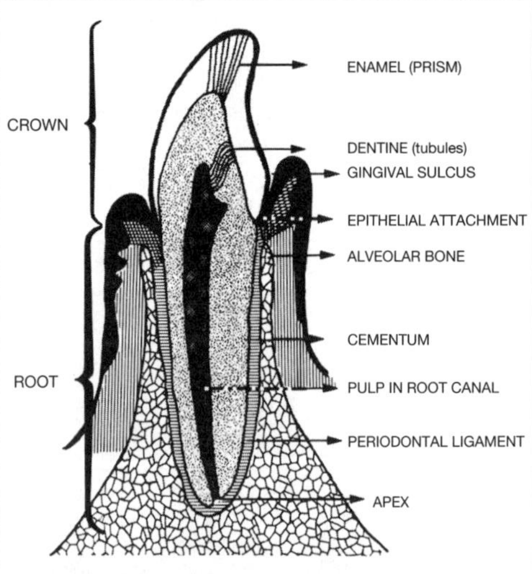

CROWN

ENAMEL (PRISM)

DENTINE (tubules)
GINGIVAL SULCUS

EPITHELIAL ATTACHMENT
ALVEOLAR BONE

CEMENTUM

ROOT

PULP IN ROOT CANAL

PERIODONTAL LIGAMENT

APEX

Figure 35.2 Masticatory mucosa – normal structures

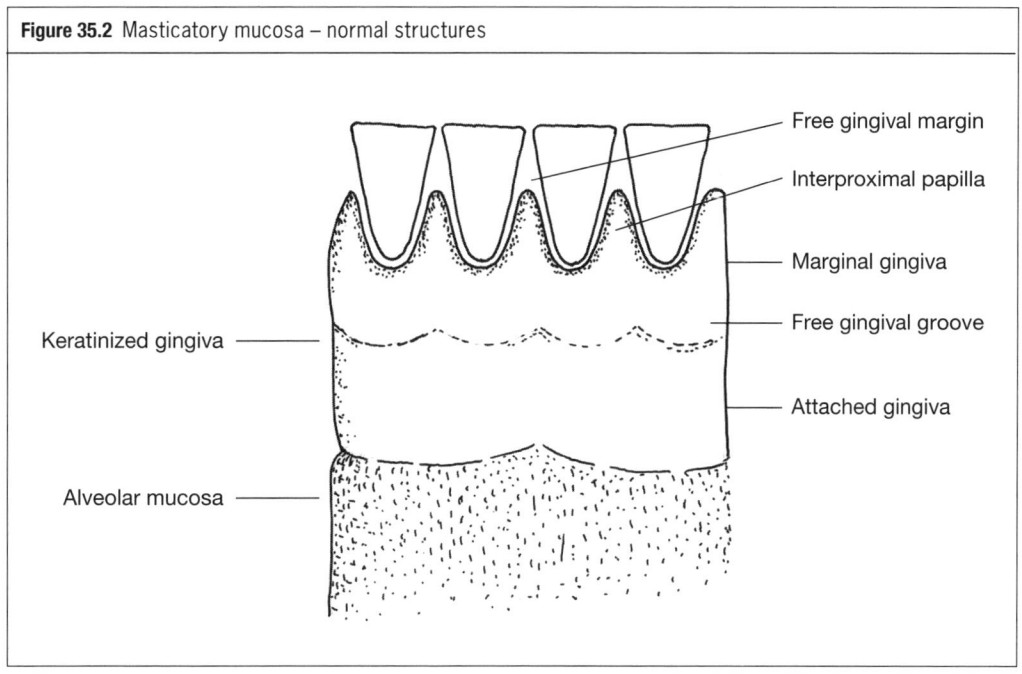

Free gingival margin

Interproximal papilla

Marginal gingiva

Free gingival groove

Keratinized gingiva

Attached gingiva

Alveolar mucosa

on the gingiva and hard palate and represents approximately 25 per cent of the oral mucosa. The dorsal surface of the tongue, with its papillae and taste buds, is a specialized mucosa and represents about 15 per cent of the total. Minor salivary glands are found in the lining, as well as in specialized mucosa and may be afflicted by various conditions that affect the major salivary glands, the parotid, submandibular and sublingual glands.

Normal dental development and tooth eruption

Dental development starts during the sixth week of fetal life. Tooth formation then continues uninterrupted until approximately 18 years, when the roots of the third molars are completed.

Tooth eruption is defined as the tooth's movement from its bony crypt, through the bone and

> Local or systemic diseases of the fetus or child, or any of a large variety of medications, have the potential to adversely affect the normal development of the teeth.

overlying oral mucosa to appear in the oral cavity and reach its opponent in the occlusal plane. This process is divided into three distinct phases: the pre-eruptive phase where the tooth germs develop and grow together with the bone of the surrounding jaws; the eruptive phase when the tooth moves from the bony crypt to the occlusal plane ('teething'); and the post-eruptive phase of tooth eruption, which is the movement of a tooth to accommodate jaw growth and various forms of dental structure wear. This last phase is a life long process. It has been shown that a tooth will move at an average rate of 1–10 μm per day when still in the bone but up to 75 μm per day once through the bone.

The dental follicle is a connective tissue sac that surrounds the developing tooth germ and, together with certain molecular determinants, has an important role in tooth eruption. The absence of a normal dental follicle or any factor that results in abnormal osteoclast formation will result in delayed or no tooth eruption at all.

Normal biologic tooth eruption occurs when approximately two thirds of the dental root has been formed. Root formation will only be completed up to two years after the tooth has erupted completely. During this time the tooth is said to have an 'open apex'. Any required dental treatment modalities are usually modified to accommodate, or even speed up, the process of closure of the root apex.

The age of tooth eruption varies but the first primary tooth to erupt is usually the mandibular central incisor at between five to eight months postnatally, and the last to erupt around 24 months is usually the second maxillary molar. (See Table 35.1.)

The permanent teeth should start to erupt from the age of six to seven years, as shown in table 35.2, and be completed by 18 years

Variations may occur and do not necessarily imply the presence of pathology. It is best to refer the child to a dentist should teeth fail to be present a year after the given times. Although all dentists are trained to attend to the oral health of children, some have a special interest in paediatric dentistry.

Teething

'Teething' is the process of tooth eruption from the bony crypt through the overlying mucosa to the occlusal plane. To diagnose teething, the gingiva should be examined and palpated for evidence of tooth eruption. Visualisation of the gums should always be part of the clinical examination of the mouth and pharynx of young children because teething, wrongly, has often been diagnosed on the basis of certain symptoms alone. It is frequently a 'scapegoat' explanation for unwelcome physical discomforts that are often found in children 6–24 months old.

Over-the-counter topical teething gels may

Table 35.1 Average age of eruption of primary teeth		
Tooth	Age of eruption (in months) Mandibular teeth	Age of eruption (in months) Maxillary teeth
First incisor	6	7.5
Second incisor	7	9
First molar	12	14
Canine	16	18
Second molar	20	24

Table 35.2 Age of eruption of permanent teeth				
	Age of eruption in years (male)		Age of eruption in years (female)	
Tooth	Maxillary	Mandibular	Maxillary	Mandibular
First incisor	8	7	7	6,7
Second incisor	9	8	8	7.3
Canine	11	10.9	9	9
First premolar	11	11	9.7	9.9
Second premolar	11.6	11.9	10.6	10.6
First molar	7.8	7.8	7	7
Second molar	12.4	12.5	11.8	11.8
Third molar	17.4	17.4	17.8	17.7

Symptoms that have been found to be significantly associated with teething from four days before to three days after tooth emergence include: congestion; irritability; decreased appetite; cough; non-facial rashes; sleep disturbances; vomiting; diarrhoea and mildly elevated temperature (less than 38.3 °C), but no specific symptom reliably predicts teething.

relieve some of the discomfort of teething, but should be used with caution. Oral ibuprofen or Paracetamol® are generally safe when not misused, but their efficacy in relieving teething symptoms is questionable. Allowing a teething child to bite and suck on a cold teething ring may soothe the discomfort and distract the child from the pain, as long as it is not a choking hazard. Parents should however be warned that frozen items may also cause cold injuries.

Natal teeth

Natal teeth are present at birth. They are rare, from 1:2000 to 1:3500 live births, with a slight female predominance. The majority of natal teeth represent the early eruption of the primary teeth, but in approximately 10 per cent of cases these are supernumerary (extra) teeth. The mandibular first incisor is most commonly affected (85 per cent) followed by the maxillary incisors (11 per cent). Natal teeth may interfere with breastfeeding and in some circumstances may become loose and may be dislodged and swallowed or aspirated during nursing or at night. Another complication is severe sublingual ulceration (Riga-Fede disease) with resultant feeding refusal. In the instance of supernumerary natal teeth, these can be removed by a dentist. Dental radiography is however, indicated before extraction, to differentiate between premature eruption of a primary deciduous tooth and a supernumerary tooth. In the case of the former, it might be wise to leave well alone if the tooth is not mobile and the dental hard structure is normal, to avoid future orthodontic problems. Early eruption of teeth is usually associated with abnormal mineralization of the dental hard tissue (enamel and dentin) which results in an abnormal, dysplastic or hypomineralized appearance and sometimes abnormal or absent root formation.

Disturbances in tooth eruption

Delayed eruption

If tooth eruption has not occurred despite the formation of two-thirds or more of the dental root, it is considered delayed tooth eruption (DTE). Tooth eruption may be influenced by various local factors as well as systemic factors. Local obstructions such as scar tissue, gingival hyperplasia and fibromatosis, supernumerary teeth, odontogenic or other tumours, injuries to primary teeth and other local factors such as lack of resorption of primary teeth or impacted teeth and ankylosis may all result in DTE. Systemic conditions such as nutritional deficiencies, endocrine disorders (most commonly hypothyroidism and hypoparathyroidism), chemotherapy and certain drugs such as phenytoin, tobacco smoke, anaemia, coeliac disease, prematurity/low birth weight, and many genetic disorders (including amelogenesis imperfecta, Apert syndrome, cleidocranial dysplasia, mucopolysaccharidosis, Down's syndrome, Gardner syndrome, Gaucher disease, Neurofibromatosis, Mc-Cune-Albright syndrome, osteopetrosis) have all been associated with DTE.

These patients should eventually be referred to a dental specialist, such as an orthodontist who is able to evaluate both the dental and craniofacial structures for further management and treatment.

Ankylosis

Ankylosis is the cessation of tooth eruption due to the anatomic fusion of tooth cementum or dentin with the alveolar bone. Ankylosis commonly affects the primary dentition and the child presents with either an absent or a 'submerged' tooth. This can follow trauma to the tooth with loss of the periodontal ligament. Management depends on each individual situation.

Oral hygiene

Tooth decay is found more frequently in infants

Even though variation in the time of normal eruption of teeth is common, significant deviations from the norm should be further investigated in view of the large number of possible aetiological associations.

and children fed a lot of sweetened drinks given by bottle, or sugar-containing food. Oral and dental hygiene is therefore mandatory from as early as eruption of the first tooth around six months of age. Brushing and cleaning of the teeth removes plaque, which contains acid-producing bacteria that stick to the teeth. A guideline based on a review of the current dental, medical, and public health literature related to infant oral health care is available online from the National Clearinghouse Guidelines at www.guideline.gov.

Regular dental check-ups should start within the first three years, preferably shortly after the first birthday. It is recommended that all primary health care professionals who serve mothers and infants should provide parent/caregiver education on the aetiology and prevention of early childhood caries. By six months of age, each infant and caregiver should obtain an oral health risk assessment from his/her primary health care provider and receive education on oral health and optimal fluoride exposure.

Fluoride supplementation

Fluoride is a highly effective way to prevent caries. Fluoride acts locally through enamel remineralization as well as by altering bacterial metabolism. When taken systemically during enamel development, the fluoride ion is incorporated into or adsorbed on the hydroxyapatite crystal, which makes it more resistant to acid dissolution. The daily fluoride exposure of an

individual through water, infant formulae, fruit juices, toothpastes and prepared food must be evaluated carefully before prescribing any fluoride supplements. Fluorosis will develop when excess amounts of fluoride are taken, with the degree of enamel abnormality dependent on the dose, duration and timing of the intake. The ameloblast (enamel-forming cell) is highly sensitive to the toxic effect of fluoride resulting in enamel that may vary from lustreless white opaque enamel that may have zones of dark-brown discoloration, to a mottled appearance with deep, irregular and brownish pits.

It is interesting to note that dental changes similar to dental fluorosis have recently been linked to amoxicillin use during early infancy.

After determining the fluoride level of the water, all other dietary sources should be taken into consideration as well before commencement of supplementation. Information on the fluoride level in the water may be retrieved from the local municipalities and the Departments of Community Dentistry at the Schools of Dentistry.

The American Academy of Paediatric Dentistry recommendation with regard to fluoride supplementation is as follows (available from www.aapd.org):

> Fluoride supplementation should be considered in all cases where the drinking water is fluoride deficient (<0.6 ppm F). When used correctly it is completely safe.

Important dental health guidance includes:

- Clean the infant's teeth with either washcloth or soft brush to reduce bacterial colonization. Parents should assist with tooth brushing up to age six.
- Restrict bottle feeding to normal meal times. Do not allow the infant to have a feeding bottle with him while sleeping. Wean from bottle to cup by one year.
- Reduce sugar intake and avoid soft drinks and fruit juices.
- Provide optimal fluoride exposure.
- Parents or caregivers should establish a dental home for infants by 12 months of age and every child should have regular dental check-ups (at least twice yearly).

Caries and pulpitis

The presence of one or more decayed, missing (because of caries), or filled tooth surfaces on any primary tooth in children up to 71 months of age is referred to as early childhood caries. Previously, additional clinical terms such as 'nursing caries' and 'bottle caries' were used to describe a form of rampant caries affecting teeth of infants and preschool children. By recent consensus, severe early childhood caries implies 'atypical', 'progressive', 'acute' or 'rampant' patterns and is defined according to the child's age and the number of decayed, missing or filled smooth tooth surfaces.

Caries may, if not treated in time, result in pulpitis or inflammation of the dental pulp. In the

Table 35.3 Recommended daily fluoride supplementation according to age and fluoride content of water

Content of F in water	<0.3 ppm F	0.3–0.6 ppm F	>0.6 ppm F
Birth-6 mo	0	0	0
6 mo–3 y	0.25 mg	0	0
3–6 y	0.50 mg	0.25 mg	0
6–16 y	1.00 mg	0.5 mg	0

case of reversible pulpitis accurate management may still save the vitality of the tooth, but in most instances, the child will either present with acute irreversible pulpitis leading to intense toothache, or chronic hyperplastic pulpitis. In acute irreversible pulpitis, endodontic treatment with removal of all the soft tissue of the pulp cavity is advised.

In chronic hyperplastic pulpitis, a unique pattern of pulp inflammation is seen and mainly affects young children. A large defect in the tooth structure is always visible and a soft tissue mass of vascular granulation tissue or mature connective tissue protrudes through the hole in the tooth crown. In most instances extraction of the tooth is indicated, as structure loss is usually so advanced that restoration after endodontic treatment is not feasible.

> It is always better, if at all possible, to keep the primary tooth as a retainer of space for the permanent tooth that will follow.

Periapical infections and cysts

During tooth development some epithelial rests of the developing tooth germ may remain behind as remnants in the periodontal ligament space surrounding the tooth root (Malassez rests) as well as in the overlying oral mucosal lamina propria (Serres rests). The epithelial rests in the periodontal ligament space at the apex of a tooth can be stimulated by inflammation to proliferate and give origin to various forms of odontogenic and inflammatory cysts. The term odontogenic refers to origin from the odontogenic apparatus of a developing tooth. With infection of the

pulp cavity, such as that caused by caries or even pulp inflammation after severe tooth trauma, the inflammation/infection may spread to and involve the periapical tissue in the jaw bone. When enough bone has been resorbed by the inflammatory process, a radiolytic lesion can be seen on dental radiographs. This consists either of vascular granulation tissue, a *periapical granuloma*, or sometimes a true epithelial lined cyst encountered from proliferation of the epithelial rests of Malassez, a radicular or periapical cyst. Typically patients with periapical cysts are asymptomatic unless there is an acute inflammatory flare-up. The treatment of a periapical cyst involves extraction of the involved tooth. These cysts can involve the deciduous teeth, especially the molar teeth and result in Turner's hypoplasia of the underlying permanent tooth. The extraction of a primary tooth should, however, be carefully planned to prevent damage to the underlying permanent tooth and a space retainer should be placed to prevent crowding of the permanent dentition later.

Chronic inflammation of the pulp cavity affecting especially the first molars in children can be complicated by osteomyelitis with *proliferative periostitis* (Garre's osteomyelitis, periostitis ossificans). The child presents with a firm swelling of the lateral and inferior border of the mandible with an 'onionskin' proliferation effect seen on radiography, due to the formation of parallel layers of new bone in the cortical area. The pathogenesis is chronic inflammation in the periosteum of the mandible, resulting in reactive bone formation. This lesion may easily be mistaken for an osteosarcoma. Management of proliferative periostitis consists of eliminating the focus of infection. The bone will remodel on its own over 6–12 months and no further intervention will usually be necessary.

Developmental defects of the oral cavity

Many developmental defects may be found in the dental structures or soft tissue and bone of the oro-facial complex deriving from the embryological origin of these structures.

Lingual thyroid

The thyroid gland develops as an epithelial proliferation in the foramen cecum area in the posterior third of the dorsal aspect of the tongue. Normally the thyroid gland descends into the anterior neck around the seventh embryonic week. Sometimes it does not descend normally and ectopic thyroid tissue may present as a mass, ranging from small asymptomatic nodules to masses large enough to block the airway anywhere between the foramen cecum and epiglottis. It is essential to determine thyroid function in all such patients.

Mucosal cysts of the newborn

These appear as small (1–3 mm) yellow-white epithelial papules on the palate or alveolar ridge of newborn babies. The palatal cysts are seen along the median palatal raphe and it has been postulated that they arise from epithelium entrapped along the line of palatal fusion. The cysts on the alveolar ridges are thought to be epithelial inclusions. As these lesions usually rupture and disappear spontaneously, no treatment is necessary.

Dental abnormalities

Developmental defects in dental structure

Amelogenesis imperfecta

Structural abnormalities of the dental enamel are due to mutations in various proteins responsible for dental development. At least 14 different hereditary subtypes have been described, with a wide variety of clinical patterns. The clinical appearance may vary from localised hypoplastic enamel to generalised thin or pitted, hypoplastic and pigmented enamel. The teeth have a higher risk for caries and are usually hypersensitive

to temperature changes. In some forms of the disease, delayed tooth eruption, tooth impaction and associated gingival inflammation may also be present. Clinical management varies according to the severity of the condition but usually involves extensive prosthodontic treatment by a specialist dentist.

Environmental alterations of teeth

Enamel defects

The ameloblast (enamel-forming cell) is extremely sensitive to a variety of external stimuli. An insult leaves a permanent abnormality because no remodelling of enamel takes place after its initial formation. Some of the factors associated with enamel defects are birth-related, such as hypoxia, premature births, breech presentations and prolonged labour, chemicals and drugs such as fluoride, antineoplastic chemotherapy, tetracyclines, thalidomide and Vitamin D, infections such as chickenpox, cytomegalovirus, measles, rubella, syphilis and tetanus. Certain metabolic disorders, malnutrition and various neurological disorders have also been associated with enamel abnormalities. Horizontal pitting or diminished enamel is a common result of pyrexia during childhood. The extent of damage is dependent on the stage of enamel development at the time of the insult, the dosage in the case of chemical insults and the duration of these. The timing of injury can accurately be determined should one wish to do this. Clinical features vary from subtle defects to hypoplastic areas and diffuse opacities with or without brownish-yellow or bluish-grey pigmentation.

Turner's hypoplasia is a frequent form of enamel defect seen in a single permanent tooth, caused by periapical inflammation or trauma of the overlying deciduous tooth. The tooth might have focal areas of abnormal enamel or sometimes extensive coronal hypoplasia.

Environmental discoloration of teeth

Intrinsic stains

Tooth colour depends on the shade, translucency and thickness of the enamel. Several different medications may be incorporated into the developing tooth structure, such as tetracycline, which is best known to cause this phenomenon. The affected teeth have a yellow-brown colour, which show bright yellow fluorescence. The fluorescence usually fades to leave a dull brown colour. Tetracyclines should not be used in childhood. Discoloration of the enamel may be due to extrinsic factors and many systemic disorders may also result in mild to severe tooth discoloration. Examples of this include hyperbilirubinemia and congenital metabolic conditions.

Physical and chemical injuries to the oral mucosa

Morsicatio buccarum (chronic cheek biting)

This is a very common condition seen mainly in adult patients, but occasionally in children who are either under stress or who exhibit some psychological condition. The lesions are usually found bilaterally and range from thickened, hyperkeratotic white areas, sometimes with a shredded appearance, to intervening areas of erythema and even ulceration.

Traumatic ulcerations (Riga-Fede disease of infancy)

This is a form of sublingual traumatic ulceration seen in babies born with natal teeth. During nursing, the anterior primary tooth/teeth ulcerate the adjacent soft tissue of the ventral tongue.

Chemical burns of oral mucosa (aspirin burn)

If pain medication, especially aspirin, is placed directly on a painful tooth, the adjacent soft tissue may sustain severe chemical burns of the gingival as well as the buccal or labial mucosa depending on the location of the sore tooth.

Gingivitis

This refers to inflammation of the soft tissue that surrounds the teeth. Plaque-related gingivitis caused by lack of proper oral hygiene is the most common form encountered in young children.

Clinically gingivitis may be diffuse or focal with loss of normal mucosal stippling, redness of the mucosa, bleeding and sometimes oedema. In the case of chronic gingivitis, significant enlargement of the gingiva may be seen. Treatment of gingivitis consists of removal of the causative factor, in this case plaque, by a good cleaning and oral hygiene instructions to the child and his/her parents.

Necrotizing ulcerative gingivitis and noma

Necrotizing gingivitis or necrotising ulcerative gingivitis is an acute opportunistic gingival infection caused by bacterial plaque. It appears more frequently in undernourished children and young adults, as well as in patients with immunodeficiency. Clinically the gingiva is highly inflamed, oedematous and hemorrhagic with necrosis, a very bad smell and sometimes excruciating pain. This condition may progress to involve the attachment apparatus of the tooth as well as adjacent bone (necrotizing ulcerative periodontitis) and may even have extensive adjacent soft tissue involvement (necrotizing stomatitis).

In cases where the necrotizing infection breaks through the skin, it is termed *noma* or *cancrum oris*. The peak age incidence of acute noma in developing countries is one to four years. Noma is especially seen in communities with poor sanitation.

Diseases that commonly precede noma include measles, malaria, severe diarrhoea, and necrotising ulcerative gingivitis. In 1998, the WHO estimated that worldwide approximately 140 000 children contract noma each year, and 79 per cent of them die from the disease and its associated complications. The WHO therefore designates noma a health priority. Clinical features include mouth pain, pronounced halitosis, bad taste, tenderness of the lip or cheek, cervical lymphadenopathy, a foul-smelling purulent oral discharge, and a blue-black necrotic discoloration of the skin in the affected area. The face

Noma results from a complex interaction between malnutrition, infections and compromised immunity. It has a high mortality. HIV/AIDS has been shown to be the predisposing factor in a substantial number of children affected by noma.

on the affected side is swollen in most cases. The lesion is unilateral in most cases but can occur bilaterally. Sequestration of the exposed bone and teeth usually occurs spontaneously after the soft-tissue slough. Treatment depends on the severity and extension of the infection and necrosis but the clinician should exclude all systemic reasons for this condition such as immunosuppression.

Correction of dehydration and electrolyte imbalance, antibiotics (penicillin and metronidazole), local wound care (irrigation of the wound with appropriate antiseptic), removal of any remaining tissue slough and sequestra as soon as the acute stage is controlled, treatment of predisposing diseases and nutritional rehabilitation, are all included in the management of these young patients.

Noma neonatorum, a necrotic lesion that generally affects the oronasal region, develops during the first month of life, and in most cases, there is evidence of infection with *Pseudomonas aeruginosa, Escherichia coli, Klebsiella spp.,* or staphylococci. Noma neonatorum affects newborn and preterm infants and clinically resembles noma in children. Preterm birth and severe intrauterine growth retardation are important predisposing factors.

Other ulcerative lesions to be considered in the differential diagnosis of noma include leishmaniasis, malignant oral lesions, midline granuloma of the face, and syphilis, but most of these are rare in children aged two to five years.

Periodontitis

The term periodontitis is used to describe a group of multifactorial diseases that result in the progressive destruction of the attachment apparatus which are the structures that support the teeth within the jaws. This includes the periodontal ligament, cementum and alveolar bone. If left untreated, this process can ultimately lead to tooth loss. Although periodontitis is usually a disease of adult patients, it can also be seen in children. By definition, these forms of aggressive periodontitis occur in otherwise healthy patients with no associated systemic disease except for one or more deficiencies in the immune response.

The child presents with bleeding gums and foul smelling breath, sometimes with complaints of pain or even mobile teeth. In this case the role of the medical caretaker is to evaluate the systemic health of the child and then to refer him/her to a specialist in periodontics for optimal management as soon as possible.

> Severe periodontitis in young individuals can be a manifestation of a serious underlying systemic disease such as HIV.

Gingival overgrowth in children

The most frequent causes of gingival overgrowth include the use of certain drugs, hereditary gingival fibromatosis, neurofibromatosis I and leukaemic infiltrates of the gingiva. Various systemic drugs can cause gingival overgrowth, aggravated by plaque and decreased by improved oral hygiene. There is an increase in the production of extracellular matrix, especially collagen, or a decrease in the normal turnover due to a decrease in collagenase activity. Phenytoin and cyclosporin have been shown to cause more severe gingival overgrowth in children than adults. Genetic factors that determine the reaction of the individual's fibroblast response to certain drugs, as well as variation of enzymatic activity of cytochrome P450 seem to play important roles. Both the primary and permanent dentitions may be affected.

The hereditary forms of gingival overgrowth are due to proliferative fibrous overgrowth of the connective tissue of the gingiva and even more so, a reduced degradation of the extracellular matrix. It is usually only the permanent dentition that is affected. Treatment of gingival overgrowth involves surgical removal of the hyperplastic tissue as well as efficient plaque control.

Infectious diseases

Herpes simplex virus (HSV) in children

Primary HSV infection is usually asymptomatic, but acute herpetic gingivostomatitis is the most common pattern of symptomatic primary infection. Following an incubation period of 1–26 days, prodromal, non-specific symptoms occur, including fever, chills, anorexia, irritability, malaise and headache. The onset of the acute phase is abrupt, and is usually accompanied by pain in the mouth, salivation, foetor oris, refusal to drink and sub-mandibular lymphadenitis. The affected mucosa develops numerous pin-head vesicles, which break down rapidly to produce numerous small, flat ulcers which may coalesce and are covered by yellow–white membranes. Lesions may involve the keratinised (gingiva, tongue and palate) and non-keratinised (cheeks, labial mucosa, ventral tongue and soft palate) mucosa. Lesions can extend into the nasopharynx and onto the vermilion and the adjacent peri-oral skin. Mild lesions usually heal within five to seven days without scar formation, but healing may take up to two to three weeks in severe cases.

During the primary infection of the oral mucosa with HSV-1, the virus is taken up by the sensory nerves and transported to the associated ganglia, especially the trigeminal ganglion, where the virus remains in a latent state until triggered again later in life. Reactivation of the virus may sometimes occur spontaneously, but this is more often secondary to exposure to UV light, inter-current infection, psychological stress, fever, cold, infection with HIV, cancer, organ transplantation, irradiation, chemotherapy, fractures, tooth extraction, sideropenia, surgery or other stress-inducing states. Recurrent herpes infection (fever blisters) usually starts as small vesicles that rupture and ulcerate in the epithelium supplied by the specific ganglion. The lip vermillion is the most common site of recurrence but any of the keratinised mucosal sites of the oral mucosa, skin of the nose, chin or cheeks may be involved in the recurrent infections. An important point to remember is that recurrent herpes is never as extensive and will not involve both keratinised and non-keratinised mucosa again in an immune competent host. When a patient presents with such an extensive infection, it is either a late presentation of primary herpetic gingivo-stomatitis or a sign of immunodeficiency, which should be evaluated carefully.

Recurrent herpes must be distinguished from recurrent aphthous stomatitis but the latter is a disease of non-keratinised mucosa only. Patients that get regular recurrences of herpes usually report prodromal signs such as pain, burning, tingling etc. in the area. Healing should occur within 7–10 days.

Treatment of primary herpes infection is usually symptomatic only, but if diagnosed early enough, acyclovir may have a significant influence on the course and length of the infection.

Human papilloma virus (HPV) infection in children

Squamous papilloma

Squamous papillomas are benign epithelial proliferations caused by HPV subtypes 6 and 11. They present as soft, painless, exophytic wart-like lesions up to 0.5 cm in diameter on lips, tongue and soft palate. The mode of transmission is still uncertain and the lesions are of extremely low virulence and have a low infectivity rate. Conservative surgical excision including the base of the lesion is the treatment of choice.

Verruca vulgaris

Verruca vulgaris is an HPV-2, 4, 6 and 40 related wart that may involve the oral mucosa due to biting skin lesions, preferentially seen on the lips and anterior tongue. The oral lesions are usually surgically excised or may be treated with laser, cryotherapy or electrosurgery.

Focal epithelial hyperplasia (Heck's disease)

Focal epithelial hyperplasia is a contagious HPV 13- and 32-induced, localised proliferation of oral epithelium. The clinical picture is characterized by multiple, circumscribed, sessile, soft, elevated whitish papules and nodules. Lesions may cluster together and sometimes give the affected oral mucosa a cobblestone appearance. The lesions are usually painless and the patients are in good general condition. Spontaneous regression is usually seen around puberty and unless the lesions cause aesthetic problems the condition can be left untreated.

HPV causes benign wart-like lesions that can also be seen inside the mouth of children.

HIV and the oral cavity

Oral manifestations are among the earliest and most important indicators of HIV infection and although specific lesions associated with HIV infection have been identified throughout the world, it is important to realise that any type of oral lesion my be encountered. Pseudomembranous candidiasis (thrush) is most commonly present. Oral ulceration and oral hairy leukoplakia, an Epstein Barr virus-related oral mucosal lesion is also seen. An increase in cancrum oris (noma) has been reported in HIV-positive children in South Africa and Zimbabwe and caries and periodontal disease are also common in these children. Many children also present with unilateral parotid enlargement. The parotid glands are usually diffusely swollen and firm without evidence of inflammation or tenderness, occasionally accompanied by xerostomia. This is often associated with lymphoid interstitial pneumonitis (LIP) and diffuse lymphadenopathy. Regular oral and dental checkups by health care workers trained in HIV-related oral diseases are mandatory.

Oral candidiasis

Infection of the oral mucosa with *Candida albicans* and some other members of the *Candida* genus are extremely common.

This organism may, due to various local and systemic factors that may alter the oral mucosal immune status, affect those with compromised immune systems as well as otherwise healthy individuals. Various clinical forms of candidiasis may be encountered in the oral cavity but only a short overview on the most commonly encountered forms will be given here.

Pseudomembranous candidiasis (thrush) is the most common form of the infection, characterised by removable white plaques on the buccal mucosa, tongue and palate, composed of masses of fungal hyphae, desquamated epithelial cells and debris. An attempt to wipe

this plaque away with a spatula leaves pinpoint bleeding sites on an erythematous background. This is the oral thrush commonly seen in infants who are bottle-fed in the first few weeks of life. Thereafter, immunosuppression, malnutrition and antibiotic therapy are the most common reasons for this form of candidiasis.

Acute atrophic candidiasis usually follows the use of a course of broad-spectrum antibiotics and presents as erythematous patches on the dorsal surface of the tongue due to loss of the normal filiform papillae. The patient may complain of a burning sensation or be unwilling to eat.

The diagnosis of oral candidiasis can easily be confirmed with a smear biopsy for direct visualisation of the candidal hyphae and yeasts under the microscope, especially in the erythematous forms of the disease. Treatment is comprised of local or systemic antifungal medication (*see* Chapter 14, Principles of infection in children).

Recurrent aphthous stomatitis

Recurrent aphthous stomatitis or aphthae is one of the most common conditions encountered in the oral cavity. It is defined as recurrent painful ulceration of the mouth, which typically appears first in childhood, is seen in the absence of systemic disease and tends to decrease by the third decade. Similar ulcers are seen in conditions such as Bechet's syndrome, gastrointestinal diseases such as coeliac disease or inflammatory bowel disease, HIV infection and cyclic neutropaenia.

Minor aphthous ulcers are 2–8 mm in diameter, heal spontaneously without scarring within 10–14 days and affect the non-keratinised oral mucosa of the lips, cheeks, ventral surface of the tongue and floor of the mouth as well as the soft palate. Diagnosis rests in the history of recurrent ulcers and the presence of extremely painful round-ovoid ulcers with yellow-white, removable fibrino-purulent membrane and

---

The mouth is commonly involved in patients with HIV infection. Oral candidiasis is most frequent, but any type of oral lesion may be encountered. Regular oral and dental checkups are mandatory.

Candida does not ulcerate the oral mucosa and should therefore never be considered a differential diagnosis for ulcerative oral conditions.

Aphthous ulcers are extremely painful, with a red erythematous halo surrounding the yellow-white ulcer on non-keratinised oral mucosa. This differentiates from recurrent oral herpes simplex infection, which is encountered on the keratinised mucosa such as the gingiva and hard palate.

a bright red erythematous halo surrounding the ulcer on non-keratinised oral mucosa. The location on non-keratinised mucosa is an important differential for recurrent oral herpes simplex infection, which is encountered on the keratinised mucosa such as the gingiva and hard palate.

The pathogenesis of aphthous ulcers is still uncertain but seems to be the result of some form of local immune dysregulation. The minor form is the most common and is seen in more than 80 per cent of cases diagnosed, while major aphthous ulceration occurs in less than 10 per cent of those affected. Treatment is usually not necessary for minor aphthous ulcerations apart from over-the-counter local anaesthetics and an antibacterial oral rinse to prevent secondary bacterial infection. In more severe cases topical steroids (e.g. Kenalog® in Orabase®) and steroid rinses may be used. Steroid rinses should however be avoided until such age where the child will not swallow it after rinsing properly.

Common salivary gland pathology

Mucocele

The mucocele or mucous extravasation cyst is a common lesion of the minor salivary glands, seen especially on the labial mucosa of the lower lip. The lesion usually follows trauma to the mucosa during physical activity or biting the lips with rupture of the minor salivary gland duct and spillage of the mucin into the adjacent soft tissue. They present as dome-shaped, bluish-translucent mucosal lesions, which may be fluctuant or firm on palpation. The lesions may rupture to leave shallow, painful ulcers. Although most are only a few millimetres in diameter, larger lesions may be seen. Many lesions may heal spontaneously and never return, but in the case of chronic lesions,

surgical excision of the cyst as well as afflicted minor salivary gland is curative.

Ranula

Ranula, meaning 'frog', is the term used for mucoceles in the floor of the mouth which develops due to trauma of the submandibular or more commonly, the sublingual salivary glands. The lesion has the same clinical features as mucoceles but is much larger and situated in the floor of the mouth. They are most commonly encountered in children and may even elevate the tongue in severe cases. Treatment consists of removal of the roof of the cystic lesion or, more commonly, removal of the feeding sublingual or submandibular salivary gland. Removal of such a gland will not significantly alter the overall saliva production of the individual. A higher incidence is seen in HIV-infection.

Common soft tissue tumours in oral cavity

Pyogenic granuloma

The pyogenic granuloma is common on the gingiva of children during orthodontic treatment when oral hygiene is even worse than normally. It is not a true granuloma, but consists of a mass of granulation tissue, which is usually the result of trauma to the oral mucosa or local irritation such as plaque due to poor oral hygiene. The lesion consists of a small to large lobulated, red-purple mass with superficial ulceration situated on the gingiva, although it may be encountered anywhere on the oral mucosa. The lesion usually bleeds easily due to its vascular nature. Conservative surgical excision, with improvement of oral hygiene is curative for pyogenic granulomas.

Odontogenic cysts and tumours

Eruption cyst

An erupting tooth is covered by a few layers of soft tissue, which include the remnants of the odontogenic epithelium from which the tooth developed and the dental follicle. In some cases fluid or blood may collect between the tooth and this surrounding soft tissue, resulting in a soft tissue cyst seen clinically as a soft, translucent to purple swelling on the gingiva overlying an erupting tooth. Treatment is usually not necessary.

Dentigerous cyst

The dentigerous cyst is the most common type of developmental odontogenic cyst encountered. The erupting tooth in this case is still enclosed in the bone. The cyst encloses the crown of the developing and/or erupting tooth and is actually attached to the neck of the tooth, also known as the cemento-enamel junction. These cysts are most commonly associated with unerupted third molars (wisdom teeth). The patient presents with a clinically missing tooth and a radiolucent lesion associated with the tooth is seen on radiographic examination. Referral to a dentist is required.

Odontoma

Odontomas are the most common type of odontogenic tumours. They are hamartomas rather than true neoplasms. A radiographic examination of a clinically missing tooth reveals a radiodense mass of tooth-like structures or mass of calcified tissue in the eruption pathway of the absent tooth.

PART 9

Procedures

36

Procedures

This chapter addresses important aspects and hazards of procedures used in paediatrics. For brevity, restraint of the child, preparation and anaesthesia have not been repeated for each procedure. Common procedures only are outlined.

Preparation

Preparation of the child and family

Explanations to the child depend on the age, developmental status and ability to understand. Parents should be informed about the need and risks but should not assist in the performance of a painful procedure. Informed consent should be obtained.

Preparation of the assistant

Adequate restraint and correct positioning are important for speed and safety. Staff who assist need guidance about the procedure and the type of restraint required.

Sedation

Sedation should be adequate. Additional analgesia is required for more painful procedures. Drug dosages in the table below are only a guideline and need to be individually titrated. Parenteral diazepam or midazolam (Dormicum®) have a rapid onset and are short-acting. Midazolam is sometimes chosen because of its amnestic effect.

Table 36.1 Drugs used for sedation in children

DRUG	ROUTE / DOSE	COMMENT
Diazepam (Valium®)	0.04–0.2 mg/kg IV	Respiratory depression*
Midazolam (Dormicum®)	0.05–0.2 mg/kg IV	Respiratory depression*
	0.5–0.75 mg/kg PO	Aggression and hallucinations may occur.
	0.2–0.3 mg/kg intranasal	Amnestic
Lorazepam (Ativan®)	0.05–0.1 mg/kg IV	Respiratory depression*
Pethidine	1–1.5 mg/kg IM or SC	Give >30 min before procedure **
Morphine	0.05–0.1 mg/kg IV	Titrate **
Ketamine (Ketalar®)	1–4 mg/kg IV over 60 seconds	Laryngospasm may occur
Chloral hydrate (Tricloryl®)	25–100 mg/kg PO	Give one hour before the procedure
Trimeprazine (Vallergan®)	3 mg/kg	Give one hour before. Older children

* Reverse with flumazenil (Anexate®) 0.2 mg IV over 15 seconds and repeated at 60 seconds as necessary to 1 mg

** Reverse with naloxone (Narcan®) 5–10 mg/kg/dose IV or IM every 3 min x 3 doses as necessary

Local anaesthesia

Lignocaine is the recommended local anaesthetic for most minor procedures in a dose not exceeding 3 mg/kg. The two main solutions available are 1% (10 mg/ml) and 2% (20 mg/ml). Preparations with adrenalin are useful to reduce bleeding but should never be used on extremities (digits, ears, penis). Occasionally regional anaesthesia may be required. Injections into inflamed or infected tissues, periosteum or liver capsule, may be followed by rapid systemic absorption with toxic side effects such as restlessness, convulsions and cardiac arrhythmias. Control of a convulsion should initially be with diazepam given rectally. Temporary respiratory support may be required.

Topical gels and creams

These are usually applied to intact skin and covered with an occlusive patch to promote absorption. Eutectic mixtures of local anaesthetics (EMLA®) needs at least 45 minutes to take effect and should not be used under one year of age. Anaesthetic gels are available for urethral catheterisation.

Technique

Aseptic technique should be followed. Hazards to the persons performing the procedure should be minimized by use of gloves and judicious use of gowns, caps, masks and goggles. The risk of needle-stick injury is reduced if used needles are not re-sheathed and are appropriately discarded immediately after use.

Ventilation

Managing the airway and breathing is critical in paediatric resuscitation. Adequate ventilation is more important than intubation and when difficulty is encountered, ventilate via an oral/nasal airway and mask.

Pharyngeal airway

The oropharyngeal (Guedel) airway is used to keep the airway between the tongue and posterior pharyngeal wall patent. The approximate size is mid-chin to angle of jaw. With an intact gag reflex there may be vomiting. In infants and small children a shortened endotracheal tube may be used as a nasopharyngeal airway.

Mask ventilation

Mouth-to-mouth and bag-valve-mask ventilation is used early in resuscitation. To open the airway the patient is positioned supine with the head extended and resting on the occiput with the chin lifted; the 'sniffing position'. After suctioning the oropharynx use a suitably sized mask and ensure a good seal to ventilate the patient. When applying pressure on the nose avoid direct pressure on the eye ball. An oropharyngeal airway may be necessary in some patients.

Endotracheal intubation

With failed mask ventilation and when there is cardiac arrest immediate intubation is indicated. Hyperextension must be avoided. Pre-oxygenate by mask or bag. Have adequate suction available. For elective intubation atropine will prevent severe bradycardia and in patients with suspected brain injury lidocaine (1 mg/kg) will blunt the rise in intra-cranial pressure.

Suggested sizes (inner diameters) for paediatric endotracheal tubes are: premature baby 2.5–3.5 mm; term newborn 3.5 mm; 3–12 months 4.0 mm; for children over 1 year the approximate inner diameter size is (Age/4) + 4 mm.

Using the left hand insert the appropriate laryngoscope (straight blade in infants) in the right corner of the mouth; by pulling the blade to the centre the tongue is lifted out of the way to obtain a view of the cords. The cords are attached to the cricoid cartilage and cricoid pressure helps push the larynx down into view and also occludes the oesophagus thereby reducing the risk of aspiration. The tube is passed through the cords for an appropriate distance (usually 2–3 cm) into the trachea. The trachea of an infant is very short and it is easy to intubate the mainstem bronchus especially with further flexion of the head. The airways of infants are small and delicate and even minimal trauma may cause oedema which may be life-threatening. Direct pressure of the laryngoscope blade onto the dento-alveolar ridge must be avoided and one must be wary of dislodging any teeth.

The position of the tube should be checked clinically and by a chest X-ray. Clinical check includes:

- Observation of chest movement
- Auscultation of chest and left hypochondrium
- Monitoring of expired carbon dioxide.

Cricothyroidotomy

This is performed as an emergency procedure in order to maintain an airway where intubation access is impossible (foreign body, hugely swollen epiglottis). The patient is placed supine with the neck extended. The gap between the thyroid and cricoid cartilages is palpated. The thyroid cartilage is grasped with thumb and middle finger and using the tip of the index finger as guide, a 14- or 12-gauge intravenous catheter is inserted downward at a 45-degree angle through the cricothyroid membrane into the larynx (Figure 36.1). A large bore needle or scalpel blade may be used. Any makeshift tube can be used but must be fixed in place to prevent it slipping through into the trachea.

Emergency tracheostomy

The patient is placed supine with support below the shoulders in order to hyperextend the head. The chin, thyroid cartilage and suprasternal notch are kept in a straight line. The operator's left thumb, second and third fingers are arched over the trachea to immobilize it, pushing the great vessels of the neck back under the sternomastoid and also keeping the skin taut. A vertical incision 2–3 cm long is made midway between the cricoid and the suprasternal notch. By blunt dissection the trachea is exposed over a distance of two or three rings. The isthmus of the thyroid should be mobilized and retracted upward if encountered. A vertical incision is made through the second and third tracheal rings. An appropriate sized tube is inserted and secured firmly but not tightly. The skin edges are loosely sutured together. Suctioning the tube in a sterile manner is important; this is done every 15 minutes for the first hour and then hourly or more frequently when required.

Complications include mediastinal or subcutaneous emphysema, pneumothorax, haemorrhage, and infection, and in the long term, ulceration of the trachea, and laryngeal or tracheal stenosis.

Injections

Intramuscular injections

It is useful to assess the depth of subcutaneous fat by pinching the skin over the injection site. For thigh injections (Figure 36.2) the area chosen

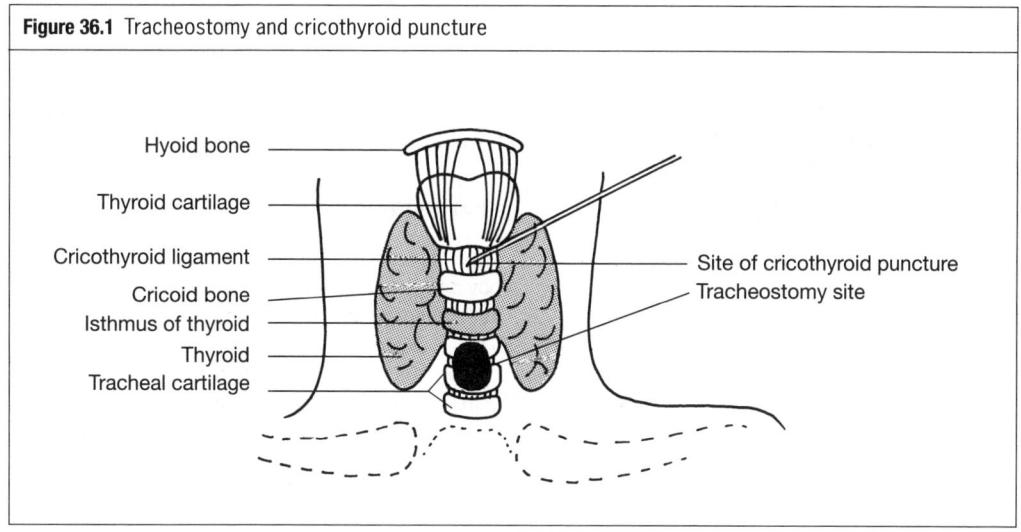

Figure 36.1 Tracheostomy and cricothyroid puncture

Hyoid bone

Thyroid cartilage

Cricothyroid ligament

Cricoid bone

Isthmus of thyroid

Thyroid

Tracheal cartilage

Site of cricothyroid puncture

Tracheostomy site

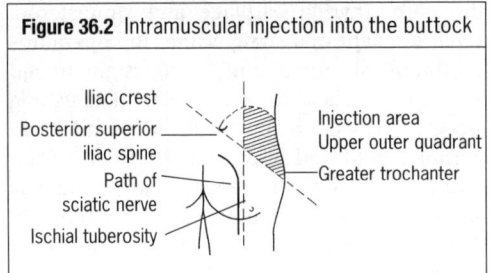

Figure 36.2 Intramuscular injection into the buttock

Iliac crest
Posterior superior iliac spine
Path of sciatic nerve
Ischial tuberosity
Injection area Upper outer quadrant
Greater trochanter

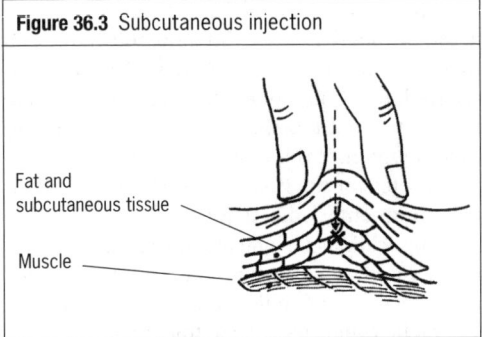

Figure 36.3 Subcutaneous injection

Fat and subcutaneous tissue
Muscle

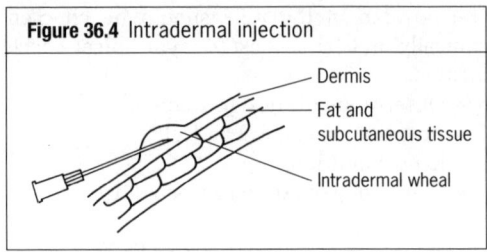

Figure 36.4 Intradermal injection

Dermis
Fat and subcutaneous tissue
Intradermal wheal

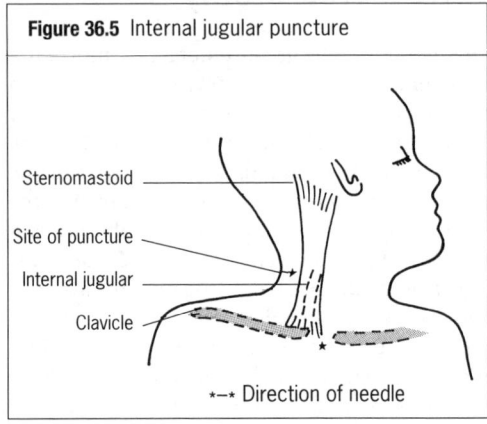

Figure 36.5 Internal jugular puncture

Sternomastoid
Site of puncture
Internal jugular
Clavicle

— Direction of needle

is on the lateral aspect, one third of the way down from the hip and into the belly of the quadriceps femoris. For buttock injections (Figure 36.3) the upper outer quadrant is chosen in order to avoid the sciatic nerve. Injections into the deltoid are given into the proximal muscle belly on the lateral aspect of the shoulder. Before injecting withdraw the plunger to ensure that the needle tip is not in a vein.

Subcutaneous injections

(Figure 36.4.)

These are given by pinching a fold of skin between the thumb and forefinger and aiming for the subcutaneous fat layer. Sites are the lower abdomen, axilla, and deltoid.

Intradermal injections

(Figure 36.4.)

These are used for vaccinations, Mantoux etc. and are performed by piercing the dermal layer of the skin at an oblique angle with the bevel of the needle pointing upwards. Avoid going through into subcutaneous tissue. On injection a wheal is raised, which has the typical *peau d'orange* appearance.

Vascular access

The superficial veins commonly used for blood sampling are the veins of the upper limb and in infants under two years of age the external jugular vein. Other sites include scalp veins (infants), internal jugular, femoral and saphenous veins. Tourniquets should be tight enough to occlude veins but not prevent arterial perfusion. It is easier to penetrate veins where they emerge through fascia or at a confluence. Puncture of the internal jugular, subclavian, and femoral veins should be avoided when there is a bleeding disorder.

External jugular puncture

This is performed with the infant held supine over the edge of bed or table with the occiput at the edge and the head tilted 15° to 20° down. The assistant holds the ipsilateral shoulder down and turns the head toward the opposite shoulder. Crying or having the vein occluded with the operator's fingers on the clavicle help to distend the vessel. The external jugular runs from the angle of the mandible to behind the middle of the clavicle over the sternomastoid muscle.

The internal jugular vein

This structure runs close to the lateral border of the carotid artery behind the sternomastoid between the sternal and clavicular heads. The positioning is similar to that for external jugular puncture. In children the high approach (Figure 36.5) is used. The needle is inserted deep to the posterior border of the sternomastoid at its midpoint and directed to just above the sternal notch. Negative pressure is applied while advancing the needle. Firm pressure is required for 3–5 minutes over the puncture site with the child in the sitting position after internal and external jugular punctures. Complications include deep neck bleeding, damage to local structures, and pneumothorax.

The femoral vein

The vein runs anterior to the hip joint, medial to the femoral artery (Figure 36.6). The femoral artery runs deep to the inguinal ligament midway between the anterior superior iliac spine and the pubic symphysis. Lateral to the artery is the femoral nerve. The artery is palpated 1–2 cm distal to the flexion crease of the thigh and the needle is advanced almost vertically 0.5 cm medial to the pulsation with negative pressure applied to the syringe.

Femoral arterial puncture

This procedure is identical to femoral vein puncture except that the needle is directed more laterally into the pulsating vessel and gentle or no negative pressure may be required. Pressure over the puncture site for 10 minutes is essential. Complications include arthritis of the hip, osteomyelitis of the femur, and compromised

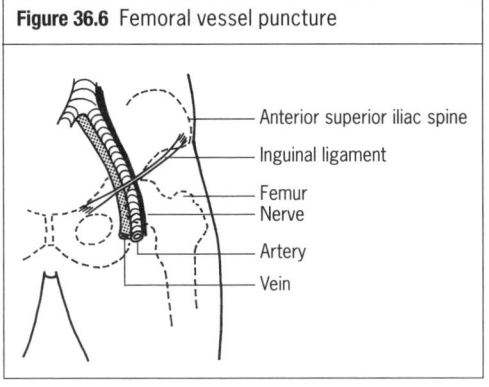

Figure 36.6 Femoral vessel puncture

- Anterior superior iliac spine
- Inguinal ligament
- Femur
- Nerve
- Artery
- Vein

circulation to the leg. If the procedure is done too high up bowel or bladder puncture may occur.

The radial artery

The vessel is preferred for arterial blood sampling but the brachial or temporal arteries may also be used. The artery is located by careful palpation and the needle is directed at a 30° to 60° angle from the horizontal into the vessel.

Saphenous vein cutdown

(Figure 36.7.) A cutdown is performed when venous access is necessary but percutaneous venipuncture is not possible. The patient is kept supine with the foot restrained in an externally rotated position. The saphenous vein is palpated just anterior to and above the medial malleolus. After infiltrating local anaesthetic, a 1.5–2 cm incision is made over the vein, which lies fairly deep and just superficial to the periosteum. The vein is exposed by blunt dissection using an artery forceps. A length of 1 cm of the vessel is freed for a distance of 1 cm and two ligatures placed underneath the vessel. The distal ligature is tied and the other is loosely knotted. While applying tension to the distal ligature the vein is incised with a small blade. A catheter filled with saline or other infusion fluid is carefully inserted into the vein via the incision. The loose proximal ligature is then tightened over the catheter and the infusion commenced. The skin incision is sutured with silk and the catheter secured with a suture and with adhesive plaster.

A subclavian vein

A catheter may be used for vascular access as well as for monitoring central venous pressure. The subclavian vein (Figure 36.8) crosses over the first rib in front of the anterior scalene muscle and continues behind the medial third of the clavicle to join the internal jugular vein and to form the innominate vein on that side. The patient is supine in a 10° to 20° Trendelenburg position with the head turned to the opposite side. A towel roll under the shoulders may be needed to hyperextend the back. Either side may be used although the right is preferred. Using aseptic techniques, local anaesthesia is injected at the entry site and the intended track, including periosteum of adjacent clavicle and first rib. The puncture site is under the distal third

Figure 36.7 Cut-down procedure

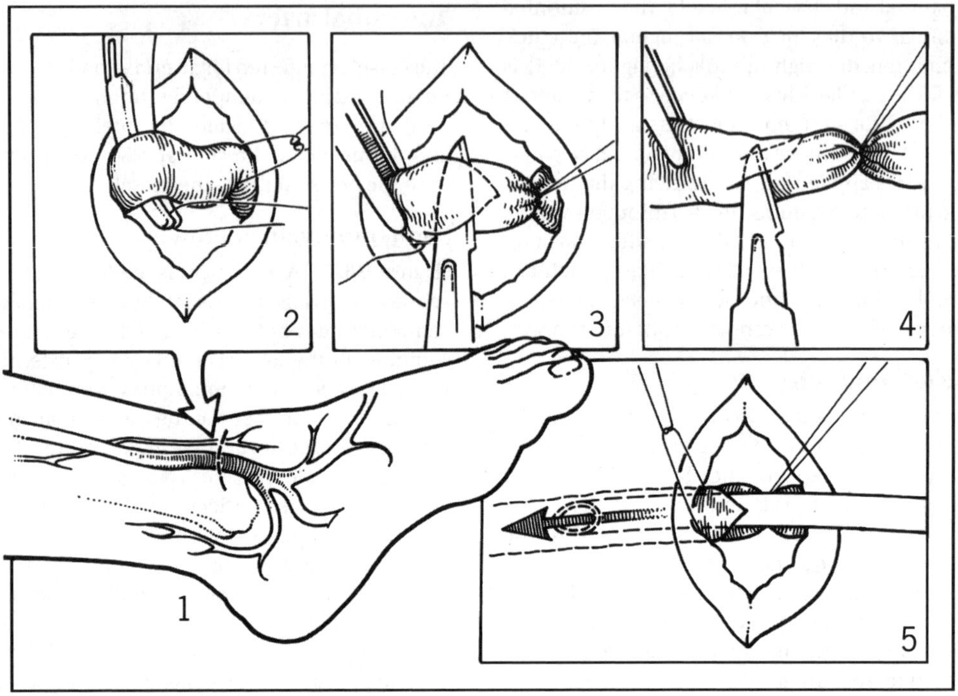

1 Selection of site for incision
2 Placing ligatures
3 Incision of vein with distal ligature tied
4 Preparation of flap
5 Insertion of catheter

of the clavicle in the depression bordered by the deltoid and pectoralis major muscles. The needle is directed beneath the clavicle at its midpoint toward the junction of the first rib and clavicle. Aspirate gently while advancing the needle with the bevel upward. When blood is aspirated advance the needle a few millimeters further. Placement of the catheter could be through the needle or over a guidewire (Seldinger technique). Keep the catheter patent using heparin (10 IU per ml). Take care to avoid air embolism and attach the iv infusion with an in-line manometer. Fix the cannula securely in place and check that blood flows back under the influence of gravity. The position of the catheter tip should be confirmed with a chest X-ray. Complications include pneumothorax, haemothorax, arterial puncture, damage to the thoracic duct, air embolism, infection and thrombosis.

Umbilical vessels

In the newborn umbilical catheterization is possible via the vein or arteries. Secure fixation of the catheter is required. The umbilical vessels comprise 2 white, thick walled arteries on the upper side and a larger thin walled vein inferiorly. To facilitate cannulation cut the umbilical stump

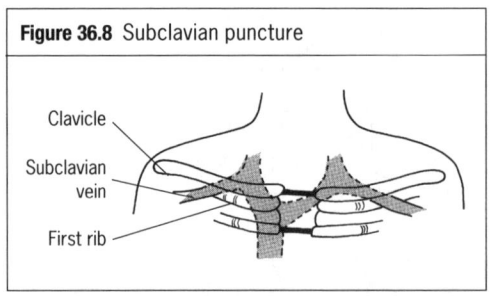

Figure 36.8 Subclavian puncture

Clavicle
Subclavian vein
First rib

1.5 to 2 cm above the abdominal wall. Place a silk tie (3-0 or 4-0) or cord ligature around the base of the umbilical stump but leave a purse-string knot untied. Locate the umbilical vessels. The vein is grasped by a pair of hooked forceps and the lumen opened with a curved probe. A catheter of appropriate size is inserted into it until there is free flow of blood (approximately half the distance between shoulder and umbilicus). The position of the catheter should be confirmed radiologically before using it for an exchange transfusion.

The procedure is similar for the arterial catheterization and the lumen is gently dilated to a depth of 1 cm. If the vessel is tortuous the stump is cut shorter. Blood should flow after passing the resistance of the bend which marks entry into the iliac artery. The knot in the ligature at the base is then tied and the catheter is securely fixed to the abdominal wall.

Intra-cardiac injection

This approach is used during resuscitation. The needle is inserted perpendicularly at the left sternal border in the fourth or fifth interspace and advanced while continually aspirating.

Intra-osseous infusion

This is indicated only when intravenous access is not available and immediate access is required on a temporary basis for infusion of crystalloid. A bone marrow aspiration needle is inserted into the marrow usually of the tibia immediately distal to the tibial tuberosity. (*See* Figure 36.9.) Hypertonic and strongly alkaline fluid should be avoided.

Exchange transfusion

Preparation for the procedure. The infant must be kept warm, adequately hydrated, and the stomach emptied prior to the exchange transfusion. Congestive cardiac failure and acidosis must be corrected where possible before commencing the procedure.

The procedure is carried out under sterile conditions, in a warm environment or in an incubator, particularly when dealing with premature or ill infants. It is advisable to use whole blood or packed cells less than 48 hours

old, preserved with citrate and warmed to room temperature. Disadvantages of this blood are that it is more acid, has a higher potassium and lower calcium content, thus predisposing the infant to acid-base and electrolyte disturbances. Heparinized blood, on the other hand, is fresh and has none of the above problems, but cannot be stored. Whole blood is most commonly used because the plasma albumin helps to bind the bilirubin, thus increasing the efficiency of the exchange transfusion. Packed cells are used more often in severely anaemic infants or those in cardiac failure.

Technique. The infant is immobilized by splinting loosely, to allow easy access to the umbilical area. The cord stump is trimmed to within 1.5 cm of the umbilicus and an 8 FG (or 6 FG in LBW infants) catheter is inserted into the umbilical vein, until venous blood appears in the catheter. A 20 ml (10 ml for LBW) deficit is established at the onset and corrected at the completion of the exchange. Aliquots of 10–20 ml are exchanged at a time. Pre- and post-exchange blood samples are taken routinely for serum bilirubin, blood cultures, full blood count, and electrolyte estimation. The volume of blood exchanged is 150–180 ml/kg. The procedure should take about 90 minutes. The infant is carefully monitored throughout for colour and temperature change, restlessness, and rising or falling pulse and respiratory rates. Cardiac and apnoea monitors may be used.

Figure 36.9 Sites for bone marrow aspirations

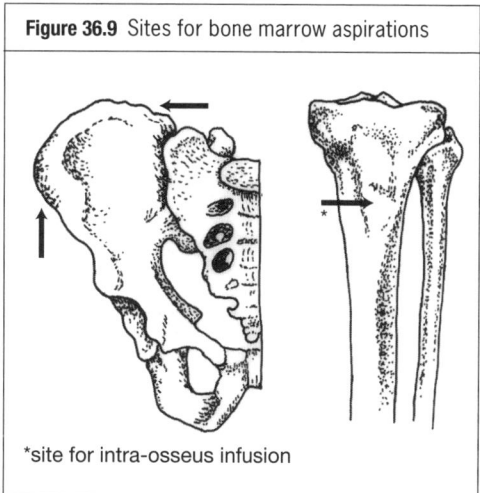

*site for intra-osseus infusion

Complications can be avoided by careful attention to detail. They relate to metabolic problems and haemodynamic alterations during the procedure. Chilling of the infant occurs readily if the blood is not warmed or the environmental temperature is too low. Heart failure from hyper- or hypovolaemia is avoided by slow, small volume exchanges. Bradycardia, arrhythmias, and cardiac arrest may occur if the donor blood is old, acidaemic, or hyperkalaemic, or if the catheter is situated in the heart. Hypocalcaemia is a risk with citrated blood. Fresh citrate-phosphate-dextrose blood, as opposed to acid-citrate-dextrose blood, will avoid most complications related to the blood itself. Air or pulmonary embolism may occur. Necrotizing enterocolitis occurs rarely, possibly as the result of haemodynamic changes transmitted to the mesenteric vessels. Septicaemia may result from a septic cord or contaminated equipment. After the exchange transfusion, blood sugars are monitored to detect hypoglycaemia, which can be prevented with a slow-running dextrose drip after the procedure.

Urine collection

Specimens may be obtained by collection bag over the genitalia, by mid-stream urine collection during voiding, by catheterization or by supra-pubic puncture. The prepuce is retracted sufficiently to expose the urethral meatus which is then cleaned with soap, saline or antiseptic solution. In the female the perineum and vulva are cleaned and the labia widely separated. The sample of urine can then be collected during voiding or into the collection bag. Any specimen obtained should be sent for culture immediately or refrigerated.

Despite aseptic technique and use of sterile equipment catheterization still caries the risk of introducing bacteria into the bladder and causing bacteraemia; this risk is increased with indwelling catheters.

Suprapubic puncture of the bladder

(Figure 36.10.)

This is a safe method to collect uncontaminated urine from infants and children less than two years old. The distended bladder at this age is primarily intra-abdominal. For children over two years catheterization is required. The bladder must be full – about 1 hour after the last voiding. Have a specimen bottle at hand to collect urine if the infant voids during the preparation. Position the child supine and restrain firmly. Insert a 22-gauge needle in the midline 1-2 cm above the symphysis with the needle directed 10-20° cephalad. Advance the needle under negative pressure. If no urine is obtained, do not remove the needle completely but re-insert the needle at an angle further away from or towards the pelvic brim. If still no urine is obtained try again

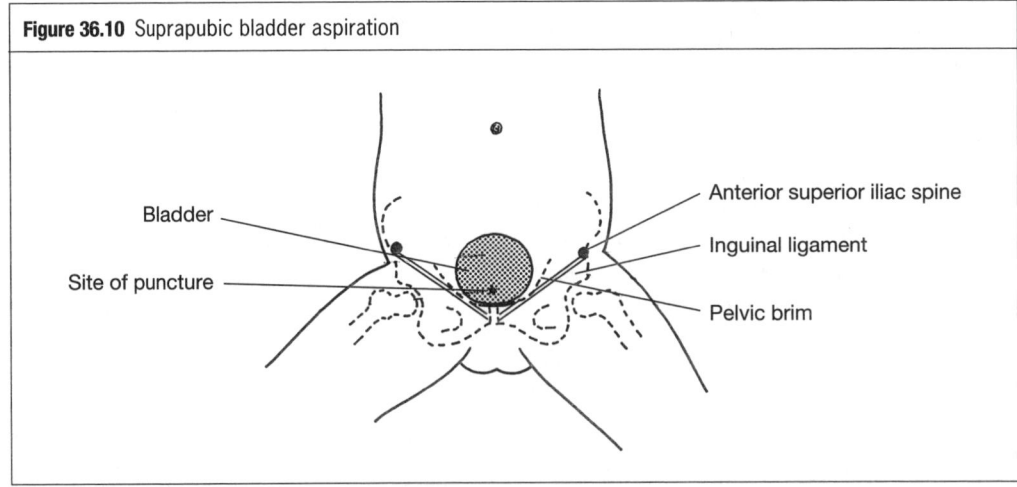

Figure 36.10 Suprapubic bladder aspiration

Bladder

Site of puncture

Anterior superior iliac spine

Inguinal ligament

Pelvic brim

Figure 36.11 Lumbar puncture: lying in the left lateral position

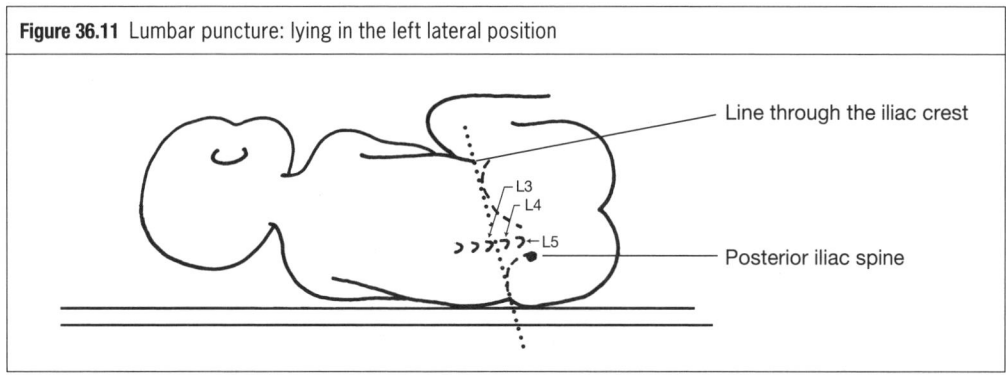

Line through the iliac crest

L3
L4
L5

Posterior iliac spine

after one hour. Microscopic haematuria virtually always occurs. Complications include gross haematuria, bowel puncture, or infection of the abdominal wall. Peritonitis is uncommon.

Lumbar puncture

This is usually done to confirm meningitis.

A lumbar puncture needle with a stylet is used. The lumbar puncture could be done in one of two positions: the left lateral position with hips, knees and spine maximally flexed without compromising the upper airway (Figure 36.11) or the seated position with maximal spinal flexion (Figure 36.12). Firmly restrain the child. The line joining the iliac crest on both sides passes over the L4

> Increased intracranial pressure, focal neurological signs with suspicion of a mass lesion or cord compression, bleeding tendency or anticoagulant therapy are contra-indications to lumbar puncture.

vertebra or the L4-L5 interspace. The L3-L4 interspace is used and the ones above and below this may also be used. The needle is advanced into the desired interspace and directed toward the umbilicus. A 'give' is felt in older patients once the dura is pierced (Figure 36.13). The needle is rotated to maximize CSF flow and the opening pressure is recorded. The foramen magnum is zero point in the sitting position and the needle level is zero point in the lateral position. Normal CSF pressure is between 50-180 mm CSF. If no CSF is obtained initially, advance the needle another millimeter or so. Aspiration of CSF with a syringe must be avoided. If bloodstained fluid is obtained, it is collected into serial containers. If the subsequent samples become clear then a traumatic tap is likely (usually because the needle has been advanced too far). Complications of lumbar puncture include headache, back pain and transient limping, radicular pain, dural leak, bleeding into the cord, infection, and in the presence of increased intracranial pressure, herniation of the brainstem or cerebellum ('coning').

Figure 36.12 Lumbar puncture: sitting position

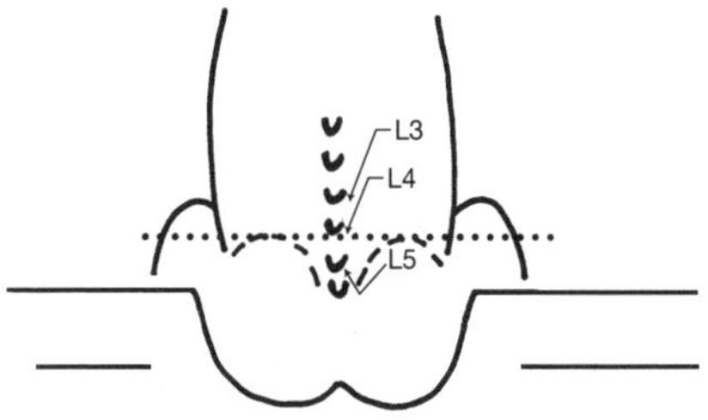

L3
L4
L5

Figure. 36.13 Lumbar puncture anatomy

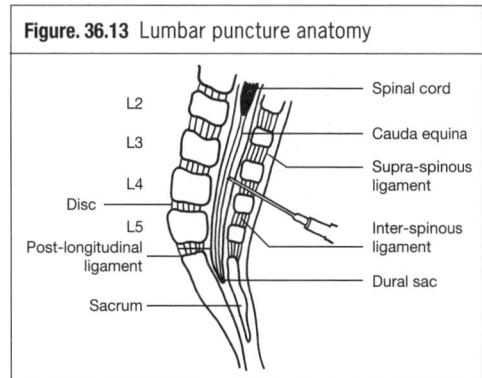

L2
L3
Disc
L4
L5
Post-longitudinal ligament
Sacrum

Spinal cord
Cauda equina
Supra-spinous ligament
Inter-spinous ligament
Dural sac

Subdural and ventricular tap

Subdural tap

Cold light transillumination of the skull may reveal a subdural fluid collection; CT scanning is confirmatory. A tap may be required to ascertain the nature of the fluid. When the sutures and fontanelle are open it is possible to tap the effusion. The area around the fontanelle is shaved and cleaned. The head should be face up (Figure 36.14) and immobilized by an assistant. The site of insertion is the lateral angle of the fontanelle or when the fontanelle is small, a point several millimeters laterally in the coronal suture. The styletted needle, preferably short bevelled, is slowly advanced perpendicular to the skin surface until there is a drop in resistance. The subdural space is very superficial and lies between the dura mater and the arachnoid. The needle normally need not be advanced more than 5–8 mm. It is quite safe to evacuate 15–20 mls of fluid from each side. The fluid should be cultured and have microscopy and chemistry checked as for routine CSF. Some infants require bilateral taps and with chronic effusions daily taps are needed. Complications include infection, subgaleal fluid collection, laceration of the superior sagittal sinus (insertion too medial) and trauma to the cerebral cortex.

Ventricular puncture

This is performed for the diagnosis of suspected ventriculitis or for relieving non-communicating hydrocephalus. Ultrasound examination helps to confirm the thickness of the cerebral cortex and the degree of ventricular dilatation. The child is prepared as for subdural tap. The needle is inserted at the lateral angle of the anterior fontanelle and then angled downwards, medially and forwards to aim at the medial canthus of the eye. Ventricular fluid is usually obtained at a depth of less than 3 cm. An atraumatic round needle with stylet is used and care should be taken not to change direction or rotate the needle in the skull to minimize damage to brain tissue. Whenever possible the right side is used in order to spare the left hemisphere (more commonly dominant and involved in speech). Normal ventricular pressure is less than 10 mm CSF. Porencephalic cyst formation along the puncture track, trauma to brain, and puncture of the superior sagittal sinus are the major complications. Repeated ventricular punctures, preferably by the same operator, should attempt to follow the previous track.

Liver biopsy

Before the procedure check the platelet count and coagulation tests and have a specimen for cross-match. Prolonged coagulation or bleeding times, an unco-operative patient, local infection, cholangitis, marked anaemia or gross ascites are contra-indications. Whenever possible the patient should practise holding the breath for about 10 seconds (full inspiration for subcostal approach and full expiration for intercostal approach). A Tru-cut® biopsy needle is used and the technique used for breast biopsy is recommended (Figure 36.15).

Spring-loaded biopsy needles are also available and are simpler to use. The operator must be familiar with the mechanics of the needle prior to the procedure. With enlarged livers the biopsy is performed in the mid-clavicular line just below the costal margin or to the right of the epigastrium (in the direction of the lower right axilla). The intercostal approach is used when the liver is not palpable. Maximal liver dullness is pinpointed between the anterior and mid-axillary lines at end-expiration and a site chosen one or two intercostal spaces below this (Figure 36.16). The needle is inserted close to the superior ridge of the rib to avoid injury to the neurovascular bundle.

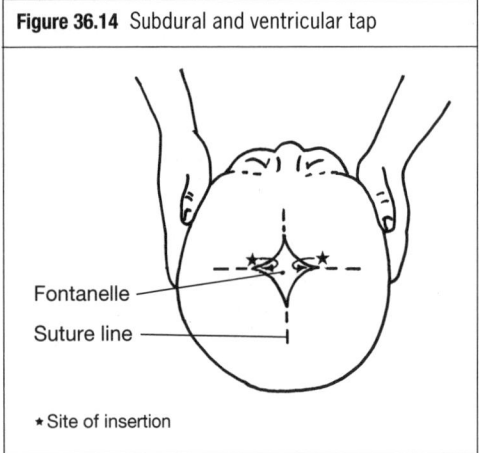

Figure 36.14 Subdural and ventricular tap

Fontanelle

Suture line

★ Site of insertion

The child is placed supine on a firm surface with the hands held above the head and legs immobilized at the knees. Local anaesthetic is infiltrated. A 2–3 mm incision is made at the desired puncture site and the procedure com-

pleted as rapidly as possible. After the procedure the patient should lie on the right side for 2–3 hours and half-hourly pulse and blood pressure checks are done. Bed rest for 24 hours is recommended. Complications include pain, bleeding, cholangitis, bile peritonitis, puncture of adjacent viscera, and pneumothorax or haemothorax.

Paracentesis

Adequate restraint and sometimes sedation is required.

Pericardial aspiration

This is performed to remove fluid, purulent exudate or blood for diagnostic or therapeutic purposes (Figure 36.17).

If the fluid is not loculated a sub-xiphoid puncture is recommended as it is extra-pleural, allows dependant drainage, and permits better stabilization of the needle. Other sites for puncture include the apical site, or the 5th or 6th interspace at the left sternal margin. The patient should be well sedated prior to the procedure and placed in a sitting posture of about 60°. Vital signs must be monitored throughout the procedure. Using an ECG monitor, ideally with a V-lead attached to the needle, watch for a current of injury.

After infiltration of anaesthetic at the angle of the left costal margin and the xiphoid, the skin is incised and the needle attached to a 3-way tap and a 20 ml syringe, is advanced until the needle reaches the inner aspect of the rib cage. The needle hub is then depressed and the tip pointed to the left shoulder and with continuous

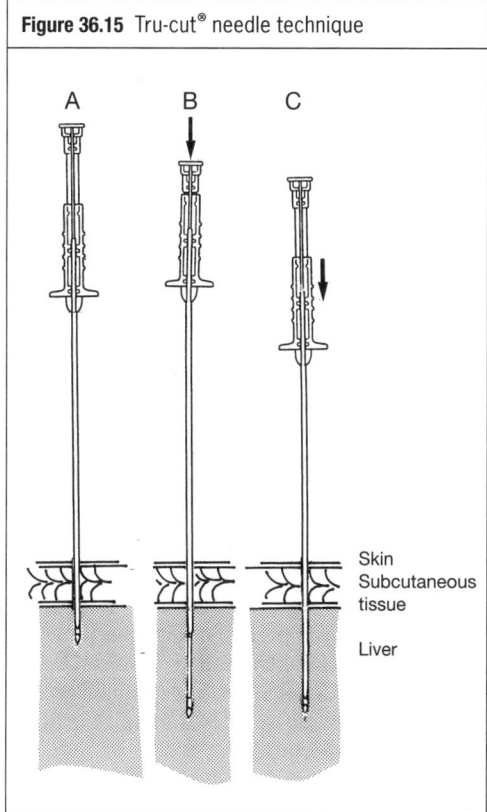

Figure 36.15 Tru-cut® needle technique

A   B   C

Skin
Subcutaneous tissue

Liver

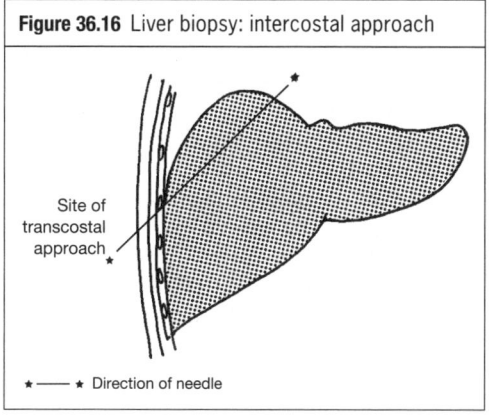

Figure 36.16 Liver biopsy: intercostal approach

Site of transcostal approach

★——★ Direction of needle

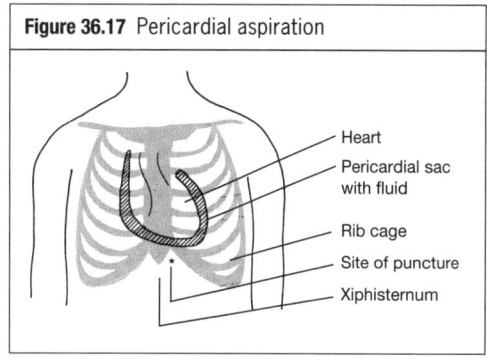

Figure 36.17 Pericardial aspiration

Heart
Pericardial sac with fluid
Rib cage
Site of puncture
Xiphisternum

aspiration, the needle is advanced in a rotatory manner as close to the inner aspect of the rib cage as possible. A 'give' may be felt with pericardial puncture. Fluid must be aspirated slowly to avoid pericardial shock. If no fluid is obtained withdraw the needle and re-direct the needle to the head or right shoulder.

A 'ventricular' ECG complex or a 'current of injury' (ST segment change and T waves) suggest myocardial penetration. Withdraw the needle and wait for return to baseline before resuming. Other complications include arrhythmias, damage to the coronary arteries, haemopericardium, pneumothorax and infection. Following the procedure there should be close observation (BP, pulse and general condition) every 15 minutes for two hours. Any complication of the procedure is unlikely to occur after this period. A follow-up chest X-ray is useful to assess size of the effusion and to exclude pneumothorax.

Thoracic paracentesis and intercostal drainage

Thoracic paracentesis (diagnostic or therapeutic) is performed with the patient seated. For tension pneumothorax the side of the chest with the pneumothorax is elevated to a near vertical position. In small infants the lateral position is used and the site used is mid to anterior axilla. With the arms elevated the puncture site is just below the lower tip of the scapula (7th intercostal space) in the posterior axillary line.

A lateral decubitus CXR will identify free fluid and an ultra-sound helps in localising loculated effusions. Assemble the equipment before inserting a drain. After anaesthetising the site an incision of 1.0–1.5 cm is made and a closed haemostat is used to penetrate the pleura. Care is taken to avoid the neurovascular bundle which lies at the inferior border of the rib. The catheter is grasped by the haemostat and directed into the pleural space. Trocar and cannula or the guidewire could also be used. The catheter is secured with a purse string suture with an underwater seal. For haemothorax and empyaema use the largest size tube that would pass through the ribs.

Peritoneal tap is performed after confirming the presence of ascites clinically. The patient is placed in a sitting or a lateral decubitus position. The puncture site could be in the midline or at a point two-thirds of the way along a line between the umbilicus and the anterior superior iliac spine.

Peritoneal dialysis

For insertion of a peritoneal dialysis (PD) catheter a site halfway between the umbilicus and the symphysis pubis is selected. Other sites are McBurney's point or a point lateral to the rectus muscles at or above the level of the umbilicus. Consider surgical placement in patients after previous surgery, or in the presence of severe colitis (e.g. with shigella dysentery), coagulopathy and when a long period of dialysis is anticipated. After sedation and local anaesthetic ensure that the bladder is empty. Fill abdomen with i.v. fluid via an i.v. catheter. A small skin incision is made and the PD catheter is inserted using the stilette. Direct the tip toward the pelvis and secure with purse string suture.

Bone marrow aspiration

Both the anterior and posterior portions of the iliac crest are suitable sites and contain cellular marrow at any age. In neonates and young infants the tibia is preferred with the puncture site being 1 cm medial and 1 cm distal to the tibial tubercle. Local anaesthetic is injected into the subcutaneous tissue down to and including the underlying periosteum.

For aspiration, the needle with obturator in place is advanced through a skin incision into the cortex of the bone with firm pressure and a slight to and fro rotation. A 'give' is felt on entry into marrow. The obturator is removed and an aspirate specimen obtained by sustained suction on a syringe. Prolonged aspiration will dilute the specimen. A 'dry tap' may be the result of faulty technique, or abnormal marrow (hyperplasia/myelofibrosis).

For a trephine biopsy the Jamshidi® or Islam® needle is used. The site selected is usually the posterior iliac crest or spine. After advancing the needle and obturator through the bony cortex, the obturator is removed and using smooth rotatory to and fro motions the needle is advanced for 1–2 cm. The needle is rotated several times and moved from side to side to separate the core of marrow and then slowly removed using slight rotatory motions. The specimen is removed through the proximal end of the needle by using the probe and after touch imprints have been made, placed into appropriate fixative.

Cardioversion

For patients in cardiac arrest or ventricular fibrillation it may be necessary to perform cardioversion before securing intravenous access or airway. Paddles used are 4.5 cm for infants (<10 kg) and 8 cm for young children. The synchronous mode must be set for direct cardioversion and the asynchronous mode for defibrillation. One paddle (apex paddle) is placed at the apex and the other just to the right of the sternum. If the paddles are too large, the left sternum and left scapula could be used as contact points (a-p placement).

Charge the unit. Choose synchronous or asynchronous mode. Apply electrode gel. Use the lowest recommended energy level initially. Clear area; ensure that operator and other assistants are not contacting patient and that patient is not contacting metal. Apply paddles firmly and apply current by pressing discharge button simultaneously for a few moments. If no response in 2–3 minutes repeat with double dose for subsequent attempts.

For synchronous cardioversion use **0.5 J/kg for initial attempt and then double** for subsequent attempts.

For asynchronous cardioversion (defibrillation) use **2 J/kg for the first attempt and then 4 J/kg** for the second and third attempts.

Bibliography

General paediatrics texts

American Academy of Pediatrics website: http://www. aap.org

Kliegman, R., Behrman, R.E., Jenson H.B. and Stanton B.F. eds. 2007. *Nelson Textbook of Pediatrics.* (18th edition). Philadelphia: W.B. Saunders & Co.

Part 1: Evaluation, growth, and development

WHO/UNICEF. IMCI Integrated management of childhood illnesses. Available from URL: http://www.who.int/child-adolescent-health/integr. htm

The WHO growth standards. Acta Paediatrica 2006, 95 (Supplement 450). Available from URL:http://www.who.int/childgrowth/standards/en/

Illingworth R.S. 1991. *The normal child.* Edinburgh: Churchill Livingstone.

London Dysmorphology Database: http://www.oup.com

Christianson, A., Howson, C.P. and Modell, B. 2006. *Global report on birth defects: The hidden toll of dying and disabled children.* White Plains, New York, March of Dimes Birth Defects Foundation. [Also available on website www.marchofdimes.com]

Gorlin, R.J., Cohen, M.M. and Hennekam, R.C.M. 2001. *Syndromes of the Head and Neck.* (4th edition). New York: Oxford University Press.

Jones, K.L. ed. 2006. *Smith's Recognizable Patterns of Human Malformation.* 6th edition. Philadelphia: Elsevier Saunders.

Rimoin, D., Connor, J., Pyeritz, R. and Korf, B. eds. 2001. *Emery and Rimoin's Principles and Practice of Medical Genetics.* 5th edition. Philadelphia: Churchill Livingstone Elsevier.

Turnpenny, P. and Ellard, S. eds. 2005. Emery's *Elements of Medical Genetics.* 12th edition. London: Churchill Livingstone Elsevier.

Part 2: Psychosocial and community paediatrics

American Psychiatric Association. 1993. *Diagnostic and Statistical Manual of Mental Disorders. (DSM-IV)* 4th edition.

Kibel, M.A, Saloojee M. and Westwood T. eds. 2007. *Child health for all: A manual for Southern Africa* (4th edition). Cape Town: Oxford University Press.

US National Academy of Sciences. 2004. *Children's Health, the Nation's Wealth: Assessing and Improving Child Health.* p5. URL: http://www.nap.edu/catalog/10886.html

Lopez, A.D., Mathers, C.D., Ezzati, M., Jamison, D.T. and Murray, C.J.L. eds. 2006. *Global Burden of Disease and Risk Factors.* The World Bank Group. URL: http://www.dcp2.org/pubs/GBD

Bradshaw, D., Bourne, D. and Nannan, N. 2003. *What are the leading causes of death among South African children?* MRC Policy Brief No. 3, December 2003. URL: www.mrc.ac.za/policybriefs/childmortality.pdf

---

Part 3: Neonatal paediatrics

MacDonald, M.G., Mullett, M.D. and Seshia, M.M. eds. 2005. *Avery's Neonatology, pathophysiology and management of the newborn.* (6th edition). Philadelphia: J.B. Lippincott & Co.

Neonatalogy website: http://www.neonatology.org

Infant and young child feeding. 2009. Model Chapter for textbooks for medical students and allied health professionals. World Health Organization. ISBN 978 92 4 159749 4

Part 4: Nutritional and metabolic disorders

American Academy of Pediatrics. 1998. *Pediatric Nutrition Handbook* (4th edition). Elk Grove Village, Ill.: AAP.

Scriver, C.R., Beaudet, A.L., Valle, D. and Sly, W.S. eds. 2001. *The metabolic and molecular basis of inherited disease.* (8th edition). New York: McGraw Hill.

World Health Organization. 2000. *Management of the child with a serious infection or severe malnutrition.* (WHO/FCH/CAH/00.1). Geneva: WHO. Website for manual: http://www.who.int/nut/manageme.pdf

Part 5: Infections in childhood

Red Book: 2006 Report of the Committee on Infectious Diseases. 2006. 27th ed. Elk Grove Village, IL: American Academy of Pediatrics.

Mandell, G.L., Bennett, J.E. and Dolin, R. eds 2005. *Principles and Practice of Infectious Diseases.* 6th edition. London: Churchill Livingstone.

Ralph, D., Feigin, M.D., Cherry, J., Demmler, G.J and Kaplan, S.L. eds. 2006. *Feigin and Cherry's Textbook of Pediatric Infectious Diseases.* 6th edition. Philadelphia, Pa: Saunders.

Hart, C.A. and Broadhead, R.L. 1992. *Color atlas of pediatric infectious diseases.* St Louis: Mosby Year Book.

Newell, M. and McIntyre, J. eds 2000. *Congenital and perinatal infections, prevention, diagnosis and treatment.* Cambridge: Cambridge University Press.

Wilson, D., Naidoo, S., Bekker, L-G., Cotton, M., and Maartens, G. eds 2008. *Handbook of HIV medicine.* 2nd edition Cape Town: Oxford University Press.

Robert Gie, for the International Union against Tuberculosis and Lung Disease, 2003. *Diagnostic Atlas of Intrathoracic Tuberculosis in Children.* (Free download – http://www.iuatld.org/index)

Guidance for National tuberculosis programs for the management of tuberculosis in children. 2006. World Health Organization. (www.who.int)

Part 6: Disorders of regulation

Brook, C.G.D., Clayton, P. and Brown, R. eds 2009 *Brook's clinical paediatric endocrinology.* (6th edition). Wiley-Blackwell

Mygind, N., Dahl, R. and Pedersen, S. eds 1996. *Essential allergy.* 2nd edition. Oxford: Blackwell Science Publications.

Pizzo, P. and Poplack, D. 2001. *Principles and practice of pediatric oncology.* 4th edition. Philadelphia: J.B. Lippincott & Co.

Stiehm, E.R., Ochs H.D. and Winkelstein, J. eds. 2004. *Immunologic disorders in infants and children.* 5th edition. Philadelphia: W.B. Saunders & Co.

The paediatric rheumatology webpage: http://www.wp.com/pedsrheum/home.html

The rheumatology webpage: http://www.serve.com/fredt/rheum.html

Part 7: System-based disorders

Keane, J.F., Fyler, D.C. and Lock J.E. eds. 2006. *Nadas' pediatric cardiology.* Philadelphia: W.B. Saunders & Co.

Chernick. V., Boat, T., Wilmott, R. and Bush, A. eds. 2006. *Kendig's Disorders of the respiratory tract in children.* 7th edition. Philadelphia: W.B. Saunders & Co.

Orkin, S., Fisher, D., Look, A.T., Lux, S., Ginsburg, D. and Nathan D. eds. 2009. *Nathan and Oski's Hematology of Infancy and Childhood.* (7th edition). Philadelphia: W.B. Saunders & Co.

Swaiman, K.F., Ashwal, S., and Ferriero, D.M. eds. 2006. *Paediatric neurology, principles & practice.* (4th edition). St Louis: C.V. Mosby Co.

Walker, W.A., Goulet, O., Kleinman, R.E., Sherman, P., Shneider, B.L. and Sanderson I.R. eds. 2004. *Pediatric Gastrointestinal Disease.* (4th edition). Hamilton: BC Decker Inc.

Rees, L., Webb, N. and Brogan, P. eds. 2007. *Paediatric Nephrology.* Oxford: Oxford University Press.

Kaplan, B.S. and Meyers, K.E.C. eds. 2004. *Pediatric Nephrology and Urology – the Requisites in Pediatrics.* Philadelphia: Elsevier Mosby.

Avner, E.D., Harmon, W.E. and Niaudet, P. eds. 2004. *Pediatric Nephrology.* (5th edition). Philadelphia: Lippincott Williams & Wilkins.

Part 8: Specialty disorders

Hutson, J.M., O'Brien, M, Woodward, A.A. and Beasley, S.W. eds. 2008 *Jones' clinical paediatric surgery.* (6th edition). Wiley-Blackwell Scientific Publications.

Solomon, L., Warwick, D. and Nayagam, S. 2001. *Apley's System of Orthopaedics and Fractures.* (8th edition). London: Arnold Publishers.

Herring, J.A. ed. 2002. *Tachdjian's Pediatric Orthopaedics.* (3rd edition). Philadelphia: W.B. Saunders & Company.

Morrisey, R. and Weinstein, S. eds 2001. *Lovell and Winter's Pediatric Orthopaedics.* (5th edition). Lippincot Williams and Wilkins.

Part 9: Procedures

Barkin, R. 1987. *Emergency pediatrics.* St Louis: C.V. Mosby Co.

Hughes, W.T. and Beuscher, E.S. 1980. *Paediatric procedures.* London: W.B. Saunders & Co.

Index